Mastery of Endoscopic and Laparoscopic Surgery

Mastery of Endoscopic and Laparoscopic Surgery

Edited by

W. Stephen Eubanks, M.D., F.A.C.S.

Assistant Professor of Surgery, Director of Surgical Endscopy, and Director of the Duke/U.S. Surgical Endosurgery Center,
Duke University Medical Center, Durham, North Carolina

Lee L. Swanström, M.D., F.A.C.S.

Director, Department of Minimally Invasive Surgery, Legacy Portland Hospital, Portland, Oregon

Nathaniel J. Soper, M.D., F.A.C.S.

Head, Minimally Invasive Surgery, Barnes-Jewish Hospital, St. Louis, Missouri

In conjunction with

Michael Leonard

Medical Illustrator, Sacramento, California

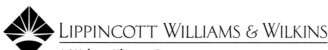

LIPPINCOTT WILLIAMS & WILKINS
A **Wolters Kluwer** Company
Philadelphia • Baltimore • New York • London
Buenos Aires • Hong Kong • Sydney • Tokyo

Acquisitions Editor: Lisa McAllister
Managing Editor: Susan Rhyner
Production Editor: Elaine Verriest
Manufacturing Manager: Tim Reynolds
Cover Designer: Sandra Mohandi
Compositor: Maryland Composition

© 2000 by LIPPINCOTT WILLIAMS & WILKINS
530 Walnut Street
Philadelphia, PA 19106-3780 USA
LWW.com

Printed and bound in China

Library of Congress Cataloging-in-Publication Data

Mastery of endoscopic and laparoscopic surgery/edited by W. Stephen
    Eubanks, Lee L. Swanström, Nathaniel J. Soper; in conjunction with
    Michael Leonard.
        p.   cm.
    Includes bibliographical references and index.
   ISBN 0-316-26865-8
    1. Endoscopic surgery.   2. Laparoscopic surgery.   I. Eubanks,
  Steve, 1959–   .   II. Swanström, Lee L.   III. Soper, Nathaniel J.
    [DNLM: 1. Surgical Procedures, Endoscopic.   2. Surgical Procedures,
  Laparoscopic.   WO 505 M423 1999]
  RD33.53.M38   1999
  617'.05—dc21
  DNLM/DLC
  for Library of Congress   98-32156
                                         CIP

---

10 9 8 7 6 5 4 3 2

Contents

SECTION I. GENERAL TOPICS

SECTION II: ESOPHAGUS AND STOMACH

SECTION III: LIVER AND GALLBLADDER

SECTION IV: ENDOCRINE

SECTION V: SMALL BOWEL, APPENDIX, AND COLON

SECTION VI: ABDOMINAL WALL

SECTION VII: CHEST

SECTION VIII: MISCELLANEOUS

Contributing
Authors

Ahmet Alponat, M.D.
Research Fellow, National University Hospital, 5 Lower Kent Ridge Road,
Singapore 0511

Wayne L. Ambroze, Jr., M.D.
Associate Clinical Professor of Surgery, Georgia Baptist Medical Center,
5555 Peachtree-Dunwoody Road, Atlanta, Georgia 30342

Charles H. Andrus III, M.D., F.A.C.S.
Chief of Surgery, Hines VA Hospital, Hines, Illinois 60141-5000

Maurice E. Arregui, M.D., F.A.C.S.
Director of Fellowship in Laparoscopy, Endoscopy and Ultrasound, Department of
Surgery, St. Vincent Hospital and Health Care Center, 2001 West 86th Street,
Indianapolis, Indiana 46260

Yutaka Atomi, M.D., Ph.D.
Professor of Surgery, Kyorin University, 6-20-2 Shinkawa Mitaka, 181 Tokyo, Japan

Mauro Bafutto, M.D.
Hospital Samaritano, Setor Coimbra, Praca Walter Santos, 01 Goiania,
Goias, Brazil 74 535-270

Garth H. Ballantyne, M.D., F.A.C.S., F.A.S.C.R.S.
Professor of Surgery, Department of Surgery, University of Medicine and Dentistry of
New Jersey, Newark, New Jersey 07103; and Director, Department of Minimally
Invasive Surgery, Hackensack University Medical Center, 20 Prospect Avenue,
Hackensack, New Jersey 07601

Timothy W. Bax, M.D.
Research Fellow, Laparoscopic Surgery, Department of Minimally Invasive Surgery,
Legacy Portland Hospital, 501 N. Graham Street, Portland, Oregon 97227

Leonard D. Benitez, M.D.
Fellow in Laparoscopic Surgery, 8720 North Kendall Drive, Miami, Florida 33176

Sunil Bhoyrul, M.B.Ch.B., F.R.C.S.
Senior Resident, Department of Surgery, Stanford University Medical Center,
Pasteur Drive, Stanford, California 94305

Luigi Bonavina, M.D., F.A.C.S.
Assistant Professor, Department of Surgery, University of Milan; and Staff Surgeon,
Ospedale Maggiore Policlinico, I.R.C.C.S., Via Francesco Sforza 35, Milan, Italy 20122

Edward J. Brennan, Jr., M.D.
Staff Surgeon, The Lankenau Hospital and Medical Research Center, 614 Penfield
Avenue, Havertown, Pennsylvania 19083

Christopher J. Bruce, M.D.
Assistant Clinical Professor, Department of Surgery, New York Medical College,
White Plains, New York 10601

L. Michael Brunt, M.D.
Associate Professor, Department of Surgery, Washington University School of Medicine, 660 S. Euclid Avenue; and Attending Surgery, Barnes-Jewish Hospital, 216 S. Kingshighway, St. Louis, Missouri 63110

Tom A. Burdon, M.D.
Assistant Professor, Cardiothoracic Surgery, Veterans Affairs Health Care Systems, Division of Cardiothoracic Surgery 112E, 3801 Miranda, Palo Alto, California 94304

Mark P. Callery, M.D., F.A.C.S.
Associate Professor of Surgery and Cell Biology and Chief, Division of General Surgery, Department of Surgery, University of Massachusetts Memorial Health Care, 55 Lake Avenue North, Worcester, Massachusetts 01655-0333

David W. Cloyd, M.D.
Director of Laparoscopy, Department of Surgery, Palomar Medical Center, 555 East Valley Parkway, Escondido, California 92025

Todd D. Cohen, M.D.
Assistant Professor of Urology, Department of Urology/Surgery, Ohio State University Medical Center, 456 West Tenth Avenue, Columbus, Ohio 43210

John A. Coller, M.D.
Department of Colon and Rectal Surgery, Lahey-Hitchcock Clinic, 41 Mall Road, Burlington, Massachusetts 01805

Geoffrey W. Cundiff, M.D.
Associate Professor, Department of Obstetrics and Gynecology, Johns Hopkins Medical Center; and Johns Hopkins Bayview Medical Center, 4940 Eastern Avenue, Baltimore, Maryland 21224-2780

Aureo L. DePaula, M.D.
Director of Surgical Laparoscopy and Endoscopy, Hospital Samaritano, Setor Coimbra, Praca Walter Santos, 01, Goiania, Goias, Brazil 74 535-270

Karen E. Deveney, M.D.
Professor, General Surgery, Oregon Health Sciences University, 3181 SW Sam Jackson Park Road, Portland, Oregon 97210-3098

Allison J. Duchow, M.D.
Associate Medical Staff, Department of Surgery, Peace Harbor Hospital, 330 9th Street, Florence, Oregon 97439

Quan-Yang Duh, M.D.
Associate Professor, Department of Surgery, University of California, San Francisco, 400 Parnassus, San Francisco, California 94143; and Assistant Chief, Surgical Service, VA Medical Center, 4150 Clement Street, San Francisco, California 94121

Titus D. Duncan, M.D., F.A.C.S.
Assistant Clinical Professor, Department of Surgery, Emory University School of Medicine, 1462 Clifton Road N.E., Atlanta, Georgia 30322; and Director, Department of Endosurgery, Georgia Baptist Medical Center, 303 Parkway Drive, Atlanta, Georgia 30312

David S. Edelman, M.D.
Division Chief, Department of General Surgery, Baptist/South Miami Hospital, 8720 North Kendall Drive, Miami, Florida 33176

Michael B. Edye, M.B., B.S., F.R.A.C.S., F.A.C.S.
Assistant Professor, Department of Surgery, Mount Sinai School of Medicine; and Attending Surgeon, Department of Surgery, The Mount Sinai Medical Center, One Gustave Levy Place, New York, New York 10029

W. Stephen Eubanks, M.D., F.A.C.S.
Assistant Professor of Surgery, Director of Surgical Endoscopy, and Director of the Duke/U.S. Surgical Endosurgery Center, Duke University Medical Center, Box 3110, Durham, North Carolina 27710

James T. Fann, M.D.
Clinical Assistant Professor, Department of Cardiothoracic Surgery, Stanford University School of Medicine, 300 Pasteur Drive, Stanford, California 94805; and Cardiovascular Surgeon, Cardiothoracic Surgery, Veterans Affairs Palo Alto Health Care Systems, 3801 Miranda Avenue, Palo Alto, California 94304

Edward L. Felix, M.D., F.A.C.S.
Assistant Clinical Professor, Department of Surgery, University of California San Francisco, 513 Parnassus Avenue, San Francisco, California 94142-0410; and Director, The Center for Hernia Repair, 6191 North Fresno Street, Fresno, California 93710

Andre Ferrari, M.D.
Hospital Samaritano, Setor Coimbra, Praca Walter Santos, 01, Goiania, Goias, Brazil 74 535-270

Aaron S. Fink, M.D.
Professor, Department of Surgery, Emory University School of Medicine, 1365 Clifton Road North East, Atlanta, Georgia 30322; and Chief, Surgical Service, Atlanta Veterans Affairs Medical Center, 1670 Clairmont Road, Decatur, Georgia 30033

Richard J. Finley, M.D., F.R.C.S.C.
Professor and Head, Department of Surgery, Vancouver Hospital and Health Sciences Center, 910 West 10th Avenue, Vancouver, British Columbia, Canada V5Z 4E3

Kenneth A. Forde, M.D.
José M. Ferrer Professor, Department of Surgery, College of Physicians and Surgeons, Columbia University, 630 West 168th Street, New York, New York 10032-3702; and Vice Chairman, Department of Surgery, New York, Presbyterian Hospital, 177 Ft. Washington Avenue, New York, New York 10032

Dennis L. Fowler, M.D., F.A.C.S.
Midwest Surgical Associates, 20375 West 151st Street, Olathe, Kansas 66061

Richard L. Friedman, M.D.
Assistant Clinical Professor, Department of Surgery, Albert Einstein College of Medicine, 1300 Morris Park Avenue, Bronx, New York 10462; and Assistant Chairman, Department of Surgery, Kings Highway Division, Beth Israel Medical Center, First Avenue at 16th Street, New York, New York 10003

William R. Fry, M.D., F.A.C.S.
Assistant Clinical Professor of Surgery, University of Colorado School of Medicine, Colorado Springs, Colorado 80918

Michel Gagner, M.D.
Clinical Professor, Department of Surgery, Mount Sinai School of Medicine and Chief, Division of Laparoscopic Surgery, Mount Sinai Medical Center, One Gustave L. Levy Place, New York, New York 10029

Gillian Q. Galloway, M.D.
San Dieguito Surgical Medical Group, 320 Santa Fe Drive, Encinitas, California 92075

Iqbal S. Garcha, M.D.
Chief Resident, General Surgery, Georgia Baptist Medical Center, 520 Bridgewater Drive, Atlanta, Georgia 30328

O. James Garden, M.D., F.R.C.S.
Professor of Hepatobiliary Surgery, University Department of Surgery, The University of Edinburgh, EH8 9AG, United Kingdom; and Honorary Consultant Surgeon, University Department of Surgery, Royal Infirmary, Edinburgh, EH3 94W, United Kingdom

W. Peter Geis, M.D.
Director, Minimally Invasive Services Training Institute (MISTI) and Chief, Minimally Invasive Surgery, Department of Surgery, St. Joseph Medical Center, 7620 York Road, Baltimore, Maryland 21204

Gary Glick, M.D.
Attending Surgeon, Department of Surgery, Mt. Sinai Hospital, 4300 Alton Road, Miami Beach, Florida 33140

Peter M. Y. Goh, M.B.B.S., F.R.C.S., M.Med.
Chairman and Associate Professor, National University Hospital, 5 Lower Kent Ridge Road, Singapore 0511

Andrew J. Graham, M.D., M.Sc., M.HSc., F.R.C.S.
Assistant Clinical Professor, Department of Surgery, University of Alberta; and Staff Surgeon, Department of Surgery, University of Alberta Hospital, 8440 112th Street, Edmonton, Alberta T6G 2B7, Canada

Frederick L. Greene, M.D.
Chairman, Department of General Surgery, Carolinas Medical Center, 1000 Blythe Boulevard, Charlotte, North Carolina 28203

Jeffrey A. Hagen, M.D.
Assistant Professor, Department of Surgery, University of Southern California, 1441 Eastlake Avenue; and University of Southern California University Hospital, 1500 San Pablo Street, Los Angeles, California 90033

Ronald A. Hinder, M.D.
Chief of Surgery, The Mayo Clinic—Jacksonville, 4500 San Pablo Road, Jacksonville, Florida 32224

Michael D. Holzman, M.D.
Assistant Professor, Department of Surgery, Vanderbilt University, D-5203 MCN, Nashville, Tennessee 37232-2577

John G. Hunter, M.D., F.A.C.S.
Professor, Department of Surgery, Emory University School of Medicine; and Director, Division of Gastrointestinal Surgery, Emory University Hospital, 1364 Clifton Road, N.E., Atlanta, Georgia 30322

Timothy G. John, M.D., F.R.C.S.Ed. (Gen)
Consultant Surgeon, Hepatobiliary Unit, North Hampshire Hospital, Aldermaston Road, Basingstoke, RG24 9NA, United Kingdom

Namir Katkhouda, M.D.
Associate Professor of Surgery, Department of Surgery and Chief, Division of Emergency Non Trauma and Minimally Invasive Surgery, University of Southern California, 1510 San Pablo Street, Los Angeles, California 90033

James Knoetgen III, M.D.
Resident in Surgery, St. Luke's-Roosevelt Hospital, Columbia University College of Physicians and Surgeons, 50 East 69th Street, New York, New York 10021

Rodney J. Landreneau, M.D.
Section Head, Thoracic Surgery, Allegheny University of the Health Sciences, 490 East North Avenue, Pittsburgh, Pennsylvania 15212

Demetrius W. M. Litwin, M.D.
Director, Minimal Access Surgery, Department of Surgery, University of Massachusetts Medical Center, 55 Lake Avenue, North Worchester, Massachusetts 01655

Thom E. Lobe, M.D.
Professor of Surgery and Pediatrics, Department of Surgery, University of Tennessee, Memphis, 777 Washington Avenue; and Chairman, Section of Pediatric Surgery, LeBonheur Children's Medical Center, 50 North Dunlap, Memphis, Tennessee 38105

William B. Long, M.D., F.A.C.S.
Clinical Professor of Surgery, Department of Surgery, Oregon Health Sciences University, 3181 S.W. Sam Jackson Park Road, Portland, Oregon 97201-3098; and Chief of Trauma Services, Shock Trauma Institute, Legacy Emanuel Hospital, 2801 N. Gantenbein Avenue, Portland, Oregon 97227

Bruce V. MacFadyen, Jr., M.D.
Professor, Department of Surgery, The University of Texas Medical School, 6431 Fannin; and Director, Minimally Invasive Surgery, Department of Surgery, Hermann Hospital, 6411 Fannin, Houston, Texas 77030

Márcio M. Machado, M.D.
Hospital Samaritano, Setor Coimbra, Praca Walter Santos, 01, Goiania, Goias, Brazil 74 535-270

Michael J. Mack, M.D.
Clinical Assistant Professor and Attending Surgeon, Medical City Dallas, 7777 Forest Lane, Dallas, Texas 75230

Maria T. Madden, M.D.
Instructor in Surgery, Northeastern Ohio University College of Medicine, 4209 State Route 44, Rootstown, Ohio 44272; and Active Staff, Department of Surgery, St. Elizabeth's Medical Center, 1044 Belmont Avenue, Youngstown, Ohio 44501

Edward M. Mason, M.D.
Assistant Clinical Professor, Department of Surgery, Medical College of Georgia, Augusta, Georgia 30912-4750; and Chief, General Surgery and Director, Endosurgery, Department of Surgery, Georgia Baptist Medical Center, 315 Boulevard Avenue N.E., Atlanta, Georgia 30312

Eli Mavor, M.D.
Chief of Surgical Unit A, Kaplan Medical Center, Rehovot, Israel

Kenneth McQuaid, M.D.
Chief, GI Endoscopy, VA Medical Center, Surgical Service 112, 4150 Clement Street, San Francisco, California 94121

Toshiyuki Mori, M.D., Ph.D.
Associate Professor and Chief of Minimally Invasive Surgery, Kyorin University, 6-20-2 Shinkawa Mitaka, 181 Tokyo, Japan

Jean Mouiel, M.D.
Professor of Surgery, Department Head, Department of Surgery, University of Nice, 8 Vallom Broge Avenue, 06000 Nice; and Chairman, Department of Surgery, Archet II, 151 Route St. Antoine, 06202 Nice, France

Alexander G. Nagy, C.D., B.Sc., M.D., F.R.C.S.C.
Clinical Professor, Head, Section of Laparoscopic Surgery, Division of General Surgery, University of British Columbia, 910 W. 10th, Vancouver, British Columbia, Canada V5Z 4E3

Margaret Napolitano, M.D.
Resident, Department of Surgery, St. Louis University, St. Louis, Missouri 63110-0250

Heidi Nelson, M.D.
Professor of Surgery, Department of Colon and Rectal Surgery, Mayo Clinic, 200 First Street S.W., Rochester, Minnesota 55905

Lucian Newman III, M.D., F.A.C.S.
Chair, Department of Surgery, Riverview Regional/Gadsden Regional, 419 South 5th Street, Gadsden, Alabama 35901

Theodore G. Obenchain, M.D.
Department of Neurological Surgery, Palomar Medical Center, 555 East Valley Parkway, Escondido, California 92025

Steven Offerman, M.D.
Assistant Unit Chief, USC University Hospital and LAC-USC Medical Center, 1510 MCC San Pablo Street, Los Angeles, California 90033

Theodore N. Pappas, M.D.
Professor, Department of Surgery, Duke University Medical Center, Durham, North Carolina 27710

Carlos A. Pellegrini, M.D.
The Henry N. Harkins Professor and Chairman, Department of Surgery, University of Washington and Attending Surgeon, Department of Surgery, University of Washington Medical Center, 1959 N.E. Pacific Street, Seattle, Washington 98195

Galen Perdikis, M.D.
Surgery Resident, Department of Surgery, Creighton University, 601 North 30th Street, Omaha, Nebraska 68132

Jeffrey H. Peters, M.D.
Associate Professor of Surgery, Department of Surgery, University of Southern California, and Chief, Department of Surgery, University of Southern California University Hospital, 1500 San Pablo Street, Los Angeles, California 90033

Quynh Pham, M.D.
Division of General Surgery, University of Toronto Mount Sinai Hospital, 600 University Avenue, Toronto, Ontario, Canada M5G 1X5

Edward H. Phillips, M.D.
Clinical Associate Professor and Director, Endoscopic Surgery, Cedars-Sinai Medical Center, 8635 West 3rd Street, Los Angeles, California 90048

Mario F. Pompili, M.D.
Clinical Assistant Professor, Department of Cardiothoracic Surgery, Stanford University Medical Center, 300 Pasteur Drive, Stanford, California 94305; and Staff Surgeon, Surgical Service, Veterans Affairs Palo Alto Health Care System, 3801 Miranda Avenue, Palo Alto, California 94304

Alexander D. Porter, M.D.
Fellow for the University of Washington Swallowing Center, Department of Surgery, University of Washington School of Medicine, University of Washington Medical Center, 1959 N.E. Pacific Street, Seattle, Washington 98195-6410

Eric C. Poulin, M.D., M.Sc., F.R.C.S.C.
Professor of Surgery, Department of Surgery, University of Toronto, Surgeon-in-Chief, St. Michael's Hospital, Wellesley Central Site, 160 Wellesley Street E., Jones Building, Toronto, Ontario, Canada M4Y 1J3

Glenn M. Preminger, M.D.
Professor, Urologic Surgery and Director, Comprehensive Kidney Stone Center, Department of Urology/Surgery, Duke University Medical Center, Baker House, Duke South, Durham, North Carolina 27710

Bruce J. Ramshaw, M.D.
Attending Surgeon and Director of Telemedicine, Georgia Baptist Medical Center, 285 Boulevard N.E., Atlanta, Georgia 30312

Robert D. Rehnke, M.D.
6450 38th Avenue North, St. Petersburg, Florida 33710

Arlene E. Ricardo, M.D.
Resident, Department of Surgery, University of Texas-Houston, 6431 Fannin, Houston, Texas 77030

William S. Richardson, M.D.
Assistant Professor, Department of Surgery, The Ochsner Clinic, 1514 Jefferson Highway, New Orleans, Louisiana 70121

Brian G. Rubin, M.D.
Assistant Professor of Surgery, Department of Surgery, Washington University School of Medicine and Barnes-Jewish Hospital, One Barnes-Jewish Hospital Plaza, Queeny Tower, St. Louis, Missouri 63110

Barry A. Salky, M.D.
Clinical Professor of Surgery, Department of Surgery, Mt. Sinai School of Medicine; and Division of Laparoscopic Surgery, Mt. Sinai Hospital, One Gustave L. Levy Place, New York, New York 10025

Philip R. Schauer, M.D.
Assistant Professor, Department of General Surgery, University of Pittsburgh Medical Center, 200 Lothrop Street, Pittsburgh, Pennsylvania 15213

Bruce D. Schirmer, M.D.
Stephen H. Watts Professor of Surgery, Department of Surgery, University of Virginia Health System, Charlottesville, Virginia 22906-0005

Brett C. Sheppard, M.S., M.D., F.A.C.S.
Physician and Surgeon, Associate Professor of Surgery, Division of General Surgery, Oregon Health Sciences University, 3181 S.W. Sam Jackson Park Road, Portland, Oregon 97201-3098

Peter W. Smiley, M.D.
Senior Clinical Instructor, Surgery Preceptor, Legacy Portland Hospital, Department of Surgery and Active Staff, Division of General and Vascular Surgery, Legacy Emanuel Hospital, 2801 N. Gantenbein, Portland, Oregon 97227

R. Stephen Smith, M.D.
Associate Professor, Department of Surgery, University of Kansas School of Medicine-Wichita; and Medical Director, Trauma Department/Surgical Intensive Care Unit, Via Christi Regional Medical Center, St. Francis Campus, 929 N. St. Francis, Wichita, Kansas 67214-3882

John T. Soper, M.D.
Associate Professor, Oncology/Obstetrics/Gynecology, Duke University Medical Center, Erwin Road, Durham, North Carolina 27710

Nathaniel J. Soper, M.D., F.A.C.S.
Professor, Department of Surgery, Washington University; and Head, Minimally Invasive Surgery, Barnes-Jewish Hospital, One Barnes-Jewish Hospital Plaza, St. Louis, Missouri 63110

Bruce C. Steffes, M.D., F.A.C.S.
Associate Clinical Professor, Department of Surgery, Duke University; and Attending Surgeon, Department of Surgery, Veterans Affairs Hospital-Durham, 5084 Fulton Street, Durham, North Carolina 27710

Thomas A. Stellato, M.D.
Professor of Surgery, Department of Surgery, Case Western Reserve University, 10900 Euclid Avenue; and Chief, Division of General Surgery, Department of Surgery, University Hospitals of Cleveland, 11100 Euclid Avenue, Cleveland, Ohio 44106

John H. Stevens, M.D.
Founder and Director, Heartport, Inc., 700 Bay Road, Redwood City, California 94063; and Consulting Associate Professor, Cardiothoracic Surgery, Stanford University School of Medicine, 300 Pasteur, Stanford, California 94305

Steven M. Strasberg, M.D.
Professor of Surgery, Department of Hepatobiliary-Pancreatic Surgery, Washington University; and Head, Hepatobiliary-Pancreatic Surgery, Department of Surgery, Barnes-Jewish Hospital, One Barnes Hospital Plaza, St. Louis, Missouri 63110

Richard S. Swanson, M.D.
Associate Professor and Chief of Surgical Oncology, Department of Surgery, University of Massachusetts, 55 Lake Avenue North, Worcester, Massachusetts 01655-0333

Lee L. Swanström, M.D., F.A.C.S.
Associate Clinical Professor, Department of Surgery, Oregon Health Sciences University; and Director, Department of Minimally Invasive Surgery, Legacy Health System, 501 N. Graham Street, Portland, Oregon 97227

Walter T. L. Tan, M.B.B.S., F.R.C.S.
Associate Professor and Head, Department of Surgery, National University of Singapore; and Chief, Department of Surgery, National University Hospital, Lower Kent Ridge Road, Singapore 119074

Claude Thibault, M.D.
Fellow in Colon and Rectal Surgery, Division of Colon and Rectal Surgery, Mayo Clinic and Mayo Foundation, 200 First Street S.W., Rochester, Minnesota 55905

Robert W. Thompson, M.D.
Associate Professor, Department of Surgery, Cell Biology & Physiology, and Radiology, Washington University School of Medicine, 4960 Children's Plaza; and Attending Surgeon, Department of Surgery, Barnes-Jewish Hospital, One Barnes-Jewish Plaza, St. Louis, Missouri 63110

Thadeus L. Trus, M.D.
Assistant Professor, Department of Surgery, Medical University of South Carolina, 171 Ashley Avenue, Charleston, South Carolina 29425

Jeffrey G. Tucker, M.D.
Attending Surgeon and Director of Metabolic Support, Georgia Baptist Medical Center, 1400 Baptist Medical Center Drive, Cumming, Georgia 30041

Juan P. Umana, M.D.
Chief Resident, Department of Surgery, Columbia University College of Physicians and Surgeons, 622 W. 168th Street; and Columbia-Presbyterian Hospital, 177 Ft. Washington Avenue, New York, New York 10032

Eric R. Van Buskirk, M.D.
Staff, Plastic Surgery Associates of Lynchburg, Inc., 1330 Oak Lane, Lynchburg, Virginia 24503

Donald Waldrep, M.D.
Assistant Unit Chief, University of Southern California University Hospital and LAC-USC Medical Center, 1510 MCC San Pablo Street, Los Angeles, California 90033

Lawrence W. Way, M.D.
Professor and Vice Chairman of Surgery, University of California San Francisco School of Medicine, 513 Parnassus Avenue, San Francisco, California 94143-0475

Stephen Wise Unger, M.D.
Attending Surgeon and Director, Surgical Endoscopy and Laparoscopy, Department of Surgery, Mt. Sinai Medical Center of Greater Miami, 4302 Alton Road, Miami Beach, Florida 33140

Foreword

"For the creation of a master work . . . two powers must conquer, the power of the man and the power of the moment, and the man is not enough without the moment."—*The Function of Criticism at the Present Time (1964)*

A decade has passed since modern endosurgery began to change the art of surgical intervention. Minimally invasive intervention now impacts most of medicine and surgery. Thus, it is time for definitive textbooks on the subject. Drs. Eubanks, Swanström, and Soper are three of the world's leaders in minimally invasive surgery. These editors have recruited remarkable contributions from many other surgical leaders to create the masterwork you are about to read. Like the quotation above, let us consider this masterwork according to two most important powers: the moment and the man.

The moment is just over 10 years since the introduction of laparoscopic cholecystectomy—the new operation that began a decade of change. Laparoscopic cholecystectomy was clearly a better choice than either traditional cholecystectomy or experimental gallstone treatments such as dissolutional agents and lithotripsy. However, traditional surgeons vehemently opposed the idea that "less exposure" might be beneficial to the patient. Private sector surgeons led the assault. Eddie Reddick, a respected private practice surgeon in Nashville, recognized the potential importance of the new technique. Along with Doug Olsen, he questioned then current surgical principles. His submissions to national meetings were repeatedly rejected. Reddick and Olsen continued to challenge tradition and principles with dollars, industry, and new educational methods.

The manuscript, "Prospective Analysis of 1,518 Cases of Laparoscopic Cholecystectomy," published in the *New England Journal of Medicine*, provided the first objective data to support this new procedure. With this manuscript, academic surgeons accepted laparoscopic procedures and began to resume leadership. Initial textbooks on endosurgery at the beginning of the decade were effective in describing the excitement of the times and telling the early history. Other texts and atlases of laparoscopic surgery have made their mark in the field; many reside upon my own bookshelves. Eddie Reddick's initial text, *Atlas of Laparoscopic Surgery*, is now sadly out of print. Karl Zucker first published *Surgical Laparoscopy* in 1991. It too is clearly a classic. Jaroslv Hulka and Harry Reich have now edited three editions of their work, *Textbook of Laparoscopy*, since it first published in 1985. Since then, much more data has been accumulated and wisdom can now be separated from excitement. Ten years after the exciting introduction of modern endosurgery, the moment is opportune for Eubanks, Swanström, and Soper to create this work.

The masters are the surgeons who write this textbook. They are now slightly graying and more wise. I am personally touched by the choice of Dr. Forde to lead the initial historical overview. Kenneth Forde was one of my earliest teachers and inspired me to become a surgeon. As the editor of *Surgical Endoscopy* for many years, Dr. Forde advocated minimally invasive procedures years before the concept became popular. He had as much to do with the initial development of minimally invasive surgery as anyone in the world.

The reader can easily identify other world leaders in endosurgery and grow enthusiastic about this book. Dr. Schauer of Pittsburgh, Pennsylvania, my second surgery fellow, describes the physiologic benefits of laparoscopic surgery. His chapter surely will become a classic. Other great minimally invasive surgeons who contributed chapters to this book include Drs. Litwin, Callery, Garden, and Hunter. All of the authors are truly masters in the field.

Mastery of Endoscopic and Laparoscopic Surgery is organized in a logical and readable way. Section I provides an initial overview of laparoscopic surgical principles. Section II focuses on diagnosis and surgery of disorders of the foregut. Section III is a master treatise on liver and biliary surgery, and Section IV reviews the techniques for solid organ surgery. Still, the most interesting section may be Section V on small and large intestinal surgeries. The remaining sections discuss in detail laparoscopic herniorrhaphy, thorascopic surgery, and minimally invasive vascular, cardiac, gynecologic, urologic, pediatric, plastic, and spine surgery. The coverage is comprehensive; the teaching value behind it is priceless.

The blend of technical information and editorial commentary in this work provides well-rounded, valuable insight into the selection of surgical procedures while elucidating various points of technical expertise. The authors have created not only an interesting perspective for students and experts, but a realistic and holistic view of the subject. Drs. Eubanks, Swanström, and Soper have seized the opportunity of the moment. They have seized the availability of the new masters to create the wonderful work you are about to read.

William C. Meyers

Preface

Few phenomena have changed the face of surgery like the widespread introduction of videoscopic technologies in the 1980s. Although flexible endoscopy and basic laparoscopy had been used for many years, it was the later ability to transmit the endoscopic image to a video monitor that allowed assistants to view the same operative field as the surgeon and freed the surgeon's hands for more complex maneuvers. Video laparoscopic surgery—using images transmitted to a video screen from the interior of the body—was a natural extension of flexible endoscopy, which viewed the interior of a natural-occurring body cavity. Although many general surgeons were woefully slow to learn and apply flexible endoscopy—either for political reasons or in the mistaken belief that it was primarily a diagnostic modality—most have become enthusiastic supporters of the subsequent "laparoscopic revolution." Ironically, many surgeons have developed a renewed appreciation for flexible endoscopy because of their laparoscopic experiences. Certainly these technologies have reinvigorated the practice of general surgery, generating enthusiasm on the part of the practitioner, involving the entire operating room staff, and causing a critical reappraisal of the effects that major incisions have on the body's homeostasis. There has also been an enhanced understanding of the physiologic and immune responses to surgery as a result of the interest in laparoscopy.

Despite the fact that more than 10 years have passed since laparoscopic cholecystectomy was first introduced in the United States, few operations other than cholecystectomy have become the "gold standard." Many practicing surgeons and, by definition, most surgical trainees remain neophytes or are in the early learning curve for many of the more advanced laparoscopic procedures. This textbook should be a valuable tool to help surmount the learning stage. We have been fortunate to assemble authors who are acknowledged authorities in the field. They are true experts, both in regard to clinical performance of endoscopic and laparoscopic procedures and in the arena of surgical education. Many were involved in the development and dissemination of the procedures they describe. We are much indebted to them for their contributions. The comments by the editors at the ends of chapters are not critiques or criticisms, but rather attempts at putting the chapters in a more global perspective or, in rare instances, to discuss even more recent developments in the field.

This textbook is a natural offshoot of the *Mastery of Surgery* text that has become one of the premier references in surgical education today. As a result, we are also indebted to Drs. Nyhus, Baker, and Fischer, who have set the high standard to which we must aspire.

We have directed this book to students of surgery at all levels—from the surgical intern to the well-established surgical practitioner. There are enough pearls of wisdom contained herein to enhance the reader's technical ability to treat patients with minimally invasive techniques. In this way, we may move closer to heeding the statement of William Osler, "Diseases that harm call for treatments that harm less."

Nathaniel J. Soper, M.D., F.A.C.S.
Lee L. Swanström, M.D., F.A.C.S.
W. Stephen Eubanks, M.D., F.A.C.S.

I

General Topics

1

History and Development of Flexible Endoscopy

Kenneth A. Forde and Juan P. Umana

Upper Gastrointestinal Endoscopy

As early as the 19th century, attempts were being made to examine the interior of the upper gastrointestinal (GI) tract by reflecting light into body cavities through a hollow cylinder, but it was not until Thomas Edison's invention of the incandescent light bulb that it became possible to perform rigid endoscopy in the late 1870s. Nevertheless, progressively smaller lamps were developed that allowed insertion into the stomach through rigid gastroscopes, but the nature of the light made it impossible to perform long or complex studies due to overheating of the instruments. In addition, the inability to adapt rigid instruments to the curvatures of the bowel permitted only limited examination of the upper GI tract and rectum due in part to patient discomfort but also to the risk of complications. In fact, most examinations required general anesthesia, which explains why these procedures were mostly performed by surgeons, such as the 19th century Polish surgeon Johann von Mikulicz-Radecki.

The era of flexible endoscopy began with the introduction of the semirigid gastroscope by R. Schindler in 1936 through work developed in collaboration with the German physician Georg Wolf. The way to the development of a flexible fiberscope was paved by Baird's demonstration in 1928 that light and images could be transmitted through a single glass or quartz fiber. Despite improvements by Hansell in the United States and Lamm, a German gynecologist, no significant progress was made until the 1950s when van Heel in the Netherlands and H. Hopkins and N.S. Kapany in England, working independently, developed usable flexible glass fiber bundles that could transmit light across relatively long distances and into body cavities. The next phase of development took place in Ann Arbor at the University of Michigan. There, physicians H.M. Pollard and Basil Hirschowitz, in collaboration with physicist C. Wilbur Peters and then physics student Lawrence Curtis, designed the first clinically usable, completely flexible endoscope. Hirschowitz and Curtis started working on this concept in 1955 by developing an instrument composed of a bundle of individual glass fibers that was, in theory, capable of transmitting light as well as images. Along the way, they encountered numerous problems, such as fiber "crosstalk," which diffused the light, making interpretation of the images impossible. This led to their invention of a glass coating for the fibers for insulation and to the development of the fiberscope. Early gastroscopes, albeit flexible, were not equipped with a steerable tip or reliable guidance system. One of the first controllable-tip gastroscopes was developed in 1962 and, in contrast to most landmark inventions, was first applied clinically and then found an industrial application in the examination of jet engines.

After trying the flexible gastroscope on himself, Hirschowitz first used it in a patient with a bleeding duodenal ulcer in February 1957. The diagnosis was successfully established, and the patient underwent operation based on Hirschowitz's observation. At that point, the clinical utility of the device was demonstrated, and it would only be a matter of time until the nonbelievers were converted to the future of diagnostic GI endoscopy. Hirschowitz's description of the negotiations that were conducted in finding a manufacturer makes for delightful reading. Several companies were in competition at that time, but only Frederick J. Wallace of American Cystoscope Makers, Inc. (ACMI, Norwalk, CT) had the combination of vision and capital to embark on the production of commercial fiberscopes, employing Peters, Hirschowitz, and Curtis as consultants. The first commercially produced fiberoptic endoscope made by ACMI was first used in 1961, and the results were published in the *Lancet* in May of that year. Once the development and widespread use of fiberoptic upper GI endoscopes became commonplace, the therapeutic potential was exploited. Experimental studies, such as those by W.D. Blackwood, S. Silvis, J.P. Papp, C. Sugawa, and others, demonstrated the feasibility and safety of endoscopic hemostasis. This has paved the way for the use of endoscopes as vehicle for numerous accessories, so that today endoscopic surgery includes methods of hemostasis, excision, ablation, dilatation, decompression, sclerosis, and foreign body removal.

Examination of the Biliary Tract

Endoscopic examination of the biliary tract began with rigid instruments. Bakes was credited with the idea and McIver with the development of the first rigid choledochoscope in 1941. During the 1950s, the Wolf company introduced an instrument that was improved upon by Karl Stroz. The first flexible choledochoscope, however, was an ACMI instrument used by Wildegans in Berlin, who reported a remarkably extensive experience by 1960. There followed several years of inactivity, with surgeons apparently reluctant to use the flexible instruments. Some thought operative time would be prolonged and the infection rate increased because use of the endoscope was not totally sterile as a result of the examiner's contact with it when looking through the eyepiece. Surgeons' lack of familiarity at that time with flexible endoscopes in general may also have had a lot to do with this reluctance. Furthermore, the inability at that time (before videocameras) to display images and communicate findings severely limited early efforts.

Meanwhile, investigators involved in developing upper GI endoscopes, primarily gastroenterologists, reached the ampullary region in their exploration of the duodenum, and McCune and colleagues in 1968 reported a 25% success rate in cannulating the pancreatic duct using an Eder duodenoscope with a cannula strapped to its back in approximately 50 patients. They used 50% Hypaque solution for pancreatography, worrying even then about producing pancreatitis. After these humble beginnings, the field of endoscopic retrograde cholangiopancreatography (ERCP) developed with the manufacture of duodenoscopes by Japanese companies (Olympus Corporation, Machida Instrument Company). I. Oi presented his experience using a specially designed sideviewing duodenoscope at the 1970 World Congress of Gastroenterology. This was an era in which both surgeons and gastroenterologists recognized the high morbidity and mortality of patients with recurrent or retained stones in the common bile duct. It is therefore not surprising that those with the new endoscopes embarked early on using these instruments for treatment, even as diagnostic expertise was being developed. There developed a new breed of aggressive, technically adept gastroenterologist-endoscopists (later to be called "interventionists"), among them, Classen and Demling in Germany and K. Kawai and S. Soma in Japan, who developed techniques of vaterian papillotomy and stone extraction. J.A. Vennes is credited with introducing ERCP in the United States, and

surgeons such as Walter Gaisford and Ali Ghazi were among the early workers in this field. Joseph Geenen and others exploited this new access to the pancreaticobiliary region to perform various physiologic studies, and more modern endoscopists now regularly employ ERCP as one approach in decompression of malignant extrahepatic biliary tract obstruction.

Examination of the Small Bowel

Once called the last frontier of flexible endoscopy, enteroscopy is now more developed, useful, and available. With few disease processes requiring direct visualization of the small bowel mucosa for their successful management and with the marked length of bowel to be traversed, it is not entirely surprising that enteroscopy came late in the evolution of flexible endoscopy and that there have been fewer workers in the development of this area. Credit must be given to early workers such as Gaisford, S.B. Lewis, and Hiromi Shinya and their coworkers in the United States and M. Tada in Japan. There have been several approaches to small bowel endoscopy. Two early methods have been virtually abandoned: One (Gaisford) involving a prototype endoscope passed over a previously swallowed string proved unreliable, and the other (Joseph Sweeting) involving a small bowel enterotomy had the potential for significant contamination of the peritoneal cavity. One approach still employed to a limited extent is intraoperative total endoscopy, in which a colonoscope, passed orally, can usually be advanced as far as the distal ileum, which can then be examined in retrograde fashion per anum (T. Bowden). Two methods for small bowel endoscopy are currently employed regularly. One is the *push* type, in which a long, thin upper GI endoscope or pediatric colonoscope is inserted directly (pushed) *per os*, usually only reaching as far as the proximal to midjejunum. The other method, called the *sonde* (French for bend) type, has been the most useful. With a distal balloon attached to a small diameter scope, this instrument is passed in fashion similar to a long intestinal tube, the inflated balloon acting as a stimulus for peristalsis, thus aiding the tube's progress down the GI tract. The small bowel is then examined while the scope is slowly pulled orad.

Examination of the Colon

Early attempts at visualizing the colon included barium enemas and rigid sigmoidoscopy. Despite this combination, many colorectal cancers were discovered late or not at all. M. Deddish and W. Fairweather proposed performing intraoperative colotomies and segmental examination of the colon using a rigid sterile sigmoidoscope, publishing their experience in 1953. The first fiberoptic sigmoidoscope (rather a misnomer) was described by Robert Turell and consisted of a rigid, large-bore sigmoidoscope to which a fiberoptic light source was attached, allowing brighter illumination of the rectum and distal sigmoid.

With advances in the field of fibergastroscopy, attempts were also being made to develop a flexible device to examine the colon. In Japan, F. Matsunaga and colleagues tried using a modification of the "gastrocamera" to study the colon. This was a fiberoptic gastroscope that allowed light transmission into the stomach, and a camera connected to the end of it permitted taking pictures from the stomach and duodenum. Its lack of a steering system and the convoluted anatomy of the colon made these attempts fruitless.

In the spring of 1961, Bergein F. Overholt, then an intern at the University of Michigan, started work on an early version of a flexible colonoscope in association with N.S. Kapany, president of Optics Technology in California. By producing a mold of the rectosigmoid colon, they were able to create a model that helped a great deal in the design of later practice models. By 1963, a flexible sigmoidoscope was successfully used by Overholt in clinical practice. At about this time in Europe, L. Provinzale and A. Revignas accomplished the first total retrograde colonoscopy using a lateral-viewing, nonsteerable Hirschowitz gastroscope. Their technique was in essence a modification of Blankenhorn's end-to-end intestinal intubation. Using soft tubing as a pulley mechanism, the gastroscope was pulled and pushed to reach the cecum. In Japan in 1963, S. Oshiba and A. Watanabe, in conjunction with Machida, developed an early colon fiberscope in competition with Olympus under the guidance of H. Niwa and T. Kanazawa.

The pioneering work of Niwa in Japan and Overholt in the United States allowed significant progress in the use of fiberoptic instruments for examining the rectum and sigmoid colon. However, it was the appearance of ACMI in this arena that permitted a giant leap forward with the manufacture of the first steerable colonoscopes in the late 1960s. At that time, colonoscopes were produced in variable sizes and lengths (86 cm, 108 cm, and 186 cm). The length of the scope was determined by the most proximal area of interest in the colon. Interestingly, all were called colonoscopes.

The concept of a specific screening instrument to be designated a "sigmoidoscope" had not yet been born. As physicians became more proficient with the longer colonoscopes and reached the cecum in a greater proportion of examinations, there came to be less need for the shorter colonoscopes. By early 1969, William I. Wolff, Director of Surgery at the Beth Israel Medical Center in New York City, along with his younger colleagues Shinya and Ghazi, developed a highly regarded program in upper GI endoscopy at that institution. This put them in an ideal position to start using the newly developed colonoscopes to intubate the colon in retrograde fashion. In the initial stages of this endeavor, they met with staunch criticism from radiologists and surgeons alike. They were wise and responsible enough to establish strict ground rules to avoid complications that would have made them vulnerable to criticism and would most likely have diminished their efforts to advance a technique that would later not only revolutionize the management of lower GI bleeding but also change the natural history of colon cancer through the discovery and regular removal of colonic adenomas. Thanks to their tenacity and, to a large extent, Shinya's technical prowess, great progress was made over the following months in developing a technique for negotiating the fiberscope around the sigmoid loop. These developments have been well chronicled by Wolff.

Colonoscopes were progressively developed to an ever higher degree of sophistication with larger ports and additional channels for air insufflation and suction. Cold light sources were developed that allowed much better quality and duration in examinations, while at the same time facilitating the performance of tissue biopsies and cytology obtained under direct vision. Initial ACMI instruments required the operator's both hands on the head of the instrument. The left hand was used for holding the instrument and controlling the air, water, and suction buttons, while the right hand was used to manipulate the "flag handle" that controlled the instrument tip. An additional person was therefore required to insert the instrument shaft. Ultimately, the flag handle was replaced by wheels that many soon learned to operate entirely with the left hand, thus liberating the right hand for instrument insertion. In 1969, Shinya designed a snare–cautery device that could be introduced into the lumen of the bowel under direct vision through the biopsy channel. The snare allowed removal of most polyps encountered by the colonoscopic route, and by 1974 the Beth Israel team was able to report on the endoscopic removal of more than 2,000 polyps with negligible morbidity. Since that time, the therapeutic potential of the instrument has been expanded. From the earliest days, the redundant, often unfixed sigmoid colon created problems by forming loops, thus inhibiting progress of the scope into the more proximal bowel. Shinya devised an overtube (external splinting device) to fix the straightened sigmoid once the splenic flexure had been reached. This requires the use of fluoroscopy for safety and so is not universally available. Prototype instruments have even been developed for special needs. Similar to therapeutic upper GI endoscopes, colonoscopes now serve as vehicles for hemostasis, excision, ablation, decompression, dilatation, and extraction.

Examination of Other Cavities

While the examination of some body cavities has remained in the realm of rigid endoscopy (e.g., arthroscopy), flexible endoscopes have enjoyed variable development in areas such as nasopharyngoscopy, laryngoscopy, bronchoscopy (including anesthesiologic use for difficult intubation), ureteroscopy, nephroscopy, and thoracoscopy.

Other Applications

Use of flexible endoscopes as vehicles for other imaging (and therapeutic) applications has been initiated with the pairing of endoscopy and ultrasonography. Initially, ultrasound probes were added to the ends of flexible gastroscopes, but smaller ultrasound probes that can be passed through one of the channels of the endoscope have also been developed.

Photodocumentation

From the earliest days of clinically useful endoscopy, it was recognized that the ability to generate permanent images would help both communication and credibility. As early as 1938, N. Henning and H. Keilhack obtained the first color images from the stomach using the semirigid Schindler gastroscope. In the purely fiberoptic era, various 35-mm-type still cameras were adapted to the eyepiece of the endoscope. The delay in film processing made instant reproduction attractive, and various Polaroid-type cameras were tested. However, the need to interrupt the procedure to attach and detach the camera proved awkward and distracting. G. Berci and colleagues developed the first miniature black-and-white and color videocameras that were attached to the eyepiece of fiberoptic instruments; these, however, proved even bulkier and less attractive than the 35-mm still camera. Videocameras were also attached to the lens of the side-viewing (teaching) adaptors to allow the operator to be undisturbed in looking through the eyepiece while permitting a televised image for others and for documentation. With the development of charge-coupled devices (or chip cameras), it has become possible to place a camera at the tip of an endoscope and transfer the images through a processor on to a high-resolution video monitor, with all the obvious advantages for efficient participation of assistants, as well as for education and training.

While much progress is still to be made in instrumentation and image quality, it is clear that the development of flexible endoscopy has been remarkable enough in less than a century to place it firmly as a strong pillar in the evolving structure of minimal-access surgery.

Suggested Reading

Berci G, Davids J. Endoscopy and television. *BMJ* 1962;1:1610.

Berci G, Schulman AG, Morgenstern L, Paz-Partlow M, Cuschieri A, Wood RA. Television choledochoscopy. *Surg Gynecol Obstet* 1985;160: 176–177.

Forde KA. Therapeutic colonoscopy. *World J Surg* 1992;16:1048–1053.

Gordon ME, Kirsner JB. Rudolf Schindler, pioneer endoscopist: glimpses of the man and his work. *Gastroenterol* 1979;77:354–361.

Hirschowitz BI. A personal history of the fiberscope. *Gastroenterol* 1979;76:864–869.

Lewis BS, Waye JD. Total small bowel enteroscopy. *Gastrointest Endosc* 1987;33:435–438.

McCune WS, Shorb PE, Moscovitz H. Endoscopic cannulation of the ampulla of vater: a preliminary report. *Ann Surg* 1968;167:752–756.

Overholt BF. The history of colonoscopy. In: Hunt RH, Waye JD, eds. *Colonoscopy: techniques, clinical practice and color atlas*. London: Chapman and Hall, 1981:1–7.

Vennes JA, Silvis SE. Endoscopic visualization of bile and pancreatic ducts. *Gastrointest Endosc* 1972;18:149–152.

Wolff WI. Colonoscopy: history and development. *Am J Gastroenterol* 1989;84:1017–1025.

2

History and Development of Laparoscopic Surgery

Alexander G. Nagy

As the 20th century draws to a close, we are witnessing the dawning of a new era in which closed body cavity operative procedures are more and more often being performed through minimal access by endoscopic visualization. This development is the result of the vision and work of many dedicated individuals over the past century. These individuals include the early pioneers of endoscopy who planted the seed, the nurturing pioneers who ensured that the benefits of the technique were publicized, and finally the modern pioneers who pushed and expanded these frontiers to the point where operative endoscopy, especially laparoscopy, has few bounds. Through the efforts of these individuals, increasingly more procedures once thought to be impossible through endoscopic access are now widely performed.

Early Developments

Few advances in medicine occur in isolation. The innate human curiosity to peer inside body cavities has been chronicled since ancient times. However, due to primitive technology and crude instruments, many of these ambitions were not realized. It is probably safe to say that the first laparoscopy would not have been performed, had it not been for the efforts of many physicians in the 19th century to develop endoscopes that would allow the examination of open orifices in the body. Thus, Phillip Bozzini in 1805 examined the urethra of a living patient using a simple tube and candlelight (Fig. 2-1). Antonin J. Des-

ormeaux in 1843 developed the first effective endoscope, which led Maximillian Nitze to perfect the cystoscope in 1879 (Fig. 2-2). Thomas Edison developed the incandescent light bulb in 1880, and it was a great improvement over Nitze's light source, an external alcohol-fueled lamp with an incandescent platinum filament on the distal tip of the cystoscope. Newman in 1883 quickly capitalized on Edison's invention, adapting it for use with a cystoscope. It was this cystoscope that George Kelling, a Dresden surgeon, used in 1901 to examine the peritoneal cavity of a living dog. He also realized that pneumoperitoneum was very important for exposure, using room air for insufflation of the peritoneal cavity. He called this procedure "celioscopy." Although apparently he used this method in two patients, this achievement was not well publicized. Also in 1901, Dimitri Oskarovich Von Ott in St. Petersburg examined a pregnant woman through a small culdotomy incision using a head mirror, naming this procedure "ventroscopy."

The term *laparoscopy* was coined by Hans Christian Jacobaeus of Sweden in a 1911 report on the results of laparoscopy and thoracoscopy in over 110 patients (Fig. 2-3). In the same year in the United States, Bertram Bernheim, an assistant surgeon at Johns Hopkins University, used a 0.5-inch proctoscope to examine the epigastric region in a deeply jaundiced patient without a pneumoperitoneum, using an electric headlamp for illumination. He was able to confirm the endoscopic findings at the subsequent laparotomy. It was quickly re-

alized that exposure was the key to the success of laparoscopy and that patient positioning was critical. S. Nordentoft described the deep Trendelenburg position to help display the pelvic organs during laparoscopy. As insertion of a needle to induce a pneumoperitoneum was cumbersome and unsafe, Otto Goetze developed an insufflating needle in 1918. Richard Zollikofer in 1924 promoted the use of carbon dioxide (CO_2) as the the most suitable insufflating gas for pneumoperitoneum because of its rapid absorption. In the United States in 1920, B.H. Ordnoff introduced a pyramidal-tipped trocar and reported its use in 42 cases of laparoscopy. The first textbook on laparoscopy and tho-

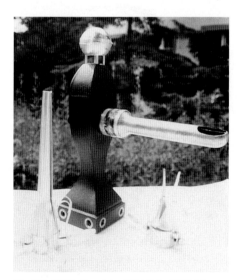

Fig. 2-1. Phillip Bozzini—"Lichtleiter" (Light conductor). (Courtesy of Grzegorz S. Litynski, Frankfurt am Main, Germany.)

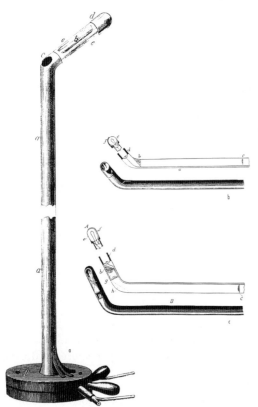

Fig. 2-2. Nitze cystoscope. (From Reuter HJ, Reuter MA. *Phillip Bozzini und die Endoskopie des 19. Jahrhunderts.* Stuttgart, Germany: Max-Nitze-Museum, 1988. Courtesy of Grzegorz S. Litynski, Frankfurt am Main, Germany.)

techniques. It was then apparent that adequate visualization and exposure would allow laparoscopic interventions.

Therapeutic and Technical Advances

In Germany in 1933, C. Fervers reported cauterizing intraabdominal adhesions, and thereafter P.F. Boesch in Switzerland and E.T. Anderson in the United States independently proposed performing laparoscopic female tubal sterilization by fulguration. However, it is claimed that the first actual laparoscopic female sterilization was performed in the United States in 1941 by Frank H. Power and Allan C. Barnes. Thus, the seeds for operative laparoscopy had also been planted. As indications expanded, so did improvements in instrumentation. John C. Ruddock in the United States designed a single-puncture operating laparoscope and accompanying instruments with which biopsies could be obtained (Fig. 2-5). Janos Veress, a Hungarian, promoted the use of a spring-loaded needle to induce pneumothorax in tuberculosis patients. The Veress needle was subsequently used to insufflate the peritoneum and remains the most frequently used pneumoperitoneum needle. The inner blunt probe of this needle protects the abdominal contents from perfor-

racoscopy was published in 1927 by R. Korbsch in Germany. The German hepatologist Heinz Kalk in the late 1920s began to promote the fore-oblique lens system (45 degrees) that allowed visualization

over the dome of the liver (Fig. 2-4). He was also the first to use an accessory port through which a working instrument could be introduced. Kalk was thus able to perform liver biopsies using laparoscopic

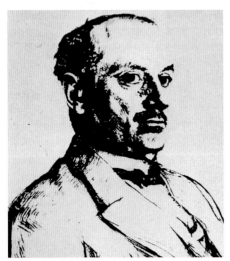

Fig. 2-3. Hans Christian Jacobeus of Stockholm, Sweden. (From Litynski, Grzegorz S. Highlights in the history of laparoscopy. *Frankfurt am Main, Germany: Barbara Bernert Verlag, 1996.* Courtesy of Grzegorz S. Litynski, Frankfurt am Main, Germany.)

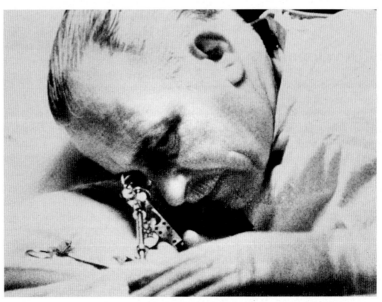

Fig. 2-4. Professor Kalk, promoter of the fore-oblique (45 degrees) lens system.

ation by the outer sharp sheath. During the 1930s and early 1940s, large numbers of successful diagnostic laparoscopies including directed biopsies were reported. Ruddock in 1937 reported 500 cases with a diagnostic accuracy of 92%. John M. Waugh from the Mayo Clinic reported 396 examinations performed over 8 years with a similarly high diagnostic accuracy. Gynecologists were a bit slower in adopting laparoscopy. During the late 1930s and early 1940s, gynecologists attempted to visualize the pelvis primarily through the cul-de-sac, using a procedure called culdoscopy. It was performed in the knee–chest position, and pneumoperitoneum was not induced.

World War II temporarily halted developments in the field of laparoscopy. The first major proponent of gynecologic laparoscopy was Raoul Palmer of Paris, who reported 250 cases in 1946. He described the use of the uterine cannula to manipulate and elevate the uterus while the laparoscopic examination is performed in the lithotomy and Trendelenburg positions. These maneuvers allowed good exposure of the pelvis. Palmer also designed special forceps for ovarian biopsy and emphasized the importance of monitoring intraabdominal pressure during laparoscopy. He is regarded as the father of modern gynecologic laparoscopy. In the 1950s, more technical advances were achieved. In 1952, N. Fourestier, A. Gladu, and J. Valmière introduced a method of transmitting light by means of a quartz rod, and Harold H. Hopkins and N.S. Kapany described the application of fiberoptics to endoscopy. These developments allowed the light source to be kept external to the peritoneal cavity, and the dangers of intraperitoneal heat due to the light source were reduced. Subsequently, in 1966, the rod-lens system was introduced by Hopkins. This system markedly improved image brightness and clarity and forms the basis for the improved laparoscopes used even today.

During this period of development, industry played a key role. Karl Storz, a German instrument maker, produced and promoted the Hopkins lens system and worked with physicians to develop other laparoscopic instruments. Also in the 1950s, H. Frangenheim in Germany embarked on improving and developing laparoscopic instruments. He is responsible for designing the first CO_2 insufflator. Al-

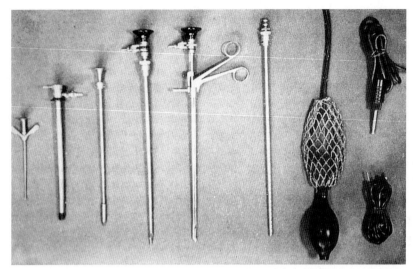

Fig. 2-5. Ruddock's peritoneoscope. (From Litynski, Grzegorz S. Highlights in the history of laparoscopy. Frankfurt am Main, Germany: Barbara Bernert Verlag, 1996. Courtesy of Grzegorz S. Litynski, Frankfurt am Main, Germany.)

though he promoted wider use of laparoscopy, he warned physicians about complications such as air embolism, hollow organ injury, and cardiopulmonary problems that may result from this procedure. He emphasized repeatedly the importance of carefully following the steps of establishing pneumoperitoneum and introducing the trocars safely after a good cushion of gas was obtained.

Acceptance of Laparoscopy by Gynecologists

Despite the achievements of these nurturing pioneers, laparoscopy failed to establish widespread acceptance among gynecologists or surgeons. This was primarily because laparoscopy was not considered a therapeutic modality. Two events occurred in gynecology in the early 1970s that lead to a dramatic increase in the use of the laparoscope. Raoul Palmer, Patrick Steptoe, R.S. Neuwirth, and W.A. Liston reported a large series of patients undergoing laparoscopic tubal sterilization. The demonstrated safety and reduced hospitalization suggested that these procedures could even be performed on an outpatient basis. K. Semm in Germany was responsible for developing many laparoscopic instruments and techniques and championed "endoscopic abdominal surgery." In 1970, V. Gomel directed the first hands-on course in gynecologic laparoscopy in Van-

couver, Canada. Several other individuals subsequently promoted gynecologic laparoscopy through similar hands-on courses, dispersing among gynecologists important information regarding therapeutic laparoscopy. In 1972, Jordan Philips founded the American Association of Gynecologic Laparoscopists (AAGL). This society widely promoted laparoscopy and disseminated rapidly developing techniques and knowledge in this field. By the late 1970s, Semm and coworkers reported on laparoscopic oophorectomies, salpingectomies, and adnexectomies. Gomel presented his initial experience with operative laparoscopy in 1973 and demonstrated the value and safety of this approach for salpingoovariolysis, fimbrinoplasty, and salpingostomy, as well as tubal pregnancy management by segmental excision. At the end of the 1970s, M.A. Bruhat described the use of the CO_2 laser for tubal surgery.

Gynecologists were well on their way with interventional laparoscopic techniques, including the use of thermal and laser energy, sharp and blunt dissection, and ligation and suturing techniques. Gynecologists were also responsible for introducing general surgeons to the use of the laparoscope, especially for evaluation of abdominal pain in young women. In this regard, Gomel promoted the use of diagnostic and operative laparoscopy among his surgical colleagues. M.M. Cohen, a staff surgeon in Gomel's hospital, subsequently reported 77 consecutive cases of diagnostic laparoscopy in general surgical patients, including biopsy procedures and staging of lymphoma. Gomel predicted the widespread utilization of laparoscopy in general surgery. In the mid-1970s, he published his vision of the utility of laparoscopy in general surgical practice in the *American Journal of Surgery*. It is ironic to note that most of the voluminous literature of the 1980s attesting to the benefits of laparoscopy was published by gastroenterologists and gynecologists.

Laparoscopy in General Surgery

As previously with gynecologists, the lack of attention given to laparoscopy by general surgeons was primarily attributable to the perception that it was only a diagnostic modality competing with other new imaging techniques such as ultrasound and computed tomography. Two pioneers of general surgical laparoscopy, however, repeatedly pointed out the accuracy of laparoscopy-guided biopsy and the inadequacy of the new imaging techniques because they could not adequately and consistently demonstrate small lesions. Alfred Cuschieri and George Berci suggested the utility of laparoscopic exploration to minimize nontherapeutic laparotomy, and applied laparoscopy in the evaluation of blunt and penetrating abdominal trauma. They also promoted interventional general surgical laparoscopy, notably, lysis of intraabdominal adhesions and laparoscopy-guided cholecystostomy. Berci was also involved in the development of video cameras to document findings in endoscopy and laparoscopy. Although some

preliminary observations regarding treatment of gallbladder disease were made with the help of the laparoscope in the laboratory setting, the first attempt to resect the gallbladder by C.J. Filipi, J. Mall, and R. Roosma in 1985 was abandoned due to inadequate exposure. Erich Mühe in Germany developed the "galloscope" to perform an early version of laparoscopic cholecystectomy in 1985 (Fig. 2-6).

A source of frustration for surgical assistants performing general surgical laparoscopy at this time was the inability to view what the surgeon was seeing through the monocular laparoscope. Although an articulated attachment to split the laparoscopic image was developed as a "teaching head," the view was inadequate and cumbersome. A major breakthrough for operative endoscopy occurred in 1986 with the introduction of the miniature solid-state camera. Once the laparoscopic image was successfully transmitted electronically to a video monitor, the entire operating team could visualize the procedure and assist in a meaningful way. Very soon after the appearance of this technology, Philippe Mouret in France performed the first laparoscopic removal of a diseased gallbladder in a patient undergoing a gynecologic laparoscopic procedure. The gallbladder was retracted cephalad to expose the cystic artery and cystic duct, and the gallbladder was dissected from the liver bed using electrocautery. The news of this achievement was initially greeted with skepticism. Francois Dubois, however, collaborated with Mouret and, after some basic animal experimentation, began to perform the laparoscopic cholecystectomy procedure as described by Mouret. Working independently in the United States and outside

the academic mainstream, Barry McKernan, a general surgeon, and William Saye, a gynecologist, performed their first laparoscopic cholecystectomy in 1988. Nearly simultaneously, two Nashville, Tennessee, surgeons, Eddie Joe Reddick and Douglas Olsen, began to routinely perform laparoscopic cholecystectomy in their institution, using the KTP laser to excise the gallbladder. Their first clinical report attesting to the safety of this procedure appeared in *Laser Medicine and Surgery News*. Thousands of North American surgeons descended on Nashville to witness laser laparoscopic cholecystectomy. It soon became apparent that laser use was not without danger and was more expensive than electrosurgery, which was equally effective for dissection and hemostasis.

Although laparoscopic interventional procedures in general surgery had to await the widespread publicity regarding laparoscopic cholecystectomy, it is noteworthy that laparoscopic appendectomy had been performed before laparoscopic cholecystectomy. In 1977, H. DeKok was the first to perform appendectomy by laparoscopy. However, he used a minilaparotomy to retrieve the appendix. In 1980, during a laparoscopic examination, Semm performed an incidental appendectomy with pretied Roeder loops and instruments he had developed. Hans Wilhelm Schreiber reported on the early experience with laparoscopic appendectomy in women in 1987. He is given credit for performing the first totally laparoscopic appendectomy for acute appendicitis. Despite publication of a large number of laparoscopic appendectomy procedures from both sides of the Atlantic and worldwide, the controversy about this procedure continues to rage, as it is difficult to demonstrate any advantages over its open counterpart.

This concern illustrates the value of prospective studies in the newly developing field of laparoscopic general surgery. These studies are difficult to organize due to their expense and the need to collect data previously ignored, such as the direct and indirect costs. The development of laparoscopic general surgery outside the usual structure of academic surgery also brought to the fore the issues of training and credentialing. Although strict guidelines are published by organizations, such as the Society of American Gastroenterological Surgeons, it is the responsibility of all surgeons to observe these guidelines before performing more advanced laparo-

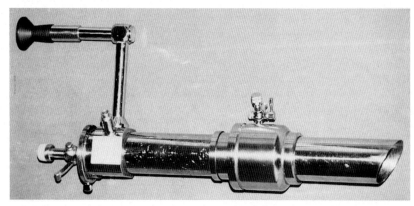

Fig. 2-6. Mühe's galloscope. (From Litynski, Grzegorz S. Highlights in the history of laparoscopy. Frankfurt am Main, Germany: Barbara Bernert Verlag, 1996. Courtesy of Grzegorz S. Litynski, Frankfurt am Main, Germany.)

scopic procedures. The many modern pioneers in laparoscopic general surgery and thoracic surgery are too numerous to name in this chapter. Expertise varies, experiences differ, safe laparoscopic instrumentation is not necessarily widely available, and new ideas are continually being developed. It is surgeons' mandate as a community to report results with an open mind and honestly. For the safe dissemination of laparoscopic procedures, surgeons must become critical of their achievements. Complications must be carefully assessed and methods to avoid them devised. New technologies must be carefully evaluated, preferably in the laboratory, before they are applied in the clinical setting. Although industry will continue to play a major role in developing laparoscopic instruments to facilitate these procedures, surgeons must take an active role in their design and evaluation. The perceived advantages of laparoscopic procedures will remain under the scrutiny of all health jurisdictions, and outcome analyses will be closely examined in the field of laparoscopic surgery during the coming years. The explosive dissemination of new techniques that occurred with laparoscopic cholecystectomy will not be repeated with other laparoscopic procedures, which will give surgeons a chance to reflect and evaluate. During the next few years, the surgical community would do well to follow an Italian saying, "chi va piano, va sano, e va lontano"—he who goes slowly, goes wisely, and goes far. This approach, no doubt, will benefit laparoscopic surgery and patients.

Suggested Reading

Berci G. Laparoscopy in general surgery. In: Berci G, ed. *Endoscopy*. New York: Appleton-Century-Crofts, 1976:382–401.

Cohen MM. Peritoneoscopy in general surgery. *Can J Surg* 1981;24:490–493.

Davis CJ, Filipi CJ. A history of endoscopic surgery. In: Arregui ME, Fitzgibbons RJ, Katkhouda N, McKernam JB, Reich H, eds. *Principles of laparoscopic surgery: basic and advanced techniques*. New York: Springer-Verlag, 1995: 3–20.

Filipi CJ, Fitzgibbons RJ, Salerno GM. Historical review: diagnostic laparoscopy to laparoscopic cholecystectomy and beyond. In: Zucker KA, ed. *Surgical laparoscopy*. St. Louis, MO: Quality Medical Publishing, 1991:3–21.

Gaskin TA, Isobe JH, Mathews JL, Winchester SB, Smith RJ. Laparoscopy and the general surgeon. *Surg Clin North Am* 1991;71:1085–1097.

Gomel V. History of laparoscopy. In: Gomel V, Taylor PJ, eds. *Diagnostic and operative gynecologic laparoscopy*. St. Louis, MO: Mosby–Year Book, 1995:1–5.

Gomel V. Laparoscopy in general surgery. *Am J Surg* 1976;131:319–323.

Gunning JE, Rosenzweig BA. Evolution of endoscopic surgery. In: White RA, Klein SR, eds. *Endoscopic surgery*. St. Louis, MO: Mosby–Year Book, 1991:3–9.

Litynski GS, Grzegorz S. *Highlights in the history of laparoscopy*. Frankfurt am Main, Germany: Barbara Bernert Verlag, 1996.

Semm K. The history of endoscopy. In: Vitale GC, Sanfilippo JS, Perissat J, eds. *Laparoscopic surgery*. Philadelphia: JB Lippincott Co, 1995: 3–11.

EDITOR'S COMMENT

Beginning nearly 200 years ago, physicians have been peering into body cavities with endoscopes. Numerous mechanical, electrical, and other technological advances were necessary to allow complex therapeutic laparoscopic operations to be performed. Many individuals deserve credit for the advances that have paved the way to our current state of *minimally invasive* surgery. Initially, endoscopes were used solely for diagnostic evaluation. The introduction of a second port that would allow rudimentary therapeutic intervention, such as the performance of liver biopsy, foreshadowed what was to come in the future. Despite the demonstrated ability to make diagnoses by looking through the eyepiece of a laparoscope, general surgeons were not interested in laparoscopic surgery until two events occurred. These were (a) the harnessing of a miniature television camera to the laparoscopic eyepiece to allow all members of the operating team to view the same image and (b) the demonstration of the ability to perform a cholecystectomy using laparoscopic guidance. It must be remembered that traditional academic surgical centers in the United States were very slow to accept laparoscopic surgery and that the force behind the rapid introduction of laparoscopic cholecystectomy emanated from the private sphere.

From 1989 to 1991, there was an unprecedented rush of general surgeons who saw the need to obtain training in laparoscopic techniques, and many courses sprang up to meet the demand. The charges to general surgeons performing advanced laparoscopic procedures today are (a) to assure that patients' best interests are maintained foremost in our practices, (b) to insist on appropriate training, certification, and maintenance of laparoscopic and endoscopic skills, and (c) to perform well planned outcome studies to clarify the precise role of minimally invasive surgery in our armamentarium for today and tomorrow.

N.J.S.

3

Preoperative and Postoperative Care of the Flexible Endoscopy Patient

Margaret Napolitano and Charles H. Andrus III

Though the vast majority of endoscopic procedures are performed on an outpatient basis, this should not minimize the importance of a methodical approach to endoscopy patients. Pre- and postprocedural care of endoscopy patients entails several facets with which the endoscopist should be familiar. Appropriate indications for the procedure must be identified to avoid the unnecessary performance of an examination that carries an inherent, albeit small, risk of complication. Adequate preprocedural evaluation that includes patients' past medical history and current systemic disturbances is necessary to determine risk assessment prior to sedation. Careful procedural and postprocedure monitoring of patients allows the detection of any adverse events. Thorough and careful documentation, beginning with informed consent and ending with the formal endoscopy report, is mandatory and prudent.

Indications

A general statement in 1992 by the American Society for Gastrointestinal Endoscopy (ASGE) discusses the conditions in which gastrointestinal endoscopy is indicated, not indicated, and contraindicated. Endoscopy is generally indicated

If a change in management is probable, based on the results of the investigation;

If an empiric trial of therapy for a suspected benign digestive disorder has been unsuccessful; or

If a primary therapeutic procedure is contemplated, in which case it is the method of initial evaluation.

Endoscopy is generally not indicated when results will not contribute to a management decision, nor is it indicated for periodic follow-up of healed benign disease, unless a premalignant condition is suspected. Contraindications to endoscopy are a known or suspected perforated viscus and inadequate patient cooperation, as well as when the risks to a patient's life and health outweigh the benefits.

Preendoscopy Laboratory Studies

The majority of patients do not require routine laboratory testing, as the results would not alter the performance of the procedure. History and physical examination can help determine which patients are considered high risk for endoscopy. Selective tests (e.g., chest x-ray, electrocardiogram [ECG], and a blood chemistry panel) can then be ordered as guided by the patient's underlying medical condition and the endoscopist's discretion. Prior to a general anesthetic, pregnancy testing is recommended and routinely performed in all potentially fertile females.

Informed Consent and Documentation

An explanation of the nature of the procedure, risks, benefits, and alternatives provides the key elements of informed consent. Legally, physicians must provide the information necessary for patients to make

an informed decision. Most endoscopy units use consent forms that require the signatures of the patient or guardian, the physician, and a witness prior to commencing the procedure. It is prudent to add a brief note to patients' records documenting that informed consent was obtained, with all the key elements addressed (indications, contraindications, possible benefits, and potential complications), and indicating their understanding of the planned examination.

Preprocedure Evaluation

All patients who undergo endoscopy should receive a brief history and physical examination. The minimum written documentation should include indications for the procedure, assessment of patients' neurologic status, cardiovascular and pulmonary systems, and abdominal fingings, and an overall preprocedure evaluation. Published data suggest that a thorough preevaluation reduces the risk of adverse outcomes from endoscopic procedures. Drug allergies or adverse reactions to sedation, current medications, and past and current medical conditions should be reviewed, as well as past surgeries. Previous endoscopy reports and any radiologic studies relevant to the planned endoscopic procedure should be available for reference and review. It is prudent to ascertain whether or not a patient has an implanted cardiac device (pacemaker, cardiac defibrillator), as dysfunction of these devices may result from the use of electrocautery. Implantable cardiac defibrillators (ICDs) are generally inactivated prior to procedures in which electrocautery may be used, and reactivated after the procedure. Electrocautery may be used in patients with a pacemaker if short, repetitive bursts are used rather than long, continuous discharges to minimize pacemaker inhibition. Patients with an ICD and pacemaker require careful monitoring of cardiac rhythm, and resuscitation equipment needs to be readily available.

Patients should receive adequate information regarding the importance of an adequate gastrointestinal preparation, as this will impact the ease and accuracy with which the procedure can be performed. For upper endoscopy, patients must have nothing by mouth (NPO) for 4 to 6 hours prior to the examination. Various bowel preparations for colonoscopy exist. For flexible sigmoidoscopy or limited (left side only) colonoscopy, two phosphate (Fleet) enemas 30 minutes before the examination are adequate. A more extensive mechanical bowel preparation is required prior to complete colonoscopy. The diet is restricted to clear liquids for 24 to 48 hours prior to the procedure. Most endoscopy units prescribe 4 L of an oral polyethylene glycol preparation (e.g., Colyte, GoLYTELY) on the afternoon prior to the procedure. These agents are favored as bowel preparation carthartics because of minimal systemic salt and water fluxes. Patients should drink the preparation over a 3- to 4-hour period. Diarrheal effluent should be clear without particulate matter. If effluent is not completely clear following oral preparation, one or two phosphate enemas can be given. Patients should remain NPO for 6 hours prior to the procedure.

Antibiotic Prophylaxis

Prophylactic antibiotics are administered intravenously to patients predisposed to the development of bacterial endocarditis. The ASGE has identified cardiac lesions at high risk for infection, including prosthetic heart valves, past history of endocarditis, surgically constructed systemic/pulmonary shunts or conduits, and synthetic vascular grafts less than 1 year old. Such patients should receive prophylaxis if they are to undergo endoscopic procedures associated with increased rates of transient bacteremia (stricture dilatation, variceal sclerosis, endoscopic retrograde cholangiopancreatography [ERCP] of an obstructed biliary tree). Data are in-

sufficient to make a definitive recommendation regarding prophylaxis prior to procedures not associated with transient bacteremia (esophagogastroduodenoscopy, variceal ligation); the decision to treat high-risk patients prophylactically prior to these procedures is left to the discretion of the endoscopist. The ASGE has also identified intermediate-risk cardiac lesions associated with an increased risk of endocarditis over the general population. Included are most congenital cardiac malformations, rheumatic and acquired valvular dysfunction despite surgery, hypertrophic cardiomyopathy, and mitral valve prolapse with valvular regurgitation. Recommendations for prophylaxis in this group of patients undergoing procedures associated with transient bacteremia cannot be made due to insufficient data, and the choice of preprocedure antibiotics is left to the endoscopist. Prophylaxis with a first- or second-generation cephalosporin is recommended in all patients prior to endoscopic percutaneous feeding tube placement to decrease the risk of soft tissue infection. Bacterial endocarditis affecting normal cardiac valves is extremely rare following endoscopy, with an estimated risk of 1 in 5 to 10 million procedures. Indiscriminate use of antibiotics in most patients is therefore unwarranted and increases the risk of adverse allergic reactions and drug-induced colitis. Data are also insufficient with regard to prophylaxis in patients with cirrhosis, ascites, and immune compromise who are to undergo procedures associated with transient bacteremia. Recommended prophylaxis for appropriate-risk patients is ampicillin sodium, 2 g intravenously, and gentamicin sulfate, 1.5 mg/kg 30 minutes prior to the procedure, followed by amoxicillin, 1.5 g orally 6 hours after the examination. If a patient is penicillin-allergic, vancomycin hydrochloride, 1 g intravenously, can be substituted.

Sedation and Analgesia

The majority of patients undergoing an endoscopic procedure find it desirable not to be fully aware during the examination and are more apt to be compliant in attending repeated endoscopic procedures if the experience is not altogether unpleasant. Amnesia plays an important role in achieving this effect. Most endoscopists utilize a benzodiazepine or a combination of a benzo-

diazepine and an opiate. The choice of agents is largely at the discretion of the endoscopist. Sedation should provide anxiolysis, analgesia, amnesia, and cooperation from the patient. The clinical goal of sedation is to allow the maintenance of cardiorespiratory functions and reflexes, eye contact, and verbal communication. Reliable intravenous access is crucial with the use of sedatives and opioids.

Generally, most patients undergoing peroral esophageal intubation receive topical anesthesia to the pharynx to reduce gagging when the scope is introduced. The topical local anesthetics benzocaine and lidocaine hydrochloride 10% (Xylocaine 10% Oral Spray) are most commonly employed.

Benzodiazepines are the drugs most capable of producing amnesia and anxiolysis. Diazepam has been the most often used drug in this capacity. It is generally administered intravenously at a dosage of 0.10 to 0.15 mg/kg (7 to 10 mg for a 70-kg patient). Diazepam's distribution half-life is 30 to 60 minutes, and plasma elimination half-life is 24 to 57 hours, which is much longer than the endoscopy procedure. The drug is metabolized by hepatic mitochondrial oxidation. Metabolites possess sedative properties and are longer-lived than the parent compound. Care must be taken with elderly patients, as many have impaired hepatic metabolism leading to longer half-lives for the drugs. Lower doses are generally recommended in this population.

Midazolam hydrochloride (Versed) is largely replacing diazepam in many endoscopy suites. Midazolam is twice as potent as diazepam on an equimolar basis and produces a more profound antegrade amnesia. The drug is administered intravenously at a dose of 1 to 2 mg for sedation and 0.05 to 0.07 mg/kg (3.5 to 5.0 mg for a 70-kg patient) as a bolus. It generally reaches peak clinical effect 3 minutes after administration. Distribution and plasma elimination half-lives of midazolam are, respectively, one-fourth and one-tenth those of diazepam. Metabolites are shorter-lived than the parent compound and possess no sedative properties. For these reasons, midazolam has become the more favored benzodiazepine in endoscopy sedation. Care must also be observed with the elderly, as the drug is almost completely metabolized by the liver, and reduced doses are recommended.

An opioid is commonly used in combination with a benzodiazepine for its anesthetic properties. This combination is known to have an additive effect on respiratory depression and hypoxemia. Commonly used opiates include meperidine hydrochloride (Demerol HCl), morphine, and fentanyl citrate (Sublimaze). The average meperidine dose is 0.7 to 0.9 mg/kg (50 to 60 mg for a 70-kg patient). If an opiate/benzodiazepine combination is to be used, the opiate should be given first followed by a reduced dose of the benzodiazepine.

Signs of oversedation or an exaggerated response to sedation are bradycardia, respiratory depression, and hypotension. Antagonists for opiates (naloxone hydrochloride [Narcan]) and benzodiazepines (flumazenil [Romazicon]) must be present in every endoscopy suite whenever opioids or benzodiazepines are administered. Indications for their use include an exaggerated response to sedation with loss of verbal contact or oxygen saturations persistently below 90% despite supplemental oxygen. The availability of these antagonists in the endoscopy suite should not minimize the need for continued clinical assessment and monitoring, nor should it permit the inappropriate overdosage of drugs.

Oxygen Supplementation

The rationale for using pulse oximetry and supplemental oxygen is to optimize arterial oxygen saturation and minimize cardiopulmonary complications known to be responsible for greater than 50% of serious adverse complications in upper endoscopy. Studies indicate that 10% to 13% of all patients who undergo upper endoscopy experience arterial desaturation (less than 90% oxygen saturation), and 15% to 18% who undergo colonoscopy experience hypoventilation secondary to sedative-induced hypoventilation. Oxygen desaturation during endoscopy procedures can be largely prevented by the administration of supplemental oxygen. It should be administered to all patients determined to be at high risk due to cardiopulmonary or other systemic disturbances. In healthy patients, oxygen should be immediately available, if not utilized routinely. Continuous pulse oximetry is more likely to detect hypoxemia than clinical assessment alone and should be used

in all endoscopy patients regardless of estimated risk, since the most important side effect of sedation is hypoventilation with declining oxygen saturation.

Oxygen can be delivered by either nasal cannulas or an oxygenating mouthpiece, which has received increased attention in the past 2 years. The actual fraction of inspired oxygen will depend on the rate and depth of respiration and oxygen mixing with room air in both of these delivery systems, classifying them as variable-performance devices. These devices are suitable for most patients, generally delivering oxygen at 2 to 4 L per minute. In patients with chronic obstructive pulmonary disease (COPD), hypercapnia is well recognized as a consequence of oxygen administration. Oxygen can still be safely administered to these patients with the use of fixed-performance oxygenating devices, such as the Venti-mask (modified to accommodate upper endoscopy), designed to deliver a specific oxygen concentration unaffected by rate or depth of respiration.

Monitoring

It has not been proven that noninvasive monitoring of sedated patients undergoing endoscopy decreases the frequency of complications. The rationale for noninvasive monitoring stems from the knowledge that more than half of serious adverse reactions in endoscopy are cardiopulmonary in nature.

Standard monitoring includes the recording of heart rate, blood pressure, respiratory rate, and oxygen saturation prior to the initiation of sedation. The heart rate, blood pressure, and oxygen saturation are generally monitored throughout the procedure in all patients. ECG monitoring is added in high-risk patients and those with a known cardiac history, although its necessity has yet to be conclusively determined in controlled trials. High-risk patients are those with previous or current cardiopulmonary disorders, renal or hepatic failure, morbid obesity, severe anemia, advanced age, or acute illness.

A well trained assistant is an important component of the endoscopy team. The assistant is responsible for verifying that equipment is functional prior to the start of the examination. Most important, the assistant can continuously monitor patients'

tolerance of the procedure while the physician can concentrate on the performance of the examination itself. Electronic equipment is a useful adjunct to patient surveillance but will never substitute for the clinical assessment of the endoscopist and endoscopy assistant.

Sedation and Anesthetic Record

Most centers have a monitoring and intravenous sedation form on which the endoscopy nurse documents vital signs and medications given. This form serves as the anesthetic record for the procedure (Fig. 3-1). Prior to the administration of any drug, a patient's allergies and specific reactions are reconfirmed. Reliable intravenous access must be established. The American Society of Anesthesiology (ASA) classification scheme for risk assessment during general anesthesia can help evaluate the potential for adverse effects from sedation. Patients are assigned an ASA score denoted by status 1 through status 5:

Status 1 Normal healthy patient
Status 2 Mild systemic disease (e.g., diabetes, controlled hypertension)
Status 3 Severe systemic disease limiting activity (e.g., COPD)
Status 4 Incapacitating disease that is a constant threat to life (e.g., congestive heart failure)
Status 5 Moribund patient not expected to survive

Following this assessment, vital signs and oxygen saturation are recorded before premedication. All medications administered are recorded by name, dose, route, time, and initials of administrator. Serial vital signs and pulse oximetry values should be recorded at 10- to 15-minute intervals at the minimum. Any significant event occurring during the procedure should be documented in the endoscopy record, as well as the intervention undertaken to address it and the patient's response.

Postendoscopy Monitoring

Following the endoscopy procedure, patients should continue to receive clinical and electronic monitoring per an established postendoscopy protocol. The effects of sedation and analgesia persist for some

MONITORING IV SEDATION

_____ Inpatient _____ Outpatient

PROCEDURE PERFORMED: _____

Preprocedure & Sedation Assessment:

Pt. has been NPO: YES   NO

Age: _____

Current Meds: _____

Specific Systems Reviewed: YES   NO

Allergies or any previous ADR to anesthesia/
sedation: _____

Alternatives to & risk of anesthesia discussed with pt: YES   NO

Consent Completed & Signed: YES   NO

Results of Relevant Diagnostic Studies Reviewed: YES   NO

ASA SCORE* (Circle One):   1   2   3   4   5

*See back of page for definition of ASA Score

Pre-Induction reassessment: _____

____ Concur with proposed Sedation/Anesthesia

____ Recommend _____ Sedation/Anesthesia

Signature of Evaluator _____   Time _____

MEDICATION	DOSAGE	TIME	ROUTE	GIVEN BY

IV FLUIDS

EKG MONITOR YES NO (CIRCLE ONE)

TIME INTER-VALS	PRE-INDUCTION								
SaO2									
250									
230									
210									
190									
170									
150									
130									
110									
90									
70									
50									
30									
10									
LOC*									

> Systolic Blood Pressure
< Diastolic Blood Pressure
Pulse
Respirations

*Use the Post Procedure Scoring Guideline for Consciousness

OP180(R) (657)
REVISED DEC 1995

SCORE SYSTEM

Post-procedure Monitoring
Minutes
0   15   30   45

Activity
Able to move 4 extremities   2
Able to move 2 extremities   1
Able to move 0 extremities   0

Respiration
Able to deep-breath & cough freely   2
Dyspnea or limited breathing   1
Apneic   0

Circulation - Postprocedure BP within
20% of preanesthetic value   2
20%-50% of preanesthetic value   1
> or < 50% of preanesthetic value   0

Consciousness
Fully awake   2
Arousable on calling   1
Not responding   0

COLOR
Pink   2
Pale, dusky, blotchy, jaundiced   1
Cyanotic   0

TOTAL

SCORE MUST BE AT LEAST 7-8 FOR PATIENTS RELEASE

COMMENTS/INSTRUCTIONS: _____
_____
_____

Status on discharge:
____ Back to baseline   ____ Other (explain): _____
DISCHARGE: After present post procedure evaluation discharge to
Mode of departure: amb   w/c   stretcher   (Circle One)

Dr. _____   Date: _____   Time: _____
RN/PA Signature
Staff member receiving patient/patient report

PATIENT IDENTIFICATION

ORIGINAL - MEDICAL RECORDS
COPY - ANESTHESIA
COPY - PROCEDURE SERVICE

Fig. 3-1. Example of a monitoring and intravenous sedation form. (Courtesy of Lois Novelin, RN, Veterans Administration Medical Center, St. Louis, MO.)

time following the procedure. For this reason, some centers require a minimum of 45 minutes of monitoring after endoscopy procedures. Following the examination, some units utilize a postprocedure scoring system to evaluate consciousness. This system evaluates activity, respiration, circulation, consciousness, and color. A score is assigned to the patient every 15 minutes for 45 minutes (see Fig. 3-1). The score enables clinicians and recovery nursing personnel to assess patients objectively and determine when they are suitable for release.

Written instructions with endoscopic findings, follow-up dates, a list of postprocedural adverse symptoms and signs, and a 24-hour telephone number for contacting help should be given to patients. A routine telephone call by endoscopy personnel 24 hours after the procedure is recommended. On the day of the procedure, patients should be accompanied by a responsible adult companion who can provide transportation. Patients should not be allowed to drive or operate machinery for 24 hours postprocedure. Resumption of oral intake is permitted 2 hours postprocedure, but patients should avoid alcohol and prescription narcotics or sedatives for 8 to 10 hours.

Endoscopy Documentation

Most endoscopy suites have preprinted report forms specific for the type of procedure performed. Patients should be identified by name, age, and medical and/or social security number. Any allergies should be listed with the reactions produced. The date and type of procedure and the names of the endoscopist and assistant performing the procedure are recorded. Relevant clinical data and procedural indications are also documented. Any imaging studies accompanying patients with findings pertinent to the planned procedure should be recorded. A diagram of the specific system studied is printed on the form, identifying the area of study at a glance. Areas that received a therapeutic intervention are indicated, as well as the type of intervention, number of times the intervention was performed, and the results. Any specimens retrieved or lost should be recorded, as well as the site of biopsy. A brief summary with impression and diagnosis is followed by specific recommendations, follow-up plans, and

patient disposition. Any complications during the procedure should be documented. The form is completed with the physician's signature. Findings of the study and follow-up plans should be discussed prior to discharge when patients are fully awake and able to comprehend the information given. Discussion in the presence of the accompanying family member or friend is recommended due to the variable duration of antegrade amnesia following conscious sedation.

Complications

Complications are inherent in any invasive procedure in medicine, no matter how minimal. Physicians and support staff must be mindful of common complications and be prepared to recognize them in flexible endoscopy patients during and after the procedure. Gastrointestinal endoscopy has enjoyed an extremely safe record, especially when performed by competent, well trained physicians. The rate of severe complications for upper endoscopy and colonoscopy approximates 0.1% and 0.2%, with complications being more likely to occur in emergency situations, the elderly with concomitant medical problems, the acutely ill, and those who undergo complex procedures (e.g., ERCP). The main complications are related to sedative respiratory depression and the nature of the therapeutic interventions, and include bleeding, perforation, and infection. With postendoscopy bleeding, patients may or may not complain of pain or develop hematemesis or hematochezia; with massive hemorrhage, patients may present with circulatory collapse. Repeat endoscopy can generally identify the site of bleeding to be from a previous biopsy or polypectomy site, which is usually amenable to electrocautery. Surgical intervention is rarely required. Perforation of a viscus may present with severe pain, circulatory collapse, and free air on radiologic examination. Depending on the location of the perforation (e.g., retroperitoneal or free intraabdominal) and clinical manifestations, patients may be treated with intravenous antibiotics and bowel rest or by operative intervention.

Hematoma formation as a result of trauma from instrumentation or biopsy has been documented in several case reports to occur in the retropharynx and duodenum.

Duodenal hematomas have been noted to be extensive, producing complete obstruction with symptoms of vomiting and abdominal pain. With large duodenal hematomas, pancreatic duct obstruction can result in pancreatitis. Treatment has been largely supportive with intravenous hyperalimentation (total parenteral nutrition), bowel rest, and nasogastric decompression. Serial imaging studies (computed tomography or ultrasound) can be used to document reduction in hematoma size. Surgery is rarely required.

Cardiopulmonary complications account for more than 50% of reported endoscopy morbidity, with the majority resulting from aspiration, oversedation, hypoventilation, airway obstruction, or vasovagal reactions. Respiratory depression is likely due to the effects of benzodiazepines with or without opiate administration. Elderly patients with a history of COPD are most susceptible to this complication. Most patients respond to gentle stimulation and arousal with oxygen supplementation. Pulse oximetry has significantly improved the detection of respiratory depression and should be used in all patients receiving intravenous sedation. It has been recommended that patients, especially those at high risk for this complication, be monitored by pulse oximetry for at least 45 minutes postprocedure because sedative effects may persist longer than the procedure. The opiate antagonist naloxone and the nonsedative benzodiazepine antagonist flumazenil are both widely available reversal agents. Indications for reversal include oversedation with loss of consciousness and respiratory depression with sustained oxygen saturation less than 90%. Following reversal, patients must be carefully observed for recurrence of respiratory depression, as the reversal agents are short-acting. Neither agent is a substitute for proper airway management and support, nor should they obviate postprocedural observation and monitoring. Support staff should be trained in cardiopulmonary resuscitation and be thoroughly familiar with the location of resuscitative equipment and additional drugs. Aspiration is minimized by performing endoscopy only when the stomach is completely empty, and an oral suction catheter for oral secretion evacuation should be available at all times. Risk of aspiration during endoscopy is increased because patients have been sedated and the gag reflex has been suppressed.

Other reactions encountered are vagally mediated responses that result from mechanical stimulation of the gastrointestinal tract. Hypotension and bradycardia are the most common manifestations. Atropine sulfate is known to diminish these effects and has been used by some to premedicate patients prior to colonoscopy, although studies have shown no significant benefit from routine atropine premedication.

Parotid swelling is a rarely documented complication following upper endoscopy and has been found to occur immediately following the procedure. Patients are noted to have a swollen gland that is tender to palpation. Several mechanisms have been proposed, including obstruction of salivary ducts by secretions, venous congestion as the result of coughing and straining, or intense parasympathetic stimulation that results in vasodilation with subsequent venous congestion of the parotid.

Conclusion

The care of flexible endoscopy patients as discussed in this chapter entails several facets of pre- and postprocedural management that allow the safe and efficient performance of the examination. Attention to the details outlined will allow the procedure to be performed for the appropriate indications, as well as providing patient comfort in a controlled setting.

Suggested Reading

American Society for Gastrointestinal Endoscopy. *Antibiotic prophylaxis for gastrointestinal endoscopy. ASGE publication no. 1028*. Manchester, MA: American Society for Gastrointestinal Endoscopy, *Gastrointest Endosc* 1995;42:622–625.

American Society for Gastrointestinal Endoscopy. Appropriate use of gastrointestinal endoscopy. In: *Policy and procedure manual for gastrointestinal endoscopy: guideline for training and practice*, rev ed. Manchester, MA: American Society for Gastrointestinal Endoscopy, 1992–1996.

Benjamin SB. Overview of monitoring in endoscopy. *Scand J Gastroenterol Suppl* 1990;179: 28–30.

Borody TJ. Methods of oxygen delivery during upper gastrointestinal endoscopy. *Endoscopy* 1994;26:320–321.

Iber FL, Livak A, Kruss DM. Apnea and cardiopulmonary arrest during and after endoscopy. *J Clin Gastroenterol* 1992;14:109–113.

Keefe EB. Sedation and analgesia for endoscopy. *Gastroenterology* 1995;108:932–933.

Mogadam M, Malhotra SK. Pre-endoscopic antibiotics for the prevention of bacterial endocarditis: do we use them appropriately? *Am J Gastroenterol* 1994;89:832–834.

Nagengast FM. Sedation and monitoring in gastrointestinal endoscopy. *Scand J Gastroenterol Suppl* 1993;200:28–32.

Plumeri PA. Informed consent for gastrointestinal endoscopy in the 90's and beyond. *Gastrointest Endosc* 1994;40:379.

Steffes CP, Sugawa C, Wilson RF, Hayward SR. Oxygen saturation monitoring during endoscopy. *Surg Endosc* 1990;4:175–178.

4

Preoperative and Postoperative Care of the Laparoscopic Surgery Patient

Stephen Wise Unger and Gary Glick

The principles of preoperative preparation of laparoscopy patients are similar to those of any general surgical patient, although attention to certain areas specific to laparoscopy will make these unique procedures safer. Care must be focused mainly on the inciting disease process and on the identification of potential sources of surgical complications. Assessment of the operative risks and maneuvers to minimize postoperative morbidity focus on the common sources of potential problems, namely, cardiovascular, pulmonary, infectious, and anatomic.

Preoperative Preparation

Primary consideration must be given to a thorough diagnostic workup and an evaluation of surgical options available to treat a patient's underlying pathology. The essence of the workup begins with a complete history, including an understanding of the time course of the disease, contributing features leading to the patient's morbidity, and their effect on individual pathophysiology (Table 4-1). Evaluation of past medical and operative histories, a medication history, and adverse reactions to both surgical and medical interventions are also important components of the preoperative evaluation. Particular attention must be directed toward ascertaining a history of previous abdominal surgery, which may impact on the performance of laparoscopy. Bleeding tendencies and coagulopathies, if uncorrected, may represent relative contraindications to laparoscopy, as well as a family or personal history of problems with anesthesia. Aller-

gic responses to medications and a patient's functional status will also contribute to the decision-making process.

The physical examination is a central part of the preoperative evaluation. After a complete inspection of the patient, including thorough examinations of the cardiac and pulmonary systems, attention is focused on the particular area of concern and its ability to be approached with a laparoscope. Very large abdominal wall hernias, diaphragmatic defects, and previous scars may affect trocar placement or be an indication for a more complex procedure to gain access to the intended laparoscopic field. Even a small umbilical hernia may alter the laparoscopic approach. Morbid obesity may increase the risks of postoperative complications, and yet many laparoscopic procedures, such as appendectomy or cholecystectomy, can actually be performed with equal or greater safety in these patients.

Ascites may complicate the laparoscopic approach. Gas-filled loops of bowel will float up toward the abdominal wall, increasing the risk of trocar injury. Ascites may be an indication of cirrhosis, which will affect the administration of anesthesia and patients' ability to coagulate. In addition, ascitic fluid may become secondarily infected if strict aseptic techniques are not undertaken, and fluid may leak from an inadequately closed abdominal wall trocar site.

Evaluation of the cardiac and respiratory systems of laparoscopic patients is mandatory to ensure a safe operation. The cardiac system is significantly affected by laparoscopy, with the mechanical effects of the pneumoperitoneum, the hemodynamic ef-

fects of the absorbed carbon dioxide (CO_2), and the volume shifts caused by patient positioning. The tendency toward decreased venous return is moderately offset by the stimulatory effect of the absorbed CO_2. Systemic and central venous pressures and venous resistance are increased during routine laparoscopy. The overall effect is a somewhat hyperdynamic response during surgery. These changes are usually well tolerated by healthy individuals but may represent significant difficulties for marginally compensated patients.

The pulmonary system is stressed during laparoscopy by absorption of the insufflated CO_2. Excess absorption, usually managed by increased ventilation, may represent a problem for patients with severe underlying lung disease unable to increase their ventilatory rate. This may lead to a respiratory acidosis. In addition, peritoneal absorption of CO_2 into the bloodstream may alter the acid–base equilibrium, produce hypercarbia, and lead to a metabolic acidosis. This acidosis may be a particularly dangerous problem in hypovolemic patients, especially victims of trauma. Finally, patient positioning on the table may be affected by past medical history. Increased abdominal pressure may restrict diaphragmatic motion and impair ventilation.

Patient preparation for a laparoscopic procedure also depends on the availability of time and the urgency of the planned operation. An individual undergoing an elective hernia repair certainly differs from an acutely ill patient who requires an emergent appendectomy. Generally speaking, acute volume deficits must be corrected to the fullest extent possible before the induc-

Table 4-1. Preoperative Checklist

History and physical examination
Evaluation of other medical problems
Evaluation of cardiac and respiratory systems
Normalization of fluids and electrolytes
Antibiotics
Deep venous thrombosis prophylaxis
Evaluation of the genitourinary system
Appropriate laboratory and radiologic studies
Informed consent

tion of anesthesia. Plasma and extracellular fluid deficits may be reversed with crystalloid solutions, but an acute or chronic anemia will require transfusion of blood products to enhance oxygen delivery and increase the safety margin of the operation. Normalization of plasma electrolytes is desirable but also depends on the urgency of the disease process. Studies have shown the relatively increased danger of the pneumoperitoneum in traumatized or ill patients who are underresuscitated at the time of surgery.

Preoperative antibiotics are used in most laparoscopic procedures. Any situation in which an infection is already established, such as cholecystitis or appendicitis, requires the administration of intravenous or intramuscular antibiotics prior to surgery as part of the treatment. In addition, procedures in which a contaminated space is likely to be encountered or opened, such as during hysterectomy or colectomy, will require antibiotic prophylaxis. If prosthetic mesh is to be used, routine prophylactic antibiotics covering skin organisms are appropriate. The choice of antibiotics should be based on culture results of infected blood or pathologic specimens, but generally a cephalosporin administered immediately before surgery is adequate for prophylaxis. Surgical techniques to minimize infection, such as good hemostasis, correct skin preparation, closed suction drainage, and gentle handling of tissues, should be stringently applied. Finally, all patients who are considered at high risk for postoperative infectious complications should be covered with antibiotic prophylaxis. This group includes diabetics, patients who are immunocompromised, the elderly, patients taking steroids, or those who have been hospitalized for a prolonged time and may have become colonized with re-

sistant organisms. Most studies show a definitive benefit from such antibiotic use.

All surgical patients are at risk for the development of deep venous thrombosis (DVT), and this should be a major consideration in the planning of a laparoscopic procedure. Several factors increase the risk of DVT, including malignancy, obesity, smoking, a history of DVT, prolonged bed rest, and positioning on the operating room table. Despite the brevity of many laparoscopic operations, all patients must be evaluated preoperatively for DVT. For prophylaxis of DVT, compression stockings on the lower extremities increase blood flow in the femoral veins and reduce the potential of stasis. The stockings are applied before surgery and are worn until patients are fully ambulatory. Intermittent pneumatic compression devices serve as an external substitute for the calf muscle venous pump. These also increase blood flow in the common femoral veins and are especially useful when anticoagulants are contraindicated. The most widely used agent for DVT prophylaxis is heparin. Its pharmacologic effect is based on its action as an antithrombin III agonist. A single 5,000-U dose is given subcutaneously several hours prior to surgery and continued every 12 hours until patients are fully ambulatory. Although bleeding is a complication of heparin administration, it is rarely significant in laparoscopic patients, assuming that adequate hemostasis is achieved. Heparin has been shown to reduce the incidence of postoperative DVT by 50% in general surgical patients.

Careful attention must be directed toward other potential sources of complications during the preoperative period. Diabetes mellitus is one of the most common endocrine disorders and is frequently present in patients undergoing laparoscopic procedures. The severity of the insulin deficiency must be assessed, with the intention of avoiding ketoacidosis, hypoglycemia, and hyperosmolar nonketonic coma. Appropriate insulin coverage must be maintained during periods of fasting, and an exogenous source of glucose must be supplied. Adequate hydration must be maintained, electrolytes should be monitored, and blood glucose levels should be checked frequently. Surgical complications, including necrotizing fasciitis, are more common in diabetics and are usually related to a lack of metabolic control, immunologic defects, atherosclerosis, and de-

layed healing. Although these complications are no more frequent in laparoscopic procedures, they must still be considered as potential postoperative problems.

Evaluation of the genitourinary system is important in laparoscopic patients. Most procedures will require insertion of a bladder catheter in the perioperative period. This is usually well tolerated if urinary symptoms, such as frequency, urgency, and nocturia, are not present. Prostatism, urinary tract infections, and renal insufficiency must be investigated preoperatively to avoid postoperative complications, and may be indications that urinary catheterization may be difficult.

Contraindications to Laparoscopy

Contraindications to laparoscopy may be considered as absolute or relative (Table 4-2). These classifications tend to change over time, but an understanding of when laparoscopy is not indicated or presents greater risks is of utmost importance. Hypovolemic shock, massive acute bleeding, and critical hemodynamic instability may be considered absolute contraindications to laparoscopy. Intraabdominal bleeding may obscure the view, may be difficult to precisely localize, and may require quicker intervention than laparoscopy will permit. Severe cardiac disease may also be an absolute contraindication to laparoscopy if insufflation and patient positioning will exacerbate underlying conditions.

Most other contraindications can be considered relative, and the extent to which each of these conditions precludes laparoscopic surgery may change over time with the development of new techniques and advanced instrumentation. Pregnancy was once thought to be an absolute contraindi-

Table 4-2. Contraindications to Laparoscopy

Absolute
  Hypovolemic shock, massive bleeding, hemodynamic instability
  Severe cardiac disease
Relative
  Peritonitis of uncertain origin
  Abdominal wall hernias
  Diaphragmatic hernias
  Uncorrected coagulopathies
  Portal hypertension
  Multiple previous surgical procedures
  Late pregnancy

cation to laparoscopy, but laparoscopic surgery has been shown to be safe and effective well into the second trimester. Peritonitis, especially of uncertain origin, usually requires a formal exploration, but laparoscopy may assist in identifying the inciting event and direct the placement of the surgical incision. Abdominal wall hernias, particularly those previously repaired with mesh, will complicate laparoscopic surgery and may lower the safety threshold. Diaphragmatic hernias may preclude adequate insufflation and should be considered by the surgeon and anesthesiologist when deciding on the surgical approach. Uncorrected coagulopathies may be a relative contraindication, and portal hypertension may lead to increased abdominal wall bleeding and complications during the surgical dissection.

Multiple prior abdominal operations with significant intraabdominal adhesions will severely impair visualization and increase the risk of intestinal injury. With careful technique, including an open placement of initial trocars, this risk can be minimized. Meticulous dissection with take-down of abdominal wall adhesions, freeing of intraloop intestinal bands, and scrupulous identification of important landmarks will convert a difficult, dangerous procedure into a straightforward case. Preoperative bowel preparation may be important in decreasing the hazards.

Prior to operation, appropriate laboratory studies should be obtained, including a complete blood cell count and measurement of electrolytes and coagulation parameters. A chest x-ray and electrocardiogram will usually be required. Patients should be instructed on what to expect in both the immediate preoperative and postoperative periods, and a fully informed consent should be obtained by the operating surgeon. This should include the possible complications of bleeding, as well as the known complications of the indicated procedure. Patients should also understand the possibility of conversion to open surgery. It is helpful to tell them that they may experience abdominal and shoulder pain postoperatively.

Postoperative Care

The postoperative care of laparoscopic patients begins immediately after the completion of the surgical procedure. Appro-

priate monitoring during the early postoperative period, usually in the recovery room, is important to ensure a smooth transition from the anesthetic. Most patients require only routine assessment of vital signs. Acutely ill patients or those with significant cardiac or pulmonary disease will require invasive monitoring in an intensive care unit. Appropriate fluids should be administered, with consideration of the duration of the inciting pathology, the extent of the dissection, the expected loss of fluid from the intravascular space, and the intraoperative blood loss. Supplemental oxygen should be provided as needed, and laboratory tests should be obtained, if needed. Unless there is a specific reason to leave the nasogastric tube and Foley catheter (if used intraoperatively) in place, they should be removed before emergence from anesthesia.

Pain management following laparoscopy is generally easier than following other, more invasive surgical procedures. Pain is generally much less with laparoscopy, one of the primary advantages of this approach. Postoperative analgesia may consist solely of oral medication or may require a combination of intramuscularly, intravenously, or epidurally administered drugs. Advanced or lengthy procedures may be accompanied by more pain than simple procedures, and patient-controlled analgesia may be appropriate. Diaphragmatic irritation is an important source of postoperative pain and may lead to complaints of shoulder or neck discomfort. The mechanism for this pain after laparoscopy may be due to irritation of the diaphragm by blood, fluid, or CO_2 or to diaphragmatic stretching. Local anesthesia (e.g., bupivacaine hydrochloride 0.25% or 0.50%) infiltrated directly into the wounds or into the peritoneum in the right upper quadrant at the conclusion of the operation will supplement systemic analgesics. By postoperative day 1, the intensity of the surgical pain generally decreases significantly, and at this point patients can be maintained on oral pain medication exclusively. Postoperative pain in excess of the anticipated degree should alert the surgeon to the possibility of a complication.

Depending on the procedure, resumption of oral intake can begin sooner than with other types of surgery. Following laparoscopic cholecystectomy or appendectomy, liquids can be provided almost as soon as patients awaken from the anesthesia. Shortly thereafter, patients are advanced to

a normal diet and prepared for discharge. Standard surgical principles should dictate when patients are capable of tolerating oral feeding. A colectomy or bowel resection may require several days of feeding restriction, but again this period is usually shorter than with comparable open procedures.

After the initial recovery period, minimal restrictions on activity are necessary. Patients are encouraged to ambulate and deep-breathe. Discharge instructions are provided, and they should include the concept of progressive rehabilitation and judicious diet selection. Staples or sutures, if placed, are usually removed at the first postoperative office visit.

Complications of Laparoscopy

Consideration of the postoperative care of laparoscopic patients must include an analysis of potential complications, particularly those unique to laparoscopy (Table 4-3). When correctly performed, diagnostic laparoscopy has a major complication rate of less than 1%, and the overall mortality is 4 to 8 deaths per 100,000 procedures. One primary advantage of the laparoscopic approach is its high safety margin and the ability to apply basic laparoscopy techniques to a wide variety of different procedures.

Laparoscopic complications can be divided into two categories: general complications of laparoscopy and complications specific to the procedure itself. General complications include those that may occur in any laparoscopic procedure and comprise complications of anesthesia, patient positioning, the pneumoperitoneum, abdominal insufflation, and the trocar site. Specific

Table 4-3. Laparoscopic Complications

General complications
  Complications of anesthesia
  Complications of the pneumoperitoneum
    Pneumothorax, pneumomediastinum
    Carbon dioxide embolization
    Hypercarbia with acidosis
  Patient positioning
  Trochar-related injuries
    Bowel injuries
    Vascular injuries
    Incisional site hernias
    Bladder injuries
  Wound infections
Procedure-specific complications

complications are unique to the individual procedure and will be considered in the appropriate procedure-specific chapters.

The complication rate of anesthesia for laparoscopic procedures is approximately 0.05%. Although local anesthesia may be used for certain diagnostic cases, most laparoscopic operations are performed under general endotracheal anesthesia. Cardiopulmonary complications, in part related to the inhalational anesthetic agents, continue to be the major cause of postoperative morbidity. Arrhythmias with both local and general agents are related to the creation of the pneumoperitoneum and are a significant cause of intraoperative and postoperative morbidity.

Complications related to the CO_2 pneumoperitoneum may present intraoperatively or postoperatively and are detailed in Chapter 5. The mechanical effects of the intraperitoneal gas may cause vagal stimulation with bradyarrhythmias, diminished venous return, and alterations in blood pressure. Pulmonary effects of the pneumoperitoneum include increased airway pressures, hypercarbia with acidosis that may persist after the surgery is completed, and hypercapnia. Gas may be introduced into the mesenteric or retroperitoneal spaces, resulting in pneumomediastinum, pneumopericardium, or pneumothorax.

Patient positioning on the operating table is critical to the success of laparoscopic procedures but has potential problems. The lithotomy position may cause femoral or peroneal neuropathy or contribute to an exacerbation of lower extremity ischemia. The Trendelenburg position may reduce pulmonary reserve, increase airway pressure, and cause gastroesophageal reflux.

Trocar-site complications may result in bowel injuries, vascular injuries, or incisional hernias. Bowel injuries most frequently involve the small intestines, followed in frequency by the colon, duodenum, and stomach. These injuries may be unrecognized at the time of surgery and present with postoperative peritonitis. Bowel injury is associated with a mortality of 5%. Direct injury can be caused by the Veress needle or by operating trocars. This is particularly significant in patients with abdominal wall hernias or prior surgery. Bowel perforation requires immediate laparotomy for repair of the injury. The trocar or sheath should be left in place to facilitate identifying the injury.

Minor perforations may not be immediately recognized and may present with delayed sepsis.

Major vascular injury during laparoscopic surgery is rare and usually occurs during pelvic procedures. Most injuries are in the vicinity of the distal aorta and its branches or the inferior vena cava or iliac veins. Early recognition of these complications is important to successful treatment. Veress needle entry into a major vessel can often be diagnosed by aspiration. If significant bleeding is seen after the insertion of a trocar or if an expanding retroperitoneal hematoma is identified, immediate exploration is mandatory. Most of these injuries can be repaired with direct suture ligation, but a patch or synthetic graft may be required for more extensive damage. Incisional hernias are rare complications caused by trocar-site fascial defects. Larger defects of 10 mm or greater carry a higher risk of postoperative complications. Omentum or bowel may become trapped and present 3 to 5 days postoperatively, sometimes as a Richter's (parietal) hernia. The incidence of incisional hernias is quite low, approximately 0.05%. Trocar insertion at an angle so that the fascial wound is not at the center of the incision decreases the risk of weakening the abdominal wall. Closing the fascia with simple or figure-of-eight sutures also reduces the incidence of herniation and should be performed in all trocar sites greater than 5 mm in diameter.

Laparoscopic injuries to the bladder may result from the Veress needle or insertion of a low abdominal trocar. The risk of bladder perforation increases with previous abdominal surgery, previous bladder surgery, or congenital anomalies. The appearance of gas in the Foley bag or unexplained urinary tract bleeding during or after the procedure should heighten suspicion of an injury. Decompression of the bladder with a Foley catheter may help reduce the risk of injury, and this should be routine before all laparoscopic procedures. Diagnosis of a urinary tract injury may be made with a retrograde cystogram, when this injury is suspected.

Wound infections following laparoscopic procedures are rare. Wound abscesses, cellulitis, and necrotizing fasciitis may occur, particularly when the subcutaneous tissue is exposed to infected material, such as an inflamed appendix or gallbladder. Judicious use of antibiotics will help prevent these unusual complications.

Conclusion

The advent of laparoscopic surgery has provided surgeons with new techniques to deal with familiar problems. Laparoscopy can reduce hospital stays, decrease postoperative pain, and hasten recovery times. The key to successful laparoscopy is appropriate patient preparation and efficient supervision after surgery. With close attention to preoperative and postoperative care, these unique procedures will be safe, effective, and enduring.

Suggested Reading

Deziel DJ. Avoiding laparoscopic complications. *Int Surg* 1994;79:361–364.

Nord HJ. Complications of laparoscopy. *Endoscopy* 1992;24:693–699.

Ponsky JL. Management of complications of laparoscopy. *Endoscopy* 1992;24:724–729.

Way LW, Bhoyrul S, Mori T. *Fundamentals of laparoscopic surgery.* New York: Churchill Livingstone, 1995.

Wolf JS, Stoller ML. The physiology of laparoscopy: basic principles, complications and other considerations. *J Urol* 1994;152:294–302.

EDITOR'S COMMENT

The ability to perform a safe laparoscopic operation is only one element in the successful outcome of a procedure. Appropriate management of patients before and after surgery is equally important, particularly in regard to minimizing the incidence of perceived and real complications. Some patients are not good candidates for laparoscopic procedures, and the surgeon must avoid elevating technical capabilities above common sense. Patients must be informed in an understandable fashion regarding the realistic expectations of surgery and the potential adverse outcomes. Inadequate preoperative communication and an adverse outcome tend to result in communication with a plaintiff's attorney! In the postoperative period, the surgeon must be alert to the potential for complications and not ignore unusual symptoms or complaints. A complication recognized early in its course will be easier to manage and will less likely result in significant untoward effects.

N.J.S.

5

Physiologic Consequences of Laparoscopic Surgery

Philip R. Schauer

Prior to the advent of laparoscopic cholecystectomy, the use of laparoscopic techniques by the average general surgeon was either nonexistent or represented a very small portion of his or her practice. Consequently, fundamental knowledge of the basic physiologic issues regarding laparoscopic surgery was understandably lacking for most general surgeons. Much of the credit for the early work in this area rightfully belongs to gynecologic surgeons and anesthesiologists, who were more frequently involved with laparoscopy. In the 1990s, laparoscopy no longer occupies a small niche in general surgery. In fact, it is estimated that currently more than 30% of all abdominal surgery is performed laparoscopically. As new laparoscopic procedures are perfected, many experts believe that within the next few decades nearly 80% of all abdominal surgery will be performed using laparoscopic techniques. As the scope of laparoscopic surgery grows, it is critically important that surgeons not only learn new laparoscopic techniques and skills but also become familiar with the basic physiologic principles of laparoscopic surgery. Since the advent of laparoscopic cholecystectomy, numerous laboratories at prestigious universities have been created, dedicated to the study of physiologic issues related to laparoscopy. Knowledge of laparoscopic physiology enables the surgeon to understand the adverse effects specific to the laparoscopic method and the principle physiologic benefits of laparoscopic versus open surgery. This information is particularly important in the assessment of risk versus benefit of a laparoscopic approach to a given clinical situation or disease process.

For example, the laparoscopic approach, compared to an open approach, may result in a superior outcome for an elective splenectomy for idiopathic thrombocytopenic purpura, but it may be exceedingly dangerous in a hypovolemic patient requiring splenectomy for a fractured spleen.

Fundamental Differences between Open and Laparoscopic Surgery

The physiologic consequences of laparoscopic surgery distinct from open surgery can be appreciated by analyzing the fundamental differences in technique between the two methods and the associated biologic responses (Table 5-1). Two major factors inherent in the laparoscopic method account for the majority of physiologic changes. The first is due to the adverse effects of creating a working space by insufflating the abdominal cavity with carbon dioxide (CO_2). In general, the physiologic effects of CO_2 pneumoperitoneum occur during the intraoperative period and resolve shortly after evacuation of the gas. These effects may have minimal physiologic consequences but may be potentially lethal. The second major difference between laparoscopic and open surgery relates to the reduction in magnitude of surgical trauma associated with the laparoscopic approach. Laparoscopic surgery is *minimally invasive* because it spares unnecessary trauma to the abdominal wall to gain access to the target in-

traabdominal organ(s). This reduction in injury has major physiologic consequences that last from the time of injury to complete recovery and essentially account for all of the benefits of laparoscopic surgery. Other factors associated with the laparoscopic approach that may have important harmful or beneficial physiologic consequences include the necessity of extreme position changes (i.e., Trendelenburg and reverse Trendelenburg) to enhance exposure, reduced visceral retraction and manipulation, less tissue desiccation, and impaired temperature regulation.

Intraoperative Physiology of Laparoscopic Surgery

As shown in Fig. 5-1, many factors may affect intraoperative homeostasis during laparoscopic surgery. Exposure methods including the CO_2 pneumoperitoneum and patient positioning are inherent to the laparoscopic method and may cause adverse physiologic changes. Often, the duration of surgery is prolonged with the laparoscopic approach, which may accentuate these adverse effects. The physiologic status of patients is equally important because it determines their ability to effectively compensate for the adverse effects specific to the laparoscopic method. In any given laparoscopic procedure, each of these factors may be operative to varying degrees; thus, a complex interplay of these factors may account for a specific adverse event. To anticipate adverse events, an understanding of these physiologic mechanisms is essential. Recently, many surgical investigators have contributed substantially to our understanding of these complex interactions; however, much still remains unknown.

Laparoscopic Exposure Methods

Various abdominal exposure techniques for laparoscopy have been devised. Insufflation of the abdomen with CO_2 has been the dominant method for many decades. Nitrous oxide (N_2O), air (80% nitrogen), oxygen, helium, and argon have also been used to create a pneumoperitoneum. The advantage of CO_2 over other gases is that it does not support combustions; it is relatively inexpensive and is rapidly absorbed. A rapidly absorbed gas such as CO_2 is less likely to produce a clinically serious gas embolism. The main disadvantage of CO_2 is that when it dissolves into solution, it becomes biologically reactive, producing many adverse effects. N_2O, the second most commonly used gas, is less preferred because it supports combustion more than room air or CO_2. Leakage of N_2O into the operating room may also adversely affect operating personnel. N_2O, however, is more suitable for laparoscopy under local anesthesia because it is associated with less peritoneal irritation than CO_2. Gasless exposure devices for laparoscopy involving abdominal wall lifting mechanisms have also been developed (see Chapter 6). Gasless systems potentially eliminate all adverse effects associated with insufflation; however, they have not become widely adopted because they provide generally inferior exposure, compared to a pneumoperitoneum.

Physiology of Carbon Dioxide Pneumoperitoneum

Since CO_2 pneumoperitoneum is the dominant method of laparoscopic exposure, its physiologic effects are most relevant to the practicing laparoscopic surgeon. Adverse effects of CO_2 pneumoperitoneum range in severity from minor to potentially lethal; these adverse effects, along with possible mechanisms, are listed in Table 5-2. Some adverse effects may be considered predictable physiologic responses. The adverse effects listed as complications are unusual or rare events. Studies of hemodynamic effects during laparoscopy

Table 5-1. Factors Possibly Accounting for Different Physiologic Responses Between Open and Laparoscopic Cholecystectomy

Factor	Open Cholecystectomy	Laparoscopic Cholecystectomy
Anesthesia	General	General
Patient position	Supine	Reverse Trendelenburg
Access method	"Open" surgery	CO_2 pneumoperitoneum
Surgical injury		
External: abdominal wall	Significant	Minimal
	1. 20-cm incision through skin, muscle, fascia	1. 1.5-cm incision and three 0.5-cm trocar incisions
	2. Retraction with static retraction apparatus	2. Stretching from pneumoperitoneum
Internal: triangle of Calot, hepatic fossa	Equivalent	Equivalent
Intraabdominal viscera retraction/manipulation	Significant (using hands, metal retractors, and sponge packing)	Minimal (retraction of viscera rarely necessary for exposure)
Tissue desiccation	Moderate (open environment promotes evaporation)	Minimal (closed environment)
Body temperature reduction	Moderate (multifactorial: evaporation, cool irrigation fluids)	Moderate (multifactorial: circulating nonheated gas, cool irrigation fluids)

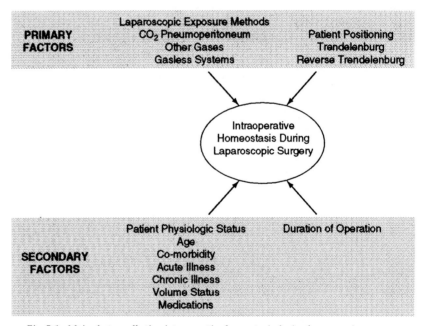

Fig. 5-1. *Major factors affecting intraoperative homeostasis during laparoscopic surgery.*

were performed in the 1970s primarily on young healthy women undergoing laparoscopic tubal ligations of brief duration. The adverse effects of laparoscopy elucidated from these studies were either clinically insignificant or well compensated by this group of patients. Patient populations and operative environments have changed significantly since then. Major abdominal operations are now performed via the laparoscopic technique on elderly and critically ill patients. The potential adverse cardiopulmonary effects of CO_2 pneumoperitoneum pose significant risks for all patients undergoing laparoscopic surgery and especially for those with cardiopulmonary disease.

The physiologic mechanisms accounting for the hemodynamic effects of CO_2 insufflation are complex and only partially understood at this time. CO_2 pneumoperi-

Table 5-2. Complications and Adverse Physiologic Effects of CO_2 Pneumoperitoneum

Complication/Adverse Effect	Possible Mechanism(s)
CARDIAC/HEMODYNAMIC	
Adverse effects	
Tachycardia	Sympathetic response to impaired venous return, hypercarbia
Hypertension	Sympathetic response to impaired venous return, hypercarbia
Increased vascular resistance	Sympathetic response to impaired venous return, hypercarbia
Increased myocardial O_2 demand	Sympathetic response to impaired venous return, hypercarbia, tachycardia, increased afterload
Decreased cardiac output	Reduced venous return, increased afterload, impaired contractility from hypercarbia
Impaired visceral blood flow	Increased resistance from increased IAP, hypercarbia-induced vasoconstriction, decreased cardiac output
Bradycardia	Vasovagal reaction to peritoneal stretching/irritation
Cardiac arrhythmias	Hypercarbia, hypoxia, catecholamine response
Hypotension	Vena caval compression, decreased venous return
Pneumomediastinum	Defect in diaphragm
Complications	
Tension pneumothorax	Diaphragm injury, dissection near esophageal hiatus, barotrauma
Myocardial infarction	Inadequate perfusion to meet increased demand
Metabolic acidosis	Inadequate tissue perfusion from reduced cardiac output, hypercarbia
Visceral organ ischemia	Impaired visceral blood flow
Venous stasis/thromboembolism	Impaired lower extremity venous return, endothelial damage from increased IAP
NEUROLOGIC	
Increased intracranial pressure	Increased cerebral blood flow from hypercarbia
Potential cerebral edema	Increased cerebral blood flow
Potential brain stem herniation	Increased intracranial pressure
PULMONARY	
Adverse effects	
Reduced lung compliance	Reduced lung volume, elevated diaphragm
Increased airway resistance	Increased intrathoracic pressure from transmitted increased IAP
Ventilation–perfusion mismatch	Reduced lung volume from mechanical effect of increased IAP
Hypercarbia/acidosis	CO_2 retention
Atelectasis	Lung bases collapsed against diaphragm
Complications	
Hypoxia	Atelectasis and reduced lung volume
Hypercarbia	CO_2 retention
Respiratory acidosis	Hypercarbia
Aspiration	Increased risk of regurgitation of gastric contents from increased IAP
OTHER PROBLEMS	
Renal failure	Impairment of renal blood flow by increased IAP and/or hypercarbia
CO_2 gas embolus	Entry of CO_2 bubbles through injured blood vessels
Hypothermia	Cooling from CO_2 gas, lengthy procedures
Subcutaneous emphysema	Insufflation into preperitoneal space
Shoulder pain	Stretching/irritation of diaphragm

IAP = intraabdominal pressure.

toneum may affect hemodynamics by multiple mechanisms. Two primary mechanisms involve the effects of increased intraabdominal pressure (IAP) and the physiologic effects of absorbed CO_2. The adverse effects of both mechanisms relate directly to the duration of the pneumoperitoneum and the elevation of IAP. Low-pressure CO_2 pneumoperitoneum (5 mm Hg or less) has minimal physiologic consequences, whereas pressures greater than 15 mm Hg may have severe consequences. Adequate surgical exposure is usually achieved at pressures at or below 15 mm Hg, so the risk of high-pressure insufflation is rarely justified. The predominant effect of increased IAP in the 10- to 15-mm Hg range is a reduction in venous return by partial obstruction of the vena cava, which normally maintains a pressure less than 5 mm Hg. Distinct from pressure effects, the CO_2 gas may be absorbed systemically and lead to hemodynamic changes related to hypercarbia. CO_2 absorption/excretion may be affected by a variety of factors, including patient pulmonary function and ventilator settings.

Cardiac/Hemodynamic Changes

Widely varying hemodynamic responses to CO_2 pneumoperitoneum have been reported because of the use of different animal models and different monitoring techniques. Most clinical studies, however, indicate that the hemodynamic effects of CO_2 pneumoperitoneum result in increases in heart rate, systemic vascular resistance (SVR), and central venous pressure, and a decrease in cardiac output. Mean arterial pressure may decrease, remain unchanged, or increase, depending on relative changes in cardiac output and SVR. Tachycardia is a compensatory sympathetic response to decreased venous return and may also result from hypercarbia. Increased SVR results from compensatory vasoconstriction and possibly hypercarbia. Increases in measured central venous pressure are artifactual and related to transmitted increases in IAP (Fig. 5-2). True preload is actually decreased because of impaired venous return, which is the primary adverse effect of CO_2 pneumoperitoneum. Although most human studies show that CO_2 pneumoperitoneum decreases cardiac output in the 20% to 40% range, some have reported no change or a slight increase. In a dog model in our laboratory using direct monitoring techniques, we demonstrated that decreased preload was the primary cause of decreased cardiac output rather than increased afterload or impaired ventricular contractility (Fig. 5-3). In that study, left ventricular contractility was quantified using the Frank-Starling relationship, which is insensitive to changes in heart rate and afterload over the normal physiologic range. Increases in cardiac workload resulting from tachycardia and increased afterload may predispose patients with coronary disease to myocardial infarction. To date, there have been no published reports of myocardial infarction directly attributable to adverse effects of pneumoperitoneum.

Strategies to prevent hemodynamic complications of CO_2 insufflation have been based on identifying patients at risk who may not tolerate these physiologic responses. Fortunately, the majority of patients who undergo laparoscopic cholecystectomy can tolerate small reductions in cardiac output associated with CO_2 pneumoperitoneum. Therefore, special considerations in young healthy patients are probably not necessary. Conversely, reduction in cardiac output may be a major concern in patients with underlying cardiopulmonary disease. Intraoperative monitoring of high-risk patients with a Swan-Ganz catheter or transesophageal echocardiography may be helpful in determining dangerously low cardiac outputs. Hemodynamic compromise may then be corrected by release of pneumoperitoneum or pharmacologic manipulation before severe consequences result. In some patients, preoperative hydration effectively attenuates the reduction in preload caused by the pneumoperitoneum.

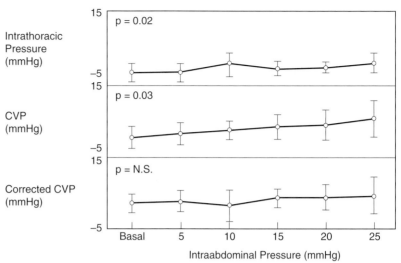

Fig. 5-2. Effect of intraabdominal pressure on central venous pressure and intrathoracic pressure in a canine model.

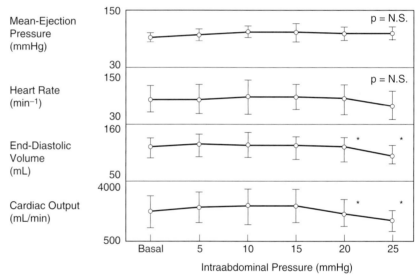

Fig. 5-3. Influences of changes in cardiac preload and afterload on cardiac output during laparoscopy at intraabdominal pressures from 0 to 25 mm Hg in a canine model.

Cardiac Dysrhythmias. Dysrhythmias occur commonly (25% to 47%) during laparoscopic surgery. Most are benign sinus arrhythmias and resolve rapidly after evacuation of the pneumoperitoneum. Hypercarbia, hypoxia, sympathetic stimulation resulting from decreased venous return, and vagal stimulation resulting from rapid stretching of the peritoneum have all been implicated in the genesis of dysrhythmias during laparoscopic surgery. Although rare, potentially lethal dysrhythmias may result from hypercarbia or abdominal pressure effects. Moderate to severe hypercarbia (P_{CO_2} of 60 mm Hg or higher) may result in ventricular irritability leading to premature ventricular contractions, ventricular tachycardia, or even ventricular fibrillation. The incidence of bradyarrhythmias resulting from vagal stimulation is as high as 30%. Rare cases of pneumoperitoneum-induced bradycardia progressing to sinus arrest have been reported. Consequently, some surgeons and anesthesiologists recommend prophylactic atropine sulfate, 0.4 to 0.8 mg, just prior to CO_2 instillation. Measures to prevent potentially serious dysrhythmias during laparoscopic procedures include close observation of the electrocardiogram, ensuring adequate oxygenation and ventilation, and specific pharmacologic therapy.

Impaired Visceral Blood Flow. Studies regarding the hemodynamic effects of elevated IAP have shown that IAP as low as 15 to 20 mm Hg may impair intraabdominal organ perfusion independent of changes in cardiac output (Table 5-3). Since pneumoperitoneum for laparoscopy requires IAP in that range, reduced organ blood flow during laparoscopy is a potential concern. Indeed, cases of pneumoperitoneum-related oliguria and renal failure have been reported. In addition to in-

Table 5-3. Effect of Elevated Abdominal Pressure on Visceral Blood Flow

| | Intraabdominal Pressure (mm Hg) | | |
| | 0 | 20 | 40 |
Organ		Organ blood flow index (10^{-3} kg)	
Omentum	0.159 ± 0.054	0.117 ± 0.036	0.056 ± 0.015†
Esophagus	0.037 ± 0.004	0.024 ± 0.004†	0.020 ± 0.002†
Stomach	0.136 ± 0.023	0.119 ± 0.021	0.060 ± 0.008†
Gastric mucosa	0.210 ± 0.033	0.122 ± 0.016†	0.076 ± 0.012†
Duodenum	0.402 ± 0.055	0.312 ± 0.037	0.285 ± 0.028*
Jejunum	0.397 ± 0.043	0.296 ± 0.034*	0.221 ± 0.029†
Ileum	0.228 ± 0.049	0.143 ± 0.025	0.142 ± 0.034
Colon	0.215 ± 0.060	0.157 ± 0.033	0.146 ± 0.038
Pancreas	0.148 ± 0.030	0.120 ± 0.022*	0.097 ± 0.019†
Gallbladder	0.122 ± 0.029	0.125 ± 0.021	0.092 ± 0.013
Liver	0.140 ± 0.029	0.105 ± 0.041	0.074 ± 0.026†
Spleen	0.754 ± 0.164	0.528 ± 0.110*	0.378 ± 0.046
Renal cortex	2.07 ± 0.19	2.31 ± 0.25	2.5 ± 0.25
Adrenal	0.619 ± 0.038	0.811 ± 0.034	1.148 ± 0.101†

Note: Mean ± SEM.
* $p < 0.05$.
† $p < 0.01$.

creased SVR related to elevated IAP, vasoconstrictive effects of absorbed CO_2 may also play a minor role in impaired visceral blood flow. The clinical relevance of reduced intraabdominal organ perfusion during laparoscopy remains unclear. Lengthy laparoscopic procedures could potentially lead to visceral ischemia and ultimately to permanent end-organ damage or increased gut-mucosal permeability to intestinal bacteria. As more patients with atherosclerosis or underlying renal disease undergo laparoscopic procedures, the potential for visceral ischemia remains a major concern. Further investigation of the effect of CO_2 pneumoperitoneum on intraabdominal blood flow is necessary before a clear understanding of its clinical relevance can be achieved. At present, urine output should be used as a gross monitor of visceral blood flow. Persistent oliguria during a laparoscopic procedure should warrant at least temporary evacuation of the pneumoperitoneum until adequate urine flow resumes.

Venous Stasis, Thrombosis, and Coagulation

Despite advances in prevention, deep venous thrombosis (DVT) and pulmonary embolism (PE) contribute significantly to perioperative morbidity and mortality. The incidence of DVT after general surgical procedures has been reported to be 14% to 33%. The risk of PE following DVT formation is 1% to 2%. Several isolated reports of DVT and PE occurring after laparoscopic cholecystectomy have been reported; however, whether the risk of DVT and PE is increased as a consequence of the laparoscopic method cannot be accurately determined from currently available studies.

Several factors specific to the laparoscopic method may either increase or decrease the risk of DVT associated with laparoscopic surgery. The increased IAP of the pneumoperitoneum partially compresses the iliac veins and inferior vena cava, resulting in reduced venous flow in the lower extremities. A 42% reduction in flow in the common femoral veins after establishment of pneumoperitoneum has been demonstrated by Millard and colleagues (1993). Impaired lower extremity venous return may potentially cause venous distention, resulting in endothelial damage that has been shown experimentally to promote thrombosis. The reverse Trendelenburg position used during laparoscopic cholecystectomy has been shown to increase intraoperative venous stasis. The duration of an operation affects the risk of postoperative thrombosis. Operative time is frequently longer for laparoscopic procedures; therefore, the laparoscopic method in this regard enhances the potential for DVT.

Thrombosis-promoting factors associated with the laparoscopic method may be at least partially negated by specific benefits of this modality. Patients are usually ambulatory within a few hours following laparoscopic cholecystectomy, while it may take several days for patients to become fully ambulatory after open cholecystectomy. Thus, enhanced mobility after laparoscopic procedures may reduce venous stasis and the risk of thrombosis. Hypercoagulability following surgery may be diminished by the reduced stress response associated with laparoscopic surgery. This condition is thought to be regulated by various cytokines of the acute-phase response, such as interleukin-6 (IL-6). These acute-phase mediators may stimulate the release or activation of the direct mediators of the coagulation and fibrinolytic system such as fibrinogen, von Willebrand factor, plasminogen activator, and plasminogen activator inhibitor-1. Attenuation of the acute-phase response after laparoscopic surgery may mitigate the postoperative hypercoagulable state. At present, however, no studies have clearly demonstrated evidence of reduced hypercoagulability after laparoscopic surgery. Whether or not the laparoscopic method may to some degree attenuate the hypercoagulable response of surgery remains to be determined. The effect of laparoscopic surgery on postoperative hypercoagulability thus deserves further investigation and prophylactic measures against DVT are advised.

At present, it is reasonable to assume that patients undergoing laparoscopic surgery are at an increased risk of complications related to DVT. The majority of North American surgeons use some form of prophylactic measures against DVT during laparoscopic operations. These generally include perioperative low-dose heparin and/or intermittent sequential pneumatic compression (ISPC). Millard and coworkers showed that ISPC can reverse reductions in common femoral vein peak flow velocity during laparoscopic cholecystectomy. Table 5-4 provides specific recommendations regarding prevention of venous thromboembolism during laparoscopic procedures.

Cerebral Blood Flow and Intracranial Pressure

The effects of CO_2 pneumoperitoneum on cerebral blood flow have primarily been attributed to hypercarbia resulting from increased absorption of intraperitoneal CO_2. It is well established that increased P_aCO_2 results in increased cerebral blood flow and ultimately increased intracranial pressure (ICP) and brain edema. For this reason, patients with head injuries or edema from brain tumors are hyperventilated to a hypocarbic state. A recent study of the effect of CO_2 pneumoperitoneum on ICP in pigs demonstrated an increase in ICP 30 minutes after onset of pneumoperitoneum. When the basal ICP was artificially increased to mimic a head injury, the pneumoperitoneum further increased ICP. In a human study using near-infrared laser spectroscopy to measure continuous intracranial hemodynamics, Kitajima and colleagues (1996) showed that CO_2 insufflation during laparoscopic cholecystectomy resulted in an increase in end-tidal (ET) CO_2 from 34 mm Hg to 53 mm Hg and markedly increased cerebral blood flow. The clinical relevance of increased cerebral blood flow during laparoscopic procedures is not known presently. Few, if any, cases of resultant brain injury have yet been reported. Nevertheless, patients at high risk for the development of elevated ICP, such as patients with head injuries or preexisting brain impairment, should be closely monitored by ET CO_2 or noninvasive methods of determining cerebral hemodynamics such as near-infrared spectroscopy. Measures to avoid hypercarbia, such as increasing minute ventilation, should be routinely exercised in these high-risk patients.

Pulmonary Function

The effect of CO_2 insufflation on pulmonary function is less controversial because most studies have similar conclusions. Impairments in oxygenation result from reduced lung volume and associated atelectasis due to cephalad displacement of the diaphragm. For similar reasons, ventilation may be impaired, resulting in retention of CO_2 and hypercarbia. Reduced pulmonary compliance, increased airway resistance, and reduced vital capacity are other untoward effects of the pneumoperitoneum. The Trendelenburg position, required for lower abdominal laparoscopic surgery, exacerbates the ad-

Table 5-4. Recommendations for Prevention of Venous Thromboembolism in Patients Undergoing Laparoscopic Surgery

Risk Category*	Recommended Modality
Low risk (no predisposing factors†)	Graduated compression stockings
Moderate risk (2–4 predisposing factors)	Intermittent pneumatic compression or low-dose heparin
High risk (>4 predisposing factors)	Intermittent pneumatic compression and low-dose heparin

* All patients undergoing laparoscopic surgery should be considered moderate risk unless they are <40 years with no predisposing factors.
† This category includes age >60 years, immobility >72 hours, history of deep venous thrombosis or pulmonary embolism, varicose veins, obesity, myocardial infarction, chronic obstructive pulmonary disease, cerebrovascular accident, operation >2 hours, venous stasis disease, malignancy, pregnancy, severe sepsis, and known hypercoagulable state.
Source: Adapted from Caprini JA, Arcelus JI. Prevention of postoperative venous thromboembolism following laparoscopic cholecystectomy. *Surg Endosc* 1994;8:741–747.

verse pulmonary effects of CO_2 pneumoperitoneum. It has been suggested that the risk of pulmonary aspiration is greater during laparoscopic procedures because of the effects of IAP and the Trendelenburg position on gastroesophageal reflux.

Management of oxygenation and ventilation during laparoscopy requires both close monitoring and early intervention. Pulse oximetry and continuous measurement of ET CO_2 are absolutely necessary for early recognition of hypoxia and hypercarbia. Adequate oxygenation can usually be maintained by increasing the inspired oxygen concentration (Fio_2) and ventilating with large tidal volumes to prevent atelectasis. Positive end-expiratory pressure may mitigate the associated reduction in vital capacity but should be used cautiously to avoid further reductions in cardiac output. Changes in ET CO_2 up to levels of 41 mm Hg may be used as an indicator of P_aCO_2. Higher levels of ET CO_2, however, may underestimate P_aCO_2; therefore, levels of ET CO_2 higher than 41 mm Hg should not be considered reliable indicators of P_aCO_2. Increased minute ventilation has generally be used as the first step in the management of hypercarbia resulting from increased peritoneal absorption of CO_2. Other maneuvers may include reduction in insufflation pressure, patient-position changes, and temporary evacuation of the pneumoperitoneum. Refractory hypercarbia may result from increased CO_2 absorption associated with massive subcutaneous emphysema resulting from slippage of a trocar into the subcutaneous space. In this situation, temporary cessation of CO_2 insufflation is usually required.

Gas Embolism

Venous gas embolism is a rare but potentially fatal complication of pneumoperitoneum. The incidence of gas embolism during gynecologic laparoscopy varies from 1 in 64,000 to 15 in 100,000 cases. The incidence for laparoscopic general surgery is unknown but is probably much higher because of the greater likelihood of major vessel injury and subsequent embolization. The pathophysiology involves entrance of the gas into the vascular system through an injured vessel. An often cited example is inadvertent Veress needle insertion into liver parenchyma and subsequent insufflation directly into hepatic veins. Gas that does not dissolve forms bubbles that become trapped in the right ventricular outflow tract, creating an obstruction. Contraction of the right ventricle against the blood–gas interface causes a characteristic "mill wheel" murmur, an important diagnostic finding. Cardiogenic shock ensues. All gases can cause a gas embolus; however, inert gases are less absorbable, and therefore entrance of small volumes can lead to shock. The lethal dose for an air embolus (80% nitrogen) is only 5 mL/kg, compared to 25 mL/kg for a CO_2 embolus.

Management of gas embolism begins with early recognition, which is often elusive. The diagnosis of a gas embolus is based on the otherwise unexplained sudden onset of hypoxia and hypotension, and the presence of a mill wheel murmur. As in all cases of cardiogenic shock, ET CO_2 will fall rapidly because of inadequate oxygen delivery and oxygen metabolism necessary for CO_2 production. Treatment should include simultaneous evacuation of the pneumoperitoneum, delivery of 100% oxygen, hyperventilation, and placement of the patient head down/right side up (Durant's maneuver) (Fig. 5-4). This position facilitates movement of the gas bubble away from the right ventricular outflow tract. Aspiration of the gas through a central venous catheter may be both diagnostic and therapeutic. The key to successful management is rapid diagnosis and prompt treatment.

Hypothermia

Numerous deleterious effects of perioperative hypothermia, defined as body core temperature less than 36°C, have been identified; they include impaired myocardial function, dysrhythmias, respiratory depression, hypokalemia, increased susceptibility to infection, negative nitrogen balance, thrombocytopenia, and depletion of clotting factors. Shivering, a compensatory mechanism to increase body temperature, may also have deleterious consequences, such as marked increases in oxygen consumption and myocardial work and an increased risk of myocardial infarction. Postoperative mortality has been shown to be five to six times greater in patients who remain hypothermic for longer than 2 hours, compared to normothermic patients.

Multiple factors in both open and laparoscopic surgery may contribute to hypothermia. Anesthetic agents disturb the normal thermoregulatory mechanisms. Patients' being unclothed in a cold operating room promotes heat loss. Iatrogenic causes of hypothermia include application of surgical skin preparations and administration of cold intravenous fluids. Evaporative water losses are enhanced in open abdominal surgery because of the increase in exposed surface area. Patient characteristics such as age, body surface area, and comorbidity may influence both the degree of hypothermia and its consequences. The risk of hypothermia also correlates with the length of the procedure.

Despite maintaining a closed environment, CO_2 pneumoperitoneum for laparoscopic procedures may have greater potential for inducing hypothermia than a laparotomy. As a consequence of the pressure drop of the compressed CO_2 in the regulator to 15 mm Hg from a range of 1,350 mm Hg to 37,600 mm Hg, the gas expands and therefore cools from room temperature to several degrees below room temperature. The cooling is dependent on the flow rate. In high-insufflator-flow systems of 10 to 15 L per minute, the cooling is more pronounced. To maintain an adequate pneu-

moperitoneum in the presence of gas leaks at trocar sites and frequent instrument exchanges, frequent periods of high gas flow are required. Thus, the potential cooling effect of CO_2 insufflation may be dramatic. A study by Ott in patients undergoing laparoscopy revealed a −0.3°C change in core temperature for each 50 L of CO_2 delivered. The cooling effect of CO_2 insufflation can be largely counteracted by the use of warmed CO_2 in the range of 30.0°C to 30.5°C. Warmed CO_2, however, may have deleterious effects, including drying of intraabdominal tissues. Further studies will be necessary to confirm the benefits of warmed CO_2 insufflation. Meanwhile, laparoscopic surgeons and anesthesiologists should take precautions to minimize all hypothermia-inducing factors that may be at work during any laparoscopic procedure. In particularly lengthy procedures with anticipated gas leaks, providing patients with a warming blanket at the outset is recommended.

Alternatives to Carbon Dioxide Pneumoperitoneum

Alternatives to CO_2 pneumoperitoneum include other gases and gasless lap-

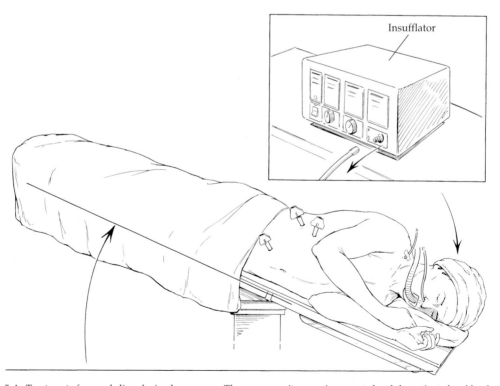

Fig. 5-4. Treatment of gas embolism during laparoscopy. The pneumoperitoneum is evacuated and the patient placed head down/right side up.

aroscopy. Gases such as helium and argon have been studied and may potentially eliminate the adverse hemodynamic and metabolic effects of CO_2 absorption. Alternative gases, however, will not eliminate those adverse effects related to elevated IAP. Gasless laparoscopy involves obtaining exposure for laparoscopy by placing an internal retracting device through a small incision and lifting the anterior abdominal wall. This method avoids both the adverse effects of CO_2 absorption and increased IAP of pneumoperitoneum. Gasless methods of access have not received wide application due to inadequate exposure for many laparoscopic procedures. Recent refinements in abdominal wall–lifting technology have improved exposure of the peritoneal cavity. Investi-gation of the potential of these methods to circumvent adverse hemodynamic changes is currently under way in multiple centers.

Patient Positioning

Because intracorporeal organ retraction is limited in laparoscopic procedures, positioning patients to achieve the maximum benefit of gravitational forces is essential. Consequently, exaggerated positions are frequently employed in laparoscopic surgery: the Trendelenburg (head-down tilt) for bowel surgery, reverse Trendelenburg (head-up tilt) for upper abdominal procedures, left lateral decubitus for splenectomy, and modified lithotomy with anal access for left-sided colectomy. Each position is associated with gravity-dependent physiologic consequences that may place patients in jeopardy. Discussion of the Trendelenburg and reverse Trendelenburg positions are most relevant because they produce the most profound physiologic changes and are also the most commonly used positions in laparoscopic surgery. Physiologic concerns pertinent to both positions primarily involve changes in cardiac filling pressures and lung volumes affecting ventilation, oxygenation, and lower extremity venous stasis.

Physiology of Positional Changes Independent of Pneumoperitoneum

Independent of pneumoperitoneum, the reverse Trendelenburg position results in gravitational pooling of blood in the lower extremities. This effectively reduces car-

diac preload and ultimately results in reduced cardiac output. In addition, the resultant lower extremity venous stasis increases the risk of DVT and PE. However, the effect of this position on the pulmonary system is generally beneficial. The gravitational pull of the viscera away from the diaphragm enhances oxygenation and ventilation. The Trendelenburg position, on the contrary, enhances venous return from the lower extremities, resulting in both increased cardiac preload and decreased risk of lower extremity venous thrombosis. The Trendelenburg position generally exacerbates oxygenation and ventilation by forcing the viscera against the diaphragm, significantly reducing lung volume.

Physiology of Positional Changes with Pneumoperitoneum

Combining the effects of CO_2 pneumoperitoneum with the Trendelenburg and reverse Trendelenburg positions should result in a hybrid effect. To further elucidate the physiologic changes associated with positional changes during laparoscopy, a swine model was used to measure hemodynamic and pulmonary changes that occurred 20 minutes after administration of CO_2 pneumoperitoneum (15 mm Hg) and placement in either the supine, Trendelenburg, or reverse Trendelenburg position. The results are summarized in Table 5-5. Based on these observations, the reverse Trendelenburg appears to exacerbate the hemodynamic impairment associated with pneumoperitoneum and should be used with caution, particularly in patients with cardiopulmonary compromise. The Trendelenburg position during laparoscopy appears to generate no further insult

to oxygenation and ventilation. Venous stasis during laparoscopy is primarily a result of the pneumoperitoneum, and neither position seems to have a significant contributory or salutary effect. These changes recognized in the swine model may not exactly extrapolate to the human condition but serve as a basis for further investigation.

Physiology of Laparoscopy during Pregnancy

The physiologic concerns of laparoscopy during pregnancy are intentionally placed at this point in the discussion because all of the preceding concerns apply. In addition, two new considerations add challenging complexities to the issue. The first involves the altered physiology of the pregnant condition that may change the biologic response to CO_2 pneumoperitoneum and positional extremes. The second involves the effects on the fetus, which maintains a physiology distinct from that of adults. At present, little is known about the effect of laparoscopic surgery on mother or fetus; however, the dominant physiologic concerns pertain to the potential of fetal acidosis and hypoperfusion.

Fetal Acidosis

Normally, the fetus maintains a state of mild acidosis thought to facilitate oxygen delivery. CO_2 is exchanged across the placenta into the maternal circulation and eventually excreted by the mother. During a laparoscopic procedure, if maternal P_aCO_2 becomes elevated secondary to CO_2 insufflation, this may impair fetal exchange of CO_2 and result in clinically severe acidosis. Several animal studies using

Table 5-5. Physiologic Effects of Trendelenburg and Reverse Trendelenburg Positions During Laparoscopic Surgery in a Porcine Model*

System	Trendelenburg	Reverse Trendelenburg
Cardiovascular	Increased central filling pressures Increased mean arterial pressure No change in cardiac output	Decreased central filling pressures Decreased mean arterial pressure Decreased cardiac output
Pulmonary	No change in oxygenation No change in ventilation	No change in oxygenation No change in ventilation
Venous stasis	No change in lower extremity venous blood flow	No change in lower extremity venous blood flow

* Intraabdominal pressure of 15 mm Hg.

a pregnant ewe model have demonstrated that fetal acidosis associated with severe tachycardia or bradycardia may occur even with mild elevations of ET CO_2. The full consequences of fetal acidosis are currently unknown.

Fetal Hypoperfusion

As described above, the compound effects of CO_2 pneumoperitoneum and the reverse Trendelenburg position may result in significant decreases (up to 40%) in cardiac output. Although such decreases may be tolerated in healthy nonpregnant patients, the effect on pregnant patients and the fetus is clearly unknown. Since CO_2 pneumoperitoneum is known to reduce visceral organ perfusion, it may likewise reduce uterine blood flow and jeopardize fetal oxygen delivery. At present, no data are available to support or refute these concerns.

Clinical Experience

More than 50 cases of laparoscopic procedures at various stages of pregnancy have been reported in the literature. Most publications involved isolated case reports or small series (two to five patients). Virtually no adverse maternal consequences have been reported; four fetal deaths have occurred. Review of the circumstances of these deaths does not clearly link the cause of death to the laparoscopic method. Yet, until proven otherwise, the laparoscopic approach must be suspect. Though many of the authors of these reports conclude that laparoscopy is safe in pregnancy, clearly outcomes in only 50 cases or even 100 cases is insufficient to support this claim. In light of the issues raised from experimental animal studies, laparoscopic surgery during pregnancy must be considered potentially hazardous. This issue will remain controversial for many years, until adequate clinical and laboratory analyses have been performed. At present, the only type of laparoscopic surgery during pregnancy that I can recommend is gasless laparoscopy. The gasless method averts all consequences related to both the pressure effects of pneumoperitoneum and absorption of CO_2. Admittedly, limitations of exposure in some cases may render a gasless method prohibitive, especially in the nearly full-term pregnancy.

Postoperative Physiology of Laparoscopic Surgery

While the adverse physiologic effects of the laparoscopic method are generally manifest only during the intraoperative period, the beneficial physiologic effects related to reduced tissue or cellular injury persist throughout the recovery period. Reduced injury includes reduction not only in abdominal wall tissue destruction but also in tissue injury resulting from organ retraction and manual manipulation of bowel. Reduced injury ultimately accounts for all the benefits of laparoscopic surgery, including reduced postoperative pain and morbidity, faster recovery, improved cosmesis, and reduced cost. In other words, the physiology of minimal invasion explains why laparoscopic surgery is (and should be) performed in many patients.

Minimal Invasion— The Concept

In the Desert Storm conflict, precise target destruction that avoided injury to surrounding innocent civilian bystanders was termed a *surgical* strike. In reality, most surgical procedures, especially abdominal operations, cannot meet this definition of surgical strike and are anything but precise because much injury is inflicted on innocent bystanders (e.g., abdominal wall). Minimally invasive surgery attempts to meet the definition of a true surgical strike. The aim of minimally invasive surgery is to eliminate or minimize all unnecessary trauma previously thought required to accomplish a therapeutic task. This concept is illustrated in Fig. 5-5. Cholecystectomy should be considered two procedures within one operation: access to the organ and the gallbladder dissection. The ultimate goal of the operation is removal of the diseased organ. Laparotomy and gallbladder dissection each have their own specific local complications, such as incisional hernia or bile leak. Yet both procedures contribute to the risk of systemic complications attributable to the stress of surgery, such as DVT, ileus, and atelectasis. The potential adverse consequences of the gallbladder dissection are necessary to achieve the surgical goal of removal of the diseased organ. However, until recently, patients have been subjected to the risks inherent in the access procedure (the lap-

arotomy) without any benefit from this portion of the operation. Advances in endoscopic techniques enable major abdominal operations to be accomplished without major injury to the abdominal wall that was previously required for the sole purpose of accessing the target organ.

Physiology of Surgical Injury: Modification of Biologic Response

The biologic response to injury, whether accidental or due to elective surgery, primarily depends on the magnitude of the insult and the organism's ability to recover. Although teleologically the biologic response is adaptive, in many instances it is in fact maladaptive. Operative morbidity and mortality can generally be ascribed to disease progression, technical failure, or an adverse physiologic response to surgical injury (Fig. 5-6). The dominant strategy for reducing operative morbidity and mortality has been to acknowledge the consequences related to the stress response and attempt to counter them by administering perioperative antibiotics, nutrition, pain control, pulmonary toilet, early ambulation, anticoagulants, and so on. Recently, strategies have changed to focus on preventive measures that minimize the magnitude of the stress response. Pharmacologically blocking or limiting the response to injury is one such strategy. General and regional anesthesia may also modify the stress response to surgery. Other agents such as perioperative steroids, intrathecal neural blockade, and postoperative cyclooxygenase inhibitors have been shown to mitigate postoperative sequelae of surgery. Minimally invasive surgery goes one step further by reducing the overall magnitude of surgical injury, thereby diminishing the stress response and consequential morbidity and mortality.

Neuroendocrine and Metabolic Consequences of Surgery

The classic hypermetabolic stress response is the dominant physiologic response to injury. This response directly or indirectly affects all other organ systems and therefore has the largest impact on the duration and success of convalescence. The stress response is classically divided into early catabolic and late anabolic phases. The hypermetabolic changes of catabolism appear to be initiated by tissue damage and

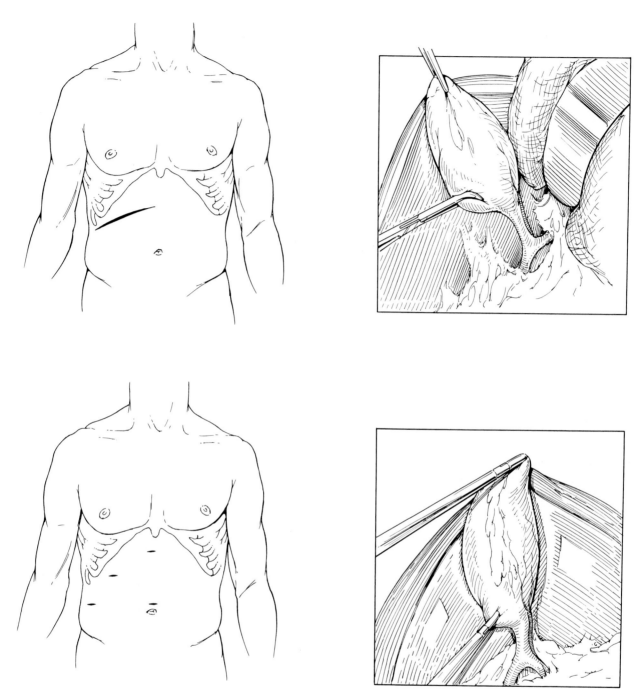

Fig. 5-5. Minimally invasive surgery—the concept.

are characterized by increased fat oxidation and marked proteolysis, causing an increased loss of nitrogen in the urine. The catabolic phase begins with the onset of injury (the skin incision) and generally lasts 24 to 48 hours for a major abdominal operation. The anabolic phase begins 3 to 6 days after a major abdominal operation and persists for 4 to 6 weeks. It has long been established that the extent, degree, and duration of metabolic changes following tissue injury depend on the severity of the injury.

Mediation of the Injury Response. The injury response begins in the wound and is primarily mediated by the central nervous system (CNS), which receives stimuli from three distinct sources: (a) afferent nerve fibers; (b) volume receptors, pressure receptors, and chemoreceptors; and (c) circulating substances. Afferent sensory nerve fibers from the wound relay the pain signal to the hypothalamus–pituitary–adrenal axis and initiate the adrenocortical response to injury. Cortisol, glucagon, and catecholamines, among others, are released in high concentrations and play a pivotal role in mediating the stress response. Fluid loss from the vascular compartment causes stimulation of volume and pressure receptors that initiates a series of CNS-mediated cardiovascular adjustments aimed at redis-

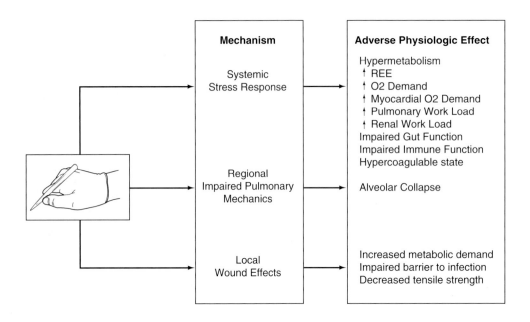

Mechanism	Adverse Physiologic Effect

Systemic Stress Response

Hypermetabolism
↑ REE
↑ O2 Demand
↑ Myocardial O2 Demand
↑ Pulmonary Work Load
↑ Renal Work Load
Impaired Gut Function
Impaired Immune Function
Hypercoagulable state

Regional Impaired Pulmonary Mechanics

Alveolar Collapse

Local Wound Effects

Increased metabolic demand
Impaired barrier to infection
Decreased tensile strength

Fig. 5-6. Physiologic response to laparotomy.

tribution of blood to vital organs. Chemoreceptors stimulated by acid–base disturbances resulting from regional hypoperfusion and anaerobic metabolism provide afferent input to vasomotor and respiratory centers, where compensatory changes are initiated. Circulating substances such as cytokines are released locally at or near the wound and may directly or indirectly stimulate the CNS or may initiate their own effects independently.

Stress Response to Laparoscopic Surgery. Studies comparing the stress response of laparoscopic surgery to open

surgery have thus far focused on comparing postoperative levels of stress indicators and mediators. The neuroendocrine response to laparoscopic cholecystectomy as indicated by postoperative catecholamine, cortisol, and glucose levels appears to be modestly attenuated at least in the immediate perioperative period (Figs. 5-7 and 5-8). Some investigators, however, applying different methodologies, have found no difference in the neuroendocrine response to open versus laparoscopic surgery. Studies specifically addressing the cytokine and acute-phase response have more consistently demonstrated different responses to open and laparoscopic

surgery. Indicators such as IL-6, C-reactive protein, leukocytosis, and erythrocyte sedimentation rate have all been shown to be lower after laparoscopic than open cholecystectomy. Collectively, these studies suggest that in the immediate perioperative period the laparoscopic method results in an attenuated neuroendocrine response and cytokine response compared to open cholecystectomy.

Perioperative Immune Function

Multiple defects in the immune system have been described following operations and trauma. Major components of cellular immunity are depressed after surgical procedures. Response to antibody also appears to be adversely affected by surgery and trauma. Other factors contributing to general immunosuppression after surgery include circulating immunosuppressive agents such as prostaglandins and cytokines. The clinical relevance of impaired postoperative immune function is the subject of intense investigation, and many believe that this impairment may be a significant contributing factor to postoperative immune-related complications such as infectious complications and tumor growth.

The above mentioned mediators of the stress response also appear to inhibit immune function. Cortisol has been found to suppress lymphocyte blastogenesis. Epinephrine and norepinephrine inhibit

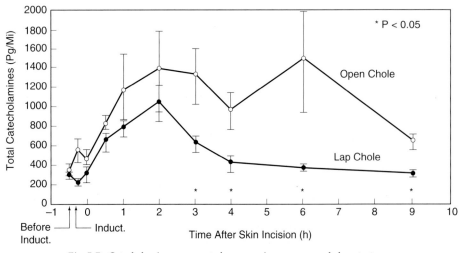

Fig. 5-7. Catecholamine response to laparoscopic versus open cholecystectomy.

neutrophil chemotaxis. Glucagon impairs neutrophil chemotaxis and bactericidal activity. Other factors such as prostaglandin E_2, endotoxin, tumor necrosis factor, proteolysis factor, and interleukin-1 have been implicated as potential mediators of the immune-suppressed state following trauma or stress. It is generally accepted that the extent of the injury is directly related to the magnitude of the stress response and consequent immunosuppression.

Since the laparoscopic method reduces tissue injury, investigators have begun to study the effects of the reduced tissue trauma of laparoscopy on perioperative immune function. Whelan and associates evaluated the effect of laparoscopic versus open colon resection on postoperative T cell–related immune function, as measured by delayed-type hypersensitivity using a swine model. Results of skin antigen testing showed that pigs undergoing laparoscopic resection had 20%-larger-diameter skin induration than the open surgery group. This same group of investigators demonstrated that rats undergoing CO_2 insufflation had no differences in response to the antigens keyhole-limpet hemocyanin and phytohemagglutinin (PHA) from control animals (no procedure performed) at 24 and 48 hours after insufflation, but animals that underwent laparotomy had a significantly diminished postoperative response to the same antigens. This group also demonstrated the clinical relevance of the preserved immune response after laparoscopic surgery by showing that tumor growth in mice was less after laparoscopy than after laparotomy (Fig. 5-9). These animal studies support the hypothesis that reduced surgical injury reduces the impairment of postoperative immune function specifically related to cell-mediated immunity.

Evidence of preserved immune function after laparoscopic surgery exists in humans as well. IL-6 and white blood cell counts have been shown to be unchanged after laparoscopic cholecystectomy, whereas they are significantly increased after open cholecystectomy. Delayed-type hypersensitivity, as determined by response to PHA, is reduced after open cholecystectomy but preserved after laparoscopic cholecystectomy. Significantly reduced monocyte and neutrophil release of superoxide anion, neutrophil chemotaxis, tumor necrosis factor, and white

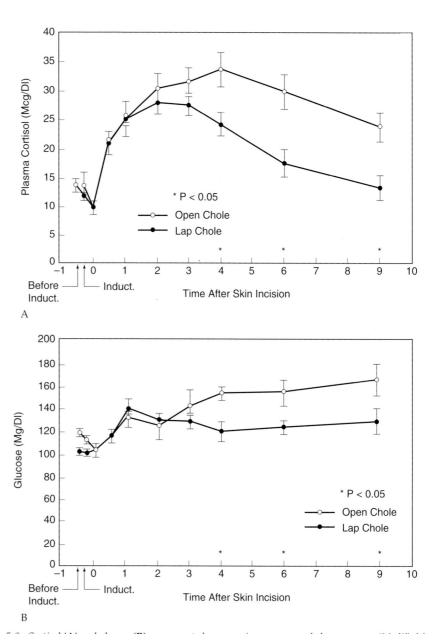

Fig. 5-8. Cortisol **(A)** and glucose **(B)** responses to laparoscopic versus open cholecystectomy. (Modified from Schauer PR, Sirinek KR. The laparoscopic approach reduces the endocrine response to elective cholecystectomy. Am Surg 1995;61:106–111.)

blood cell count have been demonstrated in laparoscopic patients compared to patients undergoing open cholecystectomy. Both animal and human studies provide preliminary and complementary evidence that immune function after laparoscopic surgery is less impaired than after open surgery.

The findings of preserved immunocompetence are particularly noteworthy in light of recent studies suggesting an increased occurrence of tumor implantation in wounds following laparoscopic surgery compared to open surgery. Although the mechanism of tumor implantation is not clear, these data supporting preserved immune function after laparoscopic surgery suggest that a technical mechanism may account for tumor implantation. Excessive tumor manipulation or shedding of tumor cells during specimen removal have been discussed as potential technical errors leading to tumor metastasis. The overall clinical significance of preservation of postoperative immune function as related to tumor metastases remains to be determined.

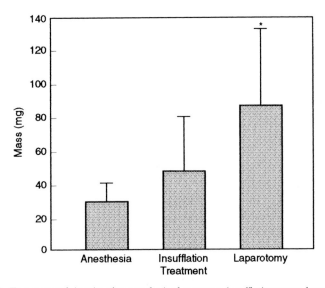

Fig. 5-9. Tumor growth in mice after anesthesia alone versus insufflation versus laparotomy.

Cardiac Function after Laparoscopic Surgery

Following surgery, cardiac performance in healthy patients, regulated by the sympathetic response, increases in the postoperative period to meet increased metabolic demands. The increase in cardiac work as a response to the hypermetabolic state, however, is detrimental to patients with compromised cardiac function and may lead to myocardial ischemia and infarction. Thus, the potential for the laparoscopic approach to reduce cardiac morbidity is significant. In a contemporary study of more than 40,000 open cholecystectomies, cardiac complications (0.6%) accounted for significant morbidity and were the most common cause of death. In a U.S. Department of Defense analysis of 5,607 laparoscopic cholecystectomies, the rate of myocardial infarction was comparatively very low (0.08%). Williams and colleagues (1993) compared the outcome of evenly matched patients undergoing 1,107 laparoscopic cholecystectomies to that of 1,283 open cholecystectomies performed 10 years previously. There was a significant decrease in cardiac complications in the laparoscopic group (0.06% vs. 1.4%). Data now available suggest that laparoscopic approaches may reduce overall cardiac morbidity; however, no definitive conclusions can be made. In addition, the potential benefit of the laparoscopic approach on postoperative cardiac function must be weighed against the detrimental intraoperative effects of CO_2 pneumoperitoneum on cardiac output.

Pulmonary Function after Laparoscopic Surgery

Significant impairment of pulmonary function after abdominal surgery and general anesthesia has been well documented. Pulmonary complications are the most common morbidity after abdominal surgery. General anesthesia produces transient impaired gas exchange as a result of decreased lung volumes, shunting, and changes in lung mechanics. The effect on pulmonary function is more pronounced and of longer duration with upper abdominal than with pelvic procedures. Pulmonary impairment may frequently persist for weeks following surgery. A restrictive pattern characterized by a 50% reduction in vital capacity and a 30% decrease in tidal volume and functional residual capacity occurs following major abdominal procedures. These changes become clinically significant when they contribute to pathologic conditions such as atelectasis, hypoxemia, and pneumonia.

Preserved pulmonary function is the most well documented benefit of the physiologic changes associated with the laparoscopic approach. Patients undergoing laparoscopic cholecystectomy have a significant improvement over open cholecystectomy patients in postoperative spirometry, total lung capacity, and oxygen saturation. Maximum voluntary ventilation, equivalent to a cardiac stress test in measuring global pulmonary function, is much less impaired after laparoscopic cholecystectomy (Fig. 5-10). Pulmonary function returns to baseline 4 to 10 days sooner after laparoscopic cholecystec-

tomy. Lower rates of pulmonary complications, including atelectasis and hypoxia, occur when the laparoscopic approach is used (Fig. 5-11). McMahon and associates (1994) showed that even when compared to the "minilaparotomy" cholecystectomy, laparoscopic cholecystectomy resulted in improvements in postoperative spirometry, better oxygen saturation, reduced analog pain scores, and reduced narcotic consumption. Many large laparoscopic cholecystectomy series have reported pulmonary complication rates of less than 0.5%, compared to 2% for contemporary open cholecystectomy. Indeed, the reduction in pulmonary morbidity is probably the most underrated benefit of laparoscopic surgery.

The reduction in postoperative pain likely plays a role in preserving pulmonary function after laparoscopic procedures. Pain resulting from deep inspiration contributes to the cascade of events resulting in chest wall splinting, reduced functional residual capacity, tachypnea, and shallow breathing, which are ultimately thought to lead to atelectasis. Atelectasis is considered the forerunner of most postoperative pulmonary complications. In addition, minimal disruption of the abdominal wall musculature, which is a component of the ventilatory pump, probably accounts for some physiologic improvement as well.

Intestinal Function after Laparoscopic Surgery

Postoperative ileus is a predictable consequence of abdominal procedures. Ileus is often the major factor in prolonging hospital stays and may account for significant morbidity related to temporary nutritional deprivation. The etiology of postoperative ileus is probably multifactorial and is incompletely understood. Sympathetic inhibition of motility is one proposed mechanism. Other possible mechanisms include bowel manipulation, release of stress-related hormones other than catecholamines (e.g., vasopressin), and postoperative narcotic usage.

Many clinical studies have demonstrated an earlier return of bowel function after laparoscopic surgery compared to conventional open surgery. Experimental studies in animals and humans evaluating intestinal myoelectric and contractile activity have yielded mixed results. Some have shown a more rapid return of normal motility following laparoscopic than open surgery, whereas others have shown

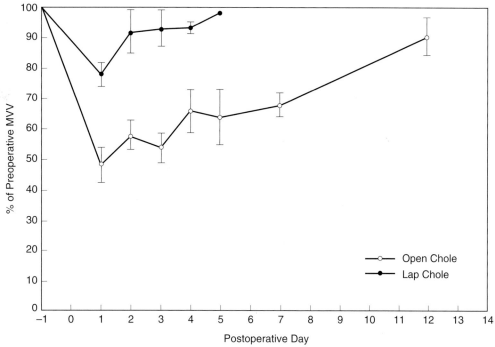

Fig. 5-10. *Maximum voluntary ventilation after laparoscopic versus open cholecystectomy.*

equivalent outcomes. It has been speculated that laparoscopic operations may be followed by rapid resolution of ileus because of minimal narcotic requirements.

Despite discrepancies in experimental motility studies, clinical indicators of bowel function have more consistently demonstrated a reduced period of ileus after laparoscopic surgery. Garcia-Caballero and Vara-Thorbeck (1993) demonstrated that the onset of flatus and bowel movement occurred sooner after laparoscopic than open cholecystectomy (10 and 36 hours vs. 60 and 96 hours, respectively). In patients undergoing colectomy, Senagore and coworkers (1995) demonstrated that laparoscopic-assisted colectomy compared to open colectomy not only resulted in a more rapid resolution of ileus but also led to an earlier return to positive nitrogen balance (Fig. 5-12). These preliminary studies overall support the hypothesis that the laparoscopic approach may positively affect postoperative ileus. More investigation of this very important clinical issue is necessary, however, before any definitive conclusions can be made.

Abdominal Adhesion Formation after Laparoscopic Surgery

Adhesion formation after abdominal and pelvic operations remains extremely com-

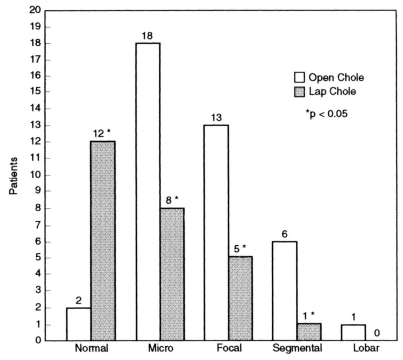

Fig. 5-11. *Atelectasis after laparoscopic versus open cholecystectomy.*

mon and is a source of considerable morbidity. Adhesions directly cause bowel obstruction, infertility, and chronic abdominal pain, and account for the major dangers of reoperative surgery. Despite a century of effort, little progress has been made in preventing or treating this challenging problem. Multiple etiologic factors contribute to adhesion formation, including mechanical trauma, thermal injury, infection, tissue ischemia, and foreign material. The pathophysiology of adhesion

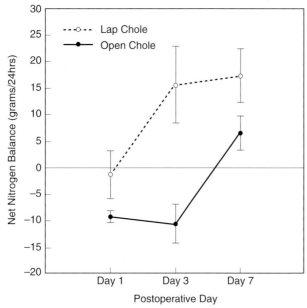

Fig. 5-12. Nitrogen balance following laparoscopic versus open colectomy. (Modified from Senagore AJ, Kilbride MJ, Luchtefeld MA, MacKeign JM, Davis AT, Moore JD. Superior nitrogen balance after laparoscopic-assisted colectomy. Ann Surg *1995;221:171–175.)*

formation is based on an inflammatory vascular response to foreign material or tissue made ischemic by injury.

Most surgeons have a clinical impression that laparoscopy results in fewer intraabdominal adhesions. However, few studies have adequately addressed this issue. Luciano and associates (1989) found that no adhesions were formed in rabbits after laser injuries to the peritoneum and uterine horn were created laparoscopically, whereas all animals had adhesions after the injuries were made via laparotomy. In a prospective, randomized clinical study, Lundorff and colleagues (1991) demonstrated that patients who underwent laparotomy for the management of ectopic pregnancy had significantly more adhesions at second-look laparoscopy than patients who initially underwent laparoscopy.

Laparoscopic surgery probably reduces adhesion formation by multiple mechanisms. Major factors include reductions in the inciting events, tissue injury, and surrounding ischemia. Visceral injury and abdominal wall injury are less during laparoscopic operations because wound retractors, packing, and bowel handling are minimized. The laparoscopic method also reduces foreign body contamination by minimizing access of glove talc or particulate matter to the abdominal cavity. A reduction in the systemic inflammatory re-

sponse may also contribute to reduced adhesion formation.

Wound Healing

Complications related to abdominal wound healing, such as hematomas, seromas, infection, dehiscence, and hernia, contribute significantly to short- and long-term postoperative morbidity. The pathophysiology of wound healing is complex, and multiple contributory factors are involved. Among the many factors related to wound complications, the size of the wound itself is an obvious but nevertheless important factor. Laparoscopic incisions commonly range from 5 to 12 mm. Wounds of this size rarely result in complications, even in high-risk patients. Multiple large series of laparoscopic cholecystectomies report overall wound-related complications much lower than would be seen with open cholecystectomy. Thus, the laparoscopic method has virtually eliminated the dreaded complications of large incisional hernias, as well as wound dehiscence and evisceration.

Effect of Laparoscopic Surgery on Morbidity and Mortality

Assessing the effect of the laparoscopic approach on overall morbidity and mortality

is inhibited by the lack of prospective, randomized studies. Furthermore, to compare rates of complications, which generally have a low frequency, large numbers of patients (in the thousands) are necessary. Accepting these limitations, there is increasing evidence to support the concept that reduced surgical injury results in reduced morbidity and mortality. Several large series clearly demonstrated a significant reduction in overall morbidity with laparoscopic techniques. At our institution, there has been a 50% reduction in overall morbidity in high-risk patients (American Society of Anesthesiologists status 3) following the introduction of laparoscopic cholecystectomy. Although the decrease in mortality with laparoscopic cholecystectomy was not statistically significant, a significant decrease in cardiopulmonary morbidity was realized. Williams colleagues (1993) demonstrated a 50% reduction in major complications in patients undergoing elective laparoscopic cholecystectomy (7.5% vs. 3.1%) and a significant reduction in mortality for patients with acute cholecystitis (2.3% vs. 0%), compared to open cholecystectomy. A statewide study of 67,537 Maryland residents who underwent open or laparoscopic cholecystectomy from 1985 to 1992 demonstrated a 30% reduction in mortality associated with the laparoscopic technique. More compelling than any other evidence, this reduction in overall morbidity and mortality reflects the net physiologic consequences of laparoscopic surgery.

Conclusion
Overall Benefit of Laparoscopic Surgery

Considering all the potential adverse effects associated with laparoscopic exposure methods and positioning together with all the potential physiologic benefits of minimal invasion, the balance is clearly in favor of the laparoscopic approach for most abdominal procedures in most patients. The physiologic and clinical data gained from the study of laparoscopic cholecystectomy suggest that minimizing abdominal wall trauma is highly beneficial to patients. Thus, the abdominal wall should be respected as a distinct entity with its own local and systemic response to injury. It is now understood that most of the morbidity of open cholecystectomy is attributed to the abdominal incision and not the gallbladder dissection. These physiologic benefits translate into faster recovery and reduced morbidity and mortality. Consequently, a paradigm shift is occurring in that the improved risk–benefit ratio of minimally invasive procedures has drastically altered the role of surgery from being reserved as a "last resort" therapy to being considered earlier in the course of a given disease process. This lowering of the threshold for operative therapy has been most clearly seen in patients with gallstones and more recently in patients with gastroesophageal reflux disease.

Which Patients Are Unlikely to Receive Benefit from Laparoscopic Surgery?

High-risk, physiologically compromised patients deserve special consideration regarding the risk–benefit ratio of laparoscopic surgery. Paradoxically, high-risk patients (e.g., the elderly, obese patients with cardiac disease) are at highest risk for a complication related to the laparoscopic technique yet also stand to gain the greatest benefit from the minimally invasive approach. In reality, the decision to proceed with a laparoscopic or an open approach is made on a case-by-case basis by the individual surgeon, depending on a variety of circumstances including expertise and local availability of ancillary support. An increased awareness and knowledge of the basic physiologic principles elucidated in this chapter will aid the individual surgeon in making the best decision for his or her patients.

Which Procedures Are Unlikely to be Improved by the Laparoscopic Approach?

Perhaps, the overall magnitude of injury (local and systemic) associated with laparotomy can be used to define the limitations of laparoscopic surgery. In operations such as cholecystectomy and Nissen fundoplication, the surgical injury required to accomplish the objective (e.g., gallbladder dissection or esophageal dissection and fundal wrap) constitutes only a fraction of the injury associated with laparotomy. In extensive abdominal operations such as pancreaticoduodenectomy,

the injury associated with laparotomy may only represent a small proportion of injury for the entire operation. Thus, the relative gains from a laparoscopic approach for a Whipple resection may be minor and not worthwhile, compared to gains for cholecystectomy or Nissen fundoplication. This concept will certainly be tested as more extensive operations are attempted using the laparoscopic technique.

Suggested Reading

Deziel DJ. Complications of cholecystectomy: incidence, clinical manifestations, and diagnosis. *Surg Clin North Am* 1994;74:809–823.

Garcia-Caballero M, Vara-Thorbeck C. The evolution of postoperative ileus after laparoscopic cholecystectomy. *Surg Endosc* 1993;7:416–419.

Kitajima T, Shinohara M, Ogata H. Cerebral oxygen metabolism measured by near-infrared laser spectroscopy during laparoscopic cholecystectomy with CO_2 insufflation. *Surg Laparosc Endosc* 1996;6:210–212.

Luciano AA, Maier DB, Koch EI, Nulsen JC, Whitman GF. A comparative study of postoperative adhesions following laser surgery by laparoscopy versus laparotomy in the rabbit model. *Obstet Gynecol* 1989;74:220–224.

Lundorff P, Hahlin M, Bjorn K, Thorburn J, Lindblom B. Adhesion formation after laparoscopic surgery in tubal pregnancy: a randomized trial versus laparotomy. *Fertil Steril* 1991;55:911–915.

McMahon AJ, Russell IT, Ramsay G, et al. Laparoscopic and minilaparotomy cholecystectomy: a randomized trial comparing postoperative pain and pulmonary function. *Surgery* 1994;115:533–539.

Millard JA, Hill BB, Cook PS, Fenoglio ME, Stahlgren LH. Intermittent sequential pneumatic compression in prevention of venous stasis associated with pneumoperitoneum during laparoscopic cholecystectomy. *Arch Surg* 1993;128:914–919.

Ott DE. Correction of laparoscopic insufflation hypothermia. *J Laparoendosc Surg* 1991;1:183–186.

Schauer PR, Sirinek KR. The laparoscopic approach reduces the endocrine response to elective cholecystectomy. *Am Surg* 1995;61:106–111.

Schauer PR, Eubanks SW, Pappas TN, Meyers WC. The effect of patient position on cardiopulmonary function and venous stasis during laparoscopy. *J Surg Res* 1998; in press.

Schauer PR, Luna J, Ghiatas A, Glen ME, Warren JM, Sirinek KR. Pulmonary function after

laparoscopic cholecystectomy. *Surgery* 1993;114:389–399.

Senagore AJ, Kilbride MJ, Luchtefeld MA, MacKeign JM, Davis AT, Moore JD. Superior nitrogen balance after laparoscopic-assisted colectomy. *Ann Surg* 1995;221:171–175.

Williams LF, Chapman WC, Bonau RA, McGee EC, Boyd RW, Jacobs JK. Comparison of laparoscopic cholecystectomy with open cholecystectomy in a single center. *Am J Surg* 1993;165:459–465.

EDITOR'S COMMENT

Although much is made of the "minimally invasive" nature of laparoscopic surgery, the term is somewhat loosely applied. In fact, most laparoscopic surgeries are "maximally invasive" yet cause minimal abdominal wall trauma due to the small incisions to gain access to the peritoneal cavity. Therefore, "minimal access" is probably the more accurate term to describe laparoscopic surgery, yet the moniker "minimally invasive" surgery is probably here to stay. Following this line of reasoning, the laparoscopic operations from which one would expect to gain most benefit compared to their open counterparts are those procedures wherein the traditional operation requires a large incision to perform a procedure in a relatively narrow operative field.

When the laparoscopic operation is performed without complications, the physiologic consequences of the operation itself should be less than its open counterpart, as discussed in this chapter. The laparoscopic surgeon must bear in mind, however, that the CO_2 pneumoperitoneum itself may lead to untoward physiologic effects due to the elevated IAP or the effect of CO_2 absorbed into the bloodstream through the peritoneal surfaces. This is particularly true in patients with significant cardiopulmonary disease, the same group in whom the commonly measured ET CO_2 may not accurately reflect the true arterial Pco_2. In these patients, it is wise to consider insertion of an arterial catheter for serial blood gas determinations, if the proposed laparoscopic procedure is expected to be prolonged. Likewise, a Swan-Ganz catheter may be beneficial to monitor preload and cardiac parameters in selected cases. Although some of the experimental data are conflicting, it appears that the body's biologic response to laparoscopic surgery is less extreme than that to traditional open operation. Consequently, this allows maintenance of a near-normal immune response, which may ultimately lead to improved oncologic outcome in patients undergoing laparoscopic operations for neoplastic disease. Furthermore, if laparoscopic surgery is truly associated with a lower incidence of adhesion formation, the long-term benefits of laparoscopic operations may be even greater than currently appreciated.

As with any operation, the development of a significant complication following a specific laparoscopic operation negates all the potential benefits of the minimally invasive approach. Therefore, although a knowledge of the physiology of laparoscopic surgery is important, the underlying tenet of the surgeon's trade—*primum non nocere* (first, do not harm)—should remain uppermost in our minds.

N.J.S.

6

Gasless Laparoscopy

Lucian Newman III

Laparoscopic instruments have evolved from relatively crude designs utilized in the early 1900s to a very complex system for surgical procedures today. Many techniques have been used to achieve the exposure required for surgical procedures. It is interesting that the techniques of laparoscopic surgery utilizing pneumoperitoneum have outpaced the development of so-called gasless surgical techniques. In the purest sense, gasless surgical procedures are a recreation of the minilaparotomy. The history of surgery includes many deviations from what is considered standard operating procedure. It has recently been recognized that one of the primary mechanisms for perioperative morbidity is the surgical wound. It is only natural that surgeons would pursue access to surgical sites through less invasive means.

Gasless laparoscopic techniques were first used by Japanese and European investigators, coincident with the explosion of laparoscopic general surgery. In fact, one the earliest laparoscopic cholecystectomies, performed by Dr. Phillippe Mouret in Lyon, France, employed a system that allowed exposure without complete pneumoperitoneum. The rationale behind the use of gasless techniques includes (a) avoiding complications associated with the establishment and maintenance of pneumoperitoneum and (b) providing a working environment within the abdominal cavity that does not limit the surgeon to specific instruments designed for laparoscopic surgery.

Most of my experience with gasless laparoscopic surgery has involved the Laparolift system developed by Origin Medsystems (Menlo Park, CA) (Fig. 6-1). Other systems are also available internationally (Table 6-1). These devices use differing means to achieve the same goal: elevation of the abdominal wall to create an intraabdominal space in which to work (Fig. 6-2). Several systems developed in Japan have targeted cholecystectomy as the only procedure for which they are intended. The Laparolift system yields greater versatility and may be used virtually anywhere within the abdominal cavity with only minor modifications and placement.

Equipment

The Laparolift system was created to become a unique intraabdominal retracting device that would allow a wide variety of laparoscopic surgical procedures to be performed without requiring insufflation. The system includes the Laparolift arm, which can be fitted to most operating room tables. The arm is driven by an electric motor, but manual operation is possible in the event of power failure. The most important aspect of the Laparolift system is the disposable Laparofan that fits into the abdominal cavity and attaches directly to the arm in dovetail fashion (Fig. 6-3). First-generation Laparofans included a simple 10- and 15-cm V-shaped fan. Second-generation fans included quadrant-specific curved fan blades, which were originally manufactured in a J shape and an S shape. The benefit of these second-generation fans was enhancement of lateral lifting. The newest lifting devices are not fan-shaped, but an inflatable balloon (Fig. 6-4). All of these lifts are introduced through an open cutdown technique using a small incision. Three access options are available for accessory port sites: (a) rigid and flexible valveless trocars that are very simple and inexpensive, (b) standard laparoscopic trocars, which are generally unnecessary, and (c) no trocar at all. My preference is the valveless trocar, which facilitates instrument exchange with minimal tissue trauma. The instruments that can be used with this system are unlimited. A surgeon may utilize standard operating equipment or any of the instruments designed specifically for laparoscopic surgery. It is this instrument flexibility that intrigues many surgeons. In the course of a gasless procedure, any number of standard instruments may be utilized, including suction and irrigation catheters, needle drivers, electrocautery probes, Metzenbaum scissors, and conventional stapling devices.

Patient Selection

The indications for gasless laparoscopic surgery parallel those considerations for similar open or pneumoperitoneum cases. Once a patient is considered to be an acceptable candidate for a given procedure, the decision is made regarding the type of access to be employed. Patients who have an increased cardiopulmonary risk with operation or those in whom anesthetic options are desired may be selected for gasless access. Just as with any open or laparoscopic procedure utilizing pneumoperitoneum, patients with a lower body mass index are more ideal. In general, female patients are preferable to male patients, perhaps because of a relatively increased distensibility of the anterior abdominal wall. This is not based on scientific proof but rather on personal experience. No significant change in perioperative management is made for patients who undergo gasless operative procedures. Some investigators utilizing gasless techniques advise

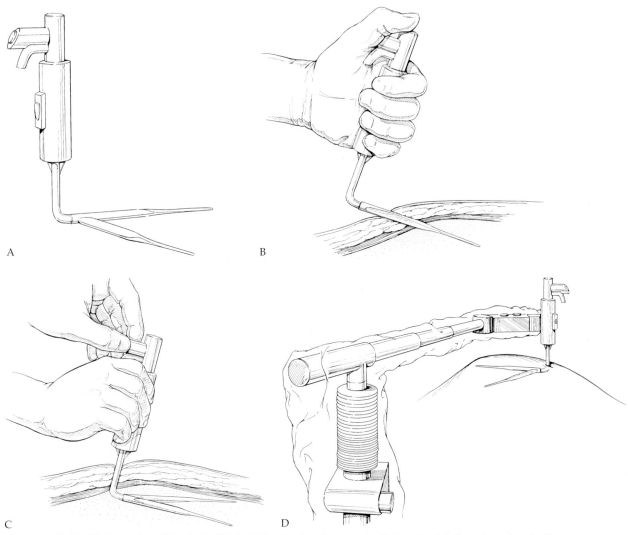

Fig. 6-1. The Laparoform lifting device (Origin Medsystems). **A:** *Fan retractor.* **B:** *Insertion into the peritoneal cavity.* **C:** *Blades separated.* **D:** *Laparofan attached to lifting arm in deployed position.*

Table 6-1. Gasless Systems

System	Type	Country of Origin
Laparolift	Planar	USA
Maher	U-shaped	Australia
Nagai	Tent lift	Japan
Hashimoto	Double-wire lift	Japan
Laparotesner	Fork-shaped fan	Italy
Omnilift/ Omnitrac	Planar	USA
Mouret Suspendeur Trois X	Circular	France
Cuschieri Sling	Sling	Scotland
Bookler Mediflex	T bar	USA
Kitano	U-shaped bar	Japan

a limited bowel preparation; however, this is not my standard practice. In the course of gasless bowel resection, however, I do perform a standard Nichols-Condon preparation. In all patients, the informed consent process includes a description of the proposed procedure and the manner in which it will occur. At this time, anesthetic options also may be discussed. The anticipated perioperative and postoperative course is discussed with patients at the time of the office visit.

One maxim that holds true is that exposure below the umbilicus with gasless surgery is easier to achieve than gasless exposure of the upper abdomen. Innovative solutions to exposure problems have been discussed relative to all surgical procedures, whether carried out in open fashion or video-assisted. Utilization of accessory lifting sites has been practiced by a number of gasless laparoscopy surgeons. It is my practice not to deviate from what I would consider the standard pneumoperitoneum access for a given procedure. Although almost any intraabdominal procedure may be carried out with gasless access, the basic aspects of exposure and behavior in five selected procedures will be described, including cholecystectomy, appendectomy, herniorrhaphy, colon resection, and pelvic procedures.

Special Considerations for Gasless Laparoscopy

Unfortunately, the presumption that pneumoperitoneum is an entirely safe modality is not true (Table 6-2). This presumption is based on the experience of a surgeon and his assumption that insuffla-

Table 6-2. Complications of Carbon Dioxide Pneumoperitoneum

Cardiovascular
    Bradycardia
    Reduced cardiac output
    Arrhythmia
    Hypotension
    Hypertension
Mechanical
    Reduced visceral blood flow
    Tension pneumothorax
    Pneumomediastinum
    Carbon dioxide embolus
    Venous thrombosis
    Subcutaneous emphysema
Pulmonary
    Reduced pulmonary compliance
    Atelectasis
    Hypercarbia
    Respiratory acidosis
    Aspiration
Renal
    Reduced parenchymal blood flow

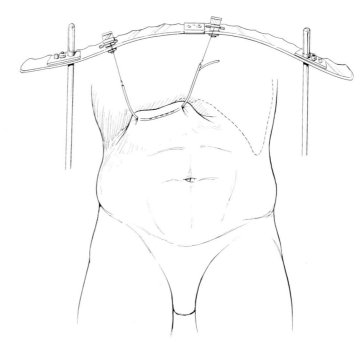

Fig. 6-2. Alternative *U*-shaped lifting device for use during laparoscopic cholecystectomy.

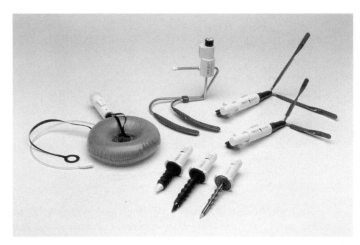

Fig. 6-3. Three basic lifting devices made by Origin Medsystems: the Airlift balloon, the quadrant-specific *J* fan, and the 10- and 15-cm *V* fans. Also shown are the flexible black and rigid clear plastic gasless trocars.

tion using pneumoperitoneum is without consequence. The risks of pneumoperitoneum can be divided into several types including those occurring (a) during the creation of pneumoperitoneum, (b) during the maintenance of pneumoperitoneum, and (c) at the termination of pneumoperitoneum. The creation of pneumoperitoneum involves the establishment of a suitable level of exposure by accessing the peritoneal cavity with one of two basic techniques: the closed or Veress needle technique and the open cutdown method. A significant number of complications are recognized with both of these techniques, including inadvertent vascular injury and/or intraabdominal visceral injury or compromise. The maintenance of pneumoperitoneum requires equipment that is not fail-safe. Cardiovascular complications related to pneumoperitoneum include gas embolism, derangements in cardiovascular output, and primary pulmonary failure related to diaphragmatic excursion. The termination of pneumoperitoneum exposes operation room personnel to expelled intraabdominal contents under pressure. The use of pneumoperitoneum in cases involving malignancy is now subject to scrutiny. Several investigators have reported studies suggesting that carbon dioxide (CO_2) pneumoperitoneum may support the viability of cancer cells in a manner not seen with standard open surgical procedures.

The complications observed with gasless laparoscopic surgery should parallel those seen with standard laparoscopic techniques and are discussed in more detail in Chapter 5. Critics of this technique cite pain at the position of the intraabdominal retractor as a specific problem. This complication has been noted in a very small number of my patients. The newest generation of abdominal wall retractors, the Airlift (Origin Medsystems/Guidant Corporation, Menlo Park, CA), was developed partially in response to this criticism. Intraoperative complications due to suboptimal exposure are best avoided by maximizing patient positioning and utilizing additional retraction options. Wound complications with laparoscopic surgery are seen, but their frequency is low. Special consideration must be given to patients with prior laparotomy and multiple intraabdominal adhesions. Complications of fan placement, such as hooking omentum or bowel, can be avoided by paying special attention to insertion of the retracting instrument at the initiation of the procedure. The postoperative care of gasless laparoscopy patients also does not deviate from the standard. The surgical wounds are closed with absorbable subcuticular sutures and dressed topically with

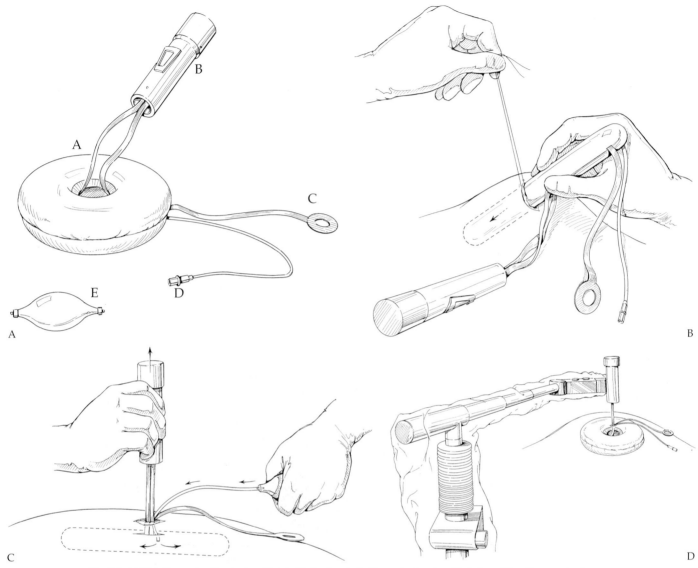

Fig. 6-4. Airlift balloon retraction system (Origin Medsystems). **A:** Elements of system (A, balloon lifter; B, connector to lifting arm; C, extraction string; D, inflation port; E, inflation pump). **B:** Insertion of deflated Airlift balloon. **C:** Inflation of Airlift balloon. **D:** Connection to lifting arm for abdominal wall elevation.

minimal dressing. For postoperative pain management, propoxy-phene hydrochloride (Darvon), ketorolac tromethamine (Toradol), or hydrocodone bitartrate may be prescribed. Patients are seen approximately 5 to 7 days after hospital discharge to monitor their progress. Postoperative nausea has not been a significant problem in these patients.

Gasless Laparoscopic Cholecystectomy

Virtually any patient who qualifies for cholecystectomy may be considered for gasless laparoscopic cholecystectomy. The problems seen with exposure in the upper abdomen may be lessened by the selection of appropriate patients. As mentioned earlier, the body habitus is taken into account. Ideal patients for gasless cholecystectomy include those with increased cardiorespiratory risk factors and a lower body mass index. There are no absolute height or weight characteristics that preclude gasless surgery in the upper abdomen; however, problems are encountered in obese patients.

In virtually all patients, the Laparolift arm is attached to the operating room bed roughly parallel to the right shoulder of the patient. Typically, the arm is attached after patients are asleep and before the abdomen is prepared. The surgeon must be prepared to move the lift mechanism cephalad or caudad, depending on where the supports are located on the side of the operating room bed. Once the lift is in place, its power supply is connected. The skin is prepared in the standard fashion, and towels are placed around the operating field. Prior to the draping of the sterile field, the sterile sheath is placed over the lift mechanism (Fig. 6-5).

After the arm mechanism is draped and in position, an open cutdown is carried out at the umbilicus in a vertical or horizontal fashion, whichever is preferable to the operating surgeon. Stay sutures are placed in the fascia lateral to the midline umbilical incision. The Laparofan is then inserted as the surgeon and assistant provide upward countertraction on the abdominal wall. Prior to insertion of the Laparofan, several maneuvers are helpful to ascertain a clear field. The first of these is a simple finger sweep to verify the absence of significant intraabdominal adhesions. The second maneuver involves simple lifting of the abdominal wall with placement of the endoscope to view the planned operative field. The Laparofan is then placed under direct vision. Once it is inserted and engaged, it is connected to the Laparolift arm. The surgeon is advised to place continued upward traction on the Laparofan to avoid catching any intraabdominal viscera while the lift mechanism is engaged. After a suitable lift has been achieved, the laparoscope is inserted inferior to the Laparofan with or without the placement of an additional trocar. Occasionally, a simple trocar sleeve is added behind the Laparofan at the umbilical incision to facilitate scope passage in and out of the abdomen. This occasionally will hinder the use of multiple instruments through the umbilical incision. In my experience, the predictor of success of a gasless laparoscopic cholecystectomy is the ability to view a small space over the liver after the lift has been achieved. If no space has been created above the liver by the abdominal lift, the gasless procedure may be quite difficult.

The patient is then positioned appropriately, including the reversed Trendelenburg position, placement of nasogastric or orogastric tubes, and ventilatory adjustments as needed. By adjustment to a lower tidal volume and a higher respiratory rate, the operative field is improved due to reduced visceral excursion with inspiration. Additional ports are placed, including two 5-mm right upper quadrant ports, which are placed under direct vision. I use the rigid gasless ports in this procedure and place an additional grasper alongside the viewing endoscope to push outward on the abdominal wall as the accessory ports are placed. After the initial cutdown, all additional port placements are done in a controlled fashion under direct vision. The epigastric port is also placed under direct vision and is generally inserted to the right of the falciform ligament. Occasionally, the body habitus may dictate placing this port in a slightly different position to the left of the midline. At this point, the gallbladder

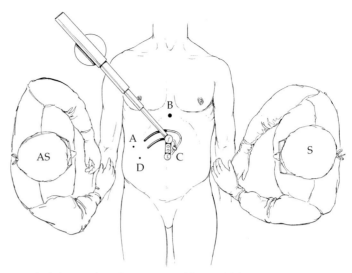

Fig. 6-5. *Laparoscopic cholecystectomy. Retractor type: J fan or Airlift; patient position: supine. (A, 5-mm port; B, 10-mm port; C, J fan or Airlift; D, 5-mm port; AS, assistant surgeon; S, surgeon.)*

is retracted cephalad, and the triangle of Calot is visualized. The surgical assistant at this point may move his or her grasping forceps along the lateral wall of the gallbladder to achieve maximal stretching and exposure of the triangle of Calot. If visualization of the triangle is suboptimal, additional retraction is placed alongside the endoscope at the umbilicus. Several instruments are satisfactory, ranging from a simple grasper to a reusable 5-mm fan retractor. Downward retraction on the duodenum stretches the common bile duct and provides the needed extra visualization of the cystic duct and cystic artery. Once these structures are properly identified, dissection is begun. In the performance of a safe laparoscopic cholecystectomy, the dissection is initiated as high on the gallbladder as possible and generally on the lateral wall of the gallbladder. After the lateral peritoneum has been opened, the cystic duct and cystic artery are exposed anteriorly. If cholangiography is anticipated, I prefer C-arm fluoroscopy to static imaging. If the arm mechanism interferes with fluoroscopy, the fan and arm can be disengaged and the arm retracted during fluoroscopic imaging. After cholangiography is completed, the gallbladder is removed from the liver bed.

During gasless laparoscopic procedures, it is apparent that cut surfaces tend to ooze more than usual. This change is attributed to the tamponade effect of the pneumoperitoneum. In my opinion, this is an additional advantage with gasless laparoscopic surgery because any bleeding at this time can be recognized and taken care of surgically before the case is completed. In the event that suction and irrigation are required during cholecystectomy, a simple bulb syringe and standard pliable plastic suction device may be inserted through the port sites, resulting in a cost savings over laparoscopic instrumentation. After the gallbladder has been removed from the liver bed and hemostasis has been assured, the gallbladder is removed from the umbilical port. Occasionally, in the presence of an inflamed or distended gallbladder, it is necessary to remove the Laparofan prior to removing the gallbladder. Once the Laparofan and the gallbladder are removed, fascial closure is carried out. It is my practice to close the umbilical fascia wound with an interrupted no.1 Vicryl stitch and the skin wounds with a 4-0 subcuticular Vicryl stitch. At this point, anesthesia is terminated, and the patient is transferred to the recovery suite for observation.

Gasless Laparoscopic Appendectomy

In the preparation of patients for gasless laparoscopic appendectomy, the Laparolift arm is attached to the operating room bed parallel to the right anterosuperior iliac crest. As is standard in any gasless pro-

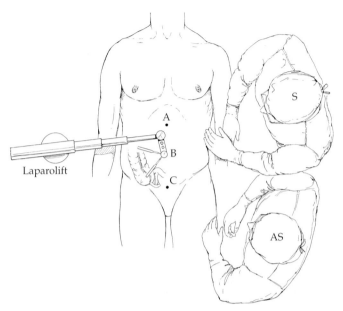

Fig. 6-6. Laparoscopic appendectomy or right colon resection. Retractor type: 20-cm *V* fan or Airlift; patient position: supine. (A, 5/10-mm port; B, 15/20-mm *V* fan or Airlift; C, 5/10-mm port; AS, assistant surgeon; S, surgeon.)

cedure, the lift arm is placed prior to preparation of the abdomen (Fig. 6-6). Sterile towels are placed, and the Laparolift arm is draped with its sterile covering. The table is then completely draped in a sterile fashion. The surgeon stands on the patient's left side, and an open cutdown at the umbilicus is carried out. This may be done in a vertical or horizontal fashion, although a vertical incision may be more easily converted to a midline incision in the event of unsuspected pathology. A 15- to 20-mm incision is made, and lateral stay sutures are placed in the fascia. Once again, a finger sweep is employed to verify the absence of significant adhesions, and the Laparofan is placed. My preference for exposure in laparoscopic appendectomy is the J fan or the Airlift balloon. The 10-cm V fan can be used alternatively; however, I

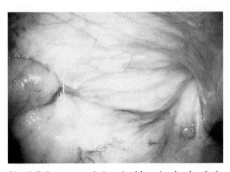

Fig. 6-7. Laparoscopic inguinal herniorrhaphy. Left lower quadrant exposure of a left inguinal hernia.

believe that the exposure is maximized with the second- and third-generation devices. After the pathology is verified, additional ports are placed in the midline. I generally place a 5- or 10-mm suprapubic port, with care taken to avoid inadvertent bladder injury. In all patients who undergo pelvic laparoscopy with infraumbilical port placement, straight drainage of the bladder is carried out prior to port placement. The third and final port for a laparoscopic appendectomy is placed in the upper midline to assist with cephalad retraction of the cecum. The appendix is dissected primarily by mobilizing the lateral and inferior attachments to the retroperitoneum. Additional retraction may be afforded using a small reusable fan retractor alongside the endoscope at the umbilicus. The mesoappendix is identified, and care is taken to identify the terminal ileum and its blood supply. A small window is created at the base of the appendix near its attachments to the cecum. At this point, the decision is made regarding the means of ligating the mesoappendix and the base of the appendix. The endoscopic 30-mm linear stapling device is used in most cases to divide both the mesoappendix and the base of the appendix. Several alternatives for vascular and visceral ligation are available. Suture ligation is simplified with the gasless techniques. A standard right-angle clamp may

be used to pass a suture of the surgeon's preference around the mesoappendix and the base of the appendix. An external knot is tied and positioned with a knot pusher placed at the umbilicus. After vascular and visceral ligation, the appendix is divided and removed from the umbilical port. It has not been necessary in all cases to employ a bag to entrap the specimen prior to removal. Hemostasis is verified, suction and irrigation are utilized, and the trocars and Laparofan are removed. The fascial wound is closed with a no.1 Vicryl stitch, and the skin edges are approximated. In the event of severe appendiceal inflammation, consideration may be given for very loose closure or open packing of the umbilicus.

Gasless Laparoscopic Inguinal Herniorrhaphy

Gasless laparoscopic hernia surgery is now utilized only in patients in whom general anesthesia must be avoided. Several different techniques are available for repairing an inguinal hernia; these include open and laparoscopic transperitoneal and extraperitoneal approaches. In the event of the preference for transperitoneal laparoscopic repair without general anesthesia, the gasless technique is excellent.

The Laparolift arm is placed parallel to the right or left anterosuperior iliac crest, generally on the side of the hernia. The arm is placed so as not to interfere with port placements and operative procedure. The procedure starts with open cutdown at the umbilicus as has been previously described. The bladder has been drained with straight catheter drainage prior to any infraumbilical laparoscopy. Draping of the Laparolift arm is carried out, and the abdomen is prepared. Open cutdown at the umbilicus is performed, and a finger-sweep maneuver is carried out. In my experience, any of the Laparofan devices, including the 20-cm V fan, the J fan, or the Airlift, are adequate for pelvic exposure. Regardless of a patient's size, exposure in the lower abdomen is nearly always easier than exposure in the upper abdomen (Fig. 6-7). Additional 5-mm lateral ports are placed under direct vision after the operating field has been established. Gasless extraperitoneal hernia repair is accomplished in a similar fashion; however, the

10-cm V fan is placed in the extraperitoneal position rather than the intraperitoneal position. In the event of a transperitoneal repair, the peritoneal flap is created on the lateral aspect of the obliterated umbilical vessels and carried high over the internal ring and laterally. When the hernia sac has been removed and the iliopubic tract, Cooper's ligament, and transversus arch are identified, the mesh is placed. The tacking device is used to secure the mesh to the appropriate ligamentous structures. When this has been achieved, the peritoneal flap is closed either with the tacking device or suture material. The ports and Laparofan are removed under direct vision, and closure is instituted as has been previously described. Because of the many other options available for laparoscopic hernia repair, gasless laparoscopic hernia repair is reserved for a small number of patients requiring anesthetic options.

Gasless Pelvic and Gynecologic Procedures

For pelvic gasless laparoscopic procedures, the Laparolift arm is placed approximately parallel with the anterosuperior iliac crest on the right or left side of the operating table (Fig. 6-8). The abdomen is prepared and sterile towels are placed. The arm of the device is draped with the included sterile sheet, and full draping is then carried out. For pelvic laparoscopy, the patient is placed in the lithotomy position with the legs in stirrups for access to the perineum. Several uterine and cervical manipulators are available, and these are placed prior to establishing the operative field. These devices are used to manipulate the position of the uterus and adnexa, if required. Open cutdown is done through a vertical or horizontal periumbilical incision. The J fan or Airlift balloon is engaged, and abdominal lift is provided. Patient positioning includes the Trendelenburg maneuver to help eviscerate the pelvis. In general, one or two additional ports are placed, either in the suprapubic or lateral abdominal positions. Visibility in the pelvis utilizing the gasless system is excellent and comparable to that during pneumoperitoneum. The reasons for this include the predominance of bony structures that are not moved in any significant manner with pneumoperitoneum and the ability to eviscerate the space by suitable

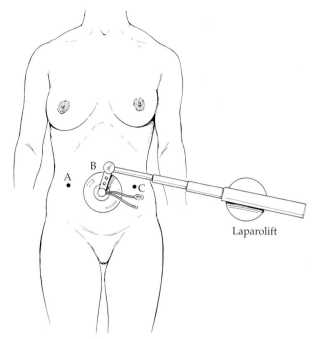

Fig. 6-8. Pelvic laparoscopy (gynecologic, hernia, colon). Fan type: Airlift or J fan; patient position: supine. (A, 5/10-mm port; B, Airlift; C, 5/10-mm port.)

positioning. Many pelvic procedures, including salpingectomy, tubal ligation, oophorectomy, and hysterectomy, as well as lymphadenectomy and pelvic colorectal procedures, are ideally suited to gasless laparoscopy.

Gasless Laparoscopic Bowel Surgery

Perhaps the best application for gasless laparoscopic procedures is resection of colon and small bowel lesions. Laparoscopy has been utilized to treat a number of intraabdominal diseases, including benign and malignant processes. The oncologic safety of colorectal surgery with pneumoperitoneum has been questioned. Gasless techniques should obviate that concern.

Gasless techniques may be used for resection of bowel lesions in virtually any quadrant of the abdomen. Perhaps the easiest procedure to accomplish is the right hemicolectomy. For this procedure, an open cutdown is initiated in a vertical fashion at the umbilicus using an incision 3 to 4 cm in length. A vertical incision is preferred here because incision enlargement can easily be achieved if required to accommodate the

specimen. The additional ports for a right hemicolectomy include midline 10-mm gasless ports, one in the epigastrium and one in the suprapubic position (Figs. 6-9 and 6-10). Anastomoses for the right colon procedure are done in an extracorporeal fashion at the umbilicus. The endoscope is transferred from the umbilical to the suprapubic position to facilitate lateral dissection of the right colon. The retroperitoneal and lateral attachments are divided using Metzenbaum scissors or electrocautery. It is important that the surgeon obtain adequate mobility of the terminal ileum prior to the anticipated anastomosis. Dissection is continued in the lateral gutter

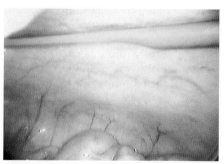

Fig. 6-9. Laparoscopic right colon resection. Exposure of the right lower quadrant is provided by the J fan.

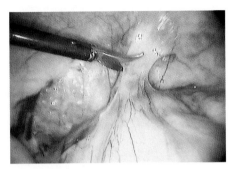

Fig. 6-10. Laparoscopic right colon resection. Gasless exposure of the hepatic flexure. Lateral peritoneal attachments are being taken down with endoscopic scissors.

by providing countertraction from instruments placed through the umbilical and epigastric ports. As mentioned earlier, multiple instruments are available to be used through the 3- to 4-cm umbilical incision. It is wise to create an incision at the umbilicus at the beginning of the operation that will accommodate the resected specimen. The hepatic flexure attachments are also taken down with cautery and occasionally require stapling or ligation. In most patients, no heroic efforts are required to mobilize the ileum and right colon. The most difficult mobilization is around the transverse colon. Occasionally, the Laparofan is removed, and the specimen is brought to the umbilicus for extracorporeal suturing as needed.

When adequate mobility has been gained and the entire right colon and hepatic flexure are mobilized, the bowel is brought to the umbilicus for division with a standard stapling device. The distal ileum is generally divided first, and its mesenteric blood supply is controlled between Kelly clamps. It is usually very easy to achieve a high vascular ligation at this point; lymph node retrievals on laparoscopic and open cases have been comparable in my experience. The middle colic artery is identified, and the specimen is taken around to this point (obviously care is taken to preserve the middle colic vasculature). A standard side-to-side anastomosis is created with the stapling device. The mesenteric defect is closed with interrupted or running fine Vicryl sutures. The bowel is returned to the abdomen and the Laparofan is reinserted to reestablish the abdominal lift. The operative field is inspected and irrigated, and when hemostasis is verified, the Laparofan is once again removed. The

umbilical fascial incision is closed with interrupted or running heavy suture, and the skin edges are reapproximated with a subcuticular 4-0 Vicryl suture.

The technique for left or sigmoid colon resection varies only with port placement. The Laparolift apparatus is affixed parallel to the left anterosuperior iliac crest. A vertical cutdown is made at or just below the umbilicus. In the event that a lower resection of the colon is anticipated, a slightly larger suprapubic vertical incision is also employed at the time of surgery. When larger incisions are used, no ports are required. This facilitates the use of standard instruments rather than specialized laparoscopic instruments. Additional retraction ports are placed either in the upper midline or the left upper quadrant. The mobilization of the colon is begun laterally and is taken as far cephalad as necessary. In obese patients, the splenic flexure can occasionally be difficult to manage. In the vast majority of patients, a sigmoid or left colectomy is possible without a great deal of difficulty.

For low anterior colon procedures, as well as abdominoperineal resection, the ports are placed in similar fashion to that of any pelvic procedure. A cutdown is used at the umbilicus and occasionally the suprapubic position. An additional left or right lower quadrant port may be required. The proximal division of bowel is accomplished after adequate vascular dissection. The ureters are identified bilaterally, and dissection is continued into the pelvis. The visibility in the pelvis is generally very good; additional retraction may be required to eviscerate the small bowel from the pelvic wall. A great benefit of pelvic procedures is the ease of suturing and ligation with the gasless technique. Ligatures can be placed with a standard right-angle device and extracorporeal knots slid into position with any knot pusher. For abdominoperineal resections, a two-team approach is utilized, with a separate team performing the perineal component of the operation. The specimen is delivered *per anum* for the abdominoperineal resection. Gasless bowel surgery is accomplished in a similar fashion to open procedures with reduced wound morbidity. Gasless laparoscopic colorectal and small bowel surgery certainly holds great promise for the future, perhaps more so than other laparoscopic operations.

Conclusion

Gasless laparoscopy requires specialized instruments to lift the abdominal wall and create a space for operating. When adequate exposure is obtained using gasless techniques, operations may be performed expeditiously using standard operating instruments and without the real and potential complications of a pneumoperitoneum. Further experience is necessary to establish the precise indications for gasless laparoscopy.

Suggested Reading

Chin AK, Eaton J, Tsoi EK, et al. Gasless laparoscopy using a planar lifting technique. *J Am Coll Surg* 1994;178:401–403.

Hashimoto D, Nayeem SA, Kajiwara S, Hoshino T. Laparoscopic cholecystectomy: an approach without pneumoperitoneum. *Surg Endosc* 1993; 7:54–56.

Kitano S, Iso Y, Tomikawa M, Moriyama M, Sugimachi K. A prospective randomized trial comparing pneumoperitoneum and U-shaped retractor elevation for laparoscopic cholecystectomy. *Surg Endosc* 1993;7:311–314.

Smith RS, Organ CH, eds. *Gasless laparoscopy with conventional instruments: the next phase in minimally invasive surgery.* San Francisco, CA: Norman Publishing, 1993.

EDITOR'S COMMENT

Several systems currently exist for performing gasless laparoscopy. These employ various slings and retractors that can be used to lift the abdominal wall away from the intraabdominal contents and thereby create a space in which to perform diagnostic and therapeutic procedures. The primary advantages of these systems are elimination of the need for a pneumoperitoneum with its potential complications and simplification of the instrumentation by obviating an airtight system. Currently, controversy exists regarding other potential detrimental effects of pneumoperitoneum, such as dispersing intraperitoneal tumor cells; gasless systems would also eliminate this potential risk. Not all patients are candidates for this type of access system, as detailed by the author. Additionally, the lifting devices may create a tent shaped space with limited exposure around the periphery of the operative field, as opposed to the rounded dome shape of the pneumoperitoneum cavity, thereby limiting visualization. With the current state of technology, gasless laparoscopy seems to be most useful for pelvic procedures and for operations on patients in whom the CO_2 pneumoperitoneum may be associated with an increased risk, such as pregnant patients, those with severe cardiorespiratory diseases, and those on whom potentially curative oncologic procedures are being performed. It will require several years and well controlled prospective trials to establish the appropriate role of gasless laparoscopy.

N.J.S.

7

Anesthesia Concerns in Surgical Endoscopy

Leonard D. Benitez and David S. Edelman

Endoscopy and peritoneoscopy have a long history of being safe and well tolerated procedures. Advances in noninvasive monitoring of patients and endoscopic equipment and techniques enable surgeons to perform more complex endoscopic and laparoscopic procedures. The range and complexity of endoscopic and laparoscopic procedures being performed are expanding. The age and severity of illness of patients undergoing these types of interventions are increasing. The goal of patients, anesthesiologists, surgeons, and nurses is the safe, uneventful, and complication-free outcome of a particular procedure. Because of the expansion of endoscopic knowledge and procedures, it is advisable that a strong level of communication exist among the surgical team—surgeon, nurse, and anesthetist. This permits appropriate selection of anesthetic technique and agents.

Preoperative Evaluation

Preprocedure assessment provides a means of preventing intraoperative and postoperative complications. Obtaining a careful medical history with special attention to the cardiovascular, respiratory, and endocrine systems is mandatory. Patients' previous experience with local, regional, or general anesthesia should be evaluated. Drugs used in the treatment of patients with cardiovascular, respiratory, and endocrine disease should be carefully reviewed during the preoperative evaluation. Although most patients resume oral intake within a day following endoscopic or laparoscopic surgery, certain procedures may delay oral intake. Withdrawal reactions should be anticipated, and the use of topical, sublingual, or parental sub-

stitutes should be considered. History and physical examination provide the most useful information, identifying underlying disease and determining operative risk.

Cardiovascular Evaluation

A murmur detected on physical examination may indicate significant valvular heart disease. Echocardiography is necessary to determine the extent of cardiovascular compromise and demonstrate mitral or aortic valve dysfunction. Aortic stenosis is a significant risk factor to anesthesia because of patients' decreased compensatory control of cardiac output. This predisposes patients to increased myocardial oxygen demand and ischemia due to the decreased systemic vascular resistance that can occur with anesthesia. Cardiac catheterization may be necessary to further evaluate valvular lesions.

Uncontrolled hypertension predisposes patients to increased perioperative risk. Exaggerated or unpredictable physiologic responses are possible during all phases of anesthesia. Labile changes in blood pressure may also occur during postoperative fluid mobilization. Congestive heart failure and cardiovascular collapse are other potential complications. End-organ disease is a possible concurrent process. Preoperative evaluation should include an assessment of end-organ perfusion and function: renal, coronary artery, peripheral vascular, and cerebrovascular. Labile changes in blood pressure occur in approximately 25% of hypertensive patients despite adequate preoperative control.

Patients with a known history of left heart dysfunction or congestive heart failure are at high risk for perioperative pulmonary edema. Interestingly, a majority of patients

in whom left ventricular dysfunction develops do not manifest preoperative signs or symptoms. Barbiturates used during induction have negative inotropic and peripheral vasodilatory side effects. Inhalational agents (nitrous oxide and halogenated ethers) also cause myocardial depression. Caution should be used when these agents are used in patients with impaired left heart function.

Unstable angina is a major preoperative risk factor. Elective surgery for patients with unstable angina should be postponed until after appropriate treatment by coronary angioplasty or coronary revascularization. Patients with recent myocardial infarction have an increased risk for reinfarction and death during the perioperative period. Studies have shown a 37% reinfarction rate in patients operated on within 3 months of infarction. This rate decreased to 16% for operation at 4 to 6 months postinfarction and to 4% to 5% for operation after 6 months. Therefore, elective surgery should be delayed until 6 months after infarction if at all possible. More recent studies have shown a decrease in the reinfarction rate to 5.7% at 0 to 3 months from infarction and 2.3% at 4 to 6 months from infarction. This is thought to be the result of invasive hemodynamic monitoring and use of newer cardiac drugs.

Multiple systems have been developed to define operative risk in patients undergoing noncardiac surgery. Goldman (1977) described a series of cardiac risk factors and a risk-stratification scale. These criteria provide a reproducible way of delineating high-risk patients. The risk factors for perioperative myocardial infarction and subsequent death are as follows:

1. Heart failure,
2. Myocardial infarction within preceding 6 months,
3. Unstable angina,
4. More than five premature ventricular contractions per minute,
5. Frequent atrial premature complexes or complex atrial arrhythmias,
6. Age greater than 70 years,
7. Illness requiring emergency procedures,
8. Significant aortic stenosis,
9. Poor general medical condition.

The risk of perioperative myocardial infarction, pulmonary edema, ventricular tachycardia, or death rises to 50% if any of the first five factors is present. A scale based on more subjective criteria was accepted by the American Society of Anesthesiologists (ASA). Patients are graded according to their state of health and severity of underlying disease as follows:

Status 1 Healthy patient
Status 2 Mild underlying disease
Status 3 Severe underlying disease with functional limitations
Status 4 Severe underlying disease that is a constant threat to life
Status 5 Moribund patient, not expected to survive 24 hours

Studies have shown that this scale, although subjective, is the best available predictor of perioperative noncardiac mortality and a good predictor of cardiac death.

Beta-adrenergic antagonists used in treating hypertensives and patients with angina should be continued through the morning of surgery. If a patient is expected to be kept from any oral intake more than a few days, longer-acting oral preparations or parenteral administration may be used. Care should be taken when stopping these agents because a rebound hyperadrenergic state with possible increased incidence of arrhythmia or myocardial infarction can occur.

Withdrawal of clonidine can cause a profound rebound hypertensive response. This response can be augmented with the concurrent use of beta-blockers. Use of transdermal clonidine preoperatively or intravenous sodium nitroprusside should be considered prior to surgery.

Assessment of fluid status should guide the judicious use of diuretics during the perioperative period. Intravenous diuretic agents offer finer control over fluid management.

Monoamine oxidase (MAO) inhibitors can potentiate a hypertensive crisis by increasing the release of norepinephrine when interacting with sympathomimetic agents and narcotics. MAO inhibitors should be stopped at least 2 weeks prior to surgery.

Antiarrhythmic agents should be continued through the morning of surgery. Digoxin therapy can be continued intravenously in the perioperative period. Intravenous lidocaine hydrochloride or procainamide hydrochloride can be used intra- and postoperatively to treat ventricular arrhythmias. Most inhalational anesthetic agents prolong the half-life of lidocaine, and therefore patients given these agents need to be monitored for signs of toxicity.

Respiratory Evaluation

The respiratory status of all patients undergoing surgery should be evaluated. Anesthesia and positioning have a significant impact on respiratory function, even in otherwise healthy patients. The increased burden placed on the respiratory system during pneumoperitoneum has been well documented. Patients with undiagnosed underlying respiratory dysfunction are predisposed to the development of serious complications. In addition to chronic obstructive lung disease, other significant risk factors for the development of perioperative pulmonary complications include obesity, history of smoking, and prolonged anesthesia time. Patients who smoke should stop at least 3 to 6 weeks prior to the operation.

The preoperative evaluation of patients identified with pulmonary dysfunction should include a baseline chest radiograph and spirometry. The type of lung disease—obstructive, restrictive, or cardiogenic—should be identified, and appropriate medical therapy and physiotherapy instituted. If a favorable response is observed during pulmonary function studies, preoperative bronchodilator therapy should be started. Obtaining an arterial blood gas measurement in the perioperative period in patients with significant disease will serve as a baseline. Preoperative incentive spirometry training is beneficial, especially in elderly patients. Inhaled beta-agonists, inhaled corticosteroids, oral corticosteroids, cromolyn sodium, theophylline, and inhaled anticholinergic agents should be continued through the perioperative period.

Patients with severe cardiorespiratory dysfunction may require a modified laparoscopic technique, such as low insufflation pressures, limited gas volume, or gasless laparoscopy. Close attention to dosing of narcotics and benzodiazepines is needed through the entire perioperative course. Administration of oxygen by nasal cannula or face mask is indicated when intravenous sedation is used, as studies have shown a decrease in blood oxygen saturation measurements.

Endocrine Evaluation

Various methods are available for managing patients with endocrine abnormalities undergoing elective surgery. Patients taking oral hypoglycemia agents should continue their dosing until the day prior to surgery. Serial fingerstick blood glucose analyses should be employed along with subcutaneous or intravenous insulin coverage in the perioperative period. The amount of insulin taken preoperatively will vary depending on patients' usual dose and the length of the operative procedure. Brittle diabetics may need continuous intravenous insulin. The normal insulin regimen is usually reinstituted once oral intake resumes.

Patients with evidence of hyperthyroidism should undergo a thorough evaluation. Beta-blockers or thyroid-ablative drugs should be used, if necessary, to establish a euthyroid state. Those patients taking oral thyroid replacement drugs can usually tolerate suspension of treatment during the perioperative period. Intravenous supplementation is available, if necessary.

It is most important to know the type, route, duration, and frequency of dosage in patients taking exogenous steroids. A daily dose of steroids equivalent to 7.5 mg of prednisone is sufficient to suppress the hypothalamic–pituitary–adrenal axis. Patients taking such a dose are at risk for adrenal insufficiency if steroid therapy is inadequate or withheld during periods of stress. Recovery from suppression may take a year or more. Provocative tests can be done to preoperatively assess the function of the hypothalamic–pituitary–adrenal axis. Appropriate patients should be placed on stress doses of parenteral steroids. A dose equivalent to 100 mg of hydrocortisone sodium succinate every 8 hours should be initiated prior to surgery and continued perioperatively. This dosage scheme represents the average output of corticosteroid from the adrenal gland in patients undergoing operative stress. Tapering intravenous steroids and resumption of maintenance dosages should be guided by the underlying disease process, duration of treatment, and patients' clinical course.

Gastrointestinal Evaluation

Patients with known gastroesophageal reflux disease are at risk of aspiration at the time of anesthetic induction. Intravenous sedation for endoscopic procedures may relax the lower esophageal sphincter. Lying supine or in the decubitus position may enhance reflux. Many general anesthetics promote emesis. An H_2-antagonist or a similar agent is recommended to neutralize gastric acid and decrease secretion in these patients to minimize the chance of aspiration.

Preoperative preparation usually includes modifying patients' diet and instituting bowel cleansing. Patients undergoing upper endoscopy require little bowel preparation and are usually placed on a clear-liquid diet the evening prior to the procedure. Oral intake is restricted 8 to 12 hours prior to the procedure. Lower endoscopy requires similar diet modification in addition to a mechanical bowel preparation. Stimulatory or osmotic cathartics and enemas are begun 1 or 2 days prior to the procedure. Those having elective laparoscopic intestinal surgery undergo both a mechanical and nonabsorbed oral antibiotic bowel preparation using the standard practices employed in open surgery.

Anesthesia Concerns in Flexible Endoscopy

Conscious Sedation

Endoscopy and endoscopic procedures (e.g., percutaneous endoscopic gastrostomy) are usually well tolerated and have a low complication rate. Although upper and lower endoscopy can be performed without any anesthesia, most patients and endoscopists prefer some form of conscious sedation. The term *conscious sedation* falls under the more general term *monitored*

anesthesia care (MAC). The primary objective of MAC is to provide for patient safety and comfort during minimally invasive procedures. What constitutes the minimal requirements of monitoring and which anesthetic drugs and techniques are used are generally left to the discretion of the anesthesiologist or endoscopist. The ASA has provided more specific guidelines.

The ASA defines MAC as the presence, with an appropriately trained physician, of an anesthesiologist or nurse anesthetist who, while a patient is undergoing a procedure using local anesthesia, intravenous sedation, or no anesthesia, is available and responsible for monitoring vital signs and medical care and determining whether or not more advanced anesthetic or medical support is necessary. It is recommended that routine patient monitoring include telemetry, pulse oximetry, blood pressure, administration of oxygen, and availability of medications such as sedatives, tranquilizers, antiemetics, analgesics, and appropriate cardiac and pulmonary agents. The type of procedure and patients' health will dictate the type of monitoring and the amount and type of medication. The goals of providing adequate analgesia, amnesia, sedation, and anxiolysis are met using a variety of agents including, but not limited to, benzodiazepines, narcotic (opioid) and nonnarcotic analgesics, barbiturates, propofol (Diprivan), and ketamine hydrochloride (Ketalar). General inhalational anesthetics are utilized in particular cases in which other agents are less effective or patients cannot tolerate the procedure by other means.

Adequate suction equipment should be available to handle excess oral or pharyngeal secretions. Readily available suction helps minimize the complications associated with vomiting and possible aspiration during sedation or as a consequence of anesthesia. This is especially important if endotracheal intubation is required.

Various levels of sedation are defined within the realm of MAC and include analgesia, local anesthesia, conscious sedation, deep sedation, and hypnosis. Conscious sedation is the most applicable to endoscopic procedures. The objectives of conscious sedation are described as follows:

1. To decrease preoperative anxiety and produce amnesia,
2. To provide analgesia (pain relief) through the use of opioid analgesics,

3. To provide adequate sedation but not impair patients' ability to communicate and follow basic commands during the procedure.

The agents of choice used in endoscopy to achieve these goals are the benzodiazepines midazolam (Versed) and diazepam and the opioid narcotics meperidine hydrochloride (Demerol HCl) and fentanyl citrate (Sublimaze).

Benzodiazepines are used alone or in combination with narcotics, depending on the particular preference of the endoscopist. Aspiration and hypoxemia are the main complications with these agents. Studies have shown that oxygen saturation decreases during endoscopy (both upper and lower). When benzodiazepines and narcotics are given together, the incidence of respiratory depression and hypoxia is greater. No correlation in the magnitude of the observed hypoxemia during endoscopy has been made regarding the type or dose of sedating agent, patient age or sex, or length of procedure. Underlying pulmonary disease has a significant effect on the extent of desaturation experienced. Investigators have done comparative studies using various sedative combinations with and without supplemental oxygen. There was a difference in the extent of the decrease in oxygen saturation between the two groups. Those with supplemental oxygen had an overall higher mean oxygen saturation and did not become hypoxic during the procedure. Those without supplemental oxygen had a lower mean oxygen saturation, with desaturation noted in the 80% to 89% range. Several studies have shown that administering both a benzodiazepine and an opioid narcotic in small titrating doses, versus bolus infusions, decreases the resultant respiratory depression and possible deleterious hemodynamic and arrhythmic responses. Therefore, the use of supplemental oxygen is advocated in patients with underlying cardiopulmonary disease.

The recent trend among endoscopists is to rely more heavily on benzodiazepines, with as little use as possible of any narcotic. This is primarily to guard against the increased incidence of respiratory depression associated with narcotic agents. Many endoscopists continue to use narcotics because they are more easily reversed with an opioid antagonist such as naloxone hydrochloride (Narcan). Respiratory depression encountered while using a benzodiazepine can be counteracted with the benzodiazepine antagonist flumazenil (Romazicon). A last advantage in using a narcotic in combination with a benzodiazepine is the smoothness of sedation and procedural amnesia. The need for diligent monitoring and careful administration of sedative and analgesic agents cannot be overemphasized.

Specific benzodiazepine characteristics are important to appreciate. Midazolam is three to four times as potent as diazepam. It produces a greater amount of periprocedural amnesia and sedation. Although the half-life of midazolam is short (2 to 4 hours), it has not been shown to have a more rapid postprocedure recovery time than diazepam. Some untoward side effects of the benzodiazepine class other than respiratory depression include phlebitis, cardiovascular depression, and a paradoxic neuroexcitatory effect. Droperidol (Inapsine) may be useful in this situation, given that it is a neuroleptic agent.

Narcotics can cause respiratory depression. Other adverse effects related to narcotic use include nausea, vomiting, peripheral vasodilatation, hypotension, constipation, urinary retention, and bradycardia. Morphine is the gold standard by which other opioid agents are measured. It produces a more pronounced vasodilatation than other opioids, such as fentanyl. Fentanyl and alfentanil hydrochloride (Alfenta) have been linked to increased postoperative nausea and vomiting.

Other agents used in upper endoscopy include the topical pharyngeal anesthetics (benzocaine derivatives). These topical agents are not used routinely by all endoscopists and have been known to induce a rare anaphylaxis in sensitive individuals. If necessary, small doses of atropine sulfate can be given during upper endoscopy to reduce the amount of oropharyngeal secretions.

In summary, the major goal of conscious sedation is to provide patient comfort while minimizing the extent of side effects in response to the various agents used. The objective is to use adequate medication to achieve the anesthetic goals necessary for completion of a meaningful diagnostic or therapeutic procedure. The dosages of the particular agents involved in achieving this goal should be dictated by continuous clinical and supportive monitoring of patients.

Monitoring

The criteria that constitute adequate monitoring for patients undergoing MAC have undergone recent changes due to advances in monitoring technologies. However, there are few studies in the literature actually comparing various monitoring configurations with their impact on reducing operative morbidity and mortality. Factors such as the amount of sedation required for a particular procedure, the anesthetic agents used, and the limitations of the particular methods of monitoring all play a role in delineating the optimal monitoring configuration for MAC. To enhance safety and lower the incidence of untoward complications, much effort has been expended by federal agencies, local and national societies, and hospitals to establish the minimum basic standards for monitoring during MAC. The ASA provides a guide to these requirements for MAC:

1. *Oxygenation*: During all anesthetics, adequate illumination or exposure of patients is necessary to assess color, or pulse oximetry should be used to ascertain adequate oxygenation, as in endoscopy usually carried out in darkened areas;
2. *Ventilation*: During MAC, adequate ventilation should be evaluated by continual observation of qualitative clinical signs (respiratory rate, chest expansion, breath sounds);
3. *Circulation*: Every patient receiving anesthesia should have an electrocardiogram (ECG) displayed from the beginning of anesthesia to the end of the procedure.

Other forms of monitoring, either noninvasive or invasive, may be necessary, depending on the needs of the endoscopist, the type and length of procedure, and patients' underlying medical state. Monitoring applications will normally be noninvasive, given the less invasive nature of the procedures done under MAC.

It is necessary to consider the cost and the technical limitations of various monitoring techniques when one elects to add to the basic requirements. Routine monitoring for endoscopy consists of ECG monitor, blood pressure cuff monitor, and pulse oximetry. The primary responsibility of monitoring patients during flexible endoscopy falls on the endoscopist and the nurse assistant. The endoscopist and nurse should monitor patients' condition and assess tolerance to the procedure from information obtained from specific monitoring modalities (ECG, pulse oximetry). Pulse oximetry is important, given the usual darkened environment during endoscopy, but careful observation of respiratory rate, pattern, and depth should be given equal weight in the continued assessment during the procedure. Signs of hypoventilation, airway obstruction, regurgitation, and aspiration should always be anticipated. At times, subtle changes in the level of consciousness and respiratory status can be noticed prior to changes appearing during monitoring. This is true when adequate ventilation is being assessed, especially since end-tidal carbon dioxide (ET CO_2) monitoring is not considered routine during MAC.

Noninvasive blood pressure monitoring, done manually or more commonly with automated devices, provides a window for assessing cardiovascular stability or perfusion. It should be kept in mind that noninvasive blood pressure monitoring can be a somewhat nonspecific indicator as to the adequacy of cardiodynamic stability. Blood pressure readings obtained from manual, automated, or Doppler blood pressure monitoring devices have potential inaccuracies. Data from these sources must be interpreted in the light of patients' clinical status.

Continuous ECG provides important data concerning heart rate, arrhythmias, conduction disturbances, and possibly ischemia. Various lead configurations can be used to more accurately detect these changes. This is especially true with regard to ischemia in the patients with known coronary vascular disease. The most common configuration is usually monitoring of leads II and V_5. Lead II is used primarily to detect changes in rhythm but may detect ST-segment changes from inferior ischemia. Lead V_5 may demonstrate anterior ischemia. Posterior or right ventricular ischemia is not as readily detected using two-lead monitoring.

In high-risk patients with possible myocardial ischemia, it may be advisable to assume a three-lead monitoring configuration. ST-segment changes or dysrhythmias may be a reflection of this myocardial derangement. It is important to confirm any suspected changes in the baseline monitored ECG with a standard 12-lead tracing. It must be kept in mind that changes in baseline telemetry can be related to monitor artifact.

Pulse oximetry has been described as the monitoring advance of the decade. Oximetry can be defined as a noninvasive measure of the oxygen-saturated hemoglobin content of arterial blood. This value can then be used to calculate the oxygen saturation expressed as a ratio of saturated hemoglobin to total hemoglobin:

$$SO_2\% = HbO_2/(HbO_2 + RHb) \times 100$$

Oximeters were initially limited in their ability to distinguish between arterial and venous saturated hemoglobin content. This problem was overcome by measuring the alternating transmissions of red and infrared light created by a pulsatile vessel (thus, the name pulse oximetry). The accuracy of this technique has widely been reported to be consistent, when compared to that of invasive methods of measuring oxygen saturation. It is important in terms of accuracy that patients are cardiodynamically stable and that oxygen saturation readings are greater than 65% to 70%. A major limitation of pulse oximetry is that it gives relatively no information concerning pulmonary gas exchange. While it gives an indication as to the state of oxygenation, adequate ventilation must also be assured via clinical assessment during endoscopy.

End-expiratory CO_2 can be measured via a sampling tube used in conjunction with a nasal cannula or a face mask. Although a good technique in theory, it is often prone to false sampling or problems in maintaining a continuous readout. The measurement of end-expiratory CO_2 levels should be reserved for those patients with known respiratory compromise who would pose a high risk for inadequate periprocedural hypoventilation.

A common theme throughout the anesthesia literature regarding monitoring is the belief that monitoring trends should always be interpreted in view of patients' clinical stability. It is the duty of the responsible physician to continually assess the clinical status of a patient, with monitoring to confirm any changes detected. Monitoring should continue into the recovery suite, with the aim of assessing the return to preprocedure baseline. The most common causes of postprocedure morbid-ity include hypoventilation, airway obstruction, hypertension, hypotension, cardiac arrhythmias, nausea, vomiting, and pain.

Anesthesia Concerns in Laparoscopic Surgery

Monitoring

Monitoring standards for patients undergoing laparoscopic surgery have been well delineated, given that a majority of these procedures are carried out under general anesthesia. The minimal requirements for patients undergoing laparoscopic procedures under local or regional anesthesia are no different from those described previously for MAC.

The baseline requirements for patients undergoing general anesthesia include continuous ECG, noninvasive blood pressure monitoring, stethoscope, pulse oximetry, temperature probe, and continuous ET CO_2 monitoring. Several of these have been discussed in the previous section.

The use of a stethoscope is one of the easiest and most effective ways of monitoring ventilatory status. Breath sounds and heart sounds can be simply, easily, and adequately evaluated. Subtle changes in patients' level of consciousness, tidal volume, and airway patency or obstruction can be readily detected.

Temperature monitoring is important. Detecting the rare complication of malignant hyperthermia and preventing the more common occurrence of hypothermia are the main goals of temperature monitoring. Hypothermia during laparoscopy is a result of the recycling of high volumes of cool CO_2 insufflator gas to maintain pneumoperitoneum. It can lead to increased perioperative pain and oxygen consumption.

During general anesthesia, ET CO_2 monitoring is the most common method of assessing ventilation and is currently considered the standard of care for patients undergoing general anesthesia. When CO_2 is used as the insufflating agent for laparoscopy, ET CO_2 monitoring is mandatory. A considerable amount of CO_2 is absorbed through the peritoneum during laparoscopy. This absorption, combined with the impaired normal mechanics of ventilation, predisposes patients to experiencing hypercarbia and acidosis. Cardiac arrhythmias are a possible sequela from hypercarbia and acidosis. Mechanical ventilation provides an adequate means of control of the resultant increased CO_2 and acidosis. Minute-by-minute adjustments in rate, tidal volume, and percentage of oxygen delivered are made with the aide of ET CO_2 monitoring.

The use of invasive monitoring during laparoscopy is generally more a function of patients' underlying medical status than the procedure's physiologic impact. As mentioned earlier, laparoscopy is being performed more frequently in patients with serious to severe comorbid conditions. Indwelling arterial, venous, and pulmonary artery lines can yield valuable and useful information. In patients with poorly controlled hypertension, coronary artery disease, or arrhythmias, invasive blood pressure monitoring should be considered. In patients with baseline pulmonary disease, the linear relationship between measured ET CO_2 and actual P_aCO_2 may be altered due to ventilation–perfusion mismatch. There may be an increase in P_aCO_2 without an appreciable change in ET CO_2. These patients would benefit from continuous arterial blood pressure monitoring and frequent arterial blood gas analysis.

Physiology of Pneumoperitoneum

The physiologic effects of pneumoperitoneum are discussed at greater length elsewhere in this volume (see Chapter 5); however, a brief review will be undertaken here. The effects of pneumoperitoneum on the cardiovascular and endocrine systems were initially evaluated in the 1960s to 1980s but have recently been extensively studied, given the advances in therapeutic laparoscopy.

Pulmonary effects of laparoscopy can be attributed to the physiologic consequence of increased intraabdominal pressure and the changes resulting from the use of CO_2 as the insufflating agent. Establishment of pneumoperitoneum results in increased intraperitoneal pressures and cephalad displacement of the diaphragm, producing a decrease in the pulmonary functional residual capacity (FRC). According to some studies, FRC is already decreased approximately 20% to 25% when patients are placed in the supine position and another 20% when general anesthesia is used. In patients with normal pulmonary function, an increase in the minute ventilation and airway pressure usually compensates for the decrease in the FRC. In patients who have compromised pulmonary function, the FRC is already decreased. With a further decrease due to general anesthesia and pneumoperitoneum, the FRC may fall below the closing capacity. This predisposes patients to ventilation–perfusion mismatch shunting. In these patients, it is important to consider using decreased insufflation pressures and gas volume, as well as increasing respiratory rates and tidal volume. It is also advisable to limit position changes, especially Trendelenburg positioning. Increased intraabdominal pressure also results in decreased vital capacity, decreased forced expiratory volume in 1 second, increased peak airway pressures, and pulmonary atelectasis. Studies have shown that a return to preoperative baseline respiratory status may take several days following laparoscopy. Morbidity as a consequence of respiratory dysfunction is low in patients with no significant pulmonary disease who undergo laparoscopy.

High-risk patients with impaired respiratory or renal function have a decreased ability to handle shifts in acid–base balance. The problems encountered with the use of CO_2, namely, hypercarbia and subsequent acidosis, are a consequence of its highly diffusible nature across the peritoneal surface. Such patients should be identified preoperatively. Modification of laparoscopic and anesthetic techniques can be used to reduce the magnitude of the problem. Therefore, small insufflation volumes with low intraperitoneal pressures (or gasless laparoscopy), arterial blood gas monitoring, and appropriate mechanical ventilation are recommended in the management of these patients.

Other insufflation agents, such as nitrous oxide (N_2O) and helium, have been studied. These agents, despite having no appreciable effect on acid–base balance, do have drawbacks of their own. N_2O, although nonflammable, does support combustion and is a concern in procedures requiring electrocautery. Helium, although inert, does not diffuse easily and is relatively insoluble in plasma, increasing the risk of gas embolism. If helium is allowed to enter into the soft tissues or retroperitoneum, subcutaneous emphysema develops, which may take weeks to resolve.

The hemodynamic effects of a pneumoperitoneum are a function of the intraperitoneal pressure attained. Multiple studies have shown that in otherwise healthy patients, insufflation pressures of less than 20 mm Hg caused hemodynamic effects but were well tolerated. These adverse effects include increases in peripheral vascular resistance, systemic blood pressure, and pulmonary vascular resistance and decreases in cardiac output and venous return. Other studies have shown that stroke volume and cardiac output remain unchanged or may decrease. This is possibly due to decreased venous return. These findings were reproducible regardless of the type of insufflation agent used. It is important to consider that the responses obtained in these various studies may be somewhat modified in the clinical setting due to the different cardiovascular effects of the different anesthetics.

Measurement of hormonal and immunologic factors in response to a laparoscopic versus an open procedure seems to confirm the decreased physiologic impact of the laparoscopic approach. Various circulating substances have been measured, including glucose, cortisol, endorphins, epinephrine, norepinephrine, and dopamine. Less inhibition of white cell function has been shown after laparoscopy in a number of studies.

Anesthetic Technique for Laparoscopic Surgery

Local Anesthesia

Local anesthetic agents can be divided into two main classes: esters and amides. The amide class comprises the most commonly used agents, with lidocaine hydrochloride being the standard of comparison. Lidocaine has a rapid onset of action and shorter duration of effect than agents such as mepivacaine hydrochloride (Carbocaine) or bupivacaine hydrochloride. The duration of effect of the latter two agents is approximately 90 to 180 minutes and 240 to 480 minutes, respectively. Shorter-acting agents are primarily used on the skin prior to making an incision. Longer-acting agents are usually injected in deep subcutaneous and fascial layers to provide adequate postoperative analgesia. A field block should be used to cover a cone-shaped area of tissue with the widest base at the parietal peritoneum to block the sensory nerves in this layer (Fig. 7-1). When this is performed properly, no painful stimuli are generated during movements of the laparoscopic trocar. The burning sensation during injection into dermal layers can be minimized by mixing the particular local anesthetic agent with sodium bi-

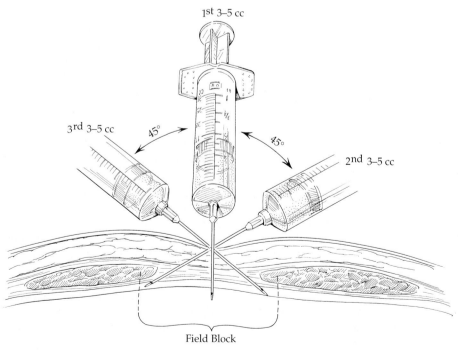

Fig. 7-1. Field block technique of local anesthesia for laparoscopic operations.

carbonate in a 5-to-1 ratio. A slow rate of injection and the smallest-gauge needle that can be safely used will help decrease the sensation of pain and burning.

In general, laparoscopic procedures that are limited to less than 1-hour duration are most amenable to local anesthetic with or without intravenous sedation. The magnitude of procedures done under local anesthesia varies greatly with patient compliance. It includes diagnostic laparoscopy, pelviscopy, staging of malignancy, liver biopsy, minor lysis of adhesions, and tubal ligations. Hernia repair, gastrostomy, jejunostomy and cholecystostomy using lidocaine with intravenous sedation have been reported.

Use of N_2O as the insufflating agent improves patient tolerance during these procedures by eliminating the peritoneal irritation due to CO_2. However, CO_2 has been safely used with most patients. Low insufflation pressures in the range of 8 to 12 mm Hg and slow instillation of peritoneal gas will also enhance patient tolerance and acceptance of tissue manipulation during the procedure.

When laparoscopic procedures using local anesthetic are attempted, care must be taken to avoid injury to the pelvic or abdominal structures as a result of patient movement or the lack of abdominal wall relaxation, since neuromuscular blocking agents are not in use. One must be especially careful when electrocautery is used in this situation.

Use of an intraabdominal topical anesthetic, such as bupivacaine, can be helpful in reducing postoperative discomfort and the need for increased postoperative analgesics. Serum levels from transperitoneal absorption of these agents have been shown to be within acceptable, safe ranges.

Regional Anesthesia

Regional anesthesia, either spinal or epidural, can be readily applied in procedures amenable to local anesthesia, as well as in slightly more invasive or therapeutic undertakings. Hernia repair, tubal ligation, lysis of adhesions, and cholecystectomy have all been accomplished using regional anesthetic techniques. As with laparoscopic procedures done under local anesthesia, it is important that patients and anesthesiologists be informed as to the extent and duration of the proposed procedure. Patient selection is an important consideration, given that a highly motivated and informed patient will better tolerate the procedure.

Much of the discomfort and resulting physiologic stress will be a consequence of the pneumoperitoneum rather than surgical-site pain. Patients are usually aware of abdominal distention and difficulty in breathing, which manifests as increased respiratory rate and work of breathing. This may be well tolerated, but if patients become uncomfortable, sedation or mask general anesthesia may be added. Conversion to endotracheal general anesthesia may be necessary if a patient cannot tolerate the procedure or if the regional block is felt to be unsatisfactory.

Physiologic changes as a result of regional techniques include vasodilatation with subsequent reflex tachycardia, hypotension, and unopposed vagal stimulation with resultant bradycardia, nausea, or emesis. Volume loading prior to beginning the regional block is helpful in preventing hypotension. Regional anesthesia produces less cardiac and respiratory depression than general anesthesia. This is a particularly desirable effect in patients with cardiac dysfunction.

Studies comparing the complication rate, morbidity, and mortality between regional and general techniques show no difference in outcome. Complications such as headache may occur after spinal anesthesia. Treatment is intravenous (or oral) hydration. Occasionally, a blood patch is necessary. Another disturbing complication is migration of the block to a higher level than anticipated, which can lead to respiratory difficulties.

General Endotracheal Anesthesia

General anesthesia can be defined as a drug-induced state characterized by amnesia, analgesia, unconsciousness, muscle relaxation, suppression of reflexes, and loss of pain sensation. It is divided into three phases: induction, maintenance, and emergence. The effects of general anesthetic agents on the central nervous system are also divided into four states: sedation, delirium with increased reflexes, steady-state anesthesia, and cardiovascular collapse.

General anesthesia allows the greatest amount of control of the cardiovascular and respiratory systems during laparoscopy. Longer, more advanced laparoscopic procedures potentiate the effects of pneumoperitoneum, as previously described. Counteracting the physiologic changes and returning patients to preoperative homeostasis are the goals in using general anesthetic techniques.

Adequate premedication establishes a smooth progression in the administration of general anesthetics. Preoperative use of a benzodiazepine and narcotic aid in decreasing patient anxiety. Anxiety-related catecholamine release increases myocardial work and myocardial oxygen demand.

Induction is usually carried out using a benzodiazepine or short-acting barbiturate with neuromuscular blockade. Inhalational agents may also be used in induction, as is the case in the pediatric population. Barbiturates (e.g. thiopental sodium [Pentothal]) have a direct negative inotropic effect on the myocardium. Benzodiazepines have a minimal effect on cardiovascular function. Patients who are hypovolemic or are being treated with a beta-blocker are prone to the development of hypotension secondary to the vasodilatory effects of barbiturates. Propofol is a short-acting agent, allowing a more rapid emergence than with barbiturates. Propofol produces far less postoperative nausea, compared to thiopental, when used in combination with inhalational agents. Propofol is an ideal choice for induction and maintenance during procedures of short duration.

The maintenance phase is a continuation of induction and is a period during which optimal operating conditions and physiologic stability are maintained. Administration of general anesthesia can involve the use of inhalational agents alone, inhalational agents with intravenous agents, and intravenous agents alone. Balanced anesthesia refers to a combination of inhalational and intravenous agents. Most procedures are accomplished by this technique. The common volatile agents used are N_2O and the halogenated ethers—halothane, enflurane, isoflurane, and desflurane. The halogenated ethers fulfill all the characteristics of a general anesthetic. All the inhalational agents produce dose-related myocardial depression. The magnitude of

8

Laparoscopic Surgery in the Complicated Patient

Demetrius W. M. Litwin and Quynh Pham

The rapid adoption of laparoscopic cholecystectomy is a significant focal event in the history of surgery. Thereafter, surgeons began to apply minimally invasive techniques to other surgical conditions. However, laparoscopic surgery is different from open surgery because the operation is restricted by trocar-insertion sites, instrumentation, and limited access. In addition, it commonly requires the establishment and maintenance of a pneumoperitoneum that can alter patients' physiology, especially in complicated patients. This chapter deals with the potential complications that may arise and the alteration(s) in laparoscopic technique that may be required when the surgeon encounters complex patients.

Patient with Neurologic Compromise

Pneumoperitoneum has been shown to increase intracranial pressure (ICP) in a live porcine model with normal or artificially raised baseline ICP. These changes are independent of changes in arterial P_{CO_2} or arterial pH. In patients with elevated ICP, pneumoperitoneum can further increase ICP and theoretically can precipitate brain herniation. Diagnostic laparoscopy has been utilized for detecting intraabdominal trauma in multiply injured patients with equivocal abdominal findings. Although there has been no clinical report of adverse neurologic sequelae, the safety of laparoscopy in patients with concurrent central nervous system trauma has not been determined. Similar risk also exists in patients with a brain tumor, abscess, or hydrocephalus. Pneumoperitoneum should be used with caution in these individuals, and apneumic (gasless) laparoscopy using abdominal wall–lifting devices may be a safer alternative. However, if hydrocephalus has been treated by placement of a one-way-valve ventriculoperitoneal shunt, there may be little risk to patients. However, we do not know whether the high pressure can override the valve, so it is most prudent to clamp the tube prior to initiating the pneumoperitoneum. Conversely, an apneumic retractor can be used with safety.

Pneumoperitoneum also decreases venous return. In patients with neurogenic shock due to spinal injury, cardiac output is reduced because of a decrease in arteriolar resistance and in venous tone, with a resultant increase in the arteriolar and venous reservoirs and ultimately a decrease in venous return to the right side of the heart. Hence, laparoscopy can exacerbate hypotension and shock. Adequate fluid administration to maintain normal central venous pressure and judicious use of vasopressors, such as phenylephrine hydrochloride, to support arterial pressure are mandatory in these individuals prior to creating the pneumoperitoneum.

Patient with Cardiovascular Compromise

The increase in intraabdominal pressure (IAP) elicited by pneumoperitoneum acts directly on the abdominal compartment and indirectly on the thoracic compartment, and modifies both circulation and ventilation. As mentioned, venous return decreases as the vena cava is compressed. The total cardiac output is decreased, but mean arterial pressure, mean pulmonary pressure, pulmonary vascular resistance, and central venous pressure are increased. Carbon dioxide (CO_2) insufflation leads to a fall in P_aO_2, an increase in arterial CO_2 with acidemia, and a hyperdynamic circulation. Healthy individuals tolerate these changes, but critically ill patients or acutely hypovolemic patients can decompensate during laparoscopic procedures. Similarly, patients with a poor left ventricle may not tolerate the afterload increase. A typical scenario to elicit caution is the elderly patient with a history of congestive heart failure who needs a groin hernia repair. A procedure without either pneumoperitoneum or general anesthetic would be preferable, and therefore conventional repair with local anesthesia must remain in the armamentarium of the general surgeon. Likewise, patients with severe coronary disease or recent myocardial infarction may be at increased risk from pneumoperitoneum. One must always remember that although the postoperative pain is less with laparoscopic surgery, the intraoperative stress can be similar to that of open surgery, together with the additional factors described above. If a patient is unfit medically, any elective surgical procedure should be delayed until the patient's condition has been optimized, and one must wait 3 to 6 months before performing elective surgery if a patient has had a recent myocardial infarction.

Preoperative optimization of hemodynamic function and intraoperative monitoring are necessary in these high-risk cardiac patients. One should augment preload by adequate fluid loading to offset the effects of increased IAP. Monitoring tools should include arterial catheter and Swan-Ganz catheter for vigilant control of hemodynamic changes, especially at initiation of insufflation. Continuous end-tidal (ET) CO_2 measurement to detect and rapidly correct hypercapnia and its associated acidemia will decrease the stress on the cardiovascular system.

Patient with Respiratory Insufficiency

The effects of laparoscopic surgery on the respiratory system are due to two main factors:

1. CO_2 pneumoperitoneum elevates arterial CO_2 and may cause acidemia;
2. IAP increases intrathoracic pressure causing (a) increased mean airway pressure and (b) an increase in effective positive end-expiratory pressure with resultant decreases in left ventricular stroke index and cardiac index.

These effects are of doubtful clinical significance in the majority of patients; most patients will benefit from the improved postoperative pulmonary function with potentially less postoperative atelectasis and pneumonia because of less incisional pain. However, in patients with severe chronic obstructive pulmonary disease, critical illness, or decreased cardiopulmonary reserve (American Society of Anesthesiologists status II or status III), severe hypercapnia and acidemia may ensue, leading to clinical deterioration. To extend the benefits of laparoscopic procedures to these patients, hemodynamic parameters and P_aCO_2 should be monitored, because measures to improve venous return, augment cardiac output, and counteract the elevation in P_aCO_2 and peak airway pressure may be required. In addition, an increase in peak inspiratory pressure may lead to pneumothorax, especially in patients with emphysematous lungs; therefore, close observation with prompt treatment for this complication is necessary.

Patient with Cirrhosis and Portal Hypertension

Several potential problems can arise in patients with hepatic insufficiency who undergo a laparoscopic procedure:

1. *Complications from trocar insertion*: Severe, difficult-to-control bleeding as a consequence of dilated umbilical and other abdominal wall veins; Postoperative leakage of ascitic fluid through trocar site(s) with the potential for bacterial seeding and subsequent peritonitis; Predisposition to the development of hernias through trocar site(s) as a result of elevated IAP generated by ascites.
2. *Complications from the surgical procedure*: Persistent and severe bleeding from dissection of the triangle of Calot and the gallbladder bed during cholecystectomy; Varices around gastroesophageal junction, rectum, and pelvis, making laparoscopic procedures in these areas extremely hazardous.
3. *Complications from hepatic insufficiency*: Hepatic failure; Renal failure and hepatorenal syndrome if a large amount of ascitic fluid is lost; Coagulopathy.

The incidence of morbidity and mortality in this population is proportional to the severity of hepatic insufficiency. Patients for elective surgery should be good to moderate risk, that is, Child's class A or B. Laparoscopic procedures decrease postoperative pain and respiratory complications, compared to conventional operations, but they may be much more challenging technically. The most common intraoperative complication is profuse bleeding uncontrollable by laparoscopic techniques; conversion to open surgery may be necessary. A transmural suture technique, insertion and then inflation of a Foley catheter, or placement of a balloon-tipped trocar may be required to stem trocar-site bleeding. Meticulous fascial closure for trocar sites 10 mm and larger is required to avoid ascitic fluid leakage and subsequent infection. Specifically for cholecystectomy, exposure may be difficult because elevation of the stiff liver is not possible due to hepatic

nodularity and fibrosis. Another trocar site for placement of an additional retractor or conversion to open surgery may be required. In extremely difficult cases, subtotal cholecystectomy may be performed to prevent massive bleeding from the gallbladder bed. This procedure involves opening the gallbladder and evacuating its contents. The cystic duct is oversewn at its origin from within the gallbladder with a figure-of-eight suture. This is greatly facilitated with a 30-degree telescope that allows one to view the cystic duct orifice. The gallbladder is then excised, with the posterior wall left attached to the liver bed. Bleeding from the remaining gallbladder edge is controlled by electrocoagulation or by suturing with a running 2-0 Vicryl suture. The mucosal surface of the posterior wall is then ablated by electocoagulation. This procedure avoids the dangerous dissection at the triangle of Calot and can be done laparoscopically, provided that the surgeon is proficient at intracorporeal suturing and has advanced laparoscopic skills. Postoperatively, these patients should be observed and treated for medical complications, such as bacterial peritonitis, bleeding, hepatic failure, or renal failure.

Patient with Previous Abdominal Surgery

Previous abdominal surgery is no longer a contraindication to laparoscopic procedures, as surgeons have become more experienced. The site of most adhesions is usually directly underneath the previous operative incision. Three approaches to entry of the abdomen are available:

Veress needle technique,
Direct cutdown with the Hasson trocar,
Conversion to formal laparotomy.

Veress Needle Technique

This is our favored strategy. The needle is placed away from the scar sites, and a 5-mm trocar is subsequently inserted at that site, provided the gas flow is adequate during insufflation with the Veress needle (Fig. 8-1). A 5-mm angled telescope is inserted through that trocar, and a clear site for an additional 5-mm trocar is selected so that it is in a favorable position to facilitate adhesiolysis. The ability to suture intracorporeally is a requirement so that accidental

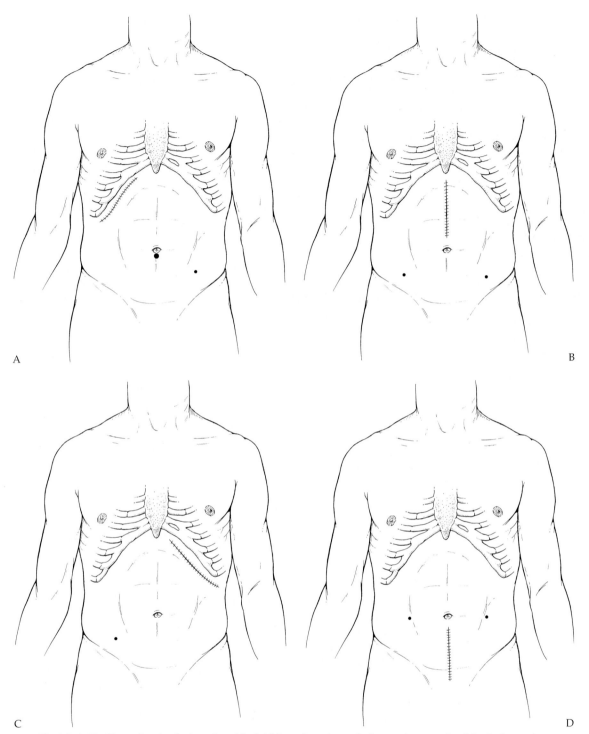

Fig. 8-1. **A–D:** *Alternative sites for insertion of the initial port in patients who have undergone prior abdominal operations.*

enterotomy can be repaired. Once an adhesion-free operative field has been created, the surgeon can then place the trocars necessary for the operative procedure. If the adhesions in the midline are dense but other locations are free, the telescope can be placed in an eccentric position. For example, during laparoscopic cholecystectomy in a patient with dense midline adhesions, the telescope is preferably placed in the right midabdomen at the lateral edge of the rectus abdominis, which will give an excellent view of the gallbladder and the right upper quadrant.

Direct Cutdown with Hasson Trocar

This technique has the disadvantage of requiring substantial dissection if the safest place for the initial trocar is away from the midline. Furthermore, entry into the abdominal cavity may still be precluded if the surgeon encounters extremely dense adhesions.

Conversion to Laparotomy

This is still the gold standard in the extremely difficult situation when entry cannot be obtained or adhesiolysis is slow and

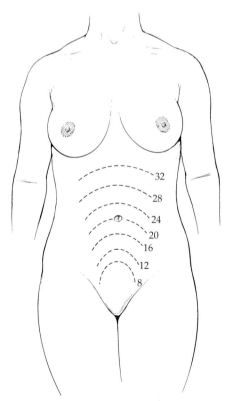

Fig. 8-2. Schematic diagram of uterine fundal height on the basis of gestational age in weeks.

arduous, especially in patients who will do well irrespective of mode of access.

Pregnant Patient

Any planned operation during gestation needs to take into consideration the risk to both mother and fetus, while acknowledging the normal physiologic changes during pregnancy. In general, nonurgent operations should be delayed until postterm, but if surgery is mandatory, it is optimally performed during the second trimester. At this time, the baby is developed and the risk of premature labor is low. Our approach to biliary colic in pregnancy has been to treat patients conservatively until delivery and then to perform laparoscopic cholecystectomy after birth. This approach has been successful in the majority of cases and does not subject the fetus to the increased risks of surgery.

If laparoscopic surgery is necessary, certain general precautionary measures need to be taken. A lead shield should be placed over the uterus to protect the fetus if any radiologic procedure is to be carried out. Perioperative and intraoperative fetal monitoring is mandatory. Because in advanced pregnancy the supine position can cause the gravid uterus to obstruct venous return by compressing the vena cava, patients need to be in slight left lateral decubitus position by tilting them on the operating table. In pregnancy, there is a significantly increased risk of thromboembolism due to venous stasis, decreased antithrombin III level, and increased fibrinogen, factor VII, and factor XII levels. Prophylactic measures should be taken to prevent deep venous thrombosis, including subcutaneous heparin or pneumatic compression devices. Laparoscopic cholecystectomy has been performed in pregnancy with results similar to those of open surgery. Use of the laparoscopic technique, however, poses two main hazards: (a) trocar insertion and (b) CO_2 pneumoperitoneum. Alterations in operative strategy must be employed.

Trocar Insertion

The gravid uterus arises from the pelvis and can be injured by the Veress needle or subsequent trocar placement (Fig. 8-2). If this technique is used, it should be performed at a site remote from the uterus. Direct cutdown with the Hasson trocar is

the safest technique for the initial trocar insertion.

Carbon Dioxide Pneumoperitoneum

Because the pneumoperitoneum will decrease maternal cardiac output, the lowest IAP that allows adequate visualization must be used (ideally less than 12 mm Hg), and adequate maternal hydration must be ensured. Furthermore, significant fetal acidosis develops with a 15-mm-Hg pneumoperitoneum, even when maternal ET CO_2 is kept within the normal range (35 to 45 mm Hg). Since arterial blood gas monitoring is the most accurate method of determining P_aCO_2 levels and the maternal P_aCO_2 level must be kept low to maintain reasonable acid–base balance in the fetus, an arterial line is mandatory. An important point to remember is that patients need good muscular relaxation throughout the period of pneumoperitoneum to avoid rapid extreme pressure rise (as high as 50 mm Hg) during light anesthesia. It is stressed that the long-term sequelae of fetal acidemia—especially neurologic sequelae, such as learning disability—are still unknown. Alternatively, apneumic retraction devices (see Chapter 6) can be used to avoid the physiologic effects of pneumoperitoneum.

Elderly Patient

In the Western world, life expectancy has steadily increased, and elderly patients have become a growing segment of the population. When treating these patients, several issues pertinent to geriatrics must be considered. Chronologic age alone should not be used as an indicator of medical fitness, yet the elderly often have significant medical illnesses such as neurovascular, cardiovascular, respiratory, and renal diseases. Each patient has to be assessed individually for the risk of surgery. One must also consider the stress of an operation, during which patients are starved, anesthetized, drugged, bled, and traumatized. Although elderly patients may carry out normal daily activity well, the stress induced by surgery may tip the balance of homeostasis with resultant decompensation. Most elderly patients will tolerate elective surgery well. However, if any complication from surgery arises, a cascade of secondary complications may develop, leading to significant morbidity. In general, emergent operations carry a significantly higher risk than elective operations in the elderly. Unfortunately, several factors exist in elderly patients that lead to delayed diagnosis. For example, acute cholecystitis and pancreatitis are more common in patients aged 65 years and older compared to the general population, and acute cholecystitis is usually more severe with a higher incidence of emphysematous cholecystitis and perforation. A delay in diagnosis and treatment can result from nonspecific symptoms in these patients and hesitancy in recommending surgery by caregivers.

Several reports have shown that laparoscopic cholecystectomy decreases the incidence of morbidity and mortality, especially pertaining to respiratory and cardiovascular diseases. However, older patients, compared to the young, are more likely to require conversion to laparotomy because of distorted anatomy from chronic disease, with resultant densely adherent, contracted, and fibrotic gallbladders. They also have a higher incidence of secondary choledocholithiasis than the young. Therefore, one should be vigilant of the risk of retained common bile duct stone, and preventive measures such as intraoperative cholangiogram should be performed liberally.

Minimally invasive surgery also has application in other conditions. Acute appendicitis can be a difficult diagnosis to make; laparoscopy and laparoscopic appendectomy can help resolve diagnostic dilemmas. Other procedures, such as laparoscopic adrenalectomy, splenectomy, colectomy, and so on, can take advantage of the decreased postoperative pain and its accompanied complications such as atelectasis, pneumonia, deep venous thrombosis, and myocardial infarction.

Patient with Abnormal Blood Coagulation

Both clotting and bleeding tendencies pose interesting problems for the laparoscopic surgeon. Patients with hypercoagulation conditions—either congenital (deficiencies in thrombosis inhibitors, e.g., protein C, protein S , antithrombin III, dysfibrinogenemias, or dysfibrinolysis) or acquired (e.g., pregnancy, thrombocythemia, erythrocythemia, systemic lupus erythemato-

sus)—are at increased risk from any surgical procedure, especially during the period of immobility under general anesthesia. Laparoscopic surgery provides the benefit of early postoperative ambulation, but this may be offset by longer operative time (therefore a longer duration of complete immobility from intraoperative muscular relaxation) and decreased venous return from the lower part of the body to the right atrium and ventricle. To date, no increased risk of thromboembolic events has been shown in the general population, but caution must be exercised in the selected patient groups described above. A full discussion of these hypercoagulation conditions is beyond the scope of this volume, but treatment generally involves both prophylaxis and specific treatment. Prophylaxis may consist of low-dose heparin, pneumatic compression, and maintenance of good hydration. Specific treatment of the disorder often involves long-term maintenance warfarin sodium (Coumadin). In these patients, oral warfarin is discontinued for several days preoperatively and replaced with intravenous heparin, which is halted 1 hour prior to the operation.

Bleeding tendencies (disseminated intravascular coagulation, hemophilia, platelet dysfunction, hepatic coagulopathy) can predispose to trocar-site bleeding and can obscure visualization of the operative site. These disorders do not contraindicate laparoscopic surgery, as long as they are corrected preoperatively.

In both of these abnormal coagulation conditions, a preoperative hematologic consultation is essential for operative safety.

Obese Patient

Obesity was initially considered to be a contraindication to laparoscopic surgery because of the fear of inadequate exposure. While it may be difficult to obtain adequate exposure, there has been no major difference in outcome in many reports of laparoscopic cholecystectomy comparing obese and morbidly obese patients to normal patients. The problem of exposure is related to the increased bulk of intraabdominal fat (e.g., omentum, mesentery, and so on). Occasionally, alterations in techniques may be required, and conversion to open surgery is mandatory if exposure is inadequate.

Pneumoperitoneum

The abdominal pannus often drapes impressively downward, and therefore the thinnest part of the abdominal wall may be above the umbilicus. Therefore, Veress needle insertion is usually safest and much more likely to gain access to the abdominal cavity through the right or left upper quadrants. In addition, improved exposure can be achieved by increasing the insufflation pressure to 20 to 25 mm Hg, although this is not routine. It is important to remember that if this increase in insufflation pressure is necessary, the anesthesia team must be informed.

Telescope Trocar

It may be necessary to place this trocar at a site closer to the operative field because the telescope may be too short to reach. For example, in cholecystectomy, this trocar should be placed above the umbilicus in the midline if the distance from the umbilicus to the right costal margin is more than the length of the telescope (Fig. 8-3). Not only will the abdominal wall entry be easier because it is away from the abdominal pannus, but the telescopic view will be improved.

Extra Trocar

An additional instrument may be required to retract surrounding bulky organs. We usually use the palpation probe for this maneuver, and it is placed at the lateral edge of the rectus abdominis on the left at the level of the umbilicus, where it can easily be handled by an assistant.

Angled Telescope

Poor visualization can be compensated by using the angled telescope to view beyond fat-ladden structures. The 30- or 45-degree scope can facilitate visualization immeasurably.

Trauma Patient

In recent years, diagnostic laparoscopy has been utilized in hemodynamically stable trauma patients with equivocal findings. A 5-mm trocar and laparoscope can be used with minimal abdominal insufflation. Some series suggest that laparoscopic examination is a highly sensitive, specific, and accurate tool for determining the presence of surgically significant abdominal

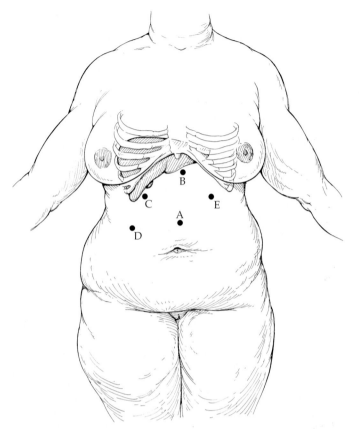

Fig. 8-3. Placement of trocars for performing laparoscopic cholecystectomy in the morbidly obese patient. (A, primary camera; B, primary op; C, dynamic retraction; D, static retraction; E, auxiliary.)

pathology and the need for therapeutic laparotomy (see Chapter 9).

Laparoscopy in trauma is not without risks. A fatal outcome of elective laparoscopy has been reported as a result of CO_2 embolism due to iatrogenic vascular injury. The potential exists for such an occurrence in trauma patients, if an intraabdominal vessel such as the vena cava, iliac vein, mesenteric vein, or pelvic vein is injured. Pneumoperitoneum can also cause acute herniation of abdominal contents through a diaphragmatic laceration into the thoracic cavity, causing respiratory distress. As mentioned earlier, pneumoperitoneum can exacerbate and potentially precipitate acute brain herniation in patients with head trauma. A final point to consider is the effect on hemorrhaging patients. Using a pig model, Ho and colleagues (1993) demonstrated that both stroke volume and cardiac index initially responded to large-volume fluid replacement after moderate hemorrhage but quickly decreased to levels comparable to those of unresuscitated animals when the abdomen was inflated with CO_2. Hence, in hypovolemic trauma patients, diagnostic laparoscopy should be used only after patients have been adequately resuscitated and have become hemodynamically stable, since it may have a deleterious effect on outcome.

Intensive Care Unit Patient

Critically ill patients are at risk for both ischemic gut and acalculous cholecystitis. The diagnosis is often difficult to establish and delayed, with resultant increased morbidity and mortality. Diagnostic tests may not be feasible to perform or may be equivocal. Laparoscopy can be a safe and accurate diagnostic tool that may spare patients multiple clinical, laboratory, and radiologic investigations, thereby avoiding a delay in diagnosis. Although laparoscopy has the potential to become a bedside procedure performed under local anesthesia with an apneumic retractor, it is most easily performed in patients already ventilated and sedated. In these patients, one cannot forget the consequences of pneu-

moperitoneum on hemodynamics and ventilation. As a caveat, it must be remembered that marginally ischemic gut can be as difficult to recognize laparoscopically as in conventional open surgery; and if there is any doubt, second-look laparoscopy is mandatory.

Conclusion

The current practice of general surgery is a continuum along which laparoscopic surgery plays an integral role. However, it is a tool that must be used with forethought and wisdom. In many instances, laparoscopy should clearly be used as the best access mode to perform an operative procedure. However, in some complicated situations, the experienced surgeon may opt for an open approach, and laparoscopy should not even be considered.

Suggested Reading

Borman PC, Terblanche J. Subtotal cholecystectomy: for the difficult gallbladder in portal hypertension and cholecystitis. *Surgery* 1985;98:1–6.

Carey JE, Koo R, Miller R, Stein M. Laparoscopy and thoracoscopy in evaluation of abdominal trauma. *Am Surg* 1995;61:92–95.

Fried GM, Clas D, Meakins JL. Minimally invasive surgery in the elderly patient. *Sur Clin North Am* 1994;74:375–387.

Ho HS, Saunders CJ, Corso FA, Wolfe BM. The effects of CO_2 pneumoperitoneum on hemodynamics in hemorrhaged animals. *Surgery* 1993;114:381–388.

Josephs LG, Este-McDonald JR, Birkett DH, Hirsch EF. Diagnostic laparoscopy increases intracranial pressure. *J Trauma* 1994;36:815–819.

Moffa SM, Quinn JV, Slotman GJ. Hemodynamic effects of carbon dioxide pneumoperitoneum during mechanical ventilation and positive-end-expiratory pressure. *J Trauma* 1993;35:613–618.

Morrell DG, Mullins JR, Harrison PB. Laparoscopic cholecystectomy during pregnancy in symptomatic patients. *Surgery* 1992;112:856–859.

Schirmer BD, Dix J, Edge SB, Hyser MJ, Hanks JB, Aguilar M. Laparoscopic cholecystectomy in the obese patient. *Ann Surg* 1992;216:146–152.

Thromboembolic problems. In: *Care of the surgical patients, Scientific American Medicine.* Chapter VII, Section 8. Scientific American, 1992:20–23.

EDITOR'S COMMENT

In most patients, laparoscopic surgery using conventional techniques and means of access to the abdominal cavity is safe and readily feasible. However, specific patients may be problematic, having complications that interfere with the normal technique for achieving access or medical conditions that may be compromised by the pneumoperitoneum. In such patients, careful planning before the operation, modification of technique, and close communication with the anesthesiologist are mandatory. The authors have highlighted several disease entities that create difficulties in patients undergoing laparoscopic surgery, a few areas of which need to be emphasized. The entire subject of therapeutic laparoscopy during pregnancy is charged with emotion, largely because of a relative dearth of scientific data clearly showing this intervention either to be safe or unsafe. The largest concern is the unknown effect of a prolonged CO_2 pneumoperitoneum on the fetus. Safe access techniques to avoid injuring the uterus, use of low levels of IAP, close periprocedural monitoring, and maintenance of low maternal ET CO_2 are ways to minimize the chance of problems, but the unknown, long-term medicolegal concerns remain daunting.

For patients with a coagulopathy, every effort should be made to correct the abnormal clotting parameters prior to operation. Brisk hemorrhage is one of the most difficult technical problems with which to deal using laparoscopic techniques. This is because the site of bleeding can be difficult to localize due to blood splashing on the scope and the loss of the pneumoperitoneum working space in the presence of vigorous suctioning. Although it may be difficult to apply direct pressure as one would in an open operative field, all attempts should be made to do this rather than applying thermal energy or hemoclips in a blind fashion.

One other class of complex patient needs to be mentioned, particularly for surgeons operating in tertiary care centers. These are patients who take exogenous adrenocorticosteroids, most commonly patients who have undergone prior organ transplantation and are administered combinations of steroids with other immunosuppressive agents, as well as patients using steroids for their antiinflammatory characteristics. Corticosteroids result in thinning and attenuation of normal body tissues, which increase the technical hazards for the surgeon. For instance, in patients who are on high-dose corticosteroids undergoing laparoscopic cholecystectomy, the gallbladder wall has occasionally torn, and the laceration has quickly extended down into the cystic duct, with subsequent difficulty closing the cystic duct stump. In these patients, meticulous dissection and gentle operative technique are mandatory.

N.J.S.

9

Surgical Endoscopy in the Trauma Patient

R. Stephen Smith and William R. Fry

Evaluation of patients with suspected abdominal injury continues to challenge the trauma surgeon despite the availability of a variety of noninvasive and invasive diagnostic modalities. Unfortunately, none of the diagnostic tools currently available is a true stand-alone technique, and sound clinical judgment is required to formulate the optimal diagnostic approach for each patient. Frequently, more than one study is required to provide adequate evaluation of a patient with potential abdominal trauma. Sonography, computed tomography (CT), and diagnostic peritoneal lavage (DPL), as well as laparoscopy and routine exploratory laparotomy, are widely used in the evaluation of injured patients. Each of these diagnostic approaches possesses distinct advantages and disadvantages that must be kept in mind when the course to follow in the evaluation of patients with potentially life-threatening injuries is decided on. As with other areas of general surgery, laparoscopy plays an important role in the evaluation and treatment of these patients, but it is not applicable or appropriate in all cases.

Sonography is inexpensive and portable and can accurately determine the presence of free fluid in the peritoneal cavity. Some organ-specific data and limited assessment of the retroperitoneum and thorax are provided by ultrasound. Unfortunately, most surgeons in the United States are not yet skilled sonographers, and the technique provides only limited organ-specific information. CT scan has been the *de facto* gold standard for the evaluation of abdominal trauma for the past decade. It has the advantage of providing detailed and accurate organ-specific information, but it is quite expensive and can miss isolated hollow viscus injuries. Additionally,

patients who are unstable are not candidates for CT due to the inherent logistic problems associated with transportation of patients to the CT suite.

DPL is extremely sensitive when used to detect even small amounts of blood in the peritoneal cavity. Unfortunately, trivial injuries such as minor hepatic or splenic lacerations will result in a positive DPL when traditional cell count criteria are used. In centers where DPL is used as the primary tool for abdominal assessment, a significant rate of negative and nontherapeutic laparotomy is accepted as a necessary evil. Additionally, DPL is an invasive technique and is associated with a definite, albeit small, complication rate.

Laparoscopy has been used sporadically over the past 25 years in the evaluation of abdominal trauma. However, this technique became more widely used in the trauma setting only after the popularity of laparoscopic cholecystectomy made modern videoscopic equipment widely available. Laparoscopy has proved useful in determining the course of anterior abdominal gunshot and stab wounds. In many instances, the wound tracts found in these patients have been demonstrated to be extraperitoneal, and therefore patients were spared a nontherapeutic or negative laparotomy. Laparoscopy has been documented by Ivatury, Fabian, and others as an excellent method for the evaluation of the diaphragm in hemodynamically stable patients who present with penetrating thoracoabdominal wounds. Experience with laparoscopic evaluation of blunt abdominal injury and with therapeutic laparoscopy in the trauma setting is more limited, but several innovative and promising techniques have recently appeared in the

literature. As laparoscopic technology continues to improve and as more trauma surgeons become skilled in videoscopic techniques, utilization of laparoscopy in the evaluation of truncal trauma is certain to increase.

Patient Selection

The majority of injured patients are not candidates for laparoscopic examination. Patients with hemodynamic instability or obvious intraabdominal injury should be prepared for immediate exploratory laparotomy with a minimum of preoperative assessment. In our experience, only 15% of patients with suspected abdominal injury will benefit from laparoscopic evaluation. Algorithms for the laparoscopic evaluation of abdominal gunshot wounds, stab wounds, and blunt trauma are presented in Figs. 9-1 to 9-3.

For patients with gunshot wounds, laparoscopy has proved most useful for evaluating the diaphragm and detecting peritoneal penetration in tangential wounds of the anterior abdominal wall. Care must be taken to prevent or immediately recognize the development of tension pneumothorax following the insufflation of pneumoperitoneum in patients with diaphragmatic injury. Timely placement of a tube thoracostomy will prevent the development of life-threatening tension pneumothorax and permit the completion of the laparoscopic examination. Discovery of peritoneal penetration or diaphragmatic injury secondary to gunshot wound should prompt the surgeon to convert to formal exploratory laparotomy without delay. Patients with midabdominal gunshot wounds are not candidates for laparoscopy, even if they exhibit hemodynamic stability, due to the very high rate (greater than 90%) of significant intraabdominal injuries associated with wounds in this location.

The percentage of patients with abdominal stab wounds who have significant intraabdominal injury is much less than that of patients with gunshot wounds to the abdomen. Therefore, a greater number of these patients are candidates for laparoscopic examination. The purpose of laparoscopy in this group of patients is much the same as for gunshot wounds: to rule out peritoneal or diaphragmatic penetration. However, since the wounding potential of a stabbing instrument is significantly less than that of a bullet, simple peritoneal penetration is not necessarily an absolute indication for conversion to laparotomy. A more extensive assessment of the diaphragm, stomach, colon, and small bowel is indicated in this group of patients. The skilled laparoscopist can perform complete examination of the peritoneum without conversion to laparotomy and can perform laparoscopic repair of some limited injuries. We have performed laparoscopic repair of several isolated diaphragmatic or gastric lacerations secondary to stab wounds with excellent results.

In our experience, the use of laparoscopy for evaluating both gunshot and stab wounds has reduced the rate of negative and nontherapeutic laparotomy. More important, laparoscopy has improved the diagnosis of occult diaphragmatic injury in patients with penetrating thoracoabdominal injury, thereby preventing the subsequent development of life-threatening intestinal herniation and strangulation.

Laparoscopy for evaluating blunt trauma is less well defined than for assessing penetrating trauma. Few surgeons would suggest that laparoscopy is the best initial method for assessing the abdomen in the blunt-trauma setting. The efficacy of sonography and CT in the diagnosis of blunt injury has limited the role of laparoscopy to that of an adjunctive technique for the further assessment of solid organ injuries that have already been identified by sonography or CT. Laparoscopy provides an excellent method for the real-time examination of hepatic or splenic lacerations to determine the presence of continued hemorrhage. When laparoscopy is performed as a prelude to exploratory lap-

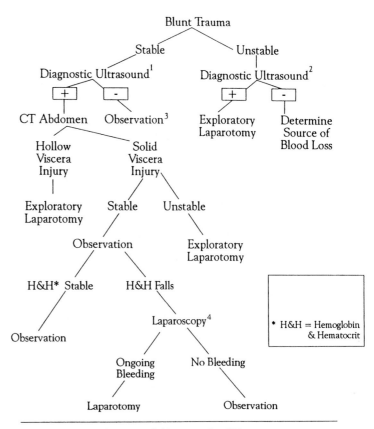

1. If diagnostic ultrasound is not available, proceed to CT scan.
2. If diagnostic ultrasound is not available, proceed to diagnostic peritoneal lavage.
3. Repeat ultrasound examination or CT scan is indicated if hemoglobin and hematocrit falls significantly.
4. Laparoscopy is used prior to laparotomy. If ongoing blood loss is found, then proceed to exploratory laparotomy.

Fig. 9-1. Laparoscopy for blunt abdominal trauma.

arotomy in patients initially treated with observation, the demonstration of hemostasis may alter the surgeon's plan to perform laparotomy in patients thought to have ongoing hemorrhage. Additionally, in patients with hemoperitoneum secondary to an isolated solid organ injury, blood may be removed from the peritoneal cavity by laparoscopy-guided suction catheters and may be processed for autotransfusion (Fig. 9-4).

Operative Technique

Standard videoscopic equipment and instruments are used in the evaluation of trauma patients. The examination is quite similar to diagnostic laparoscopy performed for the nontraumatic acute abdomen. As such, the telescope and operating ports must be located to provide optimal visualization of the entire peritoneal cavity. Insertion of a nasogastric

tube and urinary catheter aids in obtaining optimal exposure. Frequently, a physical finding such as an entrance or exit wound or a radiographic study such as a positive CT scan will permit the surgeon to focus attention on the area of the abdomen at greatest risk for injury. However, every effort must be made to fully examine the abdomen and pelvis if missed injury is to be avoided. The locations of operating ports for the optimal visualization of the respective areas of the abdomen and pelvis are presented in Fig. 9-5. Several surgeons have reported satisfactory results with the 0-degree laparoscope, but we prefer the 30 degree–angled telescope and believe it essential for the optimal visualization of the posterior aspects of the diaphragm and the lateral aspects of the ascending and descending colon.

The carbon dioxide pneumoperitoneum is initiated with a Veress needle placed through a 1-cm periumbilical position,

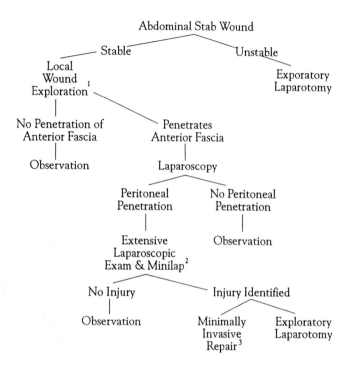

Abdominal Stab Wound

- Stable
  - Local Wound Exploration [1]
    - No Penetration of Anterior Fascia
      - Observation
    - Penetrates Anterior Fascia
      - Laparoscopy
        - Peritoneal Penetration
          - Extensive Laparoscopic Exam & Minilap [2]
            - No Injury
              - Observation
            - Injury Identified
              - Minimally Invasive Repair [3]
              - Exploratory Laparotomy
        - No Peritoneal Penetration
          - Observation
- Unstable
  - Exporatory Laparotomy

1. Local wound exploration performed in the emergency room.
2. Majority of examination is performed by laparoscopy; examination of the small bowel is performed via a 4-cm. minilaprotomy incision.
3. Limited injuries may be repaired laparoscopically depending on the capability of the surgeon.

Fig. 9-2. Laparoscopy for abdominal stab wounds.

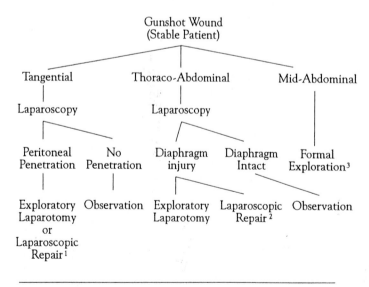

Gunshot Wound (Stable Patient)

- Tangential
  - Laparoscopy
    - Peritoneal Penetration
      - Exploratory Laparotomy or Laparoscopic Repair [1]
    - No Penetration
      - Observation
- Thoraco-Abdominal
  - Laparoscopy
    - Diaphragm injury
      - Exploratory Laparotomy
      - Laparoscopic Repair [2]
    - Diaphragm Intact
      - Observation
- Mid-Abdominal
  - Formal Exploration [3]

1. Laparoscopic repair may be performed for limited injuries, depending on the capabilities of the surgeon.
2. Posterior wounds may be more easily identified and repaired with a thorzciscopic approach. Identification of injuries of associated abdominal organs may necessitate laparotomy.
3. Gunshot wounds in this location have a greater than 90% probability of producing wounds that require definitive surgical repair.

Fig. 9-3. Laparoscopy for abdominal gunshot wounds.

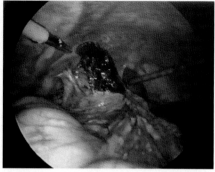

Fig. 9-4. Perisplenic hematoma following blunt abdominal trauma. Approximately 1500 mL of blood were removed from the peritoneal cavity and processed for autotransfusion. Laparoscopic observation of the hematoma documented cessation of bleeding, thereby obviating laparotomy.

limiting insufflation pressure to 8 to 10 mm Hg in patients with penetrating thoracoabdominal wounds. The rationale for this policy is to minimize the risk of tension pneumothorax, should the patient have a diaphragmatic laceration. Once these injuries have been excluded, pressures may be increased to improve exposure. In other patients, an insufflation pressure of 12 to 15 mm Hg may routinely be used. The surgeon must closely monitor patients' pulse rate, blood pressure, respiratory status, and arterial oxygen saturation during insufflation of gas. Impaired venous return caused by the combination of moderate hypovolemia and pneumoperitoneum can produce profound hypotension. Additionally, patients with intraabdominal vascular injury are at theoretical risk for the development of gas embolism. Tension pneumothorax will develop in 5% to 10% of patients with diaphragmatic perforation when pneumoperitoneum is created. Alternatively, an intraabdominal retractor system designed for isopneumic (gasless) laparoscopy may be used to provide exposure. Most of these systems remain cumbersome, but they decrease the incidence of tension pneumothorax and gas embolism. Additionally, suction and irrigation are more easily accomplished in an isopneumic environment.

After creation of the pneumoperitoneum, a 10-mm operating port is inserted through the umbilical incision. If extensive examination of the pelvis is required, the initial port should be placed in a supraumbilical position to permit optimal visualization and operative exposure. The 30-degree telescope is then introduced for initial examination of the abdomen. In patients with radiographic evidence of hemoperitoneum secondary to blunt trauma of the spleen or liver, the surgeon should expect to immediately encounter blood that must be removed prior to further examination. This may be accomplished through the use of laparoscopic suction/irrigation systems introduced into the abdomen through an additional 5-mm operating port. This additional operating port may also be used to introduce a grasper that is frequently required for manipulating the bowel or omentum.

Tangential penetrating wounds to the anterior abdominal wall are readily assessed by laparoscopy. It is important to drape patients so that entrance and exit wounds are easily accessible during the procedure. A hemostat or probe may then be gently passed through the wound tract while the area is being visualized laparoscopically. Peritoneal penetration is readily documented by this maneuver. Lateral wounds may require mobilization of the colon to determine whether or not peritoneal penetration has occurred. Posterior wounds are not reliably assessed with laparoscopy.

The liver is frequently injured in both blunt and penetrating trauma. The anterior, lateral, and medial aspects of the liver are easily visualized with a 30-degree laparoscope introduced through an umbilical port. Unfortunately, the posterior aspects of the liver are not well visualized. If injury is suspected secondary to a stab or gunshot wound, the peritoneum and diaphragm of the right upper quadrant must also be evaluated for penetration. The liver should be assessed for evidence of contusion, laceration, and hemorrhage. In the absence of associated injury, identification of a nonbleeding hepatic laceration is not an indication for conversion to exploratory laparotomy. A stable thrombus should not be manipulated or disturbed, as this may result in resumption of hemorrhage. If minor bleeding is found, hemostasis may be achieved by placing a hemostatic absorbable knitted fabric (e.g., Avitene, Surgicel) in the laceration. Cessation of bleeding must be documented prior to the completion of laparoscopy. We have frequently observed hepatic or splenic lacerations for as long as 30 minutes to assure that hemostasis was complete. Brisk or persistent hemorrhage that cannot be controlled laparoscopically is an indication for prompt conversion to an open procedure.

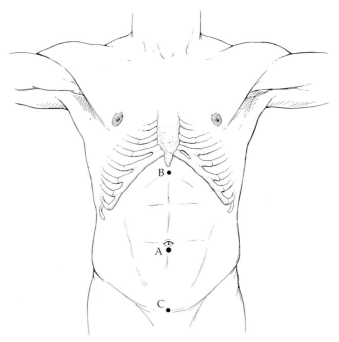

Fig. 9-5. Port sites for laparoscopy in the acute patient. For the majority of cases, use of the periumbilical port as a camera site is recommended. If the injury is in the upper abdomen, then a subxiphoid port is additionally used, usually a 10-mm port. One to two additional instrument ports should be placed, as needed, after visualization of the area of injury. These ports should be placed to allow a 30- to 60-degree separation of instruments for ease of operation. For assessment of the lower abdomen, use of a periumbilical port for the camera and a suprapubic port are generally standard, with other instrument ports being placed as needed. Inserting only two ports in a standard fashion permits flexibility for anatomic variants and minimizes the placement of unnecessary ports, should it be determined that therapeutic laparoscopy is not a viable option for the patient and that conversion to laparotomy is needed. This also keeps the incisions in the midline. If laparotomy is needed, these initial sites can be incorporated into the midline incision for open exploration. (A, camera; B, subxiphoid 10-mm port; C, suprapubic port.)

The spleen is most commonly injured when blunt force is applied to the left upper quadrant, flank, or left hemithorax. Some surgeons have reported difficulty in obtaining laparoscopic exposure of the spleen because of its posterosuperior location in the abdomen, but with proper preoperative patient positioning and the use of ancillary operating ports for retraction and suction/irrigation, we have had excellent success in obtaining complete visualization of this organ (Fig. 9-6). Prior to draping of the abdomen, a towel roll, 1-L intravenous bag, or bean-bag support should be placed to elevate the patient's left flank 30 to 45 degrees in relation to the plane of the operating table (Fig. 9-7). The patient should then be placed in the reverse Trendelenburg position so that gravity will aid in retraction of the stomach, transverse colon, splenic flexure, and omentum inferiorly. Gastric decompression via nasogastric tube is essential if optimal exposure of the left upper quadrant

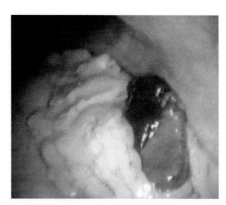

Fig. 9-6. Stable splenic hematoma visualized by laparoscopy.

is to be obtained. If exposure is still inadequate, the operating table may be rotated further to the right. Because of the location of the spleen high in the left upper quadrant, the initial 10-mm port (laparoscope) should be placed in the midline, 3 to 5 cm superior to the umbilicus. This position

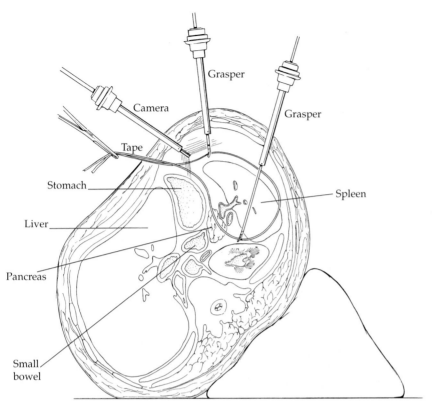

Fig. 9-7. Patient positioning for surgery. With deflation of the bean bag and rotation of the table, the patient can be quickly leveled for laparotomy if necessary. (From Koehler RH, Smith RS, Fry WR. Laparoscopic splenorrhaphy for grade III injury. Surg Laparosc Endosc 1994;4:311–315; with permission.)

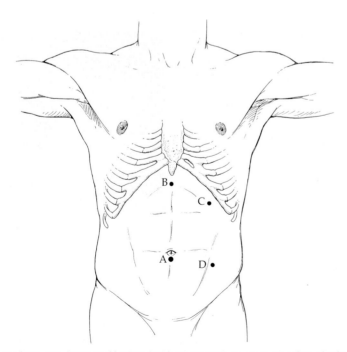

Fig. 9-8. Trocar placements. (From Koehler RH, Smith RS, Fry WR. Laparoscopic splenorrhaphy for grade III injury. Surg Laparosc Endosc 1994;4:311–315; with permission.)

gives excellent visualization of the spleen and also permits examination of the remaining quadrants of the abdomen. Additional 10-mm ancillary ports are placed in the right and left upper quadrants, respectively (Fig. 9-8). A laparoscopic Babcock clamp introduced through the right upper quadrant port is then used to retract the fundus of the stomach medially and inferiorly. An additional grasper or suction catheter may be introduced through the left upper quadrant port. These maneuvers will usually provide excellent exposure of the spleen. However, if the posterior aspects of the spleen are not visualized, two additional techniques are helpful: (a) replacing the laparoscope in the left upper quadrant port and (b) placing an umbilical tape sling around the hilum of the spleen to facilitate anteromedial retraction. Use of this exposure technique has permitted performance of laparoscopic mesh splenorrhaphy (Figs. 9-9 to 9-11). Hemostatic agents may be used for small or superficial lacerations, but a stable hematoma without evidence of ongoing hemorrhage should be left undisturbed. Failure to obtain complete hemostasis within 30 minutes should result in conversion to laparotomy.

The stomach is at risk in any patient with penetrating trauma to the epigastrium. Laparoscopic examination of the anterior wall of the stomach is easily performed by a 30-degree telescope placed through an umbilical port. Decompressing the stomach with a nasogastric tube is essential for optimal visualization. If caudal retraction is required for assessment of the gastroesophageal junction or the superior aspect of the gastric fundus, additional 10-mm ports should be placed at the level of the umbilicus lateral to the rectus muscles. Endoscopic Babcock or bowel clamps may then be used to provide the needed caudal retraction. Examination of the posterior fundus is obviously more difficult but may be done by dividing the gastrocolic ligament with cautery. While this plane is relatively avascular, ligation of identified small vessels with clips or the ultrasonic dissector should be performed. Once the lesser sac has been entered through this route, the stomach may then be retracted anteriorly with Babcock clamps. The 30-degree telescope is then used to examine the posterior wall of the stomach, the lesser sac, and the pancreas. The presence of blood, fluid, or enteric contents in the lesser sac is an indication for exploratory laparotomy. A pancreatic hematoma is also an indication for formal exploration. Laparoscopic suture or stapled repair of limited (less than 2 cm) perforations of the anterior gastric wall have been reported in the literature and appear to be both safe and expedient (Fig. 9-12). We prefer suture repair of these lacerations with 2-0 or 3-0 polytetrafluoroethylene suture. However, if these repairs are to be performed, the surgeon must first be certain that no associated injuries are present.

Complete examination of the colon and small bowel with laparoscopy is difficult in the trauma setting. The duodenum and significant segments of the colon are retroperitoneal and require extensive mobilization for adequate examination. Visualization of a hematoma in the area anterior or lateral to the duodenum is commonly associated with serious vascular, pancreatic, or duodenal injury and is therefore a finding that mandates open exploration. In patients with flank wounds, the ascending and descending segments of colon are at risk for retroperitoneal perforation. These colon segments may be adequately visualized in many patients by taking down the white line of Toldt with endoscopic scissors or electrocautery. Once this is done, endoscopic bowel clamps may be used to lift the bowel anteromedially, permitting 360-degree assessment of the bowel wall. Identification of a traumatic colon perforation is an indication for open repair.

Complete laparoscopic examination of the small intestine for the presence of small enterotomies is much more demanding than simply running the bowel in search of adhesions. Examination of the small bowel requires advanced laparoscopic skills that many trauma surgeons have not yet attained. The small bowel can be visualized in a significant number of patients by using endoscopic bowel clamps to sequentially bring loops of bowel into view. This procedure is repeated serially until the entire small intestine has been visualized. Care must be taken to examine the entire circumference of each segment of small bowel to ensure the discovery of small enterotomies. Due to the technical difficulty of small bowel examination, most reported injuries missed during trauma laparoscopy have involved the small bowel. In one early series, only 20% of small bowel injuries were identified during the initial laparoscopic examination. There-

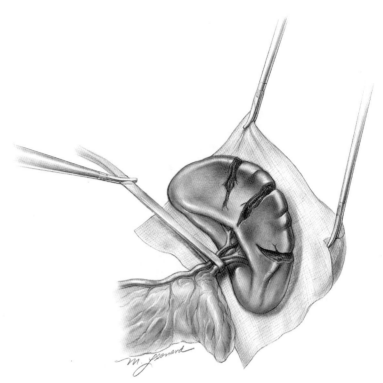

Fig. 9-9. Initial placement of mesh. The umbilical tape is utilized to apply gentle retraction on the spleen at the hilum. (From Koehler RH, Smith RS, Fry WR. Laparoscopic splenorrhaphy for grade III injury. Surg Laparosc Endosc 1994;4:311–315; with permission.)

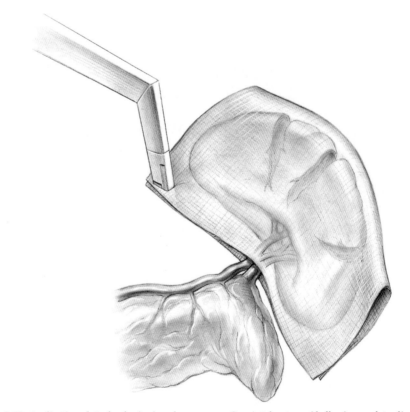

Fig. 9-10. Application of stapler, beginning along corners. Care is taken to avoid allowing mesh to slip out from underneath spleen. (From Koehler RH, Smith RS, Fry WR. Laparoscopic splenorrhaphy for grade III injury. Surg Laparosc Endosc 1994;4:311–315; with permission.)

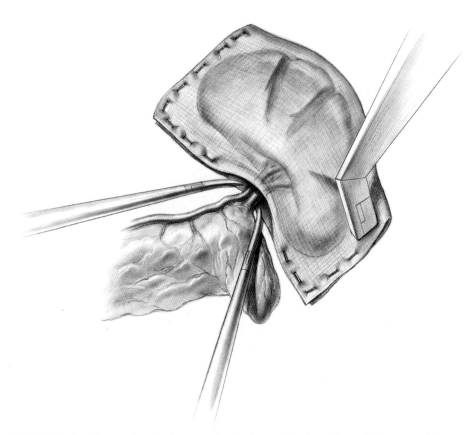

Fig. 9-11. Final application of staples. A tamponade effect is created by tightening mesh down around the parenchyma, leaving a hilar window. (From Koehler RH, Smith RS, Fry WR. Laparoscopic splenorrhaphy for grade III injury. Surg Laparosc Endosc 1994;4:311–315; with permission.)

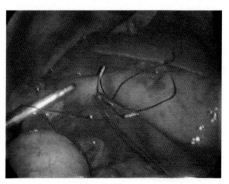

Fig. 9-12. Isopneumic laparoscopic repair of a small penetrating wound of the anterior wall of the stomach. Note the use of a conventional needle driver made possible by isopneumic exposure.

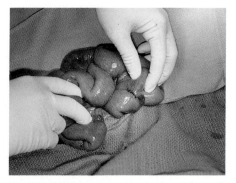

Fig. 9-13. Minilaparotomy examination of the small bowel in a patient with an abdominal stab wound. A small enterotomy was found and repaired extracorporeally.

fore, alternative techniques for examining the small bowel have been developed. We have favored a minilaparotomy approach to examine the small intestine. After a complete laparoscopic examination has failed to identify any significant injuries in a patient with a penetrating abdominal wound, the umbilical incision previously used to introduce the laparoscope is then extended to a total length of approximately 4 cm. Sequential segments of bowel 1 to 2 feet in length are then eviscerated through the minilaparotomy incision for direct examination (Fig. 9-13). This procedure provides for almost complete direct examination of the small bowel in slender patients but is more difficult to perform in the obese. Small enterotomies identified by this technique may then be repaired extracorporeally with standard suture technique. The minilaparotomy incision is then closed in standard fashion.

Cardiac Tamponade

Surgical drainage of the pericardium has been done by both the subxiphoid and the transthoracic approaches. The subxiphoid approach is used by most general surgeons when drainage of fluid alone is needed. When pericardiectomy is required for constrictive pericarditis, infected tamponade, or cardiac injury, the transthoracic approach is used to permit better exposure of the pericardium. Median sternotomy or left thoracotomy are also used when preventing contamination of the abdomen with infected material is desired or when intrathoracic injuries are undetermined.

In the acute setting, cardiac tamponade can be difficult to diagnose in the multiply injured patient. The thoracoscopic approach to hemotamponade should only be attempted when it is clear that there is no cardiac or great vessel injury. Significant bleeding from injuries to these structures can overwhelm the resources available for thoracoscopy. Cardiac and great vessel injuries require traditional open thoracotomy.

Injury to the heart and/or great vessels can be determined by transesophageal ultrasound. Ultrasound has the additional advantage of allowing direct visualization, should preoperative drainage of pericardial fluid be necessary to attempt hemodynamic stabilization prior to going to the operating room.

Other causes of tamponade such as uremic pericarditis or hemorrhage from metastatic pericardial implants can be diagnosed using transthoracic echocardiography without the need for using transesophageal probes.

Thoracoscopic Pericardiectomy to Relieve Cardiac Tamponade

The patient is placed in a right lateral decubitus position. The thoracoscope is placed in the midaxillary line at the fourth intercostal space. Two operating sites are chosen to allow approximately a 30- to 60-degree angle between operating sites. One should be placed anteriorly between the midclavicular line and anterior axillary line in the fourth to fifth intercostal space. The posterior port should be placed in the fifth to sixth intercostal space at the midaxillary line.

After deflation of the left lung, the pericardium can be well visualized in most patients. If the lung hinders visualization of the pericardium, the inferior pulmonary ligament may be incised, enabling the lung to be retracted cephalad. Being made of pleural folds, this ligament is avascular and, if desired, can be cut without need of electrocautery.

Visually, the phrenic nerve is easily identified in thin patients with little pericardial fat. However, in patients whose phrenic nerve is not visualized due to pericardial fat, blunt dissection should be carried out to identify the nerve's course to avoid injury. This dissection can be performed using graspers or dissectors to gently spread the pericardial fat to expose the nerve. Since fat tends not to dissect off the pericardium well, identification of the phrenic nerve in two to three isolated spots will suffice to determine its course over the pericardium. The phrenic nerve is generally over the posterior third of the pericardium, running in a superior to inferior course.

The pericardium should be incised anterior to the phrenic nerve to avoid injury. Since the pericardium is usually distended, it can be difficult to grasp with forceps, graspers, or hemostats. If this cannot be accomplished, a knife or a pair of scissors should be used to carefully nick the pericardium. Once the pericardium has been decompressed, it can then be grasped, pulled away from the heart, and incised for several centimeters using a pair of scissors. A defect of at least 2 to 4 cm^2 should be made by excising a portion of pericardium. Again, this should be done carefully to avoid injury to the heart and the phrenic nerve. With inflammatory pericardial processes, such as suppurative or hemotamponade from mediastinal bleeding, it is vital to excise a portion of the pericardium to prevent its edges from sealing together again.

Once the pericardiectomy has been accomplished, a chest tube can be inserted through one of the operative sites and visually placed in a dependent position. The size of the chest tube should be proportional to the thickness of the pericardial fluid. Thus, the thicker the fluid, the larger will be the diameter of the chest tube.

The chest incisions should be closed in layers. The muscle layer should be closed with an 0 to 2-0 polyglycolic acid suture. The subcutaneous layer should be closed with 2-0 to 3-0 polyglycolic acid suture. We generally close the skin with a running subcuticular 3-0 to 4-0 Monocryl suture. The chest tube should be secured with a heavy permanent suture such as 0 nylon.

Continued Thoracic Hemorrhage

In addition to damaging intrathoracic structures, penetrating chest trauma can cause injury to intercostal or internal mammary vessels. When cardiac and great vessel injuries have been ruled out, thoracoscopy is an ideal way of treating continued bleeding from injured intercostal or internal mammary vessels.

Thoracoscopy for the Evaluation and Treatment of Continued Thoracic Hemorrhage

Patient positioning is critical. The injured vessel should not be placed in a true dependent position. If it is so placed, blood will pool at the injury site, obscuring visualization and hindering treatment. Thus, a true decubitus position may not be the best for injuries close to the midline, such as internal mammary vessel injuries. In these cases, patient positioning slightly toward the posterior will obviate this potential problem.

With the patient placed in the appropriate decubitus position, placement of the camera and the operative sites must be chosen to allow the best access to the injured intercostal or internal mammary vessels. With the availability of angled and flexible thoracoscopes, it is best to chose the closest site to the expected injury for the thoracoscope. Operative access should be placed at a 45- to 90-degree angle from the injury to permit ease of operative management. Generally, two operative sites are needed, one for grasping and one for clipping and suctioning.

The lung is deflated, and the thoracic cavity is inspected for obvious sites of hemorrhage. If the main bleeding site is an un-suspected pulmonary or great vessel injury, conversion to open thoracotomy should be performed.

If the main bleeding site is an internal mammary or intercostal vessel, incision of the pleura at the site of injury may be needed, since the vessels course in an extrapleural position. The intercostal vessels are more easily visualized anterior to the axilla, coursing more directly under the pleura. Since most patients are stabbed or shot in the anterior chest, exposure is facilitated by the anatomy of the intercostal vessels in this location. Exposure can easily be achieved using a pair of scissors to incise the pleura along the inferior margin of the rib. In many penetrating injuries, the pleura has been injured to a large enough extent that combined with the dissection done by bleeding from the injured vessel the pleura will be separated from the underlying vessels. Thus, excellent exposure of the injured vessels is performed by the injury itself.

The internal mammary vessels run along the lateral margin of the sternum, usually 1 to 1.5 cm from its lateral border. Injury causing significant bleeding usually occurs at or above the fifth intercostal space, since at the sixth intercostal space the internal mammary arborizes into multiple branches.

Once the vessel or vessels have been exposed, the cut ends can be doubly clipped using an endoscopic clip applier. This is a good technique for the well developed internal mammary. Grasping the end of the vessel and applying electrocautery current may also be an effective and less expensive alternative that is useful for most intercostal vessels. Following control of intercostal or internal mammary bleeding, inspection of the rest of the thoracic cavity is done to look for other injuries. Retained blood should be evacuated. If blood clots are present that cannot be removed by conventional suction, curved and straight ring forceps are ideal for grasping and removing clot from the pleural space. Irrigation with normal saline can assist in removal of blood from recesses within the pleural space.

Closure of the thoracic incisions should be performed in layers to ensure an airtight seal. A separate muscle and subcutaneous closure should be performed with polyglycolic acid suture or an equivalent. A chest tube, usually 28 French or greater, can be inserted through one of the operative sites to evacuate retained blood. The chest tube should be secured to the chest wall with an 2-0 or 0 nylon or silk suture.

Retained Hemothorax

It is not uncommon for the initial thoracostomy tube placed for hemothorax to incompletely evacuate the hemothorax. This may become problematic because the retained hemothorax can prevent full reexpansion of the lung, become infected, causing empyema formation, and/or lead to lung collapse as it lyses. With a retained hemothorax, operative removal should be considered when the estimated volume reaches 300 to 500 mL. Consideration for thoracoscopic evacuation of the hemothorax should be made within the first 3 to 5 days. Waiting longer than this can make removal quite difficult due to hematoma organization and adherence of the clot to the pleura and lung.

Thoracoscopic Technique for Removal of Retained Hemothorax

With the patient in the appropriate decubitus position, the thoracoscope and instrumentation positions should be chosen to enter the pleural space at a point removed from the retained hemothorax. The approach should be to place the camera at a site that is far enough away from the clot that it can easily be surveyed with the thoracoscope. Thus, a thoracoscope position at third to fourth intercostal spaces above the edge of the retained hemothorax in the anterior axillary line proves to be advantageous.

Positioning of the first, and often the only necessary, operative port one to two interspaces above and posterior to the retained hemothorax provides the best operative access. Placement of the operative port should be done with thoracoscopic guidance.

After deflation of the ipsilateral lung, the lung is assessed for adherence to the clot using gentle probing and lifting of the lung away from the clot with forceps. If the lung is adherent to the retained hemothorax, direct finger dissection or use of a sponge stick with ring forceps is usually successful in separating the lung from the clot.

Curved ring forceps are best suited to grasping and removing retained clot, since they provide a large enough surface area that the clot is less likely to fragment. Use of a suction curette provides a large enough opening to aspirate clot relatively easily out of the pleural space. Normal wall suction pressure should be used, rather than the higher pressures used for therapeutic abortions, to avoid disastrous "suction biopsy" of the lung or heart. Once the majority of clot has been removed, copious irrigation with warm normal saline and repeated suctioning should remove most of the remaining small clots. The pleural space should then be inspected for sites of continued bleeding. If a bleeding site, such as an intercostal vessel, is seen, thoracoscopic therapy as described previously can be used. Significant bleeding from major vascular structures or the lung should not be repaired thoracoscopically, until advanced thoracoscopic skills are developed.

The lung should be assessed to make sure it is not restricted by chronic inflammatory reaction and rind formation. Should this be the case, the ring forceps can be used to peel away the rind, permitting full lung expansion.

The thoracic incisions should be closed in layers to ensure an airtight seal. A separate muscle and subcutaneous closure should be performed with polyglycolic acid suture or an equivalent. A chest tube, usually 28 French or greater, can be inserted through one of the operative sites to evacuate retained blood. The chest tube should be secured to the chest wall with a 2-0 or 0 nylon or silk suture.

Suggested Reading

Esposito TJ. Laparoscopy in blunt trauma. *Trauma Q* 1993;10:260–272.

Fabian TC, Croce MA, Stewart RM, Pritchard FE, Minard G, Kudsk KA. A prospective analysis of diagnostic laparoscopy in trauma. *Ann Surg* 1993;217:557–565.

Ivatury RR, Simon RJ, Stahl WM. A critical evaluation of laparoscopy in penetrating abdominal trauma. *J Trauma* 1993;34:822–828.

Ivatury RR, Simon RJ, Weksler B, Bayard V, Stahl WM. Laparoscopy in the evaluation of the intrathoracic abdomen after penetrating injury. *J Trauma* 1992;33:101–109.

Ochsner MG, Lowery RC, Frankel HL, Champion HR. Thoracoscopy: technical details and application. *Trauma Q* 1993;10:301–311.

Smith RS, Fry WR, Morabito DJ, Koehler RH, Organ CH Jr. Therapeutic laparoscopy in trauma. *Am J Surg* 1995;170:632–637.

Smith RS, Fry WR, Tsoi EK, et al. Preliminary report on videothoracoscopy in the evaluation and treatment of thoracic injury. *Am J Surg* 1993; 166:690–695.

Smith RS, Fry WR, Tsoi EK, et al. Gasless laparoscopy and conventional instruments: the next phase of minimally invasive surgery. *Arch Surg* 1993;128:1102–1107.

EDITOR'S COMMENT

The appropriate role for laparoscopy in the evaluation and operative management of trauma patients remains to be determined. The authors describe several well considered algorithms for the use of laparoscopy in this setting. Diagnostic laparoscopy in the context of abdominal trauma is hindered by several factors. Many trauma surgeons are not experienced laparoscopists, nor do many perform adequate numbers of elective laparoscopic operations to feel comfortable extending laparoscopic techniques to the therapy of traumatic injuries. Trauma patients are often hemodynamically unstable, leading to obvious time considerations and raising the specter of hypotension induced by the combination of pneumoperitoneum and hypovolemia. Furthermore, trauma patients often present to the hospital during times when experienced laparoscopic support personnel are not available. Nevertheless, laparoscopic examination bears promise in specific groups of patients, and therapeutic closure of injuries to hollow viscera and the diaphragm appears to be readily feasible. As experience with laparoscopy grows in traumatology circles, it is reasonable to expect that the role of laparoscopy in the trauma setting will increase. Similar considerations have limited the acceptance of thoracoscopy in trauma patients, and further accrual of patients and studies to define its role should be forthcoming in the near future.

N.J.S.

10

Laparoscopic Staging of Intraabdominal Malignancy

Mark P. Callery and Richard S. Swanson

The staging of cancer involves evaluating the noncontiguous anatomic spread of malignancy, usually before the institution of primary therapy. Advances in medical and surgical oncology have refined the treatments of intraabdominal malignancy. Diagnostic laparoscopy is rapidly gaining acceptance worldwide as a minimally invasive alternative to diagnostic laparotomy. In this chapter, the applications of laparoscopic staging of intraabdominal malignancy are reviewed, focusing on the anatomic areas most readily evaluated.

Laparoscopic exploration of the abdominal cavity was introduced in 1901 by G. Kelling using a cystoscope inserted under local anesthesia. Laparoscopy has since been modified and improved, and today is pivotal in the surgical management of cholelithiasis, gastroesophageal reflux, and other general surgical conditions.

Despite the availability of modern diagnostic imaging modalities, assessment of intraabdominal malignancy is often inadequate, especially in patients being considered for curative resection. Underestimation of tumor stage has resulted in many unnecessary diagnostic laparotomies. As the technology of laparoscopy has improved, so too has its value in defining the resectability of many abdominal malignancies. Laparoscopy complements current staging modalities such as transabdominal ultrasound (US), computed tomography (CT), magnetic resonance (MR) imaging, angiography and, more recently, positron emission tomography (PET). Specifically, laparoscopy has been favorably evaluated in the preoperative staging of esophageal, gastric, hepatobil-iary, pancreatic, ovarian, cervical, endometrial, bladder, and prostate carcinomas. With the recent advent of laparoscopic US, the sensitivity of laparoscopic staging of certain intraabdominal malignancies has been further improved. New laparoscopic staging techniques have evolved in parallel with both therapeutic and palliative laparoscopic and endoscopic procedures, thereby obviating formal laparotomy. While the role for therapeutic laparoscopy in surgical oncology is still early in its evolution, data are growing, supporting the use of diagnostic laparoscopy in the approach to several intraabdominal malignancies. Staging laparoscopy also has increasingly been applied as a minimally invasive method to stage thoracic and genitourinary neoplasms.

Traditional staging modalities—US, CT, and MR imaging—are usually sufficient for preoperative diagnosis and can reliably exclude patients with unresectable disease from anesthesia and futile operative diagnosis and staging. Unfortunately, traditional radiologic staging techniques have recognized limitations. As many as 30% to 40% of patients with hepatobiliary and pancreatic malignancies harbor occult metastases that cannot be imaged radiologically. Small secondary tumor deposits on the liver surface or peritoneum cannot be identified nonoperatively. Evaluation of tumor proximity to or invasion of major vascular structures is often ambiguous. Radiologic staging modalities often fail to establish a tissue diagnosis or to accurately evaluate lymphatic metastases. These procedures are expensive and time-consum-ing and have defined risks. Staging laparoscopy is intended to complement or replace traditional imaging modalities, with the goal of minimizing the understaging of malignancy.

Diagnostic Considerations

Indications

Although laparoscopic staging can alter the management of patients with intraabdominal malignancies, the specific indications for laparoscopy remain to be defined. Radiologic techniques are still preferable in the initial evaluation of intraabdominal malignancies. To make an informed decision regarding treatment approaches, one must accurately evaluate the stage of cancer prior to formal laparotomy. The positive and negative predictive values of current staging modalities must be considered. For example, an angiogram that fails to image vascular encasement for a presumed gastric carcinoma cannot rule out occult metastases that make the disease incurable. Similarly, negative laparoscopy may not rule out vascular encasement.

Staging laparoscopy appears to be indicated in intraabdominal malignancy when it can complement the positive and negative predictive values of traditional imaging modalities. Most important, staging laparoscopy is indicated when the primary malignancy may be associated with peritoneal carcinomatosis or when a preoperative tissue diagnosis for unresectable disease has not been obtained. Negative CT or US examinations do not in any way

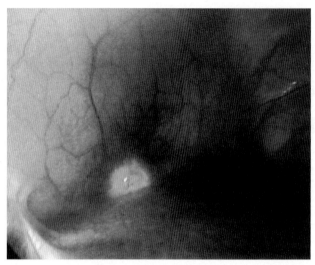

Fig. 10-1. An occult metastatic deposit from a periampullary carcinoma is seen at the junction of the falciform ligament in the left lateral segment of the liver. Small lesions of this size cannot be imaged by traditional staging modalities. (From John TG, Greig JD, Carter DC, Garden OJ. Carcinoma of the pancreatic head and periampullary region: tumor staging with laparoscopy and laparoscopic ultrasonography. Ann Surg 1995;221:156–164; with permission.)

exclude the possibility that laparoscopy may detect liver or peritoneal malignancy. Laparoscopy provides a minutely detailed view of the liver and anterior peritoneal surfaces and is the most sensitive test for detecting occult (less than 10 mm) metastases of an intraabdominal malignancy (Fig. 10-1). In addition, new laparoscopic US techniques now allow small metastases within the liver parenchyma to be identified.

Benign Disease

Diagnostic laparoscopy has long been tested in benign disease, especially gynecologic diseases. In the diagnosis of hepatic cirrhosis, laparoscopy with guided biopsy is far superior to blind percutaneous biopsy and is the procedure of choice in many centers worldwide. In the evaluation of cirrhosis and hepatitis, sampling errors for blind percutaneous liver biopsies are higher than for biopsies guided by laparoscopy. Selected patients with chronic abdominal pain syndromes also benefit from diagnostic laparoscopy. In those with focal recurrent or somatic type pain, adhesions may be causally identified and relief provided by laparoscopic adhesiolysis. Emergency laparoscopy has a growing role in the detection of intraabdominal bleeding and organ injury after blunt trauma and of abdominal wall penetration with stab wounds. Laparoscopy in acquired immunodeficiency syndrome

(AIDS) patients has recently been promoted as a means of dealing with the myriad possible diagnoses within the abdomen. Hepatic and peritoneal infections, as well as neoplasms, can be identified, avoiding unnecessary laparotomy in AIDS patients. Patients with lower abdominal pain can be nicely evaluated for acute appendicitis laparoscopically. If diagnosed, the appendix can readily be removed. Simple placement of the laparoscope accurately identifies pelvic inflammatory disease, which confounds the differential diagnosis of lower abdominal pain in women. For several benign intraabdominal conditions, laparoscopy now replaces many traditional diagnostic imaging modalities.

Malignant Disease

Diagnostic laparoscopy should be considered a complementary modality in evaluating intraabdominal malignancy. Depending on the location and site of a tumor, traditional imaging modalities may suggest a diagnosis of cancer, while others may not detect a tumor until a later stage. For example, a parenchymal lesion within the liver may be detected by CT scan. Next, laparoscopy with US can be used, if necessary, to biopsy the suspicious lesion. Surface hepatic lesions, however, are rarely apparent on CT scan but can be readily discovered and biopsied laparoscopically.

Laparoscopic staging is usually indicated to minimize understaging. In addition, radiologic staging modalities may not establish a definitive tissue diagnosis or accurately evaluate metastatic lymphatic involvement, leading to repeated imaging and attempts at invasive tissue sampling. Under these circumstances, laparoscopy appears to be useful as an alternative staging approach for intraabdominal malignancy. For example, Cuschieri and colleagues showed a 90% diagnostic yield and a 30% management benefit using laparoscopy as an adjunct to radiologic staging in pancreatic cancer. In their hands, only two patients were understaged (missed hepatic metastases and portal vein involvement by carcinoma in the head of the pancreas). These patients were evaluated before the advent of laparoscopic US, however.

Patient Selection

Laparoscopy for both diagnosis and staging of intraabdominal malignancy should be performed in careful combination with traditional imaging modalities. Patient selection and the techniques used for laparoscopy depend primarily on the diagnostic information needed to be gained from the study. Patients should be selected in light of an overall plan for their malignant disease, including the possibility of surgical resection and primary or adjuvant chemotherapy and radiation therapy. Often, patients have a preliminary diagnosis by biopsy, or a possible malignancy has been identified by preoperative staging modality. These data must be considered by the surgeon in determining the application of diagnostic laparoscopy. For example, patients with an established diagnosis of intraabdominal malignancy may require laparotomy for palliative debulking or other reasons. In these instances, laparoscopy becomes an unnecessary additional step. Conversely, if confirmation of intraabdominal metastatic disease is required, laparoscopy may be the ideal approach to avoiding a more morbid and invasive procedure.

Justification

With careful patient selection, staging laparoscopy can usually be justified. Determining the unresectability of an abdominal malignancy by minimally invasive techniques can eliminate unnecessary laparotomy. Tissue diagnosis may be obtained by laparoscopic biopsy alone or by laparoscopic US–guided percutaneous needle biopsy. Once biopsy is accomplished, patients with unresectable disease may be promptly recovered and offered appropriate chemotherapy and radiation therapy protocols. Effective palliative techniques are also now available for many abdominal malignancies without the need for formal laparotomy. For example, larger biliary stents are available that usually stay patent and functional for the remainder of life for a pancreatic cancer patient with biliary obstruction. Duodenal obstruction, if present, may also be palliated by laparoscopic gastroenterostomy.

At some centers, preoperative radiation or chemotherapy is utilized in hope of reducing intraoperative dissemination of cancers to be resected at a subsequent definitive laparotomy. Specialized surgical care is not necessarily available during initial attempts at resection. Tumors may be irrevocably violated or other adverse circumstances created for subsequent attempts at resection. Preoperative staging may therefore be more focused, and unnecessary laparotomy avoided. Patients with unresectable disease managed by minimally invasive methods benefit from lower morbidity, shorter hospital stays, and reduced costs than for cohorts undergoing open surgical therapy. Staging laparoscopy is preferred prior to open laparotomy for other purposes also. More important, patients accurately staged as inoperable may be healthier as they enter the final stages of their lives.

Contraindications

When patients with intraabdominal malignancy are evaluated, laparoscopy is contraindicated by inability to tolerate general anesthesia or formal laparotomy, uncorrectable coagulopathy, and hemodynamic instability. These contraindications are uniform for laparoscopic procedures and are covered elsewhere in this text. Relative contraindications, such as prior abdominal surgery and cardiopulmonary comorbidity, can often be managed by the experienced laparoscopist and anesthetist.

Perioperative Patient Management

Diagnostic laparoscopy for abdominal malignancy may be accomplished using general anesthesia or local infiltration with intravenous sedation in the awake patient. At our center, patients undergoing thorough diagnostic laparoscopy typically require general anesthesia to tolerate the pneumoperitoneum and allow open laparotomy, as necessary, for diagnosis and additional treatment.

After induction of general inhalational anesthesia, a bladder catheter and orogastric tube are usually placed. Decompressing the urinary bladder is necessary to optimally examine the pelvis. Preoperative antibiotics may be administered at the surgeon's discretion. Sequential compression devices should be placed on both legs and supplemented with minidose subcutaneous heparin if the risk of venous thrombosis is high. The entire abdomen is always sterilely prepared and draped suitably for open laparotomy, if required. Patients are carefully monitored with electrocardiography, pulse oximetry, blood pressure, precordial stethoscope, airway pressure, and end-tidal capnography.

Operating Room Setup

The patient is usually positioned supine on an operating table equipped for electric multiplanar movement (Fig. 10-2). Electrocautery and suction tubing are draped off the patient's left shoulder, while the fiberoptic videoscope cable and insufflation tubing are draped off the right shoulder. A sterile laparoscopic US probe is connected to its system monitor at the patient's feet. Laparoscopic video monitors are placed across from the laparoscopist and assistant. We utilize video mixer electronics to display both US and video laparoscopy images on these monitors. The instrument stand is placed at the end of the operating table with the scrub nurse.

Anatomic and Technical Considerations

A high-resolution, 10-mm, oblique-viewing (angled 30 to 45 degrees) laparoscope is always used. This maximizes lighting and increases visual field and access to most areas of the peritoneal cavity. Standard instruments required for staging laparoscopy include grasping devices, scissors, hook cautery, biopsy forceps, liver and uterine retractors, blunt probe, Babcock clamps, and a suction/irrigator probe. Access to the abdomen is usually obtained through an open insertion technique using a Hasson trocar. We prefer this safer method over the closed insertion of a Veress needle. Patients who have had previous abdominal procedures should be carefully evaluated for alternative sites of placement of the initial puncture for establishing pneumoperitoneum. The Hasson trocar is typically placed in the infraumbilical location, and following open surgical dissection to the peritoneal cavity, it is anchored with sutures placed through the fascia at the superior and inferior extent of the incision.

Pneumoperitoneum is established with insufflation of carbon dioxide to a pressure of 12 to 15 mm Hg at a flow rate of 4 to 6 L per minute. Next, the video laparoscope is placed through the Hasson trocar, and a thorough exploration of the abdomen is conducted. The peritoneal and omental surfaces are carefully surveyed for any evidence of tumor implants, which appear as dense nodules clearly distinguishable from the shiny translucent appearance of the peritoneum or fatty surface of the omentum. These implants should be biopsied, if encountered, by placing a second trocar through the abdominal wall to facilitate the introduction of biopsy forceps (Fig. 10-3).

Trocar placement depends on the type of intraabdominal malignancy being evaluated. As noted, a 10-mm trocar is inserted via open or closed technique in the standard periumbilical position through which the laparoscope is inserted. A 5-mm trocar is placed in the right midclavicular line for exposure and biopsy. A third 5-mm trocar is placed in the right midaxillary line for exposure and dissection (Fig. 10-4). Adhesions are taken down hemostatically. The entire abdominal cavity, the pelvis, the right and left pericolic gutters, and cul-de-sacs are visually evaluated. The right and left lobes of the liver are inspected to assess resectability of primary and secondary hepatic tumors and to identify any unsuspected metastatic seedlings or satellite lesions. The peritoneal undersurface of the diaphragm and the liver edge are scrutinized for evidence of metastatic disease. The omentum is inspected on both anterior and posterior surfaces. A general exploration of the remainder of the exposed intraabdominal

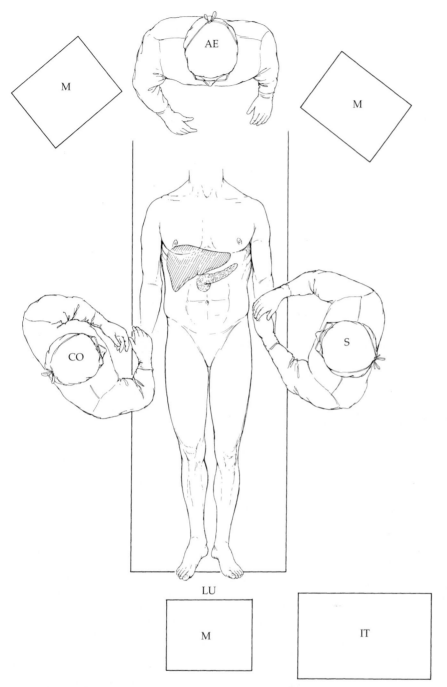

Fig. 10-2. *Schematic diagram of an operating room setup for laparoscopic staging of intraabdominal malignancy. In addition to video monitors placed at the head of the bed, a laparoscopic monitor is required and often video-mixed with the video monitors electronically. (CO, camera operator; M, monitor; AE, anesthetist; S, surgeon; IT, instrument table; LU, laparoscopic ultrasound.)*

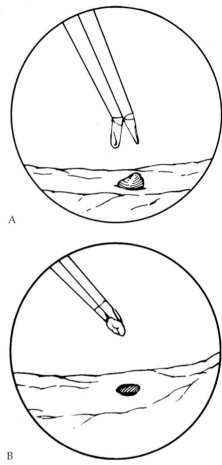

Fig. 10-3. **A,B:** *A 5-mm biopsy forceps enables the laparoscopic surgeon to both instrument-palpate and biopsy questionable metastatic lesions. In these images, surface lesions on the liver are biopsied and proven to be metastatic carcinoma.*

contents is then conducted, including the stomach, small bowel, colon, and pelvic viscera. Special evaluation is warranted in the pericolic gutters, the recesses in the upper abdomen laterally, and the deep true pelvis.

Biopsies specimens are obtained for all suspicious lesions that would preclude re-sectability. This is done under direct laparoscopic visualization using standard cup biopsy forceps through the 5-mm port. This may also be done percutaneously using a "true" cut or mechanically loaded needle technique. The needle is visualized laparoscopically as it enters the abdomen and targets the lesion. Laparoscopic US can also be used. We find it worthwhile to apply electrocautery to the needle for hemostasis within the biopsy track. This is especially worthwhile in cirrhotic livers. A laparoscopic lysis of adhesions should be directed at areas most likely to preclude resection—liver edge, peritoneum, and omentum.

Trocars should be carefully selected and positioned to optimize the use of other operating instruments during exploration. Often, a second 10-mm port is placed in the right lower quadrant, especially if laparoscopic US is needed (Fig. 10-5). If ascites is encountered, it should be aspirated and sent for cytologic evaluation. Peritoneal carcinomatosis and malignant ascites commonly occur late in the natural history of abdominal malignancies, especially carcinoma of the pancreas. Cytologic examination of peritoneal washings may also be performed for staging of intraabdominal malignancy. Normal saline (100 mL) can be instilled into the subhepatic space, agitated, and reaspirated under laparoscopic guidance. In addition to cytologic smears, stained tissue sections may be prepared for evaluation from centrifuged cell blocks. Warshaw evaluated the impact of positive peritoneal cytology on the staging of pancreatic cancer.

Esophageal Cancer

Detection of peritoneal and hepatic disease and evaluation of celiac nodal basins are very important in the staging of esophageal carcinoma. Preliminary reports evaluating the use of laparoscopy in staging esophageal cancer have been favorable. Staging laparoscopy should be considered after careful radiologic evaluation fails to disclose any gross metastatic disease, and patients are otherwise considered suitable operative candidates.

The abdomen is explored laparoscopically to visualize and biopsy any peritoneal or omental deposits. The surface of the liver is inspected, and any suspicious nodules are biopsied. Small occult metastases at these locations are not uncommon for esophageal cancer. Ascites, when found, is aspirated and sent for cytologic examina-

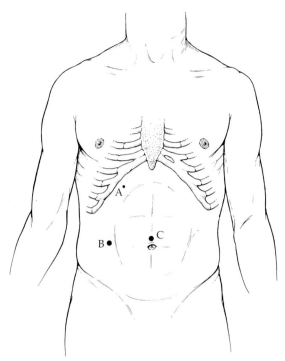

Fig. 10-4. Schematic diagram of trocar placements for laparoscopic staging of intraabdominal malignancy. A 10- to 12-mm port is placed at the umbilicus and right lower quadrant, as well as a 5-mm port in the right subcostal area. Video laparoscope and laparoscopic ultrasound probe are used interchangeably between the right lower quadrant and umbilical ports. Probes, biopsy forceps, and graspers are used during the procedure through the 5-mm subcostal port. (A, 5-mm for probe, biopsy, forceps, grasper; B/C, 10- to 12-mm for videolaparoscope, laparoscope ultrasound probe.)

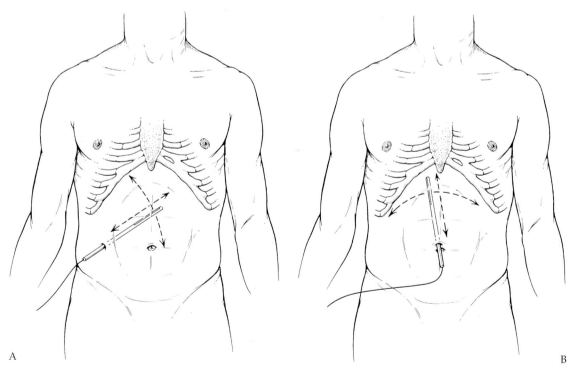

A   B

Fig. 10-5. The laparoscopic ultrasound probe is used to scan the retroperitoneal and surface parenchymal structures during laparoscopic staging. By interchanging it between the right lower quadrant (A) and the umbilical (B) ports, essentially all planes of the abdomen and especially the upper abdomen can be effectively scanned. (From Murugiah M, Paterson-Brown S, Windsor JA, Miles WFA, Garden OJ. Early experience of laparoscopic ultrasonography in the management of pancreatic carcinoma. Surg Endosc 1993;7:177–181; with permission.)

tion. Next, a 10-mm trocar is inserted under direct vision in the subxiphoid region, and a 5-mm trocar is inserted in the right anterior axillary line 2 to 3 cm below the costal margin to aid in retraction of the liver. The laparoscopic US probe is inserted through the subxiphoid port, and the superior aspect of the liver parenchyma is imaged to assess occult hepatic metastases. A retractor can then be inserted through the 5-mm port to elevate the liver superiorly to gain access to the inferior aspect of the liver including the caudate lobe. While more challenging, this area may also be imaged with the US transducer. This technique allows a nearly complete visualization of the hepatic parenchyma to exclude metastatic disease. Small metastases within the liver parenchyma can be biopsied percutaneously under laparoscopic US guidance. While certain US features may be suggestive of malignancy, no US images can confirm malignant versus benign hepatic parenchymal disease. In these situations, US-guided percutaneous biopsy is required.

After adequate examination of the peritoneal cavity and the liver parenchyma, attention is next turned to evaluating the celiac lymph nodes. A second 5-mm trocar is inserted into the left midclavicular line 3 to 4 cm below the costal margin. The lesser omentum is divided hemostatically, and the lesser curvature of the stomach is retracted laterally to the patient's left. The celiac nodes are then readily visualized adjacent to the pulsatile aorta and may be biopsied.

The intraabdominal evaluation of metastatic disease may be combined with thoracoscopy to evaluate the mediastinum for metastatic esophageal cancer. A recent study showed that minimally invasive surgical staging of esophageal cancer provides a more accurate way of assessing the extent of disease at both the primary site and lymph nodes. In fact, a multiinstitutional trial is being developed to evaluate this approach further.

Gastric Cancer

Laparoscopy has also been shown to be a valuable staging modality in gastric carcinoma, reducing the need for exploratory laparotomy. Laparoscopic staging may be considered prior to gastric resection in patients without radiologic evidence of metastatic disease (Fig. 10-6). Once again, the laparoscope is inserted through the infraumbilical Hasson trocar, and a thorough exploration of the abdominal cavity is conducted. Gastric cancer also seeds the peritoneum, hepatic surface, and omentum with occult nodules. Malignant as-

cites is also not uncommon. These findings preclude resection for cure and underscore the value of staging laparoscopy. The laparoscopic US probe is then inserted through a 10-mm subxiphoid trocar, and the superior and inferior surfaces of the liver including the caudate lobe are imaged. Any suspicious hepatic parenchymal metastases are biopsied. Node-bearing areas around the stomach may also be evaluated and biopsied as necessary. The more difficult regions to approach laparoscopically are those posterior nodal basins surrounding the stomach and pancreas and nodal basins in the retroperitoneum. Current techniques of gastric resection often include extended *en bloc* lymphadenectomies. Therefore, any search for occult lymphatic tumor spread should not delay attempts at resection. It is critical to review conventional preoperative staging studies prior to beginning a dissection of any node-bearing areas.

Solid tumors of the gastrointestinal tract may have early and significant nodal spread that may make conventional attempts at resection inappropriate in some patients. In these patients, assessment of nodal metastases is especially well suited to laparoscopic approaches. Operative and nonoperative palliative measures can be utilized in selected patients with esophageal or gastric carcinoma. Laparoscopy is almost twice as sensitive in assessing nodal involvement as conventional US and CT. In this regard, careful staging laparoscopy may detect nodal disease more thoroughly than conventional imaging modalities.

Hepatobiliary Cancer

The laparoscopic staging of hepatic and biliary tract malignancies has been extensively evaluated in recent years. The resectability of a focal liver tumor depends on size, location within the liver, relationship to major blood vessels, and the presence and location of additional tumor deposits. Extrahepatic tumor precludes resection. CT scan staging of hepatic malignancies fails to recognize extrahepatic tumor dissemination or bilobar disease in at least 8% to 16% of patients. Staging laparoscopy accurately identifies small metastases and is sensitive for staging both primary hepatocellular carcinoma and secondary metastatic tumors to the liver (Fig. 10-7). In addition to identifying bilobar or extrahepatic disease, staging

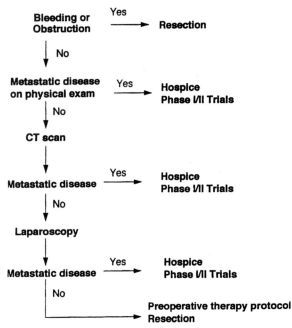

Fig. 10-6. Algorithm indicating the use of laparoscopy in the staging of gastric cancer. (From Lowry AM, Mansfield PF, Leach SD, Ajani J. Laparoscopic staging for gastric cancer. Surgery 1996;119:611–614; with permission.)

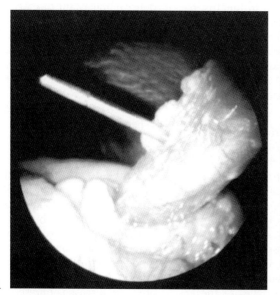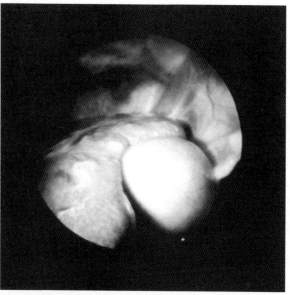

A   B

Fig. 10-7. **A:** *The round and falciform ligaments and the medial right hepatic lobe surfaces are covered with many small metastases from a gastric carcinoma. Metastases on the anterior gastric wall are shown just below the round ligament (bottom, center). All staging studies before laparoscopy, including computed tomography, indicated that disease was limited to the stomach. This laparoscopic diagnosis prevented an unnecessary laparotomy.* **B:** *The right hepatic lobe has a dark lobular pattern indicative of severe cholestasis. The gallbladder is distended and tense as a result of common bile duct obstruction; this is know as Courvoisier's sign. Along the medial margin of the right hepatic lobe are many 2- to 3-mm diameter metastases from pancreatic carcinoma, which were not detected by imaging studies before laparoscopy. Laparotomy was avoided, and an endoscopically placed biliary stent provided relief of bile duct obstruction. (From Yamada T, Alpers DH, Owyang C, Powell DW, Silverstein FE.* Textbook of gastroenterology, *2nd ed. Philadephia: JB Lippincott Co, 1995; with permission.)*

laparoscopy accurately evaluates cirrhosis, which, when present, determines operability for some patients. For example, some patients with primary hepatocellular carcinoma are deemed inoperable, based on advanced cirrhosis, unanticipated bilobar lesions, and porta hepatis lymphadenopathy identified using staging laparoscopy.

The laparoscopic technique used to adequately examine the peritoneal cavity and hepatic parenchyma has already been described. A systematic laparoscopic exploration involves visualizing the entire abdominal cavity, including the pelvis, bilateral pericolic gutters, and cul-de-sac. Both the right and left lobes of the liver must be inspected to assess resectability and identify any unsuspected metastatic seeding or satellite lesions. The peritoneal undersurfaces of the diaphragm and the edges of the liver are closely scrutinized for evidence of metastatic disease. The omentum is inspected. Biopsy specimens should be obtained for any suspicious lesions that might preclude resectability. Improved access to the gallbladder and porta hepatis may be obtained by lateral and su-

perior retraction of the right lobe of the liver using today's versatile endosurgical retractor instruments. The falciform ligament can also be used as an upward anchoring structure for the liver. The left triangular ligament is readily divided laparoscopically using electrocautery endoshears, and often aids in visualizing the left lateral segments of the liver.

There are important technical caveats to the laparoscopic staging of hepatic tumors. Many patients are evaluated following prior abdominal operations, typically for colorectal carcinoma that has metastasized to the liver. In addition to an open technique of trocar insertion, the laparoscopist must perform a meticulous laparoscopic lysis of adhesions. This is necessary to allow visualization of areas most likely to preclude resection, including the parietal peritoneum, liver edge, and omentum. When preoperative staging studies suggest tumors in the dome of the liver, laparoscopy enables the surgeon to determine whether or not there is gross invasion of the diaphragmatic surface. Finally, laparoscopy helps determine the extent of cirrhosis and the presence of dangerous intraab-

dominal varices due to portal hypertension. These critical findings contribute to the safety of planned resections and rarely are as evident on preoperative staging studies.

Laparoscopic liver biopsy is now routinely used by laparoscopic hepatobiliary surgeons. It compares favorably to other approaches of obtaining hepatic tissue. It not only provides direct visualization with an increased accuracy in obtaining abnormal tissue but also allows laparoscopic evaluation of the entire abdomen. Additionally, laparoscopy-guided liver biopsy is superior to blind percutaneous biopsy. The false-negative rate of blind percutaneous biopsy (24%) far exceeds laparoscopy-guided liver biopsy (9%). Finally, laparoscopy offers the opportunity to assess and control bleeding with cautery, laser, or the application of thrombostatic agents.

Hepatic US is commonly utilized to assess tumor extent and vascular involvement at open laparotomy. It is considered superior to manual palpation of the liver. Today, laparoscopic US complements staging laparoscopy by similarly defining intraparenchymal tumors of the liver, as well as vascular pathology such as portal vein thrombosis. Laparoscopic US provides additional staging information beyond that obtained by laparoscopy alone in many patients, and resectability rates are higher in patients who undergo both staging laparoscopy and laparoscopic US. Extrahepatic porta hepatic lymphadenopathy can be identified by laparoscopic US and targeted biopsies performed. When findings are positive, hepatic parenchymal resection offers no chance for cure. In patients with cirrhosis and primary hepatocellular cancer, laparoscopic US identifies the proximity of tumor to major vascular structures that may curtail attempts at resection on the basis of safety and hepatic functional reserve. Laparoscopic evaluation can be performed immediately prior to opening the abdomen and attempting resection.

In gallbladder cancer or primary cholangiocarcinoma, a precise image of the primary lesion, extent of local invasion, and nodal and vascular involvement may be obtained by combining staging laparoscopy with laparoscopic US. In these circumstances, it is important to retract the right lobe of the liver superiorly and laterally to the right. The duodenum, stomach, hepatic flexure of the colon, and omentum should be retracted inferiorly using laparoscopic fan retractors. This exposure brings the gallbladder and extrahepatic biliary tree into clear view and also facilitates biopsy. As always, the entire abdominal cavity should be visually inspected for occult metastases.

The laparoscopic staging of hepatic and biliary tract malignancies should be considered for all patients without radiologic evidence of metastatic disease and prior to attempt at curative resection. For these particular types of intraabdominal malignancies, laparoscopic evaluation helps considerably in avoiding unnecessary laparotomy and futile, dangerous attempts at resection.

Pancreatic Cancer

Staging laparoscopy, in our opinion, should always be performed for patients with pancreatic malignancy and without radiologic evidence of metastatic disease. This is especially true since palliation of jaundice and gastric outlet obstruction may be achieved by endoscopic and minimally invasive surgical means. The goal of

laparoscopic diagnosis is to identify patients who have occult cancer metastases noncontiguous from the primary tumor. For these patients, resection cannot be curative. Cytology washings and small amounts of malignant ascites may also prove positive for tumor cells and preclude resection.

The technique for laparoscopic staging of pancreatic cancer also begins with the general exploration of the abdomen. Initially, 5-mm trocars and instruments are positioned in upper abdominal locations. Intraabdominal adhesions should be divided hemostatically as completely as possible. A standard systematic four-quadrant video laparoscopic exploration is performed using the 5-mm instruments for both exposure and biopsy. Specifically, the peritoneal undersurfaces of the abdominal wall and diaphragm, as well as the anterior, lateral, and inferior peritoneal surfaces of the liver, are examined for evidence of occult metastatic disease. The omentum is examined and retracted superiorly, whenever possible, to evaluate the base of the transverse mesocolon. Laparoscopic cup forceps are excellent devices for biopsying suspicious firm peritoneal or liver metastases. Cytologic washings can be performed using 10 to 15 mL of saline and, when positive, correlate with both unresectability and limited survival. Usually, a preoperative CT scan will have been performed. The laparoscopist may correlate the findings with how mobile the tumor feels using the 5-mm instruments. The lesser sac is entered by dividing the gastrohepatic omentum, and evidence of multifocal pancreatic cancer, extrapancreatic spread, and bulky lymphadenopathy is sought.

When there is no evidence for inoperability, laparoscopic US should next be performed. Usually, a second 10-mm trocar is placed in the right midclavicular line at the level of the umbilicus. We utilize a linear-array laparoscopic US probe equipped with US Doppler flow imaging. This enables us to discriminate arterial and venous structures from each other and nonvascular structures. The US probe and laparoscope can be exchanged between the right lower quadrant port and the umbilical Hasson trocar to optimize evaluation of the pancreas and neighboring structures (Fig. 10-8).

The liver is systemically scanned at its anterior, lateral, and inferior surfaces for evi-

dence of metastatic disease. This examination has been described. Often, small metastatic lesions of pancreatic cancer can be found on the liver surface itself and along the triangular and falciform ligaments. Hepatic, peripancreatic, periaortic, and celiac axis lymph nodes are next evaluated visually and by laparoscopic US. When greater than 10 mm in diameter, suspicious lymph nodes are biopsied under laparoscopic guidance.

Next, the duodenum is imaged to assess for tumor invasion. For masses in the pancreatic head, mobilization of the duodenum and pancreatic head is possible laparoscopically according to the Kocher maneuver. Although rare, if tumor extends posteriorly and the avascular plane anterior to the inferior vena cava is obliterated, the disease is unresectable. For pancreatic cancers, laparoscopic US is superb for determining tumor proximity and tumor compression and invasion of the portal and superior mesenteric veins, as well as proximity to the superior mesenteric artery and celiac axis. Access to the body and tail for US can be either by the transgastric route or following opening of the lesser sac.

If a patient is deemed a candidate for curative resection after thorough laparoscopic examination, the procedure is easily converted to formal laparotomy, and resection is attempted. Otherwise, the procedure may be modified to minimally invasive palliation or terminated at the surgeon's discretion. Staging laparoscopy with laparoscopic US optimizes patient selection for pancreatic resection with curative intent (Fig. 10-9). Unnecessary laparotomies are avoided, and quality and duration of patient survival improved.

Colorectal Cancer

To date, there are no pressing indications for staging laparoscopy in the evaluation of colonic or rectal malignancies. The techniques may be chosen for selected patients as an aid to the surgeon's deciding on larger resections as opposed to local excisions (small rectal tumors). For example, identifying unsuspected occult peritoneal or liver metastases would argue in favor of limited excisions. Laparoscopy may also play a greater role in the follow-up of patients with colorectal malignancy. This may occur in parallel with the evolution of PET scanning on rises in tumor markers, such as carcinoembryonic antigen (CEA).

Concerns over intraabdominal adhesions have limited the widespread application of staging laparoscopy in these patients. In addition, the evolution of PET for detecting recurrences may ultimately limit the role of diagnostic staging laparoscopy.

Lymphoma

Laparoscopy is being used with increasing frequency for the identification of patients with abdominal involvement from Hodgkin's and non-Hodgkin's lymphomas. Through specific minimally invasive maneuvers, the pathologic staging of a lymphoma is increased in approximately 30% of patients. Laparoscopy combined with sensitive CT scans, lymphangiograms, and percutaneous biopsy techniques has made open laparotomy for staging and management of lymphomas much less common.

In addition to the general laparoscopic evaluation of the abdominal cavity summarized earlier, other techniques are important in the staging of lymphoma. A hepatic wedge biopsy is performed, as well as multiple random bilobar hepatic needle biopsies. Retroperitoneal and iliac lymph node dissections can be performed, and rarely splenectomy as well. The complementary use of laparoscopy and radiologic imaging in visualizing visceral involvement by lymphoma is improving.

While some authors advocate routine biopsy of the spleen using the laparoscope, full and adequate staging may generally be accomplished by sampling the retroperitoneal lymph nodes, hepatic biopsy, and visualization of the abdominal cavity, in association with bone marrow aspiration and biopsy. Laparoscopists must remove sufficient nodal tissue to allow the pathologist not only to make an appropriate diagnosis of lymphoma but also to fully characterize the disease according to B- or T-cell subsets by flow cytometry. Staging lymphomas requires specific histologic and immunochemical pathology techniques that have an impact on appropriate therapy, as well as predicting the natural history of the disease. Preoperatively, the laparoscopist must determine which nodal basins will yield the most sufficient amount of representative nodal tissue. This typically requires 1 to 3 g of tissue; however, this should be determined together with the responsible pathologist. As in an open staging laparotomy, every attempt should be made to

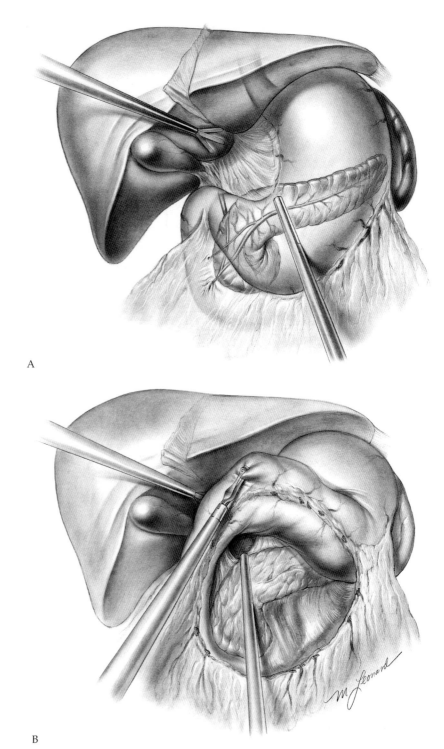

A

B

Fig. 10-8. Laparoscopic ultrasound analysis of the pancreas can be performed either transgastrically (**A**) or by opening the lesser sac and introducing the probe posterior to the stomach (**B**). This allows direct contact with the pancreatic body. The pancreatic head is usually imaged transversely and along the axis of the porta hepatis/portal vein/superior mesenteric vein junction.

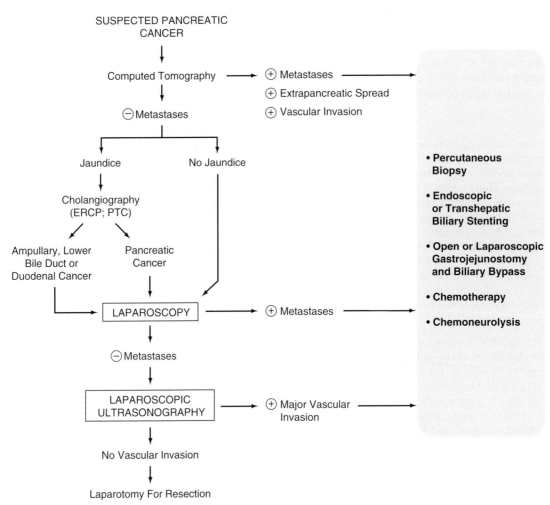

Fig. 10-9. *Role of staging laparoscopy in the management of pancreatic cancer. Laparoscopy with laparoscopic ultrasonography optimizes patient selection for definitive curative resection. This algorithm indicates the importance of scheduling laparoscopy in the patient selection for palliative care as well. The role of vascular resection, while controversial in pancreatic cancer, is not included in this algorithm.*

sample celiac, paraaortic, and hepatoduodenal ligament lymph nodes to optimize staging.

Gynecologic Cancer

Laparoscopic techniques long ago found utility in the staging of ovarian, endometrial, and cervical carcinomas. For example, in endometrial and cervical carcinomas, pelvic and paraaortic lymph node sampling can identify those with positive lymph nodes who are thereby spared laparotomy and radical hysterectomy. Radiotherapy becomes the primary therapy.

The laparoscopic techniques of pelvic and paraaortic lymph node sampling have been less well established than other minimally invasive techniques. The laparoscope is inserted via a supraumbilical position, and a general exploration of the abdomen is conducted. Smaller instrument ports are inserted in both lower quadrants and the lower abdominal midline. The patient is placed in a steep Trendelenburg position to aid in retraction of the intestine and omentum. Obvious extension of tumor into the adnexa can be discerned. Lymph nodes along the iliac vessels and distal aorta can then be meticulously dissected. Extraperitoneal techniques of lymph node sampling have also been described. In patients with cervical carcinoma, the yields of paraaortic and pelvic lymphadenectomy are generally satisfactory to guide therapy.

Initially, the surgical limits of the dissection must be established: the common iliac artery proximally, the psoas muscle laterally, the circumflex iliac vein and pubic bone distally, the obliterated umbilical artery medially, and the obturator fossa in-feriorly. The actual lymphatic resection begins after the external iliac vessels are separated from the muscle and tissues are mobilized medially. This is usually accomplished by loosely dissecting the areolar and fatty lymphatic tissue using sharp scissors and electrocautery endoshears. Deep arteries and veins should be endoclipped. The surgeon defines a systematic approach to removing all lymph node basins within these anatomic confines.

This laparoscopic pelvic lymphadenectomy may be combined, as indicated, with paraaortic lymphadenectomy. With the sigmoid colon retracted laterally and the small bowel elevated superiorly from the pelvis, the posterior retroperitoneum is opened over the right common iliac artery. The peritoneum is incised with scissors, and using mostly blunt dissection, a plane is developed between the peritoneum and the lymph node-bearing fatty tissue overlying the great vessels in the retroperitoneum. This plane is developed before the lymph nodes themselves are approached. The limits of the dissection are the bifurcation of the aorta inferiorly, the proximal part of the common iliac artery inferolaterally, and the ureters bilaterally. The superior extent of the lymphatic dissection is the third part of the duodenum or the renal vein, depending on anatomy. All lymphatic nodal tissue is removed *en bloc* in as systematic as fashion as possible. A particularly important technical point is that the dissection must be taken down to the adventitia of the aorta. Otherwise, the nodal tissue may be elevated with the small bowel mesentery and missed by the laparoscopist. For both pelvic and paraaortic lymphadenectomy, the tissues can often be removed nicely with spoon forceps through the trocar ports. This enables the laparoscopist not to disturb the architecture, optimizing pathologic lymphatic evaluation. Many feel that laparoscopic pelvic and aortic lymphadenectomy is superior to the counterpart open procedures. Patients recover much faster, and radiation therapy may be started earlier. The best results are for surgeons with advanced laparoscopic abilities who combine the systematic approach to lymphadenectomy with a clear understanding of the anatomic confines of resection.

The utility of staging laparoscopy for ovarian carcinoma lies mainly in second-look evaluation after definitive resection. The techniques are the same as for any general laparoscopic evaluation of the peritoneal cavity. Extra caution and advanced laparoscopic techniques are frequently required to gain access and adequately explore the peritoneal cavity. These patients often have dense adhesions from prior laparotomy and, in some cases, from intraperitoneal administration of chemotherapeutic agents. If there is no obvious evidence of disease, cytologic washings are taken from the pelvis, the bilateral pericolic gutters, and the hemidiaphragmatic recesses. Multiple spot biopsies are taken from all areas of the abdomen, and any residual omentum is removed. When all frozen-section biopsies are negative, the laparoscopist may proceed with paraaortic lymphadenectomy as indicated clinically.

The role of laparoscopy in the evaluation of other types of recurrent gynecologic tumors continues to be defined. Second-look staging procedures are often prompted by rises in tumor markers or CT scan or other imaging findings. These procedures seek to identify and remove residual or recurrent tumor, which will help palliate, if not cure, the patient. As noted, the application of laparoscopy in this setting can be limited because of inability to adequately identify anatomic landmarks or residual tumor due to adhesions from prior abdominal exploration.

Urologic Cancer

Laparoscopy has increasingly been applied to preoperative staging of prostate and bladder carcinomas. This typically involves pelvic and paraaortic lymph node sampling to determine suitability for radical resection. The most accurate test for metastases from the prostatic capsule is the evaluation of lymph nodes. If lymphatic tissues are found positive for metastatic prostate adenocarcinoma during staging pelvic lymphadenectomy, then the treatment changes to purely palliative. Radiation and surgery are associated with significant morbidity and mortality without any hope for cure. Open and laparoscopic pelvic lymphadenectomies have been compared in the staging of prostate cancer. Laparoscopic lymphadenectomy results in a shorter hospital stay and quicker return to normal activities at a cost of longer operating time and slightly higher complication rate early in one's experience. The techniques are quite similar to those for evaluating gynecologic malignancies and involve supraumbilical insertion of the laparoscope and general abdominal exploration.

The patient is placed in a steep Trendelenburg position to aid in bowel retraction. Smaller operative ports are inserted in both lower abdominal quadrants and the lower midline. Obvious extraanatomic extension of the primary tumor can be discerned.

Attention is next turned to lymphatic dissection along the iliac vessels and distal aorta. Extraperitoneal pelvic lymphadenectomy is also possible, should prior abdominal operation preclude transabdominal laparoscopy. By using the techniques described for laparoscopic paraaortic and pelvic lymphadenectomy, most authors agree that as many lymph nodes can be harvested during laparoscopic lymphadenectomy as during open lymphadenectomy—if not more.

Postoperative Care

Postoperative care of any patient following staging laparoscopic abdominal exploration is dictated by the patient's preoperative medical condition. Usually, if patients have a good preoperative performance status, they need only be observed in the hospital overnight. Diet is usually clear liquids, which is advanced as tolerated to a regular diet. Sequential compression devices are removed when patients are ambulatory. The orogastric tube and bladder catheter may be removed in the operating or recovery room. The most common problems encountered postoperatively are nausea and urinary retention, which are usually transient and easily dealt with. Patients can often be discharged on the day following surgery and resume normal activity within 1 week.

Surgical Complications

Most major complications, such as iatrogenic vascular or bowel injuries, should be noted at the time of operation and immediately repaired either laparoscopically or via open laparotomy. Other, delayed complications can occur, such as hernia at trocar sites where the fascia has been inadequately reapproximated. In these regards, staging laparoscopy for intraabdominal malignancy bears the same complication rate as for general laparoscopic procedures. These complications and their rates of occurrence are covered elsewhere in this volume.

Some complications, however, are specific to the procedure itself. For example, abdominal wall metastases, although rare, are a complication of laparoscopy in patients with peritoneal implants or malignant ascites. Subcutaneous abdominal wall implants can occur several months after laparoscopy at trocar sites. This phenomenon is unusual, however, and should not be a deterrent to laparoscopic examination. Management of trocar sites is very important, especially in patients with malignant ascites. Ascites may disseminate cancer and leak into the subcutaneous tissues postoperatively, if careful reapproximation of the fascia is not performed. For patients suffering from a coagulopathy secondary to malignancy, meticulous hemostasis is mandatory intraabdominally and at all trocar sites.

Staging laparoscopy for intraabdominal malignancy should be performed by experienced surgeons. In this regard, not only is the abdominal evaluation properly made from the standpoint of surgical resection, but any adverse occurrence requiring immediate abdominal exploration may be properly managed. The assurance of appropriate surgical training and experience allows for the most thorough diagnostic laparoscopy evaluation and benefits patients in terms of both thoroughness and safety.

Results

General

A plethora of literature substantiates the use of diagnostic laparoscopy for various types of intraabdominal malignancy. Esophageal, gastric, hepatobiliary, and pancreatic cancers and lymphoma all can now be routinely staged effectively with minimally invasive procedures. Gynecologic and urologic malignancies are also being evaluated more often as surgeons master laparoscopic pelvic and paraaortic lymphadenectomy.

Barnes Hospital Experience

The routine implementation of staging laparoscopy with US has recently been analyzed at a major hepatobiliary and pancreatic surgery center. This new staging modality was performed in 50 consecutive patients with hepatobiliary malignancy. All patients were considered to have resectable tumors as determined by traditional preoperative staging modalities. Primary tumors were located in the liver (n=7), biliary tract (n=11), or pancreas (n=32). Preoperative staging studies included CT (96%), alone or combined with antegrade/retrograde cholangiography (72%), arterial portography (22%), and MR imaging (14%). An average of 2.7 preoperative studies per patient were required to initially determine resectability.

Staging laparoscopy with laparoscopic US was performed under the same anesthetic as the subsequent laparotomy (70%) or as a separate staging procedure (30%). Staging laparoscopy with laparoscopic US predicted a resectable tumor in 28 patients (56%). At laparotomy, 26 of 28 patients actually had resectable tumors, indicating a false-negative rate of 4%. These techniques indicated unresectability in 22 patients—again, all considered resectable by traditional staging modalities. Laparoscopy

alone demonstrated previously unrecognized occult metastases in 11 patients (22%). For an additional 11 patients (22%) in whom laparoscopy alone was negative, laparoscopic US determined unresectability as a result of vascular invasion (n=5), lymph node metastases (n=5), or intraparenchymal hepatic tumors (n=1). All cases of unresectability due to vascular invasion were validated by laparotomy. Five of six lymph node or hepatic metastases were proven histologically by US-guided needle biopsy, obviating laparotomy. In this study, staging laparoscopy with laparoscopic US optimized patient selection for curative resection of hepatobiliary malignancy. Unnecessary laparotomy was safely avoided in patients with unresectable disease, reducing costs and morbidity.

Conclusion

Laparoscopy combined with intraoperative laparoscopic US has been demonstrated to be a valuable staging modality for the evaluation of intraabdominal malignancies. Its benefits concern the prevention of a formal laparotomy to assess resectability, thereby decreasing postoperative pain and ensuring a quicker return to normal activities and a shorter hospital stay. It may also diminish the time between determining optimum therapy and receipt of appropriate chemotherapeutic agents or radiotherapy. It may also ultimately be a more economical method of staging many intraabdominal malignancies by avoidance of both unnecessary laparotomies and redundant preoperative staging modalities.

While diagnostic laparoscopy is not a new procedure, to date laparoscopic US with the staging of intraabdominal malignancy has been tested in only the most experienced hands. The relative sensitivity of the combined laparoscopic and laparoscopic US procedures in determining vascular invasion, lymphatic spread, local unresectability, multicentricity, and occult metastases remains to be proven. In these regards, the widespread use of laparoscopic US will await prospective comparisons with traditional imaging modalities. Experienced ultrasonographers should be consulted intraoperatively by surgeons as they study and validate the potential applications of laparoscopic US. However, we now have exciting new staging modalities that continue to evolve and represent an exciting area of minimally invasive surgery.

Suggested Reading

Callery MP, Strasberg SM, Doherty GM, Soper NJ, Norton JA. Staging laparoscopy with laparoscopic ultrasonography: optimizing resectability in hepatobiliary and pancreatic malignancy. *J Am Coll Surg* 1997;185:33–39.

Cuschieri A, Hall AW, Clark J. Value of laparoscopy in the diagnosis and management of pancreatic carcinoma. *Gut* 1978;19:672–677.

Eubanks S. The role of laparoscopy in diagnosis and treatment of primary or metastatic liver cancer. *Semin Surg Oncol* 1994;10:404–410.

Forse RA, Babineau T, Bleday R, Steele G Jr. Laparoscopy/thoracoscopy for staging: I. Staging endoscopy in surgical oncology. *Semin Surg Oncol* 1993;9:51–55.

John TG, Greig JD, Carter DC, Garden OJ. Carcinoma of the pancreatic head and periampullary region: tumor staging with laparoscopy and laparoscopic ultrasonography. *Ann Surg* 1995;221:156–164.

John TG, Greig JD, Crosbie JL, Miles WFA, Garden OJ. Superior staging of liver tumors with laparoscopy and laparoscopic ultrasound. *Ann Surg* 1994;220:711–719.

Kelling G. Ueber Oesophagoskopie, Gastrokopie und Kölioskopie. *Munch Med Wochenschr* 1902;1:21–24.

Lightdale CJ. Laparoscopy for cancer staging. *Endoscopy* 1992;24:682–686.

Warshaw AL. Implications of peritoneal cytology for staging of early pancreatic cancer. *Am J Surg* 1991;161:26–29.

EDITOR'S COMMENT

The exact role of laparoscopy and laparoscopic US for staging of intraabdominal malignancy has not been determined by randomized prospective trials and is therefore controversial at the current time. Much experience with these techniques has been accrued over the last few years, occurring at the same time that advances have been made in conventional radiographic techniques (spiral or thin-cut CT scans), MR imaging (MR cholangiograms), PET (for various abdominal tumors), nuclear medicine imaging (somatostatin scans for endocrine tumors, CEA scans for colorectal cancers), and improvements in and increasing experience with endoscopic US. Obviously, technologic advancements and evolving techniques do not remain static for the convenience of assessment.

The role of laparoscopic staging will vary, depending on the individual's use of the findings gained from the examination. For instance, if one's bias is that conventional biliary and gastric bypass are the best means of managing unresectable pancreatic cancer, the utility of laparoscopy and laparoscopic US for determining resectability does not make sense. Certainly, for the assessment of hepatobiliary and pancreatic malignancies, our approach has changed dramatically over the last few years, as we have gained experience with laparoscopic staging. For patients with painless jaundice, a high-quality CT scan is performed to assess for obvious evidence of unresectability. If this is not found, we proceed directly to laparoscopy with laparoscopic US to make the tissue diagnosis and assess for resectability. Using these modalities, only patients with a high likelihood of undergoing a Whipple operation are subjected to laparotomy, whereas patients with unresectable disease undergo either laparoscopic bypass or endoscopic stent placement. We have had less experience with laparoscopic staging of esophageal and gastric malignancies, but the utility of these approaches has been well documented in this chapter. We look forward to well designed prospective, randomized trials over the next few years to guide the rational use of laparoscopy for patients with suspected intraabdominal malignancy.

N.J.S.

11

Flexible Endoscopic Ultrasonography

Toshiyuki Mori and Yutaka Atomi

Endoscopic ultrasonography (EUS) is an invaluable diagnostic tool in the management of gastrointestinal (GI) tract and pancreaticobiliary disorders. First, EUS is the only practical imaging method currently available for displaying a cross-sectional view of the gut wall and surrounding structures. Second, EUS employs higher-frequency US (i.e., 7.5, 12, 15, and 20 MHz), compared with conventional extracorporeal ultrasonography (US) (i.e., 3.5, 5, and 7.5 MHz). In general, the higher the frequency of US used, the more image resolution increases and depth of penetration decreases. It is therefore especially useful when a lesion is in close proximity to the gut wall. In the diagnosis of GI tract cancers, EUS can clearly display the depth of invasion of malignant tumors. In the era of minimally invasive surgery, this capability is of great importance because local excision or other less invasive management by minimally invasive surgery for early cancers can be justified by this information without any compromise of cure. Other examples include lesions in the head of the pancreas, which are best imaged by EUS from the duodenum, and findings can sometimes be definitively diagnostic. Since the area being imaged by high-frequency US is small, it is useful when a relatively small area is concerned. Thus, EUS is not suitable for screening purposes. The aim of this chapter is to provide an overview EUS technology, technical tips for use of EUS, and image interpretation.

Instrumentation

Several types of US probes are currently available. A standard EUS system is a transducer attached to a conventional endoscope. Mechanically rotating (360 degree) or linear-array (90 to 180 degree) transducers with or without Doppler capabilities are on the market and/or under clinical investigation. Also available are US transducers incorporated into the tip of small-diameter, flexible, nonguided plastic catheters. They are used either freely or through the working channel of a standard flexible endoscope (i.e., miniature probes). Other EUS probes include a nonoptic endoscopic linear probe, a mechanical rotating probe, and an intraductal imaging catheter. These probes have an advantage over earlier types of probes only on specific occasions. Currently, an EUS probe with the capability of aspiration biopsy under US observation is also available.

Standard Endoscopic Ultrasonography System

The first commercially available instrument was the Olympus EU-M3 system (Olympus America Inc., Melville, NY). This dedicated system consists of a console that contains the US controls, display, and imaging unit. Endoscopes are connected to this unit. The GF-EUM3 endoscope is a side-viewing endoscope with a 1.3-cm diameter transducer attached to its tip. A balloon attached to the transducer can be filled with water through a special port. This instrument provides a 360-degree field of view orthogonal to the long axis of the scope. Both 7.5- and 12-MHz images can be obtained; the frequencies are switched from a console control and do not require removing the instrument. Depth of field is a maximum of 7-cm radius at 7.5 MHz and 3-cm radius at 12 MHz. The axial resolution is 0.2 mm for the 7.5 MHz and 0.12 mm for the 12 MHz instrument. This resolution is usually sufficient to image the gut wall and surrounding lymphatic drainage areas. Also available at this time are the GF-UM20, JF-UM20, and CF-UM20. The GF-UM20 has forward oblique–viewing optics (45 degree) and a slightly smaller transducer (Fig. 11-1). The JF-UM20 has side-viewing optics and is especially useful for the diagnosis of the pancreaticobiliary region from the duodenum. The CF-UM20 has forward-viewing optics and is slightly thicker, designed for use in the colon. These systems acquire digitized information, allowing processing and postprocessing of images.

Miniature Probe

Miniature probes are available from several companies (Fig. 11-2). The US system consists of an US probe and an US generator, processor, and display. A small US transducer with a frequency of either 15 or 20 MHz is incorporated in the side of the probe tip. Dimensions of these probes are 8 French for 15 MHz and 6 French for 20 MHz; they are 192 cm in length. The probe is inserted into a sheath filled with water to eliminate air that could interfere with transmission of the US beam and is rotated at a speed of 900 rpm. A standard forward-viewing gastroendoscope has a working channel 2.8 mm in diameter. Through this channel, probes with a sheath can be passed down to reach the area of concern. A 360-degree real-time image is generated orthogonal to the probe.

Gastrointestinal Tract

EUS is the only method that can display a cross-sectional view of the gut wall; thus, it is the only method that can display the origin and the nature of submucosal tumors of a wide variety. In the management of GI tract cancer, EUS is invaluable for obtaining locoregional information, including depth of invasion, lymph node involvement, and direct invasion of adjacent organs. If a tumor is superficial enough to predict no or only local lymph node involvement by accumulated oncologic data, local excision or less invasive treatment may be the method of choice. In advanced cancer, EUS is useful in staging, avoiding unnecessary exploratory thoracolaparotomy.

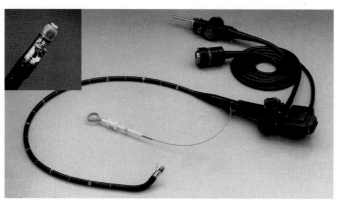

Fig. 11-1. The Olympus GF-UM20 ultrasonic endoscope. The transducer at the tip of the instrument is mechanically rotated by a cable connected to an electric motor in the handle, producing a 360-degree image orthogonal to the instrument axis. A button in the handle can switch from 7.5- to 12-MHz ultrasound.

Normal Gut Wall Structure

The frequencies employed in EUS typically display the gut wall as a structure composed of layers (Fig. 11-3). The image of the normal gut wall obtained with conventional EUS comprises five or seven layers. The reflected echo nearest the transducer is named the first, and that farthest from the transducer the fifth or seventh. The derivation of the sonographic image of the gut wall is relatively complex. Fortunately, it turns out that for practical purposes the first (echogenic) layer and the second (echo-poor) layer correspond to the interface echo and the mucosa. The third (echogenic) layer corresponds to the submucosa. The fourth (echo-poor), fifth (echogenic), and sixth (echo-poor) layers correspond to the muscularis propria, with the fifth layer representing the interface echo and connective tissue between the inner circular muscle (fourth layer) and the outer longitudinal muscle (sixth layer). The seventh (echogenic) layer corresponds to the subserosa and serosa or adventitia. When the muscularis propria is not separated into three layers, the entire gut wall displays five layers. When optimum resolution is obtained with a high-frequency US probe, thin echogenic and echo-poor layers are seen on the submucosal layer, corresponding to the interface echo and the lamina muscularis mucosae. In such cases, the gut wall displays nine layers in all.

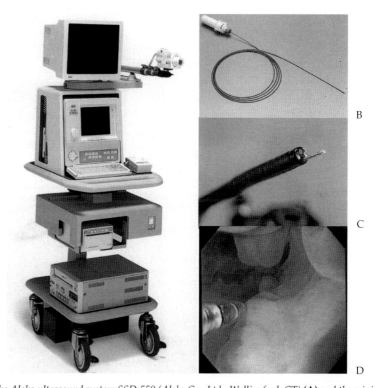

Fig. 11-2. The Aloka ultrasound system SSD-550 (Aloka Co., Ltd., Wallingford, CT) **(A)** and the miniature probe MP-PN15 **(B)**. **C:** The probe can be inserted through the channel of an endoscope. **D:** The lumen of the gut is usually filled with water and the probe is placed on the lesion of concern under endoscopic observation.

Staging

Tumor (T) Stage

Using the usual five-layer pattern of the gut wall seen at 7.5 to 12 MHz, EUS divides the tumor into four stages, matching the tumor-node-metastasis (TNM) classification (Fig. 11-4):

uT1	Tumor without disruption of the middle echo-rich layer
uT2	Tumor disrupting the middle layer
uT3	Tumor disrupting the outer echo-rich layer
uT4	Tumor invading adjacent organs

Node (N) Stage

In most studies, patients are staged as N0 or N1 according to the presence or absence of metastatic nodes. EUS criteria for evaluating lymph nodes include size, shape, margins, echo density, and homogeneity.

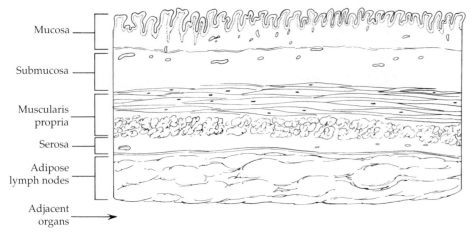

Fig. 11-3. *Layers of the gut wall. Thickness of each layer varies by sites. Note that a thin echogenic layer can be seen in the fourth (hypoechoic) layer. [Mucosa (first high-echoic and second low-echoic layers); submucosa (the third echo-rich layer); muscularis propria (the fourth echo-rich layer); serosa or adventitia (the fifth high-echoic layer); adipose tissue (high echoic); lymph nodes (low echoic).]*

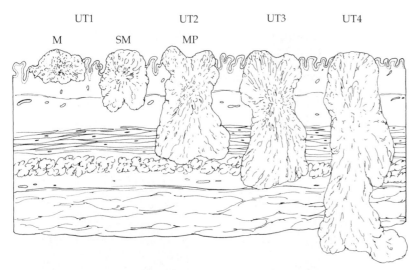

Fig. 11-4. *It is important to distinguish tumors invading only the mucosa from those invading the submucosa, which can be achieved by EUS more accurately than any other imaging modality.*

EUS interpretation of lymph nodes, however, is quite subjective (Fig. 11-5).

Several studies have compared the uTNM (ultrasound) and pTNM (pathology) staging after esophageal resection. High accuracy is found for all T stages, the most difficult to recognize being T2. Studies evaluating nodes site by site are difficult to perform, as correspondence between nodes seen at EUS and at pathology is hard to ascertain. On the whole, EUS accuracy for N-staging is somewhat lower than for T-staging, and is higher in pN1 than pN0 patients. Metastatic lymph nodes must be searched for in uT1 tumors, where they are infrequent but affect the prognosis. EUS accuracy is as low as 50% in this

indication due to the poor visualization of very small lymph nodes, the small area of invasion in visualized nodes, or both.

Submucosal Tumors

The term *submucosal lesion* is used to describe any lesion protruding into the lumen of the gut and covered by normal-appearing mucosa. These lesions include a wide variety of tumors, including those arising in the submucosa or within the muscularis propria. These lesions include even external compression. EUS has shown that the appearance of submucosal lesion has many possible causes, thus ex-

panding and refining knowledge of these lesions. Yasuda and colleagues (1990) described EUS findings in a large series of submucosal tumors (n=308). Cysts are imaged as echo-free structures in the submucosa or as extrinsic impressions. Leiomyoma and leiomyosarcoma are described as hypoechoic structures arising from the fourth (hypoechoic) layer (Fig. 11-6), corresponding to the muscularis propria. Improvement is needed in the definition of these widely various lesions by EUS.

Distinguishing leiomyosarcoma from leiomyoma by EUS can be problematic. Previously, the most important clinical criterion for malignancy was size; that is, the larger the lesion, the more likely it is malignant. Researchers have reported distinguishing features of leiomyosarcomas. On EUS, these tumors appear as a nonhomogeneous, hypoechoic mass that is relatively large and has sharply demarcated or irregular margins; occasionally, there is a central ulcer or fistulous tract. In contrast to the pattern of benign tumors, these sarcomas destroy the sonographic layers of the wall and may exhibit irregularly shaped sonolucent areas corresponding to liquefaction necrosis, indicative of leiomyosarcoma. These distinctive findings are seen only in large tumors; there are no distinctive EUS findings for small leiomyosarcomas. The only reliable sign of malignancy rests on the biologic behavior of the tumor (invasion of adjacent organs or distant metastases). In this regard, careful follow-up or, occasionally, surgical resection will be needed until a method is available for obtaining a biopsy specimen for histologic evaluation (i.e., EUS-guided needle biopsy).

Esophageal Cancer

Although comparative studies have shown that EUS is more accurate than computed tomography (CT) for N- and T-staging of esophageal carcinoma, EUS is indicated when locoregional staging may alter the treatment options. Patients with esophageal cancer can be grossly divided into three groups (Fig. 11-7):

Group 1 includes patients with metastases, evident invasion of adjacent organs, or very poor status (20%) for whom a cure is impossible and only palliative treatment is indicated. CT and US provide enough information, and EUS is of little interest.

Group 2 includes patients with large tumors at endoscopy, no clear invasion of adjacent organs, and no metastases (70% to 75%). These patients are suitable for surgery or aggressive medical treatment. Cure is highly improbable, but long-term survival can be improved, with a good quality of life. EUS provides more information than CT for staging, but CT remains the primary examination due to its ability to detect metastases. Notably, EUS can provide information on celiac lymph nodes (M stage) or intraluminal lymphatic metastases. If more accurate staging could alter the treatment option, EUS is mandatory.

Group 3 includes patients with small tumors with superficial patterns at endoscopy (5% to 10%) who have the best chance for cure. EUS is highly accurate in distinguishing T1 from more invasive carcinomas that are treated in the same way as those in group 2. Recent studies have shown that T1 tumors contain heterogeneous groups with regard to N status. The risk of nodal metastases increases from 0% in epithelial cancer to 50% when the tumor invades the entire thickness of the submucosa. It is therefore necessary to differentiate tumors invading only the mucosa (i.e., mucosal cancer) from those invading the submucosa (i.e., submucosal cancer). Fortunately, high-frequency US probes (15 and 20 MHz) allow a distinction between mucosal and submucosal tumors. In patients with esophageal cancer invading the submucosa, operative therapy is potentially curative, if general medical status allows surgery. Patients with mucosal tumors can be treated nonsurgically without any compromise of cure.

Gastric Cancer

It is practically impossible to distinguish malignant from benign gastric lesions, including ulcer and polyp, based on EUS images alone (Fig. 11-8). The differential diagnosis should be made by ordinary endoscopy and biopsy. Although EUS can classify gastric cancer into four stages, precise uT classification is of less importance for several reasons. First, endoscopic findings alone can provide information on the depth of invasion as accurately as EUS. Second, stage T1 includes both mucosal and submucosal cancers. In mucosal cancers, lymph node metastases are extremely

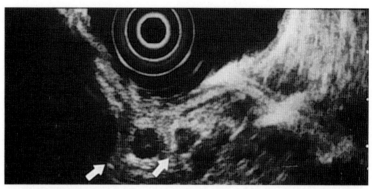

Fig. 11-5. *Although interpretation is quite subjective, EUS can detect lymph node swelling. Note low-echoic, round lesions outside the gastric wall. Metastases were ascertained by pathologic examination of the resected specimen.*

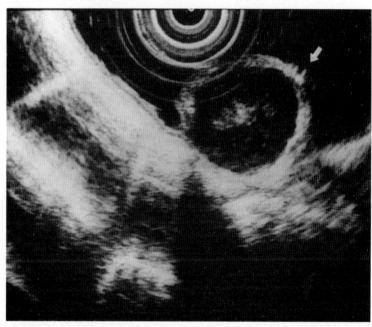

Fig. 11-6. *Leiomyosarcoma of the stomach. A round-shaped, low-echoic tumor is observed that is continuous with the muscularis propria. Internal echo of the tumor is inhomogeneous.*

rare, and endoscopic therapy is often indicated. In submucosal cancers, local lymph node involvement is common, and standard surgery is indicated if general status allows. Differentiation between mucosal and submucosal cancers is thus a critical problem, and EUS is the only modality that can make the differential diagnosis. If cancer is located near a peptic ulcer or its scar, classification of the lesion, as described above, is difficult to make. The major factor complicating the diagnosis of invasive cancer is the influence of peptic ulceration; the layered structure of the wall is modified by ulcerative changes. In addition, fibrous proliferation during the process of ulcer healing cannot be distinguished by EUS from fibrous proliferation

accompanying invasive cancer. The presence of inflammatory cell infiltration also complicates the diagnosis of invasion. If a peptic ulcer near a tumor looks to be confined to the mucosa, it may be safer to regard it as submucosal or more advanced.

EUS is capable of detecting lymph node involvement along the lesser and greater curvatures of the stomach and around the celiac axis. It is, however, of little importance in the management of gastric cancer because these lymph nodes would usually be dissected in a standard operation for advanced gastric cancer regardless of the EUS findings. Palliative gastrectomy may be indicated when lymph node involvement is found in a distant area, such as the

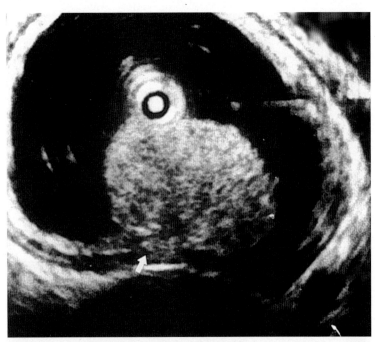

Fig. 11-7. Esophageal cancer (stage uT2). Note that the tumor is disrupting the middle echo-rich layer (arrow).

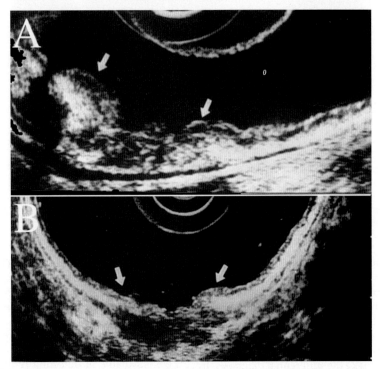

Fig. 11-8. **A:** Early gastric cancer. Note that the low-echoic tumor is invading the submucosa. The continuity of the third echo-rich layer is not disrupted. **B:** Advanced gastric cancer. The continuity of this layer is disrupted in the middle of the lesion, spreading into the fourth and fifth layers.

paraaortic region or hepatoduodenal ligament, that is out of reach of EUS detection. CT can provide more information in this regard.

In this era of minimally invasive surgery, EUS is potentially of great importance in the management of early gastric cancer. As mentioned, EUS is capable of accurately distinguishing mucosal from submucosal lesions, and for mucosal tumors less invasive treatment, such as endoscopic mucosal resection or laparoscopic local excision of the gastric wall, may be offered. However, more clinical parameters must be considered in this regard. Examples include the shape and maximum diameters of the lesion and the degree of differentiation of cancer cells. In general, the larger the lesion is, the more frequently lymph node involvement occurs. Depressed-type cancer is more likely to be associated with metastatic lymph nodes than the protruded-type if size is similar. Cancers composed of poorly differentiated cells (e.g., poorly differentiated adenocarcinoma, signet ring cell and mucinous cancers) tend to have microscopic submucosal invasion, compared to tumors with well differentiated cells (e.g., papillary and tubular adenocarcinomas), even if the EUS diagnosis is a mucosal lesion. Accumulated oncologic data from Japan show that, for well differentiated mucosal gastric cancers, local resection is the treatment of choice, without any compromise of cure, if a depressed-type lesion is less than 15 mm in diameter or a protruded-type lesions is less than 20 mm in diameter.

Colorectal Cancer

As in the management of gastric cancer, EUS is of value only in regard to whether or not less invasive treatments are curative of colonic cancer. EUS can differentiate mucosal from submucosal tumors more accurately than standard colonoscopy. Patients with mucosal cancer often have no lymph node involvement, and endoscopic mucosal resection may therefore be indicated for relatively small (less than 20 mm in maximum diameter) mucosal cancers. In addition, reports indicate that further classification by EUS of submucosal tumors into moderate submucosal and massive submucosal may be of value. Colonic cancers invading less than halfway through the submucosal layer have about a 10% chance of local lymph node metastases along the long axis of the colon, never exceeding 5 cm from the lesion (Fig. 11-9). Laparoscopic local colonic resection should be sufficiently curative of these tumors, since local lymph nodes would also be removed together with the colon if the 5-cm surgical margin, both oral and anal, is kept. Since colonic cancers invading more than halfway through the submucosal layer may accompany more extensive lymph node metastases, standard surgery should be performed to improve patients' survival.

Pancreaticobiliary Disorders

EUS of the pancreas is performed from the second and third portions of the duodenum distally to the gastric body proximally. The pancreas head is in immediate contact with the duodenal sweep, allowing visualization of the head and uncinate process. The body and tail of the pancreas are in close relation to the gastric body and fundus, which are readily visualized using the water-filled stomach as an acoustic window. Relationships are somewhat confusing in this area because the transducer undergoes multiple changes in the plane of orientation. In some cases, the image may be reversed. It is therefore important to be aware of these relationships at all levels.

In the head of the pancreas, the most important relationship is the junction of the common bile duct and the pancreatic duct. This relationship defines the ampullary region. At the junction of the head and body of the pancreas, defining the medial aspect of the uncinate process, is the junction of the splenic and superior mesenteric veins. The body and tail of the pancreas are readily visualized through the greater curvature of the stomach. The pancreatic duct can be reproducibly seen and measures approximately 1 mm at the level of the body of the pancreas. As the common bile duct and the gallbladder are in close proximity to the bulb and the second portion of the duodenum, they are usually well displayed by a scan from the duodenum.

Pancreatic Cancer

Primary Diagnosis

Data on sensitivity and specificity of EUS in the primary diagnosis of pancreatic tumors show high accuracy rates in the detection or exclusion of a pancreatic mass lesion. In this regard, EUS is superior to US

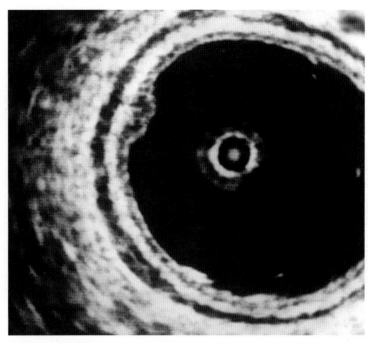

Fig. 11-9. Mucosal cancer of the sigmoid colon. Note that the third layer is intact. This tumor was removed by endoscopic mucosal resection. The preoperative diagnosis of invasion depth was confirmed by pathologic examination of the specimen.

and CT and equal or superior to endoscopic retrograde cholangiopancreatography (ERCP) (Fig. 11-10). This is especially true for smaller lesions. EUS, however, would not contribute to improving the early detection and prognosis of patients with pancreatic cancer, since it is not a first-line procedure in the diagnosis of pancreatic carcinoma and at present cannot be used as a screening procedure. It has also been shown that in the primary diagnosis of pancreatic tumors, a combined evaluation of US, CT, and ERCP is of similarly high diagnostic sensitivity as EUS. At present, an established role for EUS in the primary diagnosis of pancreatic cancer is only complementary to ERCP in those smaller pancreatic carcinomas with ductal signs on ERCP but without tumor visualization on US and CT.

Differential Diagnosis

In the differential diagnosis of a given pancreatic or ampullary tumor, EUS is much less reliable in distinguishing malignant from inflammatory lesions. Earlier reports listed features distinguishing malignant tumors from inflammatory change; for example, echo-poor masses with irregular borders are malignant. Later, larger series, however, showed EUS to be only 67% accurate. Analysis of the echo patterns of

these patients did not reveal any significant differences between malignancy and focal chronic pancreatitis.

Staging

Local staging of pancreatic cancer involves assessment of tumor size and spread into parapancreatic structures, mainly large vessels, and prediction of the T and N stages. Resectability can be deduced from these parameters. In several studies using surgical exploration and/or angiography as the gold standard, EUS was shown to be highly accurate in the detection of portal venous involvement and in the prediction of the T and N stages, but less reliable in determining arterial invasion than angiography. Resectability can thus be correctly predicted in more than 80% of patients. Detection of distant metastasis is not possible using the EUS due to its limited penetration depth, and therefore US, CT, or laparoscopic examination are necessary to diagnose distant tumor spreading. EUS should only be applied for locoregional staging in those patients who are fit for surgery and have no evidence of distant metastases. It could replace angiography in the assessment of the portal venous system. EUS might save some of these patients from unnecessary explorative laparotomy.

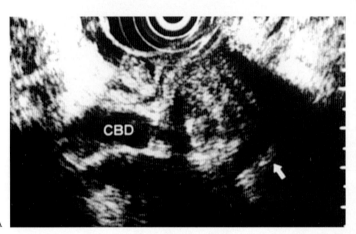
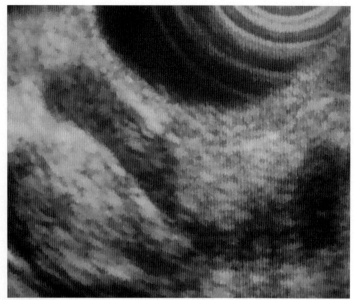

A

B

Fig. 11-10. Pancreatic cancer. **A:** *EUS from the second portion of the duodenum could detect the tumor in the head of the pancreas, while conventional US and CT examination failed to image this tumor.* **B:** *EUS is also useful for detecting portal vein invasion by pancreatic cancer, which may eliminate the need for angiography.*

Other Pancreatic Disorders

Other clinical indications for EUS evaluation in pancreatic disorders include tumors other than pancreatic cancer, such as endocrine tumors, mucin-producing pancreatic neoplasm, and malunion of the pancreatic and biliary duct. Although these disorders are rare, EUS is the most sensitive means of detecting small tumors, and findings are often diagnostic.

Endocrine tumors, mainly insulinoma, are often small when they produce clinical symptoms, and escape detection by US and CT in 40% to 60% of patients. As described in several case reports and smaller series, EUS seems to be highly accurate in this respect. This was confirmed by a recent collaborative study of six different centers showing an 80% accuracy in detecting small endocrine tumors, which were not visualized by US and CT. EUS has also been shown to be superior to angiography.

Biliary Tract Tumors

Staging of Biliary Tumors (Bile Duct and Gallbladder)

Only a few recent studies have concentrated on the role of EUS in the staging of biliary tumors. It was mainly T.L. Tio's

group that showed high accuracy rates for EUS in predicting the T and N stages in distal as well as in proximal bile duct carcinoma. The same group previously reported an 80% accuracy rate for EUS in predicting resectability in bile duct malignancy. If T- and N-staging, as well as proximal extension of Klatskin tumors into both hepatic ducts, are considered, the value of EUS might be restricted due to limited penetration depth. Whether EUS staging results will have an impact on the management of these patients has yet to be shown. A recent series from Japan reports on the high accuracy of EUS in staging gallbladder cancer, which might also be another important indication for EUS.

EUS has also been reported to be the most accurate modality in the differential diagnosis of gallbladder polyps. It might become mandatory in patients with gallbladder polyps found incidentally with conventional US, avoiding unnecessary cholecystectomy (Fig. 11-11).

Cancer of the Papilla of Vater

Studies comparing EUS to histopathologic findings of resected specimens, as well as to other imaging procedures, showed high accuracy rates in predicting the T and N stages of ampullary tumors. The clinical impact on the management of cancer of the

papilla of Vater is less impressive, since most of these tumors are locally resectable. Estimation of a patient's prognosis and differentiation of ampullary from pancreatic head carcinoma are clinically useful indications for EUS.

Conclusion

EUS is more accurate than conventional US and CT in locoregional staging of cancers of the gut. It should be performed when detailed staging may alter the therapeutic options. It has been shown that stage T1 includes heterogeneous groups with regard to lymph node metastases. It may be worthwhile to subdivide T1 into mucosal and submucosal cancers by EUS, since we now have more therapeutic options than ever, including endoscopic intervention and laparoscopic surgery. It is also certain that EUS will change our concepts of GI submucosal lesions and current approaches to the management of these tumors.

Although EUS has repeatedly been shown to be highly accurate in the primary diagnosis of pancreatic tumors (carcinoma, endocrine tumors) and in the preoperative staging of pancreatic, ampullary, and biliary malignancies, the clinical impact of these findings is obvious in only a few of these indications. Further studies must show to what extent EUS can change the management of patients with pancreaticobiliary disorders, compared with other diagnostic procedures.

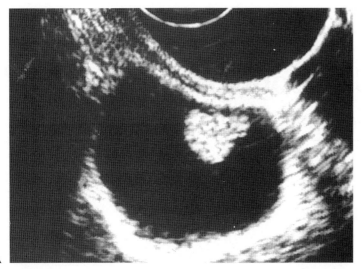 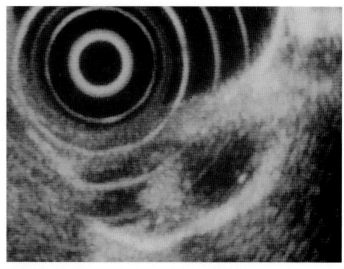

Fig. 11-11. **A:** *Cholesterol polyp. EUS from the duodenum reveals a pedunculated polyp 13 mm in diameter. An aggregation of echogenic spots with echopenic areas seen in this lesion is characteristic of a cholesterol polyp.* **B:** *Cancer of the gallbladder. EUS reveals a granular-surfaced, homogeneously echogenic pedunculated mass 14 × 9 mm in size. Histologic findings showed adenocarcinoma limited to the mucosa of the gallbladder.*

Suggested Reading

Botet JF, Lightdale C. Endoscopic ultrasonography of the gastrointestinal tract. *Gastroenterol Clin North Am* 1995;24:385–412.

Rosch T, Lovenz R, Braig C, Classen M. Endoscopic ultrasonography in diagnosis and staging of pancreatic and biliary tumors. *Endoscopy* 1992;24 Suppl 1:304–308.

Rosch T, Braig C, Gain T, et al. Staging of pancreatic and ampullary carcinoma by endoscopic ultrasonography: comparison with conventional sonography, computed tomography, and angiography. *Gastroenterology* 1992;102:188–199.

Sugiyama M, Atomi Y, Kuroda A, Muto T, Wada N. Large cholesterol polyps of the gallbladder: diagnosis by means of US and endoscopic US. *Radiology* 1995;196:493–497.

Tio TL, Tytgat GN, den Hartog Jager FC. Endoscopic ultrasonography for the evaluation of smooth muscle tumors in the upper gastrointestinal tract: an experience with 42 cases. *Gastrointest Endosc* 1990;36:342–350.

Yasuda K, Cho E, Nakajima M, Kawai K. Diagnosis of submucosal lesions of the upper gastrointestinal tract by endoscopic ultrasonography. *Gastrointest Endosc* 1990;36:S17–20.

12

Laparoscopic Ultrasonography

Timothy G. John and O. James Garden

Intraoperative ultrasonography (US) facilitates high-resolution real-time imaging of the abdominal organs because of the surgeon's ability to position an US transducer in direct contact with the underlying tissues. The beneficial impact of intraoperative US on operative decision making is now well established, and many hepatobiliary and pancreatic surgeons regard it as an indispensable part of their operative armamentarium. The principles of intraoperative US have been exploited during laparoscopy where adequate palpation of tissues is often impossible and the view of solid organs and retroperitoneal tissues restricted.

Laparoscopic US was first performed by Japanese investigators as early as the 1950s. However, their prototype probes employed primitive A-mode scanners that were of limited practicality. In the 1980s, prototype B-mode laparoscopic US systems were developed, and there were reports of their utility in generating high-resolution cross-sectional images of the abdominal organs, facilitating the diagnosis of previously unsuspected liver and pancreatic tumors. Renewed interest in diagnostic and therapeutic laparoscopy, coupled with advances in miniaturized US technology, has stimulated the development of a range of commercially available laparoscopic US systems. Furthermore, increasing recognition of the limitations of conventional radiologic imaging techniques in assessing intraabdominal pathology has led laparoscopic surgeons to rediscover the benefits of intraoperative US during minimal-access surgical procedures.

Indications

Liver Disease

Laparoscopic US is indicated whenever laparoscopic assessment of the liver is undertaken. Although focal lesions are visible at the liver surface during laparoscopy in two-thirds of patients, information is not available regarding the presence of deep-seated intrahepatic lesions that might otherwise be detected by the surgeon's palpating hands at open operation. Furthermore, in the absence of surface anatomic markings, laparoscopic US is required to define the relationships between liver lesions and intrahepatic vascular and biliary structures. Laparoscopic inspection of the liver is commonly performed as a diagnostic procedure to ascertain the nature of diffuse or focal liver disease, and facilitates safe and accurate liver biopsy. Staging laparoscopy is increasingly employed as a method of assessing the resectability of primary and secondary liver tumors because of its sensitivity in detecting extrahepatic and bilobar liver lesions. Laparoscopic US further improves the detection of multifocal disease and regional lymphadenopathy, and allows the surgeon to plan the extent of hepatic resections. Many surgeons also regard staging laparoscopic assessment of the liver and peritoneal cavity as an indispensable prelude to laparotomy in patients with a variety of primary tumors. In Edinburgh, staging laparoscopic US in the preoperative assessment of patients presenting for consideration of hepatic resection yielded staging informa-

tion in addition to that derived from laparoscopy in 42%. Furthermore, adoption of this technique was associated with a reduction in the rate of unnecessary laparotomy from 42% to 7%.

As the indications for laparoscopic resection of intraabdominal malignancies are extended, proper evaluation of the liver for metastatic involvement should be performed to allow meaningful interpretation of results as novel techniques and adjuvant therapies are adopted. In particular, the presence of occult hepatic metastases has been shown to be an important determinant of prognosis in patients with colorectal carcinoma. During laparoscopic colorectal resections for malignant disease, laparoscopic US is able to fulfill the role formerly provided by intraoperative US and manual palpation in routine screening of the liver for metastases.

Biliary Tract Disease

Laparoscopic US is a rapid and noninvasive alternative to laparoscopic intraoperative cholangiography in detecting common bile duct calculi during laparoscopic cholecystectomy. To date, experience with the technique has shown it to be at least as sensitive as intraoperative cholangiography, and less liable to technical failure. However, its role in defining variations in biliary anatomy and lessening the risk of bile duct injury is less well defined.

Pancreatic Disease

Laparoscopic US enhances staging laparoscopy in patients with pancreatic or periampullary malignancy by demonstrating precisely the tumor and its relationships with retroperitoneal vascular, ductal, and visceral structures. Laparoscopic mobilization and dissection of the peripancreatic tissues is rendered unnecessary, and the appearance of the liver and regional lymph nodes may be assessed. The adoption of staging laparoscopy with laparoscopic US improves patient selection for surgery or nonoperative palliation of pancreatic malignancy. Having identified "occult" intraabdominal metastases by laparoscopy in 35% of patients considered to have potentially resectable peripancreatic cancers, our own experience with staging laparoscopic US showed additional factors confirming tumor unresectability in 53% of patients. The decision regarding tumor resectability was modified on the basis of laparoscopic US in 25% of cases. Avoidance of unnecessary laparotomy in patients with unresectable tumors reduces morbidity in patients with reduced life expectancy, and more efficient use of operating time has obvious health economic implications.

In instances of diagnostic doubt, characterization and biopsy of pancreatic lesions may be performed. Laparoscopic localization of pancreatic neuroendocrine tumors, especially insulinoma, may be achieved with the same high sensitivity as for intraoperative US during laparotomy. However, apart from excluding intraabdominal malignant dissemination, a laparoscopic approach to the diagnosis of neuroendocrine tumors is justified only if a minimal-access approach to tumor resection is proposed, rather than at open operation.

Gastroesophageal Diseases

The beneficial role of staging laparoscopy in demonstrating peritoneal, nodal, and hepatic malignant dissemination in the preoperative assessment of patients with gastroesophageal malignancy has been reproducibly demonstrated. The adoption of laparoscopic US allows further evaluation of the extent of local invasion of stomach tumors and staging of regional lymph node status.

Miscellaneous Indications

Laparoscopic US is a useful technique for guiding a variety of laparoscopic drainage procedures. Accurate delineation of liver cysts, pancreatic pseudocysts, and perigraft lymphoceles following renal transplantation permits the judicious siting of incisions away from regions of overlying parenchyma and blood vessels. The application of laparoscopic US during pelvic operations, such as lymphadenectomy and endometrial ablation, and for identification of the ureter or mesenteric vessels in obese patients during laparoscopic colorectal operations has been described.

Operative Technique

Equipment

Laparoscopic US systems consist of a probe, which is inserted into the abdominal cavity through a standard 10-mm-diameter laparoscopic port, and the scanning machine, which is positioned near the operating table. The laparoscopic US probe is a rigid wand that houses the US transducer, the scanning surface of which is placed in contact with the target tissues. Various types of transducer may be employed during laparoscopic US: Linear-array transducers have a flat side-viewing footprint that generates rectilinear-shaped sonograms over a distance of approximately 4 cm; curved linear-array transducers generate a divergent scanning field that appears sector-shaped; rotatory sector scanners incorporate an oscillating piezoelectric crystal mechanism within the tip of the probe that produces a 90- to 360-degree sectoral field of view from a small surface area of transducer contact. Multielement linear- or curved linear-array laparoscopic US transducers are in most frequent usage, operating with frequencies of 5 to 10 MHz that provide a resolution of less than 1 mm and tissue penetration of 3 to 7 cm. Some laparoscopic US probes incorporate articulating joints, operated by levers from the handpiece, that allow the transducer to be flexed in multiple planes to facilitate transducer contact with variations in organ contour.

The probe is sterilized by immersion in glutaraldehyde solution or by exposure to ethylene oxide gas, and is connected to the scanner by a cable. The laparoscopic US images are displayed on the integrated monitor of the portable scanning machine. However, use of an audiovisual mixing device is recommended to permit simultaneous picture-in-picture demonstration on the operating room monitors of the laparoscopic camera view and the laparoscopic sonograms. When a sterile remote-control handset is not available, an assistant is required to operate the various controls displayed on the scanning machine under instruction of the operator (e.g., magnification/zoom, measuring calipers, image gain/power, Doppler controls). Additional features include Doppler sampling and color Doppler flow analysis, which allow vascular and ductal structures to be rapidly distinguished.

General Considerations

Laparoscopic US is performed under general anesthesia with muscle relaxation. Access to the peritoneal cavity is achieved by a direct cutdown approach to the parietal peritoneum immediately superior or inferior to the umbilicus. This allows blunt introduction of a 10-mm-diameter port with high-flow insufflation of carbon dioxide through a side port to achieve a 12- to 15-mm Hg pneumoperitoneum. Despite the presence of adhesions associated with previous abdominal operations, this safe and rapid approach to achieving pneumoperitoneum rarely fails. Use of disposable ports is recommended to minimize the risk of damage to the vulnerable laminated transducer surface during its passage through the spring-loaded metal valves that are a feature of most nondisposable ports.

Laparoscopic US requires the insertion of at least two ports to facilitate accurate positioning of the probe over the target tissues under direct vision. Although "blind" laparoscopic US through a single port is feasible, this technique is not recommended because of the risk of tearing adhesions. The laparoscopic US probe and camera may be alternated between ports so that scanning may be performed in a variety of planes. The sites of insertion of additional ports depend on the primary laparoscopic procedure and the area under investigation. In general, it is convenient to consider laparoscopic US scanning using a rigid linear-array probe inserted via the umbilical port as providing images in a predominantly sagittal plane, whereas scanning takes place in a predominantly transverse plane when the probe is operated from a lateral port. In reality, scanning occurs in a full range of oblique "cuts" that enables the laparoscopic ultrasonographer to appreciate three-dimensional anatomic detail in real-time from a sequence of two-dimensional images. Flexible probes and sectoral transducers permit greater variation in the available range of scanning angles without altering port position.

Laparoscopic US examination of upper abdominal organs is facilitated by decompression of stomach gas by nasogastric suction. A supine reverse Trendelenburg position encourages exposure of the porta hepatis and peripancreatic region. The thin film of moisture covering the abdominal organs is sufficient to permit high-resolution contact US. However, instillation of up to 500 mL of crystalloid solution into the peritoneal cavity optimizes "acoustic coupling" and minimizes the amount of down pressure required to achieve satisfactory transducer contact with the under-lying tissues. The fluid may also be used as a "standoff" to facilitate laparoscopic US examination of lesions situated superficially in the "near-field" of the transducer. Peritoneal washings may also be retrieved for cytologic examination following diagnostic or staging laparoscopy in cases of intraabdominal malignancy. Peritoneal cytology, however, is rarely positive in the absence of peritoneal or hepatic carcinomatosis, and provides little additional information apart from signifying a grave prognosis.

Laparoscopic Ultrasonography of the Liver

A complete laparoscopic US examination of the liver is achieved in most patients using a single 10-mm-diameter port inserted at the umbilicus (Fig. 12-1). Evaluation of the liver may therefore be performed during most minimal-access therapeutic procedures without the requirement for additional ports. A second port placed laterally in the right flank provides the best access for full evaluation of the right hemiliver, although the siting of additional ports may depend on the presence of adhesions. Laparoscopic US is performed following laparoscopic inspection of the peritoneal cavity, porta hepatis, and liver surface. It is important to inspect the underside of the left hepatic lobe and the caudate lobe through the lesser omentum by elevating the left lobe with a probe.

If a reference hepatic lesion has been identified either by laparoscopic inspection of the liver or by preceding investigations, characterization of its sonographic appearance should be performed initially to facilitate comparison with any other abnormalities. Thereafter, a systematic anatomic survey of the liver is undertaken so that

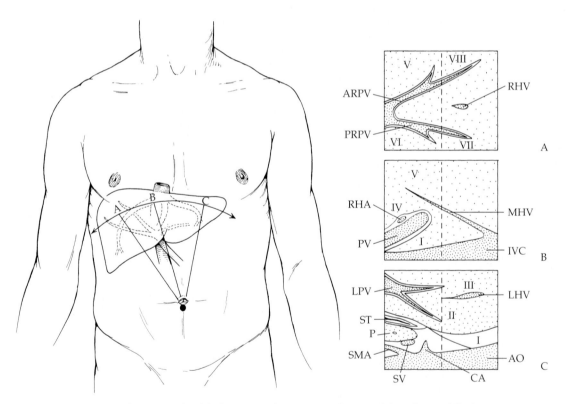

Fig. 12-1. Laparoscopic ultrasonography of the liver using a linear-array probe inserted through an umbilical port. Diagrammatic representation showing the segmental hepatic anatomy and sonographic anatomic landmarks. **A:** Examination of the right hemiliver demonstrates the bifurcation of the right portal vein into its anterior (ARPV) and posterior (PRPV) sectoral branches perpendicular to the plane of the right hepatic vein (RHV). **B:** Sagittal section in the midline of the liver demonstrates the hilar structures anteriorly and the course of the middle hepatic vein (MHV) to its confluence with the inferior vena cava (IVC). **C:** Examination of the left hepatic lobe demonstrates branches of the left portal vein (LPV) to segments II and III, separated by the plane of the left hepatic vein (LHV) posteriorly. The left lobe also acts as an acoustic standoff for examination of the stomach (St), pancreas (P), and paraaortic region (AO, aorta; CA, celiac axis; SMA, superior mesenteric artery; SV, splenic vein).

the precise pattern of liver involvement is documented and no "blind" areas of parenchyma are neglected. The anatomic survey relies on the recognition of intrahepatic vascular landmarks, given the paucity of surface markings on the liver capsule (see Fig. 12-1). Sonographically, the liver parenchyma normally has a fine homogenous texture of medium echogenicity. Portal tracts are characterized by their hyperechoic fascial sheaths and diverging course away from the hilum. Laminar blood flow may be observed within the prominent portal vein branches, but the intrahepatic arterial and biliary radicles are less obvious. The hepatic veins converge in a posterosuperior direction toward the inferior vena cava, have attenuated walls, and may exhibit the fluctuations of the central venous pulse.

An understanding of hepatic segmental anatomy, as described by the French surgical anatomist Claude Couinaud and later popularized by Bismuth, is a fundamental requirement (see Fig. 12-1). The eight hepatic segments are divided into those constituting the right hemiliver (V to VIII), the left hemiliver (II to IV) and caudate lobe (I). The right and left hemilivers are divided by the plane of the principal fissure that passes between the gallbladder fossa and the inferior vena cava. This plane has no external markings but is defined by the course of the middle hepatic vein, which should be identified at the outset of the anatomic survey with the probe placed on the diaphragmatic surface of the liver. Advancement of the probe in a posterior direction traces the course of the middle hepatic vein to the confluence of the hepatic veins with the inferior vena cava. Anteriorly, the structures of the hepatoduodenal ligament are identified traversing the liver hilum. This plane represents an important anatomic landmark from which a systematic survey of the right and left hemilivers is performed. The survey is performed with smooth, slow sweeps and subtle rotatory movements of the probe over the liver capsule.

The left hemiliver comprises hepatic segment IV (the quadrate lobe) and the left hepatic lobe (segments II and III) (see Fig. 12-1). These entities are separated by the insertion of the falciform ligament and ligamentum teres. Examination of the left hepatic lobe requires repositioning the laparoscopic US probe to the left of the falciform ligament, and if this is prevented by left upper abdominal adhesions, incision of the falciform ligament may provide access to the left subphrenic space. Scanning through hepatic segment IV identifies the left hepatic pedicle, which gives branches to segments I to IV near the ligamentum teres insertion. The boundary between segments II and III is defined by the course within the left lobe of the left hepatic vein, which converges with the middle hepatic vein to form a common trunk before entering the inferior vena cava. The fascia of the hepatic insertion of the lesser omentum is identifiable as a well defined hyperechoic plane that demarcates the caudate lobe, the inferior vena cava, and the paraaortic region from hepatic segment II posteriorly.

The right hemiliver is divided by the transverse course of the right hepatic vein into anterior (segments V and VIII) and posterior (segments VI and VII) sectors (see Fig. 12-1). This plane has no surface markings and is best appreciated with the laparoscopic US probe inserted through a right flank port along the right paracolic gutter and right lateral subphrenic space. Scanning in the predominantly coronal plane of the right hepatic vein is achieved from this position. The anterior sector comprises segment V inferiorly, easily identified adjacent to the gallbladder fossa, and segment VIII, situated superiorly and forming the dome of the liver. The posterior sector comprises segment VI, overlying the right kidney inferiorly, and segment VII, being least accessible and concealed beneath the bare area posterolaterally. The anterior and posterior sectoral divisions of the right portal pedicle are identified, bifurcating perpendicular to the plane of the right hepatic vein, and their respective segmental branches can be defined.

Diffuse abnormalities of the hepatic parenchyma in patients with cirrhosis and steatosis appear coarse and hyperechoic during laparoscopic US. Diffuse malignant infiltration, especially when due to multifocal hepatocellular carcinoma, may be difficult to diagnose when the tumor is of similar echogenicity (isoechoic), compared with background cirrhosis. A patchy texture may be appreciated sonographically, but ultimately biopsy is required to distinguish areas of tumor from benign regenerating nodules. Intrahepatic duct dilatation due to extrahepatic biliary obstruction may impede examination of the parenchyma when grossly dilated lakes of anechoic bile with posterior acoustic shadowing dominate the scanning field. Conversely, relief of biliary obstruction by stent insertion or biliary enteric anastomosis results in pneumobilia that may cause bright areas of acoustic interference.

Focal hepatic abnormalities are characterized as hyperechoic, isoechoic, or hypoechoic, compared with the background parenchyma (Fig. 12-2). Benign lesions most commonly encountered include simple hepatic cysts, areas of fatty infiltration, and hemangiomas. Simple cysts are anechoic, lack a defined wall, and cause posterior acoustic enhancement. Fatty infiltration is commonly observed adjacent to the ligamentum teres insertion and gallbladder fossa in segments IV and V, appearing as a circumscribed but irregular hyperechoic area. Hemangiomas are round, circumscribed hyperechoic lesions, discovered incidentally in 5% to 10% of patients. Hemangiomas do not cause posterior attenuation of the US beam (shadowing), and posterior acoustic enhancement is frequently observed (Fig. 12-2). This is an important discriminating feature from metastases of gastrointestinal origin, which, although often hyperechoic, also cause posterior acoustic attenuation.

In patients with suspected focal hepatic malignancy, a careful and systematic search for malignant focal lesions is performed, with reference to the sonographic appearance of the reference lesion, where possible. Malignant liver tumors vary in their echogenicity, the presence of cystic or necrotic areas, calcification, and the presence of daughter nodules. However, the presence of an anechoic halo immediately surrounding a lesion is pathognomonic for metastases; this appearance is termed a *bull's-eye* or *target* lesion. The number, size, site, and spatial relationships of the tumor with important vascular structures are defined so that, where appropriate, anatomic liver resections may be planned with adequate tumor clearance to achieve the best chance of long-term survival. Occlusion or stenosis of the portal veins, hepatic veins, or inferior vena cava may be apparent, and the proximal extent of isoechoic intraluminal tumor thrombus within the portal venous trunks may affect resectability in cases of hepatocellular carcinoma. The hilar and paraaortic regions should be scrutinized for extrahepatic disease in the form of malignant regional lymphadenopathy.

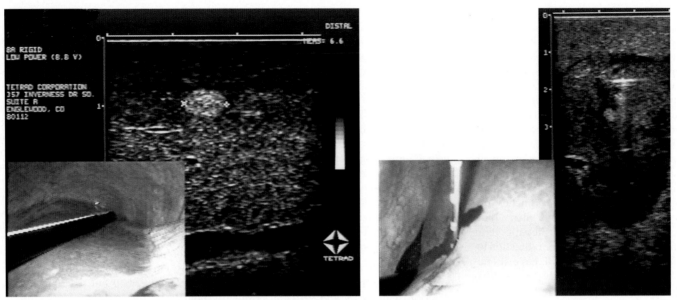

A

B

Fig. 12-2. Laparoscopic ultrasonography of the liver. **A:** Incidental finding of a hemangioma measuring 6.6 mm in maximum diameter. Note its hyperechoic appearance with no posterior acoustic enhancement. The lesion is situated between segments IV and V, anterior to the middle hepatic vein. **B:** Laparoscopic ultrasound–guided needle biopsy of a 5-cm-diameter hypoechoic metastasis of colorectal origin situated in hepatic segment V. The oblique pass of the needle tip gives a linear hyperechoic signal.

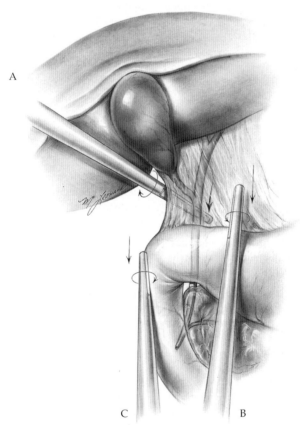

Fig. 12-3. Diagrammatic representation of the technique for laparoscopic ultrasound examination of the biliary tree during laparoscopic cholecystectomy. A: Scanning in a perpendicular plane to the bile duct is achieved with the probe operated from the subxiphoid port and the transducer in contact with the free edge of the hepatoduodenal ligament. B: Longitudinal scanning of the structures of the hepatoduodenal ligament is performed with the probe operated from the umbilical port. C: Scanning in a coronal plane is performed with the probe operated from the umbilical port and the transducer displacing duodenal contents to demonstrate the distal bile duct.

Laparoscopic Ultrasonography of the Biliary Tree

Laparoscopic US of the biliary tree should routinely be preceded by an examination of the liver to identify intrahepatic duct dilatation, incidental pathology, or malignant involvement in patients with cholangiocarcinoma or gallbladder cancer. Examination of the proximal biliary tree and gallbladder in patients with suspected malignancy is usually best performed with the probe inserted through an umbilical or right flank port and with the transducer positioned on the diaphragmatic surface of hepatic segments IV and V using the intervening liver as an acoustic standoff (Fig. 12-3). The gallbladder wall normally exhibits three distinct echo layers and is examined for mural thickening, tumor mass, or mucosal polyps. The number and size of contained gallstones or the presence of echogenic debris or crystals within biliary sludge are observed.

Local staging of proximal cholangiocarcinomas using laparoscopic US may reveal occlusion or stenosis of the portal or hepatic arterial pedicle, with regional intrahepatic duct dilatation. However, cholangiocarcinomas are often isoechoic and poorly circumscribed, and staging information obtained during laparoscopic US may consist simply of confirmation of the patency of the main portal vein and hepatic artery and the absence of hepatic metastases.

Screening of the biliary tree for choledocholithiasis during laparoscopic cholecystectomy is rapidly mastered. Using a linear-array probe, laparoscopic US may be performed in a predominantly sagittal plane using an umbilical port (see Fig. 12-3). Alternatively, transverse scanning of the duct throughout its length may be achieved with the probe inserted through a subxiphoid port with the transducer placed perpendicularly alongside the free edge of the hepatoduodenal ligament. Either technique or both may be employed early in the course of laparoscopic cholecystectomy before the presence of metal clips or gas in the dissection planes causes interference with the images. Common duct stones are strongly suspected when a crescentic hyperechoic signal from the surface of the calculus and/or a dense posterior acoustic shadow are evident (Fig. 12-4). The common duct may also be dilated, and its maximum internal diameter is measured using electronic calipers, or estimated using the graduated scale in millimeters that appears alongside the sonogram.

Laparoscopic sonograms obtained in the longitudinal axis of the hepatoduodenal ligament identify the common bile duct, hepatic artery, and portal vein as parallel tubular structures separated from the inferior vena cava in the cephalad direction by the wedge-shaped caudate lobe of liver (see Fig. 12-1B). Having defined the portal vein by its posterior position, lack of pulsatility, and visible luminal blood flow, the hepatic artery and duct are distinguished by the anteromedial position and visible pulsation of the former and the anterolateral position, relatively thicker wall, absence of luminal flow, and confluence with the cystic duct of the latter. Laparoscopic US Doppler sampling is a convenient method for distinguishing rapidly among portal, arterial, and inferior vena caval blood flow. No flow is detected when ductal structures are examined.

Transverse scanning obtained with the probe placed perpendicular to the hepatoduodenal ligament produces cross-sectional images of the portal vein, hepatic artery, and common duct, which have been likened to a Mickey-Mouse silhouette (Fig. 12-5). This maneuver is facilitated by

elevating the gallbladder with fundal grasping forceps after division of adhesions where necessary. The instillation of fluid into the subhepatic space optimizes acoustic contact and reduces any tendency to compress the duct by inadvertent transducer pressure.

Irrespective of which approach is used, slow sweeps of the transducer along the length of the hepatoduodenal ligament, gastric antrum, and duodenum permit the course of the common duct to be visualized from the hepatic duct confluence as far as its termination at the papilla. It is particularly important to visualize the duct throughout its distal divergent course away from the portal vein as it traverses the plane between head of pancreas and inferior vena cava. Gentle probe pressure may be required to displace duodenal gas, which may degrade the image and cause confusing bright signals and acoustic shadowing in the peripapillary region (see Fig. 12-3). Some investigators have suggested instilling crystalloid solution into the common duct via a cystic duct cholangiogram cannula to distend the distal duct, although we have never found this to be necessary.

Laparoscopic Ultrasonography of the Pancreas

The pancreas is examined in a predominantly sagittal plane with the linear-array probe operated from an umbilical port, and in a predominantly transverse plane with the probe in a right flank port (see Fig. 12-5). The pancreatic parenchyma appears homogenous and of similar echogenicity to that of the liver. An anatomic survey of the pancreas and peripancreatic structures is important to achieve orientation and correct interpretation of the laparoscopic sonograms, especially when the anatomy is distorted by pancreatic disease. The structures of the hepatoduodenal ligament are relatively constant features and should be examined as part of an initial survey of the liver and biliary tree whenever laparoscopic US of the pancreas is performed.

With the probe operated in a sagittal plane via an umbilical port, the long axis of the portal vein is followed posterior to the pancreatic neck as the probe is withdrawn

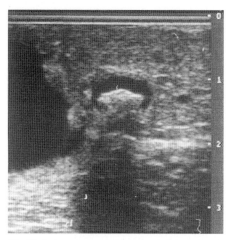

Fig. 12-4. An unsuspected calculus is demonstrated within the distal intrapancreatic portion of the common bile duct and adjacent to the papilla by laparoscopic ultrasonography.

inferiorly over the gastric antrum and first part of the duodenum (Figs. 12-5 and 12-6). This is the key position for examination of the pancreatic head and uncinate process to the right of this plane and of the body and tail of the gland to its left. This position of reference should always be regained if orientation is lost. The pancreatic neck is a relatively thin structure, measuring 10 mm or less, and conveys the main pancreatic duct, which is identified in transverse section and normally measures 3 mm or less in diameter. Slight rotation or displacement of the transducer to the right surveys the head of the pancreas and the convergent courses of the pancreatic duct and common bile duct anterior to the inferior vena cava. The echo layers of the duodenal wall demarcate the lateral extent of the pancreatic head, and fluid may be appreciated within the duodenal lumen. Inferiorly, the uncinate process extends posterior to the superior mesenteric vein. Scanning to the left of the plane of the portal vein and neck of pancreas identifies the superior mesenteric artery, with its origin from the aorta immediately inferior to the celiac axis and its anteroinferior course into the root of the mesentery. The body and tail of pancreas are identified in a series of oblique sonograms as the probe is swept laterally and superiorly over the stomach toward the spleen. The demarcation between the pancreatic borders and the retroperitoneal tissues may be indistinct, and the main pancreatic duct and splenic vessels are convenient points of reference that identify the parenchyma of the distal pancreas.

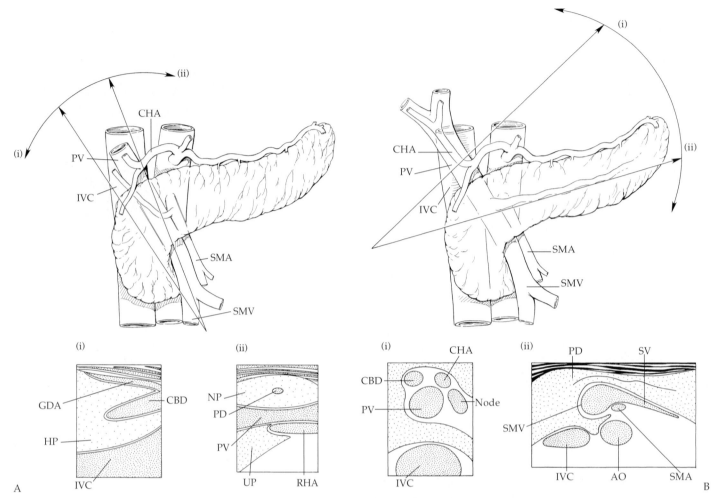

Fig. 12-5. Laparoscopic ultrasonography of the pancreas. Diagrammatic representation shows sonographic anatomic landmarks identified during laparoscopic ultrasound examination of the pancreas using a linear-array transducer in sagittal **(A)** and transverse planes **(B)**. (IVC, inferior vena cava; AO, aorta; PV, portal vein; SMA, superior mesenteric artery; CHA, common hepatic artery; RHA, aberrant right hepatic artery arising from the SMA; GDA, gastroduodenal artery; SV, splenic vein; HP, pancreatic head; NP, pancreatic neck; PD, pancreatic duct; UP, uncinate process; SAL, saline used for acoustic coupling.)

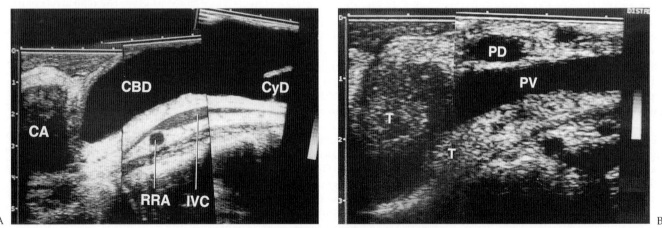

Fig. 12-6. Carcinoma of the pancreatic head. **A:** Laparoscopic sonogram in the sagittal plane shows a hypoechoic carcinoma (CA) causing obstruction of the common bile duct (CBD). The common duct measures 20 mm in maximum diameter, and its confluence with the cystic duct (CyD) is shown to be free from tumor invasion. The inferior vena cava (IVC) is compressed due to probe down pressure (RRA, right renal artery). **B:** Unresectable carcinoma of the pancreatic head. Laparoscopic sonogram in the sagittal plane shows a cut through the pancreatic neck. Invasion of the portal vein (PV) by hypoechoic tumor (T) has been demonstrated. A dilated pancreatic duct (PD) is shown traversing the neck of the pancreas. (From John TG, Garden OJ. Intraoperative ultrasonography. In: Trede M, Carter DC, eds. Surgery of the pancreas, 2nd ed. Edinburgh: Churchill Livingstone, 1997:173–180; with permission.)

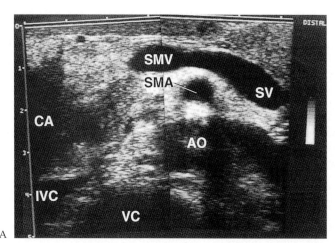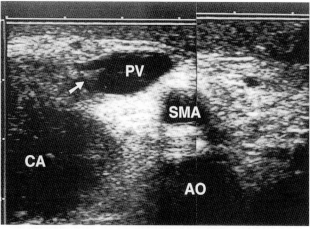

Fig. 12-7. *Unresectable carcinoma of the pancreatic head. Laparoscopic sonogram in the transverse plane demonstrates a hypoechoic 3-cm-diameter carcinoma (CA) with irregular margins within the pancreatic head.* **A:** *A cut taken at the level of the splenoportal-mesenteric venous junction shows the superior mesenteric vein (SMV) and artery (SMA) to be clear of tumor invasion.* **B:** *Scanning in the cephalad direction demonstrates direct invasion of the lateral wall of the portal vein (PV) by tumor (arrow) (SV, splenic vein; AO, aorta; IVC, inferior vena cava; VC, vertebral column). (From John TG, Garden OJ. Intraoperative ultrasonography. In: Trede M, Carter DC, eds.* Surgery of the pancreas, *2nd ed. Edinburgh: Churchill Livingstone, 1997: in press; with permission.)*

Viewed in transverse section, the spleno-portal mesenteric venous junction, superior mesenteric artery, aorta, and inferior vena cava are the key vascular landmarks that delineate the posterior limits of the pancreas, while the walls of the stomach and duodenum beneath the transducer demarcate the gland anteriorly (Figs. 12-5 and 12-7). As the transducer is swept superiorly, the portal vein is followed as it emerges from the superior pancreatic border to enter the hepatoduodenal ligament. At this level, the common hepatic artery is identified arching over the portal vein, with the gastroduodenal and superior pancreaticoduodenal arteries emerging to pass superficially between the pancreatic head and duodenum. Inferiorly, the parallel courses of the superior mesenteric vessels into the mesenteric root are apparent. The longitudinal course of the pancreatic duct within body and tail of the gland may be traced distally by advancing the probe over the stomach. An accessory or replaced right or common hepatic artery arising from the superior mesenteric artery or aorta may be identified in 20% to 30% of patients and should be suspected whenever an artery is identified passing posterior to the neck of pancreas and portal vein. Confirmation of its presence is achieved by tracing it inferiorly to its origin below the celiac trunk.

Focal pancreatic abnormalities often cause secondary changes that are apparent dur-ing the anatomic survey. A grossly dilated common bile duct may initially be confused with the portal vein, but closer scrutiny reveals its lateral position within the hepatoduodenal ligament, the confluence with a distended, tortuous cystic duct, intrahepatic duct dilatation, a thickened hyperechoic wall, and a sediment of luminal biliary sludge (see Fig. 12-6). The artefactual hyperechoic flashes of a biliary stent may mark the course of a collapsed bile duct, which should be traced distally to localize the distal obstructing lesion when this is not immediately apparent. Lesions of the pancreatic head or peripapillary region also cause dilatation of the pancreatic duct, whose tortuous, sacculated appearance is typically accompanied by marked atrophy of the surrounding parenchyma in the pancreatic neck, body, and tail.

Ductal carcinoma of the pancreas typically appears as a predominantly hypoechoic mass with irregular margins that may cast a dense posterior acoustic shadow (see Figs. 12-6 and 12-7). However, the tumor is often heterogeneous with patchy areas of mixed echogenicity and cystic components, and it is impossible to differentiate pancreatic malignancy from focal chronic pancreatitis on sonographic appearances alone. Peripapillary carcinomas arising from the distal common bile duct, papilla, duodenum, or pancreatic head may appear isoechoic, compared with the adja-cent pancreas, and may be identified prolapsing into the duodenal lumen or extending proximally within the lumina of dilated pancreatic and/or bile ducts.

Once the primary pancreatic abnormality is characterized, its resectability should be assessed in terms of local tumor invasion. Tumor invasion of the portal vein is the main consideration in determining local resectability of pancreatic or peripapillary cancer, although it is recognized that criteria of resectability for cure vary among surgeons and institutions. The interface between the tumor and the vein is examined in detail. Sonographic features of portal vein invasion include obliteration or thrombosis of the vein, fixed stenosis of the vein wall, loss of the hyperechoic vessel–tumor interface, or envelopment of the vein with tumor (see Figs. 12-6 and 12-7). Care must be taken to avoid artefactually creating the impression of portal vein compression by excessive probe pressure. The superior mesenteric artery should similarly be examined, although arterial invasion is rare in the absence of portal vein invasion. The margins of the tumor are examined for evidence of local infiltration of the hepatic artery and hepatoduodenal ligament superiorly and the mesenteric root inferiorly.

Regional lymph node enlargement is commonly observed in patients with suspected pancreatic or periampullary cancer. Unfortunately, no reliable sonographic criteria exist that differentiate enlarged reactive nodes from metastatic nodes, although confirmation of massive malignant hilar or retroperitoneal lymphadenopathy is readily obtained by guided needle biopsy.

Laparoscopic Ultrasonography of the Stomach

In addition to an umbilical port, a second 10-mm-diameter port is inserted on one side of the midline or the other to allow access to the intraabdominal portion of the upper gastrointestinal tract, regional lymph node fields, and the liver. After examination of the liver parenchyma for metastases, an assessment of regional lymph node involvement is performed. The liver is conveniently used as an acoustic window for laparoscopic US examination of the porta hepatis, peripancreatic region, and paraaortic lymph node fields. In patients with gastroesophageal malignancy, laparoscopic US has high sensitivity and specificity when a diameter of 10 mm or greater is adopted as a sign of metastatic lymph node involvement. Morphologic sonographic criteria also differentiate benign from malignant nodes. Malignant nodes appear hypoechoic and exhibit a sharply demarcated border, compared with the blurred outline and increased echogenicity of reactive nodes.

The wall of the entire gastrointestinal tract has a characteristic sonographic appearance, comprising five alternating hyperechoic and hypoechoic bands (Fig. 12-8). Laparoscopic US of the stomach is facilitated by the evacuation of gas by nasogastric suction, following which the anterior and posterior walls are separated with the introduction of crystalloid solution into the gastric lumen. The entire stomach is visualized from the distal esophagus to the pylorus, with the left hepatic lobe as a standoff to visualize the collapsed distal esophagus and gastroesophageal junction anterior to the supraceliac aorta and adjacent to the caudate lobe. Elevation of the left hepatic lobe with the probe allows inspection of the lesser sac and identifies an anomalous left hepatic artery arising from the left gastric artery, when present, in 10% to 15% of patients. The probe is then gently swept over the anterior serosal surface of the stomach.

Tumors of the stomach are identified as abnormal masses disrupting the normal echo pattern of the stomach wall (Fig. 12-9). Local tumor staging is performed by assessment of the depth of penetration of the tumor within the stomach wall, and the extent of its lateral spread proximally and distally is assessed to plan the extent of surgery. In particular, invasion through the serosal surface to involve adjacent organs such as the pancreas is defined by loss of the most superficial hyperechoic layer of the gastric wall overlying the tumor.

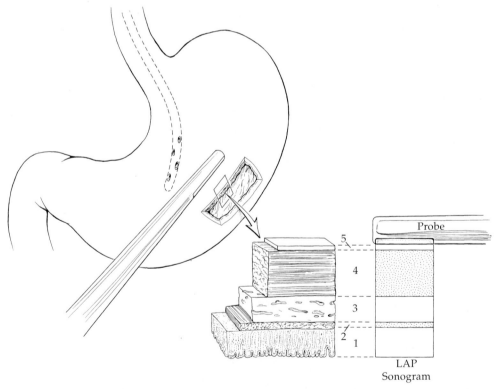

Fig. 12-8. Laparoscopic ultrasonography of the stomach. Diagrammatic representation shows five distinct sonographic zones of the stomach wall and the corresponding histologic layers: 1, hyperechoic band—interface between lumen and mucosa; 2, hypoechoic band—lamina propria and muscularis mucosae; 3, hyperechoic band—submucosa; 4, hypoechoic band—muscularis; 5, hyperechoic band—interface between muscularis and serosa.

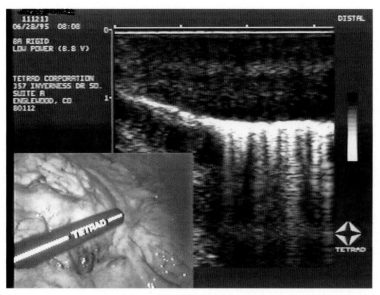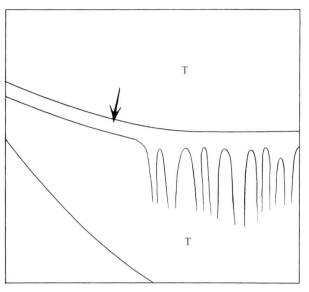

Fig. 12-9. Laparoscopic sonogram obtained with a linear-array probe placed on the body of the stomach. Hypoechoic tumor (T) has replaced the anterior and posterior stomach walls, with obliteration of the normal banded echo pattern. Repeated endoscopic biopsies failed to confirm the presence of tumor, which did not breach the hyperechoic mucosa–lumen interface (arrow). Laparoscopic ultrasound guided–needle biopsy confirmed the diagnosis of adenocarcinoma and resolved the diagnostic dilemma.

Laparoscopic Ultrasound–guided Biopsy

A two-puncture, "freehand" technique is currently utilized for laparoscopic US–guided needle biopsy of lesions in the liver, pancreas, stomach, or retroperitoneum. Prototype laparoscopic US probes have been developed that incorporate an axial biopsy channel within the probe shaft for accurate guidance of a needle to a precise point within the sonographic field, and this goal has also been attempted using a transducer channel for guidance of externally introduced biopsy needles. Unfortunately, such probe designs are not commercially available at present.

Light abrasion of the tip of the biopsy needle with a scalpel blade facilitates identification of its passage through the tissues because of the resultant hyperechoic flashes. The site of needle puncture must be chosen carefully to allow access to the desired target and to anticipate the angle of the needle within the sonographic field. Care must be exercised in the vicinity of large blood vessels, the bile ducts, and gallbladder, and laparoscopic US is especially useful when the target lesion is situated near the porta hepatis. The needle appears as a hyperechoic point when the needle enters perpendicular to the sonographic cut, and as a hyperechoic linear signal when the needle is inserted along the same plane as the US beam (see Fig. 12-2B). Slight rotatory or sideways displacement of the transducer helps maintain the three-dimensional orientation of the ultrasonographer during the biopsy procedure.

It is important to exercise judgment and restraint when biopsy of focal lesions of the liver or pancreas is contemplated. Needle biopsy of potentially resectable tumor is contraindicated because of the risk of malignant seeding into the peritoneal cavity, to the port site, or to the needle track. It is an avoidable catastrophe when potentially resectable disease is disseminated in this way, as laparoscopic US findings of focal liver tumor in an anatomically resectable location and in the absence of extrahepatic dissemination warrant exploratory laparotomy with a view to liver resection. Histologic proof of malignancy is rarely required under these circumstances, as the likely diagnosis is usually apparent from imaging findings, serum biochemical assays, and the clinical context of the case.

Increasing interest in the treatment of unresectable hepatic malignancy using laparoscopic US–guided ablation techniques such as interstitial laser therapy, cryotherapy, and injection of cytotoxic substances will stimulate further refinements in integrated laparoscopic US–guided biopsy systems.

Complications and Postoperative Care

Laparoscopic US is essentially a noninvasive refinement of laparoscopy, and apart from the recognized complications associated with the establishment of a pneumoperitoneum, this technique is not associated with any specific immediate problems. However, needle biopsy of the liver or other upper abdominal organs is associated with a small risk of hemorrhage or bile leak, and a high index of suspicion should be observed if signs of peritoneal irritation persist in the postoperative period.

All laparoscopic procedures in patients with intraabdominal malignancy carry a risk of malignant port-site seeding. This distressing complication occurs more frequently following therapeutic laparoscopic procedures, where there may be breach of the tumor, shedding of malignant cells into the peritoneal cavity, and delivery of the tumor specimen through the port site. This has proven to be a rare event following diagnostic or staging laparoscopic US for malignancy, and is then usually associated with established malignant dissemination.

Suggested Reading

Bemelman WA, de Wit LT, van Delden OM, et al. Diagnostic laparoscopy combined with laparoscopic ultrasonography in staging of cancer of the pancreatic head region. *Br J Surg* 1995;82: 820–824.

Bismuth H, Kunstlinger F, Castaing D, eds. *A text and atlas of liver ultrasound*. London: Chapman & Hall, 1991.

Garden OJ, ed. *Intraoperative and laparoscopic ultrasonography*. Edinburgh: Blackwell Science, 1995.

John TG, Garden OJ. Liver assessment during laparoscopic colorectal surgery. In: Monson JRT, Darzi A, eds. *Laparoscopic colorectal surgery*. Oxford: Isis, 1995:162–184.

John TG, Garden OJ. Ultrasonography in laparoscopy. In: Brooks D, ed. *Current review of laparoscopy*, 2nd ed. Philadelphia: Current Medicine, 1995:77–95.

John TG, Greig JD, Carter DC, Garden OJ. Carcinoma of the pancreatic head and periampullary region: tumor staging with laparoscopy and laparoscopic ultrasonography. *Ann Surg* 1995;221:156–164.

John TG, Greig JD, Crosbie JL, Miles WFA, Garden OJ. Superior staging of liver tumors with laparoscopy and laparoscopic ultrasound. *Ann Surg* 1994;220:711–719.

Röthlin M, Largiadèr F. The anatomy of the hepatoduodenal ligament in laparoscopic sonography. *Surg Endosc* 1994;8:173–180.

Röthlin MA, Schlumpf R, Largiadèr F. Laparoscopic sonography: an alternative to routine intraoperative cholangiography? *Arch Surg* 1994; 129:694–700.

EDITOR'S COMMENT

With the enthusiasm for therapeutic laparoscopic surgery, several technical problems remain to be solved. One of these is the loss of the haptic sense—that is, the ability to touch and feel the tissue. Associated with this is the limitation of video laparoscopy in viewing only the surface of visible areas within the cavity being examined. The application of intracorporeal-contact US with laparoscopy allows the surgeon to see beyond the visible surface. The authors describe the primary current uses for laparoscopic US, a tool that should be increasingly applied over the foreseeable future. To realize the full potential of this new technology, surgeons must become interested in US and learn as much as possible about its principles and applications. Once an appropriate probe is available for intraoperative use, it may be worthwhile to familiarize oneself with the probe and its images during laparoscopic cholecystectomy to rapidly build up experience. We have found screening laparoscopic US to be an excellent way to clear the common bile duct during laparoscopic cholecystectomy, taking on average only 3 to 5 minutes rather than the 15 to 20 minutes required for cholangiography. Once one masters the nuances of the access, tissue contact, and interpretation of the basic images, myriad potential uses become readily apparent. The application of US to staging laparoscopy is a natural fit and should diminish the incidence of nontherapeutic laparotomy in patients with hepatobiliary and pancreatic malignancies. It is also worthwhile for scanning the retroperitoneum for pathology such as lymphadenopathy, localization of adrenal masses, and even localization of aneurysms in the splenic vasculature. The imagination is the only limitation on applications of this technology. As surgeons, we must learn and apply nontraditional techniques such as US that should facilitate and extend the scope of laparoscopic surgery.

N.J.S.

13

Intraoperative Endoscopy

Thomas A. Stellato

Intraoperative endoscopy refers to the *combined* use of intraluminal endoscopy (flexible or rigid) and either open or laparoscopic surgery. Until the advent of laparoscopic cholecystectomy, which definitively incorporated laparoscopy into general surgical clinical practice, intraoperative endoscopy consisted mainly of the evaluation of the small intestine using flexible endoscopes during celiotomy, most commonly to evaluate for unexplained sources of gastrointestinal (GI) hemorrhage. This use for endoscopy remains valid today; however, myriad creative applications combining endoscopy and laparoscopy have been developed and continue to be developed. Thus, this discussion will arbitrarily segregate the use of endoscopy during celiotomy from its combination with laparoscopic general surgery.

Endoscopy during Celiotomy

Intraoperative Localization of Bleeding Sites

With the advent of fiberoptic flexible endoscopy, the interior of the esophagus, stomach, duodenum, and colon became accessible for both evaluation and treatment. Since most neoplasms and mucosal vascular anomalies occur in these portions of the GI tract, an accurate preoperative localization of lesions contributing to GI hemorrhage is usually possible. Nonetheless, at least 1% of GI bleeding originates from the relatively inaccessible portions of the small intestine, making the evaluation complex, time-consuming, and costly. One of the most important contributions of intraoperative endoscopy is the evaluation of the small bowel to identify the source of obscure GI hemorrhage. Since small bowel sources for bleeding are rare, all patients must undergo a thorough preoperative evaluation of their upper and lower GI tracts. This evaluation necessitates esophagogastroduodenoscopy and colonoscopy. Barium contrast studies will fail to disclose most mucosal lesions and also cannot identify whether a lesion is responsible for the bleeding or simply an "innocent bystander," such as diverticulosis coli in the presence of lower GI bleeding secondary to arteriovenous malformation. Once careful evaluation by upper and lower endoscopy is completed, the following diagnostic modalities are most commonly used to study the small intestine:

I. Barium studies
   A. Upper GI with small bowel follow through
   B. Enteroclysis
   C. Barium enema with small bowel reflux
II. Radionuclide scans
   A. Technetium Tc 99m (^{99m}Tc) sulfur colloid
   B. ^{99m}Tc-labeled red blood cells
   C. ^{99m}Tc pertechnetate (Meckel scan)
III. Angiography
IV. Enteroscopy (preoperative)
V. Percutaneous abdominal ultrasound
VI. Computed tomography
VII. Long-tube small bowel intubation with serial aspiration to assess for the presence of blood

Despite the availability of all of the above, the etiology and precise location of small bowel bleeding not uncommonly remains obscure. Intraoperative endoscopy provides the following advantages:

1. Precise visual localization of bleeding sites,
2. Identification of additional pathology,
3. Confirmation or exclusion of lesions identified by preoperative studies,
4. Guide to the extent of resection.

Careful preparation before intraoperative endoscopy improves the likelihood of a successful outcome. When possible, mechanical bowel cleansing is performed; at times intestinal lavage can be undertaken even with active bleeding, provided that the patient is stable. Antibiotic prophylaxis is administered because bowel resection is anticipated. Intraoperative endoscopy can be accomplished *per os, per anum,* or per enterotomy. If there is any possibility that per enterotomy will be utilized, the endoscope must be sterilized; similarly, use of the colonoscope for upper endoscopy mandates sterilization of the equipment. Successful intraoperative endoscopy can be performed using either a fiberoptic endoscope or video endoscope. Video endoscopy has the advantage of allowing the entire surgical team, including the surgeon, to view the endoscopy (Fig. 13-1). When the endoscope is introduced by mouth, it should be advanced into the duodenum *prior* to the celiotomy. The intact abdominal wall prevents looping in the stomach and excessive insufflation. A nasogastric tube can help eliminate air from the stomach during the procedure. Once the duodenum is intubated, the celiotomy can be performed, and the endoscope can be guided by the surgeon. Using the palm of the hand along the greater curvature of the stomach and the C-loop of the duodenum, excessive stretching of these areas can be avoided.

In contrast to routine preoperative endoscopy, in which much of the examina-

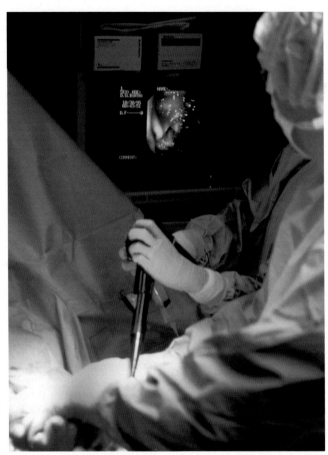

Fig. 13-1. *Intraoperative small bowel endoscopy to evaluate the etiology of bleeding. Video endoscopy allows all members of the operating team to view the small bowel mucosa.*

tion takes place during withdrawal of the scope, intraoperative endoscopy mandates a careful visual inspection throughout the insertion, since mucosal trauma secondary to the procedure is common and can be misinterpreted as pathology. Before the endoscope is advanced beyond the duodenum, the surgeon should lyse all adhesions and perform a careful exploration. The small bowel should be managed as individual segments of 10 to 20 cm. By pinching the distal border of the segment, excess insufflation is avoided. The endoscope is gently advanced into each segment under direct vision, guided by the surgeon. Insufflation is kept to a minimum, and all areas of the mucosa are inspected. When an area of pathology is identified or suspected, the operating room lights should be dimmed so the segment can be transilluminated. Each area of suspected pathology is thus examined by *direct inspection, transillumination,* and finally *palpation.* After these three maneuvers are performed, the lesion can be

marked on the serosal surface if still felt to be abnormal. Marking the serosa before completion of all three maneuvers may induce an artefact. To examine the full length of the small intestine, the intestine must be telescoped over the shaft of the endoscope. As indicated above, care must be undertaken to avoid mucosal trauma or mesenteric hematoma. The entire small bowel may be evaluated in this manner; if the distal ileum cannot be examined, the endoscope should be gently removed, and intraoperative colonoscopy should be performed with intubation of the ileum via the ileocecal valve. This endoscope *cannot* be introduced by an enterotomy because it is now contaminated.

Because intubation of the colon may be necessary in these patients, positioning the patient in dorsal lithotomy position at the initiation of the operative procedure simplifies the endoscopy from below. Intraoperative colonoscopy at celiotomy can be more difficult than routine colonoscopy.

Once again, excess insufflation should be avoided. The surgeon should guide the endoscope through the sigmoid colon to prevent looping. Everting the ileocecal valve into the cecum with a finger placed in the ileum will allow easier intubation of the terminal ileum. The actual management of pathology identified during intraoperative endoscopy will depend on the nature and extent of the pathology, as well as the experience of the surgical team. Management may consist of resection, enterotomy with ligation or local means of destruction, or endoscopic removal or destruction under surgical guidance. The technique described above can similarly be used for lesions in the remainder of the GI tract, as well as the small intestine. Although endoscopy *per os* or *per anum* has appeal because it avoids the contamination associated with the introduction of the endoscope via the enterotomy, there are advantages to the latter. It is less technically demanding than the former, and the surgeon can directly advance the endoscope. A shorter and thus smaller-diameter instrument can be used. If a small bowel lesion is palpated or suspected and endoscopy by enterotomy is planned, the enterotomy should be made a short distance from the suspect lesion so that it does not interfere with its inspection. A purse-string suture may be placed at the enterotomy to minimize the risk of contamination. The bowel should be examined both proximally and distally (Fig. 13-2). The technique follows the same principles as those outlined above.

Other Uses of Endoscopy during Celiotomy

The most common indication for intraoperative small bowel endoscopy is evaluation of GI hemorrhage. Various other indications exist, including the diagnosis and treatment of small bowel polyps and tumors, management of intestinal webs and stenoses, and evaluation of inflammatory bowel disease and radiation enteritis. Since colonic pathology is much more frequent than small bowel disease, intraoperative colonoscopy is especially useful when open resection is necessary for polyp disease and the lesion cannot be accurately identified as to location by inspection and palpation during celiotomy. Intraoperative colonoscopy can prevent incorrect, inadequate, or excessive resection. Upper endoscopy can be used in a similar fashion.

Rigid and flexible endoscopy can be used to evaluate the integrity of anastomoses. Low anterior resection has the highest rate of anastomotic disruption of all colonic anastomoses. Once the anastomosis is completed either by suturing or stapling, a simple intraoperative maneuver to test its integrity relies on the presence or absence of air leakage through the anastomosis. The pelvis is filled with sterile saline or water so that the newly constructed anastomosis is submerged. The colon is pinched closed proximal to the anastomosis. A rigid or flexible endoscope is then introduced into the rectum via the anus but not allowed to traverse the anastomosis. Insufflation via the endoscope causes the bowel to distend; if bubbling is seen in the pelvic fluid, an anastomotic leak is present. The anastomosis is also visually inspected in this manner. Anastomoses in the upper GI tract can be evaluated in a similar fashion by introducing a gastroscope into the esophagus.

Endoscopy during Laparoscopy

The marriage of intraluminal endoscopy and laparoscopy has allowed a creative approach in the management of both benign and malignant GI diseases. This union occurred early in the evolution of laparoscopic surgery. In 1937, John C. Ruddock authored a paper entitled "Peritoneoscopy," published in *Surgery, Gynecology and Obstetrics*. Ruddock described the technique for examining the stomach for suspected malignancy using laparoscopy and an endoluminal tube fitted with a light and a channel for insufflation (Fig. 13-3). Although not truly an endoscope, this special tube allowed transillumination and distention of the gastric (or sigmoid colon) wall during laparoscopy. Gastric or intestinal wall that distended was identified as not being infiltrated by tumor. In that same year, E.T. Anderson also published a report entitled "Peritoneoscopy" in the *American Journal of Surgery*. He described a special instrument for use during laparoscopy called a "gastrodiaphane." This instrument carried light intraluminally and allowed for insufflation. In addition to the uses described by Ruddock, Anderson suggested that this instrument could be used to balloon the sigmoid colon while inspecting it during laparoscopy. These two examples, although not endoscopy and laparoscopy in the strict sense, represented ingenious attempts to merge two separate technologies to enhance the diagnostic power of laparoscopy.

The modern era of laparoscopy began with the introduction of laparoscopic cholecystectomy. Once laparoscopic cholecystectomy became established, the need to address common bile duct stones during this

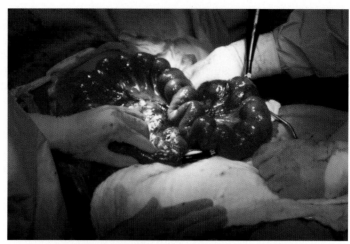

Fig. 13-2. Small bowel endoscopy by enterotomy. Contamination can be minimized by the use of a purse-string suture, surgical pads, and careful technique.

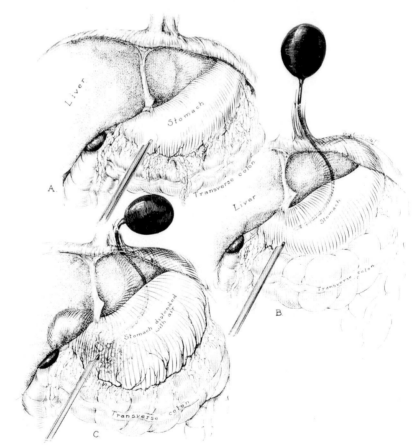

Fig. 13-3. Operability of gastric malignancy. A: Visualizing the stomach, liver, and adjacent tissues and localizing the malignancy. B: Unfolding the stomach under vision with air. C: Transillumination of the inflated stomach. (From Ruddock JC. Peritoneoscopy. Surg Gynecol Obstet 1937;65:623–629; with permission.)

procedure followed. Flexible choledochoscopy with stone extraction during laparoscopic cholecystectomy represents one of the most common intraoperative endoscopic examinations performed during laparoscopy (see Chapter 30). As expertise in both laparoscopy and flexible endoscopy increased, with concomitant improvement in technical support such as multiple video monitors and video mixers to produce simultaneous images, various other creative combined laparoscopic and endoscopic procedures have followed. For the sake of convenience, I have called this combination of simultaneous laparoscopy and endoscopy "endolap." Endolap is truly a surgical technique in evolution, and consequently what follows represents some examples of the direction and potential of the union between laparoscopy and endoscopy.

Applications of Endolap

Localization of Tumors and Lesions

As discussed earlier, intraoperative colonoscopy may at times be helpful during celiotomy, when accurate localization of lesions cannot be defined by palpation. Since palpation is even less sensitive during laparoscopy, intraoperative gastroscopy and colonoscopy can be invaluable for localization of lesions. It is also possible to perform laparoscopic-assisted enteroscopy to localize sources of obscure GI hemorrhage, duplicating the techniques described above during celiotomy (Fig. 13-4). Other examples include using flexible endoscopy to localize a lesion during laparoscopy and then employing a lift-and-resect technique with laparoscopic staplers, thus performing both excisional biopsy and simultaneous closure of the viscus. Alternatively, a lesion could be resected by the endoscope under laparoscopic control. If a full-thickness defect is created, it can be repaired by either laparoscopic suturing or stapling. I have found these techniques most helpful in managing sessile cecal polyps, which cannot be safely removed by colonoscopy alone.

Control of Upper Gastrointestinal Bleeding

Several endolap procedures have been devised to control upper GI bleeding. Kitano and associates reported a creative technique for intragastric insertion of the laparoscope for direct control of a bleeding lesion (Fig. 13-5). The lesion is initially localized intraoperatively with gastroscopy, and if it is posterior in location, laparoscopic cannulas are introduced directly into the stomach. This provides access for laparoscopic suturing and clipping of the bleeding vessel. Another ingenious method utilizes the transil-

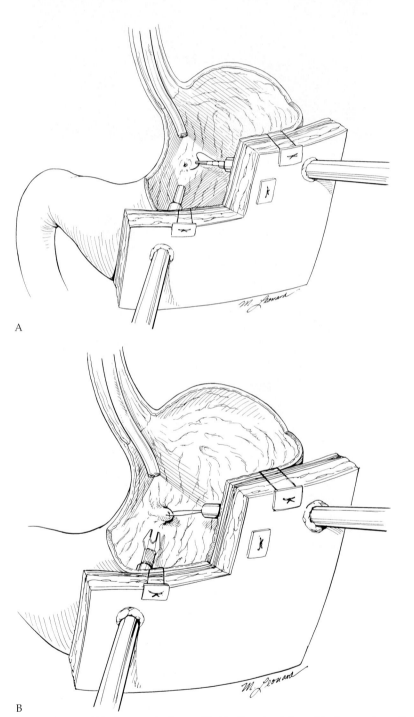

Fig. 13-4. Suture ligation of bleeding gastric ulcer. **A:** The bleeding ulcer is located in the posterior wall of the stomach as viewed laparoscopically. **B:** Suturing of the bleeding ulcer was done under laparoscopic guidance. (continued)

lumination of the gastric wall at the bleeding site provided by the gastroscope. Laparoscopy is used to define the feeding vessel on the serosal surface of the stomach. The vessel is then clipped proximally and distally with laparoscopic clips.

Gastric Tumor Excision

Introduction of the laparoscope directly into the stomach has been used to resect small posterior tumors (Fig. 13-6). The gastric lesion is identified by intraoperative gastroscopy, and then under gastroscopic control trocars are inserted directly into the anterior gastric wall. The lesion is then excised using laparoscopic techniques.

Laparoscopic Hepaticogastrostomy

Creation of an internal fistula to relieve obstructive jaundice when a malignancy encases the porta hepatis has been accomplished with a creative application of intraluminal endoscopy, interventional radiology, and laparoscopy (Fig. 13-7). This procedure illustrates the integration of multiple less invasive techniques to provide a result (palliation of obstructive jaundice) that would otherwise entail complex hepatobiliary surgery. This endolap procedure incorporates percutaneous intubation of the biliary tree using the Seldinger technique, laparoscopy, gastroscopy, and finally a variant of the technique of percutaneous endoscopic gastrostomy.

Conclusion

One may debate whether or not the sum of all of these minimally invasive procedures is truly less invasive than open surgery for this procedure, as well as other procedures. It is appropriate to be critical in the evaluation of each of these new procedures. By the nature of the problems that these operations address, there will be few instances in which these procedures can be critiqued in prospective, randomized trials. Reintroduction of endoscopy and laparoscopy into general surgical practice has unquestionably rejuvenated the disciple and expanded its horizons. It is hoped that the disciples of surgery can honestly and critically guide this growth for the betterment of patients and medicine.

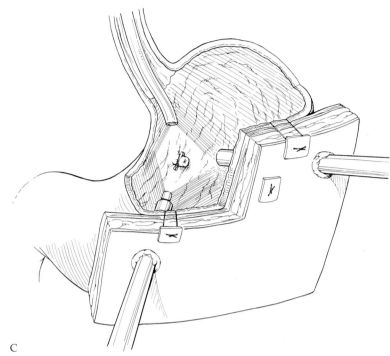

C

Fig. 13-4. (Continued) **C:** *The suture was pulled outside, and an endoclip was placed under endoscopic guidance. Bleeding from the gastric ulcer ceased. (Modified from Kitano S, Kawanaka H, Tomikawa M, Hirabayashi H, Hashizume M, Sugimachi K. Bleeding from gastric ulcer halted by laparoscopic suture ligation.* Surg Endosc 1994;8:405–407.)

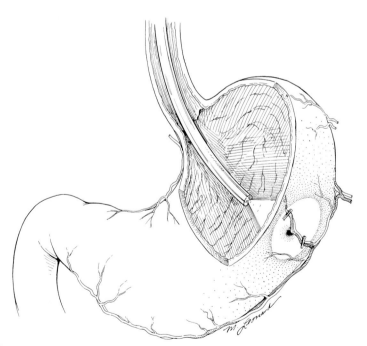

Fig. 13-5. *Gastroscope used to illuminate the gastric wall at bleeding site. Laparoscopy was used to define the feeding vessel on the serosal surface of the stomach. The vessel was then clipped proximally and distally with laparoscopic clips.*

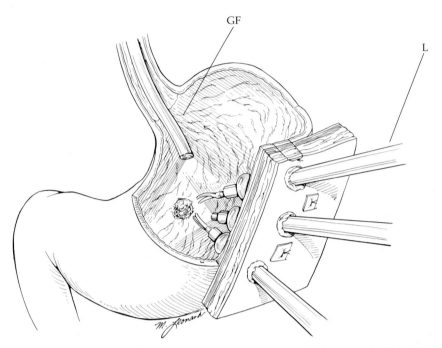

Fig. 13-6. Schema of laparoscopic intragastric surgery (GF, gastrofiberscope; L, laparoscope). (Modified from Ohashi S. Laparoscopic intraluminal (intragastric) surgery for early gastric cancer: a new concept in laparoscopic surgery. Surg Endosc 1995;9:169–171.)

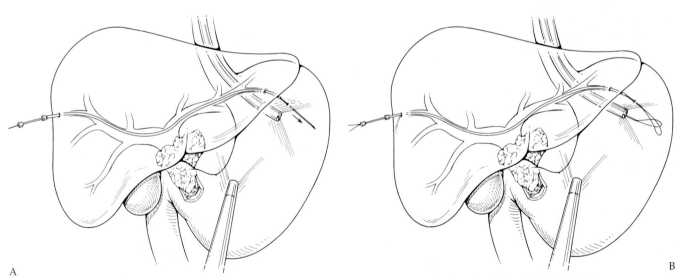

A

B

Fig. 13-7. Technique of peripheral biliary diversion. **A:** A 0.38-gauge flexible needle (3) is introduced through a 5-French (2) catheter to perforate the stomach. **B:** The snare is then introduced through a catheter into the stomach. (continued)

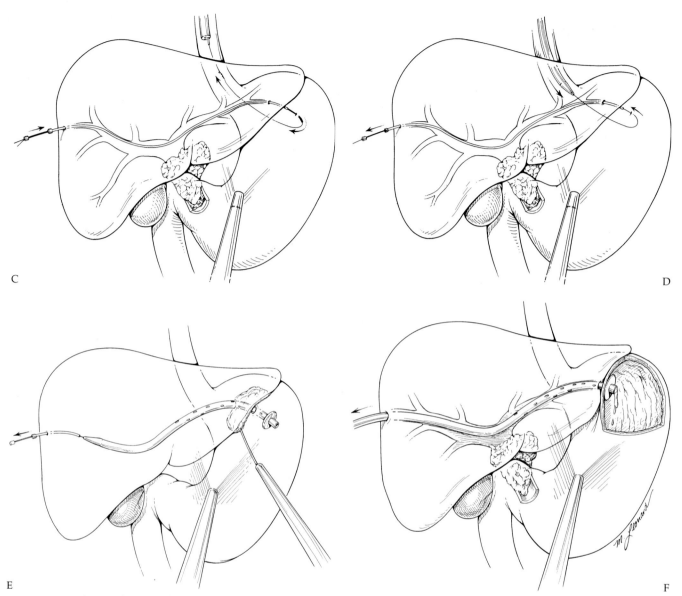

C   D

E   F

Fig. 13-7. (Continued) **C:** *The snare is grasped by the endoscopist and pulled through the patient's mouth.* **D:** *The snare is bound to a 20-French percutaneous endoscopic gastrostomy tube (8). The radiologist then pulls the wire previously positioned across the transhepatic tract, and the gastrostomy tube is gently drawn into the stomach by the surgeon.* **E:** *Stomach and inferior surface of the left hepatic lobe are coated with fibrin glue (10) by the surgeon.* **F:** *Anastomosis is maintained by tight traction on the tube, which is affixed to the skin to prevent bile leakage. (1, 8.5-French catheter; 2, 5-French catheter; 3, 0.38-gauge flexible needle; 4, endoscope; 5, laparoscope; 6, percutaneous snare; 7, endoscopic snare; 8, 20-French silicone percutaneous endoscopic gastrostomy tube; 9, flexible catheter for application of fibrin glue; 10, fibrin glue.) (Modified from Soulez G, Gagner M, Therasse E, et al. Malignant biliary obstruction: preliminary results of palliative treatment with hepaticogastrostomy under fluoroscopic, endoscopic and laparoscopic guidance.* Radiology 1994;192:241–246.)

Suggested Reading

Anderson ET. Peritoneoscopy. *Am J Surg* 1937;35:136–139.

Bowden TA Jr. Endoscopy of the small intestine. *Surg Clin North Am* 1989;69:1237–1247.

Bowden TA Jr. Intraoperative endoscopy of the gastrointestinal tract. In: Dent T, Strodel W, Turcotte J, eds. *Surgical endoscopy.* Chicago: Year Book Medical Publishers, 1985:167.

Flickinger EG, Stanforth AC, Sinar DR, MacDonald KG, Lannin DR, Gibson JH. Intraoperative video panendoscopy for diagnosing sites of chronic intestinal bleeding. *Am J Surg* 1989;157: 137–144.

Lau WY, Yuen WK, Chu KW, Poon GP, Li AK. Obscure bleeding in the gastrointestinal tract originating in the small intestine. *Surg Gynecol Obstet* 1992;174:119–124.

Kitano S, Kawanaka H, Tomikawa M, Hirabayashi H, Hashizume M, Sugimachi K. Bleeding from gastric ulcer halted by laparoscopic suture ligation. *Surg Endosc* 1994;8: 405–407.

Ruddock JC. Peritoneoscopy. *Surg Gynecol Obstet* 1937;65:623–629.

Stellato TA. Flexible endoscopy as an adjunct to laparoscopic surgery. *Surg Clin North Am* 1996; 76:595–602.

Stellato TA. History of laparoscopic surgery. *Surg Clin North Am* 1992;72:997–1002.

EDITOR'S COMMENT

Intraoperative endoscopy is an example of several individuals cooperating during an operative procedure to allow multiple simultaneous interventions in a given patient, thereby improving the outcome of the operation. One's imagination is the only limitation on the types of procedures that can be performed, based on this concept. Established procedures include those described in this chapter, as well as those for the combined therapy of common bile duct stones described in other chapters. Preoperative planning, coordination of the different surgeons, and appropriate patient preparation with bowel cleansing and positioning on the operating table are mandatory. In the future, newer combinations of intraluminal and extraluminal endoscopy will allow therapies heretofore unimagined. The surgeon with experience and the technical capabilities to perform these various modalities of endoscopy will be ideally suited to direct the operating team of the next millennium.

N.J.S.

II

Esophagus and Stomach

14

Diagnostic Upper Gastrointestinal Endoscopy

Bruce V. MacFadyen, Jr. and Arlene E. Ricardo

Esophagogastroduodenoscopy (EGD) can be a very challenging procedure, even in the hands of the most experienced endoscopist. It is essential to have a complete understanding of not only the instruments and their operation but also the indications, contraindications, preparation, potential hazards, and complications of EGD, as well as the appropriate technique for evaluating the upper gastrointestinal (GI) tract in a comprehensive manner while maintaining patient safety.

Although radiologic contrast studies continue to be an initial step in the evaluation of many GI complaints, actual visualization of the esophagus, stomach, and duodenum increases the accuracy of correctly identifying many pathologic lesions, including strictures, ulcers, masses, inflammatory changes, and foreign body. In addition, under direct visual examination, tissue specimens can be directly obtained by biopsy, brushings, or cytology.

It should be stressed that each endoscopist may have his or her own technique to perform EGD and that alternative techniques are available. There are several ways to navigate the endoscope through the upper GI tract by knowledge of different maneuvers. Special maneuvers are particularly helpful when dealing with difficult or altered anatomy. Even in these complicated cases, a safe and effective evaluation can still be performed.

Indications and Contraindications

One of the most important decisions an endoscopist has to make is to decide whether or not an EGD examination is indicated for a patient. Although the procedure is relatively safe, that does not necessarily equate to being appropriate in every case.

Diagnostic EGD is indicated for evaluating upper GI disorders (Table 14-1). It can provide early histologic evidence of malignancy by identifying and allowing biopsy of mucosal lesions. Symptoms of acid reflux, such as burning epigastric pain or vague abdominal and back pain, may indicate peptic ulcer disease and require a complete EGD evaluation. Melanotic stools usually indicate an actively bleeding source, whereas occult blood *per rectum* is more indicative of slower, more chronic bleeding. Any suspicion of upper GI bleeding should promptly be assessed with EGD, and therapeutic intervention performed, if necessary. Dysphagia and odynophagia are suggestive of esophageal pathology and are usually present for some time before patients present for evaluation. In such cases, it is important to perform an endoscopic examination as soon as possible. Abnormal radiographic studies, such as those suggestive of a mass lesion, ulcers, or strictures, require further endoscopic evaluation and biopsy. In addition, indeterminate radiographic examinations not yielding sufficient information require further evaluation. Other indications for EGD include the surveillance of premalignant conditions such as Barrett's esophagus and monitoring of healing or improvement of gastroduodenal ulcers.

There are also a few potential contraindications to performing EGD (Table 14-2). Lack of adequately trained personnel can make EGD more dangerous to patients and should not be performed unless a qualified endoscopist and assistant are available. Despite its necessity and a full understanding of the procedure and its risks and benefits, competent patients can still refuse a procedure. If there is any suspicion of perforation, patients require immediate surgical intervention, rather than delaying definitive treatment to perform an endoscopic examination. Similarly, ingestion of caustic materials can destroy the mucosa and weaken the intestinal wall, making EGD a dangerous examination in the acute period. Endoscopic evaluation in these cases should be delayed until the risk of perforation has diminished. If there is evidence or history of coagulopathy, such as a decreased platelet count or increased prothrombin or partial thromboplastin times, or if the patient is taking any medications that alter coagulation, the examination should be postponed until coagulation abnormalities are corrected and have returned to normal.

Instrumentation

Flexible endoscopes come in a variety of diameters and lengths and are either direct-viewing or video. The primary endoscope used for upper endoscopy is a 0-degree, forward-viewing endoscope, whereas the duodenoscope visualizes the GI tract at 90 degrees to the shaft. Side-viewing endoscopes are primarily used in the duodenum to visualize the ampulla of Vater, but they may also be used in the stomach. A major limitation of side-viewing endoscopes is that they pass blindly through the posterior pharynx and esophagus, unable to visualize these areas during the examination. Which endoscope to use depends on the examination to be done. All endoscopes are either video or fiberoptic, and all have a control head. In

Table 14-1. Indications for Diagnosis Esophagogastroduodenoscopy

Upper abdominal symptoms/signs suggesting malignancy

Gastroesophageal reflux refractory to appropriate medical therapy

Assessment of potential sites of acute or chronic upper gastrointestinal bleeding

Evaluation of symptoms of dysphagia or odynophagia

Abnormal or indeterminate radiographic studies

Previous upper gastrointestinal tract surgery or procedure with continued symptomatology

Follow-up of previous lesions that underwent therapeutic interventions

Surveillance for malignant lesions in high-risk patients

Table 14-2. Contraindications for the Performance of Esophagogastroduodenoscopy

Suspected or known perforation

Ingestion of caustic materials

Evaluation of lesions responding to medical management

Known or suspected coagulopathy

Refusal of procedure by competent patient

Uncooperative patient

Inadequately trained personnel

the fiberoptic units, an eyepiece is present for either direct visualization or for a video attachment. The shaft of the endoscope is flexible, especially at the distal tip, which has deflection capabilities ranging between 90 and 240 degrees in the up/down positions and 100 degrees in the right and left directions. The diameter of the insertion tube can range between 5.5 mm at the distal tip to 11 mm for a therapeutic endoscope, whereas the duodenoscope ranges between 11.5 and 12.5 mm.

The controls for maneuvering the deflection tip are located on the control head, with the larger, inner knob producing the up or down deflection and the smaller, outer knob producing a left or right deflection. Two depressable buttons are located adjacent to these deflection knobs, and, when pressed, the top button produces suction that may be necessary during the examination. The lower button serves two additional functions. Air insufflation occurs by simple placement of a finger over the lower button without applying pressure. When this button is depressed, a small amount of water is released from the tip of the endoscope that is useful for cleaning the lens tip during the examination, should it become dirty (Fig. 14-1). In video endoscopes, video control buttons on the top of the control head are used to freeze an image on the video screen or to save an image for printing.

The flexible shaft is usually 110 to 120 cm in length. These endoscopes contain a working channel that varies between 2 mm in pediatric endoscopes to 3.7 mm in therapeutic gastroscopes. On the other hand, the instrument channel in the duodenoscope varies from 3.2 to 4.2 mm. Biopsy forceps, cytology brushes, or other diagnostic instruments are passed through the accessory channel. A double-lumen therapeutic endoscope is also available for more advanced therapeutic endoscopy.

The flexible endoscope is connected to a light source that is either a 300-W xenon arc lamp or a halogen-tungsten lamp. In addition, air and water pumps for insufflation, suction, and irrigation are connected to the endoscope via the light source unit and controlled using the control buttons. If a video monitor is being used, this is also connected to the endoscope through the light source.

Proper hand positioning and manipulation of the flexible endoscope is key to performing an efficient examination. Most endoscopists will hold the control head of the endoscope in the left hand, with the thumb on the up/down knob and the index and middle fingers on the suction and air/water buttons. The thumb and index finger are then used to control the deflection tip during the examination. The right hand of the endoscopist is used to hold the flexible shaft for insertion, withdrawal, and rotation during the examination (Fig. 14-2).

Preoperative Preparation

During the initial office or clinic visit, all aspects of a patient's case should be reviewed by the endoscopist. The history and symptoms should be carefully reviewed to ensure that the an EGD evaluation is truly warranted. If radiologic contrast studies have been obtained, it is essential that the endoscopist review the films personally because they can provide valuable anatomic information, as well as warning of potential hazards, such as the presence of a stricture or a Zenker's or epiphrenic diverticulum.

A full explanation of the procedure and what patients can expect will greatly aid the endoscopist, since many fears or misconceptions can be eliminated in anxious patients. Many physicians will also give patients an information pamphlet or instruction document that will also answer questions. Most centers require that an informed consent document be signed by

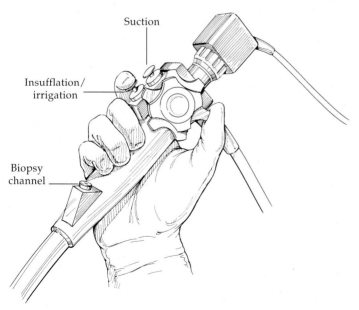

Suction

Insufflation/ irrigation

Biopsy channel

Fig. 14-1. Controls of a modern video upper endoscope.

patients or their representative prior to the procedure, indicating that they have received the appropriate and necessary information regarding the examination including its benefits and potential risks and agree to undergo the evaluation. Routine laboratory values may be obtained, especially a platelet count and coagulation studies, if any diagnostic or therapeutic procedures are anticipated.

Patients should be instructed not to take any food or liquid by mouth within 8 to 12 hours of the procedure. However, necessary medications such as antihypertensives, antiarrhythmics, or hypoglycemic agents may be taken with some water.

On the day of the procedure, patients should present themselves at least 1 hour before the scheduled examination time and should be accompanied by someone who can take them home afterward because sedation is usually given. Patients should then have an intravenous catheter placed through which sedative medications can be administered. The intravenous line is typically placed in the right hand or arm because patients are usually placed in the left lateral decubitus position. Hemodynamic monitoring devices should be applied to obtain blood pressure, heart rate, and oxygen saturation determinations. Real-time electrocardiogram monitoring may be necessary in patients with an extensive cardiac history. Supplemental oxygen should be readily available in the event of oxygen desaturation. The oral cavity should be inspected, and any dentures or prostheses removed, along with removal of eyeglasses and contact lenses. Mechanical problems during the evaluation can be hazardous to patients or interfere with the assessment and interpretation of findings. For this reason, the endoscopy nurse or assistant should ensure that the instrument chosen for the examination is functioning properly. All controls should be tested, and the water channels and suction apparatus should be checked for proper connection and operation. Once the examination is ready to begin, patients are placed in the left lateral decubitus position.

Sedation

To facilitate passage of the endoscope through the oropharynx, local pharyngeal anesthesia (i.e., benzocaine spray) is administered to the back of the oropharynx

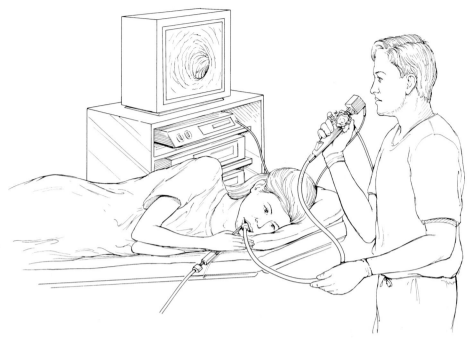

Fig. 14-2. Setup and patient positioning for diagnostic endoscopy.

to suppress the gag reflex. The physician can test the degree of anesthesia by placing his finger into the back of the throat and checking the gag reflex.

Most endoscopists use some sort of conscious sedation when performing an EGD. Sedation not only makes patients more comfortable but also enables the endoscopist to perform a more complete examination in a safer manner. Several different medications are used in endoscopy suites, and the agent or combination of medications chosen depends primarily on physician preference (Table 14-3). Initially, diazepam was the preferred medication; however, its association with thrombophlebitis has led to the increased use of other agents. Midazolam hydrochloride (Versed) is more potent than diazepam and has a more pronounced amnesic effect. These medications, however, can cause some degree of respiratory depression and should be used with close respiratory monitoring. With the combination of an opiate analgesic with the medication regimen, smaller doses of a benzodiazepine may be required, decreasing the risk of respiratory compromise. The addition of meperidine hydrochloride (Demerol HCl), for example, helps suppresses the gag reflex and produces a euphoria in anxious patients. Smaller initial doses of all medications are used in elderly, debilitated, and pediatric patients. Additional

Table 14-3. Medications Available for Conscious Sedation

Benzodiazepines
  Diazepam (Valium)
  Lorazepam (Ativan)
  Midazolam (Versed)
Opiate Analgesics
  Meperidine hydrochloride (Demerol HCl)
  Morphine
  Fentanyl citrate (Sublimaze)
  Butorphanol tartrate (Stadol)
Antihistamines
  Diphenhydramine hydrochloride (Benadryl)
  Promethazine hydrochloride (Phenergan)
Reversing Agents
  Naloxone hydrochloride (Narcan)
  Flumazenil (Romazicon)

doses of these medications can be given, as needed, throughout the examination. Some antihistamines, such as diphenhydramine hydrochloride (Benadryl) and promethazine hydrochloride (Phenergan), also have sedative properties, but they do not result in respiratory compromise and can be added during the procedure, if necessary. Reversal agents for both benzodiazepines and opiates—flumazenil (Romazicon) and naloxone hydrochloride (Narcan), respectively—must be readily available in case of respiratory depression or hypotension.

Endoscopic Technique

It is wise to develop a systematic routine for examining the entire esophagus, stomach, and proximal duodenum during EGD; this will reduce the potential for an incomplete evaluation. With patients in the left lateral decubitus position, pharyngeal anesthesia and intravenous sedation are administered. Once sedation is felt to be adequate, a bite block is placed in the patient's mouth to avoid inadvertent biting on the endoscope, which can damage the optic and mechanical apparatus.

Advancing the endoscope into the posterior pharynx to enter the esophagus can be very challenging, even for the experienced endoscopist. Three different techniques

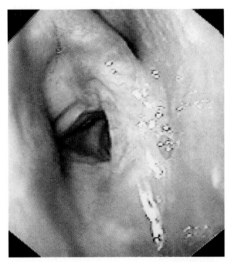

Fig. 14-3. The posterior pharynx with the vocal cords and cricoarytenoid cartilages visualized.

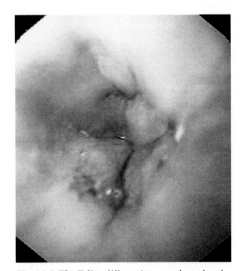

Fig. 14-4. The Z-line differentiates esophageal and gastric mucosa.

for esophageal intubation can be utilized, and it is important to know all three methods. Should one method fail, switching to another may prove successful. The first and safest method is using direct vision. With the light source and camera on, the endoscopist can visualize the structures of the posterior pharynx. As the tongue is passed, the uvula briefly comes into view. As the base of the tongue is passed, the epiglottis can be visualized, and finally the vocal cords and cricoarytenoid cartilages are seen (Fig. 14-3). To facilitate reaching this part of the pharynx, it is useful to angle the tip of the endoscope downward. To enter the first portion of the esophagus, the tip must pass below the cricoarytenoid cartilage on either side. The patient is asked to swallow, and with insufflation of some air, the upper esophageal sphincter will relax and open, allowing the instrument to slide into the esophagus. The esophageal lumen is now in view, and the endoscope is slowly advanced.

Another method for passing the instrument through the oropharynx is blind tip manipulation. With the tip of the endoscope held in the right hand, the instrument is passed over the tongue to the back of the mouth. With downward deflection of the tip, slight forward pressure is applied, and the patient is asked to swallow when the 20-cm mark is just outside the bite block. When the cricopharyngeal sphincter relaxes, resistance is lost, and the instrument passes into the esophagus.

The third method is to advance the endoscope past the posterior pharynx using finger guidance. The bite block is first passed over the endoscope, instead of being placed in the patient's mouth. With the fingers of the left hand placed over the back of the tongue to aid in keeping the instrument in the midline, the right hand pushes the tip of the endoscope to the back of the mouth. The fingers of the left hand are then removed, and the bite block is slipped into the patient's mouth. The patient is again asked to swallow, which should relax the sphincter, allowing the endoscope to pass into the esophagus. This method can be dangerous because patients may inadvertently bite on the endoscopist's fingers or on the endoscope prior to placement of the bite block.

Once the esophageal lumen is intubated, the instrument should be advanced while the lumen is kept in direct vision. The esophagus is lined by what appears to be

pale-pink squamous mucosa, and at the gastroesophageal junction, the pale mucosa changes to darker-red gastric mucosa. This junction is termed the *Z-line* (Fig. 14-4). This zone of mucosal transition is normally located at 38 to 40 cm from the incisors and approximately 1 cm above the diaphragmatic hiatus. Alterations in these measurements may give the examiner some indication that pathology exists in this area.

The tip of the endoscope usually passes easily through the lower esophageal sphincter into the cardia with the aid of some insufflation. At this point, some examiners choose to rapidly advance to the pylorus and into the duodenum, performing the majority of their evaluation on withdrawal

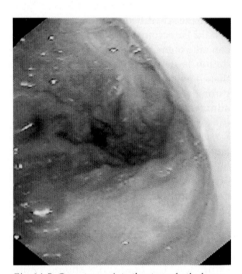

Fig. 14-5. On entrance into the stomach, the lesser curvature is on the right, and the fundus on the left. This helps identify the area of the antrum.

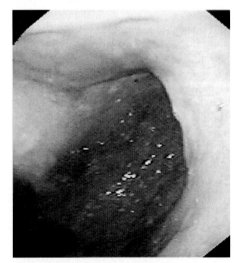

Fig. 14-6. The incisura on the right will indicate the direction of the pylorus.

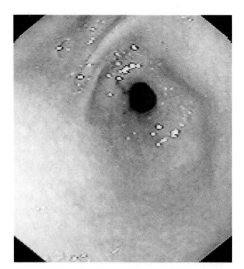

Fig. 14-7. Once in the antrum, the pylorus can be seen directly ahead.

of the instrument, whereas others choose to evaluate the stomach entirely prior to proceeding into the duodenum. Whichever method is chosen, the examiner should adopt a systematic approach so that no areas or lesions are missed.

Once the endoscope has passed into the stomach, its tip angles posteriorly, and the lesser curvature is now visualized. With counterclockwise rotation of the endoscope, turning of the tip to the right with the control knobs and insufflation of some air, the endoscope will be placed in the correct axis of the lumen. Again, the endo-

scope should never be advanced without having direct vision of the lumen. At this point, the view obtained should have the smooth surface of the lesser curvature on the right and the rugae of the fundus on the left (Fig. 14-5). The incisura can be seen demarcating the two, indicating the direction that must be taken to reach the pylorus (Fig. 14-6). Gastric juices, if present, can be aspirated; however, caution should be taken not to aspirate on the mucosa because this can create minor trauma or a "suction polyp" that can be confused with a pathologic lesion. To avoid this, the tip of the endoscope should be positioned just at the level of the fluid or just above it prior to aspiration. If there are excessive gas bubbles obscuring the mucosal view, a solution containing simethicone can be instilled through the working channel and subsequently aspirated.

The endoscope should be advanced slowly to the antrum and toward the pylorus (Fig. 14-7). The antral mucosa can be inspected, and the motor activity of the pylorus visualized. To complete the gastric survey, retroflexion of the endoscope is necessary to visualize the fundus and cardia and evaluate for the presence of a hiatal or paraesophageal hernia. Complete 180-degree upward angulation is obtained by deflecting the tip all the way up using the control knobs. The instrument is now seen passing through the gastroesophageal junction (Fig. 14-8), and by clockwise and

counterclockwise rotation of the endoscope along its axis, this area of the stomach can be completely visualized. Paradoxically, close-up views can be obtained by slowly withdrawing the endoscope from the mouth. After this portion of the examination, the endoscope is placed in the neutral position, and the examination is resumed.

Cannulating the pylorus can be a frustrating maneuver if there is a lot of motor activity at the pyloric channel. Using the control knobs, the tip of the endoscope is placed at the pyloric opening (Fig. 14-9). When the peristaltic activity of the stomach reaches the pylorus and it relaxes, the opening widens, and with gentle pressure the endoscope can pass into the duodenal bulb. Once through the pylorus and in the first portion of the duodenum, the control knob is turned to the right, and the scope is rotated clockwise along its axis. Upward movement of the tip also is often needed to fully visualize the duodenal lumen (Fig. 14-10). Since the endoscope can loop in the stomach, it may be difficult to manipulate or advance once it is in the duodenum. To correct this, the scope can be straightened by slow withdrawal, which will give the endoscopist better control of it.

The duodenum is then inspected methodically in a circumferential manner using the control knobs while the endoscope is slowly withdrawn back into the pyloric

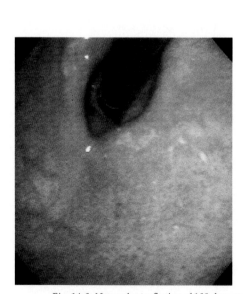

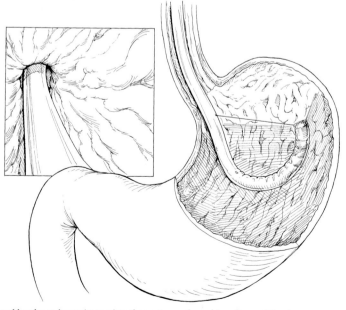

Fig. 14-8. Upward retroflexion of 180 degrees enables the endoscopist to view the gastroesophageal junction and fundus.

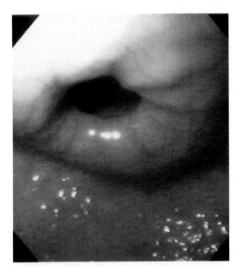

Fig. 14-9. Close-up of the pyloric opening.

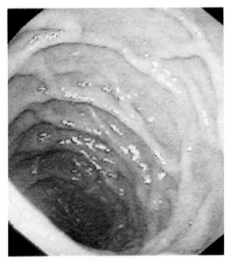

Fig. 14-10. Identification of the plica circularis confirms that the endoscope is in the duodenum.

channel. Several passes throughout the pylorus may be necessary to completely examine the pyloric channel and duodenal bulb. Once the evaluation of the duodenum is felt to be adequate, the endoscopic evaluation resumes in the stomach to complete the inspection of areas not previously visualized.

Once the entire EGD has been completed, any specimens can now be taken for histologic examination. It is important to take specimens after the visual evaluation because there is an increased risk of perforation if specimens are taken and the wall of the organ is compromised.

After all specimens have been obtained, the endoscope is returned to the neutral

position at the gastroesophageal junction. All excess air is aspirated to make the patient more comfortable during the recovery period. When this is accomplished, the instrument is withdrawn as the lumen is kept in view.

Diagnostic Procedures

During the EGD examination, biopsies, brushings, and aspirates are easily obtained. Typical lesions routinely evaluated by biopsy are esophageal strictures, mass lesions, gastroduodenal ulcers, gastroduodenitis, and polyps. Diagnostic yield increases when multiple specimens are taken of any suspicious lesion. If one suspects a malignancy, six biopsy specimens and cytology will increase diagnostic accuracy to better than 90% to 95%. Lesions arousing any suspicion for being varices should not be biopsied, as this can lead to significant bleeding.

Biopsy forceps come in many shapes and sizes (Fig. 14-11). The biopsy instrument is passed through the working channel, and once the tip is visible, the jaws are opened, pushed into the mucosa, closed, and then quickly pulled back, bringing with them an adequate specimen. Biopsy forceps containing a spike can be used to obtain multiple specimens without having to remove it from the endoscope. Biopsies of gastric ulcers should typically be taken in all four quadrants and at the base of the ulcer. The

transition zone between the ulcer and surrounding mucosa is the area that most likely contains increased mitotic activity in malignant ulcers, and therefore biopsy of this region improves diagnostic yield. Biopsies of submucosal masses can have limited yield because the submucosal location is not easily reached. To improve diagnostic yield, several biopsy specimens in the same location can be taken; however, caution is the rule because the area can become weakened and be at risk for perforation. Esophageal strictures, such as those from chronic acid reflux, may also demonstrate dysplasia or malignant transformation, and specimens should be obtained.

Polyps in the stomach or duodenum can also be cancerous and should be sampled. Either hot or cold biopsy forceps can remove diminutive polyps less than 5 mm in diameter, whereas a snare is best for larger polyps. The snare is placed at the base of a pedunculated polyp, and the polyp is removed in piecemeal fashion. Japanese investigators have developed techniques for lesion removal whereby a suction apparatus is passed through the endoscope and the lesion grasped with suction. A snare is then placed around the base of the lesion and closed tightly, and removal of the specimen is then possible. If significant bleeding results, standard coagulation techniques can be employed.

Cytology brushings can be taken during endoscopic examination as well. These

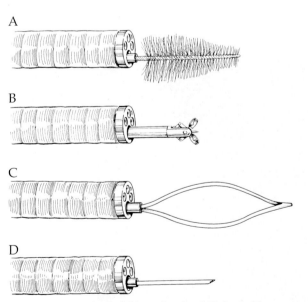

Fig. 14-11. Diagnostic tools for upper endoscopy. [A, cytology brush; B, jumbo biopsy grasper with spike; C, cautery snare; D, cytology needle (fine-needle aspiration).]

specimens are useful for diagnosing malignancies, fungal infections (candidiasis), and viral infections (cytomegalovirus). The brush is passed through the working channel of the endoscope and is then advanced along the surface of the lesion. The brush is then removed, the specimen is smeared on a slide, and a fixative is applied.

Aspirates are likewise easily obtained during EGD by instillation of sterile saline through the working channel and subsequent suctioning of the fluid back. To avoid contamination by other material previously aspirated, the fluid should be collected into a clean container with a trap attached to the suction apparatus. Both cytology and microbial examination can be performed on the collected material.

Gastric specimens from the antrum can be obtained by biopsy to test for *Helicobacter pylori*, which has a high correlation with the presence of peptic ulcer disease. When collected, these specimens are placed into specific kits prepared with chemical indicators to test for urease activity present in these bacteria (CLOtest*, Draper, UT).

Potential Problems

Occasionally during EGD evaluation, the endoscopist may come across some difficulties in completing the evaluation. Getting lost during EGD can be very frustrating. Slow, methodical progression of the examination is essential, and one must remember to always keep the lumen in view prior to advancing the instrument. The first maneuver to perform when one is unsure of one's location is to withdraw. This will usually put the lumen back into view and enable the endoscopist to confirm the location. Altered anatomy, such as that caused by previous surgery, can also often distort the remaining structures. This again emphasizes the need for knowing patients' full history and the importance of viewing prior radiographic studies. If there is still difficulty in proceeding with the evaluation, rotating the instrument or trying another direction or angle is often helpful.

Difficulty with visualization and disorientation in patients with normal anatomy can be due to insufficient insufflation. Problems with the air pump should have been identified prior to the start of the procedure. Adequate insufflation in the organ should allow the lumen to be visualized, but caution should be taken to avoid over-inflation, as this can become painful to patients or, in an extreme circumstance, lead to perforation. Perforation can also occur when force is applied either while the lumen is not visualized or when significant resistance is encountered, such as with a stricture. If the endoscope does not easily pass through an area, a smaller pediatric instrument can be tried, or the procedure terminated.

Retained food in the stomach can prevent viewing the entire mucosa and should either be washed away with saline through the working channel or aspirated to allow complete evaluation. Large particles or quantities of retained food should be lavaged with a large-bore orogastric tube first, and then the endoscopic evaluation can proceed.

Patient agitation can pose a serious problem during endoscopy by endangering the safety of patients and all involved in the examination. Patients should be securely restrained. Administering small quantities of additional sedation will usually allow the procedure to continue. Occasionally, the agitation is paradoxical, and in these instances the examination should be terminated and rescheduled. In some cases, general anesthesia is required in patients who are extremely difficult to sedate or in children. Respiratory distress in patients given too much sedation is infrequently encountered if the endoscopist is familiar with the side effects of the medications being used and if patients have the appropriate respiratory monitoring. All intravenous medications should be titrated slowly to obtain the desired level of sedation. Most important, reversal agents should be readily available and used if the need arises.

Complications

Bleeding occurs infrequently after a mucosal biopsy is obtained. Any history of prior bleeding or coagulation disorder, together with a list of current medications, should have been obtained prior to the examination. Checking the platelet count, prothrombin time, and activated partial thromboplastin time during the initial office evaluation will also alert the endoscopist to any potential bleeding problems.

These laboratory values should be routinely obtained, especially if biopsy or therapeutic procedures, such as stricture dilatation or stent placement, are anticipated.

Although perforation is rare, it can be life-threatening. All levels of the upper GI tract are vulnerable to perforation, but it occurs most commonly in the cervical and distal esophagus. Perforation is also associated with blind instrument passage. A perforation usually causes immediate pain; however, if it occurs in the stomach or duodenum, it is not always immediately apparent, and diagnosis may be delayed until the patient exhibits signs of either mediastinal, peritoneal, or retroperitoneal irritation. If there is any suspicion of perforation during EGD, the procedure should be terminated, and a chest x-ray and an abdominal series should be obtained. In most cases, perforation can be avoided by observance of some basic rules of endoscopy:

Pass the endoscope only with direct vision of the lumen;
Do not force the endoscope if resistance is encountered;
Do not use the endoscope as a dilator.

If it is determined that perforation has indeed occurred, emergent surgical intervention may be necessary.

Postprocedure Management

After EGD is completed, patients should be observed for a minimum of 1 hour. Hemodynamic and respiratory monitoring should continue until patients are fully awake and the effects of the sedation have sufficiently resolved. Signs of abdominal discomfort may be due to excess air left in the stomach or may be an indication of unsuspected perforation. Obtaining a plain-film radiograph of the abdomen (with either a standing or a lateral decubitus film) may be useful for identifying free air in the peritoneum, retroperitoneum, or even the mediastinum. If there is still a question regarding perforation, an esophagram and upper GI series utilizing meglumine diatrizoate (Gastrografin) contrast should be obtained. When patients are ready for discharge, an instruction sheet should be given, indicating diet, further follow-up, and a phone number to call if any questions or emergencies arise.

Conclusion

With the advent of flexible endoscopy and technologic advances in instrumentation, EGD has become a mainstay in the evaluation of upper GI pathology. Although the examination is relatively easy to perform and is usually the first endoscopic examination learned by training physicians, it can still be a very challenging procedure. A systematic method of endoscopic survey is necessary for proper and complete evaluation of the upper GI tract, with patient safety always kept in mind.

Suggested Reading

Andrus CH, Dean PA, Ponsky JL. Evaluation of safe, effective intravenous sedation for utilization in endoscopic procedures. *Surg Endosc* 1990;4:179–183.

Baillie J, ed. *Gastrointestinal endoscopy: basic principles and practice*. Oxford: Butterworth–Heineman, 1992:27–61.

Cotton PB, Williams CB, eds. *Practical gastrointestinal endoscopy*, 3rd ed. Oxford: Blackwell Science, 1990:23–55.

Fleischer D. Monitoring the patient receiving conscious sedation for gastrointestinal endoscopy: issues and guidelines. *Gastrointest Endosc* 1989;35:262–266.

Green FL. Esophagogastroduodenoscopy: indications, technique, and interpretation. In: Greene FL, Ponsky JL. eds. *Endoscopic surgery*. Philadelphia: WB Saunders, 1994:27–35.

Jaffe PE. Technique of upper gastrointestinal endoscopy. *Gastrointest Endosc Clin N Am* 1994; 4:501–521.

EDITOR'S COMMENT

Flexible endoscopy has become the diagnostic gold standard for many surgical diseases of the upper GI tract. It is particularly valuable for upper abdominal pain, GI bleeding, dysphagia, and peptic complaints. In addition, it is a valuable surveillance tool for diagnosis, staging, and follow-up of upper GI cancers or premalignant conditions.

Improvements in medication and technology have combined to make EGD a very benign and increasingly effective procedure. Short-acting sedatives with improved amnesia effect have made the procedure much more patient-friendly and safe.

The coupling of video technology to flexible endoscopes has also improved the procedure. The ability of the endoscopy staff to watch with the surgeon makes the procedure safer, quicker, and more effective. The improved lighting and magnification of the video monitor makes it less likely that small lesions or subtle mucosal changes will be missed.

Ease of use and portability mean that video endoscopy is an available tool for all aspects of surgical patient care. This includes use in the emergency and trauma rooms, in the surgical intensive care unit, and in operating room suites in combination with open or minimally invasive surgeries, as well as postoperatively as part of patient follow-up. As such, it should be an essential part of every GI surgeon's operative repertoire.

L.L.S.

15

Interventional and Therapeutic Upper Gastrointestinal Endoscopy

Thadeus L. Trus and Aaron S. Fink

Since its introduction at the turn of the 20th century, upper gastrointestinal (GI) endoscopy has progressed from a cumbersome exercise using large, rigid instruments to an integral component in the diagnosis and treatment of GI disorders. Esophagogastroduodenoscopy (EGD) has superseded barium meal as the diagnostic tool of choice for upper GI disorders. Beyond diagnosis, EGD allows biopsy, foreign body removal, stricture dilation, and direct control of bleeding lesions with diathermy, sclerotherapy, and laser coagulation. This chapter aims to review interventional and therapeutic measures available in upper GI endoscopy.

Foreign Body Removal

The majority of foreign body ingestions occur in the pediatric population, primarily in children 1 to 5 years of age. Foreign body ingestion in the adult population is generally associated with inebriation or psychiatric disorders or is performed intentionally for secondary gain, as in the case of incarcerated individuals. Fortunately, most (85% to 90%) objects will pass through the GI tract spontaneously. Approximately 10% require endoscopic removal, and approximately 1% require surgical intervention.

Indications for immediate extraction are respiratory distress and inability to handle secretions. Sharp objects such as small bones, toothpicks, pins, and glass should be removed expeditiously because of the risk of local or distal perforation. Generally, objects longer than 5 cm or thicker than 2 cm are unlikely to pass through the pylorus and should be removed. Airway protection is of utmost importance when foreign bodies are removed endoscopically. General anesthesia and endotracheal intubation are often used in pediatric patients but are generally not necessary in adults, provided one uses adequate sedation. Placing patients in Trendelenburg position decreases the likelihood of the object's falling into the trachea during removal. An endoscopic overtube may protect the esophagus from perforation when sharp objects are removed. If possible, extraction rehearsal should be performed *ex vivo* using a similar foreign body.

Coins are by far the most common foreign body ingested by children. The majority (95%) lodge in the cervical esophagus and are easily seen radiographically. If the coin is lodged in the cervical esophagus, its edge is seen on the lateral view, and the flat surface on posteroanterior view. The views are reversed if the coin is lodged in the trachea. If there is more than an hour delay between the diagnostic radiograph and endoscopy, or a sudden disappearance of symptoms, repeat studies should be performed to rule out migration. The longer the foreign body remains in the esophagus, the greater will be the risk of respiratory symptoms, as well as pressure necrosis and fistula.

Endoscopic removal can be achieved using alligator forceps, tenaculum forceps, or occasionally a polypectomy snare. Blunt removal with a Foley catheter is not recommended, since it does not provide adequate control of the foreign body. After adequate patient preparation, the endoscope is gently introduced into the cervical esophagus. The coin, usually seen immediately on entry into the cricopharyngeus, is grasped and removed with the endoscope. If it has migrated into the distal esophagus, it can be removed or pushed into the stomach and left to pass spontaneously. If it is not initially seen, the posterior esophageal wall should be carefully inspected in case the coin is hidden by a mucosal fold. Intraoperative radiography is seldom necessary to locate the object.

Meat impaction is the most common foreign body in the adult population. Contrast studies are rarely necessary and often make subsequent endoscopy more difficult. If patients are able to handle secretions, urgent endoscopy is not necessary. In fact, the food bolus may pass spontaneously after administration of mild sedation. These patients should still undergo endoscopy to rule out esophageal pathology, which is usually present, although rarely neoplastic. The impacted bolus can often be gently pushed into the stomach through the point of obstruction. If necessary, extraction can usually be achieved with a polypectomy snare. Occasionally, the meat will fragment and require removal in piecemeal fashion; in the latter situation, an esophageal overtube may be helpful because multiple reinsertions of the endoscope will be necessary (Fig. 15-1). Meat tenderizing agents such as papain are not recommended.

Whatever the object, successful removal should be followed by careful endoscopic examination of the esophagus. Peptic stricture can be dilated immediately, provided that tissue reaction or edema is not excessive.

Esophageal Stricture Dilation

Esophageal strictures narrow the esophageal lumen as a result of scar contracture or abnormal tissue deposition. Three pathogenic mechanisms lead to stricture formation: epithelial injury, motility disorders, and malignant degeneration. The latter is an obvious etiology that is discussed in subsequent chapters.

The most common cause of epithelial injury is gastroesophageal reflux of acid. Other causes include bile reflux, caustic ingestion, contact injury from foreign bodies or pills, and radiation injury. Epithelial injury leads to inflammation and subsequent repair with collagen deposition and fibrosis. Circumferential scar tissue, in turn, can narrow the esophageal lumen. Key to successful stricture management is prevention of further exposure to the offending agent (e.g., acid, pills) and early, aggressive dilation. Rigid, noncompliant scar tissue may not be dilatable by usual means and may require surgery.

Esophageal dysmotility can also result in stricture formation. Poor esophageal clearance of even small amounts of refluxed acid can lead to prolonged mucosal exposure with subsequent epithelial damage. Similarly, poor peristalsis results in prolonged esophageal exposure to ingested food and liquids, some of which may cause mucosal injury. Finally, failure of lower esophageal sphincter relaxation in achalasia results in delayed esophageal emptying due to functional distal esophageal narrowing.

Esophageal strictures present clinically with symptoms of dysphagia, odynophagia, regurgitation, and occasionally bleeding. Most diagnoses can be made from the clinical history. Physical examination should be performed with a view to signs of connective tissue disease (e.g., scleroderma) or malignancy. Barium studies are useful to identify stricture location, length, and caliber. Endoscopy with cytologic brushings and/or biopsy should then be performed to identify the nature of the stricture. If possible, complete upper GI examination should be performed after dilation to rule out any associated disorders.

Strictures can be graded as follows:

Grade I Strictures with a diameter of 12 mm or greater, allowing passage of a 36-

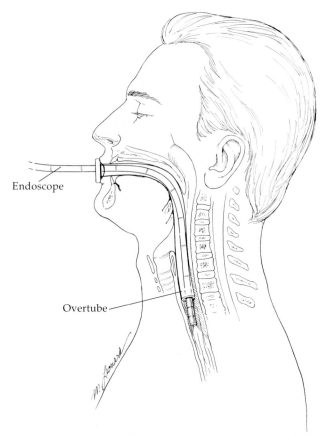

Fig. 15-1. Esophageal overtube is useful for procedures needing multiple scope introductions.

Endoscope

Overtube

All sharp objects should be removed before they pass through the pylorus, since up to one-third will perforate the bowel distally (usually around the ileocecal valve). Extraction of sharp objects may be particularly challenging. Extreme caution must be used to prevent the potentially fatal complication of esophageal perforation. Safety pins can be particularly troublesome. If the sharp point is directed orad, it can be pushed into the stomach, regrasped, and removed with the sharp point trailing, thus avoiding perforation. Large-pin or razorblade removal is facilitated by an esophageal overtube.

Many small electronic devices are powered by small alkaline button batteries. These small (less than 2 cm) batteries usually pass through the GI tract without problem. If lodged, however, batteries may cause injury by pressure necrosis, direct corrosion, or low-voltage burns. If one encounters difficulty in grasping the battery, it can be pushed in the stomach where retrieval may be easier or abandoned to allow for spontaneous passage. One must carefully inspect the esophagus

after the battery is removed to ensure that the mucosa is not damaged.

Cocaine trafficking has created another cause of foreign body ingestion. The cocaine is often packaged in condom packets that are swallowed to avoid detection. These packets *should not* be removed endoscopically because of the risk of package rupture. These are best managed expectantly or surgically.

Radiolucent objects such as fish bones, glass, or wood are often not visualized radiographically. Thin barium may be used to outline the object prior to endoscopic extraction. If patients remain symptomatic but no foreign body is identified by contrast radiography, endoscopy should be performed.

If extraction was in any way difficult or patients develop signs and symptoms of perforation, water-soluble swallow with meglumine diatrizoate (Gastrografin) should be performed immediately. Perforation is a potentially fatal complication that must be treated aggressively with antibiotics and often with surgical repair.

French (36-F) (12 mm) endoscope without difficulty

Grade II Strictures with a diameter between 10 and 12 mm, allowing passage of a 36-F endoscope with some difficulty

Grade III Strictures with a diameter less than 10 mm, not allowing passage of a 36-F endoscope

Dilation is usually achieved using one of three types of dilators: (a) flexible, mercury-filled rubber dilators with either a blunt tip (Hurst) or a taper tip (Maloney) (Fig. 15-2); (b) semiflexible taper-tipped polyvinylchloride dilators with a hollow core, allowing guidewire passage (Savary), or (c) balloon dilators passed either through the scope or over a guidewire. The more rigid, olive-tipped dilators (Eder-Puestow) are no longer recommended.

Maloney dilators range in size from 12- to 60-F (4 to 20 mm) and are often preferred over Hurst dilators because of their tapered tip. These dilators are generally reserved for patients with short, mild-to-moderate chronic strictures in a relatively short esophagus. Patients should be placed in a sitting position to allow gravity-assisted dilator passage (Fig. 15-2). Little or no intravenous sedation is given; topical pharyngeal anesthesia may be used.

The initial dilator size should be smaller than the stricture. A well lubricated dilator is then introduced into the posterior pharynx for the patient to swallow. Gentle pressure is used to advance the dilator with swallowing. Excessive force should never be used, as it may result in esophageal perforation. Successive dilators should increase in size by three or four French with each passage. Some advocate that no more than three dilators of successive size be used at each session. Others continue successive dilation to a size of 50-F or until pain, resistance, or blood staining of the dilator is encountered. Multiple sessions are frequently required to alleviate dysphagia and maintain a patent lumen. The frequency of dilation depends on stricture severity and patients' symptoms.

Savary dilators are available in 70- or 100-cm length (70 cm is adequate for esophageal dilation) and range in size from 5 to 15 mm. As mentioned, they contain a hollow core, allowing passage over a guidewire. These dilators are somewhat

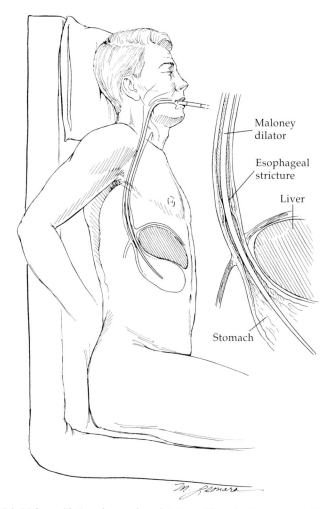

Fig. 15-2. Maloney dilation of an esophageal stricture. The patient is in an upright position.

more rigid than mercury-filled bougie dilators and are used more frequently in long, narrow, and/or firm strictures. Guidewires can be passed through the strictured segment using endoscopic and/or fluoroscopic guidance. Many advocate routine fluoroscopy for guidewire placement and dilator passage to ensure that the wire does not migrate during dilator changes. Fluoroscopy is particularly useful when dealing with an esophagus that is tortuous or contains a diverticulum.

Savary dilation is performed with the patient mildly sedated and in the left lateral decubitus position (Fig. 15-3). Endoscopy is performed, the wire is passed beyond the strictured segment, and the endoscope is then removed. Guidewire position is confirmed fluoroscopically. The dilator is then passed over the guidewire beyond the strictured segment (Fig. 15-3). An assistant holds the guidewire and tries to prevent its migration during dilator pas-

sage. Repeat fluoroscopy is helpful to ensure that the guidewire remains in the proper position. It is generally recommended that one should not exceed the initial dilator size by more than three sizes. The appearance of blood on the dilator is also an indication to terminate the current dilation session.

Balloon dilation is an alternative technique of stricture dilation. Balloon dilators may be passed through the scope or over a guidewire. As implied, the former are placed through the stricture under direct endoscopic visualization (Fig. 15-4), whereas the latter are passed over an endoscopically or fluoroscopically placed guidewire. Through-the-scope dilators are available in sizes from 18- to 54-F (inflated, outer diameter); although these may be passed through a 2.8-mm biopsy channel, a 3.5-mm working channel is preferred. Over-the-guidewire dilators are available in sizes up to 60-F.

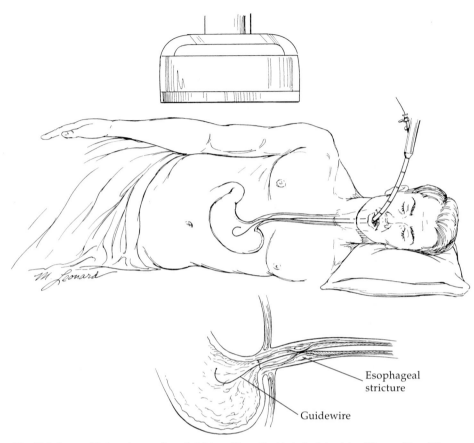

Fig. 15-3. Savary dilation of an esophageal stricture. The patient is in the lateral decubitus position. Wire position is confirmed fluoroscopically prior to dilator passage.

Esophageal stricture

Guidewire

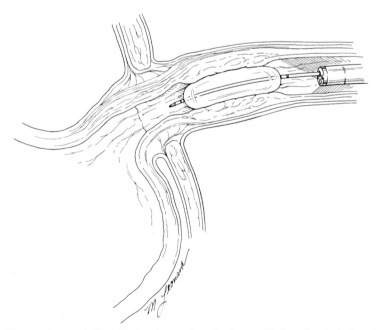

Fig. 15-4. Through-the-scope balloon dilation of an esophageal stricture with the patient in the lateral decubitus position. The deflated balloon is passed through the operating channel of the endoscope and positioned across the stricture under direct vision, thus eliminating the need for fluoroscopy in most cases.

Through-the-scope dilators do not require fluoroscopy because the entire process is performed under direct vision. Patients are sedated and placed in the left lateral decubitus position. Endoscopic placement of the deflated balloon is achieved, and then the balloon is inflated with water. A pressure gauge is used to avoid excessive inflation pressure that might cause balloon rupture. The balloon is inflated for several 1-minute intervals; occasionally, several balloons of increasing size may be required to achieve the desired dilation. Over-the-guidewire balloon dilators have fluoroscopic markers to assist balloon positioning within the stricture. Dilation is monitored by following the disappearance of the balloon's waist created by the stricture.

Compared to techniques using tapered dilators, balloon dilation provides decreased mucosal injury and slightly lessened patient discomfort. Unfortunately, the balloon's theoretical advantage of evenly distributing force around the stricture surface has not translated into a significant clinical advantage over other dilation techniques. In fact, balloon dilators may actually be less effective with particularly rigid strictures. Familiarity should be acquired with the various dilation techniques because they are frequently used in combination.

Overall success rates of peptic stricture dilation approach 80% to 90%. Approximately 50% of these patients gain long-term relief with only one dilation, whereas 50% require multiple dilations. Factors influencing long-term success include stricture character, as well as control of the underlying reflux either medically or surgically. Optimal dilator size and dilation frequency should be decided on an individual basis. Occasionally, steroid injection of the strictured segment, coupled with dilation, is helpful when dealing with strictures resistant to dilation alone. Failure to achieve prolonged relief of dysphagia after repeated dilations is an indication for surgical intervention.

While complications infrequently follow stricture dilation, they can be fatal if misdiagnosed or improperly treated. Significant bleeding is rare. In experienced hands, perforation rates are 0.01% to 0.25%. Forceful pneumatic balloon dilation (used to stretch and rupture the circular lower esophageal sphincter muscle in achalasia) carries a slightly higher perforation rate than those described above. Eder-Puestow dilators are also associated with a higher perforation risk than more commonly used dilators, and thus are not recommended. Stricture character also influences the perforation risk: Caustic stricture dilation carries a significantly higher risk of perforation than peptic stricture dilation.

Since the signs and symptoms of perforation may be quite subtle, one should have a high degree of suspicion, and aggressively investigate and treat any patient with postdilation complaints. Persistent pain and tachycardia in the postdilation period is often the earliest symptoms. The presence of subcutaneous emphysema is diagnostic. Late signs and symptoms include fever, dysphagia, odynophagia, and pleuritic or retrosternal pain. Since plain radiographs are normal in approximately one-third of patients, contrast esophagram is the investigation of choice. Water-soluble contrast should be used first, and if findings are normal, this should be followed by dilute barium, which can detect small leaks not visualized with water-soluble contrast. False-negative rates for contrast esophagrams have been reported as high as 10%; thus if clinical suspicion remains high, computed tomography should be performed.

Initially, esophageal perforations cause a chemical mediastinitis, are usually contained within the mediastinum, and drain back into a nonobstructed esophagus; therefore, early perforations can often be treated conservatively. Conservative management consists of *nil per os*, total parenteral nutrition, nasogastric suction, and broad-spectrum antibiotics for 10 to 14 days. Surgical drainage and/or repair should be used liberally in patients who fail to improve or whose perforation was not diagnosed early, allowing development of mediastinal sepsis. Malignant stricture perforation should be treated surgically with excision and reconstruction.

Gastric Polyps

Gastric polyps are relatively uncommon and most often asymptomatic, usually being discovered incidentally during endoscopic or radiographic investigations of the upper GI tract. Most (75%) are hyperplastic and do not carry a significant risk of malignant potential. On the other hand,

25% of polyps are adenomatous and carry a malignant potential relative to their size.

All gastric polyps should be biopsied, and pedunculated polyps or those causing bleeding or obstruction should be removed. If the biopsy reveals that the polyp is hyperplastic, excision is not recommended. Adenomatous polyps, however, should be excised. Patients with adenomatous polyps should undergo endoscopy annually until no further polyps are found at consecutive examinations. Surveillance endoscopy should then be performed every 3 years. If polyps are sessile, multiple, or larger than 2 cm, partial gastrectomy should be considered.

Nonvariceal Upper Gastrointestinal Bleeding

The most common causes of upper GI bleeding are listed in Table 15-1. While the first priority in patients with upper GI hemorrhage is adequate resuscitation and stabilization, early endoscopic evaluation plays a crucial role in their management. Upper GI hemorrhage is often self-limiting. A nonbleeding period following an acute bleed provides an excellent window of opportunity to intervene and possibly prevent recurrent bleeding. Whenever possible, the upper GI tract should first be lavaged of blood and clots with a large-bore tube to allow adequate endoscopic visualization.

Intervention should be performed in actively bleeding lesions and in those lesions likely to rebleed (Table 15-2). Between 80% and 90% of actively bleeding or oozing le-

Table 15-1. Endoscopically Diagnosed Causes of Upper Gastrointestinal Bleeding

Bleeding Source	Incidence (%)
Peptic ulcer disease	36
Acute gastric mucosal lesions	33
Esophageal varices	13
Mallory-Weiss tear	7
Other	11

Table 15-2. Endoscopic Findings Predictive of Rebleeding

Massive hemorrhage
Posterior duodenal bulb ulcer
High lesser curve ulcer
Active bleeding or oozing ulcer bed
Visible vessel or pigmented protuberance
Adherent clot
Positive Doppler signal

sions will continue to bleed or rebleed. The presence of a sentinel clot or a visible vessel within a nonbleeding ulcer crater is also a strong (approximately 50%) predictor of rebleeding (Fig. 15-5). A black protuberance or black spot may represent pseudoaneurysm of an underlying vessel; its ability to predict rebleeding is less than those mentioned above. The location and size of a lesion are also predictors of rebleeding; an ulcer of the inferoposterior wall of the duodenal bulb is much more likely to rebleed than a prepyloric lesion because the former often overlies a branch of the gastroduodenal artery.

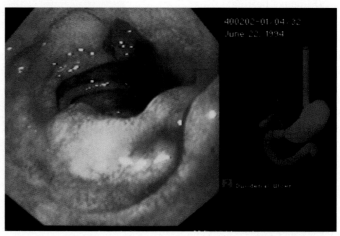

Fig. 15-5. Presence of a visible vessel in a duodenal ulcer.

Several options for hemostatic control are available to the endoscopist. The more common means are thermal coagulation and injection therapy. Mechanical devices and topical agents have also been used.

Early techniques of thermal coagulation employed monopolar electrocautery. The device transfers electric current from a generator to the tissue and subsequently to a grounding pad. The high-density current is converted to heat at the tissue level, resulting in protein coagulation and tissue (vessel) shrinkage. The probe is placed approximately 2 mm from the vessel and activated for approximately 2 seconds. The process is repeated circumferentially around the area. Successful coagulation rates have been reported to be 80% to 95%. Unfortunately, the depth of tissue injury is difficult to control, leading to a significant perforation rate. Monopolar hemostasis devices have been abandoned with the development of safer methods.

Bipolar or multipolar electrocoagulation limits tissue injury depth to a maximum of 3 mm, thus making perforation less likely than with monopolar devices. Current passes between electrodes arranged around the probe tip, alleviating the need for a grounding pad. Power settings may be varied up to 50 W, delivering power either in 1- or 2-second intervals or continuously. Power delivery and irrigation are controlled with a foot pedal. Large probes (3.2 mm) have been found to achieve better hemostasis than smaller ones. The endoscopist should place the probe firmly against the lesion to encourage coaptive coagulation and fire the probe at a high power for several 2-second bursts. If this method is unsuccessful, a lower-power, continuous-output (i.e., 5 to 10 seconds) method is employed to provide deeper heating.

The heater probe contains a polytef (Teflon)-coated, aluminum-encased heater coil at its tip that can achieve extremely high temperatures. The probe is somewhat rigid to allow coaptive coagulation. Irrigation of the target lesion through channels within the probe prevents tissue adherence to the probe tip (Fig. 15-6). Coagulation is achieved by heat conduction without passage of any electrical current through patients. Thermal energy delivery and intensity of irrigation are both adjustable.

A variety of techniques may be used to achieve coagulation. Generally, firm pressure should be applied to tamponade ac-

tive bleeding, after which several energy pulses are applied circumferentially around the lesion's edge and to any visible vessel. Others advocate bleeding-point coagulation alone. Regardless of technique, successful hemostasis can be achieved in over 90% of patients with a very low perforation rate (Fig. 15-7).

Laser light, the final thermal coagulation method, is delivered to the tissue through its probe's quartz fibers; the probe also allows passage of water or carbon dioxide to prevent overheating at the tip. Both argon and neodymium:yttrium-aluminum-garnet (Nd:YAG) lasers have been used successfully in the treatment of GI hemorrhage. The argon laser generates a blue-green light that is strongly absorbed by hemoglobin; thus, this laser has a minimal depth of tissue penetration, resulting in a relatively shallow coagulative effect. Argon lasers are often used preferentially for treating vascular malformations, but not ulcers. The Nd:YAG laser, on the other hand, emits light in the near-infrared portion of the spectrum that is poorly absorbed by tissue chromophores. This results in maximal light scattering and a wider, deeper area of tissue coagulation and injury.

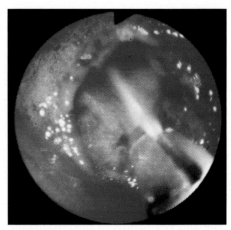

Fig. 15-6. *Irrigation of an ulcerated area immediately following coagulation with a heater probe.*

Laser coagulation of upper GI hemorrhage is equivalent to other forms of coagulation. Unfortunately, laser units are large and costly and require a significant amount of training for their use. Conversely, other coagulation and injection techniques are just as effective, more portable, and much less expensive. These differences have limited laser use to fairly specialized situations (i.e., pigmented lesions).

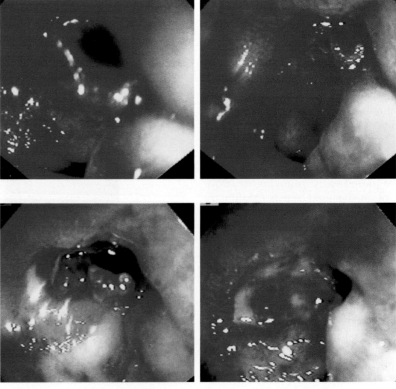

Fig. 15-7. *Duodenal ulcer before and immediately after treatment with a heater probe.*

Although developed primarily for bleeding esophageal varices, injection techniques have increasingly been used in nonvariceal hemorrhage. Table 15-3 lists various sclerosing and vessel-constricting agents available and their recommended dosages. Therapy is performed through a 23- or 25-gauge retractable 5-mm needle that is passed through the endoscopic operating channel. The goal is to view the lesion *en face* and to inject submucosally at three or four sites circumferentially around any bleeding vessel, as well as at additional circumferential sites approximately 1 cm away. Injection volumes are variable and should be large enough to achieve tamponade without extensive tissue damage. Vessel constriction and/or sclerosis may be induced, depending on the nature of the sclerosant. No agent has been shown to be superior, all offering 85% to 95% efficacy with very low complication rates.

Topical agents such as tissue glues, clotting factors, and collagen hemostatic agents have been used with varying degrees of success. Early experience with mechanical devices such as endoscopically applied clips or metal sutures has been encouraging. However, experience is limited and proper trials of their use remain to be performed.

Complication of established hemostatic techniques are relatively rare. These include perforation, tissue necrosis, induction of bleeding, and delayed hemorrhage. Perforation is reported in 1% to 3% of patients and is more commonly seen with monopolar cautery and Nd:YAG laser use. Tissue necrosis has been associated with ethanolamine oleate injection but is rare. Induced bleeding from a visible vessel occurs in 5% to 30% of patients and is more commonly seen with thermal coagulation. These rebleeds can usually be controlled with repeated endoscopic therapy.

Upper Gastrointestinal Varices

Most variceal hemorrhages originate from the distal esophagus; approximately 10% originate from the gastric fundus. The in-

hospital mortality of bleeding esophageal varices approaches 30%, with a greater than 60% rebleeding rate among survivors. Acute sclerotherapy controls bleeding and reduces transfusion requirements but does not significantly influence

Table 15-3. Sclerosing Agents Available for Injection Therapy of Upper Gastrointestinal Hemorrhage

Sclerosing Agent	Recommended Dose (mL)
Absolute ethanol (98%)	0.5–1
Epinephrine (1:10,000)	6–12
Epinephrine (1:10,000) + polidocanol (1%)	5–12 + 5
Hypertonic saline (3.6%) + epinephrine (1:20,000)	9–12
Morrhuate sodium (5%) + (thrombin + dextrose [50%])	3 + 2
Thrombin (100 IU) in 3 ml of saline (0.9%)	10–15

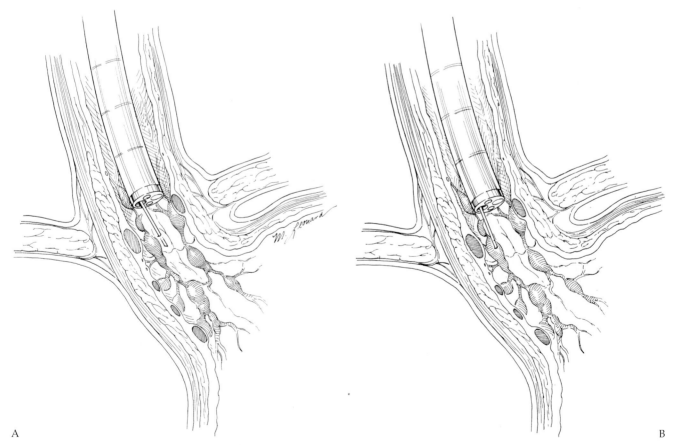

A   B

Fig. 15-8. Variceal injection sclerotherapy. **A:** *Paravariceal injection sclerotherapy. Small aliquots of sclerosant are injected beside the varix to induce fibrosis but maintain venous flow.* **B:** *Intravariceal injection sclerotherapy. Sclerosant is injected directly into the varix to cause thrombosis.*

long-term survival. Newer methods of variceal banding may improve these results.

Endoscopy should be performed as soon as possible after adequate resuscitation. Tracheal intubation should be used liberally for airway protection. An esophageal overtube may facilitate multiple endoscope insertions, lavage of blood, and airway protection in nonintubated patients. Rarely, in situations of massive hemorrhage, a Sengstaken-Blakemore tube may be necessary for 12 to 24 hours prior to endoscopy.

Various sclerosing agents are available, none of which has been shown to be superior in comparative trails. The most commonly used agents in the United States are 0.7% to 3.0% sodium tetradecyl sulphate and 5% morrhuate sodium. Ethanolamine is more commonly used in Canada and Europe. Total volumes of injected sclerosant vary according to the agent and the nature of the varices (generally 18 to 30 mL).

There are two schools of thought as to the optimal injection site. Paravariceal injection is used to develop a fibrous cover around the varices, preventing bleeding while allowing them to serve as collaterals for portal venous decompression (Fig. 15-8A). Multiple injections of less than 1 mL of sclerosant are made at 1-cm intervals on either side of the varix in the distal 5 to 10 cm of esophagus. This process should be performed circumferentially. Intravariceal injection (Fig. 15-8B) is used to induce varix thrombosis (Fig. 15-9). Injections of 1 to 5 mL are made directly into the varix at

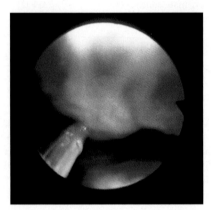

Fig. 15-9. Endoscopic view of an intravariceal injection of sclerosant to cause thrombosis.

or just proximal to the gastroesophageal junction; distention and blanching of the varix should occur. If active bleeding is encountered, an injection should be attempted below the bleeding site. Further injections may be made at 2- to 3-cm intervals more proximally until small-caliber vessels are encountered. Both techniques appear to be equally effective in most studies. Only one study has demonstrated superiority with intravariceal injection.

After resolution of acute bleeding, a second sclerotherapy session should be performed 5 days later. Subsequent sessions should be repeated at 1- to 3-week intervals until variceal ablation is achieved. Successful control of bleeding is achieved in approximately 85% of acute bleeding episodes. Recurrent bleeding may decrease with serial sclerotherapy sessions.

Complication rates are significant. Pulmonary complications may be as high as 60%, although major complications (e.g., aspiration pneumonia, adult respiratory distress syndrome) can be minimized with aggressive pretreatment airway protection. Fever and chest pain occur in 5% to 10% of patients following sclerotherapy.

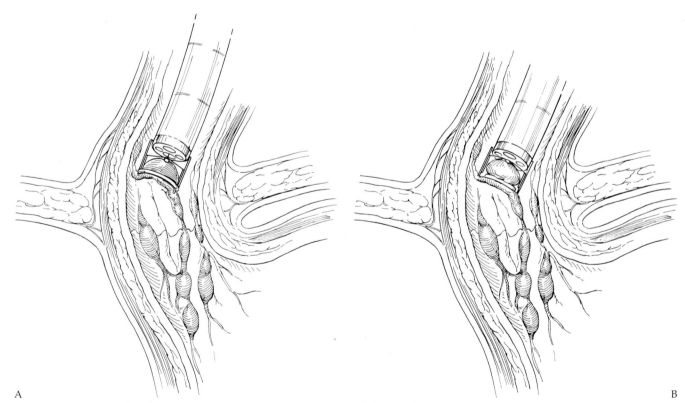

A

B

Fig. 15-10. Endoscopic variceal ligation. **A:** *After the varix is encircled with the ligating device, suction is applied to draw the varix into it.* **B:** *A tripwire is pulled to release the ligating band.* (continued)

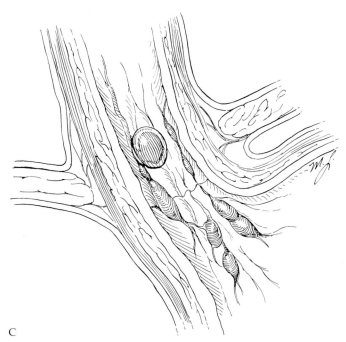

C

Fig. 15-10. (Continued) **C:** *A ligated varix. The endoscope is removed, the device is then reloaded, and the process is repeated with other varices. Generally, five to eight varices are ligated per session.*

Injection site ulceration is very common: 2% to 13% will bleed, 10% to 20% will develop stricture following multiple sessions, and 1% to 6% of patients may experience esophageal perforation. Prophylactic sclerotherapy is not recommended in patients who have not experienced an initial variceal bleeding episode.

An alternative method of variceal eradication is endoscopic ligation using elastic bands similar to those used for hemorrhoidal ligation. Initial endoscopic examination is performed through an endoscopic overtube. The scope is then removed, and a ligating device is attached. Beginning distally, the end of the ligating device should be positioned so as to encircle the varix. Suction is then used to draw the varix into the device, after which the device is fired by pulling a tripwire, releasing the band around the variceal base (Fig. 15-10). Suction is then released, and the scope is removed and reloaded, as needed, to repeat the process. Five to eight ligations can be performed during the initial treatment.

Early reports suggest endoscopic variceal ligation may be associated with a significantly lower complication rate than sclerotherapy and is at least as effective. It also appears that fewer treatments may be required, and rebleeding rates may be less. Combination therapy of ligation and low-dose sclerotherapy has shown promising results in several small clinical trials.

Conclusion

Endoscopy is an invaluable tool for the diagnosis and treatment of a variety of upper GI disorders. It behooves surgeons to become familiar with the indications for and proper use of the various endoscopic interventions currently available. New horizons in interventional technology include the combination of laparoscopic instrumentation and flexible endoscopy, allowing the performance of increasingly complex intraluminal surgery.

Suggested Reading

Adams DB. Endoscopic management of esophageal stricture. In: Greene FL, Ponsky JL, eds. *Endoscopic surgery*. Philadelphia: WB Saunders, 1994:36–54.

Cook DJ, Guyatt GH, Salena BJ, Laine LA. Endoscopic therapy for acute nonvariceal upper gastrointestinal hemorrhage: a meta-analysis. *Gastroenterology* 1992;102:139–148.

Hughes R. Diagnosis and treatment of gastric polyps. *Gastrointest Endosc Clin N Am* 1993;2:457–467.

Sarin SK, Nanda R, Sachdev G, Chari S, Anand BS, Broor SL. Intravariceal versus paravariceal sclerotherapy: a prospective, controlled, randomized trial. *Gut* 1987;28:657–662.

Steigmann GV, Goff JS, Michaletz-Onody PA, et al. Endoscopic sclerotherapy as compared with endoscopic ligation for bleeding esophageal varices. *N Engl J Med* 1992;326:1527–1532.

EDITOR'S COMMENT

Flexible endoscopy has moved well beyond its role as a simple diagnostic tool to become a true therapeutic modality, even to the extent of replacing many traditional surgical procedures. This chapter points out that flexible endoscopy has become the mainstay of treatment for both esophageal strictures and upper GI foreign bodies, which are often associated with the same underlying pathology. Although the vast majority of both strictures and foreign bodies can be managed with conservative therapy, the endoscopist is occasionally needed to treat these conditions. With foreign bodies in particular, conservative therapy is often sufficient and should include giving patients a smooth muscle relaxant such as glucagon (1 mg intravenously), and reassurance that these objects will pass spontaneously in the majority of cases. Treatment of strictures often is less important than dealing with their underlying etiology, whether it is from chronic untreated reflux, esophageal motor disorders, or caustic ingestion. Finally, the use of rigid endoscopy for the treatment of foreign bodies is a fast-vanishing art still practiced and advocated at certain centers, particularly for the pediatric population. Advocates argue that the rigid scope allows the use of a broader spectrum of grasping and manipulating instruments and therefore ensures easier recovery of foreign bodies. This is less true today with the increasing sophistication of flexible endoscopic instrumentation.

Flexible endoscopy is increasingly effective in treating upper GI bleeding. For the majority of interventions, a multimodel approach is the most effective. Typically, this involves injecting vasoactive substances or sclerosants and treating with cautery or banding. New developments such as hemostatic clips, flexible argon-beam coagulators, and multiple-band applicators provide additional means of controlling bleeding sources whether from varices or ulcerations. The result is a decreased need for operative intervention.

The most exciting development in endoscopic therapies of the upper GI tract is the ability to perform complex surgical interventions. These include techniques for ablating premalignant mucosal changes of the stomach and esophagus, including Barrett's epithelium, either by photodynamic therapy, resection, or thermal ablation. Similar techniques of mucosal stripping have been described as a curative therapy for early gastric and esophageal malignancies. Finally, the possibility of performing endoscopic antireflux surgery is being explored at several centers both in animal models and in early clinical trials. This introduces a whole new era of endoluminal surgery that will offer therapeutics in the least invasive manner possible.

L.L.S.

16

Flexible Endoscopy and Enteral Access

Quan-Yang Duh and Kenneth McQuaid

Indications for Enteral Access and Choice of Procedures

Nutritional status is one of the best predictors of survival of patients in the hospital. Appropriate nutritional support improves the prognosis of acutely ill patients and is required for many chronically ill patients. Enteral nutrition—feeding through the gut—is superior to parenteral nutrition and causes fewer infections. Enteral feeding promotes better immunity, maintains the integrity of the gut, and is cheaper and easier to administer. In general, if the gut is functioning, it should be used for nutrition.

The technique of choice for providing enteral nutrition depends on how long nutritional support is needed and whether or not the stomach is functional. If enteral nutrition is needed for less than 30 days, one should use a nasogastric (NG) or a nasojejunal feeding tube, which is minimally invasive and inexpensive. For uncooperative patients, however, interruptions in feeding because of tube dislodgement may lead to unpredictable intake. If enteral nutrition is needed for more than 30 days, we usually place a gastrostomy or jejunostomy to facilitate nursing care and improve patient comfort.

A gastrostomy and jejunostomy can be placed using endoscopic, laparoscopic, interventional radiologic, or open laparotomy approaches. The approach is usually chosen in accordance with the availability of local expertise and the preference of the physician caring for the patient. The three most common techniques for establishing access for chronic enteral feeding are percutaneous endoscopic gastrostomy (PEG), laparoscopic gastrostomy (Lap-G), and laparoscopic jejunostomy (Lap-J). Due to the success with these techniques, we rarely perform an open laparotomy for enteral tube placement. Similarly, we rarely use interventional radiology to place feeding tubes because it is more expensive and the success rate less guaranteed. Although a jejunal feeding tube can be threaded through an existing PEG tube to create a so-called percutaneous endoscopic jejunostomy (PEJ), we find this technique to be cumbersome and prone to easy tube dislodgement.

In general, a gastrostomy is preferred (PEG or Lap-G) over a Lap-J when patients have a functioning stomach. Gastrostomy is easier for nursing care because the tubes are larger and less likely to clog and permit bolus feeding. Jejunostomy is indicated when there is insufficient amount of stomach (gastrectomy), when the stomach does not function (gastroparesis in a diabetic), when the gastric outlet is obstructed (duodenal ulcer), or when gastroesophageal reflux is present and patients are at risk for aspirating gastric contents.

Patients with pharyngeal dysfunction are at risk for aspirating oropharyngeal secretions. Whether or not they should have a feeding jejunostomy instead of a gastrostomy is controversial. On the one hand, neither tube can prevent patients from aspirating oropharyngeal secretions. On the other hand, the risk of aspirating gastric contents may be higher for those with gastrostomy, since many of them do not have a functioning upper esophageal sphincter and rely only on the lower esophageal sphincter to prevent aspiration of gastric contents. Although one can argue that placing the tube in the jejunum in these patients lowers the risk of aspiration, this contention is not supported by any controlled, randomized study.

Preoperative Patient Management

Informed Consent

Informed consent should be obtained before placement of an enteral feeding tube. This is important not only because of the potential risks of the procedure and subsequent tube feeding but also because of the ethical implications for initiating enteral feeding in patients who may subsequently wish to terminate feeding. Not uncommonly, patients who require a feeding tube may have neurologic problems, such as stroke, that preclude informed consent. In such cases, family and primary care physician will need to be consulted and consent obtained from a legal guardian.

Prophylactic Antibiotics

Although the acid in the stomach prevents growth of most bacteria, patients requiring feeding tubes usually have concomitant illness and not infrequently receive antacid prophylaxis or treatment. We therefore routinely give prophylactic antibiotics to almost all patients undergoing gastrostomy (PEG or Lap-G). All patients undergoing jejunostomy also need prophylactic antibiotics. We give a single dose of a first-generation cephalosporin within 1 hour before tube placement.

Recurrent Aspiration Pneumonia

Recurrent aspiration pneumonia is a common problem for patients who require a feeding tube, especially those with stroke or head and neck cancer. Pneumonia should be treated, and patients' pulmonary function should be optimized before the procedure. Because most patients will require conscious sedation and a few may require general anesthesia, these patients are at risk for aspiration during the procedure and worsening of existing pneumonia.

Operative Techniques
Percutaneous Endoscopic Gastrostomy

PEG is usually performed with intravenous sedation, most commonly with a

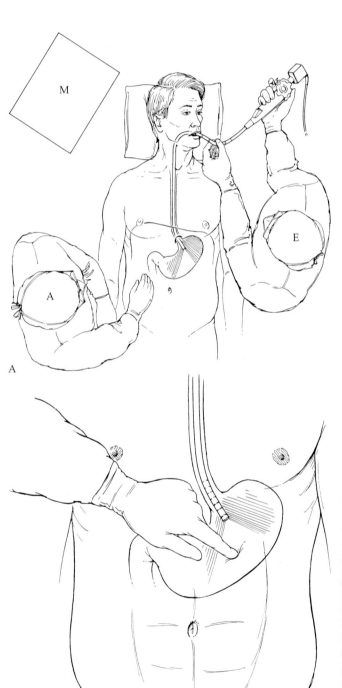

A

B

Fig. 16-1. **A:** *The endoscopist stands to the left of the patient; the assistant stands to the right of the prepared abdomen. (A, assistant; M, monitor; E, endoscopist.)* **B:** *The insertion site is identified by endoscopic transillumination.* **Left:** *The left upper quadrant of the abdominal wall is indented with a finger from the outside.* **Right:** *The indentation is viewed endoscopically to determine the site for the gastrostomy.*

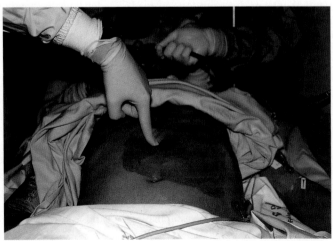

narcotic and a short-acting benzodi-azepine. Patients are monitored during the procedure with an electrocardiogram monitor, automatic blood pressure cuff, and pulse oximeter. Patients are placed in a slight sitting position with the upper abdomen exposed, supine but with the face slightly turned to the left. The endoscopist stands to the left of a patient's head, watching the procedure on the monitor to the right. The assistant stands to the patient's right (Fig. 16-1A).

Push or Sacks-Vine Technique

The push or Sacks-Vine technique is most commonly used. The endoscope is inserted, and a full upper gastrointestinal endoscopic examination is performed to rule out unexpected diseases such as reflux esophagitis or pyloric stenosis, which may contraindicate a gastrostomy.

After the scope is pulled back from the duodenum, with the stomach fully insufflated, the scope is pointed anteriorly to identify the site for the gastrostomy in the body of the stomach. The light from the scope transilluminates the abdominal wall. The site of maximal light transillumination is indented by the assistant with a finger (usually in the left upper quadrant halfway between the umbilicus and the midcostal margin), and the indentation on the stomach wall is in turn identified by the endoscopist (Fig. 16-1B).

Once the site of gastrostomy is selected, the abdominal wall is prepared and draped sterilely. The gastrostomy site should be at least 2 cm from the costal margin to avoid pain and future difficulty in caring for the tube. The transilluminated gastrostomy site is infiltrated with local anesthetic and then incised with a scalpel. The incision should be large enough (1 to 1.5 cm) to allow drainage around the gastrostomy tube to avoid infection. An 18-gauge trocar needle is then inserted through the incision into the stomach under endoscopic visualization. A snare is passed through the endoscope's biopsy channel to encircle the needle. A guidewire is inserted through this needle into the stomach. The snare is then loosened, slipped off the needle, and closed securely around the guidewire. The scope and the wire are then pulled as a unit out through the mouth as the assistant advances the wire through the trocar into the stomach (Fig. 16-2).

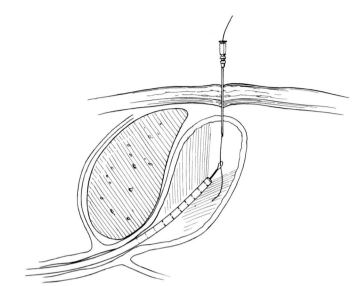

Fig. 16-2. After a skin incision is made in the center of the transilluminated area, an 18-gauge needle is inserted through the abdominal wall into the stomach under endoscopic view. A wire is inserted through the needle and is snared through the endoscope.

Enough wire is pulled out of the mouth so that the full length of the gastrostomy tube can be slid over it. As the endoscopist controls one end of the wire and the assistant the other end, the gastrostomy tube is pushed through the mouth, down the esophagus, and into the stomach. As the tapered end of the gastrostomy tube emerges from the stomach through the skin of the abdominal wall, the gastrostomy tube is grabbed by the assistant and pulled out of the abdominal wall. Once the assistant has pulled the entire gastrostomy tube through the wall and the bumper tip is seated next to the gastric mucosa, the wire is removed (Fig. 16-3).

The endoscope should be reintroduced into the stomach to visually confirm proper positioning of the gastrostomy tube. The bumper of the gastrostomy

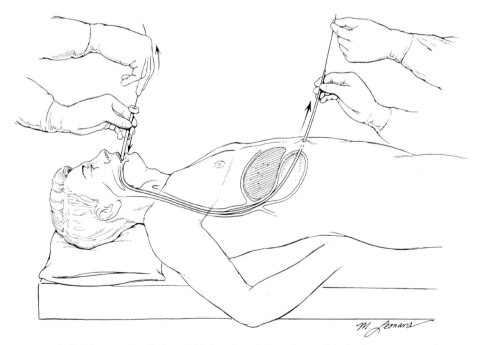

Fig. 16-3. Sacks-Vine or push technique. With the wire pulled taut from both ends, the gastrostomy tube is slid over the wire.

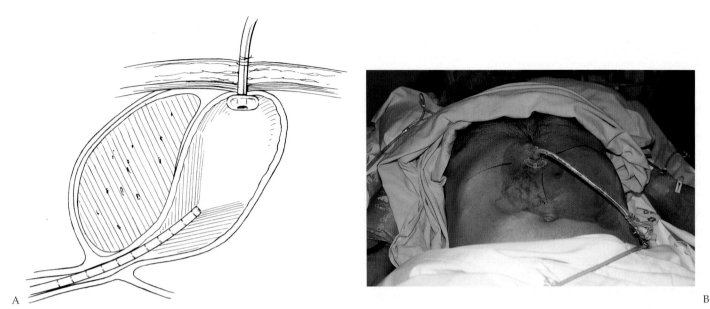

Fig. 16-4. Sacks-Vine or push technique. **A:** Schematic internal view. **B:** Intraoperative photo. The gastrostomy tube is held in placed by friction and anchored by the bumper inside the stomach and the skin disk. Repeat endoscopy confirms appropriate placement and tension on the gastronomy tube.

should be pulled as close to the gastric mucosa as possible without causing excessive pressure (Fig. 16-4). This can be checked by confirming that the bumper rotates freely as the tube is rotated externally. The tube is then fastened by a suture or by friction with a skin disk (Fig. 16-4), which will maintain apposition of the bumper against the gastric mucosa. The external tube may then be cut to a desired length.

Pull or Ponsky Technique

The pull or the Ponsky technique was the originally described technique. The end of the gastrostomy tube is tied to a sturdy suture that has been introduced percutaneously through a trocar needle or angiocatheter into the stomach, snared, and pulled out of the mouth. The tube is pulled via this suture by the assistant toward the stomach and out through the abdominal wall (Fig. 16-5).

Introducer or Russell Technique

The introducer or the Russell technique uses a peel-away introducer and a balloon catheter to place the tube retrograde through the abdominal wall instead of antegrade through the mouth. A guidewire is inserted into the stomach through a trocar needle. Progressive dilators are then passed. A peel-away-sheath introducer is then slid over the wire into the stomach (Fig. 16-6). The wire and the introducer are removed. A balloon-tipped catheter is then inserted into the stomach through the peel-away sheath. The balloon is inflated to anchor the tip of the tube in the stomach, and the sheath is then peeled away to remove it (Fig. 16-7).

Laparoscopic Gastrostomy

Lap-G can be performed under general anesthesia or local anesthesia with intra-

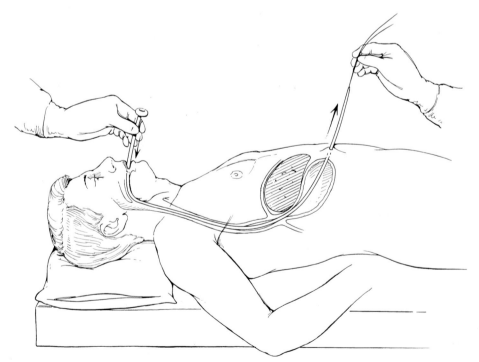

Fig. 16-5. Ponsky or pull technique. The suture that has been snared, pulled out of the mouth, and tied to the end of a gastrostomy tube is used to pull the end of the tube from the mouth, into the stomach, and out through the abdominal wall.

venous sedation. We have found a continuous intravenous infusion of propofol (Diprivan) without endotracheal intubation an excellent anesthetic technique for simple laparoscopic procedures such as gastrostomy or jejunostomy. A prophylactic antibiotic is given. An oral or NG tube is very helpful because it can be used to decompress the stomach for laparoscopy and insufflate the stomach for the procedure. A urinary catheter and sequential compression stockings are not necessary because this procedure rarely takes longer than 30 minutes.

The abdominal wall is prepared and draped sterilely. The surgeon and the camera holder stand to the patient's right side, facing the patient's left shoulder. The laparoscopic monitor is placed above the patient's left shoulder (Fig. 16-8).

A standard subumbilical port is established either with the closed Veress needle technique or with the open Hasson trocar technique (Fig. 16-9). A diagnostic laparoscopy is performed. Trocars larger than 5 mm are not necessary for Lap-G or Lap-J; smaller trocars also avoid the risk of future trocar-site hernia. The 5-mm scope achieves adequate resolution for tube placement. It is more important to use a 30-degree scope instead of a 0-degree scope. The 30-degree scope allows the surgeon to look down on the anterior stomach wall from the subumbilical port and to look around the tube once it is placed.

The anterior surface of the stomach is identified laparoscopically. This is facilitated by placing the patient in a reverse Trendelenburg (head up) position and by insufflating the stomach through the oral or NG tube with carbon dioxide, with the pressure set slightly above that of the pneumoperitoneum.

The pneumoperitoneum is decreased to 6 to 8 mm Hg to bring the anterior stomach wall closer to the anterior abdominal wall. We determine the position of the gastrostomy tube by pressing on the abdominal wall with a finger and viewing the indentation laparoscopically. The gastrostomy tube should enter the body of the stomach approximately one-third of the way from the greater curvature to prevent injury to the gastroepiploic or short gastric vessels near the greater curvature or perforation of the posterior wall when the catheter is too close to the lesser curvature.

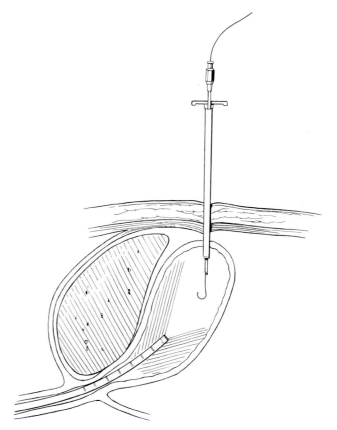

Fig. 16-6. Russell or introducer technique. Under endoscopic guidance, a J-guidewire has been inserted into the stomach through a needle. After dilation of a tract, a peel-away-sheath introducer is placed into the stomach over a guidewire.

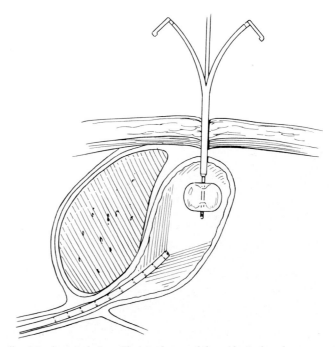

Fig. 16-7. Russell or introducer technique. The introducer and the guidewire have been removed, and a balloon-tipped catheter has been inserted through the peel-away sheath. The balloon is inflated. The sheath is then peeled and removed.

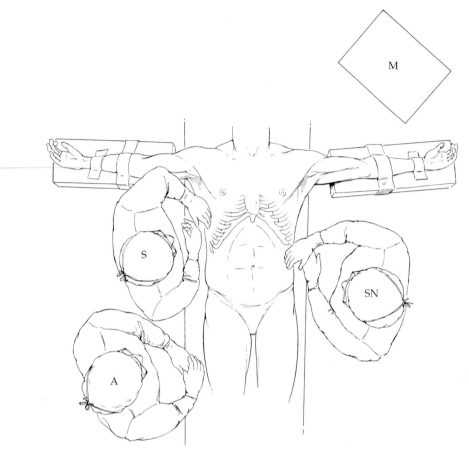

Four T-fasteners are used to retract the anterior stomach wall to the anterior abdominal wall. The T-fasteners are placed sequentially in a square configuration 4 cm apart. Correct placement of the first T-fastener is crucial because it determines how the subsequent T-fasteners are placed. The T-fastener farthest away from the scope should be inserted first. Thus, as the anterior stomach wall is retracted by the first T-fastener, one has an *en face* view to place the remaining three T-fasteners (Fig. 16-10). After each T-fastener is inserted into the stomach, it is pulled up against the anterior abdominal wall, leaving only a 1- to 2-cm gap. This prevents misalignment of the T-fastener sites on the stomach wall versus the abdominal wall. Pulling the stomach wall too close to the abdominal wall, however, would obscure the view and make tube placement more difficult.

Occasionally, a grasper is needed to lift the anterior surface of the stomach to facilitate the T-fasteners' placement. This is usually necessary if the stomach cannot be insufflated via an oral or NG tube. This grasper is inserted through a 5-mm trocar in the right upper or left lower quadrant of the abdomen.

After the anterior stomach wall is retracted with the 4 T-fasteners, the gastrostomy tube is placed through the center of this 4-cm square. The skin is generously incised to allow drainage around the gastrostomy tube to prevent local infection. An 18-gauge needle is inserted through the skin incision and into the stomach (Fig. 16-11). Correct placement is confirmed by insufflation of air into the stomach with a syringe. A J-guidewire is then inserted through the needle into the stomach, and the needle is removed. Over this wire, dilators serially increasing in size are passed to enlarge the gastrostomy tract up to 22 French (22-F). Pulling on the T-fasteners provides countertraction to help insert the dilators.

An 18-F balloon-tipped catheter is inserted over the wire. The balloon is insufflated with 20 mL of saline, and then the guidewire is removed. Letting loose the T-fasteners and pulling on the balloon catheter with the stomach deflated will demonstrate the intragastric placement of the tube. The placement can also be confirmed by insufflating the stomach with air. The risk of leakage around the tube or

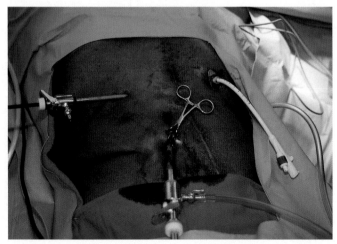

Fig. 16-9. Laparoscopic gastrostomy. Positioning of the trocars and gastrostomy tube.

perforation through the posterior stomach wall is very low. If it is a concern, this complication can be ruled out by injecting dilute methylene blue and looking for staining, or by injecting radiologic contrast followed by a roentgenogram or fluoroscopy.

The T-fasteners are immobilized by crimping on the aluminum crimpers. This should be done in the same sequence as for the initial placement, starting from the one farthest away from the laparoscope. Using barely enough retraction on the T-fasteners to appose the anterior stomach wall to the anterior abdominal wall will prevent tissue necrosis. The balloon tip is gently pulled against the anterior stomach wall, and the catheter is immobilized by the skin disk (Fig. 16-12).

Laparoscopic Jejunostomy

The patient is prepared and positioned in a manner similar to that for Lap-G. The surgeon and camera holder stand on the patient's right side, and the monitor is placed above the patient's left shoulder (see Fig. 16-8).

The subumbilical port is established as for Lap-G, and diagnostic laparoscopy is performed with a 5-mm 30-degree laparoscope (Fig. 16-13). Two atraumatic bowel graspers are inserted through 5-mm trocars in the right upper and the left lower quadrants of the abdomen (Fig. 16-13). The transverse colon is lifted away from the small bowel. The proximal jejunum is identified by running the small bowel with the graspers. We place the jejunostomy about 20 cm from the ligament of Treitz, where the mesentery is long enough to allow the jejunum to be pulled up to the abdominal wall.

The pneumoperitoneum is decreased to 6 to 8 mm Hg, and the abdominal wall is indented with a finger to identify the site for jejunostomy. This site is usually more lateral and caudal than that for a gastrostomy.

Four T-fasteners are inserted in a diamond configuration 3 cm apart through the antimesentery border of the proximal jejunum (Fig. 16-14). A skin incision is made, and an 18-gauge needle is inserted through this incision, through the center of the T-fasteners, into the proximal jejunum. Intraluminal placement is confirmed by

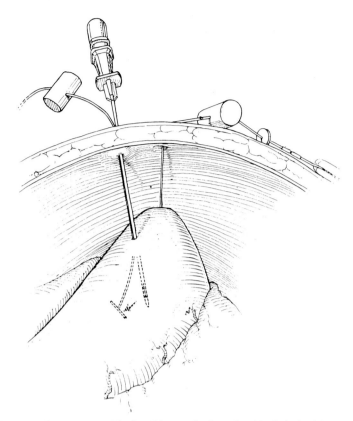

Fig. 16-10. Laparoscopic gastrostomy. The first T-fastener has been placed in the body of the stomach and is used for traction. The second T-fastener has been inserted, and the metal T piece is ejected into the stomach.

injecting some air and watching for bowel distention. A J-guidewire is then inserted through the needle into the lumen of the small bowel.

A peel-away sheath–covered dilator/introducer is then inserted over the J-wire into the jejunal lumen. The wire and the introducer are then removed, leaving the peel-away sheath. A 10-F jejunostomy tube is then inserted through the sheath, which is pulled apart and removed, leaving the jejunostomy catheter in place (Fig. 16-15).

The intraluminal position of the jejunostomy catheter is once again confirmed by rapidly insufflating 12 mL of air and seeing the bowel distend. Leakage around the tube or puncturing of the bowel away from the catheter site are very rare but can be ruled out by infusing dilute methylene blue or radiologic contrast followed by roentgenogram or fluoroscopy.

The four T-fasteners are then tightened and fixed by crimping the aluminum

crimpers. Minimal traction is used to just pull the bowel against the abdominal wall (see Fig. 16-16).

A balloon catheter should not be used for jejunostomy because of the obvious risk of obstruction and migration. The catheter is immobilized by suturing the skin anchor to the skin. The anchor holds the jejunostomy catheter in place by friction. As with a gastrostomy, the position of the catheter should be noted so that if it migrates, it will be noticed and corrected.

Surgical Complications and Postoperative Care

Feeding through the gastrostomy or the jejunostomy tube can be started as soon as the sedation or the anesthesia has resolved and there is no ileus. It is usually possible to begin feeding the morning after the procedure and to advance rapidly if tolerated. The tube is irrigated with 30 mL of saline

(text continues on page 142)

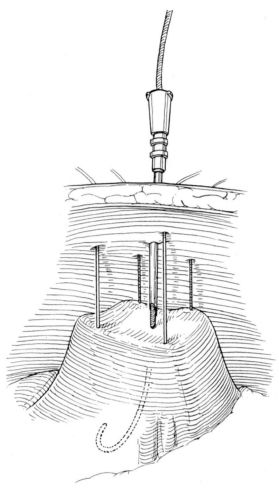

Fig. 16-11. Laparoscopic gastrostomy. The anterior abdominal wall has been retracted upward by the four **T**-fasteners. A **J**-guidewire is inserted into the stomach using a needle through the center of the T-fasteners.

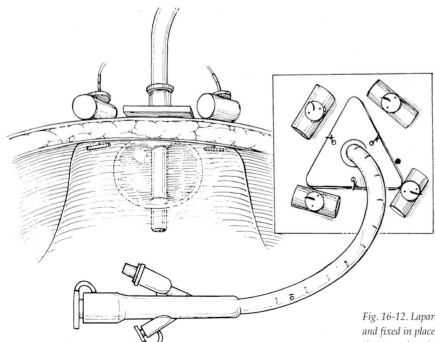

Fig. 16-12. Laparoscopic gastrostomy. The four **T**-fasteners have been crimped and fixed in place. The gastrostomy catheter is immobilized by the balloon inside the stomach and the skin anchor.

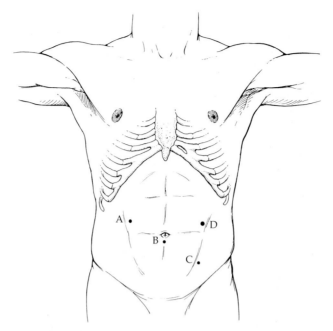

Fig. 16-13. Laparoscopic jejunostomy. Port placement and typical tube placement sites. (A, 10-mm trochar; B, 5 mm [camera]; C, 5 mm; D, jejunostomy site.)

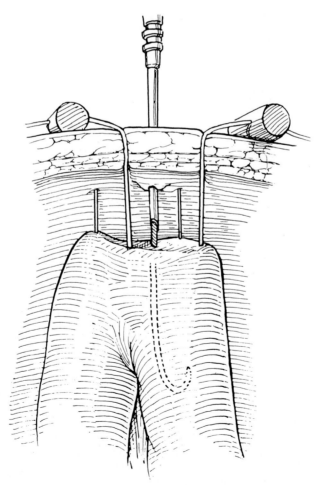

Fig. 16-14. Laparoscopic jejunostomy. The proximal jejunum is retracted by four T-fasteners, through the center of which a needle and then a J-wire are inserted. Atraumatic graspers can be used to stabilize the bowel during insertion.

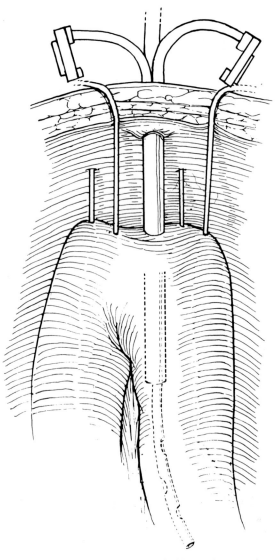

Fig. 16-15. *Laparoscopic jejunostomy. The jejunum is retracted upward with the four T-fasteners. The jejunostomy tube has been inserted, and the peel-away sheath is being removed.*

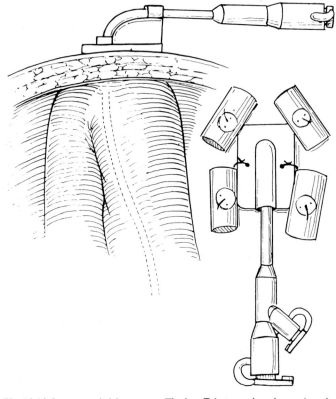

Fig. 16-16. *Laparoscopic jejunostomy. The four T-fasteners have been crimped and fixed in place, and the proximal jejunum has been immobilized to the abdominal wall. The jejunostomy catheter is immobilized by an anchor that is sutured onto the skin.*

every 4 hours while not in use to prevent clogging.

Peritonitis from perforation of the bowel is possible, and patients should be examined after the procedure. The transverse colon is especially at risk during PEG, the posterior stomach wall is at risk during Lap-G, and the small bowel is at risk during Lap-J.

Tube site infection is possible, especially if the skin incision is insufficient to allow drainage around the tube. Necrotizing fasciitis can complicate local infection and should be watched for.

Dislodgement of the catheter is a nuisance for the nurse and can be life-threatening,

especially if a balloon-tipped catheter is used without fixing the stomach to the abdominal wall. The T-fasteners used in Lap-G and Lap-J act as a safety device and keep the stomach or the jejunum against the abdominal wall, even if the tube is dislodged. The tube can be reinserted at bedside followed by a radiologic contrast study to confirm placement, or it can again be reinserted under laparoscopic guidance. If a Russell PEG tube is dislodged from a stomach that has not been anchored by the T-fasteners, we perform a diagnostic laparoscopy and reinsert the gastrostomy tube under laparoscopic guidance.

The T-fasteners are removed in 2 weeks by cutting the nylon suture at the skin surface

and letting the metal T piece drop into the lumen.

Removing the Feeding Tubes

After 2 weeks, the feeding tube can be electively removed. Russell balloon-tipped devices are the easiest to discontinue, requiring only deflation of the balloon and gentle traction. Some types of button-tipped tubes are designed to be removed by moderate traction. This causes the button to collapse and come out through the tract. Occasionally, this type of tube will break at the skin level, or one may encounter an older, noncollapsing design. These tubes should be removed under upper endoscopic visualization, with the button being snared and removed to avoid the small, but real, chance of bowel obstruction if it is left to pass through the gastrointestinal tract.

Suggested Reading

Duh QY. Laparoscopic access to the gastrointestinal tract. *Laparosc Surg* 1995;2:141–197.

Duh QY, Senokozlieff-Englehart AL, Siperstein AE, et al. Prospective evaluation of the safety and efficacy of laparoscopic jejunostomy. *West J Med* 1995;162:117–122.

Gauderer MWL, Ponsky JL, Izant RJ Jr. Gastrostomy without laparotomy: a percutaneous endoscopic technique. *J Pediatr Surg* 1980;15:872–875.

Moore FA, Feliciano DV, Andrassy RJ, et al. Early enteral feeding, compared with parenteral, reduces postoperative septic complications: the results of a meta-analysis. *Ann Surg* 1992;216:172–183.

Sangster W, Hunter JG. Surgical access for enteral nutrition. In: Hunter JG, Sackier JM, eds. *Minimally invasive surgery.* New York: McGraw-Hill, Inc., 1993:113–121.

Strong RM, Condon SC, Solinger MR, Namihas BN, Ito-Wong LA, Leuty JE. Equal aspiration rates from postpylorus- and intragastric-placed small-bore nasoenteric feeding tubes: a randomized, prospective study. *J Parenter Enteral Nutr* 1992;16:59–63.

EDITOR'S COMMENT

Flexible endoscopic feeding tube placement is undoubtedly today's gold standard for enteral access. Until recently, this was confined to the placement of gastrostomy tubes (PEG). More recently, transgastric jejunal tubes (PEJ) and direct endoscopy jejunostomy placement have been described. These have not been as enthusiastically embraced because of their greater difficulty, potential for dislodgement, and higher complication rates.

Laparoscopic placement of feeding tubes, either gastric or jejunal, is certainly more invasive but is indicated in certain settings:

When one cannot do flexible endoscopy because of patient habitus, disease, or unavailability of endoscopic equipment;

When patients need laparoscopy for other reasons—a situation more frequently encountered as laparoscopic surgery becomes increasingly utilized;

When there is an absolute need for a feeding jejunostomy.

Certain patient groups cannot tolerate gastric feedings or are at high risk of aspirating gastric contents (e.g., those with severe strokes, gastroesophageal reflux disease, and head injuries). The failure rate of PEJ tube placement is quite high, and a surgical gastrostomy offers the greatest assurance that enteral feeds will stay out of the stomach.

This chapter demonstrates how straightforward the laparoscopic approach is, even describing a good experience with procedures done under local anesthesia. Dr. Duh is known for the innovative use of T-fasteners to fix the stomach or small bowel to the abdominal wall, and certainly this is a great advance for the placement of gastric tubes. I have some reservations with the use of T-fasteners in the small bowel, however, as these nylon sutures transit the lumen of the small bowel, subcutaneous tissue, and skin. After dividing these from the outside, do they indeed pass into the lumen of the small bowel, or remain as potentially contaminated foreign bodies in the subcutaneous tissue? An alternative method is to use interrupted sutures to fasten the stomach or the small bowel to the anterior abdominal wall. Once the surgeon becomes skillful in laparoscopic suturing, this is a fast and cost-effective technique to achieve laparoscopic enteral access.

L.L.S.

17

Laparoscopic Nissen Fundoplication

William S. Richardson and John G. Hunter

Laparoscopic Nissen fundoplication has become the most common antireflux operation performed in the United States, but exact procedure numbers are hard to come by. It is likely that 50,000 to 70,000 of these procedures are performed annually. The open Nissen fundoplication is reported to provide complete relief of reflux with few significant side effects in 85% to 95% of patients followed for 10 to 20 years. The short-term success with laparoscopic Nissen fundoplication has been slightly better, but follow-up is shorter. Compared to open fundoplication, laparoscopic Nissen fundoplication offers a shorter hospital stay, less pain, a good cosmetic result, and rapid rehabilitation. The popularity of laparoscopic Nissen suggests that it is a much more attractive option than open fundoplication, based on its perceived "patient-friendly" characteristics.

Although many modifications to Dr. Nissen's fundoplication have been made through the years, the "floppy" Nissen fundoplication is today the standard to which other antireflux operations are compared. Nissen's first fundoplication, performed in 1937, was used to protect a gastroesophageal (GE) anastomosis done after a proximal gastrectomy for a perforated ulcer in the cardia. The patient's long-standing gastroesophageal reflux (GER) symptoms were found to be totally relieved postoperatively. Nineteen years later, he performed his first "Nissen fundoplication" in a patient with GER. It was a 360-degree, 6-cm long imbrication of the gastric fundus around the distal esophagus. Today, most surgeons perform a short (2 cm), floppy wrap around a 50- to 60-

French (F) dilator. The equivalent fundoplication is performed laparoscopically.

Incidence of Gastroesophageal Reflux

In a Gallup survey, 44% of American adults experienced heartburn once a month, and 7% experienced it daily. Many of these patients self-medicate with over-the-counter (OTC) medications for these symptoms. Oral antacids and H_2-blockers, which are now available in OTC formulations, are widely used, and many patients take them without seeking medical advice.

Although the majority of patients complain of classic heartburn and/or regurgitation (water brash), many patients also have atypical symptoms that can include chest pain, dysphagia, odynophagia, vomiting, hoarseness, nocturnal choking, chronic cough, asthma, pneumonia, upper esophageal dysphagia (globus hystericus), or excessive salivation. Some patients suffer with these atypical symptoms only and may have been worked up and even treated for other illnesses mimicking GER. This is particularly true in patients who have chest pain or asthma. Some medications such as calcium channel blockers and theophylline used to treat these patients may actually increase symptoms because they decrease lower esophageal sphincter pressure.

Further confusing the spectrum of GER is the fact that only 50% to 65% of patients with GER symptoms have esophagitis on endoscopy. Conversely, 35% of patients

who have inflammation on endoscopy and 25% of patients with Barrett's esophagus have no GER symptoms. Of patients who have esophagitis, 20% will have had one or more complications, including Barrett's esophagus in 10% to 15%; 4% to 20% will have esophageal stricture, 2% to 7% esophageal ulcer, and 2% hemorrhage. The goal of therapy then is to resolve symptoms, improve quality of life, and decrease the incidence of complications.

Indications for Operation

Because of increasing patient and doctor satisfaction with laparoscopic antireflux procedures, more and more patients are being referred for surgery. Indications for operation include failure of conservative measures to control symptoms (alteration in dietary habits, weight loss, sleeping with head of bed elevated) and persistent symptoms, esophagitis, or complications of GER (esophageal ulcers, strictures, Barrett's esophagus) with maximal medical therapy (usually acid suppression with proton pump antagonists); noncompliance or inability to tolerate medical therapy; and patients who prefer surgery rather than adapting their lifestyle or accepting lifetime medical treatment to control GER (Table 17-1).

It is difficult to determine the actual medical cost of treating a patient with GER because of the broad spectrum of the disease. Patients who require proton pump antagonists to control GER often can never be taken off medication and may require increasing doses. The cost of omeprazole

Table 17-1. Indications
for Laparoscopic Nissen Fundoplication

Failure of medical therapy
   To control symptoms
   To prevent complications (Barrett's
      esophagus, stricture, ulceration)
Inability to take medical therapy
   Reaction to medication
   Poor compliance
   Unable to afford medication
Preference for surgery

(Prilosec), 20 mg per day, is approximately $1,200 per year. As time goes on, some of these medications may become less expensive, or they may not. Charges for laparoscopic fundoplication with a 2-day hospital stay vary from $10,000 to $25,000, averaging approximately $15,000 at our institution. Costs for surgery are significantly less ($3,000 to $7,000).

Preoperative Evaluation

The success of fundoplication depends partly on the underlying cause of patients' symptoms and partly on their expectations of symptom relief. Typical symptoms such as heartburn and regurgitation reliably improve after a properly constructed fundoplication. Atypical symptoms do not improve to the same extent as typical symptoms after fundoplication. This may be due to one of three possibilities:

1. Symptoms are not caused by reflux.
2. Patients have associated illnesses, such as asthma, that may be worsened with reflux but not completely improved after an antireflux procedure.
3. Permanent changes have occurred as a consequence of GER that only partially heal after reflux is stopped.

Patient workup includes a careful history and physical examination. Conditions that mimic GER such as cholelithiasis, gastric ulcer, gastric dysmotility, and associated illnesses are carefully ruled out.

Esophagogastroduodenoscopy (EGD) is an extremely important test. Esophagitis is scored endoscopically by the Savary-Miller score in which

Grade I is mild erythema;
Grade II is isolated ulcerations;
Grade III is confluent severe ulcerations;
Grade IV is complication secondary to esophagitis, such as Barrett's esophagus or strictures.

The presence and type of hiatal hernia and the esophageal length are also best assessed with endoscopy. If Barrett's esophagus or a stricture is found, careful biopsy is done to rule out high-grade dysplasia and/or esophageal cancer. Esophageal manometry is performed in all patients to assess esophageal body and lower esophageal sphincter function. Esophageal body motility is helpful in determining whether total (Nissen) fundoplication or a partial fundoplication ought to be performed. Patients with severely weak esophageal contractions or aperistalsis may require alternative therapy. Lower esophageal sphincter pressure, sphincter length, and location with respect to the diaphragm, as well as relaxation of the sphincter, are also assessed with motility. Twenty-four-hour ambulatory acid–base studies are performed in all patients without erosive esophagitis and all patients with dominant atypical symptoms. Barium swallow is useful for assessing mechanical reasons for dysphagia, such as strictures, rings, webs, and best demonstrates the size and configuration of hiatal hernias. Most of these tests should be repeated if they were performed more than 1 year prior to operation. Endoscopy should certainly be repeated if a patient had Barrett's esophagus or previous endoscopy was performed more than 6 months previously. Radionuclide gastric emptying studies are done when patients have symptoms of slow gastric emptying, diabetes, or peptic ulcer. In addition, patients with significant reflux on 24-hour pH study and a manometrically normal lower esophageal sphincter need close assessment of their gastric function. In patients who have greater than twice normal delayed gastric emptying, we perform hand-sewn pyloroplasty at the time of fundoplication. Some reports suggest that gastric emptying may improve after fundoplication, and therefore patients with low-normal or mild emptying disorders are probably best treated with fundoplication alone.

Contraindications to laparoscopic fundoplication include the inability to tolerate general anesthesia, uncorrectable coagulopathy, and severe chronic obstructive pulmonary disease. We have had some success with attempting laparoscopic fundoplication in patients who have had previous upper abdominal surgery or even previous antireflux surgery, but these operations are quite difficult and should only be done if the surgeon has extensive experience in such cases. Morbid obesity with a large fatty liver may make it impossible to perform laparoscopic fundoplication because of the difficulty of exposing the GE junction. Morbidly obese patients are put on a diet prior to surgery and not operated on until their weight is within 75 pounds of ideal body weight. Esophageal shortening greater than 5 cm associated with an esophageal stricture and poor peristalsis is a difficult problem. If we cannot mobilize the esophagus well enough to allow 2 to 3 cm to reside tension free below the diaphragm, we have performed a laparoscopic Collis-Nissen repair. Alternatively, an esophagectomy may be indicated. Otorhinolaryngologic and other specialty consultations are liberally used, as indicated, to evaluate patients' disease and appropriateness for surgery.

Operative Technique

Preoperative Preparation

Routine laboratory studies are obtained 1 week before operation, and patients enter the hospital on the day of surgery. After induction of general anesthesia, patients are placed in the supine position with the legs abducted on straight leg boards (Fig. 17-1). There is no flexion of the hips or knees, as this may increase the risk of deep venous thrombosis. This also allows the operating surgeon to work from between the legs, which is ergonomically easier. A nasogastric tube, Foley catheter, and pneumatic compression boots are appropriately placed. Prophylactic antibiotics are generally unnecessary.

Operative Technique

A Veress needle is placed periumbilically, and a pneumoperitoneum to 15 mm Hg is established with carbon dioxide. If there is a contraindication to the Veress needle, the

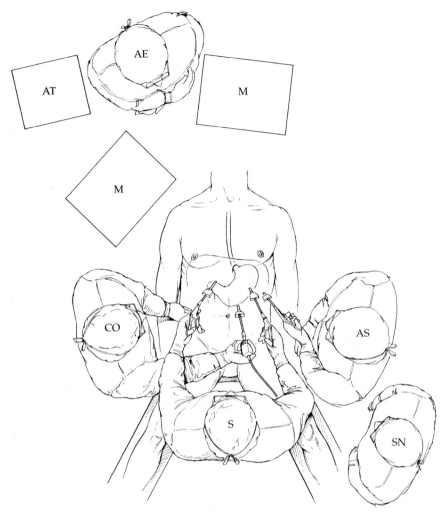

Fig. 17-1. After induction of general anesthesia, the patient is placed in the supine position, with the legs abducted on straight leg boards. (S, surgeon; CO, camera operator; M, monitor; AT, anesthesia table; AE, anesthetist; AS, assistant surgeon; SN, scrub nurse.)

Hasson trocar technique is used. A 10-mm port is placed 15 cm below the xiphoid, to the left of the umbilicus, and medial to the inferior epigastric artery (Fig. 17-2). A 45-degree telescope with a high-definition three-chip video camera is essential. The patient is placed in a steep reverse Trendelenburg position, and the location and size of the liver are assessed for optimal port placement. The size of all trocars depends on the instrumentation that will be used. A 10-mm trocar is placed at the left subcostal margin approximately 10 cm from the xiphoid. A 5- or 10-mm trocar is placed approximately 15 cm from the xiphoid underneath the right costal margin, depending on the diameter of the liver retractor. A second 5-mm port is placed 10 cm from the xiphoid underneath the right costal margin and immediately below the edge of the liver. A 5-mm port is placed approxi-

mately 20 cm from the xiphoid below the left costal margin. A sixth port is occasionally used under the xiphoid to further assist in liver retraction or in the left hypochondrium to assist in retraction of omental fat and exposure of lesser sac bleeding sites.

A 5-mm articulated liver retractor (Endoflex, DSP Worldwide, Tucker, Georgia) is used through the right lateral port to elevate the left lobe of the liver. This is attached to the operating table to hold it in place (Bookwalter Endoscopic Instrument Holder, Codman, Piscataway, New Jersey). Dissection starts at the GE junction. An atraumatic bowel clamp (Hunter Grasper, Jarit Instruments, Hawthorne, New York) is placed by the first assistant through the left lateral port and grasps the epiphrenic fat just below the GE junction,

pulling down toward the left foot and thereby exposing the gastrohepatic ligament of the stomach at the GE junction. This retracting clamp and the camera are held in position by assistants. We frequently use a robotic arm (AESOP, Computer Motion, Goleta, California) to assist in holding the camera. The operating surgeon then takes an atraumatic bowel clamp in the left hand and electrosurgical scissors in the right hand and operates through the highest right and left subcostal ports.

The operation begins by opening the lesser omentum (gastrohepatic ligament) above the vagal branches to the liver and preserving them if possible (Fig. 17-3). Dividing the vagal branches to the liver may increase the risk of cholecystitis in the future. In addition, a replaced left hepatic artery will occasionally be found in this region. This should be preserved, if at all possible. The caudate lobe of the liver is seen once this thin membrane has been incised. The dissection is taken across the esophagus, preserving the anterior vagus nerve. The peritoneum can be lifted off the esophagus using an atraumatic bowel clamp and then incised with scissors. This is carried out over the left crus of the diaphragm. An atraumatic bowel clamp is then taken in the surgeon's right hand, and with two atraumatic bowel clamps and judicious use of cautery, the right and left crura are dissected free. By dissection of the crura far posteriorly instead of searching for the esophagus, esophageal perforation may be avoided. Once the right and left crura are cleaned back to their junction posteriorly, blunt dissection can be carried out behind the esophagus. All tubes and esophageal probes must be removed prior to posterior esophageal dissection. With the surgeon's right hand, the esophagus is lifted anteriorly from the right side with the atraumatic bowel clamp. Posteriorly, blunt dissection is carried out, watching for the posterior vagus nerve, which in most patients is left attached to the esophagus. Dissection can continue from both sides of the esophagus in a similar manner. With the use of blunt dissection, a window is created around the posterior esophagus (Fig. 17-4). Often, the spleen can be seen through this window from the right side. A 10-cm, 5-mm Penrose drain is then brought around the esophagus and clipped to itself anteriorly (Fig. 17-5). The assistant grasps the drain with a ratcheted clamp and retracts it inferiorly left and

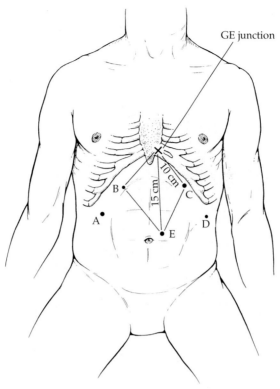

Fig. 17-2. *Technical success and optimal ergonomics is achieved by using a diamond approach to the gastroesophageal junction. (A, 5 mm; B, 5 mm; C, 10 mm; D, 5 mm; E, 10 mm.).*

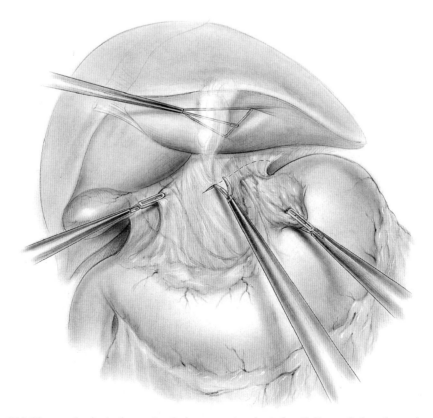

Fig. 17-3. *The operation begins by opening the lesser omentum (gastrohepatic ligament) above the vagal branches to the liver, preserving them if possible.*

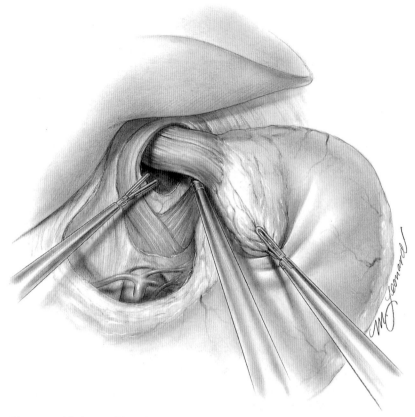

Fig. 17-4. *With the use of blunt dissection, a window is created around the posterior esophagus.*

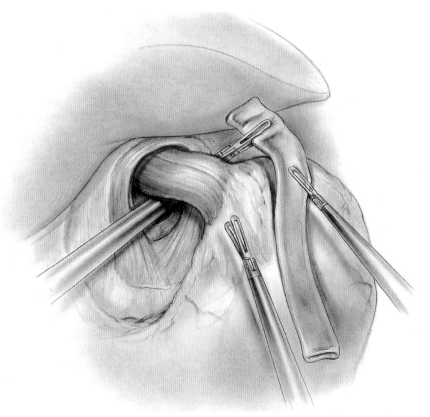

Fig. 17-5. *A 10-cm, 5-mm Penrose drain is then brought around the esophagus and clipped to itself anteriorly.*

right as the surgeon mobilizes the esophagus from the mediastinum. This is carried out both bluntly and with the ultrasonic coagulating shears (Ethicon-Ultracision, Smithfield, Rhode Island) until 2 to 3 cm of abdominal esophagus can be easily brought into the abdomen. The short gastric vessels are taken down starting one-third of the way down the greater curvature (Fig. 17-6). Exposure is obtained by grasping the stomach with the left hand, retracting it to the right, and asking the assistant to grasp the gastrosplenic omentum and retract it to the left. With the ultrasonic coagulating shears, the surgeon completely mobilizes the fundus of the stomach. If the short gastric arteries are extremely large (greater than 4 mm), they are also clipped for added security. The gastric fundus is mobilized all the way down to the base of the left crus to prevent potential kinking when the fundus is brought around the esophagus. If the crural opening is enlarged, it is then closed with simple sutures of size 0 nonabsorbable material (Nurolon, Ethicon, Cincinnati, Ohio) (Fig. 17-7). If this opening is extremely wide and these sutures are going to be under some tension, Teflon pledgets are used. The fundoplication is then pulled posteriorly around the esophagus (Fig. 17-8). If it does not easily remain in place when released, further mobilization should be carried out.

To provide an internal stent for the wrap construction, a 56-F to 60-F bougie is carefully advanced into the stomach. If the patient has a history of stricture, a smaller dilator should be used, but generally 10-F greater than the largest previous dilation. The fundoplication is then sutured in place with three 2-0 nonabsorbable sutures (Nurolon), taking full-thickness bites of stomach and partial-thickness bites of esophagus with each suture. The first suture is placed 2 cm above the GE junction, and two additional sutures are placed 8 to 10 mm apart distally along the esophagus for a length of no greater than 2 cm, with care to avoid the anterior vagus nerve (Fig. 17-9). Instead of securing the fundoplication to the diaphragmatic crura, which have little ability to prevent displacement during violent retching, we now suture the cardia of the stomach and the esophagus to the left side of the fundoplication to keep it from slipping. The Penrose drain is then cut and removed. The area of the fundoplication and left upper quadrant is then irrigated. The patient is given three

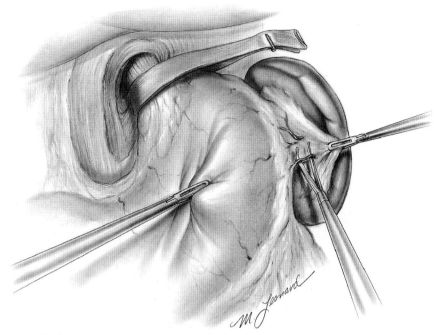

Fig. 17-6. The short gastric vessels are taken down all the way down to the base of the left crus, so that there will be no kinking when the gastric fundus is brought around the esophagus.

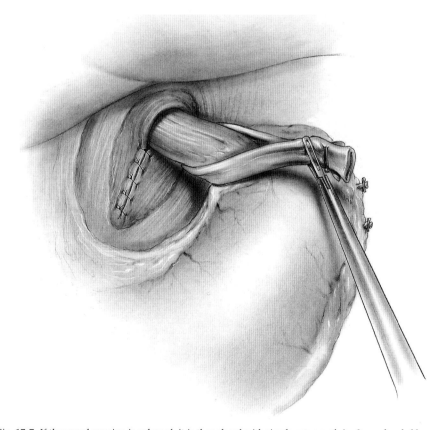

Fig. 17-7. If the crural opening is enlarged, it is then closed with simple sutures of size 0 nonabsorbable material (Nurolon).

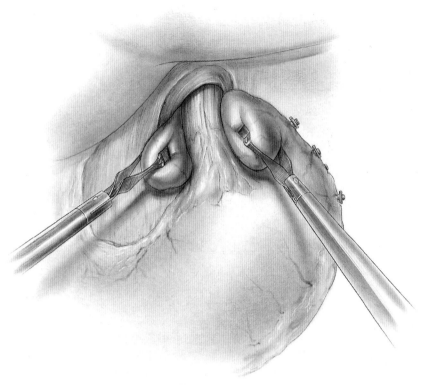

Fig. 17-8. The fundoplication is then brought around posteriorly to the esophagus.

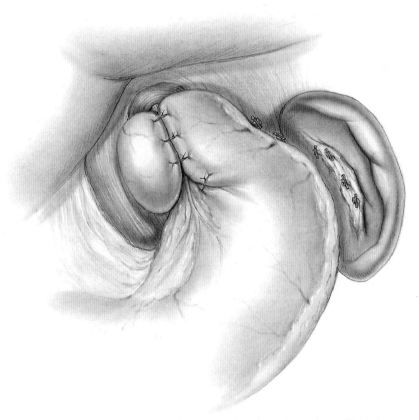

Fig. 17-9. The first suture is placed 2 cm above the gastroesophageal junction, and two additional sutures are placed 8 to 10 mm apart distally along the esophagus for a length of no greater than 2 cm, with care to avoid the anterior vagus nerve.

large manual breaths to help assist in deflating the pneumoperitoneum and pneumomediastinum completely, and the ports are removed under direct vision to make sure that none of the sites is bleeding. Fascial closure is not routinely necessary if the ports have been placed obliquely through the muscle layers. The skin is closed with absorbable sutures, and Steristrips are placed.

Postoperative Care

The Foley catheter is removed in the recovery room, and clear liquids are started the day of surgery, as soon as patients are awake and alert. A mechanical soft diet is started on the next day. Occasionally, patients are discharged on the first postoperative day, but usually they are discharged on postoperative day 2. A soft diet is continued for approximately 3 weeks to allow edema at the GE junction to resolve. Patients may return to work when ready.

Results

Nissen fundoplication is the most commonly employed fundoplication procedure in the United States, with long-term favorable results in 85% to 95% of patients. Laparoscopic Nissen fundoplication has been performed since 1991, and long-term results are not known, although short-term results have demonstrated efficacy comparable with that of open fundoplication (Table 17-2). No long-term, randomized, controlled trials have compared open with laparoscopic Nissen fundoplication, and it is unlikely that such a trial will ever be performed. One retrospective comparative trial demonstrated significantly more postoperative dysphagia and limited lower esophageal sphincter relaxation following laparoscopic Nissen fundoplication than following open Nissen fundoplication.

We recently reviewed the first 300 patients referred to our institution for laparoscopic treatment of GER. Mean operative time in this series was 185 ± 51 minutes, and this was shortened to 154 ± 30 minutes in the last 20 cases. This is slightly longer than reported series for open fundoplication. Mean length of stay was 2.2 days with a range from 1 to 32 days.

Patients who had moderate to severe symptoms of heartburn and regurgitation

Table 17-2. Comparative Results of Laparoscopic Nissen Fundoplication Series

Reference	n	Conversion	Hospital Stay (days)	Wound Infection	Incisional Hernia	Perforated Viscus	Fundoplication Herniation	Repair Disruption	Bleeding	Pneumothorax	Dysphagia	Gas Bloating	Recurrent Symptoms
Hinder et al. (1994)	198	2.0	3	—	—	2	0	1	1	1	6	13	1
Hunter et al. (1996)	252	1.0	2	—	—	2.8	0.3	—	3	1	4	11	3
Jamieson et al. (1994)	155	12.3	2.6	—	1.3	—	—	—	—	1.3	17.6	0	1.2
Weertz et al. (1993)	132	3.3	2.8	—	1.5	2.3	—	0.8	0	—	5.4	—	0.8

Percentages unless otherwise specified.

were nearly universally free of these symptoms following operation. One year following laparoscopic fundoplication 93% of patients are symptom-free, 4% have occasional symptoms, and 3% have frequent symptoms of heartburn. Nearly 50% of patients in our series had moderate to severe regurgitation preoperatively, and postoperatively only 3% of patients had more than rare regurgitation. Most patients with moderate to severe recurrent heartburn or regurgitation had acid–base probe abnormalities and stretched or disrupted fundoplications.

Atypical symptoms do not improve as well as typical symptoms after fundoplication. Patients whose major symptom was asthma, hoarseness, chest pain, or cough did not improve to the same extent as patients with heartburn only. The difference between response of atypical and typical symptoms to laparoscopic fundoplication may be that the atypical symptoms were only in part a result of GER, whereas typical symptoms were entirely a result of GER. In our series, we found that most patients who suffered bloating postoperatively actually had these symptoms before operation. Fifteen percent of patients are unable to belch postoperatively, and all patients have some degree of hyperflatulence, presumably because aerophagic habits persist postoperatively and are not compensated by frequent belching. Gas bloating and hyperflatulence may also be a result of the extremely competent valve formed by the Nissen procedure. Fortunately, true gas bloating is very rare. Gastroparesis or dumping may result from injury to the vagus nerves during the procedure, although this is usually self-limited and resolves in weeks to months.

Conversion from laparoscopic to open Nissen fundoplication should be considered good surgical judgment and not a complication. In our series of 300 laparoscopic fundoplications, there were three conversions. Two of these were caused by severe adhesions, and one was caused by an enlarged liver in an obese patient.

Intraoperative Complications

One of the most feared complications is esophageal perforation. This should occur less than 1% of the time and may be a result of severe periesophagitis making it difficult to find the tissue planes. Patients with severe esophagitis should be treated aggressively medically before surgery is attempted. To prevent this injury, one should start dissection by identifying the crura, instead of dissecting directly around the esophagus. Prior to dissecting posterior to the esophagus, all esophageal tubes should be removed. Circumferential dissection should be done under direct vision with an angled (30 degree or 45 degree) laparoscope. Spreading dissection utilizing two blunt graspers works well. For retraction, epiphrenic fat should be grasped instead of directly grasping the stomach or esophagus. Simple perforations may be closed laparoscopically with interrupted sutures. If possible, the repair should be covered with the fundic wrap. More complex injuries or injuries in an area difficult to access justify conversion to an open repair.

Bleeding has been an uncommon complication during or after laparoscopic fundoplication. Most large series have described a 0% incidence of the need for transfusion. Some bleeding may occur when the short gastric vessels are taken down to mobilize the gastric fundus, but this is easy to control with the use of the harmonic scalpel or the occasional clip. Fracture of the liver can easily occur during retraction. It is important to use an atraumatic retractor and helpful to attach these to static, table-mounted instrument holders. Most hepatic and splenic hemorrhage can be stopped by direct pressure or with topical hemostatic agents. During dissection around the esophagus, small-volume bleeding may obscure tissue planes. Bleeding vessels may be clipped or coagulated. To avoid severe hemorrhage, gentle and meticulous surgical technique is needed, particularly around the liver and spleen and in the area of the short gastric vessels.

Clinically significant pneumothorax rarely occurs. It is reported in the literature approximately 1% to 5% of the time and is caused by inadvertent entry into the pleura when the esophagus is dissected in the mediastinum. Pneumothorax is usually well tolerated during surgery because positive pressure ventilation is greater than intraperitoneal pressure. To avoid this problem, dissection should be performed as close to the esophagus as possible when it is deep in the mediastinum, and posterior dissection of the esophagus should occur below the left crus of the diaphragm. Postoperatively, patients should be given several vital capacity breaths to allow complete venting of the pneumoperitoneum through the trocar sites. If a pneumothorax has been identified, a red rubber catheter can be slipped into the chest through the hiatus and pleural vent. At the conclusion of the procedure, the end of the tube is pulled through a trocar hole and placed under water while the anesthetist administers several vital capacity breaths by hand bagging. Postoperative chest x-rays are not routinely obtained, unless a patient is having respiratory problems in the recovery room. Carbon dioxide pneumothorax is rapidly reabsorbed, usually in less than 1 hour.

Subcutaneous and mediastinal emphysema are often noted during laparoscopic Nissen fundoplication. When there is extensive dissection of the mediastinum, such as required when reducing a large hiatal hernia, subcutaneous emphysema may be extensive. Although this particular complication requires no specific treatment, it can cause elevated Pco_2 from tissue absorption that may extend the need for ventilatory support, especially in patients with underlying pulmonary disease.

Postoperative Complications

Solid food dysphagia is the most frequent and troublesome postoperative problem. It occurs very frequently in the early postoperative period, and in some series can be as high as 34%. In our series, it occurred 17% of the time in the early postoperative period; however, only 4% of patients experienced long-term dysphagia. Early postoperative dysphagia is probably a result of edema or hematoma at the GE junction

and will resolve in days to weeks. Dysphagia that does not resolve may be caused by twisting or kinking of the fundoplication, by an excessively long or tight fundoplication, or by poor esophageal motility. In patients with poor esophageal peristalsis, consideration should be given to performing a partial fundoplication, such as the Toupet procedure (a 270-degree posterior wrap) to help avoid postoperative dysphagia. Prolonged dysphagia may also be due to technical errors during surgery. It is critical to completely mobilize the entire upper gastric fundus from one-third of the way down the greater curvature up to the left crus, including the posterior attachments, and to create a 2-cm floppy Nissen around a 60-F dilator. Failure to adequately mobilize the fundus can put torsion on the wrap, causing it to twist the distal esophagus postoperatively. Making the wrap too long or placing it around too small a dilator also creates outflow resistance and subsequent dysphagia. If solid food dysphagia persists beyond 6 weeks postoperatively, dilation may be helpful. If three or four dilations in 3 months do not cure dysphagia, reoperation will be necessary. In our series, this has been required less than 1% of the time. Thorough testing should be obtained to define the cause of dysphagia, especially since an unrecognized esophageal dysmotility disorder, such as achalasia, may be the actual cause.

Early and late reoperations for complications of fundoplication such as suture-line failure, paraesophageal hernia, slipped Nissen, and constricting (too tight) fundoplication have recently been reported. In these case reports, these complications are sometimes associated with an acute perioperative episode of intense vomiting or coughing. Precautions must be undertaken to avoid such episodes with the use of strong antiemetic agents, including droperidol (Inapsine) and ondansetron hydrochloride (Zofran). To help avoid the possibility of a slipped Nissen, esophageal bites should be taken with every suture used in the fundoplication, and the fundoplication should be sutured to the stomach on the left side of the fundoplication. To help avoid paraesophageal hernia, we close the crura snugly behind the esophagus. Good results have been described with redo laparoscopic fundoplications under these circumstances, but the best results are always achieved with the first operation.

Conclusion

GER is a common disease, and despite improvements in medical therapy, a significant number of patients require surgical treatment. Nissen fundoplication is the simplest procedure to perform laparoscopically and the easiest to teach and learn. Although long-term results of laparoscopic Nissen fundoplication are unknown, we expect them to be similar to those of open Nissen fundoplication and expect excellent results. Excellent results are obtained by appropriate patient selection and preoperative evaluation and by good operative technique that requires appropriate training and adherence to recognized operative protocol.

Suggested Reading

Cuschieri A, Hunter J, Wolfe B, Swanstrom L. Multicenter prospective evaluation of laparoscopic antireflux surgery: preliminary report. *Surg Endosc* 1993;7:505–510.

DeMeester TR, Bonavina L, Albertucci M. Nissen fundoplication for GERD: evaluation of primary repair in 100 consecutive patients. *Ann Surg* 1986;204:9–20.

Hinder RA, Filipi CJ, Wetscher G, Neary P, DeMeester TR, Perdikis G. Laparoscopic Nissen fundoplication is an effective treatment for gastroesophageal reflux disease. *Ann Surg* 1994;220:472–483.

Hunter JG, Trus TL, Branum GD, Waring JP, Wood WC. A physiologic approach to laparoscopic fundoplication for gastroesophageal reflux disease. *Ann Surg* 1996;223:673–687.

Jamieson GG, Watson DI, Britten-Jones R, Mitchell PC, Anvari M. Laparoscopic Nissen fundoplication. *Ann Surg* 1994;220:137–145.

Nissen R. Gastropexy and "fundoplication" in surgical treatment of hiatal hernia. *Am J Dig Dis* 1961;6:959–961.

Peters JH, Heimbucher J, Kauer WKH, Incarbone R, Bremner CG, DeMeester TR. *J Am Coll Surg* 1995;180:385–393.

Spechler SJ. Comparison of medical and surgical therapy for complicated gastroesophageal reflux disease in veterans. The Department of Veterans Affairs Gastroesophageal Reflux Disease Study Group. *New Engl J Med* 1992;326:786–792.

Spechler SJ. Epidemiology and natural history of gastro-oesophageal reflux disease. *Digestion* 1992;51(suppl):24–29.

Watson DI, Jamieson GG, Devitt PG, Mitchell PC, Game PA. Paraesophageal hiatus hernia: an important complication of laparoscopic Nissen fundoplication. *Br J Surg* 1995;82:521–523.

Weerts JM, Dallemagne B, Hamoir E, et al. Laparoscopic Nissen fundoplication: detailed analysis of 132 patients. *Surg Laparosc Endosc* 1993;3:359–364.

EDITOR'S COMMENT

The importance of mastering the technical details of laparoscopic Nissen fundoplication cannot be overstressed. The price of cutting corners in the evaluation, performance, and follow-up of this procedure is an unacceptable incidence of postoperative dysphagia, gas bloating, and intraoperative complications that can be truly devastating. Certainly, the end result of a poorly performed Nissen is an unhappy or damaged patient and, secondarily, an unhappy referral source. Dr. Richardson and Dr. Hunter mention a number of important points that deserve emphasis since they explain their excellent outcomes.

Thorough preoperative evaluation of patients is critical. In my experience, as many as 30% of patients will have their operative approach modified, based on results of preoperative testing. A point of difference with Dr. Hunter's group is the importance of 24-hour pH testing preoperatively. The use of 24-hour pH testing has great value in objective assessment of the severity of disease and symptom correlation. In addition, without a preoperative baseline, it is difficult to assess patients who have complaints postoperatively. There is a large difference between a patient with postoperative symptoms and an abnormal De-Meester score of 20 who had a preoperative score of 25 versus a preoperative score of 150. Intraoperative technique is especially important. Atraumatic retraction, use of safe energy sources, and use of an angled scope to allow dissection under direct vision are all critical. I agree with the authors that division of the short gastrics and full mobilization of the fundus will minimize postoperative dysphagia and wrap failure. In fact, surgeons will find that the added effort in mobilizing the fundus is more than compensated by the subsequent ease of performing the wrap. A short, floppy Nissen is of course the ultimate goal. An esophageal dilator can help achieve this goal, but caution must be used in placing the bougie. Careless advancements of the dilator can easily result in perforation of the esophagus. Coordination with anesthesiology and liberal use of Savary guidewire dilators are important.

Finally, patients with a shortened esophagus must be approached carefully. It is easy, through the laparoscope, to convince oneself that an adequate length of intraabdominal esophagus has been obtained, when in fact repair is either being done around the upper stomach or under tension. Both will lead to a high failure rate. Selective use of the laparoscopic or open Collis procedure should be considered in these cases.

L.L.S.

18

Laparoscopic Partial Fundoplication

Richard J. Finley and Andrew J. Graham

Gastroesophageal reflux disease (GERD) is due to an excessive exposure of the esophageal lining to gastric juices. The functional abnormalities of the upper gastrointestinal (GI) tract known to produce GERD are a mechanical defect of the lower esophageal sphincter, inefficient esophageal pump function causing decreased esophageal clearance of refluxate, increased concentrations of acid or alkali in the refluxate, decreased gastric motility, or gastric outlet obstruction leading to increased gastric pressure and reflux. These functional disorders must be identified with accurate testing before effective treatment can be prescribed. A barium swallow is usually obtained in patients with typical GER symptoms who fail to respond to antacids or changes in lifestyle. This test investigates a variety of differential diagnostic possibilities, including hiatal hernia, gastric emptying disorders, gastric ulcer, and duodenal ulcer, as well as GER. Documentation of an irreducible hiatal hernia suggests that significant shortening of the esophagus may be present, making an abdominal approach more difficult. Upper GI endoscopy should be performed to evaluate the possibility of Barrett's esophagus, to grade the degree of esophagitis, and to evaluate esophageal or gastric ulceration. Endoscopy can also aid in detection of esophageal shortening. Significant esophageal shortening is likely to be present if the esophagogastric junction is greater than 5 cm proximal to the crural impression. Currently, 24-hour esophageal pH monitoring is the best way of objectively measuring exposure of the esophagus to gastric juices. If surgery is contemplated, esophageal pump function and functional defects of the lower esophageal sphincter can be evaluated by

esophageal manometry. A functional gastric disorder can be diagnosed by gastric emptying scintigraphy.

A functional gastric disorder is suspected if patients complain of excessive postprandial fullness or early satiety. These extensive investigations prior to surgery are required to ensure the best possible outcome from the chosen therapy. Antireflux surgery is considered for patients who have clearly documented GER and who have failed a trial of medical therapy that includes lifestyle alterations and acid-reduction medication. Surgery is a cost-effective antireflux treatment in patients younger than 55 years with a mechanically defective cardia, as defined by a lower esophageal sphincter pressure of less than 6 mm Hg, short overall lower esophageal sphincter length (2 cm or less), or short intraabdominal lower esophageal segment (1 cm or less), and with normal function of the stomach and the body of the esophagus.

In 1956, Nissen discovered that a gastric fundoplication prevented reflux when he studied a patient many years after a partial esophagectomy in which the initial aim was to protect the anastomotic area rather than prevent reflux. Fundoplication has subsequently become the most widely used form of antireflux surgery, the efficacy of which has been established by clinical and endoscopic follow-up and esophageal pH monitoring. DeMeester clarified the understanding of the antireflux operation by observing three important technical features that all successful operations have in common:

1. Closure of the diaphragmatic crura,
2. Anchoring of 4 to 5 cm of tubular esophagus in the abdomen,

3. Wrapping of the lower esophagus with a partial or total fundoplication.

Using these principles, a Nissen fundoplication is generally very effective in controlling GER. However, the prevention of reflux alone does not always provide an optimum result for patients. Persistent postoperative symptoms can jeopardize an otherwise excellent result in a significant group of patients after these procedures in the form of dysphagia, inability to belch and vomit, postprandial fullness, bloating and pain, and flatulence. Skinner classified failures after antireflux surgery as indication problems, wrong choice of operative procedure, and insufficient surgical technique during the procedure itself. Incorrect indications for surgery or the wrong choice of a certain operative procedure often originate from an unclear understanding of the physiologic situation of a particular patient.

The decision whether to perform a total or a partial fundoplication depends on the identification of the functional defects producing GERD. If a patient with reduced quality of life and GER symptoms has a classic functional situation with hypotensive lower esophageal sphincter, normal esophageal peristalsis, and normal gastric function, a short, "floppy" Nissen fundoplication can be expected to prevent GERD in 90% of patients after 5 years. Fully mobilizing the fundus by taking down all the short gastric vessels, wrapping the fundus over a 60-French (60-F) Maloney bougie, and decreasing the length of the total fundoplication to 1 cm has decreased the rate of early temporary dysphagia from 83% to 39%, the rate of long-term dysphagia from 21% to 3%, and the incidence of gas bloating symptoms from 8% to 4%. In GERD patients with impaired esophageal peristalsis, a partial rather than total fundoplication decreases the incidence of postoperative dysphagia. Gas bloating symptoms are also decreased with partial fundoplication.

The term *partial* fundoplication means less than 270 degrees of the esophageal circumference has been encircled by a gastric fundus wrap. The most widely studied partial fundoplication is the Belsey Mark IV operation that requires a transthoracic approach. This chapter discusses only transabdominal partial fundoplication and, in particular, the laparoscopic performance of this procedure.

Transabdominal partial fundoplication was first described in the early 1960s. In 1962, Jacques Dor described an 180-degree anterior fundoplication following esophageal myotomy for achalasia. In 1963, A. Toupet described a posterior partial fundoplication, again in conjunction with an esophageal myotomy. In 1965, James Lind proposed a transabdominal modified Belsey operation, and more recently A. Watson has developed an anterolateral fundoplication. Reduction in the incidence of postoperative complications of dysphagia and gas bloating symptoms is the principal reason that partial rather than total fundoplication is used. Various techniques for performing partial fundoplication have been described (Table 18-1).

Surgeons favoring total fundoplication believe that long-term GER control is poorer with partial fundoplication, based on R. Belsey's long-term follow-up that showed a symptomatic recurrence rate of 6% in 219 patients followed for at least 5 years with objective evidence of recurrence in 11%. However, three prospective, randomized studies have compared transabdominal

Table 18-1. Partial Fundoplication Techniques

PARTIAL WRAPS

Dor	90–150-degree anterior wrap
Thal	90-degree anterior wrap
Belsey IV	270-degree transthoracic anterolateral wrap
Toupet/Lind	200-degree posterior wrap

ESOPHAGOGASTROPEXY

Hill repair

Watson repair

partial fundoplication with total fundoplication. These studies suggest equivalent symptomatic relief of GER with slightly fewer postprandial side effects in the partial fundoplication groups.

A few reports describing laparoscopic partial fundoplication have been published. McKernan (1994) reported on 14 laparoscopic posterior fundoplications compared with 14 laparoscopic total fundoplications, noting a marked decrease in incidence of postoperative dysphagia in the partial fundoplication group. Watson and colleagues (1991) reported on 23 patients who underwent laparoscopic 120-degree anterolateral partial fundoplication, with two patients requiring dilation and no incidents of gas bloating symptoms. In our experience with early anterior partial fundoplication follow-up on 18 patients, 16 have had good results with no gas bloating symptoms. One patient required a single dilation following surgery, and another complained of intermittent epigastric pain without demonstrated recurrent reflux. A. Cuschieri and coworkers (1993) reported on a multicenter trial in which laparoscopic posterior partial fundoplication provided equivalent reflux control with a decreased incidence of gas bloating syndrome and dysphagia compared to those undergoing laparoscopic total fundoplication, although the study was not specifically designed to examine for this difference. To maximally decrease postoperative complications following total fundoplication, all short gastric vessels must be divided, the fundus totally mobilized, and a short fundoplication carried out over a 60-F Maloney bougie. Complete laparoscopic mobilization of the fundus has resulted in occasional injury to the spleen, resulting in conversion to open laparotomy for control of bleeding from the spleen. The advantage of anterior partial fundoplication is that not all of the short gastric vessels need to be divided to carry out an adequate fundoplication. However, posterior partial fundoplication usually requires division of the short gastric vessels and complete mobilization of the fundus of the stomach.

Indications for Operation

Laparoscopic partial fundoplication is the procedure of choice for patients with GERD and significant esophageal dys-

motility. It is also recommended following laparoscopic Heller myotomy and is an appropriate procedure, in the place of laparoscopic total fundoplication, for patients with normal esophageal motility with the expectation of less postoperative dysphagia and gas bloating symptoms. Long-term conclusive studies are not available to determine the efficacy of laparoscopic partial fundoplication in controlling GER (Table 18-2).

Contraindications to partial fundoplication include a short esophagus with the esophagogastric junction 5 cm or more above the diaphragmatic crura on endoscopy, an irreducible hiatal hernia on barium swallow, delayed gastric emptying or gastric outlet obstruction, and a normal or hypertensive lower esophageal sphincter (Table 18-3). A history of upper abdominal surgery is not a contraindication to an attempt at laparoscopic antireflux operation, but we have found that previous dissection at the hiatus usually results in a laparotomy.

Perioperative Management

Patients are kept on proton pump inhibitors during and for 2 weeks following the operation to avoid rebound hyperacidity during the immediate postoperative period. All patients receive deep vein thrombosis prophylaxis in the form of subcutaneous heparin and pneumatic compression stockings prior to and during the operation. Patients with esophageal stenosis are dilated up to a 56-F Maloney bougie prior to the operation. They also receive a single dose of a first-generation cephalosporin on entering the operating room.

Operative Technique

Under general anesthesia, the patient is placed into the lithotomy position with the hips at 30-degree of flexion. A urinary catheter is placed in the bladder following induction of anesthesia and removed prior to anesthetic reversal. Pneumatic compression stockings are placed on all patients prior to the start of the anesthetic. An endotracheal tube is placed to the left side of the mouth to facilitate insertion of a bougie during the procedure. An 18-F orogastric tube is placed in the stomach to ensure

**Table 18-2. Indications
for Laparoscopic Partial Fundoplication**

Primary esophageal motility disorders
    Achalasia
    Scleroderma
    Chagas' disease
    Diffuse esophageal spasm
Secondary esophageal motility disorders
    Hypomotility secondary to chronic reflux
    Hypomotility secondary to Barrett's disease
Inability to tolerate postfundoplication side
    effects
    Aerophagia
    Chronic nausea
    Revision of obstructing Nissen wrap

**Table 18-3. Contraindications
to Laparoscopic Fundoplication**

Shortened esophagus
Contraindication to general anesthesia
Previous fundoplication
Gastric outlet obstruction

gastric decompression. Video monitors are placed on either side of the patient's shoulders (Fig. 18-1), and the anesthetic machine is placed to the right of the patient's head. The abdomen and lower anterior chest are prepared and draped. The clamp for the Omni self-retaining retractor (Pillings-Wecle Co., Scarborough, Ontario, Canada) is placed on the right side of the table at the level of the patient's arm, with careful padding to avoid injury to the ulnar nerve. The surgeon operates between the patient's legs to optimize spatial orientation to the hiatus and video monitors and provide the surgeon with a comfortable position and the best mechanical advantage for suturing.

Pneumoperitoneum is achieved using the Veress needle placed into the peritoneal cavity at the umbilicus to avoid injuring the liver. In patients who have had previous abdominal surgery, the Hasson trocar is used instead of the Veress needle. Once the pneumoperitoneum is achieved, a 10-mm trocar is placed in the medial border of the left rectus sheath approximately 15 cm below the base of xiphoid. A 30-degree laparoscope is inserted, and under direct vision a 12-mm port is inserted below the right subcostal margin 15 cm from the base of xiphoid. The laparoscope is then temporarily inserted via the right subcostal

port to allow direct visualization for the insertion of 10-mm left subcostal port 10 cm from the xiphoid. A 5-mm port is inserted through the right rectus muscle approximately 10 cm below the xiphoid. A 10-mm port is then inserted through the right rectus muscle approximately 15 cm from the xiphoid (Fig. 18-2).

The left lobe of the liver is retracted, with placement of a fan retractor through the right subcostal port to a position beyond the falciform ligament. The fan blades are then opened with the convex surface against the left lobe of the liver. The convex surface is used to minimize puncture injuries to the liver. The left lobe of the liver is then retracted cephalad to expose the hiatus. The retractor is then clamped to the Omni retractor or held by an assistant. Adequate exposure of the esophageal hiatus with retraction of the left lobe of the liver is a prerequisite to proceeding laparoscopically. The table is placed in 25-degree reverse Trendelenburg position to produce caudal migration of the intraabdominal organs. A Babcock grasper is then

placed via the 10-mm port on the patient's right side to retract the fundus of the stomach inferiorly, completing exposure of the hiatus.

Dissection of the Esophageal Hiatus

Dissection of the hiatus is now begun by dividing the peritoneum and phrenoesophageal ligament overlying the anterior esophagus and left crus, with care taken not to injure the anterior vagus nerve. Attachments between the fundus of the stomach and the inferior diaphragm are taken down with sharp dissection. The left crus of the diaphragm is dissected down as far as possible to expose the retroesophageal space on the left side. Dissection is carried out with a grasper in the right 5-mm rectus port and insulated dissecting scissors in the left 10-mm subcostal port.

Dissection of the right side of the esophagus and right crus is begun by retracting the esophagus to the patient's left side using the Babcock grasper. The gastrohepatic

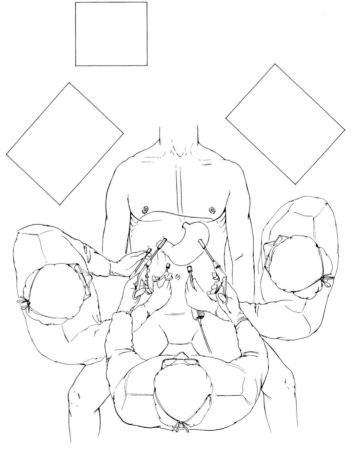

Fig. 18-1. Operative setup.

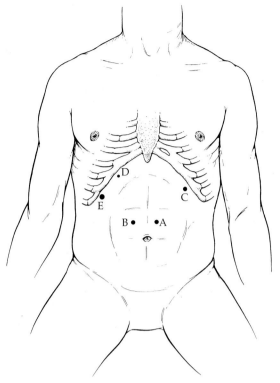

Fig. 18-2. Port placements. (A,B,C, 10-mm port; D, 5-mm port; E, 12-mm port.)

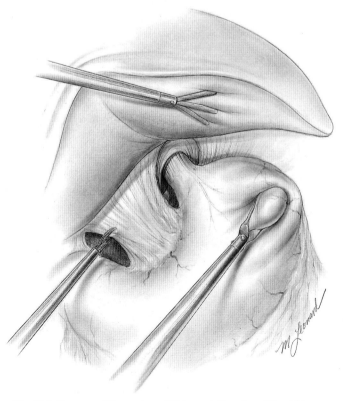

Fig. 18-3. Exposure of the esophageal hiatus and dissection of the right crus.

ligament is opened up, with care taken not to injure the hepatic branch of the vagus nerve (Fig. 18-3). An aberrant left hepatic artery may also be found within the gastrohepatic ligament in 7% to 10% of patients. Attempts are made to preserve the vessel, but if the aberrant vessels need to be divided, the vessel should be compressed with a clamp for at least 15 minutes before division to ensure that the patient does not develop hepatic necrosis or lactic acidosis. The vessel may then be clipped or suture-ligated and divided. Dissection of the anterior phrenoesophageal ligament is then completed. Occasionally, branches of the inferior phrenic vein need to be divided to adequately mobilize the anterior esophagus. Dissection of the phrenoesophageal ligament is then carried down onto the right crus of the diaphragm. Care is taken not to mistake the inferior vena cava for the right crus of the diaphragm at this stage of the operation. The 30-degree laparoscope is particularly advantageous when dissection of the retroesophageal space is begun. The posterior vagus nerve is visualized and dissected with the esophagus. Using careful hemostasis and blunt dissection, the retroesophageal space is dissected between the posterior aspect of the esophagus and the inferior border of the left crus of the diaphragm. If the left crus has been well dissected from the front, the retroesophageal space is easily opened into the left upper quadrant. The grasper is placed through the right 5-mm rectus port into the left upper quadrant, with care taken not to injure the short gastric vessels or the spleen. A vascular loop is passed through the left 10-mm subcostal port into the grasper. The vascular loop encircling the posterior vagus nerve, the esophagus, and the anterior vagus nerve is held by a ratcheted grasper placed through the right 10-mm rectus port after removal of the Babcock grasper.

To deliver at least 5 cm of tubular esophagus, dissection of the esophagus is now performed up into the mediastinum for at least 5 to 6 cm using either the insulated scissors or a cherry dissector. Care is taken not to injure the vagus nerve or the parietal pleura to avoid a pneumothorax.

Closure of the Crura

The crura are closed in all cases to reduce the chance of intrathoracic migration of the fundoplication (Fig. 18-4). The crural

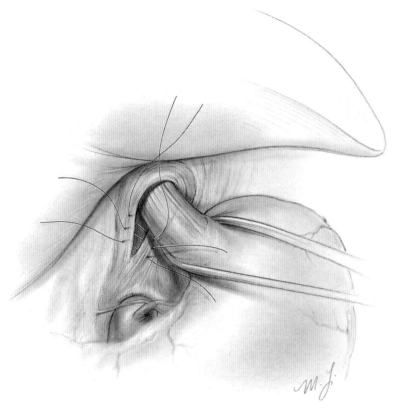

Fig. 18-4. Closure of the crura. A vascular tape retracts the esophagus to the left. Three 0 silk sutures approximate the crura posteriorly.

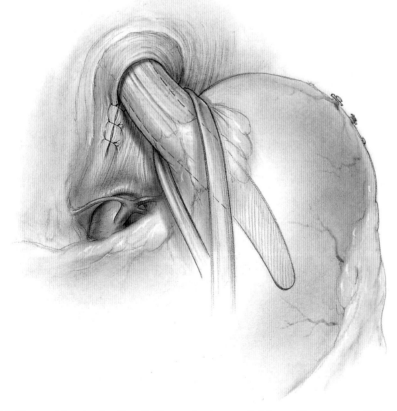

Fig. 18-5. Closure of the crura (continued). The crural sutures are tied down with a 56-French Maloney bougie in the esophagus.

sutures (0 silk) are inserted through the 10-mm left subcostal port. The crura are approximated inferiorly to superiorly using interrupted 0 silk sutures tied intracorporeally. Prior to the most superior suture's being tied down, the orogastric tube is removed after aspiration of the stomach, and a well lubricated 56-F Maloney bougie is inserted into the stomach (Fig. 18-5). This avoids an excessively tight crural closure. The bougie is withdrawn into the thoracic esophagus following hiatal closure to avoid tearing the esophagus during anchoring of the esophagus in the abdomen. The above steps are common to both the anterior and posterior fundoplication. The anterior and posterior fundoplication are described separately.

Anterior Partial Fundoplication

We prefer to use the anterior fundoplication, as we believe that it most closely achieves the principles of the Belsey Mark IV operation, which are to close the crura, anchor 4 cm of tubular esophagus below the diaphragm, and partially wrap the esophagus with the fundus of the stomach. It has also been our experience that a tension-free anterior fundoplication can more often be achieved without division of all of the short gastric vessels, thus avoiding injury to the spleen. The anterior fundoplication is begun by closing the angle of His, as well as fixing 4 to 5 cm of tubular esophagus in the abdomen. The first 2-0 silk suture is passed through the medial aspect of the lower fundus, through the left crus, and into the left side of the esophagus, with care taken not to injure the anterior vagus nerve. The second suture passes through the upper aspect of the medial fundus and the left crus and is anchored into the left side of the esophagus (Fig. 18-6). The vascular loop is removed. The next component of the operation is to anchor the right side of the phrenoesophageal ligament to the inferior aspect of the right crus of the diaphragm, with care taken not to injure the anterior or posterior vagus nerves (Fig. 18-7).

A trial mobilization of the fundus to the right crus is performed. If any tension exists, sequential short gastric vessels are divided until the fundoplication is tension-free over a 56-F Maloney bougie. The fundus is sewn to the anterosuperior aspect of the crura with a 2-0 silk suture (Fig. 18-8). The fundus is then rolled over the

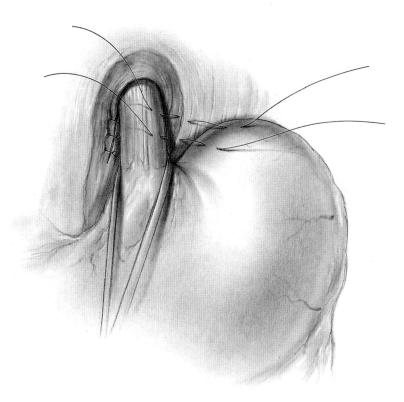

Fig. 18-6. Closure of the angle of His. The fundus is sutured to the left crus of the diaphragm and the left side of the esophagus, with care taken not to injure the anterior vagus nerve.

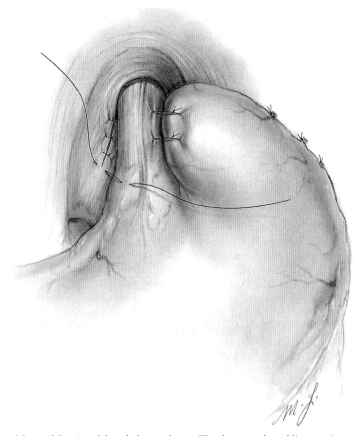

Fig. 18-7. Intraabdominal fixation of the tubular esophagus. The phrenoesophageal ligament is sewn to the inferior aspect of the right crus, with care taken not to injure the vagus nerve.

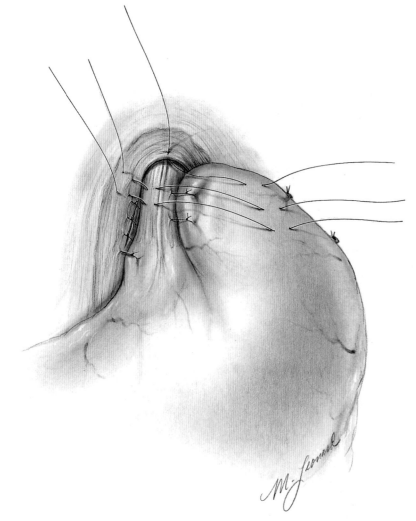

Fig. 18-8. Fixation of the anterior fundoplication. The superior aspect of the fundus is sewn to the anterior aspect of the hiatus with a 2-0 silk suture.

taken not to injure the anterior vagus nerve (Fig. 18-12).

Posterior partial fundoplication requires considerably more time as a result of the multiple sutures required. We have been reluctant to substitute the stapler for suture, as we are uncomfortable controlling the depth of application of the staples.

Closure

Following completion of the fundoplication, the field is systematically inspected. The spleen and left lobe of the liver are inspected for hemostasis, and the colon and stomach are also examined to detect any injuries that may have occurred out of the visual field. The ports are then removed under direct vision. The fascial defects are closed using an 0 polyglycolic suture. The skin is closed using absorbable subcutaneous sutures.

Postoperative Care

A nasogastric tube is not used, unless the patient requires gastric decompression for relief of nausea or abdominal distention. This occurs in fewer than 5% of the patients. Parenteral antiemetics are given, as required. Clear liquids are started the morning following surgery and advanced to a dental soft diet as tolerated. Patients are usually discharged after the second or third postoperative day and remain on a dental soft diet for 2 weeks before returning to a normal diet. An upper GI endoscopy (Fig. 18-13) and barium swallow (Fig. 18-14) show the anatomy of an anterior partial fundoplication.

Complications

Complications of laparoscopic partial fundoplication presenting in the intraoperative or early postoperative phase are common to any form of antireflux surgery. Injury to the spleen has not occurred in our series, but is usually recognized intraoperatively and often necessitates conversion to an open procedure. The usual splenic preservation techniques should be utilized to avoid splenectomy, if possible. Occasionally, splenic injury may not be recognized until the early postoperative period when it may present as hypotension or anemia.

anterior aspect of the stomach and sewn to the lateral aspect of the esophagus and the right crus of the diaphragm using two 2-0 silk sutures. The lower part of the fundus is sewn to the lower right crus with a 2-0 silk suture (Fig. 18-9). This creates approximately a 220-degree wrap. The bougie is then reinserted into the stomach to ensure that the wrap is not overly tight.

Posterior Partial Fundoplication

The technique of posterior partial fundoplication utilized is modeled on the Boutelier and Jonsell (1982) modification of the Toupet partial fundoplication. After mobilization of the esophagus and closure of the crura, the fundus is mobilized by dividing the short gastric vessels. The posterior partial fundoplication is begun by placing a Babcock grasper through the right 10-mm rectus port behind the esophagus to grasp the fundus. The fundus is retracted through the retroesophageal space, and the vascular loop around the esophagus is removed. At this time, the 56-F Maloney bougie is inserted into the stomach, and a trial application of the posterior fundoplication is carried out. The fundus must encompass 200 degrees of the esophagus in a tension-free manner. The bougie is withdrawn to the midesophagus, and the fundus is fixed to the left crus using two 2-0 silk sutures (Fig. 18-10). The fundus is sewn to the right crus using three 2-0 silk sutures (Fig. 18-11). It is important to ensure that 4 cm of the esophagus are anchored within the abdomen. To achieve this, the esophagus is then sutured to the fundus anteriorly in two locations on both the right and left lateral aspects of the esophagus, with care

(text continues on page 163)

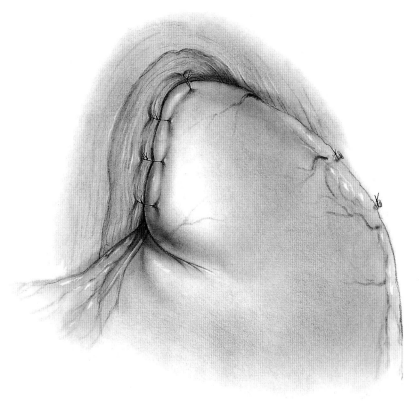

Fig. 18-9. Fixation of the anterior fundoplication (continued). The fundus is sewn to the right crus of the diaphragm.

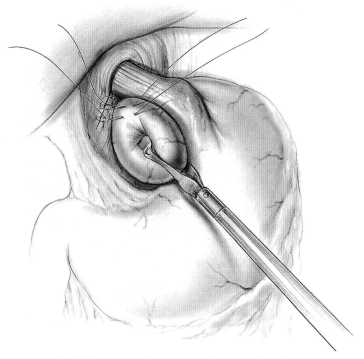

Fig. 18-10. Posterior fundoplication. Fixation to the left crus.

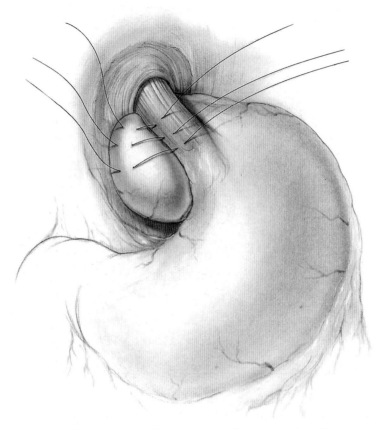

Fig. 18-11. Posterior fundoplication (continued). Fixation to the right crus.

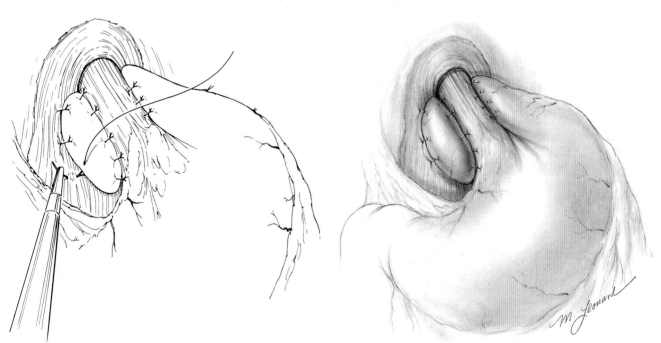

Fig. 18-12. Posterior fundoplication (continued). Intraabdominal anchoring of the tubular esophagus.

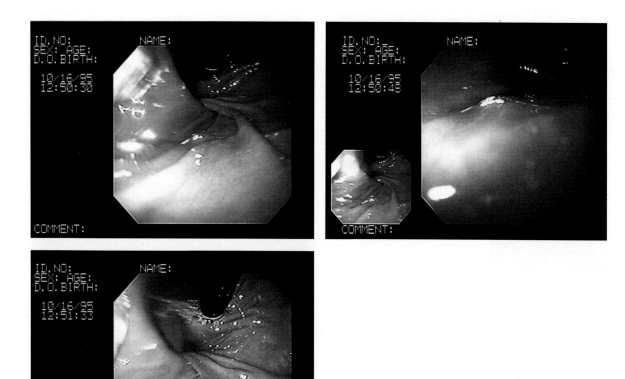

Fig. 18-13. Upper gastrointestinal endoscopy shows an anterior partial fundoplication.

Esophageal perforation has not occurred in our series but may be recognized intraoperatively. If this occurs, the bougie should be removed and a nasogastric tube inserted into the stomach prior to closure of the perforation; this tube remains in place postoperatively until water-soluble contrast studies confirm adequate healing of the perforation. It is appropriate to attempt laparoscopic repair of the perforation. The length of the mucosal defect should be visualized and closed with absorbable interrupted sutures. The muscle defect is closed with nonabsorbable interrupted sutures. The site of perforation is covered with the fundoplication. Late recognition of esophageal perforation may be difficult, but it must be excluded with a water-soluble contrast swallow if a postoperative fever or ileus develops. Late perforation should be managed with open laparotomy, operative closure of the defect, and clean out of the contaminated abdomen and mediastinum.

The development of gastric ileus is rare following laparoscopic partial fundoplication but should be suspected when patients complain of excessive epigastric pain or nausea. A nasogastric tube should be inserted when this is suspected to avoid forceful vomiting and potential disruption of the fundoplication.

Intrathoracic migration of the fundoplication has been reported following laparoscopic antireflux surgery in up to 14% of patients if the crura are not closed. This complication has not been observed in our series but usually presents as epigastric pain or recurrence of reflux symptoms. Recurrence of symptoms requires careful reevaluation including contrast studies, endoscopy, and 24-hour pH studies to carefully document the cause for the symptoms.

Persistent postoperative complaints of hyperflatuence or abdominal distention associated with epigastric pain, that is, gas bloating symptoms, can usually be managed with simple measures. Counseling patients regarding air swallowing and the likely transient nature of the problem is often sufficient. If these measures fail to resolve the problem, a prescription for simethicone and a consultation with a speech therapist to alter swallowing techniques may be required. Finally, if gas bloating symptoms persist, delayed gastric emptying should be ruled out by a gastric emptying study.

The causes of persistent dysphagia following laparoscopic antireflux surgery are multiple. These include (a) unrecognized preoperative esophageal stricture, achalasia, and hypomotility of the body of the esophagus; (b) tight crural repair; (c) twisting of the lower esophagus, particularly with the Rossetti-type total fundoplication; and (d) tight fundoplication, particularly if the short gastric vessels are not divided.

The management of persistent dysphagia following laparoscopic fundoplication involves (a) maintenance of nutrition with blended high-calorie and high-protein diet, (b) esophageal dilation up to a 60-F Maloney bougie, (c) barium swallow with and without solids to determine the exact site and cause of obstruction, (d) repeat esophageal manometry to rule out achalasia, dysmotility, or tight fundoplication,

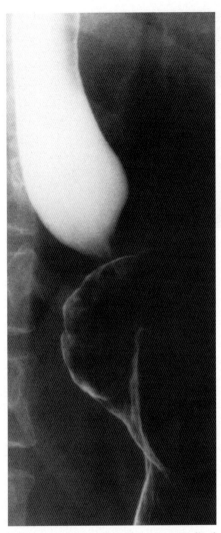

Fig. 18-14. Barium swallow shows a contrast-lined anterior partial fundoplication around 4 cm of air-filled intraabdominal esophagus.

and (e) reoperation to correct the underlying cause if dysphagia persists for more than 2 months.

Suggested Reading

Bauer AE, Belsey RHR. The treatment of sliding hiatus hernia and reflux esophagitis by the Mark IV technique. *Surgery* 1967;62:396–406.

Boutelier P, Jonsell G. An alternative fundo-plicative maneuver for gastroesophageal reflux. *Am J Surg* 1982;143:260–264.

Crookes PF, DeMeester TR. Does Toupet fundo-plication out-perform the Nissen procedure as the operation of choice for gastroesophageal reflux disease? *Dis Esophagus* 1994;7:265–270.

Cuschieri A, Hunter J, Wolfe B, Swanstrom LL, Hutson W. Multicenter prospective evaluation of laparoscopic antireflux surgery: preliminary report. *Surg Endosc* 1993;7:505–510.

Hemming AW, Finley RJ, Evans KG, Nelems B, Fradet G. Esophagogastrectomy and the variant left hepatic artery. *Ann Thorac Surg* 1992;54: 166–168.

Lundell L. Management of gastro-esophageal reflux disease 1995: the role of semifundoplica-tion in the long-term management of gastro-esophageal reflux disease. *Dis Esophagus* 1994;7: 245–249.

McKernan JB. Laparoscopic repair of gastroe-sophageal reflux disease: Toupet partial fundo-plication versus Nissen fundoplication. *Surg Endosc* 1994;8:851–856.

Mir J, Ponce J, Juan M, Garrigues V, Ibanez JL, Berenguer J. The effect of 180 degree anterior fundoplication on gastroesophageal reflux. *Am J Gastroenterol* 1986;81:172–175.

Watson A, Jenkinson LR, Ball CS, Barlow AP, Norris TL. A more physiological alternative to total fundoplication for the surgical correction of resistant gastro-oesophageal reflux. *Br J Surg* 1991;78:1088–1094.

Watson A, Spychal RT, Brown MG, Peck N, Callander N. Laparoscopic "physiological" an-tireflux procedure: preliminary results of a prospective symptomatic and objective study. *Br J Surg* 1995;82:651–656.

EDITOR'S COMMENT

The high interest in laparoscopic antire-flux surgery is primarily related to the per-ception that it offers a low-morbidity, cost-effective surgical alternative to prolonged and expensive medical therapy. In expert hands, open or laparoscopic fundoplica-tion certainly yield excellent results, and yet the Nissen procedure in particular has gained a reputation as a surgery of desper-ation associated with side effects and com-plications. Some have long felt that the side effects associated with Nissen fundo-plication—gas bloating, inability to belch, dysphagia—are too common to be accept-able. These practitioners advocate the use of a partial fundoplication to minimize the side effects associated with a 360-degree wrap. This argument has been amplified to some degree in the era of laparoscopic antireflux surgery. Patients, as consumers, and health care purchasers (insurance companies and capitated primary care providers) are unwilling to pay for *morbid* surgical alternatives to medical therapy. On the other hand, they are interested in low-morbidity, cost-effective, well toler-ated surgical interventions. Laparoscopy has certainly played a key role in this de-velopment. Dr. Finley and his group have been keen practitioners of alternative fun-doplications for some time. His group de-scribes a procedure that has some ele-ments in common with other partial wraps, such as the Dor or Toupet proce-dures, and some elements in common with the Hill procedure. In general, the relative benefit of these procedures is that they provide less esophageal outflow restric-tion with correspondingly less reverse-flow characteristics. There is no doubt that this minimizes the incidence of dysphagia following surgery, as well as allowing pa-tients a high chance of being able to belch postoperatively, thereby minimizing the chance of gas bloating and other uncom-fortable side effects. On the other hand, one must question whether this comes at the cost of long-term, antireflux preven-tion, which is, after all, the primary goal of this surgery. Answers to these questions await results from well constructed, long-term outcome studies. Until then, there is little doubt that partial fundoplications play a valuable role in the repertory of an-tireflux surgery. To date, the primary indi-cations are for patients with esophageal motility disorders and for those unable to tolerate a standard 360-degree repair. In the future, partial fundoplications may play a greater role in providing a well tol-erated, low-morbidity alternative to chronic medical therapy for GERD.

L.L.S.

19

Laparoscopic Paraesophageal Hernia Repair

Galen Perdikis and Ronald A. Hinder

Postempski performed the first diaphragmatic hernia repair in 1889. However, paraesophageal herniation was only described for the first time in 1926 by Akerlund, who noted that it is a relatively uncommon form of hiatal hernia. Hiatal hernias are commonly classified into three types:

Type I   Classic sliding hiatal hernia, in which the gastroesophageal (GE) junction migrates cephalad through the esophageal hiatus

Type II True paraesophageal or rolling hernia, in which the fundus herniates into the mediastinum relative to a normally positioned GE junction

Type III Combined hernia, in which both the GE junction and a large part of the fundus herniate into the thorax

In type III hernias, the entire stomach may herniate into the chest (Fig. 19-1). Type II hernias, or true paraesophageal hernias, are very rarely seen, and type III hernias, which behave pathophysiologically like the other two types, are commonly classified as paraesophageal (Fig. 19-2). Overall, paraesophageal herniation constitutes 5% of all hiatal hernias.

A sliding hiatal hernia develops because of a weakening of the phrenoesophageal ligament and loss of attachment of the GE junction to the preaortic fascia and median arcuate ligament. Paraesophageal hernias develop differently. There is a consistently seen widening of the hiatus anterior to the esophagus, possibly congenital in origin. Occasionally, a portion of the crus is defective, and the defect extends across into the left leaf of the diaphragm. In a type II hernia, the GE junction remains fixed in its normal position; however, the gastrosplenic and gastrocolic ligaments are lax. This leads to herniation of the fundus, which rolls into the thorax in front and to the left of the esophagus. This can be associated with organoaxial rotation of the stomach around its longitudinal axis (Fig. 19-3A). Occasionally, mesentericoaxial volvulus around the transverse axis occurs, but this is less common (Fig. 19-3B). A type III hernia develops when an anterior defect is associated with loss of fixation of the GE junction.

Iatrogenic paraesophageal herniation may occur following antireflux procedures, esophagomyotomy, esophagogastrectomy, and other procedures at the esophageal hiatus. Pathogenetic mechanisms include breakdown of crural repair, inadequate crural repair, disruption of the phrenoesophageal ligament by operative dissection, postoperative gastric dilatation, and failure to recognize shortening of the esophagus. Children, particularly younger than 1 year, undergoing Nissen fundoplication are especially prone to the development of a paraesophageal hernia, with a reported incidence of 16.8%.

Clinical Presentation

Many patients are totally asymptomatic, and the hernia is found incidentally on chest radiography. When symptoms are present, they are usually vague, with epigastric or substernal chest discomfort being the most common. Symptoms of postprandial fullness, nausea, and dysphagia can be due to twisting of the stomach around the GE junction and therefore can be an early sign of strangulation. Bleeding due to vascular engorgement or gastric ulceration leads to anemia from chronic insidious blood loss or frank hematemesis. The incidence of gastric ulceration is approximately 23% in giant paraesophageal hernias. These ulcers typically occur at the level of the esophageal hiatus, are related to mechanical irritation, and are known as Cameron's ulcers. Respiratory complications include dyspnea due to the mechanical effect of a large hernia in the chest and repeated aspiration if the hernia results in delayed esophageal emptying. Other organs such as the spleen or colon may also herniate into the mediastinum, leading to bowel obstruction, infarction, or perforation. GE reflux symptoms and esophagitis occur in patients who have a type III hernia associated with incompetence of the lower esophageal sphincter.

One-fifth of patients with a paraesophageal hernia present as an acute surgical emergency with profuse bleeding, incarceration, volvulus, strangulation, or perforation. Incarceration heightens patients' symptoms, which then become continuous. Volvulus leads to increased pain associated with obstruction. If the blood supply is compromised, necrosis and perforation with resulting sepsis and shock may ensue. The mortality rate at this stage of the disease approaches 50%.

Investigations

An upright radiograph of the thorax will often demonstrate a retrocardiac air–fluid level, which indicates the diagnosis (Fig. 19-4). Contrast radiographic studies almost always successfully demonstrate a paraesophageal hernia. If upper en-

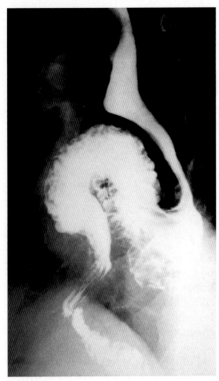

Fig. 19-1. Contrast radiography demonstrates a completely intrathoracic stomach.

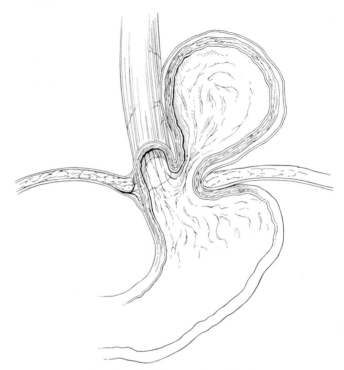

Fig. 19-2. Type II paraesophageal hernia.

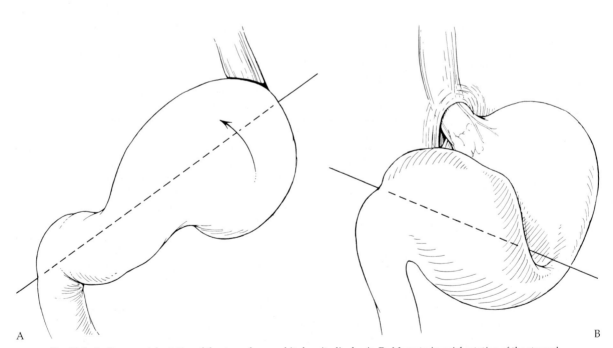

Fig. 19-3. **A:** Organoaxial rotation of the stomach around its longitudinal axis. **B:** Mesentericoaxial rotation of the stomach around its transverse axis.

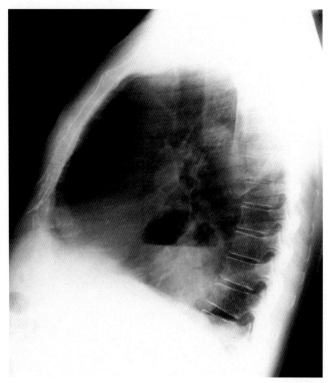

Fig. 19-4. Lateral chest radiograph demonstrates a retrocardiac air–fluid level indicative of a paraesophageal hernia.

doscopy is performed with the endoscope retroflexed in the stomach, a second orifice adjacent to the GE junction with gastric rugae ascending into the hernia is diagnostic of a paraesophageal hernia (Fig. 19-5). There is often difficulty in identifying normal gastric anatomy and the pylorus due to the great distortion of the stomach. Twenty-four-hour pH monitoring and stationary manometry are only necessary if patients complain of reflux symptoms, are candidates for surgery, and do not present as an emergency.

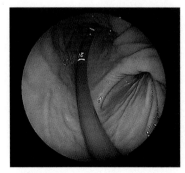

Fig. 19-5. Retroflexed endoscopic view of a paraesophageal hernia. Note the gastric rugal folds ascending into the paraesophageal hernia.

Therapy

Considering the severity and frequency of complications associated with paraesophageal hernias, elective surgical repair is advocated. There is no consensus as to whether or not an antireflux procedure should be included in the operation. Some base their decision on preoperative testing in patients undergoing elective repair. We feel that to perform an adequate repair, the esophagus must be extensively mobilized, particularly posteriorly, disrupting the phrenoesophageal ligament and hence leaving the lower esophageal sphincter unsupported and prone to reflux. We therefore routinely perform an antireflux procedure such as the Nissen fundoplication. Ellis and colleagues (1986) and Hill and Tobias (1968) described an anterior repair of the hiatal defect and leaving the posterior esophageal attachments intact during open laparotomy; hence, no fundoplication was required. A gastrostomy may be used to hold the stomach from migrating into the chest. This approach has also been applied laparoscopically. The argument for doing an antireflux procedure is that up to 18% of patients will experience reflux symptoms after a simple

anatomic repair. It is also easier to obtain a satisfactory intraabdominal segment of esophagus with a posterior repair because of the oblique angle of the plane in which the crura lie. We have also found that there is less tension when the repair is carried out posteriorly. Furthermore, while a true anterior repair leaves the posterior attachments intact, the dissection associated with adequate excision of the paraesophageal hernia sac, particularly if the hernia is large, disrupts these attachments.

Laparoscopic Technique

The procedure is performed under general anesthesia with the patient in the lithotomy position. The knees should be kept extended, so as not to interfere with the surgeon's arm movements. Sequential compression devices are placed on both legs to prevent deep venous thrombosis. A nasogastric tube is passed, and the stomach contents are aspirated, after which the tube is removed. A urinary catheter is usually not necessary. The surgeon stands between the patient's legs, and assistants stand on either side of the patient. The operating table is placed in a steep reverse Trendelenburg position, which aids in exposing the esophageal hiatus (Fig. 19-6).

A carbon dioxide pneumoperitoneum is established by insertion of a Veress needle into the peritoneal cavity through a vertical 1-cm incision placed 2 to 3 cm above the umbilicus. Once the pneumoperitoneum is established, a 10-mm port is placed through the same incision. After exploratory laparoscopy, a second 10-mm midline port is placed 3 to 4 cm inferior to the xiphoid process. Right and left sub-

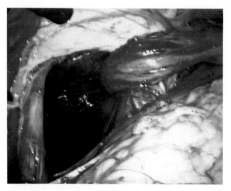

Fig. 19-6. Laparoscopic view of a paraesophageal hernia.

costal 10-mm ports are placed in the respective midclavicular lines. A fifth 10-mm port is placed in the far left lateral subcostal position. The subxiphoid and left subcostal ports are used by the surgeon; the right subcostal port is used for liver retraction by an assistant, who also controls the laparoscope (Fig. 19-7). A 30-degree laparoscope may be used, but a 0-degree laparoscope is easier for a junior assistant to use and provides more than adequate visualization. The second assistant assists the surgeon via the left lateral subcostal port. The subsequent procedure can be broken into four parts: (a) hernia reduction, (b) sac excision, (c) crural repair, and (d) fundoplication.

Hernia Reduction

A fan retractor is placed through the right subcostal port and used to retract the left lobe of the liver. The large hernia is easily visible. The herniated abdominal organs are returned into the abdomen using atraumatic graspers. This usually consists of the stomach and not infrequently the transverse colon. The hernia at the hiatus should now be easily discernible, especially anteriorly. The gastrohepatic omentum is divided to visualize the right crus of the diaphragm more easily (Fig. 19-8). Most of the dissection is best performed with a hook cautery. Hemostasis must be meticulous, and small segments of tissue are cauterized at a time and under direct vision. No tearing of tissue with the hook cautery should occur. The hook cautery is useful in lifting tissues away from the esophagus and stomach, thus preventing cautery injuries. Care should be taken to preserve intact an aberrant left hepatic artery, seen in 13% to 25% of patients.

Excision of the Hernia Sac

The sac is dissected off the crural edge using the hook cautery beginning at the inferoposterior pole of the right crus. Dissection is taken up along the right crural edge and across the hiatus anteriorly (Fig. 19-9). Much of the sac over the left crus anteriorly is then dissected free. Dissection of the sac off the inferoposterior edge of the left crus is awkward and is best left until the rest of the sac has been reduced from the mediastinum. Once a plane of dissection is found, the sac is gently peeled away from the mediastinal structures using atraumatic graspers until the whole sac is in-

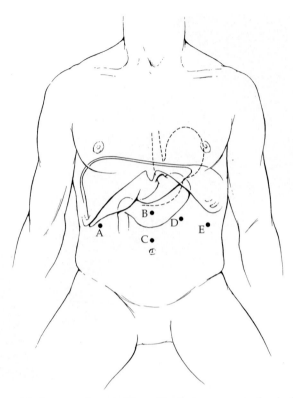

Fig. 19-7. Port placement for laparoscopic repair. The port for the laparoscope is placed a few centimeters above the umbilicus. (A, 10-mm port with fan retractor; B, 10-mm port with scissors; C, 10-mm camera port; D, 10-mm port with grasper; E, 10-mm port with babcock.)

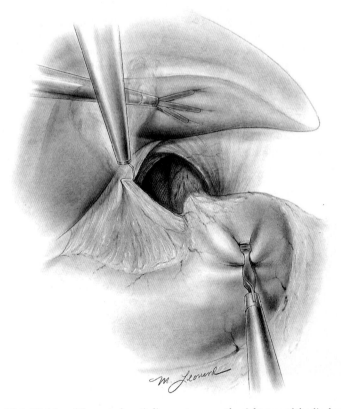

Fig. 19-8. Division of the gastrohepatic ligament exposes the right crus of the diaphragm.

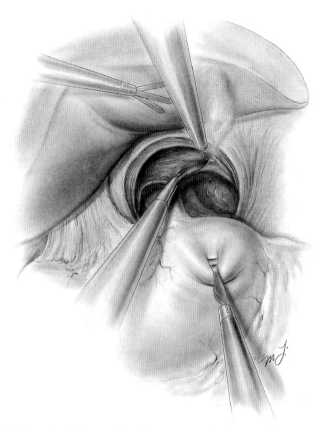

Fig. 19-9. *Dissection of the sac off the right crus is continued across the hiatus anteriorly.*

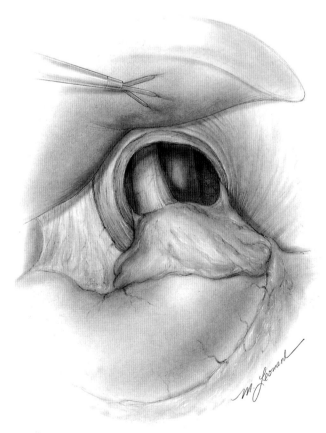

Fig. 19-10. *Dissection of the sac off the mediastinal structures.*

verted into the abdomen (Fig. 19-10). Inadvertent entry into the pleura must be avoided. If it does occur, the surgeon and anesthesiologist must be vigilant in observing for the development of a tension pneumothorax. If this occurs, immediate release of the pneumoperitoneum will usually reverse the situation. Conversion to an open procedure may be necessary. Because of the extensive mediastinal dissection, subcutaneous emphysema may occur, which is usually of no consequence. The sac is finally dissected off from behind the esophagus, with care taken not injure the esophagus, aorta, or fundus of the stomach. There is no need to excise the sac by dividing it at its attachment to the GE junction. The first assistant provides exposure by retracting the stomach via the left lateral port using a Babcock grasper.

Crural Repair

To facilitate the crural repair and the fundoplication to follow, it is necessary to mobilize the esophagus posteriorly. This can be difficult because the redundant sac makes it difficult to find the correct planes, especially between the esophagus and the left crus. This dissection needs to be done with utmost care. A bougie can be passed into the esophagus to facilitate where to dissect, but dissection should not proceed with the bougie in place, as this increases the likelihood of esophageal injury. An endoscope can also be used for this purpose. Posterior dissection begins by gentle dissection the right crus off the esophagus. Careful dissection of the mediastinal esophagus includes dividing the small vessels posteriorly while avoiding esophageal and posterior vagus nerve injury (Fig. 19-11). Once a space behind the esophagus is secured, a Babcock grasper with its jaws closed is passed from the left lateral port through the window to sweep the esophagus upward. This important maneuver allows excellent access to the area posterior to the esophagus. Any bleeding must be dealt with meticulously. Careful dissection by pushing the esophagus upward and its soft tissue attachments posteriorly eventually takes the dissection across to the left side. It is important to direct this dissection inferior to the left crus and not up into the chest. This may be difficult, especially if the sac has not been adequately freed off the left crus. The posterior vagus nerve is identified and dissected away from the esophagus. In the dissection behind the esophagus, care must be taken not to injure the fundus of the stomach or the esophagus it-self. The window is enlarged so that it is able to easily accept a portion of the fundus for the fundoplication. The crura are then repaired with several interrupted 2-0 Pro-lene sutures placed posteriorly (Fig. 19-12). The first stitch is placed inferoposteriorly almost in the preaortic fascia. The size of the hernia defect will dictate the number of sutures necessary. An extracorporeal method is used to tie the knots. A 58-French bougie is then passed down the esophagus into the stomach to assess the size of the hiatal repair and ensure that the repair is not too tight. Extreme care must be taken when the bougie is being passed into the stomach, as perforation may occur. Ax-ial traction on the stomach at the time of passing the bougie decreases the risk of perforation. The bougie is then withdrawn into the proximal esophagus.

Oddsdottir and associates (1995) reported a series of 10 patients in whom the laparo-scopic approach was used to repair a paraesophageal hernia. In this series, pled-geted sutures were used to close the hiatus both anteriorly and posteriorly. An ante-rior repair is feasible laparoscopically, but further reports are awaited. An anterior re-pair, however, precludes the addition of a fundoplication. Polypropylene mesh has been used to bridge a large hiatal defect af-ter the stomach is reduced and the sac is left in place. This approach is doomed to fail and should not be used.

Fundoplication

In some cases, the short gastric vessels need to be divided along the upper 10 cm of fundus to ensure a floppy Nissen fun-doplication. The stomach is often so mo-bile in association with a paraesophageal hernia that this step is not required. A Bab-cock grasper is passed from the right port behind the esophagus inferior to the re-paired crura to grasp the mobilized fun-dus, which is gently pulled through the window posterior to the esophagus. The fundus forms the posterior segment of the fundoplication. An anterolateral portion of the stomach is chosen to form the ante-rior portion of the fundoplication. At this stage, the bougie is passed back into the stomach. The two portions of stomach are approximated to assess the adequacy of the proposed fundoplication. The bougie is removed, and a U-shaped stitch of 2-0 Prolene supported with two polytef (Teflon) pledgets is used to secure the fun-

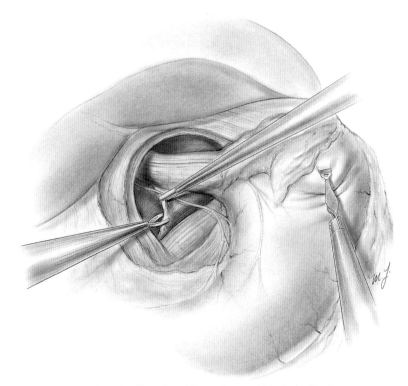

Fig. 19-11. *Posterior dissection of the esophagus within the mediastinum.*

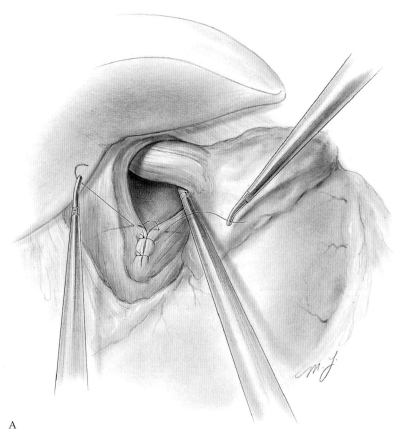

A

Fig. 19-12. **A,B:** *Crural repair posterior to the esophagus. A grasper is used to elevate the esophagus anteriorly.* (continued)

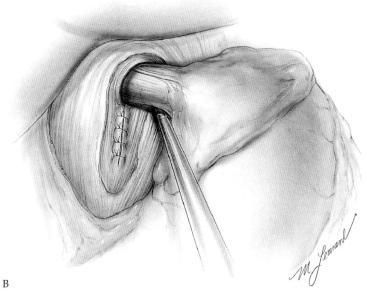

B

Fig. 19-12. (Continued)

doplication. The suture incorporates both portions of stomach and the right anterolateral portion of esophageal muscle (Fig. 19-13). Full-thickness bites through the stomach decrease the chance of the U-stitch tearing out with disruption of the fundoplication. An additional one or two sutures may be placed above or below the

U-stitch, as necessary. The fundoplication is then tacked to the diaphragm on both sides using 2-0 silk suture.

Following inspection of the crural repair and fundoplication, the pneumoperitoneum is released, and the ports are removed under vision. The port sites are

closed using a fascial 2-0 Vicryl stitch. The skin is closed with subcuticular absorbable sutures and Steri-Strips.

Postoperatively, no nasogastric decompression is required, and patients are encouraged to ambulate soon after surgery. A postoperative chest radiograph may be obtained if a large mediastinal dissection was necessary. Intravenous analgesia may be required for 24 hours, following which liquid oral analgesia suffices. Patients are allowed to drink fluids later in the day after recovery from anesthesia and advanced to a soft diet as tolerated. The hospital stay is usually 1 to 2 days. Mild dysphagia may be temporary due to postoperative edema. Patients should be instructed to avoid meats and fresh bread for 2 or 3 weeks. A normal diet is resumed by 6 weeks.

Role of Gastropexy

Gastropexy by various methods may be a useful adjunct to repair of a paraesophageal hernia. Johnson and colleagues (1994) described a method for laparoscopic mesh repair of hernias, together with anterior gastropexy through a left upper quadrant incision. However, the hernia sac was not dissected out, thus predisposing patients to recurrence and seroma formation. Placement of a gastrostomy laparoscopically is also an option. The gastrostomy prevents gastric volvulus and recurrent migration into the chest by anchoring the anterior surface of the stomach to the abdominal wall. This type of gastropexy may be useful in elderly or acutely ill patients who would not tolerate a long procedure. In addition, it may be a convenient route for initial gastric decompression and later nutrition for patients who have prolonged feeding problems after reduction of a large paraesophageal hernia. If patients are healthy and the procedure is elective, we do not suggest using a gastrostomy. An alternative to a gastrostomy is a suture gastropexy (Fig. 19-14). Interrupted sutures are placed from the greater curve of the stomach to the anterior abdominal wall. These are tied extracorporeally while the abdominal insufflation is decreased.

Results

Between 1991 and 1995, 42 patients have been operated on laparoscopically for paraesophageal hernia at Creighton Uni-

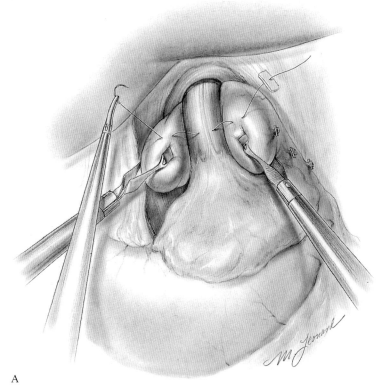

A

*Fig. 19-13. **A,B:** Fundoplication using pledgeted suture.* (continued)

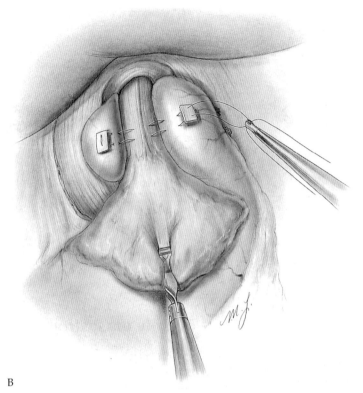

B

Fig. 19-13. (Continued)

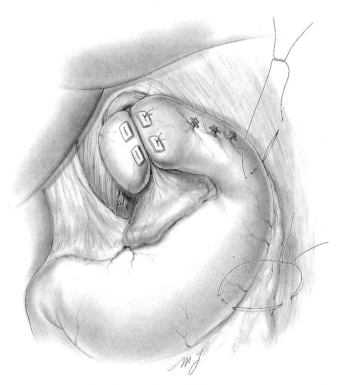

Fig. 19-14. Suture gastropexy may be used as an adjunct to help prevent recurrent paraesophageal herniation.

versity. Most patients had type III hernias. Eight of 11 patients who underwent preoperative manometry had a defective lower esophageal sphincter. Intraoperative complications included three cases of stomach perforation. This was managed laparoscopically in one patient and by open laparotomy in two patients due to initial inexperience. This would not be considered necessary at this stage of our experience. Postoperatively, at a mean follow-up of 13 months (range, 1 to 36 months), one patient had an asymptomatic recurrent paraesophageal hernia, and two patients had mild reflux symptoms controlled with acid suppression. There was a significant reduction in preoperative symptoms.

Numerous other small series reporting on the laparoscopic approach in paraesophageal hernia have been published, showing good short-term results; however, no consensus has been reached as to the best technique. Further long-term studies are required to evaluate the results obtained with these techniques and the long-term success of laparoscopic repairs.

Conclusion

The laparoscopic approach offers a minimally invasive means of repairing paraesophageal hernias. If the principles of the open approach are employed, similarly satisfying results should be obtained with the laparoscopic approach. This operation is challenging and requires advanced laparoscopic skills with extensive previous experience in laparoscopic GE surgery.

Suggested Reading

Congreve DP. Laparoscopic paraesophageal hernia repair. *J Laparoendosc Surg* 1992;2:45–48.

Edelman DS. Laparoscopic paraesophageal hernia repair with mesh. *Surg Laparosc Endosc* 1995; 5:32–37.

Ellis FH Jr, Crozier RE, Shea JA. Paraesophageal hiatus hernia. *Arch Surg* 1986;121:416–420.

Hill LD, Tobias JA. Paraesophageal hernia. *Arch Surg* 1968;96:735–744.

Johnson PE, Persuad M, Mitchell T. Laparoscopic anterior gastropexy for treatment of paraesophageal hernias. *Surg Laparosc Endosc* 1994;4:152–154.

Koger KE, Stone JM. Laparoscopic reduction of acute gastric volvulus. *Am Surg* 1993;59: 325–328.

Oddsdottir M, Franco AL, Laycock WS, Waring JP, Hunter JG. Laparoscopic repair of paraesophageal hernia: new access, old technique. *Surg Endosc* 1995;9:164–168.

Perdikis G, Hinder RA. Paraesophageal hiatal hernia. In: Nyhus LM, Condon RE, eds. *Hernia*, 4th ed. Philadelphia: J.B. Lippincott Co, 1995: 543–554.

Pitcher DE, Curet MJ, Martin DT, Vogt DM, Mason J, Zucker KA. Successful laparoscopic repair of paraesophageal hernia. *Arch Surg* 1995;130: 590–596.

Skinner DB, Belsey RHR. Surgical management of esophageal reflux and hiatus hernia: long-term results with 1,030 patients. *J Thorac Cardiovasc Surg* 1967;53:33–54.

Streitz JM Jr, Ellis FH Jr. Iatrogenic paraesophageal hiatus hernia. *Ann Thorac Surg* 1990; 50:446–449.

EDITOR'S COMMENT

Paraesophageal hernia repair holds a unique place in esophageal surgery. Considered an absolute indication for surgical intervention, paraesophageal hernia is frequently asymptomatic and found only on routine x-rays obtained for other reasons. Even when symptomatic, patients seldom present with the classic feared symptom of acute gastric strangulation (the incidence of which is probably much lower than has been described). On the other hand, numerous other problems including chronic anemia, chest pain, early satiety, and dysphagia associated with paraesophageal hernia can dramatically decrease patients' quality of life. Laparoscopic repair remains a difficult procedure fraught with many technical hurdles and more prone to failure and complications than a simple laparoscopic antireflux procedure. Preoperative evaluation of patients should include a barium swallow, upper endoscopy, and motility testing at a minimum. Twenty-four-hour pH testing is optional and is probably beside the point for these patients, as an antireflux procedure is typically added routinely. Attention to surgical detail is critical. As outlined by by Dr. Perdikis and Dr. Hinder, this is a procedure best described as mediastinal sac reduction, as opposed to gastric reduction. It should be remembered that this sac includes both a large anterior component and a smaller posterior component and that both must be reduced to prevent herniation postoperatively. The majority of giant type III paraesophageal hernias will present with a shortened esophagus, and as many as 15% of these have an irreducible GE junction. Adequate mobilization of the esophagus is very important to achieve a tension-free repair and, if the GE junction cannot be reduced by mediastinal dissection, the patient would probably benefit from an esophageal lengthening procedure (Collis gastroplasty) performed either laparoscopically or by conversion to an open procedure.

Finally, we agree that the tendency of giant paraesophageal hernias to recur justifies the use of multiple maneuvers to prevent reherniation: pledgeted posterior crural closure, addition of a fundoplication, an esophageal lengthening procedure when indicated, and a gastropexy either with a gastrostomy tube or anterior greater curvature suture gastropexy. The use of mesh or other prosthetic materials to replace hiatal closure is best avoided, except in extraordinary circumstances.

L.L.S.

20

Surgical Endoscopy for Achalasia and Esophageal Motility Disorders

Alexander D. Porter and Carlos A. Pellegrini

The advent of thoracoscopic and laparoscopic techniques for esophageal surgery in the late 1980s provided surgeons with a novel means for treating esophageal motility disorders. Prior to this time, most esophageal surgery, including myotomy, required a thoracotomy or laparotomy. These operations were successful, but the incisions caused considerable pain, and the procedures were associated with potentially significant postoperative morbidity and long hospital stays. Hence, until the introduction of the newer video endoscopic myotomy techniques, most patients opted for less effective medical treatments, such as medications and bougie or balloon dilations. The newer, minimally invasive alternatives, which appear to be as effective as the open procedures, have resulted in a resurgence of the surgeon's role in treating esophageal motility disorders.

Minimally invasive procedures offer other advantages over formal thoracotomy and laparotomy, in addition to decreased pain, morbidity, and hospital stay. First, video endoscopy magnifies the operative field. Thus, surgeons can operate with greater accuracy in determining muscle layers and other important structures such as the vagus nerve, blood vessels, and so on. Second, the minimally invasive approach requires virtually no movement of the esophagus from its bed. This factor minimizes the trauma caused by the operation, therefore limiting postoperative complications. Last, these advantages, when combined with intraluminal endoscopy, afford the surgeon the ability to perform the operation with greater ease. In particular, the endoscope helps identify the esophagus in

the initial stages of the procedure, thus allowing the surgeon to tailor the operation to each patient.

Anatomy

The esophagus begins at the base of the hypopharynx just below the cricopharyngeal muscle and some terminal fibers of the inferior laryngeal constrictor muscle. Together, these two muscle groups form the upper esophageal sphincter at approximately the level of the C-6 vertebra posteriorly and the cricoid cartilage anteriorly. As the esophagus leaves this region, it deviates slightly to the left of the midline until it reaches the tracheal bifurcation, where it returns to the midline. After the bifurcation, the esophagus continues down and deviates anteriorly and toward the left in preparation for passing through the diaphragmatic hiatus. As it passes through the hiatus, the esophagus is attached to the hiatus by the phrenoesophageal membrane, which is a fusion of the endoabdominal fascia with the peritoneum. The hiatus comprises a left and right crus, originating from the top of the L-3 to L-4 vertebrae and joining in front of the esophagus. The phrenoesophageal membrane is composed of descending and ascending layers. The descending layer covers the periesophageal fat pad and serves as an external marker for the gastroesophageal junction.

The esophagus maintains a close proximity to many important structures as it traverses the thoracic cavity. Some of the more prominent structures include nerves,

blood and lymphatic vessels, the heart, and the lungs. The most prominent nerves are the left and right vagus nerves, which travel laterally to the esophagus as far as the lower thoracic region, where they rotate to an anterior and posterior position, respectively. Another neighboring nerve is the left recurrent laryngeal nerve, which travels cephalad for a short distance near the superior portion of the esophagus. The aorta runs lateral and slightly anterior to the esophagus above the level of vertebrae T7-8, but more posteriorly below this juncture. Other important vessels near the esophagus are the azygos vein and thoracic duct, which lie right posterolaterally and posteriorly, respectively, for most of thoracic cavity. The heart and lungs lie anterior and lateral to the esophagus, respectively.

Indications and Preoperative Evaluation

Thoracoscopic or laparoscopic myotomy is indicated to treat patients with achalasia and diffuse esophageal spasm (DES) refractory to medical therapy. Nutcracker esophagus (NE), another motility disorder, may also respond to surgical intervention.

To fully characterize a patient's disease, four tests are usually needed: (a) barium upper gastrointestinal (UGI) study, (b) UGI endoscopy, (c) esophageal manometry, and (d) ambulatory 24-hour pH monitoring. In particular, a barium-contrast UGI study helps confirm a diagnosis by demonstrating a bird's-beak pattern in patients with achalasia (Fig. 20-1), as opposed to the corkscrew configuration characteristic of DES. In addition, a UGI study provides information about the esophagus by identifying strictures, the pressure of severe dilatation (sigmoid) of the esophagus, esophageal shortening, and so on. Preoperative intraluminal endoscopy is used to examine the interior for evidence of other pathology, such as cancer and strictures. Twenty-four-hour pH monitoring with esophageal manometry is used to evaluate the competency of the lower esophageal sphincter (LES) and rule out peptic stricture. Manometry is also used to diagnose motility disorders; in achalasia patients, it typically shows an absence of peristalsis, deficient relaxation of the LES, and increased intraesophageal basal tone. The manometric patterns in DES or NE show an increase in the presence of simultaneous waves or an increase in the peak peristaltic pressure, respectively. More significantly, manometry can dictate the approach of the operation by showing the surgeon where the esophagus is most affected by the motility disorder. Thus, for patients with a greater problem in the mid- to upper esophagus, a right-sided thoracoscopic approach offers the best view and access. Conversely, problems in the vicinity of the

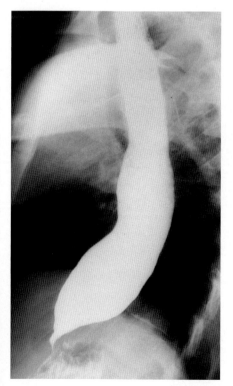

Fig. 20-1. *Lateral view of barium x-ray shows the classic bird's-beak pattern of achalasia.*

LES or high-pressure zone are best handled through a left-sided approach. These technical points are discussed later in the operative description sections.

In addition to the above tests, a thorough preoperative evaluation requires an assessment of patients' cardiac and pulmonary function and general health. To assess these, further testing may be required. In particular, pulmonary function studies are almost mandated in every thoracoscopic patient due to intraoperative single-lung ventilation. Likewise, patients may need an electrocardiogram, echocardiogram, and so on for cardiac function assessment.

Preoperative Preparation

Prior to surgery, the surgeon should advise patients to remain on a liquid diet during the 2 to 3 days preceding the operation. This step prevents having solid particles in the esophagus during the operation and decreases the risk of aspirating such material during intubation. Antibiotics are given just prior to the operation to reduce the risk of infection in the event of a mucosal perforation.

The surgeon must ensure that the proper equipment is available. The equipment used in laparoscopic surgery can be used in thoracoscopic operations. However, these instruments are often too long and thus cumbersome in thoracoscopic surgery. Hence, it may be preferable to use shorter equipment in the chest. A straight (0 degree) scope and a 30- or 45-degree angled telescope should be available for all video endoscopic procedures, as the operation frequently requires visualization of the operative field from different views. This is particularly true in the abdomen, where the posterior location of the esophagus makes the 30- to 45-degree scope useful. With proper preparation and equipment, minimally invasive surgery becomes easier, and therefore excellent results can be obtained with shorter operative times in most cases.

Heller Myotomy

History

In 1914, Heller described a procedure for the treatment of what was then known as

cardiospasm with dilation of the esophagus. In his original work, he performed extramucosal myotomies on the anterior and posterior distal esophageal walls. The immediate results were spectacular, with complete relief of patients' dysphagia. However, the postoperative course was often marked by reflux disease and recurrence of dysphagia due to peptic stricture. In addition, the open operation was associated with significant morbidity. Over the intervening years, many surgeons have attempted modifications of the Heller myotomy with variable success. Unfortunately, these modifications did little to modify the associated morbidity, and hence surgery was often not chosen by patients or their primary care physicians. However, in the late 1980s, advances in video and computer technology allowed A. Cuschieri and colleagues to perform one of the first laparoscopic Heller myotomies and furthermore to find a decrease in postoperative morbidity and convalescence time. In 1993, Pellegrini and associates published one of the earliest series of patients treated by thoracoscopic or laparoscopic esophagomyotomy. In their study, they found that 21 (88%) of 24 patients treated by a minimally invasive approach had an excellent to good outcome several months postoperatively. In addition, they noted that 22 patients were eating by the second postoperative day and discharged by the third postoperative day. This published series, as well as some subsequent series, helped establish minimally invasive procedures as excellent alternatives to open procedures. Furthermore, these studies illuminated some of the advantages of a thoracoscopic or laparoscopic approach in terms of postoperative feeding and hospitalization.

Since then, many surgeons have adopted a minimally invasive approach, either thoracoscopic or laparoscopic, for treating achalasia. In the following sections, we outline both thoracoscopic and laparoscopic approaches.

Thoracoscopic Approach to Heller Myotomy

The patient is intubated with a double-lumen catheter and placed in the right lateral decubitus position. The left lung is then allowed to collapse, and the thoracoscopic ports are placed in a diamond pattern (Fig. 20-2). The diamond pattern has four vertices (ABCD) and one extraneous point (E) on one side. The center of the diamond lies over the sixth to seventh intercostal space (ICS) at the posterior axillary line, which corresponds to the esophagus at the level of the LES.

The actual sequence of placement begins with port A, which is inserted anterior to the posterior axillary line in the third or fourth ICS after the skin is incised and blunt dissection through the subcutaneous tissues is performed. The telescope is then placed in port A, and the thoracic cavity is examined and evaluated for adequacy of lung collapse and positioning of the remaining ports. Port B is usually inserted at the fifth to sixth ICS behind the posterior axillary line and serves as the permanent port for the telescope. Ports C and D are inserted one ICS below and above port B, respectively. Port C should lie anterior to the posterior axillary line, and it serves as the port for the left hand of the surgeon. Port D is positioned anterior to the anterior axillary line and is used by the first assistant. The last port (E) is placed below port A, usually at the fourth ICS and anterior to the posterior axillary line. This port is used by the right hand of the surgeon. Port A during the operation is used for lung retraction. Prior to their creation, the intended port sites for B, C, D, and E are checked by inserting a spinal needle that

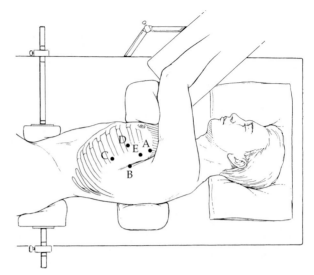

Fig. 20-2. Port placement for thoracoscopic procedures from a left approach.

can be seen internally by telescope and evaluated for best positioning. A hazard associated with port placement is the possibility of disrupting the intercostal artery or vein; the resulting bleeding can obscure the view. Most often, this event can be managed by placing a larger port in the site or by suture ligation.

After the diamond-plus-one pattern has been completed, exposure of the esopha-

gus is begun by using the lung retractor to pull the lung upward. The inferior pulmonary ligament is exposed and placed under tension by this maneuver (Fig. 20-3). The ligament is divided by hook electrocautery or scissors, thus exposing the pleura overlying a groove between the pericardium and the aorta, which is also divided. The esophagus is located within the groove, and its identification is simplified by tilting the head of the endoscope

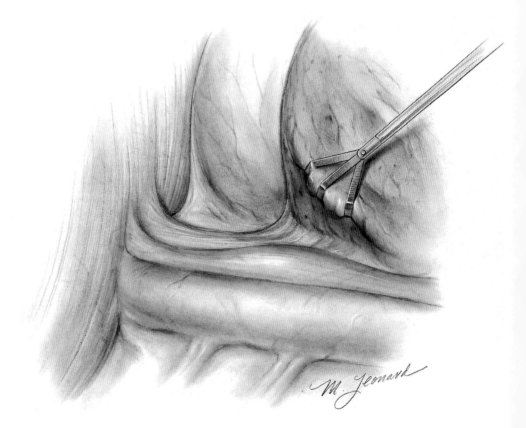

Fig. 20-3. The lung is retracted, exposing the inferior pulmonary ligament.

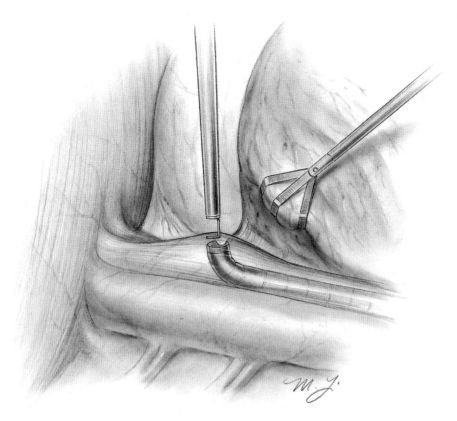

Fig. 20-4. The endoscope is seen within the lumen, aiding the surgeon by showing the location of the esophagus.

upward and toward the left. In this manner, endoscope light is used as a beacon for the esophagus (it may be necessary to dim the telescope light first). However, more important, the endoscope has moved the esophagus toward the surgeon, lifting it out of the groove (Fig. 20-4). The pleura and mediastinal tissues can then be bluntly swept away from the esophagus to fully expose it.

At this point a 6- to 7-cm-long superficial line is marked onto the esophagus using the elbow of the hook electrocautery. The mark is extended from the left inferior pulmonary veins to the diaphragm and provides orientation during the surgery. The line is then deepened for a length of 2 to 3 cm through the longitudinal layer. At this point the circular layer becomes apparent. This layer is dealt with by first lifting individual fibers away from the mucosa with the hook of the electrocautery and then dividing them with a short burst of current. After the first five or six fibers have been cut, the submucosal plane is exposed, and the rest of the myotomy can easily be carried out (Fig. 20-5).

The myotomy is then extended from the inferior pulmonary veins to the di-

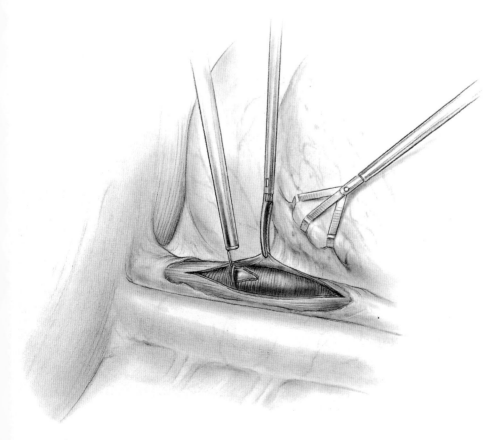

Fig. 20-5. The circular muscle fibers are first retracted from the esophagus and then divided.

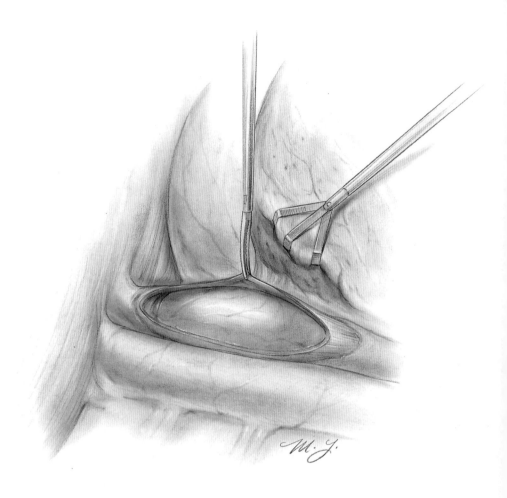

Fig. 20-6. *The submucosal space is entered, and the muscle layers are bluntly dissected from the mucosa, exposing the latter. Approximately 40% of the circumference should be exposed.*

aphragm; occasionally, it is necessary to evacuate gastric air through the endoscope to keep the diaphragm from encroaching on the operative field. Throughout the myotomy, transillumination provided by the endoscope plays a key role by helping identify muscle fibers, thus ensuring complete division of the muscle fibers.

To complete the myotomy, the incision must be carried through the cardioesophageal junction. The junction is first exposed by pushing the diaphragm down while pulling upward on the myotomy edge away from the diaphragm. The cardioesophageal junction is usually identified by an overlying fat pad, the appearance of stomach serosa, and a sudden change in vascularity to a richer network of vessels. After identification, the junction is divided until the endoscopist (through the endoscope) suddenly sees the lumen become widely patent. Dissection of the junction is done cautiously, for here the muscular wall is thinner and is often difficult to clearly identify. In addition, the mucosa is also thinner and can be easily injured.

With the myotomy completed, the surgeon then focuses on lifting the myotomy edges from the mucosa by blunt dissection. Again, the endoscope is used to facilitate the maneuver; here, gentle insufflation helps push the mucosa out and the edges up (Fig. 20-6). At least 40% of the mucosal circumference should be exposed to prevent closure of the myotomy (Fig. 20-7).

Once the surgeon and the endoscopist are satisfied that there are no unattended mucosal injuries, the ports are removed under direct vision, and the trocar sites are sutured. A small, 26-French (26-F) angled chest tube is left in the lowest trocar site under waterseal and is removed the next day.

Laparoscopic Approach to Heller Myotomy

Unlike the thoracoscopic approach, a laparoscopic Heller myotomy requires division of the phrenoesophageal membrane and disruption of many of the supporting structures of the antireflux mechanism. In

addition, it requires a pneumoperitoneum. These factors lead to the incorporation of two changes in the overall approach. The first involves the addition of an antireflux procedure that is directed at minimizing the chance of postoperative reflux caused by disruption of the antireflux mechanism; this is discussed in more detail at the end

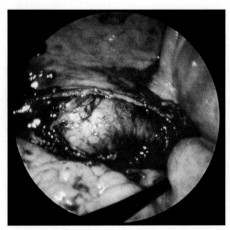

Fig. 20-7. *Thoracoscopic myotomy completed. The mucosa can easily be seen.*

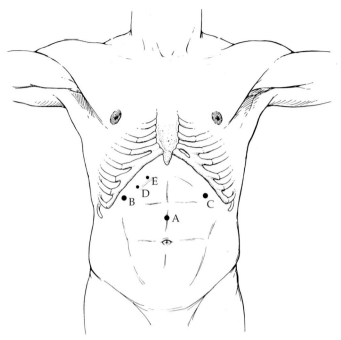

Fig. 20-8. Trocar placement for the laparoscopic approach.

of this section. The second change involves the use of sealed ports and longer instruments due to the presence of a pressurized and distended abdomen. With the exception of the antireflux procedure and use of a pneumoperitoneum, most of the steps in a laparoscopic myotomy are closely matched by similar steps in the thoracoscopic approach.

With the patient supine, the operation is begun with port placement in the abdominal wall. After satisfactory induction of the pneumoperitoneum, port A is placed at a midline location about 3 to 5 cm above the umbilicus. The telescope is placed through this port. Two ports, B (10 mm) and C (10 mm), are placed one finger breadth below the costal margins on the left and right in the midclavicular line, respectively. Two additional ports, D and E, both 5 mm, are required to help with liver and gastric retraction by instruments handled by assistants (Fig. 20-8).

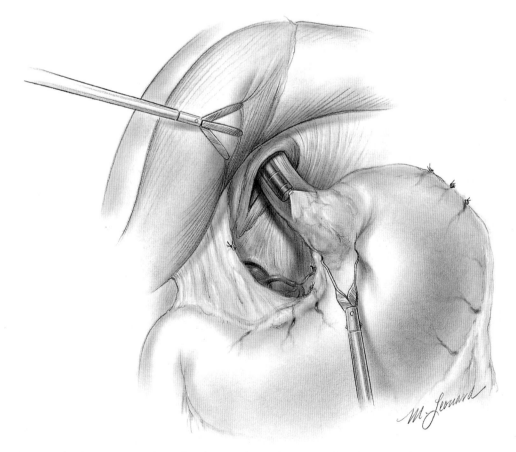

Fig. 20-9. A Babcock retractor is used to pull on the stomach near the gastroesophageal junction, while the liver retractor pushes up on the liver and diaphragm. These maneuvers expose the lower esophagus for the procedure. With the endoscope in the esophageal lumen, the myotomy can be evaluated for its adequacy.

After trocar placement, exposure of the esophagus is started by lifting the liver out of the operative field with an atraumatic fan retractor and placing a Babcock clamp near the cardioesophageal junction. The junction is then gently pulled down, and the peritoneum overlying the esophagus is thus exposed and divided. The endoscope tip is placed through the hiatus and tilted anteriorly, thereby pushing the anterior surface of the esophagus into view (Fig. 20-9). Alternatively, and more recently, we have omitted the use of an endoscope. In our experience, there has been no problem with this change. At this point, the anterior vagus nerve is identified, and the esophagus is bluntly dissected from both diaphragmatic crura. The anterior surface of the esophagus is cleaned to the left of the anterior vagus, and the fat overlying the gastroesophageal junction is resected.

Once the esophagus has been exposed for a distance of 6 to 7 cm, a lighted esophageal bougie is passed transorally.

The bougie replaces the endoscope in our more recent procedures and provides a surface on which the incision of the muscle can be carried out. At this point, the anterior surface of the esophagus is marked with the hook electrocautery elbow for 6 to 7 cm to the right of the anterior vagus. As in the thoracoscopic approach, the mark is deepened in one portion for 2 to 3 cm until the circular fibers are seen. The circular fibers are then divided as previously described. The mucosa is then exposed, and the myotomy is extended toward the inferior pulmonary veins and through the cardioesophageal junction, following the submucosal plane as described above. It is important for the surgeon to remember that the esophageal muscle wall is thinner and more difficult to identify at the junction and that the fibers should be lifted away from the wall prior to dividing them. With completion of the myotomy as determined by the endoscopist, the myotomy edges are bluntly dissected from the mucosa.

At this point, some practicing surgeons feel that the operation is complete. However, it is our view that an antireflux operation should be performed in all cases because the risk of trading one problem (reflux) for the correction of another (achalasia) is too great. In addition, reflux in an achalasia patient, if unrecognized, could have long-term sequelae in the form of severe erosive esophagitis, stricture, and epithelial dysplastic changes. We therefore perform a Dor fundoplication with all Heller myotomies done through this approach.

The Dor fundoplication is achieved by suturing the anterior wall of the gastric fundus to the edges of the myotomy (Fig. 20-10). The surgeon must avoid closing the myotomy during this procedure. Thus, we include the left crus of the diaphragm in our first suture. Similarly, after completing the left side, we incorporate the right crus in the right-sided suture. By incorporation of the crura, the edges of the myotomy are kept separated.

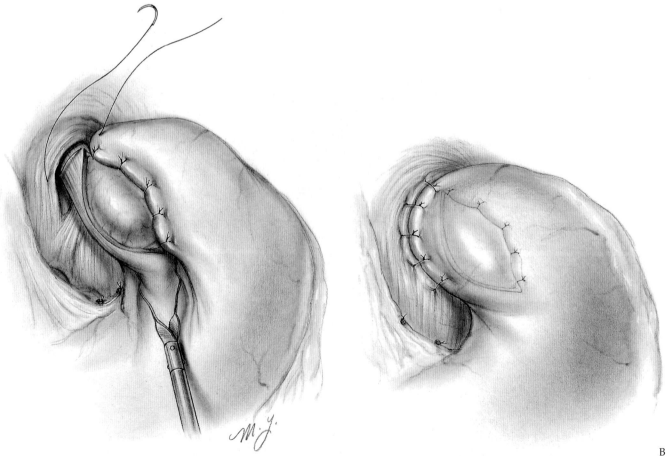

A   B

Fig. 20-10. **A,B:** *The Dor fundoplication involves suturing the anterior fundus to the edges of the myotomy.*

The Dor fundoplication incorporates several features that have made it a very attractive addition to the Heller myotomy. First, it is a partial wrap and therefore less prone to cause postoperative dysphagia in achalasia patients who have virtually no peristalsis. Second, a Dor fundoplication helps prevent closure of the myotomy by suturing of the anterior portion of the stomach to the myotomy edges. Third, it provides protection and support for the exposed mucosa.

Thoracoscopic Long Myotomy

Left Approach

In patients whose preoperative studies implicate the lower esophagus as the site of disordered motility, the left approach is used because it is easier to access the lower esophagus, particularly the LES, from this side. The procedure is very similar to that of the thoracoscopic Heller myotomy described above. The major differences are that the myotomy is carried up to the aortic arch and the muscle at the cardioesophageal junction is divided only if necessary (i.e., studies implicate its involvement or it appears tight clinically). A good myotomy of approximately 10 to 11 cm can be made from this side.

Right Approach

The right approach is used when the primary site of esophageal involvement is located in the mid- or upper esophagus. This side offers virtually complete accessibility to the esophagus with the exception of the cardioesophageal junction.

The right approach begins with the patient being placed in the left lateral decubitus position. Port placement is higher (approximately one to two ICSs) in this approach than in the left approach or the thoracoscopic Heller myotomy. In particular, port A is placed anterior to the posterior axillary line in the third or fourth ICS. The telescope is then placed in port A, and the thoracic cavity is examined. Port B is usually inserted at the fourth or fifth ICS behind the posterior axillary line and serves as the permanent location for the telescope. Ports C and D are inserted one to two ICSs below and one above port B, respectively. Port C should lie anterior to the posterior axillary line and serves as the

port for the right hand of the surgeon. Port D is positioned anterior to the anterior axillary line and is used by the first assistant. The last port (E) is placed below port A, usually at the fourth ICS anterior to the posterior axillary line. This port is used by the left hand of the surgeon. Port A during the operation is used for lung retraction. As above, the intended port sites for B, C, D, and E are checked with a spinal needle seen internally for best positioning. The overall goals in positioning should be to maintain a good distance between ports C and E (the surgeon's right and left hands) and to position the diamond's center over the posterior axillary line near the fifth ICS.

After trocar placement, the collapsed right lung is retracted anteriorly and pushed medially, thus exposing the esophagus and azygos vein. Unlike in the left approach, the esophageal dissection is simplified because there is no deep groove. Hence, the division of the pleura overlying the esophagus can begin immediately on a line 3 to 4 mm below and parallel to the azygos vein. The line is extended up to the point at which the azygos vein crosses over to the left side. If necessary, the pleura above the cross-point can also be incised, and the azygos vein gently dissected from the wall of the esophagus. Occasionally, it will be necessary to divide the inferior pulmonary ligament on this side to fully expose the esophagus.

After exposure, the myotomy is carried out in a manner similar to that discussed above for the left approach. Once completed, a myotomy should be approximately 18 to 20 cm in length, if extended above the azygos vein. As described above, the results are checked with the endoscope. At the end of the operation, the ports are removed under direct vision, and the trocar sites are sutured. A small, 26-F angled chest tube is left in the lowest trocar site under waterseal. Usually, this tube is removed the next day.

Postoperative Care

Patients are left fasting for 12 to 24 hours postoperatively, after which a soft-food diet is started. In addition, during this time, the chest tube is removed and antibiotics are discontinued. In the case of an esophageal perforation and repair, patients are usually kept fasting for an addi-

tional 36 to 48 hours and checked with a meglumine diatrizoate (Gastrografin) swallow, before starting a diet.

After approximately 2 to 3 days, patients can be discharged home with follow-up instructions. The follow-up should include clinic visits and postoperative manometry and 24-hour pH monitoring within a few weeks of the surgery. We believe that the follow-up studies provide invaluable information about possible postoperative reflux. Due to their poor motility and potentially impaired LES postoperatively, this is of particular concern in myotomy patients who have not had an antireflux procedure.

Complications

Operative Complications

Operative complications associated with the above procedures can be grouped into two categories: trocar-related and myotomy-related. Complications associated with trocar placement are varied and common to other thoracoscopic and laparoscopic procedures. A detailed account of this group is beyond the scope of this chapter. The two most common complications associated with the myotomy are bleeding and mucosal injury.

The typical sites for bleeding are the trocar sites, the lung surface, or a periesophageal vessel. The bleeding can obscure the field but can usually be controlled endoscopically. However, significant ongoing blood loss is unacceptable and requires conversion to an open procedure.

Mucosal injuries can occur either early or late. Early injuries result from completely traversing the esophageal wall during the myotomy. Whereas late perforations can develop in areas that were damaged by heat during the operation, these areas can then slowly necrose postoperatively. The typical time interval between injury and perforation is approximately 1 week for late perforations. Regardless of the exact time of injury, all mucosal perforations typically occur near the gastroesophageal junction. In this region, the esophagus is thinner, and the muscle layers are more difficult to distinguish. However, with vigilant use of the telescope and the endoscope, these early injuries can be caught and repaired endoscopically, depending on the surgeon's expertise with the procedure. The mucosal defect should be repaired with a 4-0 or 5-0 silk suture, and the repair can be buttressed with the stomach if the hole is close to the junction, as it usually is. Follow-up in these patients consists of good clinical observation and a postoperative UGI study with meglumine diatrizoate within the first postoperative week, prior to discharge.

Postoperative Complications

Postoperative complications besides late perforation are generally related to the lung that had been collapsed during the operation. The possibilities range from mild atelectasis and lobar collapse to pneumonia and adult respiratory distress syndrome. For the most part, patients do well; however, the surgeon must be vigilant in managing these patients, as the potential for severe complications always exists.

Suggested Reading

Ancona E, Anselmino M, Zaninotto G, et al. Esophageal achalasia: laparoscopic versus conventional open Heller-Dor operation. *Am J Surg* 1995;170:265–270.

Filipi C, Hinder R. Thoracoscopic esophageal myotomy—a surgical technique for achalasia, diffuse esophageal spasm and "nutcracker esophagus." *Surg Endosc* 1994;8:921–926.

Esophageal disease. In: Kaiser LR, Daniel TM, ed. *Thoracic surgery*, 1st ed. Little Brown and Company, 1993.

Pellegrini CA. Myotomy and resections. In: *Esophageal surgery*. New York: Churchill Livingstone, 1995.

Pellegrini CA. Achalasia of the esophagus: management by videoendoscopic surgery. In: Debas HT, sect ed. *Operative surgery: surgery of the upper gastrointestinal tract*, 5th ed. London: Chapman & Hall, 1994.

Raiser F, Perdikis G, Hinder RA, et al. Heller myotomy via minimal-access surgery: an evaluation of antireflux procedures. *Arch Surg* 1996; 131:593–598.

Sinanan MN, Pellegrini CA. Videoendoscopic procedures of the esophagus, stomach, duodenum. In: Zuidema GD, Ritchie WP, eds. *Shackelford's surgery of the alimentary tract*, 4th ed. Columbia, MD: WB Saunders, 1995;11: Vol. 11.

EDITOR'S COMMENT

Endoscopic treatments have been available as a minimally invasive treatment for achalasia for several decades. Unfortunately, flexible endoscopic balloon dilation and, more recently, botulinum toxin injection of the LES has not been totally satisfactory. Both approaches have a high rate of recurrent dysphagia that necessitates repeat procedures at added cost and the potential for morbidity (perforation, scarring, or inducement of reflux). Surgical myotomy has always offered the best success rate, and the introduction of thoracoscopy and laparoscopic approaches by surgical pioneers such as Dr. Pellegrini have allowed this to be done with minimal-access morbidity. Whether this is best done thoracoscopically or laparoscopically remains somewhat of a controversy, but, barring a hostile abdomen, the laparoscopic approach is probably preferred because it offers simpler anesthesia and excellent exposure and it allows the surgeon to perform an antireflux procedure to minimize the chance of late dysphagia from peptic stricture. The choice of the Dor anterior partial fundoplication or the Toupet posterior partial wrap, both originally described in conjunction with the Heller myotomy, is the the surgeon's choice, based on relative (theoretical) pros and cons for each. The main concern with using the Dor wrap is closure of the myotomy when the wrap is pulled anteriorly. This can be avoided with very careful technique. The benefit of the Dor procedure is the fact that it is easy to perform. The Toupet repair is technically more difficult but has the benefit of providing a better antireflux mechanism, and by the nature of its attachments to the myotomized edges of the esophagus, it guarantees that the myotomy will be open. A complete wrap is contraindicated in these patients because of the severity of accompanying esophageal motility disorder. Patients with other esophageal motility disorders, diffuse esophageal spasm, or nutcracker esophagus should be approached only when all other conservative measures fail, as the results from long myotomy are not as satisfactory as the results from myotomy for more localized problems such as achalasia. Finally, caution should be used in performing this procedure with monopolar electrocautery. Monopolar current runs the risk of burning the esophageal mucosa, allowing a delayed perforation. This could be disastrous, and the use of bipolar cautery or ultrasonic coagulation—or no cautery at all—is probably preferable.

L.L.S.

21

Flexible Endoscopy for Palliation of Esophageal Cancer

Frederick L. Greene

Flexible upper gastrointestinal endoscopy plays a major role in the diagnosis of malignant esophageal stricture and is currently the primary diagnostic test, having supplanted radiographic studies, which were unable to provide tissue confirmation of the malignancy. The ability to assess the size of an esophageal cancer and its distance from the upper incisors and to utilize photography and videoscopic data-keeping make flexible endoscopic assessment mandatory in the development of a treatment plan for esophageal cancer patients (Fig. 21-1). In addition to being a diagnostic tool, the flexible upper endoscope may be used as a palliative vehicle for patients who either may eventually undergo surgical resection or are treated nonsurgically using combinations of radiation chemotherapy or stenting.

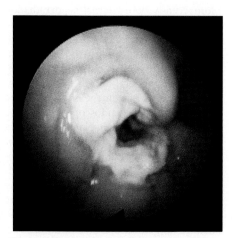

Fig. 21-1. Endoscopic view of squamous cell carcinoma of the thoracic esophagus.

Bougienage for Relief of Dysphagia

Frequently, the initial use of flexible endoscopy after diagnosis is in the application of bougienage to relieve significant dysphagia associated with advanced esophageal cancer; dilation of the strictured segment may be required. The principle of dilating an esophageal stricture with a bougie was introduced in the 16th century. The initial technique was to use a wax taper to blindly dilate the narrowed area of the esophagus. The word *bougie* is derived from the Arabic name of Boujiyah, Algeria, which was a medieval center known for its wax candle trade. Current principles of endoscopic treatment were developed more than 100 years ago when the English physician J.C. Russell introduced a balloon dilator similar to those used today. Samuel Mixter of Boston developed the concept of passing a bougie over a string that served as a guide to avoid perforation. The patient would initially swallow the string, and once the string became anchored in the small intestine, a dilating bougie was passed. Sir Arthur Hurst introduced the mercury-filled flexible bougie in 1915. Utilizing these ancient and more recent concepts, the introduction of both rigid and flexible endoscopy were well adapted to the techniques of bougienage and served to make them safer.

Current advances in dilation include balloon techniques and tapered bougies that can be safely passed over a guidewire (Savary-Guillard bougies) (Figs. 21-2 and 21-3). Strictures may occur in any area of the esophagus, but they are most common in the middle and distal segments. This corresponds to the most frequent locations of both squamous cancer and adenocarcinoma of the esophagus. Use of dilating techniques is appropriate in patients who have previously been treated with external-beam radiation or current intracavitary techniques using high-dose-rate brachytherapy, which occasionally results in nonmalignant strictures and dysphagia. The flexible endoscope also serves as an excellent tool for performing biopsies to rule out the presence of ongoing tumor in treated patients.

Esophageal dilation under direct visualization can be done by a hydrostatic balloon system that may be passed directly through the instrument channel of most flexible esophagoscopes (Fig. 21-4). These balloon systems are available with diameters of 8 to 15 mm. Balloons are much safer than blindly placed bougies or even those inserted with the assistance of a guidewire. Contrast agents may also be instilled into the balloons to confirm the location of these devices radiographically or fluoroscopically. Repeat dilation is frequently needed for patients with strictures secondary to tumor. Postirradiation strictures may also need redilation if dysphagia redevelops.

Another use of flexible upper endoscopy is to serve as a vehicle for both laser tumor ablation and the delivery of endoluminal regional irradiation. Contact ablation using a neodymium:yttrium-aluminum-garnet laser has been effective in relieving malignant obstruction if a patient has an

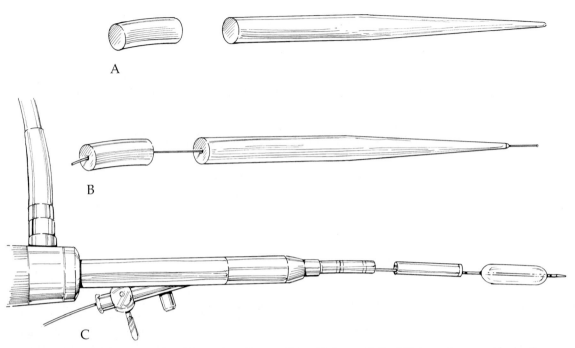

Fig. 21-2. **A:** *Tapered bougie for blind dilation of a malignant stricture.* **B:** *Savary-Guillard dilator used over a guidewire.* **C:** *Hydrostatic balloon dilator passed through an endoscope.*

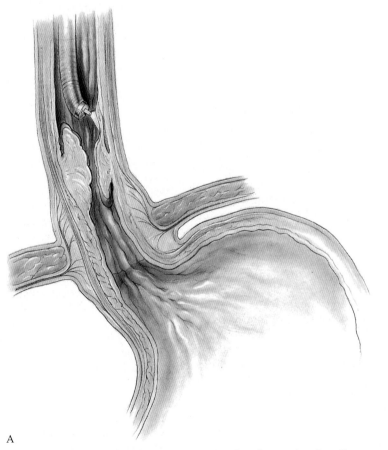

A

Fig. 21-3. **A:** *Laser ablation of circumferential esophageal tumor.* (continued)

identifiable lumen through which the laser fiber may be passed. Initially, placement of a guidewire and subsequent dilation of the esophagus may be needed prior to passing the laser fiber. Several applications of the contact laser may be needed to create an appropriate esophageal diameter to mitigate dysphagia.

Palliation of Malignant Strictures

More recently, both external-beam radiation and endoluminal radiation utilizing flexible endoscopic techniques have enabled palliation of malignant strictures. Patients can generally be treated as outpatients and seldom require general anesthesia. The technique involves placement of a guidewire through the flexible endoscope to guide the passage of a 16-French plastic tube. This tube serves as an afterloading receptacle for either iridium or cesium seeds that will generate 500 to 1,000 rad (5 to 10 Gy) of radiation energy to a small segment of the esophageal tumor. This technique has the advantage of avoiding radiation effects to adjacent lung tissue and surrounding structures that are often damaged by external-**beam** therapy. The endoscopist must work

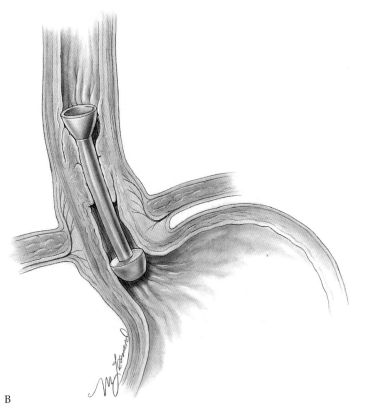

B

Fig. 21-3. (Continued) **B:** *Rigid endoluminal esophageal stent is placed using flexible endoscopic technique.*

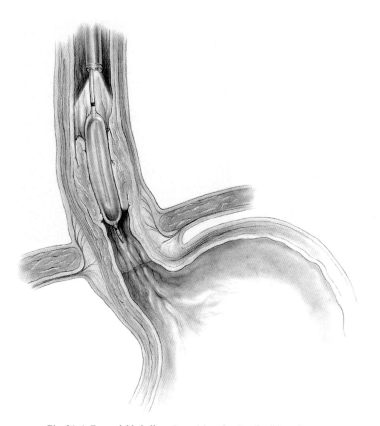

Fig. 21-4. Expandable balloon is positioned using flexible endoscopy.

in close association with the radiation oncologist to ensure that the afterloading device is placed at the appropriate level to encompass the entire length of esophageal tumor and to calculate dosimetry. Postendoscopy chest x-ray must be obtained prior to application of radiation to ensure appropriate placement of the afterloading device. Intraluminal stents, such as Celestin tubes, have been available for several decades for palliation of esophageal cancer.

Intraluminal stents have recently been developed that allow safe placement utilizing flexible endoscopic techniques (Fig. 21-5). These stents are collapsible, permitting easy placement across the esophageal tumor; after placement they can be expanded to create a lumen that will allow a patient to eat a soft diet (Fig. 21-6). These stents are made in variable lengths ranging from 7 to 15 cm and are either self-expanding or require balloon expansion. The endoscope serves as the vehicle for proper stent placement and may be also be needed to insert a balloon to dilate the stricture once the stent is properly placed (Fig. 21-7). Stents are useful for palliation of intraluminal tumors and relief of obstruction caused by extraluminal disease. Even patients with tracheoesophageal fistula may have solid stents placed to serve as a buttress between the esophagus and trachea and allow some protection from chronic aspiration (see Fig. 21-3B). The long-term effect of expandable stents has not been fully defined, but most reports suggest that they are better tolerated than older stents made of thick rubber that required open surgery to place. Endoscopic placement of expandable stents allows patients to be treated in an outpatient setting, adding to improved overall quality of life for patients who face only a few months more of life.

Complications

Palliation of carcinoma of the esophagus using endoscopic techniques can be fraught with significant complication, including perforation and bleeding, particularly when performed by endoscopists inexperienced in their use. Passage of flexible endoscopes through an area of narrowed friable tumor is a high-risk situation for perforation. Direct visualization of the lumen must be maintained at all times. Use of dilators compounds the risk of complication, particularly bleeding or perforation. Dilators that

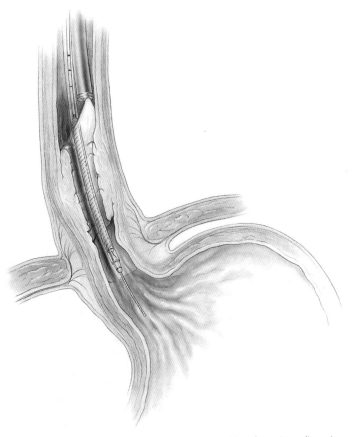

Fig. 21-5. Placement of expandable esophageal stent with endoscopic confirmation.

are inserted over guidewires or via balloon dilation are probably optimal in this high-risk group. Lasers or thermal devices may create acute perforation of the esophagus into the mediastinum or pleural space that can be difficult to recognize. These potential complications also apply to newer techniques of endoscopic stent placement. It is important to obtain a chest film following any manipulation of an esophageal tumor to look for air extending outside the esophageal lumen. Fluoroscopy during these procedures and x-ray confirmation following stent placement with or without dilation are mandatory to minimize perforation. Long-term complications of esophageal stricture may occur in patients with perforation, especially after the use of intracavitary irradiation. Follow-up esophagoscopy and biopsy should be performed to ensure that any stricture is not a result of recurrent tumor.

Conclusion

The flexible endoscope is an important diagnostic and therapeutic tool for assessing patients with esophageal cancer and for palliating obstructive symptoms caused

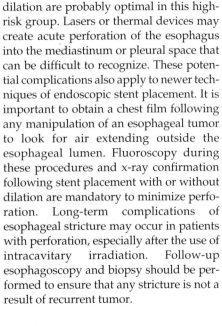

B

Fig. 21-6. **A:** Expandable stent in position. **B:** Endoscopic view of deployed metal stent.

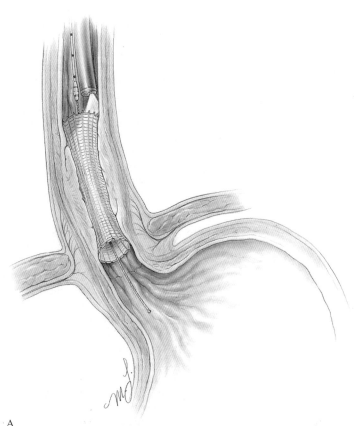

A

by this disease. In patients who have undergone esophageal resection, endoscopic surveillance of the remaining esophagus or the esophagogastric or esophagocolic anastomosis is appropriate and may identify early recurrent disease. Techniques such as dilation or stenting may be used if anastomotic strictures occur and further serve as a method for palliation of patients with significant malignant processes.

Suggested Reading

Adams DB. Endoscopic management of esophageal stricture. In: Greene FL, Ponsky JL, eds. *Endoscopic surgery*. Philadelphia: WB Saunders, 1994:36–54.

Fleisher D. Endoscopic laser therapy for carcinoma of the esophagus. *Endosc Rev* 1984;1:37–41.

Greene FL, Boulware RJ, Bianco J. Role of esophagogastroscopy in application and follow-up of high-dose-rate brachytherapy (HDRB) for treatment of esophageal carcinoma. *Surg Laparosc Endosc* 1995;5:425–430.

Goldin E. A new self-expandable nickel titanium coil stent for esophageal obstruction: a preliminary report. *Gastrointest Endosc* 1994;40:64–68.

Wu WC. Silicone-covered self-expanding metallic stents for the palliation of malignant esophageal obstruction and esophagorespiratory fistulas: experience in 32 patients and a review of the literature. *Gastrointest Endosc* 1994;40:22–33.

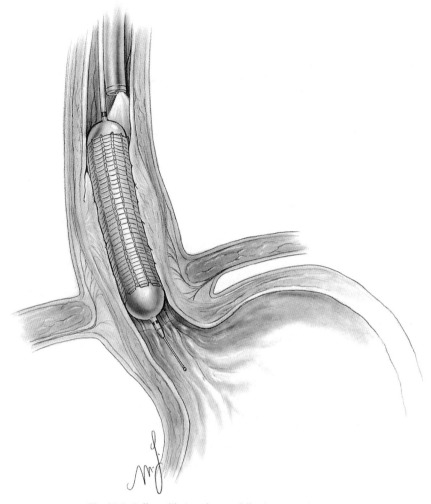

Fig. 21-7. Balloon dilation of tumor following stent placement.

EDITOR'S COMMENT

Though seldom mentioned as a primary concern of surgeons, the palliation of unresectable cancers is one of the great achievements of surgical care. End-stage esophageal cancer has tremendous morbidity and impact on quality of life for patients. Formal surgical resection of the cancer often has high morbidity for a group of patients who have a very limited life expectancy. Fortunately, flexible endoscopy permits several methods of effective palliation (mostly for dysphagia) to be performed with a minimum of access morbidity. Dr. Greene nicely outlines the many flexible endoscopic techniques for palliation of patients with profound dysphagia from obstructive esophageal malignancy.

Unfortunately, flexible endoscopic techniques for palliative treatment are meeting with resistance in this era of managed care and cost consciousness. Techniques such as bougienage or balloon dilation require frequent repeat endoscopies to maintain long-term palliation. Stents, with their longer interval success, are currently quite expensive and still require maintenance endoscopy for patency. The future of palliative treatment of esophageal malignancy is unclear. Flexible endoscopy certainly plays a major role in the diagnosis and staging of these cancers, especially with the addition of endoscopic ultrasound. More invasive endoscopic palliation techniques are well tolerated and have a low morbidity, but are not complication-free and require frequent visits. In spite of the obvious advantages of flexible endoscopy for the palliation of esophageal cancer, it may be necessary to compare these techniques to other new techniques, such as laparoscopic esophagectomy, to determine what is truly the most effective and most cost-effective treatment for these patients.

L.L.S.

22

Surgical Endoscopy for Esophageal Resection

Aureo L. DePaula, Márcio M. Machado, Andre Ferrari, and Mauro Bafutto

Indications

One of the most traumatic procedures in the field of digestive surgery is esophagectomy. Early efforts at surgical removal of the esophagus were restricted because of its thoracic location. In the beginning, efforts were centered in the cervical esophagus due to its anatomic position. Albrecht Theodor Middlekorp (1824 to 1864) was the first surgeon to perform an esophageal resection for a carcinoma of the proximal esophagus. The first attempts to perform esophagectomy for more distal lesions utilized an extrapleural approach because it was impossible to perform a thoracotomy at the time. With the development of more sophisticated anesthesia and surgical techniques, the transthoracic approach was finally feasible and subsequently became the most frequent way to perform esophagectomy. The technique of transhiatal esophagectomy was developed later as a less invasive procedure, and it represents a valid alternative for patients with both benign and malignant esophageal disorders.

Laparoscopic surgery has become the latest option for the surgical approach to a number of digestive diseases. The advantages of this new approach include a shortened hospital stay, more rapid recovery, and less perioperative discomfort for patients.

The indications for thoracoscopic and laparoscopic transhiatal esophagectomy include patients with both benign and malignant esophageal diseases.

Benign Diseases

Thoracoscopic and laparoscopic esophagectomy is indicated for patients with end-stage achalasia (sigmoid esophagus) and ex-

tensive nondilatable strictures from esophageal reflux, as well as for a selected group of patients with failed antireflux and Heller operations or with long caustic strictures. Elective esophagectomy should also be recommended to reflux patients with high-grade dysplasia documented in Barrett's esophagus, as more than 40% will have occult adenocarcinoma. The first option for these patients is the laparoscopic transhiatal approach. Thoracoscopic esophagectomy is an option when the transhiatal approach proves to be not technically viable.

Esophageal Carcinoma

The laparoscopic approach has been selected for patients with esophageal carcinoma, based on the location of the tumor, local invasion, general clinical condition, and preoperative staging. Thoracoscopic esophagectomy is the best option for those with carcinoma of the upper and middle third of the thoracic esophagus and also for those lesions suspected to have significant local invasion. Transhiatal esophagectomy is indicated for carcinoma of the cervical esophagus, carcinoma of the lower third of the thoracic esophagus, and early esophageal carcinoma, as well as for high-risk patients, especially cirrhotics and those with advanced cardiopulmonary disease.

Preoperative Evaluation

A careful preoperative evaluation must be performed because patients are usually elderly and undernourished and have several concomitant disorders. Special emphasis is given to the cardiac evaluation, pulmonary function (P_{ao2} − forced expiratory volume in 1 second), and hepatic and

renal function. Cancer patients must be thoroughly staged preoperatively.

Benign Diseases

Evaluation should include a barium meal examination, upper digestive endoscopy, biopsy, esophageal manometry, and 24-hour esophageal pH monitoring. The esophagogram of patients with advanced esophageal achalasia typically demonstrates dilation of more than 7 cm in diameter, loss of the longitudinal orientation of the organ, an air–fluid level, and significant stasis (sigmoid esophagus). Important endoscopic findings include mucosal edema, retained food, loss of the typical vascular pattern, and stasis esophagitis. Esophageal manometry usually shows absence or incomplete relaxation of the lower esophageal sphincter (LES), high or normal LES pressure, and aperistaltic waves of the esophageal body. In these patients, the esophagus must be emptied and cleaned through a large-caliber nasoesophageal tube before surgery to avoid aspiration at the beginning of anesthesia and reduce the risk of intraabdominal contamination if esophageal perforation occurs during surgery. The colon is routinely prepared as well.

Upper endoscopy with biopsy is the most important test for patients with refractory gastroesophageal reflux strictures to exclude the possibility of concomitant carcinoma. Esophageal manometry typically shows severe changes characterized by inadequate (or sometimes absent) esophageal contractility and decreased LES pressure.

Esophageal Carcinoma

Preoperative evaluation should include barium meal, upper digestive endoscopy with biopsy, computed tomography of the chest and abdomen, bronchoscopy, ultrasonography, and endoscopic ultrasound.

Operative Technique

Laparoscopic Transhiatal Esophagectomy

The procedure is performed with the patient supine and the legs in gynecologic straps; a reverse Trendelenburg of approximately 30 degrees is used, and the patient's head should be turned to the right. The surgeon stands between the patient's legs, with the first assistant on the patient's left. The second assistant stands on the patient's right and holds the camera (Fig. 22-1). A pneumoperitoneum is established through an incision in the midline 3 to 4 cm above the umbilicus, where a 10-mm trocar is introduced. A 30-degree telescope is routinely used. Intraperitoneal pressure is maintained at or below 12 mm Hg. Two 5-mm trocars are placed near the right and left subcostal margins in the midclavicular line, and a 10-mm trocar is placed below the xiphoid. A 12-mm trocar is introduced somewhere between the left subcostal trocar and the telescope. The surgeon's right hand works with this last trocar, while the left hand controls the graspers and bipolar devices positioned through the trocar placed just beneath the right costal margin. The subxiphoid trocar is used by a liver retractor or a grasper to help exposure of the greater curvature, and the last trocar placed below the left costal margin accommodates a grasper (Fig. 22-2).

The first step is to perform a pyloroplasty or an extramucosal pyloromyotomy (Fig. 22-3). Next, the gastrocolic omentum and the short gastric vessels are clipped and divided, preserving the right gastroepiploic artery. Liberal use of a bipolar grasper usually makes this part of the procedure faster. The left gastric artery and vein are divided between silk ligatures and clips close to their origin. Thus, the stomach remains vascularized via the right gastroepiploic and right gastric arteries (Fig. 22-4). The phrenoesophageal membrane is opened, and the connective tissue attachments between the esophagus and crus are divided. For patients with esophageal carcinoma, a meticulous dissection is performed at the celiac axis, hepatic artery, and splenic artery to retrieve the nodes usually found at this level. The upper part

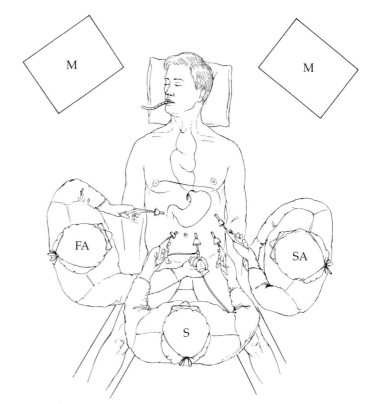

Fig. 22-1. Operating room setup for totally laparoscopic esophagectomy. (S, surgeon; FA, first assistant; M, monitor; SA, second assistant.)

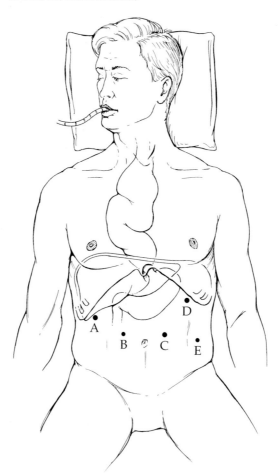

Fig. 22-2. Trocar placement for totally laparoscopic esophagectomy.

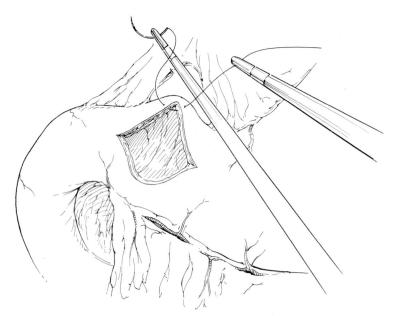

Fig. 22-3. *Laparoscopic pyloroplasty.*

of the lesser curvature and part of the fundus are divided using a linear stapler. This resection starts at the level of the fourth vessel along the lesser curvature (Fig. 22-5). Sutures are placed between the end of the divided esophagus and the apex of the gastric fundus. This kind of oncologic resection is also used for patients with benign disease in order to have a longer gastric tube.

The esophagus is then mobilized from its mediastinal bed laparoscopically using instruments passed through the hiatus. This largely consists of blunt dissection, but a few small vessels are clipped before being cut. The dissection from below is continued as far as the aortic arch 2 to 3 cm beyond the tracheal bifurcation (Fig. 22-6). It is unnecessary to enlarge the esophageal hiatus in any of these operations, although enlargement may be used for selected patients.

An incision is made in the neck parallel to the anterior border of the left sternomastoid muscle (Fig. 22-7). The prethyroid muscles are divided, and the recurrent laryngeal nerve is identified. The upper thoracic and cervical esophagus is bluntly dissected from its mediastinal attachments far enough down to meet the esophageal dissection from below. At this point in the operation, the esophagus has been completely detached from adjacent structures. Traction is placed on the esophagus from above, which will draw the entire stomach into the mediastinum and the apex of the fundus into the neck. The esophagus is extracted through the cervical incision. A cervical esophagogastric anastomosis is performed in one layer using interrupted sutures of 4-0 Prolene (Fig. 22-8). A feeding laparoscopic jejunostomy is done. The jejunostomy tube is positioned through one of the lateral trocars, and a purse-string of absorbable suture is made in the appropriate loop of jejunum. A small enterotomy is created, and the feeding tube is advanced at least 15 cm into the jejunum. The purse-string is tied intracorporeally, and three additional sutures are used to fasten the small bowel to the abdominal wall at the site of the feeding tube.

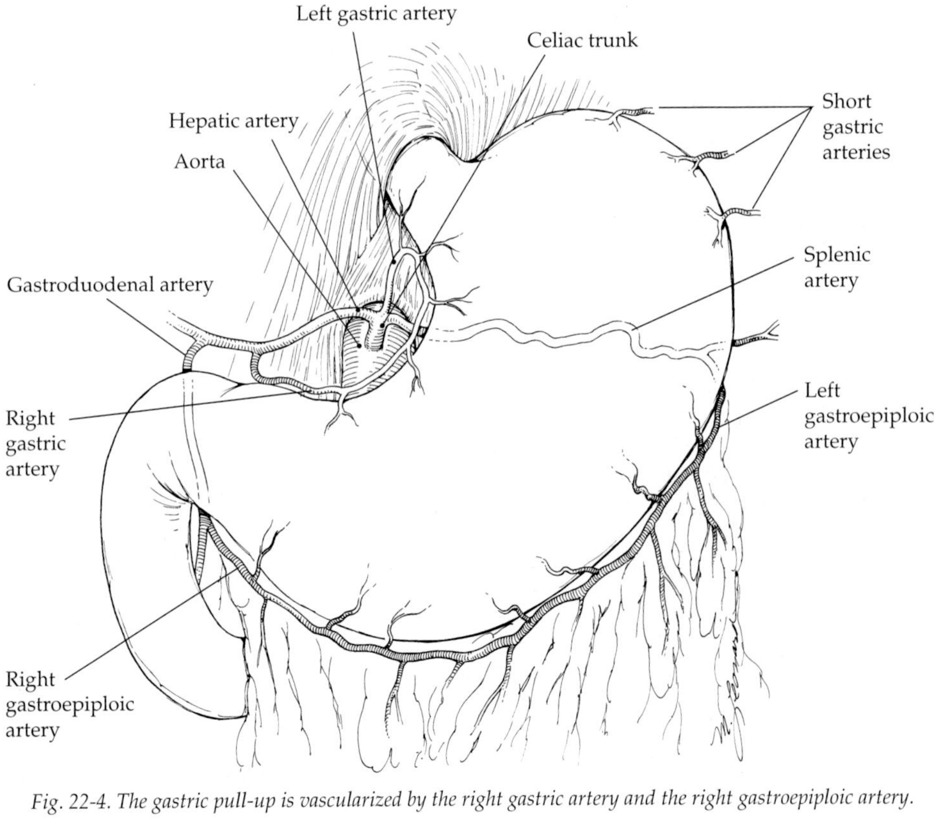

Thoracoscopic Esophagectomy

After double-lumen endotracheal intubation, the patient is placed in the left lateral decubitus position (Fig. 22-9). Five trocars are introduced into the right thoracic cavity. The first one, for the 0-degree telescope, is placed through the sixth intercostal space in the posterior axillary line. The second 10-mm trocar is positioned in the seventh intercostal space in the midaxillary line. The third trocar (5 mm) is placed in the fifth intercostal space in the midaxillary line. Two additional 5-mm trocars are positioned in the sixth and fourth intercostal spaces in the anterior axillary line (Fig. 22-9).

The right lung has already been collapsed. The first step is to divide the azygos vein between ligatures. This is followed by dissec-

Fig. 22-4. *The gastric pull-up is vascularized by the right gastric artery and the right gastroepiploic artery.*

tion of the upper esophagus, which is encircled with a Penrose drain. Another Penrose drain is placed around the inferior esophagus, and the esophageal dissection is done under traction of the two Penrose drains (Fig. 22-10). Curved instruments are used to detach the left side of the esophagus. The extent of the dissection is as large as possible. The most difficult part of this portion of the procedure is the dissection of the left recurrent laryngeal nerve. The pleura attached to the esophagus and azygos vein is retrieved together with the esophagus. For patients with benign disease, the dissection is made as close as possible to the esophageal wall. Two tubes are left in place after esophageal mobilization has been completed.

The patient is then positioned supine, with the head turned to the right. Abdominal trocars are placed, and the gastric mobilization is performed as described above for laparoscopic transhiatal esophagectomy. Care should be taken to complete the intraabdominal dissection before the esophageal attachments are divided close to the crura, to avoid the loss of the pneumoperitoneum. The cervical dissection and the esophagogastric anastomosis are the same as described previously.

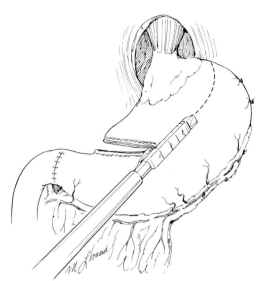

Fig. 22-5. Multiple endoscopic linear stapler firings are used to divide the gastric pull-up.

Results, Complications, and Follow-up

Benign Diseases

From July 1992 to December 1995, 28 patients underwent a laparoscopic transhiatal esophagectomy, and three patients a thoracoscopic esophagectomy. Mean age was 57.6 years (range, 19 to 78 years); mean weight was 51 kg. Serious complications included the following:

Duodenal perforation in two patients, who needed conversion to laparoscopic pyloroplasty.
Unilateral pneumothorax in nine patients and bilateral in four. Concomitant pneumoperitoneum was well tolerated by the

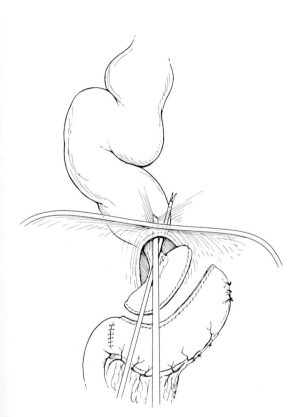

Fig. 22-6. Transhiatal dissection.

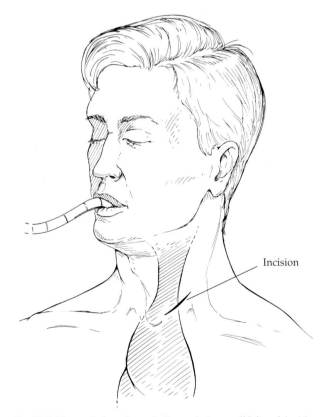

Incision

Fig. 22-7. The cervical esophagus is dissected via a small left neck incision.

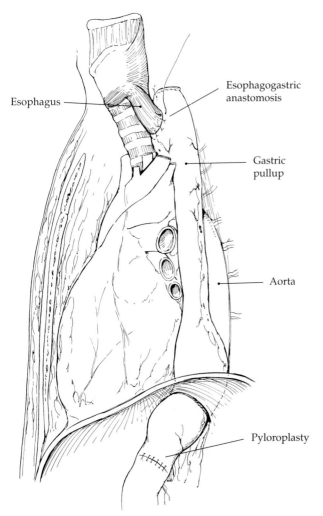

Fig. 22-8. *A single layer anastomosis is performed between the gastric pull-up and the cervical esophagus.*

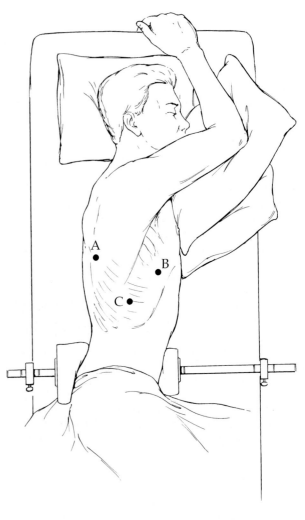

Fig. 22-9. *Port placement for a right thoracoscopic esophageal dissection. For thoracoscopic esophageal mobilization, the patient is positioned as for right thoracoscopy. (A, dissector/retractor; B, retractor; C, camera.)*

majority of patients. Due to hemodynamic changes, four patients required interruption of the pneumoperitoneum, intraoperative chest drainage, and use of a mechanical abdominal wall suspension for the procedure to be completed. Tracheal laceration during the cervical dissection in one patient.

One patient was converted to open surgery because of a large left liver lobe, and another was converted to the thoracoscopic approach because of extreme esophageal dilation. Two patients needed blood transfusion (500 mL each).

Mean operative time was 225 minutes. Mean hospital stay was 7.2 days. Postoperative complications included pleural effusion in 10 patients (42%), transitory dipho-

nia in four (16.7%), delayed gastric emptying in two (8.4%) (requiring endoscopic dilation of the pylorus), and anastomotic leak with spontaneous resolution in one (4.2%). There was no mortality. After a mean follow-up of 18 months (range, 2 to 32 months), relief of dysphagia was observed in 92.2% of patients, and slight and occasional dysphagia in 7.8%.

Esophageal Carcinoma

From July 1991 to September 1995, 40 patients were submitted to laparoscopic transhiatal esophagectomy and 16 patients to thoracoscopic esophagectomy. Mean age was 62.3 years (range, 44 to 78 years); mean weight was 53.2 kg. Forty-seven patients had squamous carcinoma and nine adenocarcinoma.

Intraoperative complications included the following:

Pneumothorax in 30 patients, including bilateral pneumothorax in seven. In this last group, three patients required interruption of the pneumoperitoneum, intraoperative chest drainage, and mechanical abdominal wall suspension.
Duodenal perforation during pyloromyotomy in two patients.

Four patients needed blood transfusion (500 mL each). Mean anesthetic time was 312 minutes and mean operative time 256 minutes. The average time in the intensive care unit was 28 hours. Mean hospital stay was 12.9 days (range, 6 to 45 days). Two patients required conversion to open surgery and two to the thoracoscopic approach. Both had lesions invading adjacent mediastinal structures.

Four patients were stage I, five stage IIa, nine stage IIb, 34 stage III, and four stage IV. The average number of dissected lymph nodes was 11 for transhiatal esophagectomy and 18 for thoracoscopic esophagectomy.

Postoperative complications for the transhiatal approach included pleural effusion in 26 patients (65%), transitory dysphonia in three (7.5%), anastomotic leak in eight (20%), pneumonia in four (10%), delayed gastric emptying in two (5%) and myocardial infarction in one (2.5%). Five patients (12.5%) died. In those who underwent a transthoracic procedure, pleural effusion developed in five (31.3%), transitory dysphonia in three (18.8%), and anastomotic leak in two (12.5%); one patient (6.3%) died. Due to short postoperative follow-up, evaluation of the survival rate is not yet possible.

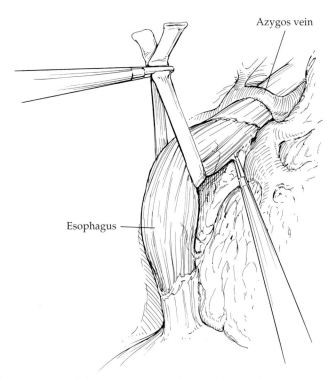

Fig. 22-10. *Adequate retraction facilitates thoracoscopic dissection of the esophagus and surrounding tissues.*

Azygos vein

Esophagus

Suggested Reading

Akiyama H, Tsurumara M, Kawanura T, Ono Y. Principles of surgical treatment of carcinoma of the esophagus: analysis of lymph node involvement. *Ann Surg* 1981;194:435–446.

DePaula AL, Hashiba K, Ferreira EAB, Paula RA, Grecco E. Laparoscopic transhiatal esophagectomy with esophagogastroplasty. *Surg Laparosc Endosc* 1995;5:1–5.

Dexter SPL, Martin IG, McMahon MJ. Radical thoracoscopic esophagectomy for cancer. *Surg Endosc* 1996;10:147–151.

Gossot D, Cattan P, Fritsch S, Halimi B, Sarfati E, Celeriere M. Can the morbidity of esophagectomy be reduced by the thoracoscopic approach? *Surg Endosc* 1995;9:1113–1115.

Jagot P, Sauvanet A, Berthoux L, Belghiti J. Laparoscopic mobilization of the stomach for oesophageal replacement. *Br J Surg* 1996;83:540–542.

el Nakadi IE, Houben JJ, Gay F, Closset J, Gelin M, Lambilliotte JP. Does esophagectomy cure a resectable esophageal cancer? *World J Surg* 1993; 17:760–765.

Orringer MB. Transhiatal esophagectomy without thoracotomy for carcinoma of the thoracic esophagus. *Ann Surg* 1984;200:282–288.

Sadanaga N, Kuwano H, Watanabe M, et al. Laparoscopy-assisted surgery: a new technique for transhiatal esophageal dissection. *Am J Surg* 1994;168:355–357.

Swanstrom LL, Hansen P. Laparoscopic total esophagectomy. *Arch Surg* 1997;132:943–949.

EDITOR'S COMMENT

Use of laparoscopy and thoracoscopy for esophageal resection has failed to gain widespread acceptance over the past several years since it was first described. The reasons for this are concerns about adequate oncologic resections and the high technical demands of laparoscopic esophageal resections. Pioneers such as Dr. DePaula have demonstrated that laparoscopic or thoracoscopic resections are possible and well tolerated by patients. On the other hand, these procedures do require special instrumentation (longer instruments) and commitment to a long operative time and steep learning curve on the part of the surgeon. The potential benefit of performing esophageal resections endoscopically include the ability to stage the patient before committing to a full operation and the hopes of decreasing the metabolic and cardiopulmonary impact of this major surgery. Early series reported in the literature have indeed indicated that while hospital stays are almost the same, compared to those with open procedures, there seems to be less need for postoperative intensive care unit care and ventilatory support and an early return to gastrointestinal continuity. This also would lead one to theorize that there would be decreased immunosuppression from the surgical insult, which may eventually be shown to improve the dismal cure rates for esophageal resections for cancer. On the other hand, adequacy of margins, the ability to perform wide node resections, and the possibility of access-port wound metastases remain valid concerns that will need close scrutiny before acceptance of these techniques is widespread. One positive aspect of the use of endoscopy in esophageal resections is the ability to approach this in a staged fashion, and several investigators have described performing Ivor Lewis–type techniques with either the abdominal portion of the dissection performed laparoscopically or the thoracic portion performed thoracoscopically. This may serve as an intermediate step toward full endoscopic resection of the esophagus and thereby lessen the learning curve and operative times for this procedure.

L.L.S.

23

Surgical Endoscopy for Peptic Ulcer Disease

Barry A. Salky and Michael B. Edye

Anatomy

A thorough understanding of the esophageal hiatus, the gastric attachments, and the vagal anatomy are key to the ability to perform highly selective vagotomy (HSV). The dissection technique and anatomy are closely related to laparoscopic surgery for gastroesophageal reflux disease. For peptic ulcer surgery, the dissection plane is closer to the stomach and esophagus, especially in HSV, than it is in fundoplication. The relationship of the anatomic structures to each other is easily demonstrated. The nerve of Latarjet runs along the lesser curvature in the lesser omentum. The nerve can be seen as a thin, white string coursing from cephalad to caudad following the lesser curvature of the stomach (Fig. 23-1). Each branch of the nerve follows the arterial and venous branches of the left gastric vessels. The last branch of the nerve of Latarjet enters the stomach between 5 and 7 cm from the pylorus, just above the "crow's foot" (Fig. 23-1; color inset). This can be identified even in obese patients. It is important that these antral branches be preserved to maintain proper pyloric function. Figure 23-1 demonstrates the proper line of dissection once these nerve branches are identified. There are several techniques for keeping the main nerve out of harm's way. It is not necessary to place a suture or loop around the nerve of Latarjet, as traction injury to the main trunk can easily occur. Instead, one identifies the trunk and keeps the dissection close to the lesser curvature of the stomach wall.

The phrenoesophageal ligament must be dissected to mobilize the distal 5 cm of esophagus. As described later, the dissection plane is kept close to the esophagus and the gastroesophageal junction. The surgical dissection is 2 to 3 cm more cephalad than that done for fundoplication. A complete HSV cannot be accomplished without adequate esophageal mobilization. The anterior and posterior vagus nerve trunks, both crura of the diaphragm, and the angle of His have to be identified to stay in the proper surgical plane.

The nerve branches from the main trunk of Latarjet and vascular supply from the left gastric artery and vein lie in two distinct anterior and posterior omental "leaves" along the lesser curvature. However, there is also a less distinctive intermediate plane that will require division.

Hemostasis is critically important during this dissection. Small amounts of blood can stain the tissues and make identification of the nerve branches difficult. These blood vessels are thin and are easily avulsed during the dissection. Bleeding also makes perforation of the stomach or esophagus more likely as the dissection is very close to both.

Diagnostic Considerations and Indications for Procedure

Esophagogastroduodenoscopy (EGD) is considered the first-line test for the diagnosis of peptic ulcer disease. Recent documentation of *Helicobacter pylori* as a causative factor in gastroduodenal ulcer has had a dramatic effect on the medical treatment of this common disease. *H. pylori* can be diagnosed by biopsy (EGD) or by serum assay. If findings are positive, treatment and eradication with triple-antibiotic therapy and bismuth should occur before surgical consideration. EGD also has the advantage of determining response to medical therapy. Upper gastrointestinal radiographs are sometimes useful, mainly in obstructive disease. Hypersecretory states such as Zollinger-Ellison syndrome must be excluded with serum gastrin levels, if clinical suspicion exists. Maximal acid output and basal acid output are helpful tests to obtain in patients whose diagnosis is not clear-cut or who have recurrent disease. They also provide good baseline information for surgeons to follow up their operative results.

In spite of improvements in medical management, surgery has a role in the treatment of chronic peptic ulcer disease. The two most common procedures performed are bilateral truncal vagotomy with antrectomy (in the United States) and HSV (in Europe and Australia). Both of these procedures can be accomplished using laparoscopic techniques. As gastrectomy is covered elsewhere in this volume, this chapter focuses on HSV only. Although outside the scope of this chapter, laparoscopic surgery also has a role in the performance of drainage procedures for obstructive peptic ulcer disease (vagotomy and gastrojejunostomy) and for perforated peptic ulcer disease (closure and omental patch).

All laparoscopic treatments of peptic ulcer disease require advanced skills including knot-tying, two-handed dissection, and suturing abilities.

Adequacy of Vagotomy

Intraoperative testing for the completeness of vagotomy is a controversial subject. The traditional approach of vital dye (Congo red) and Burge (gastric body mo-

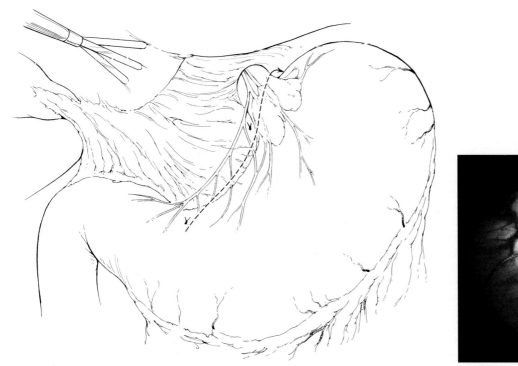

Fig. 23-1. *The nerve of Latarjet is identified as a thin, white filament descending on the lesser curve in the lesser omentum. The upper blue thread Dissection stays to the left (stomach) side of the nerve. The line of dissection passes from the lower stitch cephalad, hugging the stomach wall and passing to the left of the upper stitch toward the angle of His.* **Color inset:** *The crow's foot is demonstrated by the lowermost blue thread, with accompanying antral branches that must be protected. Dissection begins just proximal to the crow's foot.*

tor denervation) testing is very unwieldy in the laparoscopic setting. Many surgeons who performed it routinely during open procedures discarded testing as their familiarity with the anatomy improved. It is unlikely that large numbers of surgeons will gain enough experience with laparoscopic vagotomy to enjoy this luxury, especially when learning the operation. A case can be made for routine intraoperative testing for the surgeon's early experience and in a teaching setting. There is no specific equipment for laparoscopic use, although an endoscopic Congo red test is easily performed.

Instrumentation

Several instruments are essential for safe performance of the surgery:

1. Reliable sharp endoscopic scissors;
2. Pointed grasper (Maryland) for precise dissection;
3. Gently curved, angled dissector (endoscopic Lahey or Mixter);
4. Atraumatic grasper to retract the stomach (Babcock or 5-mm Glassman

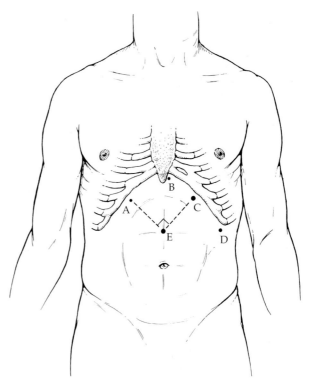

Fig. 23-2. *Cannulas must be inserted high in the upper abdomen. The main operating cannulas (two and three) should be sited at least 8 cm from the laparoscope site (cannula one) and they form a right angle with it to give an optimal operating angle. [A, 5 mm; B, 5 mm port; C, 10 mm port; D, 5 mm port; E, 10-mm camera port (A and C are 90 degrees from E).]*

grasper); the requirement is that the instrument will not tear the stomach and yet will hold tissues securely;

5. Laparoscopic ultrasonic shears (Ultra-Cision, Smithfield, Rhode Island); recent experience has shown this to be a major advance for dissection of the perigastric tissues, and it is an instrument that will considerably speed the operation.

Operative Technique

A modified lithotomy position with thigh abduction allows comfortable midline access for the operator. The video monitor is placed above the patient's head. Five cannulas are required with the sites identical to those for hiatal surgery (Fig. 23-2). The first cannula for the laparoscope is inserted after insufflation at a point at least 5 cm above the umbilicus. Cannulas two (10 mm) and three (5 mm) are inserted just below the costal margin on the left and right, respectively, so that they form a right an-

gle with cannula one at least 8 cm or more away. The size of the inverted pyramid thus formed is dependent on the distance between the xiphisternum and umbilicus and the angle between costal margins, and can be increased by inserting cannula one closer to the umbilicus. It is important to keep as high as possible, as this improves the angle at which the stomach is viewed. A 45-degree telescope is preferred, as it can compensate for cannula's one being placed too low and provides superior visualization in all cases. This cannula distribution allows the surgeon to operate at a comfortable angle, with the scissors (cannula two) in the right hand and the grasper (cannula three) in the left. The stomach is retracted through cannula four (5 mm), inserted below the costal margin as far laterally as possible by the assistant/camera operator who stands to the patient's left. The liver is elevated by a second assistant standing on the right. A smooth, round probe or grasper is inserted through cannula five (5 mm), sited at the left edge of

the xiphoid process. This cannula should be as high as possible so that its handle does not clash with instruments in cannulas one or two with the liver fully retracted.

A marking stitch is placed just to the left of the anterior vagus nerve where it appears from under the peritoneum and the phrenoesophageal ligament at the gastroesophageal junction (Fig. 23-3). A second stitch is placed at the lower limit of the planned vagotomy, usually at the level of the first branch of the crow's foot (Fig. 23-4). These two stitches are invaluable landmarks if the tissues become stained with blood or a hematoma spreads into the lesser omentum.

The direction of dissection is from caudad to cephalad, keeping medial to each stitch and extending over the anterior aspect of the cardia to the angle of His and as far posteriorly as the lateral aspect of the left crus (Fig. 23-5). Dissection of the lesser curvature vessels must be performed with extreme care to avoid tearing them, as they are fragile and thin-walled. The gastrohepatic ligament should be completely incised, and a hole made through the peritoneum above and below each vessel. This permits the insertion of a curved scissors or a gently curved, angled dissector behind the vessel. Each vessel with its accompanying nerve must be clipped and divided. The tip of each clip should be visible beyond the vessel after its closure to ensure security. Hemostasis is critically important, as small amounts of blood can stain the tissues, making subsequent identification of the neurovascular pedicles difficult. The dissection hugs the wall of the stomach and esophagus, and therefore injury to either viscus is possible if the surgical field is not kept free of blood.

All anterior leaflet vessels are clipped in this way and then divided, leaving the anterior leaf completely opened from the crow's foot to the angle of His (Fig. 23-6). This saves time by reducing repetitive changes of dissector, clip applier, and scissors. Ultrasonic shears can solely coagulate and divide these vessels without fear of heat or current propagation involving the vagus nerve trunks or stomach wall.

Smaller intermediate leaflet vessels can be controlled by simple electrocautery, allowing the lesser curve to roll anteriorly. To prevent injury to the anterior and posterior vagus nerves contained in the lesser omentum on the patient's right and in the

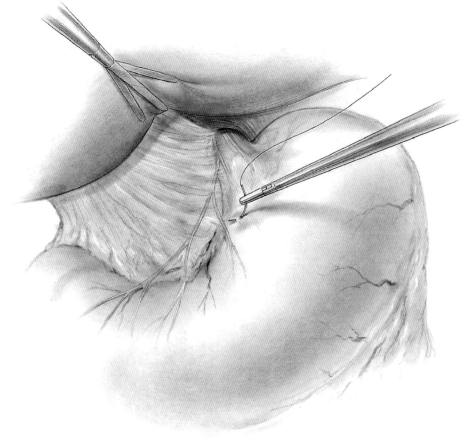

Fig. 23-3. A stitch marks the site where the anterior gastric nerve appears from under the phrenoesophageal attachments.

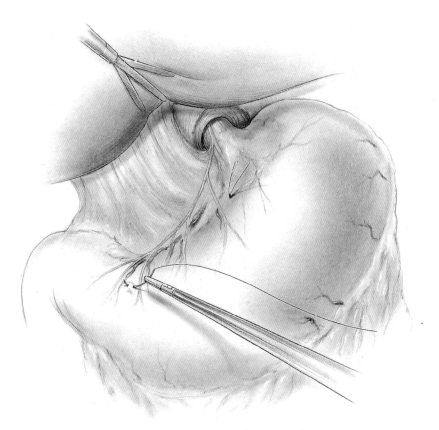

Fig. 23-4. *A second stitch is placed just after the first branch of the crow's foot.*

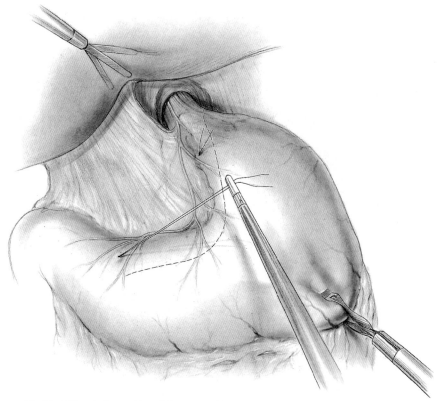

Fig. 23-5. *The relative position of the two marking stitches is seen with traction on the stomach.*

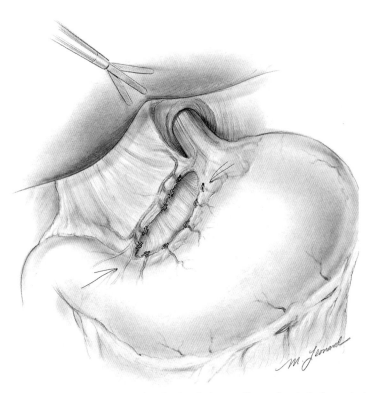

Fig. 23-6. *The anterior leaf dissection is complete, leaving the intermediate and posterior leaves (not seen) yet to be dissected.*

progressively denuded lesser curve to the left, it is essential to stay precisely on the gastric serosa and no deeper.

To begin the division of the posterior leaflet, gentle blunt dissection at a right angle to the plane of the lesser omentum is used to create a window into the lesser sac just above the lower limit of dissection of the crow's foot (Fig. 23-7). Using an atraumatic clamp, the greater curve of the stomach is next elevated, causing the omentum to hang like a curtain (Fig. 23-8). The omentum is incised, and several filmy avascular layers posterior to this are divided with scissors to create an opening into the lesser sac.

This exposes the posterior aspect of the stomach, which can then be regrasped with atraumatic forceps to elevate the greater curve and expose the posterior crow's foot. The posterior vagus nerve is visible crossing an arcade of vessels at this point (Fig. 23-9). The vessel marking the lower end of the posterior dissection is selected and, following dissection, is clipped and divided. Higher up in the lesser sac

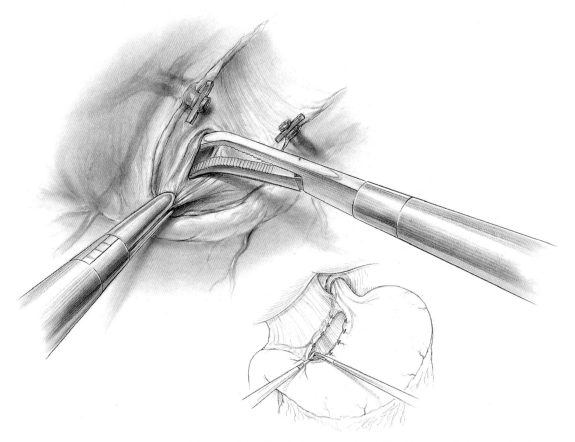

Fig. 23-7. *By hugging the lesser curve of the stomach just above incisura, gentle blunt dissection opens the lesser sac from in front.*

under a thin peritoneal fold is a fairly constant communication between the left gastric and splenic arteries that should also be clipped and divided.

A length of Penrose drain is looped around the distal stomach at the crow's foot to allow downward traction (Fig. 23-10). The Penrose also defines the completed lower limit of the dissection.

Dissection then proceeds cephalad, starting at the free edge of the divided lesser omentum and separating it from the lesser curve of the stomach. The posterior leaf will contain two to four large pedicles that should be dissected, clipped, and divided (Fig. 23-11).

By this stage, it is a simple matter to pass a grasper, held in the left hand, posterior to the esophagus but in front of the left crus to the angle of His, where the peritoneum has previously been opened anteriorly. Another short length of Penrose drain is used to encircle the esophagus, and it is secured with a clip to allow esophageal traction (Fig. 23-12).

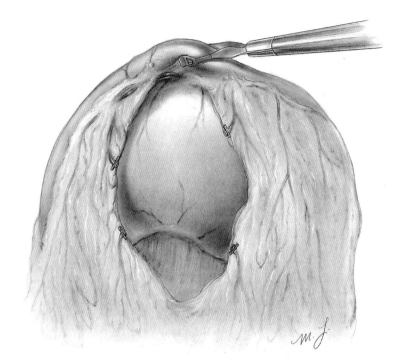

Fig. 23-8. A Babcock instrument elevates the stomach, exposing the lesser sac that has been opened by dividing fat and vessels of the omentum hanging below the stomach.

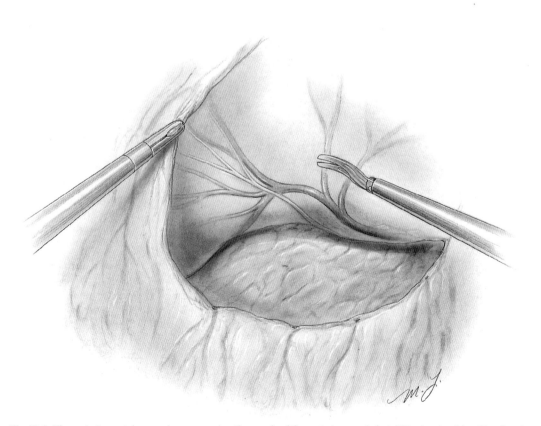

Fig. 23-9. The posterior gastric nerve is seen crossing the vessels of the posterior crow's foot. This view is achieved by elevating the posterior wall of the stomach.

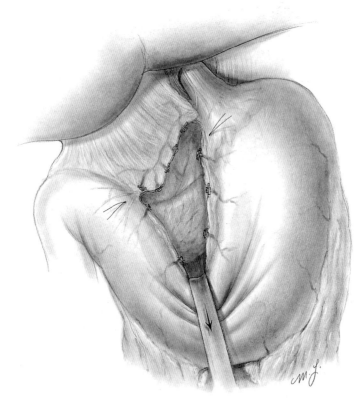

Fig. 23-10. Appearance of the lesser curve with downward traction using a Penrose drain at the lower limit of the vagotomy dissection.

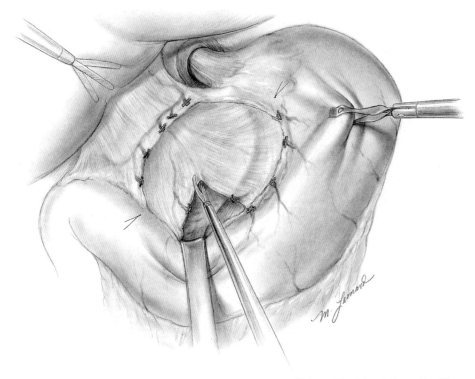

Fig. 23-11. The longitudinal fibers of the denuded lesser curve are well shown. The Babcock forceps is rolling the lesser curve anteriorly to expose the posterior aspect, thereby placing the nerve and vascular elements on traction. Small intermediate vessels can be electrocoagulated.

The stomach is lifted away from the diaphragmatic hiatus, and the peritoneal folds are divided. Gentle upward traction on the upper Penrose allows access to the under side and posterior aspect of the esophagus, which is carefully cleaned of vagal fibers under direct vision (Fig. 23-13). Five centimeters of distal esophagus should be cleared of any branches from the truncal vagus (Fig. 23-14). The epiphrenic fat pad that envelopes the cardia and lower esophagus and contains the anterior and posterior vagal nerves and left gastric vessel pedicle and its branches is gently displaced medially and cephalad. Little or no dissection is required in the mediastinum.

The gastric body becomes progressively more flaccid during the dissection due to the division of secretomotor fibers. The resulting operative field should now consist of the gastric body, still attached along the greater curve by intact short gastric vessels to the spleen. The lowermost 5 cm of the esophagus, cardia, and lesser curve have been denuded extending down to the partially divided crow's foot. The back of the stomach is completely liberated from the posterior abdominal wall, and the lesser curve vessels and the accompanying vagal fibers have been ligated and divided. Even though the distal esophagus is mobilized and the crura exposed, if not formally dissected, no antireflux procedure is usually necessary.

Intraoperative Testing

Intraoperative testing for completeness of vagotomy can be a valuable tool. There are several techniques for determining completeness of vagotomy, including intragastric electrodes, stimulated acid secretion assay, or the use of mucosal vital dyes.

Vital dye testing, most often using Congo red dye, is the most commonly used test because of its simplicity and accuracy. Congo red dye is pH-sensitive, going from red to black in the presence of an acidic pH. To perform the Congo red test, an atraumatic clamp is applied gently across the proximal antrum to close off the distal stomach. Pentagastrin, 6 μg/kg, is administered subcutaneously by the anesthesiologist about 30 minutes prior to this to stimulate acid production from the parietal cells. Next, 200 mL of a 0.5% sodium bicarbonate solution is instilled into the stomach, which is vigorously agitated to neutralize residual acid mixed with mucus in the gastric rugal folds. The sodium bicarbonate solution is aspirated and replaced with 200 mL of 0.3% Congo red in 0.5% sodium bicarbonate solution, which is again agitated to distribute it well. Intraoperative gastroscopy is then performed, the dye solution aspirated, and the stomach wall inspected for telltale areas of black pigment. The stomach should be well distended to flatten out the rugae. Air leakage can be minimized by gentle tightening of the upper Penrose loop around the esophagus and endoscope. If an area of incompletely denervated mucosa is identified, the responsible nerve branch must be found and divided. Special attention should be given to the left posterior quadrant of the gastric fundus. Evidence of acid secretion in this area indicates persistent innervation from small branches of the main vagus trunk ("criminal nerves of Grassi"). If the dye turns black in the lower fundus or antrum, it indicates persistent innervation from the lower vagus or from vagal branches following the gastroepiploic vessels. Additional dissection is indicated with division of the gastroepiploic arcade 6 cm proximal to the pylorus.

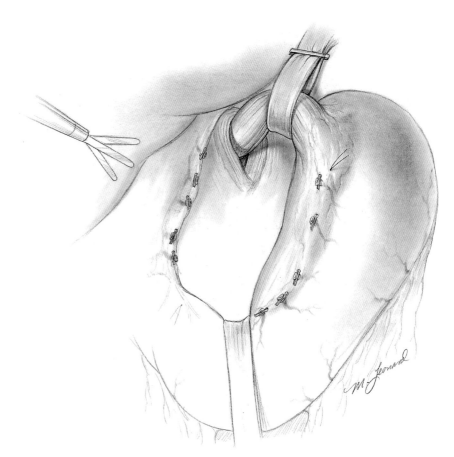

Fig. 23-12. *Elevation of the esophagus with the Penrose loop helps in the exposure of the bare area of the posterior aspect of the stomach.*

Postoperative Care

All patients are ambulated the same day as surgery. A urinary catheter or nasogastric tube is not routinely inserted. Injectable pain medication (meperidine hydrochloride [Demerol HCl]) is utilized for the first 12 hours. Oral pain medication (oxycodone or acetaminophen) is begun on the first postoperative morning along with clear fluids. By the second day, patients should be tolerating solid foods and can be discharged.

Complications

Problems related to the laparoscopic part of the procedure declare themselves early. Those specifically related to the vagotomy can become apparent early or late. Bleeding after laparoscopic surgery is distinctly uncommon but can occur either from the dissection field or from the trocar sites. All wounds should be inspected for active

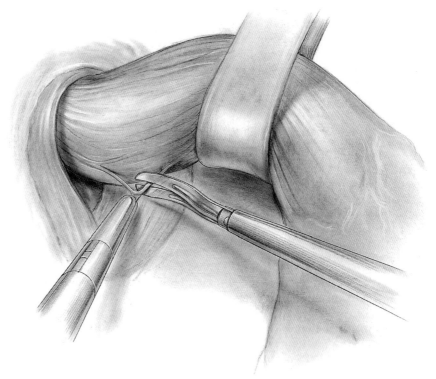

Fig. 23-13. *The esophagus is meticulously dissected for 5 cm of its intraabdominal course to divide any small vagal filaments passing in the fascial bands, seen here in the scissors blade.*

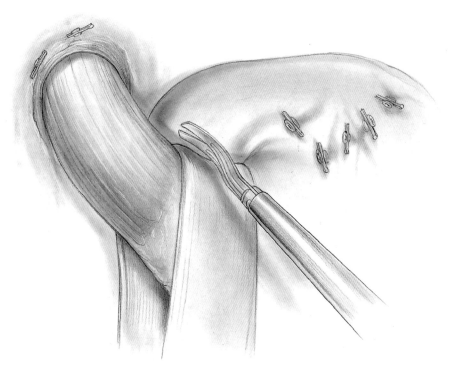

Fig. 23-14. Traction downward and to the right gives access to the lateral aspect of the esophagus and fundus of the stomach, which must be completely freed from the crura.

bleeding from within during cannula removal. All puncture sites 10-mm and larger should be sutured at the fascial level to prevent herniation and subsequent obstruction. Any clinical signs of obstruction require immediate relaparoscopy and visualization of all trocar sites as the first step. A hematoma in the abdominal wall can manifest itself by abnormally severe pain and swelling at the cannula site and should be treated with pressure and icepacks, if noted early, and with local heat, if detected late.

Persistent nausea and upper abdominal fullness or distention may signal an acute gastric dilatation secondary to gastroparesis, and requires prompt passage of a nasogastric tube. This complication is extremely uncommon after laparoscopic gastric procedures but needs to be treated early.

As with most laparoscopic surgery, patients' clinical course is usually benign. Any deviation from the norm deserves rapid investigation. A low-grade fever is common for the first 24 hours but unusual after the first day, its significance depending on the clinical state of the patient. Wound infection is rare but urinary, pul-

monary, or perigastric infections need to be considered if fever and pain persist.

Injury to a hollow organ should be minimal with good laparoscopic technique. Dissection should be a meticulous and hemostatic, and the stomach should only be grasped with atraumatic instruments. It is not necessary to "reperitonealize" the lesser curve, a meddlesome procedure of no proven benefit in the prevention of lesser curve necrosis. This complication is due more likely to incorporation of the full thickness of the gastric wall in a suture ligature with subsequent transmural necrosis and perforation than to true ischemic necrosis from devascularization.

Delayed complications of HSV are due to incomplete vagotomy or injury of both nerves of Latarjet. The former will be manifest by recurrent peptic ulcer disease that may be managed medically. If this fails, reoperation may be indicated. Loss of the nerves of Latarjet results in impaired gastric emptying. Prokinetic drugs are the first line of treatment for this problem. If prokinetic drugs fail, balloon dilation of the pylorus can improve gastric transit. If that is unsuccessful, an operative drainage procedure is needed.

Suggested Reading

Cadiere GB, Himpens J, Bruyns J. Laparoscopic proximal gastric vagotomy. *Endosc Surg Allied Technol* 1994;2:105–108.

Dallemagne B, Weerts JM, Jehaes C, Markiewicz S, Lombard R. Laparoscopic highly selective vagotomy *Br J Surg* 1994;81:554–556.

Goligher JC. A technique for highly selective (parietal cell or proximal gastric) vagotomy for duodenal ulcer. *Br J Surg* 1974;61:337–345.

Johnston D, Wilkinson A. Selective vagotomy with innervated antrum without drainage procedure for duodenal ulcer. *Br J Surg* 1969;56:626.

Stabile BE. Current surgical management of duodenal ulcers. *Surg Clin North Am* 1992;72:335–356.

Wilkinson JM, Hosie KB, Johnson AG. Long-term results of highly selective vagotomy: a prospective study with implications for future laparoscopic surgery. *Br J Surg* 1994;81:1469–1471.

EDITOR'S COMMENT

The development of effective treatments for *H. pylori* infection has made elective surgery for peptic ulcer disease an unusual procedure. Emergency surgery for complications of peptic ulcer disease remain a fairly frequent occurrence, and there are some patients who have resistant disease in spite of the current improvements in medical therapy. For these patients, a less invasive method of surgical treatment is ideal. Laparoscopic access has allowed the application of the full spectrum of antipeptic surgical procedures, including vagotomy and antrectomy, vagotomy and pyloroplasty, completion vagotomy transthoracically, subtotal gastrectomy, and variants of HSV.

HSV has proven to be a successful and well tolerated alternative to more radical resectional ulcer surgery. If it is performed well, the ulcer cure rates are good (greater than 85%), and, most important, the potential side effects of dumping, bile reflux, or marginal ulceration are less. Minimization of these side effects of ulcer surgery are increasingly important to patients, physicians, and third-party payers.

Early reports of laparoscopic HSV utilized alternative procedures, such as posterior truncal vagotomy with anterior leaflet dissection or posterior truncal vagotomy with anterior seromyotomy (Taylor procedure), that were uniquely amenable to the laparoscopic approach. These procedures performed open had a sound theoretical basis and were championed by a few surgeons, although they had not achieved widespread adoption. This created concerns that surgeons were letting the access dictate the operation and potentially compromising patient outcomes. As laparoscopic tools improved and laparoscopic surgeons became more comfortable with complex dissections, many surgeons began performing laparoscopic HSV using the same methods described for the open procedure.

Dr. Salky and Dr. Edye have also followed this precept, nicely describing the technique of formal laparoscopic HSV in this chapter. They stress the importance of a thorough preoperative evaluation and workup, including endoscopy with biopsy and upper gastrointestinal contrast studies when indicated. They emphasize the importance of a thorough dissection of the vagus nerves done in a safe and atraumatic manner to prevent injury to the nerve trunks, stomach, and esophagus. Their technique is performed in much the same way as open HSV, using meticulous dissection, clips, and division of vascular and nervous structures. Other authors have described using alternative technologies such as ultrasonic coagulating shears to achieve the same results with less operative time. The authors also stress the importance of intraoperative testing to assure the completeness of the vagotomy, and I would agree with this as well. Congo red testing, while not perfect, offers fairly reliable intraoperative assessment of the completeness of vagotomy and should be performed, when possible. In my experience, the test reveals that innervated gastric mucosa requiring additional nerve division remains in 18% of patients.

Adoption of time-proven procedures and meticulous technique will ensure a place for surgery for ulcer disease in the small patient population that continues to require such treatment.

L.L.S.

24

Totally Intraabdominal Laparoscopic Billroth II Gastrectomy and Gastric Bypass Procedures

Peter M. Y. Goh, Ahmet Alponat, and Walter T. L. Tan

The use of laparoscopy to perform major gastric resections and reconstructions was first described in 1992. These procedures have slowly been adopted around the world using various techniques. It is no surprise that the Billroth II type of gastrectomy has been the most frequently described procedure, as this operation lends itself well to reconstruction by stapling. The laparoscopic approach has also been described for other gastric operations, including Billroth I gastrectomy, wedge resection, and total gastrectomy. In addition to totally laparoscopic gastric resections, procedures using gasless techniques (elevating the abdominal wall with mechanical retractors and avoiding insufflation of the abdomen with carbon dioxide) have been described by several authors. The indications for laparoscopic gastrectomy have recently been expanded to include early gastric cancer and palliative resections for advanced gastric cancer. Although the number of operations done worldwide for cancer is small, preliminary results are quite encouraging.

The techniques described in this chapter focus on a totally laparoscopic gastric resection with Billroth II reconstruction as would be done for a benign ulcer at the incisura of the stomach. This demonstrates the basic techniques and instruments required for any laparoscopic or laparoscopic-assisted gastric resection.

Indications and Contraindications

Indications for laparoscopic gastrectomy include the following:

1. Failure of gastric peptic ulcer to heal af-

ter 3 months of well supervised, intensive medical treatment. Biopsies must be performed to exclude malignancy.
2. Gastric ulcer that continues to bleed after failure of endoscopic control.
3. Perforated gastric ulcer with minimal soilage.
4. Failure of chronic duodenal or pyloric channel ulcer to heal after *Helicobacter pylori* eradication, or other complications of ulcer disease such as recurrent bleeding or ulcer complicated by stricture.
5. Early gastric cancer or palliative resection in advanced gastric carcinoma.

Relative contraindications to laparoscopic gastrectomy include the following:

1. Patients with previous upper abdominal surgery,
2. Patients with cardiopulmonary disease who would not tolerate prolonged carbon dioxide pneumoperitoneum,
3. Patients with gastric malignancy other than very early or very late stages that would benefit from radical lymph node clearance,
4. Very old (greater than 80 years) or very ill patients.

Laparoscopic gastrectomy is absolutely contraindicated in patients with multiple medical problems such as cardiac, pulmonary, or end-stage hepatic diseases who are therefore unfit for general anesthesia.

Patient Positioning, Team, and Instruments

Surgery is performed under general anesthesia with intubation and muscle relax-

ation. At induction, a third-generation cephalosporin is given for antibiotic prophylaxis, as the operation is potentially contaminated. The patient is positioned supine with the legs apart supported by flat leg supports. The arms are also extended on both sides on arm boards. A nasogastric tube and urinary catheter are inserted. The operating table is positioned at a 20-degree reverse Trendelenburg position. The surgeon stands between the legs with one assistant on each side. Two monitors are placed over the patient's shoulders. The scrub nurse stands on the right side next to the patient's right leg (Fig. 24-1).

Trocar Placement

Positioning of the trocars may be varied in each individual case, depending on the configuration of the body and the type of procedure being performed. Generally, it follows the approximate locations indicated in Fig. 24-2. Five trocars are usually sufficient for a Billroth II gastrectomy. The first 10-mm trocar used for the laparoscope is inserted using the open technique at the umbilicus. The other four trocars are all 12 mm and are positioned in each quadrant as illustrated.

Operative Technique

A 30-degree 10-mm laparoscope attached to a three-chip charge-coupled device camera is inserted via the umbilical port. The abdomen is surveyed, and the site of the ulcer is identified. If the external signs of ulcer or cancer are not distinct enough to recognize, which happens occasionally, flexible gastroscopy is helpful in locating

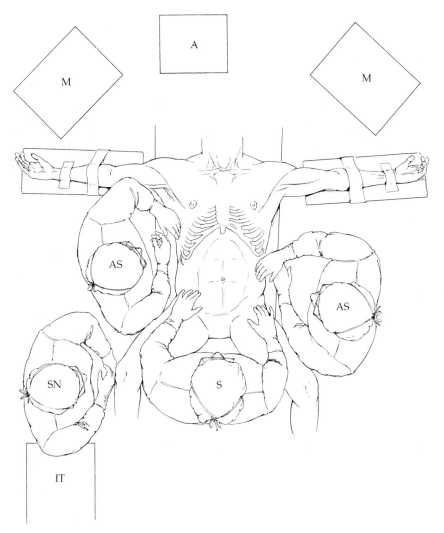

Fig. 24-1. Operating room setup. (S, surgeon; IT, instrument table; SN, scrub nurse; AS, assistant surgeon; M, monitor; A, anesthesia.)

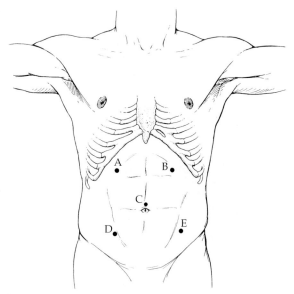

Fig. 24-2. Position of the trocars. (A, 12 mm; B, 12 mm; C, 10-mm camera; D, 12 mm.)

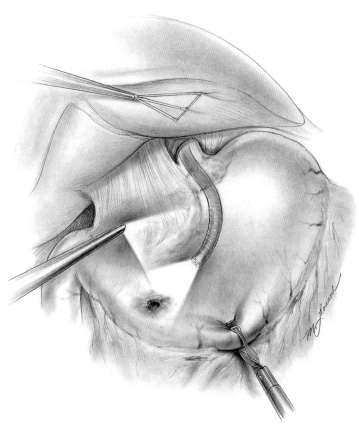

Fig. 24-3. Use of flexible endoscopy to identify the lesion and final landmarks.

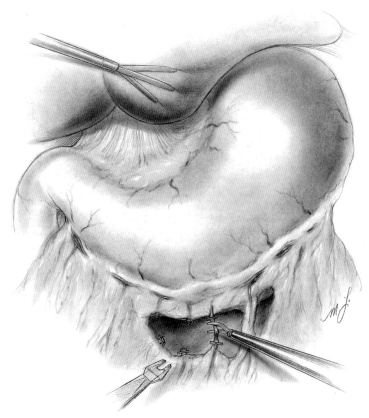

Fig. 24-4. Mobilization of the greater curve.

the pathology (Fig. 24-3). It can also help determine the level of resection and identify the pylorus, and therefore should always be available for these procedures.

Dissection of the Greater Curve

Dissection begins on the greater curve of the stomach. Two endoscopic Babcock forceps are inserted through both hypochondrial trocars. The greater curve is grasped and lifted anteriorly. Mobilization of the distal two-thirds of the greater curve is performed by means of sharp dissection and monopolar electrocautery. Alternatively, an ultrasonic coagulating shears (UltraCision, Smithfield, Rhode Island) can simplify this process by simultaneous sealing and transecting of vessels smaller than 5 mm in size. Large branches of the gastroepiploic vessels are secured with Endoclips (United States Surgical Corporation, Norwalk, Connecticut) before division (Fig. 24-4). In thinner individuals with less fat in the greater omentum, the dissection can be kept outside the epiploic arcade in the avascular plane, avoiding the time-consuming dissection and multiple clipping of small feeding vessels required with dissections along the greater curve of the stomach.

Mobilization of the Duodenum and Lesser Curve

Mobilization of the duodenum is started along its inferior border. A number of small vessels at this border and posterior to first part of duodenum are connected to the pancreas. Dissection in this area should be done slowly and very carefully by a combination of electrocautery and careful, sharp dissection with cautery scissors (Fig. 24-5). Alternatively, ultrasonic coagulating shears may be used for any vessels up to 5 mm in size. The vessels larger than 5 mm should be clipped. Securing the vascular supply of this area is mandatory before dividing the duodenum. The posterior aspect of the duodenum is handled in the same manner. Application of too many clips on the duodenal transection line should be avoided because they may interfere with endoscopic stapling (Endo GIA) during subsequent transection.

Transection of the Duodenum

After the inferior and posterior aspects of the duodenum have been fully mobilized, a small window is opened in the lesser sac just above the superior aspect of the duodenum to enable the 30-mm endoscopic stapler to be applied across the proximal duodenum (Fig. 24-6). Before stapling, it is imperative that the entire first part of the duodenum is free circumferentially. If it is not transected with a single stapler application, a second staple load should be applied. The stapler will transect the duodenum and seal each end of the resection margin with three rows of staples. Mobilization then proceeds by dividing the avascular plane between the stomach and the liver using the same technique as with the greater curve dissection. Care must be taken in dissecting the thickened area of lesser omentum adjacent to the incisura angularis, which is vascular and prone to bleeding. The dissection should preferentially be made through the less vascular area close to the liver. Alternatively, this area, including the descending branch of left gastric artery, can be divided with the 30-mm endoscopic stapler using a vascular-staple load.

Transection of the Stomach

The level of gastric resection is chosen proximal to any lesions, and the resection line is drawn by superficially cauterizing the anterior surface of the stomach at this level. An endoscopic Babcock is inserted via the left lower trocar, and the greater curve is held just distal to the resection line and stretched downward to ease the application of an endoscopic stapler. The stapler is inserted via the left hypochondrial trocar, and the transection is accomplished with four or five applications, starting from the greater curvature to the lesser curvature along the previously marked transection line (Fig. 24-7). Applications of the subsequent staple loads must be started at the apex of the resection line. Alternatively, the transection can be performed with two applications of a 60-mm endoscopic stapler. However, this instrument requires a larger port (15 mm), and when it is inserted through the left hypochondrial trocar, which gives the best angle for application, there is often not enough room to open the jaws. If the stapler is inserted through the left lower quadrant trocar, the resulting resection line may be too vertical and cause a narrowing of the gastric outlet. After division, the gastric specimen is placed into a specimen bag and left above the right lobe of the liver.

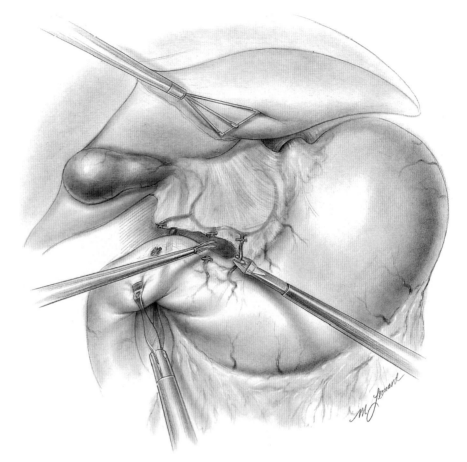

Fig. 24-5. Mobilization of the duodenum and lesser curvature.

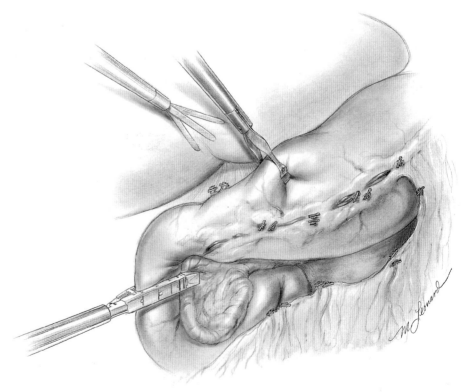

Fig. 24-6. Transecting the duodenum.

Construction of the Gastrojejunal Anastomosis

The laparoscope is inserted in the lower abdominal trocar. An endoscopic Babcock is inserted via the right hypochondrial trocar, and the transverse colon is retracted cephalad with the patient in a steep Trendelenburg position. The ligament of Treitz is identified, and a point 20 cm distal to the junction is brought superiorly anterior to the transverse colon to create an antecolic anastomosis. The patient is then placed in a steep reverse Trendelenburg. The jejunal loop is held against the gastric remnant with a Babcock, and the position is adjusted to facilitate the creation of a gastrojejunostomy anastomosis without tension or kinking. The anastomosis can be either isoperistaltic (afferent loop on the greater curve) or antiperistaltic (efferent loop on the greater curve). However, the possibility of narrowing of the efferent limb of the anastomosis is probably reduced if the antiperistaltic technique is used. Two intracorporeal stay sutures are placed to hold the gastric stump and jejunum together. Two small openings are created with electrocautery, one on the anterior wall of the stomach close to the lesser curve and proximal to resection line and one on the antimesenteric aspect of the jejunum (Fig. 24-8). The anastomosis is created from lesser curve to greater curve. During stapling, the surgeon changes his position to the patient's right and the camera operator moves between the legs. The 30-mm endoscopic stapler is inserted via the right hypochondrial trocar and then positioned with one jaw in each of the enterotomies (Fig. 24-9). If there is difficulty in placing the jaws into the enterotomies, additional stay sutures can be placed to align the enterotomies better. The stapler creates an anastomosis between the stomach and the jejunal loop. This anastomosis is enlarged to 6 cm with a second firing of the stapler across the apex of the V of the first staple line. During this step, it is important to pull the stab wound margins against the hilt of the stapler to maximize the anastomotic length (Fig. 24-10). The anastomosis can alternatively be done with the 60-mm endoscopic stapler if one is willing to change the trocar to a larger 15-mm port. The common openings then become a single defect that can be closed by additional applications of the stapler across it. An alternative is to close the common enterotomies with one or two layers of running absorbable sutures (2-0 Vicryl or Polysorb) on a 30-mm curved nee-

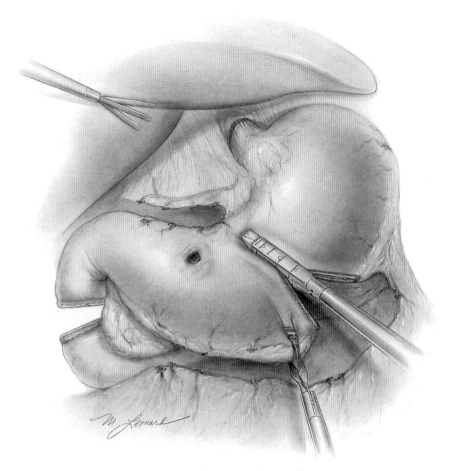

Fig. 24-7. Transecting the stomach.

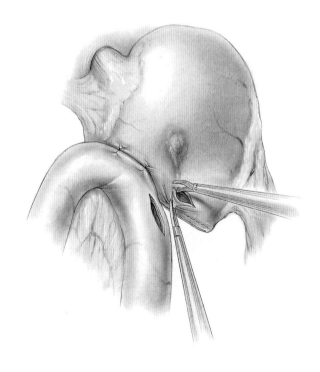

Fig. 24-8. Creating small openings for stapler application.

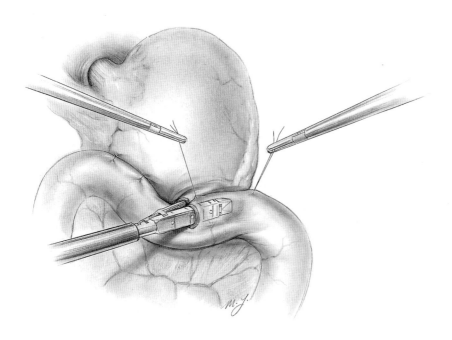

Fig. 24-9. Stapled gastrojejunostomy.

ated using either endoscopic scissors or a hook and cautery. Cautery is necessary, as bleeding, particularly from the gastric wall, may be troublesome. Therefore, electrocautery should be used to divide all layers of the stomach, and hemostasis at the gastrotomy site should be obtained by precisely picking up the tiny bleeding points with fine coagulating forceps. Once the gastrotomy and enterotomy are completed, the anastomosis is completed in two layers of continuous sutures (Fig. 24-12). As suturing is ergonomically easier working toward oneself, each layer is completed with a separate suture working in the same direction. To avoid time-consuming end-knotting, absorbable suture clips (Lapra Ty, Ethicon, Cincinnati, Ohio) can be used for securing both the proximal and the distal ends. The Endostitch device promises to facilitate rapid continuous suturing.

Modifications for Performing Gastroenterostomy without Gastrectomy

Performing a gastric bypass without gastrectomy is very similar to the procedure described above. First, a dependent site is identified on the greater curve of the stomach. The anastomosis may be made on ei-

dle either by intracorporeal suture technique or by Endostitch (United States Surgical Corporation, Norwalk, Connecticut). It is important to staple or suture this defect transversely to create a "plasty" effect to prevent the narrowing that could occur with simple closure (Fig. 24-11).

Totally Hand-sutured Anastomotic Technique

Although hand-suturing is time-consuming, it is significantly cheaper. We prefer a continuous, two-layered anastomosis using a parrot-beaked needle holder and flamingo-beaked knotting forceps (Karl Storz, Tutlingen, Germany). It is recommended that the surgeon stand on the patient's right and the camera operator move

to between the legs. The left lower quadrant and right lower quadrant trocars are used for the needle holders. As a first step, two stay sutures are placed at the proposed anastomosis, and a posterior seromuscular layer is created with a running 3-0 Vicryl suture on a 30-mm curved needle. The gastrotomy and enterotomy are cre-

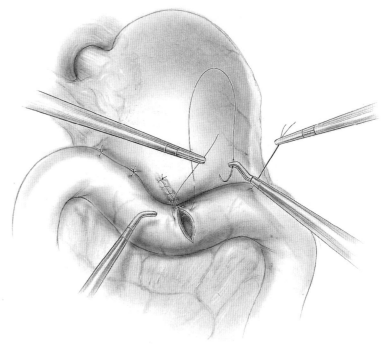

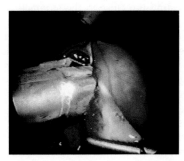

Fig. 24-10. Stages of performing gastrojejunostomy.

Fig. 24-11. Suturing the common stab wound.

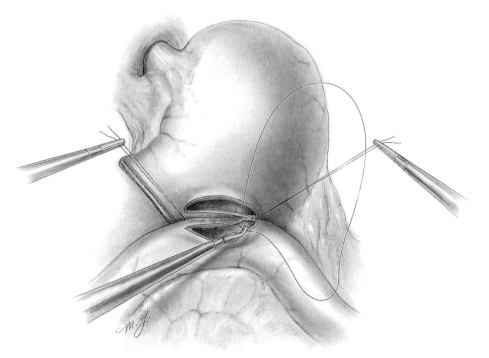

Fig. 24-12. Hand-sutured anastomosis.

ther the anterior or the posterior wall and should be positioned about 1 to 2 cm away from the vessels entering the greater curve. If a posterior wall anastomosis is preferred, it is necessary to detach part of the greater omentum using the techniques described for gastrectomy. It is only necessary to detach enough for the posterior wall of the stomach to be visualized easily and the anastomosis to be constructed. The appropriate loop of jejunum is located by running the small bowel and is attached to the site of anastomosis on the stomach using two intracorporeal stay sutures. Again, the surgeon may do an iso- or antiperistaltic anastomosis and either an ante- or retrocolic one, as he or she prefers. Two short enterotomies are created on one side of the anastomotic line, and the endoscopic stapler is applied with one jaw in each hole. If the 30-mm stapler is used, a second or even a third application may be necessary. The minimum size of the anastomosis is 6 cm. The remaining common enterotomy is then closed with a running intracorporeal suture line of 2-0 absorbable suture material, as described above.

Checking the Anastomosis

At the completion of the procedure, upper gastrointestinal endoscopy is performed to check for leakage and ensure the patency of the anastomosis. Air is insufflated through the scope to distend the stomach while the anastomosis is bathed with saline irrigation. The laparoscopic team looks for bubbles coming through the anastomotic line, indicating a leak. The endoscopy is also done to visualize the patency of both afferent and efferent limbs of the jejunal loop.

Extraction of the Specimen

The umbilical port site is enlarged to 2 cm by incising the fascia vertically. The specimen is grasped by the duodenal end and extracted through the umbilical opening using a spiral-twisting motion. Removal of the specimen in a plastic bag is not needed in ulcer cases; however it is mandatory in cancer surgery. To perform extraction using a bag, the specimen is first placed above the left lobe of the liver. A large retrieval bag is introduced through the enlarged umbilical port and held open by the assistant while the specimen is inserted. The neck of the bag is then withdrawn through the umbilical site. The specimen can then either be grasped within the bag and extracted or morselized and removed. Morselization may, however, compromise the ability of the pathologist to interpret margins. The trocar wounds are closed in two layers and bupivacaine hydrochloride

1% is infiltrated around the wounds for postoperative pain relief.

Laparoscopic-assisted Gastrectomy

For this technical variation, dissection and transection of both duodenum and stomach are completed laparoscopically. A small incision is then made in the upper abdomen over the site of the proposed anastomosis, and the jejunal limb and gastric stump are brought out. The anastomosis can then be completed as in open surgery by either hand-suturing or standard stapling technique. This technique saves a number of stapler applications and is attractive where cost and time factors are paramount.

Postoperative Care

Laparoscopic gastrectomy patients have a somewhat shorter recovery period than patients following an open gastrectomy. There is less pain, and patients are ambulatory on the first postoperative day. Since gastrointestinal function returns more quickly after laparoscopic surgery, patients can usually take fluids by the third day and a regular diet by the fifth day. Discharge from the hospital is usually within 1 week if there are no complications.

Complications
Bleeding

Meticulous hemostasis is vital in laparoscopic gastrectomy as it is in all laparoscopic interventions. Once bleeding occurs, the resulting accumulated blood obscures the view and frustrates the surgeon. Furthermore, it absorbs light and darkens the video image. Bleeding is often related to the wrong choice of dissection planes or too great a dependency on endoscopic staplers.

Dissecting too close to the stomach edge, where there are more vessels, should be avoided. Close dissection of the stomach edge is necessary only where the transection will occur. The majority of the greater curve mobilization is best confined to the avascular plane outside the epiploic arcade. It is tempting to use endoscopic staplers to divide the mesentery along the lesser and greater curvature, but these staplers are not adequately hemostatic, and much time will be spent trying to control bleeding from the staple line. Meticulous and patient dissection and control of individual vessels by ligatures or clips are preferable. The ultrasonic coagulating shears has simplified some of this tedious dissection by allowing the surgeon to boldly cut through the perigastric vascular fatty tissue without excessive bleeding. There is, however, a limit to the size of the vessel that can be controlled by this device. Vessels greater than 1.5 mm or so probably should be clipped or ligated.

Anastomotic Obstruction

Compromise of the gastric pouch can easily occur when a 60-mm endoscopic stapler is used. The best angle for transection is achieved using the left subcostal trocar. Unfortunately, the 60-mm endoscopic stapler cannot be opened when inserted through this trocar. There is simply insufficient space between the abdominal wall and the greater curve of the stomach to allow enough of the stapler to be inserted to open the jaws. The 60-mm endoscopic stapler works best when inserted through the left iliac trocar, but this vertical angle may result in transecting the stomach higher on the lesser curve than intended, resulting in a small gastric pouch or even compromising the esophageal lumen (Fig. 24-13). To avoid this, it is preferable to use the 30-mm stapler through the left upper port.

Either the afferent or efferent loop may be narrowed when the common enterotomies of the gastrojejunostomy are closed with a stapler. This complication is best avoided by suturing the common stab wounds in a transverse fashion with a fine, running suture line. If a narrowing is detected on intraoperative gastroscopy, the anastomosis can be revised, or if only one limb is restricted, a side-to-side jejunojejunostomy can be constructed with an 30-mm endoscopic stapler or hand-suturing. Alternatively, a quicker but more invasive technique would be to expose the narrowed anastomosis and construct the jejunojejunostomy by open surgical technique through a minilaparotomy located precisely over the site by laparoscopic localization. Attention should also be paid to the positioning of the jejunal loop. Additional interrupted sutures may be needed to prevent afferent or efferent limb kinking.

Anastomotic Failure

Misfiring of a stapler or inadequate suturing (thankfully rare) can lead to defects in

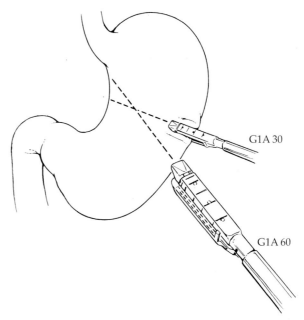

Fig. 24-13. Use of the 60-mm endoscopic stapler may result in a bad angle for gastric resection.

the anastomotic line and result in catastrophe. This can occur at the duodenal stump or at the gastrojejunostomy anastomotic site. The anastomotic line should be carefully checked intraoperatively by gastroscopy or by instilling methylene blue via a nasogastric tube; any defects are repaired using an endoscopic suturing technique. If the operator is not adept at endoscopic techniques, the repair can be sutured through a small incision using open surgical techniques. Rarely, defects can be closed by the imaginative use of staplers. The new Endo TA stapler device (United States Surgical Corporation, Norwalk, Connecticut) can be very effective in these situations.

Incidental Findings of Malignancy

Although multiple biopsies have been taken to exclude malignancy before operation, an unexpected area of malignancy may be discovered in the ulcer after resection. In most cases, the laparoscopic gastrectomy itself is curative, depending of course on the stage and type of the cancer. In patients with invasive cancer, a subsequent open surgical resection and lymphadenectomy should be performed for cure. Data reported from Japanese experience with local resection for stages I and II gastric cancers do not support the need for radical lymphadenectomy and may indi-

cate that laparoscopic resections are adequate for cure.

Discussion

Laparoscopic gastrectomy and reconstruction have been adopted and performed in many centers throughout the world with satisfactory results. With advances in the medical treatment of gastric ulcers (particularly the ability to eradicate *H. pylori*), the indications for surgery seem to have decreased. Nevertheless, there remain many complications of gastric ulcer that occasionally warrant gastrectomy. In North America, where vagotomy and antrectomy have remained the standard operation for complicated duodenal ulcers, there is certainly a place for laparoscopic resections of this sort. It is a natural extension of this patient-friendly procedure to take the next step into the realm of cancer surgery. There are some centers in Europe where radical cancer resection is being actively pursued using this technique with the addition of a radical lymphadenectomy. Some reasonable early result have been produced in Italy and Belgium. It has even been possible to perform total gastrectomy with the aid of endoscopic circular staplers. Esophagogastrectomy for proximal gastric tumors has also been performed with a thoracoscopic anastomosis in the chest. In Asia, where many stomach cancers are discovered early, there may also be a role for laparoscopy in the treatment of these early gastric cancers by laparoscopic wedge resection or a partial gastrectomy, as described.

The main constraints to the widespread adoption of this procedure is the cost of stapling and the technical demands on the surgeon. This is certainly not an operation for the novice laparoscopic surgeon. Increasing experience with advanced laparoscopy and improvement in instrumentation and technique will of course change this in time.

Conclusion

There are certainly advantages to laparoscopic gastrectomy. It offers the promise of less pain, less immobility, quicker alimentation, shorter hospitalization, fewer wound and respiratory complications, and earlier return to normal daily activities. Indications for this technique are expanding to include early gastric cancer and palliative resection for late gastric cancer. The main drawbacks of this technique are its cost and technical difficulty. Most costs, however, are related to the expense of the stapling devices, and these are optional. Almost all anastomoses can be hand-sutured if one has adequate instruments and experience. With sufficient experience, the average operation time can be between 2.5 and 3.5 hours.

Surgeons will be inspired by the prompt recovery and superior mobility profile in their early cases. However, the real benefit of this procedure will not be scientifically proven for some time due to the rarity of suitable cases and the resulting small series. To fully evaluate this procedure, we need long-term follow-up of all patients and well constructed studies looking at the results for gastric malignancies.

Suggested Reading

Anvari M, Park A. Laparoscopic-assisted vagotomy and distal gastrectomy. *Surg Endosc* 1994; 8:1312–1315.

Azagra JS, Goergen M. Laparoscopic total gastrectomy. In: Meinero M, Melotti G, Mouret PH, eds. *Laparoscopic surgery*. Milan: Masson, 1993: 289–296.

Goh P. Laparoscopic Billroth II gastrectomy. *Semin Laparosc Surg* 1994;1:171–181.

Goh P, Kum CK. Laparoscopic Billroth II gastrectomy: a review. *Surg Oncol* 1993;2(suppl 1): 13–18.

Goh P, Tekant Y, Kum CK, Isaac J, Shang NS. Totally intra-abdominal laparoscopic Billroth II gastrectomy. *Surg Endosc* 1992;6:160.

Johanet H, Cossa J, Hamdan M, Marmuse J, LeGoff JY, Benhamou G. Laparosocpic gastrectomy for obstructing duodenal ulcer. *J Laparoendosc Surg* 1994;4:447–50.

Kitano S, Shimoda K, Miyahara M, et al. Laparoscopic approaches in the management of patients with early gastric carcinomas. *Surg Laparosc Endosc* 1995;5:359–362.

Kitaoka H, Yoshikawa K, Hirota T, Itabashi M. Surgical treatment of early gastric cancer. *Jpn J Clin Oncol* 1984;14:283–293.

Llorente J. Laparoscopic gastric resection for gastric leiomyoma. *Surg Endosc* 1994;8:887–889.

Lointer P, Leroux S, Ferrier C, Dapoigny M. A technique of laparoscopic gastrectomy and Billroth II gastrojejunostomy. *J Laparoendosc Surg* 1993;3:353–364.

Melotti G, Meinero M, Tamborrino E. Gastric resection for cancer. In: Meinero M, Melotti G, Mouret PH, eds. *Laparoscopic surgery*. Milan: Masson, 1993:273–282.

Uyama I, Pgiwara H, Takahara T, Kato Y, Kikuchi K, Iida S. Laparoscopic and minilaparotomy Billroth I gastrectomy for gastric ulcer using an abdominal wall-lifting method. *J Laparoendosc Surg* 1994;4:441–445.

Van Houden CE. Laparoscopic bilateral truncal vagotomy, antrectomy, and Billroth I anastomosis for prepyloric ulcer. *Surg Laparosc Endosc* 1994;4:457–60.

Watson DI, Devitt PG, Game PA. Laparoscopic Billroth II gastrectomy for early gastric cancer. *Br J Surg* 1994;82:661–662.

EDITOR'S COMMENT

Laparoscopic partial gastrectomy and reconstruction techniques are procedures that were pioneered by Dr. Goh and associates. These complex procedures are technically difficult and should only be attempted by experienced laparoscopic surgeons. The technical difficulty of these procedures lies in the large size of the organ and multiple resection lines and anastomoses required for reconstruction. As Dr. Goh has mentioned, one must take care not to compromise lumen size by improper angulation of the endoscopic stapling devices, which is easy to do in the laparoscopic environment. Improvement in laparoscopic tools, such as angulated stapling devices and ultrasonic coagulating shears, have made laparoscopic gastrectomy easier and safer to perform. In addition, other endoscopic techniques may be helpful in gastric resections. Gasless techniques, as pioneered by S. Kitano, A. Cuschieri, and others, allow the introduction of larger stapling devices through the access site that are needed at some time for removal of the specimen. Early availability of the access incision also permits an extracorporeal anastomosis to be performed. New findings also seem to indicate that there may be less risk of tumor dissemination with gasless laparoscopy for resection of gastrointestinal tumors. Another new technique that may be useful in this procedure is the pneumosleeve for hand-assisted laparoscopy. We have found this especially useful when dealing with large organs such as the stomach.

Laparoscopic treatment of gastric cancer should be approached cautiously. On one hand, the use of laparoscopy in the staging of gastrointestinal malignancy, particularly with the addition of intraoperative ultrasound, has been well demonstrated and may have a valuable place in the treatment of gastric cancer. However, it is becoming increasingly accepted that an extensive lymphadenectomy is helpful in stage T2 or greater gastric cancers. Whether or not this can be accomplished laparoscopically with the same thoroughness as it can with an open procedure remains to be discovered.

L.L.S.

25

Endoluminal Surgery

Sunil Bhoyrul and Lawrence W. Way

Since the description of laparoscopic cholecystectomy in 1987, advances in both technology and skill have enabled surgeons to perform a wide array of procedures. These operations depend on maintaining adequate exposure using a combination of pneumoperitoneum, patient position, retraction of viscera, and surgical technique that emphasizes traction and countertraction of the tissue adjacent to the area of dissection. Once surgeons develop these skills (including suturing and knot tying), the range of procedures that can be performed within the abdomen is virtually unlimited. The next technical challenge for minimally invasive surgeons has been performing surgery within the lumen of the gut, where gaining adequate exposure while maintaining the integrity of the organ is more difficult. Early attempts were made to perform pancreatic cystogastrostomy laparoscopically, but this required making a large anterior gastrostomy that had to be sutured closed and posed potential problems associated with spillage of luminal contents into the peritoneum. Furthermore, the time taken to complete these procedures was lengthened by the time taken to close the gastrostomy. The aim of this chapter is to describe the considerable advances in technology and techniques over the last few years that have made it possible to perform laparoscopic surgery within the lumen of the gut (endoluminal surgery) with adequate exposure while still maintaining the integrity of the organ.

The success of endoluminal surgery has been aided by unique trocars that allow the surgeon to insert laparoscopic instruments into the gut and maintain a tight seal around the trocar. Conventional cutting trocars are unsuitable, as the bowel wall stretches after the initial incision, leading to a loss of anchoring of the trocar and leakage of air and luminal contents from around the trocar, and a subsequent loss of exposure. One suitable endoluminal trocar is the Radially Expanding Device (RED) (Innerdyne Medical, California).

The RED consists of an 18-gauge needle used to puncture the anterior surface of a hollow organ (Fig. 25-1). The needle is encased in a silicone sheath. Once the needle enters the lumen, it is removed, leaving the sheath in place. A 5- or 7-mm cannula is then deployed through the center of the sheath, which stretches the tract in the wall of the viscera. The result is a self-sealing cannula through which 5- or 7-mm laparoscopic instruments may be passed. The integrity of the organ is maintained throughout, and on completion of the procedure, the cannulas are removed, leaving small holes on the anterior surface of the organ that usually require only a single interrupted suture for closure. Other technologies for gaining access to hollow viscera have been described, such as using a Malencot-type cannula or balloon cannula to anchor the trocar to the bowel wall.

Indications and Contraindications

Using REDs, it is possible to gain laparoscopic access to almost any lesion within the lumen of the gastrointestinal tract. Patients should of course be suitable candidates for laparoscopic surgery. Although the presence of intraabdominal adhesions is not a contraindication to laparoscopic surgery, dense adhesions on or close to the anterior surface of the organ of interest make the endoluminal operation technically more demanding and is a relative contraindication. To date, most endoluminal operations have been performed within the lumen of the stomach or duodenum. The greatest experience has been with pancreatic cystogastrostomy for patients with pancreatic pseudocysts, but there have also been reports of resection of gastric leiomyoma and diagnostic duodenoscopy. In addition, we have developed an animal model for drainage of the common bile duct via an antegrade sphincterotomy using a 5-mm laparoscope within the duodenum to visualize and direct the procedure. Others, such as Hunter, Swanstrom, Gagner, Geis, and Mori, have also performed procedures such as treatment of bleeding ulcers (Dieulafoy's vascular malformation), resection of gastric mucosal tumors, and enteroscopy of the small and large bowel. An important anatomic consideration for laparoscopic endoluminal surgery is the site of the lesion. As the rigid endoluminal trocars enter the abdomen through the anterior abdominal wall, they must also penetrate the lumen of the bowel through its anterolateral surface. This essentially limits endoluminal procedures to operating on lesions on or close to the posterior wall of the stomach. The presence of a lesion on the anterior wall is less of a problem if the organ is suspended by its own mesentery and is therefore mobile. Another technical consideration is that intracorporeal suturing is technically more demanding (because of the awkward port positions and the reduced working space) than it would be if the patient had a large enterostomy and instruments were placed directly into the lumen of the organ. Therefore, if suturing is a major part of the procedure, this

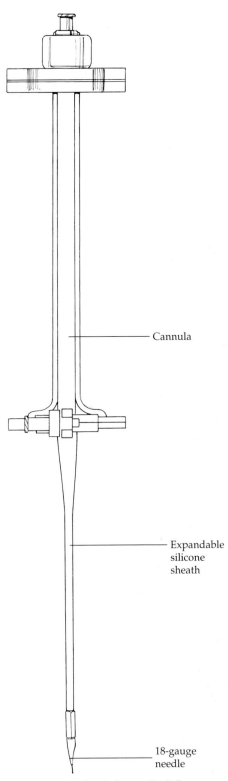

Fig. 25-1. *An intraluminal trocar (Radially Expanding Device) used to gain access to the lumen of the gut. Once the cannula is deployed using radial expansion, the balloon is used to anchor the device.*

Cannula

Expandable silicone sheath

18-gauge needle

may be a relative contraindication to a completely endoluminal operation, depending greatly on the surgeon's experience in performing endoluminal suturing. However, as discussed later, electrocautery, ultrasonic energy, and extracorporeal knot-typing techniques are sometimes acceptable alternatives to intracorporeal suturing.

Preoperative Tests

In addition to any tests specific to the lesion being treated, computed tomography (CT), endoscopy, and occasionally barium studies are used to localize the lesion as accurately as possible before surgery. This is necessary (a) to ensure that the pathology is amenable to endoluminal access (taking into account the constraints described in the previous section) and (b) to guide the surgeon in placing the first trocar through the wall of the gut. In pancreatic cystogastrostomy, the preoperative CT scan should be carefully studied to ensure that the pancreatic pseudocyst is well adhered to the posterior surface of the stomach. If the cyst is not well adhered, a posterior gastrostomy would result in an entrance into the lesser sac and would require difficult placing of sutures in the small space between the posterior wall of the stomach and the anterior wall of the pseudocyst. The pseu-

docyst may be more likely to be separate from the posterior wall of the stomach if it is a posttraumatic pseudocyst rather than one from a previous episode of acute pancreatitis. In addition to any preoperative tests, intraoperative ultrasound and flexible endoscopy may be helpful in localizing the lesion before puncture of the hollow organ with an endoluminal trocar.

Operative Technique

Patients should be prepared for a conventional laparoscopic procedure with general anesthesia, complete muscle relaxation, antibiotic prophylaxis, and avoidance of nitrous oxide as the inhalant anesthetic. The supine position is suitable for operations in the gut, but an electric table is desirable, as frequent repositioning may be required to assist in exposure. A list of additional instruments that should be made available for an endoluminal procedure is shown in Table 25-1.

One early unsuccessful modification of the endoluminal technique was to use a flexible endoscope instead of a rigid laparoscope to view and guide the surgery. Successful endoluminal surgery, however, depends on mimicking the natural eye–hand axis that the surgeon uses in open surgery and indeed in everyday life,

Table 25-1. Special Instruments Required for Endoluminal Surgery

Instruments	Notes
Radially expanding devices, 5 mm	Other intraluminal trocars, such as Malencot or balloon trocars may also be suitable
Additional insufflator and tubing	Have a connecting piece for attaching the tubing to the nasogastric tube
Rigid laparoscopes, 5 mm	Both the 0- and 30-degree laparoscopes are useful
Spinal needle	Useful to aspirate contents of pancreatic pseudocyst to confirm location
Electrocautery device, 5 mm	One with built-in suction is preferable to avoid build of smoke
Ultrasonic dissector, 5 mm	Alternative to electrocautery
Suturing instruments	Required for closing defect made by the endoluminal trocars
Extracorporeal sutures and knot pusher	Simplest way of closing defects inside the bowel
Endoloop or other performed knot	Useful for resection of pedunculated tumors
Flexible endoscopy	Useful in localizing lesion and removal of bulky specimen
Laparoscopic or endoscopic ultrasound	Useful in localizing lesion

and the surgeon soon learns the importance of placing operating ports within a 30- to 45-degree axis of the port used for the laparoscope. The loss of this relationship, as occurs when a flexible endoscope is used, makes the eye–hand coordination an unnatural and difficult one. Furthermore, the view gained from using a rigid laparoscope with a Hopkins lens (or similar) system is far superior to that using a flexible scope with the image reconstituted from a finite number of fiberoptic cables.

Access into the peritoneum with a 10-mm trocar is followed by diagnostic laparoscopy and identification of the target organ. CT scans and other preoperative tests are usually reviewed intraoperatively to assist in placing the first endoluminal trocar (RED) directly opposite the lesion. Before placement of this first RED, it is necessary to distend or splint the organ to ensure that the trocar does not perforate its posterior wall. In the case of the stomach, a second carbon dioxide insufflator should be hooked up to the nasogastric tube, and the stomach insufflated to 15 to 30 mm Hg. Distention of the stomach is facilitated by reducing the intraperitoneal pressure to 5 to 8 mm Hg. For organs other than the stomach, the wall should be steadied with a grasper to avoid perforation of the opposite wall. It is not necessary to occlude the duodenum to maintain the distention of the stomach, but performing endoluminal surgery within the small bowel may require placing a bowel clamp distal to the area of interest to maintain distention of the bowel lumen. Once the area of interest is identified, the bowel wall is punctured with the RED, with care taken not to perforate the opposite wall, and a working cannula is then deployed into the lumen of the bowel (Fig. 25-2). The insufflator tubing is then connected to the RED to maintain distention of the lumen, and the abdomen is desufflated to facilitate this distention. A 5-mm rigid laparoscope is inserted through the RED, and a diagnostic enteroscopy is performed to ensure that the opposite wall of the bowel is intact and also to localize the lesion. A 0-degree laparoscope is adequate to view the areas opposite the point where the RED enters the lumen, but it is necessary to use a 30-degree laparoscope to look at most other areas, as corners often have to be navigated and a circumferential view of the lumen cannot be gained by using the 0-degree scope. In some instances, such as localiz-

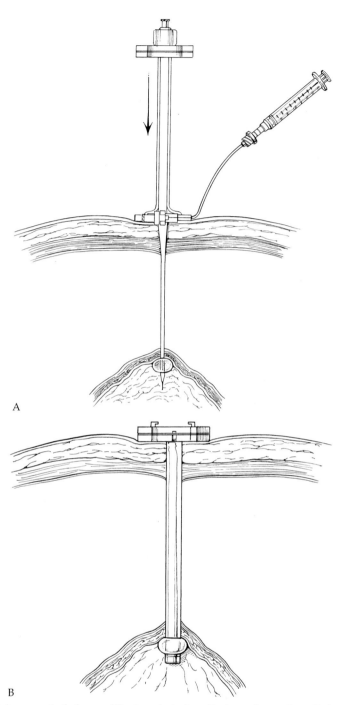

A

B

*Fig. 25-2. Gaining access to the lumen of the stomach. **A:** A needle pierces the anterior wall of stomach after the stomach has been distended with carbon dioxide instilled through the nasogastric tube. **B:** Radial expansion used to deploy cannula.*

ing a tumor or bleeding point before a planned resection of a segment of bowel, this may be all that is required from the endoluminal part of the procedure. More often, however, an additional one or two REDs are deployed into the lumen to place surgical instruments and commence the therapeutic part of the procedure. The sit-

ing of these additional trocars with respect to the lesion is critical. These cannulas should be positioned on either side of the one used for the laparoscope, and ideally so that they subtend an angle of 60- to 90-degrees with each other at the target area (Fig. 25-3). This arrangement will facilitate any technically demanding maneuvers, such as intracorporeal knot tying. In the case of a pancreatic cystogastrostomy, only one additional RED is required, but for tumor resections, two additional REDs should be deployed.

Pancreatic Cystogastrostomy

For pancreatic cystogastrostomy, a useful maneuver in localizing the cyst is to pass a spinal needle through the posterior wall of the stomach in the suspected location of the cyst. Aspiration of cyst contents confirms the location of the cyst. The site of the pseudocyst is usually suspected by a bulge on the posterior wall of the stomach.

Several surgical instruments may be used to perform the surgery. For pancreatic cystogastrostomy, we have used monopolar electrocautery on coagulation setting. We have not encountered any cases of bleeding from the edge of the cystogastrostomy that could not be controlled with monopolar electrocautery and, in our series of 21 cases so far, have never placed sutures and have not had any trouble with postoperative bleeding from the edge of the cystogastrostomy. In one case, we successfully used the hook ultrasonic dissector instead of the monopolar cautery device. Once the initial incision through the posterior wall of the stomach is made, it should be lengthened so that the opening in the pseudocyst is at least half the diameter of the cyst itself to prevent the likelihood of early closure. Gauging the size of the incision from outside the cyst alone can be misleading due to the magnification of the laparoscopic image. The direction in which to enlarge the incision is best decided by placing the laparoscope inside the cyst and judging the extension of the cyst. The cyst contents are aspirated and debrided, and any suspicious areas of the cyst wall should be biopsied if pancreatic cancer is suspected from the patient's history. The cyst contents either can be removed via the REDs or can even be placed into the duodenum. A technical pitfall is to extend the incision in the stomach beyond the edge of the cyst, in which case a hole is created into the lesser sac that has to be closed. This can be done by regaining the laparoscopic view, dividing the gastrocolic omentum, and placing sutures from behind the stomach to close the hole between the stomach and the lesser sac.

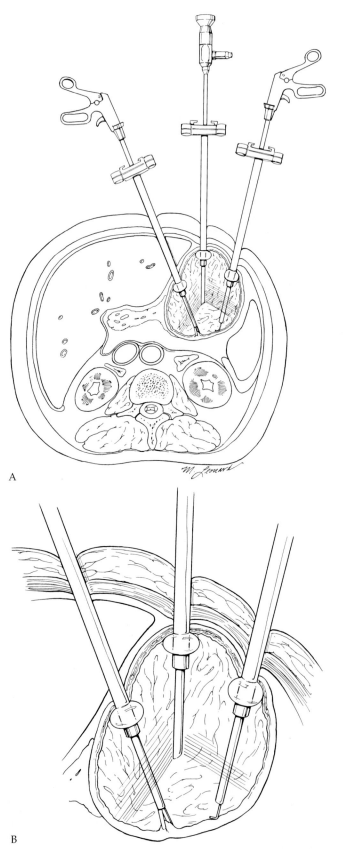

Fig. 25-3. **A:** *Ideal positioning of intraluminal trocars to restore normal eye–hand axis and facilitate technically demanding maneuvers.* **B:** *Close up of positioning.*

Benign Gastric Tumors

For removal of pedunculated benign gastric mucosal tumors, the tumor is grasped with an atraumatic grasper, and two preformed extracorporeal knots ("endoloops") are placed snugly at the base of the lesion (Fig. 25-4); the tumor is then amputated above the suture line using monopolar electrocautery. This technique should also be applicable to pedunculated tumors in other parts of the bowel. For resection of gastric tumors, we have used a flexible endoscope to retrieve the resected specimen, as this avoids having to enlarge the 5-mm puncture in the anterior wall of the stomach. In practice, these cases are usually the ones that cannot be treated with flexible endoscopy techniques.

Biliary Sphincterotomy

Laparoscopic biliary sphincterotomy using endoluminal techniques is also feasible. DePaula and Gagner have both previously described antegrade sphincterotomy of the sphincter of Oddi using a sphincterotome fed over a guidewire inserted through the cystic duct. For these cases, endoluminal visualization of the sphincter is used to guide the procedure (Fig. 25-5), and localization of the sphincter is aided by passing a guidewire antegrade through the duodenum. Although a flexible gastroscope may be used to guide the antegrade sphincterotomy (Fig. 25-6) performed at the time of laparoscopic cholecystectomy, this may be awkward with the patient supine, and additional personnel may be required to control the flexible scope. The endoluminal approach overcomes both these problems at the expense of an additional enterostomy that is to be sutured. We feel that it should be possible to perform a complete exploration and drainage of the common bile duct laparoscopically and have successfully performed the sphincterotomy in pigs using a RED placed through the duodenum and a 5-mm rigid laparoscope to view the procedure. In humans, the retroperitoneal position of the duodenum would require either a Kocher maneuver to mobilize the duodenum or preferably placement of the RED through the distal antrum and using either a 30-degree rigid 5-mm laparoscope or a flexible choledochoscope placed through the RED to view the sphincter and guide the procedure. The advantage of this somewhat invasive approach is that it en-

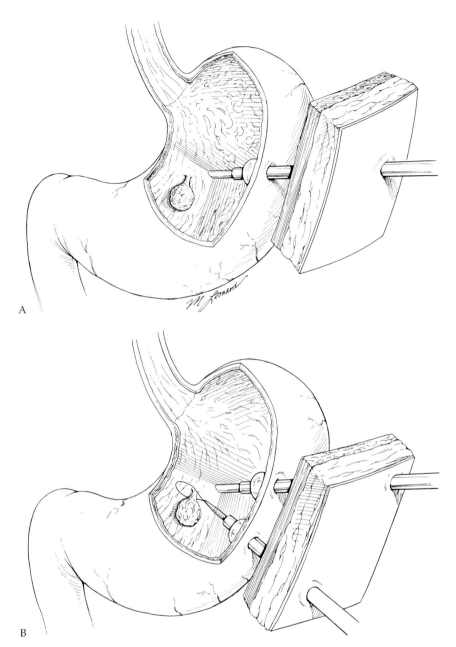

Fig. 25-4. *Identification of benign gastric tumor* **(A)** *and placement of an extracorporeal knot across its pedicle* **(B)**.

ables a single surgeon to take care of every aspect of the management of gallstone disease without having to subject the patient to a second procedure, while still maintaining all the benefits of a minimally invasive procedure.

Other Procedures

Experience with other endoluminal procedures is sparse, but the principles of exposure, tissue dissection, resection, and specimen retrieval are the same as in the stomach. Potential sites amenable to endoluminal surgery include the colon, small bowel, and esophagus.

Closure of Enterostomies

On completion of the endoluminal procedure, the REDs are removed, and the defects on the surface of the bowel closed with inverting interrupted sutures. This is easiest to accomplish if additional abdom-

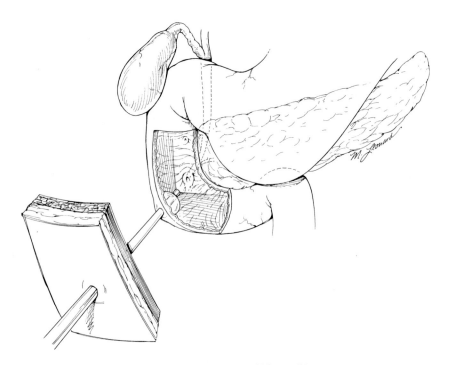

Fig. 25-5. Endoluminal visualization of biliary sphincterotomy.

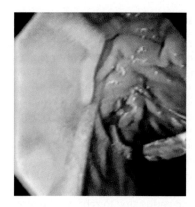

Fig. 25-6. Endoscopic view of antegrade sphincterotomy of the common bile duct performed during laparoscopic cholecystectomy. (Courtesy of Dr. DePaula).

First, it is possible to lacerate or even perforate the wall of the hollow organ opposite the site of entry of the first endoluminal trocar. If this injury occurs, it is usually possible to close the perforation with a single extracorporeally tied suture. Second, the loss of anchoring of one of the intraluminal trocars, due to either perforation of the balloon used to anchor the device or accidental pulling out of the trocar, leads rapidly to a loss of distention of the working space and a loss of exposure. This can usually be prevented by testing the anchoring mechanism of the trocar before it is inserted. If a trocar slips out or its anchor has been damaged, it is preferable to insert a larger one through the same defect so that the subsequent friction between the new trocar and the tissue is enough to anchor the trocar in place.

We have not experienced any complications associated with distention of the lumen of the stomach with carbon dioxide, but have noticed that the small bowel does become distended with gas, although this has not been to the extent that it interferes with the surgery.

Hemostasis during endoluminal surgery is a potential concern. During pancreatic cystogastrostomy, we have created the communication with the cyst using monopolar electrocautery on a high-power (60 W or greater) setting in the coagulation waveform. This has always been adequate for hemostasis, and we have never experienced postoperative bleeding from the site of the cystogastrostomy. Splenic artery bleeding from the base of the cyst is a recognized complication from this procedure, the incidence of which is probably not altered by performance of the procedure in an endoluminal fashion.

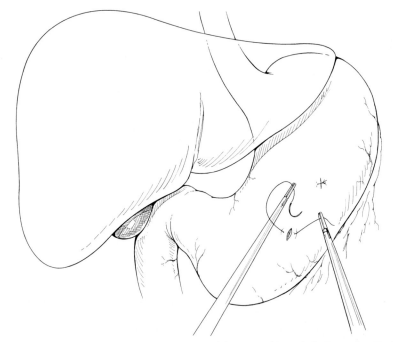

Fig. 25-7. Single interrupted sutures are used to close defects created by Radially Expanding Devices.

inal trocars are placed to pass the suturing instruments, but it is also possible to close the holes by passing the suturing instruments through the REDs after they have been removed from the lumen of the bowel but are still left in place in the abdominal cavity (Fig. 25-7).

Surgical Complications

Complications associated with endoluminal surgery are similar to those associated with laparoscopic surgery in general. In addition to these, there are several technical complications specific to endoluminal surgery.

Postoperative Care

The postoperative care of these patients is along the same principles for other elective laparoscopic patients. In general, patients are commenced on a light diet within 4 to 6 hours of surgery, and early ambulation is encouraged. During their hospital stay, patients are closely observed for the first 2 to 4 hours for signs of shock, following which their observation is less rigorous. Pain control in the acute postoperative period is usually adequate with intravenous or subcutaneous opiates. Patient-controlled analgesia is more expensive and not routinely indicated. Patients are soon managed on regular oral analgesics. Foley catheters and intravenous fluids are discontinued before patients leave the postoperative area, unless they are unable to take oral fluids. No postoperative blood tests or x-ray examinations are performed, unless specifically indicated because of either a possible complication during the surgery or the development of symptoms or signs suggestive of a complication. Routine chest x-ray films to exclude pneumothorax are not indicated. Unless patients have a prior acute illness or other morbidity, it is reasonable to expect discharge within 24 hours and resumption of normal activities within 1 week.

Suggested Reading

Bhoyrul S, Way LW. Intraluminal gastric surgery. In: Duh Q-Y, ed. *Laparoscopic surgery: laparoscopic access to the gastrointestinal tract.* Decker Medical Publications, 1995:189–197.

Filipi CJ, Perdikis G, Hinder RA, DeMeester TR, Fitzgibbons RJ Jr, Peters J. An intraluminal surgical approach to the management of gastric bezoars. *Surg Endosc* 1995;9:831–833.

Geis WP, Baxt R, Kim HC. Benign gastric tumors: minimally invasive approach. *Surg Endosc* 1996;10:407–410.

Mori T, Bhoyrul S, Way LW. Laparoscopic pancreatic cystogastrostomy: the first operation in the new field of endoluminal laparoscopic surgery. *Surg Endosc* 1994;8:448.

Ohashi S. Laparoscopic intraluminal (intragastric) surgery for early gastric cancer: a new concept in laparoscopic surgery. *Surg Endosc* 1995;9:169–171.

Potvin M, Gagner M, Pomp A. Laparoscopic transgastric suturing for bleeding peptic ulcers. *Surg Endosc* 1996;10:400–402.

EDITOR'S COMMENT

As advanced laparoscopic procedures gained increasing acceptance in the early 1990s, several pioneers utilized the improved technologies of endoscopic surgery to push the frontiers of surgery forward. Among these were Dr. Bhoyrul and Dr. Way, who early on established the feasibility of moving the laparoscopic environment and all of its advantages to the interior of hollow viscera. This chapter describes the use of laparoscopic instruments and techniques for the treatment of a variety of diseases of the lining of the stomach, duodenum, and intestines.

These are techniques still in the development stage, as the technical difficulties of accessing the lumen of an organ by traversing the abdominal cavity are still not fully worked out. Even such devices as the RED are not fully developed or foolproof. Many questions remain with regard to the appropriate fixation trocars and the appropriate instruments to operate in a very small, confined space, and these subjects continue to be investigated. Since many of the possible indications for endoluminal surgery are for urgent bleeding, foreign body removal, impacted common bile duct stones, or oncologic indications (e.g., submucosal cancer resections, nonendoscopically resectable colon lesions, periampullary tumors), its exact role remains undefined and somewhat controversial. Still, the potential offered by positive-pressure insufflation, good illumination, and high magnification remains very appealing. In summary, endoluminal endoscopic surgery represents another wave of possible minimally invasive surgery being defined with the goal of benefiting patients.

L.L.S.

26

Laparoscopic Bariatric Procedures

Bruce D. Schirmer

Indications for Bariatric Surgery

Severe obesity, defined as being at least twice ideal body weight or having a body mass index (BMI) of greater than 40, is a major health problem affecting at least 4 million people in the United States. This condition predisposes to many associated health problems. Such patients are often referred or self-referred because of complications of one of these medical problems, which cannot be adequately addressed without associated weight loss.

Successful treatment of severe obesity is difficult to achieve, and nonsurgical treatments are subject to a 95% or greater failure rate. A recent National Institutes of Health consensus conference confirmed that surgical therapy is the most successful long-term treatment for this problem. However, it should be considered only when nonsurgical means of weight loss have failed. Demonstration by a patient of a willingness to undergo a medically supervised diet reinforces his or her ability to make a long-term commitment of effort to the problem, since this will ultimately be required postoperatively. Patients who are unwilling to do this or who feel surgery will be a "quick fix" to their problem are unlikely to have a successful result.

Gastric stapling procedures have been the most successful operations for treating severe obesity. The principle of restricting the volume of oral intake is the basis of all gastric stapling operations, and two have proven most effective: the vertical banded gastroplasty (VBG) and the Roux-en-Y gastric bypass (RYGBP). A third procedure, amenable to a laparoscopic approach, is silicone gastric banding (SGB).

This chapter deals with all three procedures, but the reader is cautioned that SGB is currently a very new procedure and therefore has not been subjected to rigorous scrutiny as to its long-term efficacy and safety.

Of the three procedures, RYGBP has proved to be the most effective in producing long-term weight loss in severely obese patients. Weight loss after RYGBP has generally ranged from 48% to 74% of excess weight after 5 years of follow-up and more than 50% after 9 years. RYGBP has achieved equivalent or better short-term and better long-term weight reduction results than the VBG in prospective comparison series. An advantage of RYGBP over VBG is the tendency for patients with RYGBP to have dumping and therefore to avoid sweets and high-calorie liquid foods. This has made RYGBP the procedure of choice for patients with a preoperative history suggesting high sugar or sweets intake. It has also been the most effective procedure for superobese patients (more than 200 lbs over ideal body weight).

Patients undergoing VBG lose approximately 45% to 60% of excess weight at 1 year after surgery. However, long-term follow-up shows a significantly greater tendency for patients to regain lost weight after this operation. Patients have shown a tendency to convert their eating habits to a diet high in sweets, high-calorie liquids, and ice cream, causing the regain of weight. The operation does not alter the route of food through the digestive tract and allows continued access to the distal stomach and duodenum. There are no long-term metabolic consequences of the procedure. VBG is technically easier and faster to perform than RYGBP.

Few data concerning weight loss after laparoscopic bariatric surgery are available. These data show that weight loss has been nearly the same for these procedures as for the corresponding open procedures.

SGB has been shown to produce successful short-term weight loss, when performed via celiotomy, although complication and reoperation rates have been high. The results after laparoscopic SGB from one center with extensive experience have initially been successful, with a reported 90% loss of excess weight.

Indications and Preoperative Evaluation

Patient selection is key to postoperative success. Basic eligibility criteria for weight reduction surgery are that patients must be severely obese, have attempted a medically well supervised diet, be under age 60 years, be strongly self-motivated to undergo the operation, and be free of any psychiatric problems. Patients must be sufficiently intelligent to grasp the changes in diet and eating habits that the operation will entail.

In the preoperative evaluation of patients, it is important to involve the opinions of the primary care physician, dietitian, and psychiatrist or psychologist. The opinion of each of these is important for ruling out significant contraindications to surgery from the point of view of each of these disciplines.

The basic preoperative medical evaluation should include a complete history and physical examination. Pertinent questions in the history should include a weight history, dietary habits, motivation, social situation, and evidence of comorbid medical diseases. Screening laboratory blood tests include a complete blood cell count, chem 20 (serum chemistries, electrolytes, and liver function tests), measures of iron, vitamin B_{12}, and cortisol, thyroid panel, arterial blood gases, urinalysis, electrocardiogram, and chest x-ray. Ultrasound of the gallbladder and upper endoscopy are also routinely done. Patients with cardiorespiratory conditions must have these evaluated preoperatively and treated optimally.

Shortly before the scheduled operation, patients should again be thoroughly counseled as to the risks and expected benefits of the operation. Videotaping consent sessions is not inappropriate in this patient population. With laparoscopic VBG or RYGBP, the still limited experience with this approach in performing these procedures must be emphasized, as should the high possibility for potential laparotomy to complete the operation in a traditional fashion should any aspect of the laparoscopic approach be unsatisfactory.

Currently, I recommend that patients must meet several additional criteria before being considered for laparoscopic (as opposed to traditional open) bariatric surgery. Weight should not be much greater than 300 lbs, and the abdominal girth should not be excessive (BMI greater than 45). Patients should have had no previous upper abdominal surgery. Another contraindication is hypoventilation syndrome of obesity. Finally, ultrasound examination should not show an excessively large left lobe of the liver. Current instrumentation and technology contraindicate laparoscopic bariatric surgery for the superobese, particularly early in the surgeon's experience.

For patients who have a proclivity for eating sweets, the RYGBP will produce greater weight loss due to the effects of dumping created by the gastrojejunostomy. Patients with known peptic ulcer disease, gastric polyps, antral gastritis, or significant iron or vitamin B_{12} deficiencies are good candidates for a VBG. In my experience, most patients will be better suited for an RYGBP due to their eating habits. This makes laparoscopic bariatric surgery even more difficult, since currently the largest experiences of successful laparoscopic bariatric surgical procedures are somewhat inversely proportional to the long-term success of their corresponding open procedures. It has been my policy

to recommend the operation that best suits a patient's long-term needs, regardless of whether or not it can be done laparoscopically, and only then to consider a laparoscopic approach if the patient is enthusiastic about this and is an appropriate candidate.

Finally, all patients must be informed that rapid weight loss is associated with at least a 30% incidence of gallstone formation postoperatively. Patients are therefore advised either to have a simultaneous prophylactic cholecystectomy or to take prophylactic ursodiol (Actigall) for 6 months postoperatively.

Perioperative Management

Severely obese patients are a technical challenge for the anesthesiologist in terms of venous access and safe intubation. Peak airway pressures may be increased due to a patient's size. Ventilation volume, medication doses, and anesthetic doses must all be adjusted for increased patient size. Careful monitoring of end-tidal carbon dioxide is essential, as is monitoring of arterial blood gases intraoperatively for all patients with significant cardiopulmonary disease who are undergoing laparoscopic surgery.

Modifications in laparoscopic instrumentation to accommodate the special needs of severely obese patients have been inadequate. Extra-long 10-mm trocars are available, but the 30-mm trocar through which the endoscopic circular stapler is passed has too short a length and must be sutured to the abdominal wall to prevent dislodgement by the pneumoperitoneum. The 30-mm trocar also predisposes to subcutaneous emphysema, causing conversion to laparotomy in any procedure not completed expeditiously.

For laparoscopic VBG, an airtight endoscopic circular stapler (31 mm), a 30-mm trocar, a 60-mm endoscopic linear cutting stapler, an abdominal wall body retractor as used in gasless laparoscopy, and a good set of laparoscopic instruments including needle drivers and atraumatic graspers are required. An atraumatic liver retractor that can be affixed to some form of static external retractor is useful. A flexible upper gastrointestinal endoscope is quite helpful for use as a calibrating instrument along the lesser curvature. A 30-degree telescope is needed.

For a laparoscopic RYGBP, the above equipment is necessary as well, together with a 21- or 25-mm endoscopic circular stapler. A harmonic scalpel can also be helpful for dividing the mesentery to create the Roux limb. Both an endoscopic linear cutting stapler and a 60-mm linear cutting stapler are required.

Operative Technique for Vertical Banded Gastroplasty

For all laparoscopic bariatric procedures, the patient should be secured to the operating table as well as possible to allow reverse Trendelenburg positioning. A foot board is helpful. The surgeon stands on the patient's right, the first assistant on the left. The camera operator can stand on either side of the table, depending on telescope placement. The video monitor is placed near the left shoulder. The abdominal wall retractor is placed above the left shoulder (Fig. 26-1).

The principle of reproducing the open procedure identically is followed in performing a laparoscopic VBG. Performance of this procedure should only be undertaken by surgeons who have extensive laparoscopic surgical experience.

Suggested port placement is shown in Fig. 26-2. This is simply a recommendation, but certain considerations are almost mandatory. These include generally high placement of the ports, particularly several near the xiphoid and upper costal margin areas. The port for the telescope needs to be well above the umbilicus. The liver retractor is generally best placed in the lower portion of the right upper quadrant to allow retraction of the liver. One additional port on the right side of the midline is needed to allow good visualization of the posterior surface of the stomach. These latter two ports can subsequently be used if the patient has requested and requires a prophylactic cholecystectomy. Often, simply the addition of one additional 5-mm trocar in the right upper quadrant (not shown in Fig. 26-1) is needed to allow performance of this additional procedure.

The operation begins with creation of the pneumoperitoneum. An abdominal wall retractor (as used in gasless laparoscopy) is then placed to lift the abdominal wall and allow a steep reverse Trendelenburg

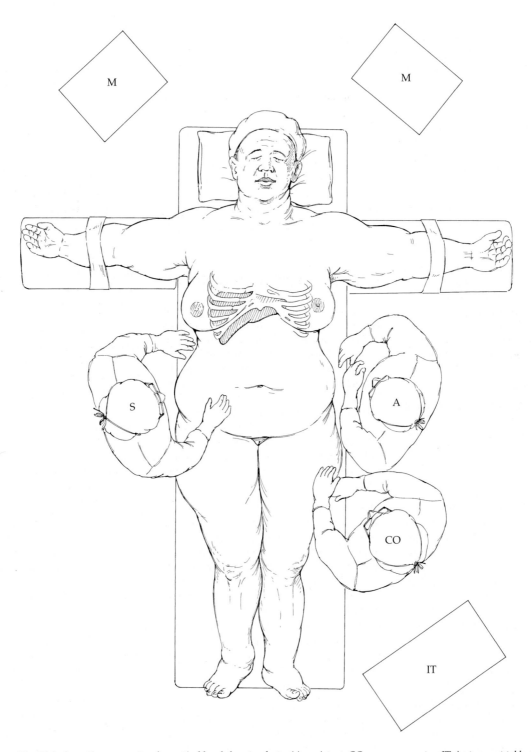

Fig. 26-1. Operating room setup for vertical banded gastroplasty. (A, assistant; CO, camera operator; IT, instrument table; M, monitor; S, surgeon.)

position. The retractor should be placed carefully and under laparoscopic vision to avoid trauma to internal organs. Often, division of the round and falciform ligaments is necessary to allow safe placement of the retractor.

Division of a portion of the triangular ligament of the left lobe of the liver with cautery scissors may be necessary to permit optimal exposure of the gastroesophageal (GE) junction area. The liver retractor is then placed for additional exposure.

The peritoneal attachments near the angle of His are incised. Visualization here often requires using one of the upper ports for temporary placement of the 30-degree telescope. Only the peritoneal attachments need be divided; short gastric vessels should be left intact. The gastrohepatic ligament is then opened in its avascular portion. The stomach is elevated and the telescope repositioned from the right-sided port so that the posterior surface of the stomach is visible. Some careful sharp and blunt dissection may be necessary to develop a sufficiently wide passage for clear visualization of the upper posterior stomach (Fig. 26-3).

The intended site for placement of the endoscopic circular stapler, approximately 6 cm down from the gastroesophageal (GE) junction near the lesser curvature, is determined. The endoscopic stapler anvil is optimally positioned so that its lateral edge, closest to the lesser curvature, permits only the passage of a 32-French tube along the lesser curvature (Fig. 26-4). A therapeutic upper endoscope, which is approximately this size, is advanced perorally to lie along the lesser curvature and allow calibration of the site. The endoscope has the advantage of having an illuminated end for easier visualization by the surgeon, as well as allowing intragastric monitoring of the procedure. Excess air should not be used to insufflate the stomach, and a noncrushing clamp on the proximal jejunum or duodenum minimizes the introduction of air into the gastrointestinal tract.

Once the site for the center of the endoscopic stapler defect is chosen, a straight needle and heavy suture are passed transgastrically at that point from anterior to posterior, and the suture is tied to the tip of the endoscopic stapler anvil (see Fig. 26-4). The suture guides passage of the anvil

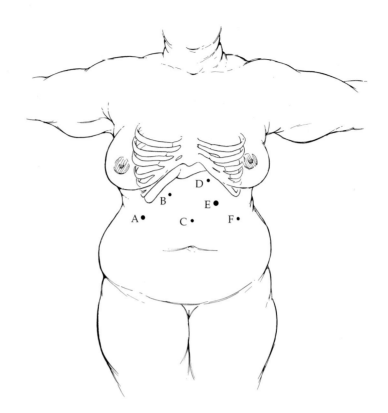

Fig. 26-2. Port placement for vertical banded gastroplasty. (A, 10-mm liver retractor; B, 10-mm telescope/graspers; C, 10-mm telescope/dissector; D, 10-mm graspers/needle holder/dissector; E, 33-mm trocar for endoscopic circular stapler/endoscopic linear cutting stapler; F, 5/10-mm graspers/needle holder.)

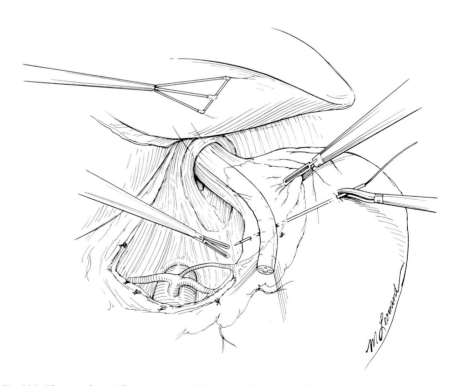

Fig. 26-3. The gastrohepatic ligament is opened in its avascular portion. Under direct visualization, a suture is passed through anterior and posterior gastric walls at the site intended for circular stapling.

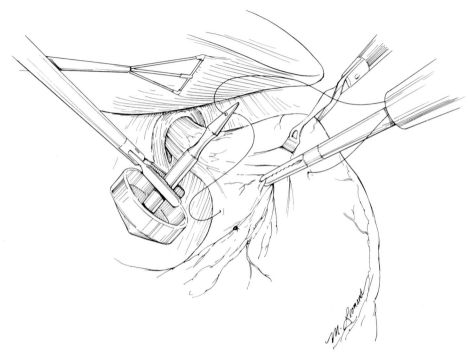

Fig. 26-4. A suture guiding the circular stapler anvil in place.

transgastrically. This is technically one of the more difficult portions of the operation, as the grasping forceps must have a good hold on the anvil, the orientation of the anvil spike must be correct, and the suture must be heavy enough not to break during the trauma of passage through both walls of the stomach. A small amount of incising or cutting of the anterior gastric wall with electrocautery at the point where the anvil spike is to pass through can be helpful, but care should be taken to avoid cutting the suture or injuring the gastric wall over an area outside the margins of the circular staple line that will not be resected (Fig. 26-5).

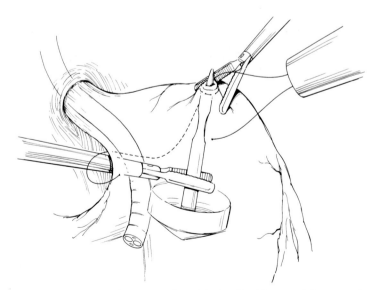

Fig. 26-5. The anvil of a circular stapler is passed through both walls of the stomach from posterior to anterior direction.

The spike from the anvil is removed. The endoscopic circular stapler shaft is passed through the 30-mm trocar and attached to the anvil. The stapler is closed and fired, producing a large transgastric circular defect (Fig. 26-6).

With the endoscope remaining in place, the endoscopic linear cutting stapler is advanced into the peritoneal cavity, and the stomach is divided from the 12-o'clock position in the endoscopic circular stapler ring up toward the angle of His. This may take two applications of the stapler. Care should be taken to be certain that the endoscope, as well as any nasogastric or other tubes, are removed from the path of the linear cutting stapler.

Once the gastric pouch is completed, the surgeon may oversew the staple line at any point along its length as desired (Fig. 26-7). The vertical band is then introduced into the peritoneal cavity after a space is first cleared along the lesser curvature corresponding to the 9-o'clock position of the circular staple line ring. Here, again, the dissection must be done carefully to avoid troublesome bleeding. The band is passed around the outflow tract and sewn to itself using several interrupted 2-0 nylon sutures. Rather than using a precalibrated length of band, as with open surgery, I have found it technically easier to make the band approximately 7.5 cm long to facilitate passage around the outflow tract, and then to cut the excess band after sewing the band at the appropriate tightness around the dilator (Fig. 26-8).

Finally, the endoscope is removed, the stomach inspected, and the operation completed with closure of the port sites. Port-site closure in severely obese patients is often well accomplished only if specially designed hook-ended instruments are used to pass sutures, under laparoscopic vision, through the abdominal wall at the incision site to effectively close the peritoneum.

Operative Technique for Roux-en-Y Gastric Bypass

Laparoscopic RYGBP is more difficult than laparoscopic VBG. The only group in the United States with any current significant experience with this procedure is that of A.C. Wittgrove and associates in San Diego, California. Since my experience

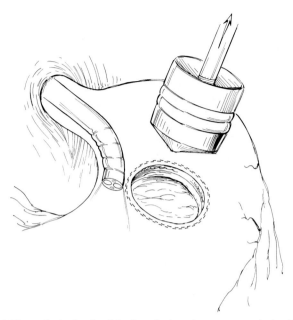

Fig. 26-6. *The stapler is closed and fired, producing a large transgastric circular defect.*

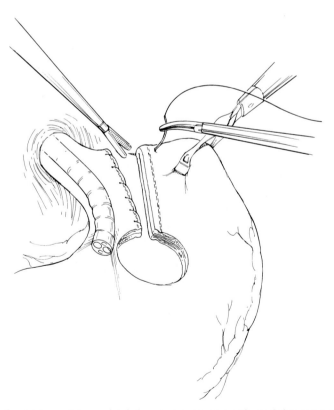

Fig. 26-7. *Once the gastric pouch is completed, the surgeon may oversew the staple line at any point along its length as desired.*

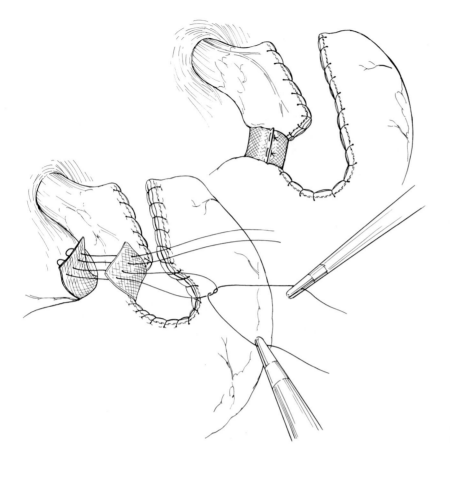

Fig. 26-8. The band is passed around the outflow tract and sewn to itself using several interrupted 2-0 nylon sutures.

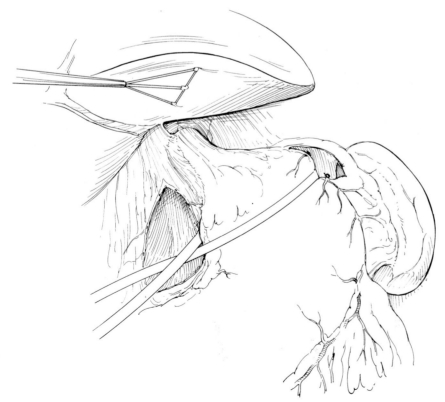

Fig. 26-9. The gastrohepatic ligament is opened.

with laparoscopic RYGBP is limited, the description that follows is based on the operation as done via celiotomy.

The same considerations for patient setup and positioning are needed as for VBG. Similarly, ports are mainly positioned in the upper abdomen. An abdominal wall lifter is necessary to support the patient in the reverse Trendelenburg position. A liver retractor is also necessary.

Division of the peritoneum at the angle of His is accomplished just as for VBG. The gastrohepatic ligament is similarly opened (Fig. 26-9). A space adjacent to the lesser curvature of the stomach, approximately 5 cm down from the GE junction, is cleared through the lesser curvature mesentery to allow the passage of an endoscopic linear cutting stapler for gastric division (Fig. 26-10). The harmonic scalpel can be useful for hemostatically clearing the area through the lesser curvature mesentery.

At this point, the intended location of the staple line to divide the stomach is envisioned, and often marking the anterior gastric wall with a few sutures is helpful in maintaining this orientation. Two or more applications of the endoscopic stapler are often needed to completely divide the stomach, creating a 20- to 30-mL proximal gastric pouch that has a sufficiently large enough surface on its anterior gastric wall to allow creation of the gastrojejunostomy.

With the patient now in the Trendelenburg position, attention is turned toward creation of the Roux limb. This is done from the first loop of jejunum distal to the ligament of Treitz, where a good vascular arcade is visible. The bowel is divided with the endoscopic linear cutting stapler, and then the mesentery is serially divided with either endoscopic ligatures, the endoscopic linear cutting stapler with vascular staples, or the harmonic scalpel (which can safely divide vessels up to 3 mm in diameter). The Roux limb is passed retrocolically through a defect created in the transverse colon mesentery and gastrocolic ligament (Fig. 26-11). I have brought the Roux limb up in an antegastric position, but Wittgrove's group has favored a retrogastric approach for the Roux limb for anastomosis. Both approaches are proven acceptable using an open approach. The passage of the Roux limb is one of the most difficult portions of the laparoscopic procedure, although it is not difficult during celiotomy because palpation and blind passage are often incorporated during the latter. However, with laparoscopy, a passage for the Roux limb must first be created under laparoscopic vision, and then a Penrose drain is placed through the passage. The bowel is sutured to the drain, and then the drain is pulled back through the passage, bringing the bowel with it. Care must be taken that the mesentery of the Roux limb is not twisted.

I have favored creating the gastroenterostomy with a 25-mm endoscopic circular stapling device. A gastrotomy is made in the lesser curvature lateral surface of the proximal gastric pouch sufficiently large enough to allow passage of the anvil of the endoscopic circular stapler into the lumen of the pouch. The spike of the endoscopic stapler anvil is brought through the anterior wall of the gastric pouch toward the greater curvature side (Fig. 26-12). The end of the Roux limb is opened, allowing placement of the main shaft of the endoscopic stapler into the lumen of the Roux limb. The spike of the stapler shaft is used to penetrate the antimesenteric wall of the jejunum about 10 cm proximal to the open-

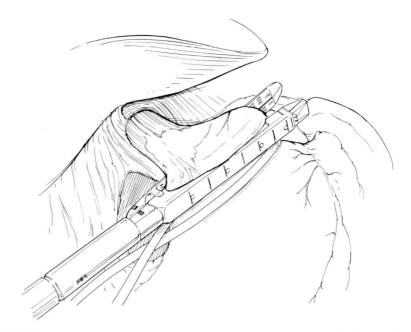

Fig. 26-10. The endoscopic linear stapler is passed around the stomach just low enough to allow creation of a small proximal pouch.

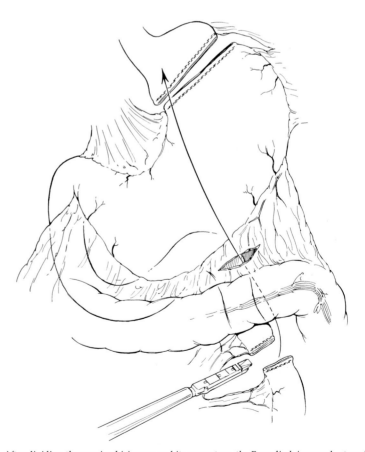

Fig. 26-11. After dividing the proximal jejunum and its mesentery, the Roux limb is passed retrocolically through a defect in the transverse colon mesentery.

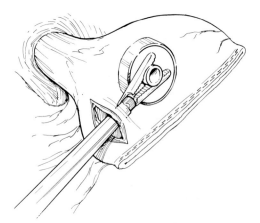

Fig. 26-12. *The spike of the endoscopic circular stapler anvil is brought through the anterior wall of the gastric pouch.*

ing made in the end of the jejunum. The anvil and shaft of the endoscopic circular stapler are connected, and the stapler is fired (Fig. 26-13). The gastrotomy along the lesser curvature of the gastric pouch is closed with a linear cutting stapler, and the excess Roux limb is removed by dividing the bowel with an endoscopic linear cutting stapler. The circular staple line can be reinforced with a circular continuous suture of 3-0 nylon, if desired, but I recommend first passing a dilator through the anastomosis to prevent narrowing if this is to be done.

Wittgrove's group has used an endoscopic approach to place the anvil of the circular stapler into the gastric pouch. The anvil is placed in a similar manner to placement of a percutaneous gastrostomy device using a wire loop passed into the lumen of the proximal gastric pouch under laparo-scopic guidance; the wire loop is then retrieved by the endoscopist and used to pull the anvil of the endoscopic circular stapler down to and through the anterior wall of the gastric pouch. The circular stapler shaft is inserted through an enterotomy made in the Roux limb 10 cm distal to its proximal end, and an end-to-end stapled anastomosis is performed with the gastric pouch. Afterward, the enterotomy is closed with the endoscopic linear cutting stapler.

An enteroenterostomy is performed 90 to 100 cm distal to the gastroenterostomy using the endoscopic linear cutting stapler. The mesenteric defect in the small intestine at the enteroenterostomy must be closed and the Roux limb sutured to the transverse colon mesentery to prevent postoperative herniation (Fig. 26-14).

Operative Technique of Silicone Gastric Banding

SGB incorporates an adjustable inflatable band placed around the proximal stomach to limit oral intake. I have no personal experience with this procedure, but the general approach and anatomic considerations for performing it are very similar to those for laparoscopic VBG. The setup and positioning of the patient can be done similarly, and again emphasis is on allowing a safe steep reverse Trendelenburg position and good visualization of the proximal gastric pouch.

M. Belachew, a surgeon experienced in this procedure, has emphasized that creation of the passage for the band around the proximal stomach should be done through the lesser curvature mesentery and along the posterior surface of the proximal stomach. He favors using curved instruments to facilitate the dissection. Once a passage is created, the inflatable band is placed around the proximal stomach to create a 15- to 25-mL proximal gastric pouch. The band is secured in place by imbricating a portion of the stomach over the band and sewing stomach to stomach.

Band restriction is adjustable by means of adding or removing saline from the inflatable band itself. This is done by use of a reservoir system of saline attached to the band and accessible through a port attached via a catheter to the band. The port is placed subcutaneously in the anterior abdominal wall after the band is secured around the stomach.

Postoperative Care

The postoperative course of patients undergoing bariatric surgery is usually uncomplicated, provided that good surgical technique has been used. Prophylaxis for deep venous thrombosis is recommended. Prophylactic intravenous antibiotics are used. Nasogastric tubes are removed either in the recovery room or within 24 hours. Ice chips are given the day of surgery. An oral liquid diet (blenderized foods) is initiated on the second or third postoperative day after a meglumine diatrizoate (Gastrografin) swallow examination. This diet is continued for approximately 2 weeks, at which time solid food is begun. Ambulation is begun within 24

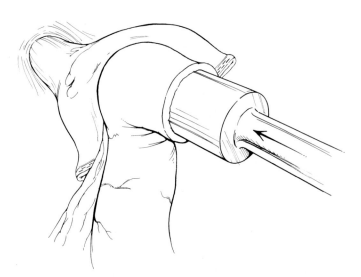

Fig. 26-13. *The anvil and shaft of the endoscopic circular stapler are connected, and the stapler is fired.*

hours of surgery. Discharge is usually 4 to 5 days postoperatively for patients undergoing celiotomy but can be less for laparoscopic procedures.

Complications

Operative mortality for RYGBP and VBG done via celiotomy is in the 1% range. Overall morbidity rate, including late complications, is in the 40% range, with well over one half of morbidity arising from delayed postoperative complications, the most common of which are incisional hernias. Incisional hernias have occurred in approximately 20% of patients in my experience. Using a laparoscopic approach to these procedures should decrease the incidence of this problem.

Immediate postoperative complications for both procedures done via celiotomy include wound infection or seroma (2% to 10%), urinary tract infection (1% to 4%), atelectasis (5% to 10%), wound dehiscence (1%), deep venous thrombosis (1% to 3%), anastomotic leakage (1% to 3%), marginal ulceration (1% to 6%), and cardiovascular complications (1% to 4%). Serious, lift-threatening morbidity is in the 3% range. Wound infections and seromas, the most frequent problems after celiotomy for these procedures, should also be significantly decreased using a laparoscopic approach.

Long-term complications for VBG include stricture formation at the anastomosis (5% to 17%) and regain of weight (significant in up to 50% of patients). However, severe GE reflux may also arise following VBG, and this has been reported in the initial experience of Belachew with laparoscopic SGB, occurring in 10% of patients. The reoperation rate after VBG can be considerable, reported from 17% to 36% for past series. However, much of that was due to staple line disruption from failure to initially divide the stomach, which is now routinely done as described above. Pouch or stoma enlargement are also reasons for reoperation for weight regain.

Patients undergoing RYGBP also suffer from postoperative anastomotic strictures (5% to 12%), marginal ulcers (4% to 8%), severe dumping (requiring medication in 1% to 2%), and internal herniation of bowel with obstruction (1%). RYGBP predisposes to micronutrient deficiencies, particularly iron, vitamin B_{12}, folate, and

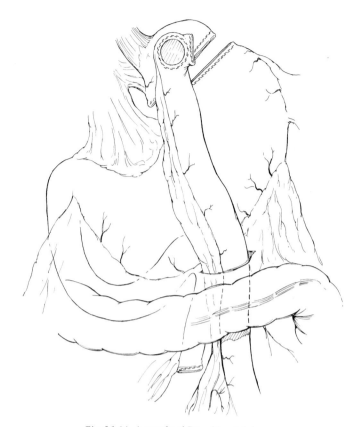

Fig. 26-14. A completed Roux Y gastric bypass.

calcium. Iron or vitamin B_{12} deficiency anemias occur in at least 20% of patients in the long term after RYGBP. Iron deficiency can usually be corrected with oral supplementation, while vitamin B_{12} deficiency may require parenteral supplementation.

Complications reported thus far with SGB include a high incidence of readjustment of the band after initial experiences with the procedure done via celiotomy, reported as 35% to 50% within 6 months in several series. In one series, 20% of patients required reoperation for posterior herniation of the stomach upward inside the band with obstruction. An additional 12.5% of patients requested removal of the band. In another series, there was a 15% incidence of inadequate early weight loss due to poor positioning of the band.

In the only significant series of laparoscopic SGB reported thus far, there was a 2% incidence of early postoperative complications and a 1% mortality. There was only a 4% incidence of food intolerance due to band tightness.

Since the anatomic arrangement of SGB is essentially the same as that of the VBG, the same postoperative problems are likely to occur in the future as long-term follow-up increases; these problems include reflux esophagitis, alterations of diet to include high-caloric liquids, and regain of weight.

Selected Reading

Belachew M, Legrand MJ, Defechereux TH, et al. Laparoscopic adjustable silicone gastric banding in the treatment of morbid obesity. *Surg Endosc* 1994;8:1354–1356.

Brolin RE. Critical analysis of weight loss and quality of data. *Am J Clin Nutr* 1992;55(suppl 2): 577S–581S.

Brolin RL, Robertson LB, Kenler HA, Cody RP. Weight loss and dietary intake after vertical banded gastroplasty and Roux-en-Y gastric bypass. *Ann Surg* 1994;220:782–790.

Gastrointestinal surgery for severe obesity. NIH consensus development conference consensus statement. *Ann Intern Med* 1991;115:956–961.

Mason EE Gastric surgery for morbid obesity. *Surg Clin North Am* 1992;72:501–513.

Pomerri F, Liberati L, Curtolo S, Muzzio PC. Adjustable silicone gastric banding for obesity. *Gastrointest Radiol* 1992;17:207–210.

Sugerman HJ, Kellum JM, Engle KM, et al. Gastric bypass for treating severe obesity. *Am J Clin Nutr* 1992;55(suppl 2):560S–566S.

Sugerman HJ, Starley JV, Birkenhauer R. A randomized prospective trial of gastric bypass vs. vertical banded gastroplasty for morbid obesity and their effects on sweets vs. non-sweets eaters. *Ann Surg* 1987;205:613–624.

Wittgrove AC, Clark GW, Tremblay LJ. Laparoscopic gastric bypass, Roux-en-Y: preliminary report of five cases. *Obes Surg* 1995;4:353–357.

Wolfel R, Gunther K, Rumenapf G, et al. Weight reduction after gastric bypass and horizontal gastroplasty for morbid obesity: results after 10 years. *Eur J Surg* 1994;160:219–225.

EDITOR'S COMMENT

In the United States, bariatric surgery has gained a reputation as a "bad surgery." This is a result of the high number of complications and what is perceived as a high failure rate described in early experiences with weight loss procedures. This reputation is not deserved. Morbidly obese patients represent a very high-risk population both for surgical complications and poor long-term outcome of the antiobesity surgery. As the psychologic underpinnings of this disease and the physiologic effects of various weight loss surgeries are better understood, the results have improved. In addition, early morbidity rates have shown improvement, except for a continuing high rate of wound complications and pulmonary problems. The ability to perform bariatric surgeries laparoscopically would be a tremendous benefit to the outcomes of these procedures, both real and perceived. The laparoscopic approach would essentially eliminate postoperative wound complications, which are seen in as many as 20% to 50% of patients. In addition, the decrease in postoperative pain associated with laparoscopy should make pulmonary toilet, early ambulation, and rapid recovery accessible to bariatric surgery patients, further decreasing the postoperative complication rate.

Dr. Schirmer has effectively described the laparoscopic approaches corresponding to current open antiobesity procedures. As yet, there is no consensus as to what is the best open bariatric procedure, with various centers preferring one approach over another. Obviously, one key element of this procedure is that it be done on patients with access to a comprehensive program that can provide dietary counseling, psychologic support when indicated, and medical management. This is probably more important than which particular procedure is used. As has been demonstrated in many other laparoscopic procedures, any gastrointestinal procedure that can be done openly can probably be accomplished laparoscopically. It would seem logical that centers that have gained experience and comfort with a particular antiobesity procedure should adapt it to the laparoscopic approach. Without a doubt, over the next several years, the laparoscopic approach will become the gold standard of treatment for obesity, and it is hoped that this will lead to a better perception of this surgery and its wider application in this chronically ill patient population.

L.L.S.

III

Liver and Gallbladder

27

Diagnostic and Therapeutic Endoscopic Retrograde Cholangiopancreatography

Maurice E. Arregui and Maria T. Madden

Endoscopic retrograde cholangiopancreatography (ERCP) was introduced into clinical practice in 1968 by W.S. McCune, an Ohio surgeon. Endoscopic sphincterotomy (ES) followed in 1974. The advantage of ERCP over other radiographic modalities is that a pancreatogram and a cholangiogram can be obtained, and a variety of therapeutic measures can be employed as well. ERCP can be done on an outpatient basis and is associated with a low morbidity and mortality. With ES, the risks are a little higher; reports show a 10% complication rate and a mortality of 1% to 1.5%.

Although ERCP was initially a valuable diagnostic tool, it has currently become a widely available therapeutic tool that has largely supplanted open surgery in the management of many pancreatic and biliary diseases, both benign and malignant. Unfortunately, very few surgeons perform ERCP. Most often, it is performed by gastroenterologists, who are relatively new to this field and have much less experience than surgeons. Although the American Board of Surgery and the American College of Surgeons recommend endoscopy as part of a surgical residency, most programs in the United States do not adequately prepare surgeons in endoscopy, and only rare programs provide ERCP training. ERCP is a valuable surgical tool that should be in the surgeon's armamentarium.

Anatomy of the Sphincter of Oddi

The earliest recognition of the distal part of the common bile duct (CBD) was in 1542 by Vesalius, who described the CBD as a "vesicle that travels down . . . and is implanted in duodenal jejunum." F. Glisson was the first to describe a sphincter, but credit goes to Ruggero Oddi, who as a medical student identified the sphincter and extensively described its physiologic properties. Oddi suggested that the sphincter played a major role in the control of the flow of bile and pancreatic juice and that abnormalities in the sphincter could give rise to a variety of maladies. We are still attempting to understand Oddi's sphincter to this day.

It was not until 1937 that Boyden provided an extensive anatomic description of the sphincter of Oddi (SO). He described it as a conglomeration of smooth muscle fibers that encircle the terminal ends of the CBD and the pancreatic duct, as well as the ampulla of Vater, named the sphincter choledochus, sphincter pancreaticus, and sphincter papillae. This would imply three separate muscle group functions; however, we now know that manometrically the SO behaves as a single unit independent of duodenal activity. This would make sense, since the SO develops from specialized mesenchymal tissue independent of the duodenum.

Anatomically, the relationship of the ducts is such that the major duct of Wirsung is caudal and medial to the CBD. The union of the CBD and the pancreatic duct at the papilla varies. Approximately 80% of the time the two ducts form a common channel that drains into the duodenum through the papilla of Vater. About 20% of the time there is virtually no common channel, but there is a small common entry through the papilla. In the remainder, both ducts enter completely separately at the papilla. The papilla itself is located medially in the second portion of the duodenum. The cylindrical protuberance is covered by a triangular duodenal fold. The epithelium of the terminal portion of the CBD and common channel covers long papillary fronds that may branch and extend beyond the ostium of the papilla, called valvules or valvulae, a frequently noted occurrence at ERCP. Anatomic and immunohistochemical investigations have demonstrated that the SO is 4 to 6 mm in length and is richly innervated by cholinergic, adrenergic, and peptidergic neurons and that there are neural connections between the sphincter, gallbladder, and proximal gastrointestinal tract.

Physiology of the Sphincter of Oddi

SO motor activity helps regulate bile flow and pancreatic flow. The exact characteristics of this mechanism are still not completely understood. It is generally believed that the SO contributes to gallbladder filling by offering resistance during fasting periods. Studies done by cinefluorography and endoscopic manometry indicate that the SO inhibits the flow of bile from the CBD to the duodenum. Other actions of the SO have been more controversial. For example, some feel that the SO functions as a propulsive pump (first proposed by Toouli), where the SO segment is allowed to fill with bile during a relaxation phase and this is then squeezed out by a contraction. The opposing theory is that the SO merely releases bile on demand. The other accepted action of the SO is to prevent reflux of duodenal contents into either the CBD or the pancreatic duct.

SO motor activity is thought to be regulated by a complex neurohormonal system composed of both sympathetic and parasympathetic innervation. Multiple enteric peptides are also thought to control SO motor function. Of these, cholecystokinin (CCK) is the most extensively studied. CCK appears to abolish phasic activity and inhibit SO basal pressure, allowing SO relaxation. Glucagon, vasoactive intestinal polypeptide, secretin, neurotensin, neuropeptide Y, somatostatin, gastrin-releasing peptide, and pentagastrin are all involved to varying degrees in SO activity. The SO is also probably influenced by the migrating motor complex, although this is not universally accepted. Various pharmacologic agents have been shown to have an influence on SO activity. Morphine in particular has a marked effect on the SO, causing an increase in frequency and amplitude of contractions.

Indications for Endoscopic Retrograde Cholangiopancreatography

Common Bile Duct Stones

Particularly in the era of laparoscopic cholecystectomy, ERCP has played a major role or has at least been the subject of much debate with regard to the treatment of choledocholithiasis. ERCP with ES and stone extraction is now an accepted modality in the treatment of CBD stones, with a success rate of around 85% to 95%. From November 1989 to March 1995, we performed 99 ERCPs for known or suspected choledocholithiasis. The procedure was performed preoperatively in 60 patients, intraoperatively in four patients, and postoperatively in 35 patients. ERCP with ES and stone extraction was successful in 17 of 25 instances of choledocholithiasis identified preoperatively, for a success rate of 68%. Five patients were successfully cannulated, but the stones could not be completely cleared in four patients and not at all in one patient. Two patients had stones that were too large to extract endo-

scopically, and in two instances the stones were impacted in the CBD. These five patients then underwent laparoscopic CBD exploration with complete extraction of all stones. Therefore, our combined clearance rate with ERCP and laparoscopic CBD exploration was 88%. One patient had both preoperative and postoperative ERCP to completely clear CBD stones, and an additional three patients underwent open CBD exploration. This was early in our experience, before we became proficient in the technique of laparoscopic CBD exploration. As laparoscopic equipment and methods become more widely available and known, we feel most CBD stones will be managed in this manner. The four intraoperative ERCPs were successful. In the 35 patients examined postoperatively, 21 had CBD stones and all of these were cleared with ERCP.

Many authors have attempted to identify laboratory and or ultrasound data that successfully predict the likelihood of CBD stones. This would be important, given the high cost of ERCP and its potential risks. Still, approximately 8% to 10% of patients with CBD calculi have normal liver chemistries and a normal-size CBD.

Our approach has been to perform preoperative ERCP with ES and stone extraction (if CBD calculi are present) in instances when multiple factors indicate the possibility of choledocholithiasis in a high-risk patient or on an urgent basis to relieve CBD obstruction in cases of cholangitis. Additionally, patients with severe life-threatening and worsening pancreatitis due to CBD stones may benefit from endoscopic stone removal. With regard to gallstone pancreatitis, ES is potentially a safe and effective means of alleviating CBD obstruction and preventing recurrent pancreatitis. The problematic issue is that of timing. Several studies have shown that early ERCP and ES are safe and effective, with a lower complication rate than conservative treatment and possibly an improved clinical outcome and shorter hospital stay in patients with severe pancreatitis. In cases of mild pancreatitis, conservative treatment until the pancreatitis resolves followed by an elective operation is still recommended. Most patients with uncomplicated gallstone pancreatitis will pass the stone by the time of surgery. We usually wait 2 to 3 days before performing laparoscopic cholecystectomy. Our operative approach is to routinely assess the CBD

with either laparoscopic ultrasound or cholangiography at the time of laparoscopic cholecystectomy and then, if needed, perform transcystic CBD exploration or laparoscopic choledochotomy. If laparoscopic removal of CBD stones is felt to increase the operative risks or is technically too difficult, intraoperative or postoperative ERCP is performed.

Sphincter of Oddi Dyskinesia

A discussion about diagnostic ERCP would not be complete without mentioning the value of biliary manometry and its usefulness in patients with SO dyskinesia. There are a host of terms used to describe patients either with or without a gallbladder who have biliary-type symptoms. These include biliary dyskinesia, dystonia, sphincterismus, SO dyskinesia, biliary dysmotility, postcholecystectomy syndrome, and so on. Whatever the term, these patients typically have right upper quadrant pain, back pain, nausea, and/or vomiting. They may have abnormal liver enzymes, a dilated CBD, or delayed emptying of the CBD at ERCP. Some of these patients may have papillary stenosis that may be discernible at the time of ERCP. Frequently, however, there is a paucity of objective findings. In these instances, manometry can be of great diagnostic value. The technique involves using a triple-lumen catheter with side holes 2 mm apart hooked up to a multichannel recorder (Fig. 27-1). No narcotics or other agents that may affect the SO may be given prior to or during the manometry. One measures physiologic sphincter length, the duodenal pressure, CBD basal pressure, and SO pressure. Normal values are an SO basal resting pressure 5 to 15 mm Hg above the CBD or pancreatic duct pressure and 15 to 30 mm Hg above the duodenal pressure. Superimposed on the basal pressure are high-amplitude phasic wave contractions that occur two to six per minute, measure 100 to 180 mm Hg in amplitude, and last approximately 4 seconds. Up to 10% of these contractions can be retrograde in normal patients. Criteria for an abnormal study include sustained basal SO pressure of 40 mm Hg or more, peak SO pressure greater than 240 mm Hg, more than 50% retrograde contractions, absent inhibition of the SO following CCK infusion, and wave frequency of more than eight per minute (tachyoddi). Cur-

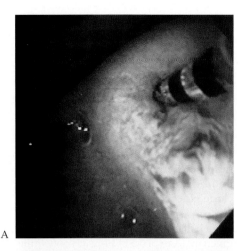

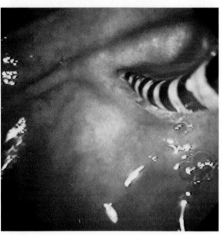

Fig. 27-1. **A:** *Manometry catheter entering papilla.* **B:** *Manometry catheter with gradations 2 mm apart.*

rently, ES is considered the treatment of choice. Many studies now have concluded that upwards of 90% of patients with pain and an increase in SO pressure on manometry will benefit from ES. The mortality of ES in patients with SO dyskinesia is 0.4%, which compares favorably with surgical sphincteroplasty (0.6% to 6.0%).

The limitations of manometry are that it is technically very challenging and requires the cooperation of many to perform the endoscopy and accurately record the pressure readings. There may be much subjective variability in interpretation, and artifact can easily be introduced into the system by air in the tubing, incorrect positioning of the catheter, and duodenal contraction. In addition, the manometry is done over a brief period of time only in the fasting state and may not accurately reflect actual SO activity. Pancreatitis is the most frequently associated complication with manometry.

Trauma

Pancreatic duct rupture can be very difficult to discern in the multiple-trauma victim either by routine imaging tests or at the time of surgery, secondary to extensive retroperitoneal hematoma. Missed pancreatic duct rupture results in increased morbidity and mortality. Both peritoneal lavage and computed tomography (CT) have been reported to miss the diagnosis of pancreatic duct rupture in trauma victims. Hence, ERCP may be very useful as a reliable means of detecting duct rupture.

Pancreatic Disorders

In young nonalcoholic patients with a first attack of pancreatitis in whom there is no discernible etiology, ERCP is useful for ruling out an anatomic cause such as pancreas divisum. Pancreas divisum is a congenital nonunion of the ventral and dorsal buds of the pancreas. It occurs in approximately 6% of the population and can only be demonstrated by ERCP. Pancreatitis in cases of pancreas divisum is theorized to result from a relative outflow obstruction through the minor papilla. Treatment includes ES and/or stenting of the minor papilla.

Other potential pathologic findings demonstrated by ERCP include pancreatic stones, undetected gallstones, papillary tumors, choledochocele, or pancreatic pseudocyst. Few cases of pancreatic cancer initially present as pancreatitis.

In patients with pancreatic pseudocyst, ERCP may provide useful information for planning the operation, such as instances of pancreatic duct obstruction or dilatation. Drainage should be performed as soon as possible after ERCP to avoid pancreatic sepsis. Depending on the anatomic conditions, most pancreatic pseudocysts can be drained endoscopically using a variety of endoscopic methods, specifically, cystogastrostomy, cystoduodenostomy, and transpapillary drainage using a pancreatic stent. Surgery is seldom required.

Malignant Obstruction

For malignant biliary tumors, a primary resection should be undertaken in appropriate candidates. Again, ERCP is helpful in planning the surgery. In unresectable cases, several endoscopic options are available to palliate the biliary obstruction.

The first endoscopic placement of internal plastic stents took place in 1980. Since then, placement of endoprostheses for palliation of malignant biliary tumors has become the procedure of choice. Stents range in size from 7 to 12 French (F). Patency is longer the larger the stent diameter. If proximal obstruction is present, two stents may be needed, one each in the left and right hepatic duct. The plastic stents generally remain patent for 3 to 6 months, depending on their size. They need to be changed regularly or whenever the patient shows signs of cholangitis or obstruction. Large, expandable wire-mesh stents are also available that are permanent and achieve sizes up to 30 F (Fig. 27-2). The only disadvantage of the metal stent is that it cannot be removed; therefore, the patient's life expectancy should not exceed that of the stent.

Treatment of Complications from Laparoscopic Cholecystectomy

An assortment of surgical complications has been described in conjunction with laparoscopic cholecystectomy. Many of these, such as CBD stricture, accessory duct leak, and cystic duct leak, are successfully treated with ERCP, ES, and/or CBD stenting. Recently, we treated two such patients, both of whom responded successfully to endoscopic and/or percutaneous drainage measures. The first patient underwent an uneventful laparoscopic cholecystectomy at another institution. Postoperatively, she developed a biloma and returned to surgery for open suture ligation of an accessory duct. When she developed a biloma again, she was referred to our institution for further evaluation. We first did an ultrasound-guided drainage of the biloma. Because of a hepatic iminodiacetic acid (HIDA) scan that showed filling of the gallbladder fossa, we studied her with ERCP, which showed a cystic duct leak (Fig. 27-3). She was successfully treated with ES and stent placement for 2 months (Fig. 27-4).

In the second patient, jaundice developed 4 weeks after laparoscopic cholecystectomy. Ultrasound in our office revealed a 12-mm CBD. ERCP showed a tight stricture of the distal common hepatic duct just proximal to the cystic duct–hepatic duct

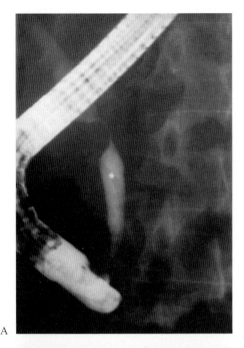

A

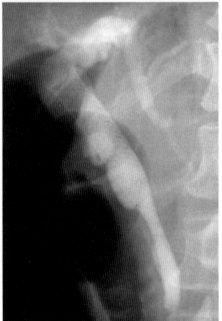

B

Fig. 27-2. **A:** *Cholangiogram of common bile duct (CBD) with stricture from neoplasm.* **B:** *Same CBD with wall stent placed successfully across stricture.*

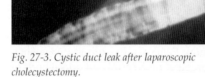

Fig. 27-3. *Cystic duct leak after laparoscopic cholecystectomy.*

Fig. 27-4. *Plastic stent within common bile duct.*

junction. This was successfully stented, and her jaundice has since cleared (Fig. 27-5). The injury here may have been from electrocautery, since no clips were identified in the area of the stricture. Treatment with ES or stenting is not uniformly successful. On one occasion, we have had to perform laparoscopic peritoneal lavage and placement of a drain in a patient who

had persistent bile leakage in spite of an endoscopically placed biliary stent.

Technical Aspects

ERCP is performed in the fluoroscopy suite with the patient in the prone posi-

tion. A scout film is taken to ensure proper positioning and to look for calcifications or other x-ray densities that could represent pancreatic or CBD stones or obscuring barium from previous studies. Conscious sedation consisting of a narcotic such as meperidine hydrochloride (Demerol HCl) and an amnestic such as midazolam hydrochloride (Versed) is administered; the dosages will vary, ranging from 25 to 150 mg for meperidine and up to 5 to 10 mg for midazolam. Other medications used include glucagon and hyoscyamine sulfate to decrease duodenal motility. Glucagon has a half-life of 3 to 6 minutes and can be given in doses of 0.5 to 1 mg. Hyoscyamine sulfate has a longer onset to action and a half-life of 2 to 3 hours. Recommended doses range from 0.2 to 0.5 mg, but this agent should be used with caution or avoided altogether in patients with glaucoma, cardiac disease, or intestinal ileus or obstruction. Patients must also be appropriately monitored with electrocardiography, interval blood pressure, and continuous oxygen saturation. Oxygen and other emergency equipment should be available in the event that patients have respiratory or cardiac problems during the procedure.

Because the duodenoscope is a side-viewing scope, a certain amount of conceptualizing the endoscope in three dimensions is required to pass the scope through a patient's oropharynx, pharynx, and esophagus. The duodenoscope is usually passed blindly into the upper esophagus. Once in, the pale wall of the esophagus is seen to slide by. Once in the stomach, the scope is positioned to slide along the greater curvature until the pylorus in encountered. It is important to aspirate any secretions pooled in the stomach. Since this is a side-viewing scope, the pylorus must be placed at the 6-o'clock position to pass the scope through. Once in the pylorus, the endoscope is turned all the way to the right, and the tip is deflected down to reach the second portion of the duodenum. This maneuver leaves the scope in a big loop or what is termed the *long-scope* position. To *short-scope* the duodenoscope, the shaft is twisted to the right or clockwise and the tip is deflected upward and withdrawn until the papilla is seen *en face*. In the short-scope position, the shaft of the duodenoscope is positioned on the lesser curve of the stomach. A view of the papilla is maintained with very gentle small movements of the tip of the scope.

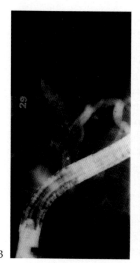
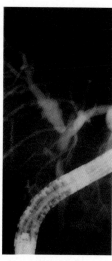
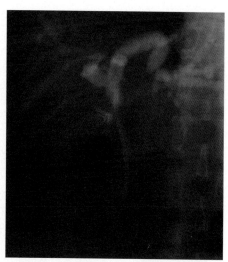

Fig. 27-5. **A:** *Stricture of the proximal common bile duct after laparoscopic cholecystectomy.* **B:** *Stent placed across the stricture.*

A diagnostic 7-F catheter is used first to cannulate the desired duct and identify the suspected pathology. The direction of the catheter determines which duct is cannulated. The CBD is usually located at the 11-o'clock position and angled acutely upward; occasionally, a mucosal shelf has to be elevated to cannulate the CBD selectively. The pancreatic duct is at less of an angle and more in the 3- or 4-o'clock position.

ES is used for a variety of indications and therapeutic measures. Various papillotomes are available in various sizes, wire lengths, and designs. Sphincterotomy is achieved using a papillotome with a diathermy wire with cutting current. We favor a papillotome with a short tip and 2-cm cutting wire. Ideally, the wire is positioned at 11 to 12 o'clock, with the wire bowed so that the sphincter muscle is taut against it. Placing a guidewire in the CBD will help maintain position. About one-third of the diathermy wire should be exposed to control the incision length. The current should also be delivered in short bursts in a stepwise fashion, redirecting or repositioning between cuts as needed (Fig. 27-6).

The amount of current will depend on the type of wire (monofilament or braided) and the amount of tissue fibrosis. As mentioned, we prefer a cutting current, but some prefer a blended current. The length of the cut is also determined by what procedure needs to be done. Incising to the first transverse duodenal fold is the maximum; however, if the procedure to be performed is to extract small stones from the CBD or to place a small stent, a 2- to 5-mm incision is all that is needed.

In some patients, anatomic variations or impacted stones make cannulation impossible. In these instances, a precut papillotomy can be performed. The tip of this papillotome has an extremely short cutting wire at the tip and is used in such a way that the papilla is unroofed, facilitating cannulation with a standard catheter or papillotome. The other option is to use a needle-knife technique. This instrument has a longer wire at the tip. Here, the wire is applied to the apex of the papilla and directed downward to the orifice. Once access to the sphincter is obtained, the needle knife is exchanged for a standard sphincterotome. These methods should only be used by very skilled and experienced endoscopists.

In the difficult sphincterotomy, a needle knife can also be used to incise over the top of a stent placed in the CBD or pancreatic duct. In patients with a Billroth II gastrectomy, other tricks include using a standard gastroscope or a special Billroth II papillotome. In this case, access to the papilla is obtained by entering the proximal jejunal limb. The papilla is seen from below. Cannulation is performed with a standard diagnostic cannula, but a special Billroth II papilltome is required for sphincterotomy.

In special situations in which the CBD is obstructed by tumor and proximal cannulation cannot be achieved due to a tight stricture, a rendezvous technique can be used. Access to the biliary tree is gained by a percutaneous transhepatic approach. A guidewire is then maneuvered through the obstructing tumor. Because there is a shorter, more direct route of passage of a guidewire through the CBD, a better angle and more direct pressure often allow a wire to pass a stricture from above. We usually perform this in the operating room with ultrasound guidance and fluoroscopic imaging.

On rare occasions, a sphincterotomy of the pancreatic duct may be required. This is best achieved after performing a biliary sphincterotomy that exposes the septum between the pancreatic duct and CBD. Pancreatic duct sphincterotomy is associated with a higher incidence of pancreatitis and other complications, but is indicated in rare instances of pancreatic duct stones or pancreatic duct stenosis.

ES is fraught with potential dangers. Proper positioning, selective cannulation, and taking care not to extend the cut beyond the first transverse duodenal fold should avoid perforation. Selective cannulation and minimal manipulation of the pancreatic duct are employed to avoid pancreatitis. When a cholangiogram or pancreatogram is obtained or confirmation of position is desired, the injection must be done very slowly so as not to overdistend the ducts and induce a pancreatitis. Hemorrhagic complications depend on how carefully the ES is done. When bleeding is encountered, it is frequently self-limited and rarely requires any intervention. Infectious complications generally occur only if the CBD is inadequately drained.

An ES allows extraction of CBD stones with the introduction of a variety of instruments through the working channel of the endoscope. Balloon catheters and Dormia baskets are frequently employed to extract stones (Figs. 27-6 to 27-8). If the stones are too large, an electrohydraulic lithotriptor or pulsed dye laser can be used first to fragment the stones. These methods require passage of a daughter scope through the channel of the therapeutic duodenoscope directly into the CBD to visualize the stones being fragmented. Other alternatives include mechanical lithotripsy, in which the stone is crushed in a reinforced, specially designed wire basket. This latter technique is less expensive and more widely available. In cases in

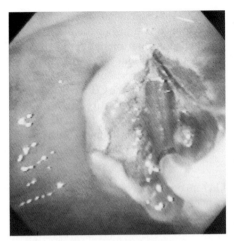

Fig. 27-6. Papillotome in ampulla of Vater after sphincterotomy completed without complication.

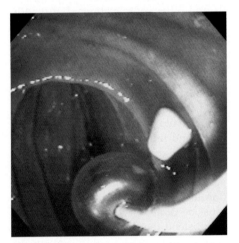

Fig. 27-7. Biliary balloon catheter used to extract a common bile duct stone.

which the duct is not completely cleared, a stent or nasobiliary catheter should be left in the duct to allow adequate drainage until complete clearance can be achieved. The latter is somewhat problematic for patients but does allow delivery of litholytic agents effective on cholesterol stones only. Extracorporeal shock wave lithotripsy has also been used in the treatment of CBD stones.

Endoprostheses are frequently used in the treatment of malignant obstruction. Stent placement is less hazardous than by percutaneous methods and offers patients palliation without surgery and its concomitant morbidity and mortality. Stents can be placed with or without ES, but we have found that placement is frequently easier with ES. Once a catheter or a papillotome is positioned in the CBD, a guidewire is maneuvered through the ob-

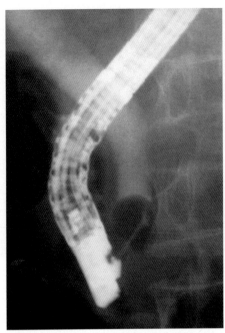

Fig. 27-8. Large common bile duct (CBD) stone in distal CBD.

struction using fluoroscopic guidance. The catheter is then removed, leaving the wire in place. With malignant obstruction, we try to place the largest stent possible. An overtube is placed over the guidewire, allowing some stiffening and support for the large stent. Over the wire and overtube, the appropriate length stent is placed, and using fluoroscopic guidance, an 11.5-F pushing tube is used to position the stent at the site of the obstruction (Fig. 27-9). The size of the stent selected should be as large a diameter as possible and long enough to traverse the obstruction and still have a few millimeters exposed in the duodenum. The plastic stents have a flange on each end to prevent either distal or proximal migration. Pancreatic duct stenting is done in a similar fashion. These stents are smaller and have side perforations to allow drainage of pancreatic juice.

Peroral cholangioscopy can provide a direct picture of the CBD. As mentioned above, a "baby scope" is introduced through the working channel of the duodenoscope and used to cannulate the CBD, allowing stones or tumors to be seen and potentially biopsied directly.

Complications

Certain anatomic factors such as juxtapapillary diverticula and history of Billroth II

gastrectomy were thought to increase the risk of complications, but more recent evidence indicates that these conditions do not predispose to increased risk, although they do have a higher failure rate secondary to difficulty in cannulation. Factors associated with more complications are sphincterotomy in a normal-size CBD and the use of precut sphincterotomy. Specific complications include pancreatitis, infection, perforation, and bleeding.

Pancreatitis

The incidence of significant pancreatitis is approximately 0.5% to 2% for diagnostic ERCP, but potentially much higher for therapeutic ERCP for which incidences as high as 26% have been reported. The variable frequency of pancreatitis probably reflects diversity in the definition of pancreatitis, which can vary from an asymptomatic hyperamylasemia to a clinical syndrome with chemical evidence of pancreatitis. Several factors may be involved in the etiology of post-ERCP pancreatitis. These include mechanical, chemical, hydrostatic, enzymatic, microbiologic, thermal, and patient factors, which have been outlined by Sherman and Lehman.

Mechanical factors are largely related to cannulation trauma that creates papillary edema and possibly SO spasm. This in

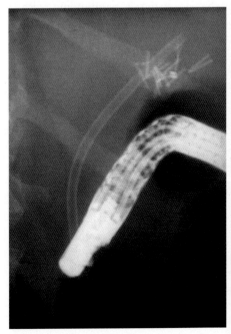

Fig. 27-9. Stent in the common bile duct.

turn may restrict flow of pancreatic juice and result in pancreatitis. The same sequence of events can follow a submucosal injection. Mechanical trauma seems a likely culprit, since an increased incidence of pancreatitis has been observed after repeated cannulations of the pancreatic duct and with pancreatography more so than with cholangiography and pancreatography or cholangiography alone.

Chemical factors mostly depend on the type of contrast medium used. Low-osmolality contrast appears to have a minimal advantage in reducing pancreatitis over conventional agents. Given the high cost of low-osmolality contrast, we recommend its use only in patients at high risk for developing pancreatitis.

A high hydrostatic pressure on injection is probably the most common cause of pancreatitis. Elevated pressure may disrupt cellular membranes or tight junctions between cells and cause backflow of intraductal contents into the interstitial space. Acinarization and urographic visualization are associated with an increased incidence of post-ERCP hyperamylasemia and pancreatitis.

The most common organisms causing bacteremia after ERCP are enterobacteria, fecal streptococci, *Staphylococcus epidermidis*, and *Bacteroides* organisms. Scope contamination has also been implicated in infectious complications of ERCP. This will be discussed further later in this chapter. Sphincterotomy creates edema that can obstruct the flow of pancreatic juice and cause pancreatitis. To avoid this, care should be taken to apply cutting current only, since this creates less tissue injury, and to place the diathermy wire in exactly the 11- to 1-o'clock positions. Correct positioning should maintain a few millimeters between the pancreatic orifice and the edematous tissue.

Extreme care should be taken in patients with a history of pancreatitis, SO dyskinesia, or papillary stenosis. The incidence of pancreatitis has been shown to be much higher in patients with chronic pancreatitis who undergo manometry in particular.

The management of pancreatitis is the same despite the etiology. Conservative measures should be employed first, but surgery may be indicated if there is clinical deterioration or evidence of infected pancreatic necrosis.

Infection

Cholangitis occurs in 0.6% to 0.8% and is the most common cause of death following ERCP. The incidence of sepsis is higher in malignant obstruction than in benign disorders. In one series, hilar strictures were more frequent in septic patients and may need combined percutaneous and endoscopic methods for complete drainage to avoid cholangitis. Lack of complete drainage is the most common etiologic factor in cases of post-ERCP sepsis. Therefore, when stones cannot be removed, a nasobiliary drain or stent should be placed. A diagnostic ERCP should be avoided in patients with suspected obstructive jaundice if decompression can not be done soon afterward, and antibiotics should be continued until the bile duct is completely decompressed.

Various antibiotics are recommended for prophylaxis. It is generally agreed that patients with obstructive disease of the pancreas or biliary tree should be treated with a broad-spectrum antibiotic prior to ERCP and/or ES. An antibiotic is also recommended for patients with valvular prostheses, a history of bacterial endocarditis, or valvular heart disease. The standard recommended antibiotic prophylaxis consists of gentamicin sulfate, a penicillin active against gram-negative bacteria and enterococci, or a cephalosporin. We generally use a second-generation cephalosporin, unless there are culture results indicating another antibiotic would be more effective. *Candida albicans* is a rare pathogen in the biliary tract, but patients who are immunocompromised or on total parenteral nutrition and/or prolonged antibiotics are at risk. The same principles apply to patients with pancreatic pseudocyst undergoing ERCP. Just as the obstructed biliary tree requires immediate drainage after ERCP, so does a pancreatic pseudocyst to avoid pancreatic abscess.

Hemorrhage

The incidence of bleeding is reported at around 2.5% to 5%, with a 0.3% mortality. Most bleeding stops spontaneously, while other cases require injection with epinephrine, balloon tamponade, coagulation, or angiographic embolization. Operation for bleeding is rare and usually consists of converting the ES to a sphincteroplasty. The coagulation status of each patient should be routinely checked. In our practice, we accept an international

normalized ratio (INR) of less than 1.8 to 2.0 for sphincterotomy. Aspirin and nonsteroidal antiinflammatory agents should be withheld around the time of the ERCP, if possible.

Perforation

The incidence of perforation varies from 0.4% to 2.5%. Retroduodenal perforation occurs in approximately 1% of patients undergoing ES. Intraperitoneal perforation is extremely rare. The diagnosis is usually obvious at the time of sphincterotomy with findings of air or contrast outside the CBD and duodenum. Early CT to assess the extent of the contamination is recommended. Most cases can be managed conservatively with nasogastric suction and antibiotics. Adequate biliary drainage is a must for this approach to work. The challenge is to predict which patient will not respond to these measures and will require operative management. The operation may consist of T-tube drainage of the bile duct and retroperitoneal drainage or retroperitoneal drainage alone. Each case must be managed on an individual basis.

Unusual Complications

Brief mention should be made of some of the rarer complications associated with ERCP, since a general awareness of these mishaps may lead to earlier diagnosis and treatment. Many of these are case reports, such as a case of biloma after ERCP from a ruptured distal biliary radicle or air in the portal vein. Others include cases of CBD perforation, impaction of endoprotheses, gallstone ileus, medication reactions, and cardiac complications.

Splenic injury has been reported in association with esophagogastroduodenoscopy, colonoscopy, and ERCP. The proposed mechanisms have included traction on the stomach and short gastrics, direct trauma to the hilum of the spleen, or traction on ligaments, mesentery, or adhesions. Complaints of localized pain in the left upper quadrant or hemodynamic instability should lead to further investigative studies and/or operation.

Conclusion

ERCP is a powerful diagnostic and therapeutic tool that has greatly reduced the need for open surgery in the management of benign and malignant pancreatic and hepatobiliary diseases. Most of these are surgical problems. Surgeons should include ERCP in their therapeutic armamentarium.

Suggested Reading

Arregui ME, Davis CJ, Arkush AM, Nagan RF. Laparoscopic cholecystectomy combined with endoscopic sphincterotomy and stone extraction or laparoscopic choledochoscopy and electrohydraulic lithotripsy for management of cholelithiasis with choledocholithiasis. *Surg Endosc* 1992;6:10–15.

Barkun AN, Barkun JS, Fried GM, et al. Useful predictors of bile duct stones in patients undergoing laparoscopic cholecystectomy. *Ann Surg* 1994;220:32–39.

Becker JM. Physiology of motor function of the sphincter of Oddi. *Surg Clin North Am* 1993;73:1291–1309.

Carr-Locke DL. Role of endoscopy in gallstone pancreatitis. *Am J Surg* 1993;165:519–521.

Cotton PB, Lehman G, Vennes J, et al. Endoscopic sphincterotomy complications and their management: an attempt at consensus. *Gastrointest Endosc* 1991;37:383–393.

Flati G, Flati D, Porowska B, Ventura T, Catarei M, Carboni M. Surgical anatomy of the papilla of Vater and biliopancreatic ducts. *Am Surg* 1994;60:712–718.

Hixson LJ. Biliary obstruction: nonsurgical treatment with endoscopic and radiologic techniques. *Postgrad Med* 1993;94:61–62.

Lai ECS, Lo CM. Acute pancreatitis: the role of ERCP in 1994. *Endoscopy* 1994;26:488–492.

Niederau C, Pohlmann U, Lubke H, Thomas L. Prophylactic antibiotic treatment in therapeutic or complicated diagnostic ERCP: results of a randomized controlled clinical study. *Gastrointest Endosc* 1994;40:533–537.

Parikh NJ, Geenen JE. Current role of ERCP in the management of benign pancreatic disease. *Endoscopy* 1992;24:120–124.

Ponsky JL, Scheeres DE, Simon I. Endoscopic retrograde cholangioscopy: an adjunct to endoscopic exploration of the common bile duct. *Am Surg* 1990;56:235–237.

Sherman S, Troiano FP, Hawes RH, O'Connor KW, Lehman GA. Frequency of abnormal sphincter of Oddi manometry compared with the clinical suspicion of sphincter of Oddi dysfunction. *Am J Gastroenterol* 1991;86:586–590.

Tang E, Stain SC, Tang G, Froes E, Berne TV. Timing of laparoscopic surgery in gallstone pancreatitis. *Arch Surg* 1995;130:496–500.

Toouli J, Baker RA. Innervation of the sphincter of Oddi: physiology and considerations of pharmacological intervention in biliary dyskinesia. *Pharmacol Ther* 1991;49:269–281.

EDITOR'S COMMENT

In the past 25 years, ERCP has become increasingly utilized as a means of diagnosing and treating biliary and pancreatic disorders. Endoscopic access to the ampulla of Vater allows precise anatomic characterization of the biliary and pancreatic ducts and, with the application of manometric techniques, has increased our understanding of the pathophysiology of the sphincteric mechanism. With the advent of laparoscopic cholecystectomy, many surgeons relegated the treatment of CBD stones to gastroenterologists performing ERCP due to a perceived inability to remove CBD stones laparoscopically. Therapy of choledocholithiasis has long been in the surgeon's purview; with knowledge and application of laparoscopic and endoscopic techniques, CBD stone disease can return to the surgeon's fold.

Although most patients with "soft" signs of choledocholithiasis at the time of laparoscopic cholecystectomy may be spared preoperative ERCP, certain indications remain. These include severe acute biliary pancreatitis, stone-induced cholangitis, and persistent jaundice, as tumors will be found to be the cause of jaundice in over one-third of the patients. ERCP following laparoscopic cholecystectomy should be among the first tests performed when there is suspicion of ongoing pathology of the CBD due to retained stones or possible CBD injury. If the surgeon does not perform his or her own ERCP, it is critical to learn the outcome of ERCP examinations performed by the local expert, as ERCP is a technically demanding procedure. Individuals whose cannulation rate is low and incidence of complications exceeds that of the norms established in this chapter should probably not be counted on for postoperative treatment of CBD stones discovered at the time of laparoscopic cholecystectomy. Rather, the surgeon should treat those stones intraoperatively or place a CBD catheter through the cystic duct that will facilitate cannulation in the postoperative period using the rendezvous technique.

N.J.S.

28

Laparoscopic Cholecystectomy

Edward M. Mason and Titus D. Duncan

It has been said that the development of laparoscopic cholecystectomy is the single most important event in general surgery in the last 30 years. This is due to the emergence of an entirely new approach to surgery and the realization that incision size does affect postoperative recovery. Publicity about laparoscopic bile duct injuries has threatened the acceptance of this operation, and surgeons must use safe and meticulous dissection techniques to minimize such unwanted outcomes.

Anatomic Considerations

The classic anatomy of the biliary tree occurs in only 30% of individuals, so it may be said that anomalies are the rule, not the exception. It is of utmost importance that the surgeon has extensive knowledge of the anatomy and the various anomalies. This is even more important in the remote, two-dimensional laparoscopic setting. Only when one has this understanding will complications and misadventures decline.

Cystic Duct

The cystic duct may join the common bile duct at an acute angle, travel parallel to the common duct for several centimeters prior to insertion, insert into the right hepatic duct, or be congenitally absent. Perhaps, the most challenging consideration is a short cystic duct, for it is in this setting that the common duct is most likely to be injured.

Cystic and Hepatic Arteries

The cystic artery arises from the right hepatic artery. One must be absolutely sure that the cystic artery is visualized entering the gallbladder wall, for often the right hepatic artery will loop up onto the surface of the gallbladder, and a very short cystic artery will arise. If this dissection is incomplete, then the likelihood of ligating the right hepatic artery is great. There can be early branching of the cystic artery, with the other branch often found in a posterior location. Occasionally, the cystic artery can be found to the right of the cystic duct.

Common Bile Duct

The common bile duct (CBD) begins at the junction of the cystic duct and the common hepatic duct and traverses inferiorly to the ampulla of Vater. Its normal diameter is less than 6 mm, although it may be larger in elderly patients and those with biliary obstruction.

Triangle of Calot

This is the area formed by the gallbladder and the cystic duct to the right, the common hepatic duct to the left, and the margin of the right lobe of the liver superiorly. Careful dissection of this area will minimize the chance of injury and complications.

Accessory Hepatic Ducts

Small bile ducts may enter the gallbladder directly from its bed (ducts of Luschka). There may also be small biliary radicles in the superficial liver parenchyma of the gallbladder bed. If these ducts are damaged during the dissection and not ligated at the time of surgery, a postoperative biloma will develop.

Indications

Almost all agree that patients with symptomatic gallstones should undergo cholecystectomy. Failure to do so usually leads to complications. When medical conditions contraindicate surgery, temporizing measures such as percutaneous cholecystostomy can be performed until definitive surgery can be achieved. There may be some rationale for performing laparoscopic cholecystectomy for asymptomatic gallstones in certain patients, such as *Salmonella* carriers, immunocompromised individuals, or those who are frequently removed from modern medical care. The appearance of a porcelain gallbladder is an indication for cholecystectomy due to the increased incidence of cancer.

In recent years, there has been an effort to expand the indications for surgery to patients with biliary dyskinesia. This diagnosis is made in patients who have biliary pain, but all diagnostic studies (ultrasonography, computed tomography [CT]) are unrevealing. A hepatobiliary scan is performed with cholecystokinin injection, and the ejection fraction of the gallbladder is measured. Less than 35% ejection is considered abnormal, thus suggesting biliary dyskinesia. Although postoperative pain relief is the rule when cholecystectomy is performed for typical biliary colic in the presence of an abnormal scintiscan, patients should understand that preoperative discomfort may not be relieved by operation.

With the advent of laparoscopic cholecystectomy, the number of cholecystectomies performed has dramatically increased. Controversy exists as to whether unnecessary procedures are being performed or whether the increase is transient in nature, occurring as a result of patients previously unwilling to have an open procedure undergoing laparoscopic cholecystectomy. Departmental quality-management committees should monitor this situation closely to ensure that unnecessary procedures are not performed.

Contraindications to laparoscopic cholecystectomy, other than medical conditions precluding general anesthesia and laparoscopy, primarily relate to the experience of the surgeon. That is, more experienced surgeons will generally convert to an open procedure less often than surgeons with limited experience. It must be clearly understood that performing an open cholecystectomy or converting to an open procedure is not a complication or failure, but rather prudence for less experienced surgeons. The "hostile" abdomen may be a contraindication, but again this is more a case of a surgeon's experience. Third-trimester pregnancy is certainly a contraindication to laparoscopic cholecystectomy, whereas an early pregnancy may be a relative contraindication in a medicolegal sense, as published reports support its safety.

Diagnostic Considerations

The only preoperative study necessary in patients with typical biliary colic is an ultrasound examination revealing gallstones. A hepatobiliary scan in the absence of stones is useful for revealing cystic duct obstructions or diminished ejection fraction. Other diagnostic measures, such as oral cholecystogram, inspection of bile for cholesterol crystals, CT scan, and endoscopy or contrast studies of the upper gastrointestinal tract, are reserved for patients in whom the diagnosis is uncertain or confounding considerations exist.

Perioperative Patient Management

Patients are assessed by the anesthesiologist to determine coexisting diseases and their effect on anesthetic management during surgery. Of importance in the preoperative workup is a biochemical profile with particular emphasis on the liver function studies. Marked elevations in these tests may be an indication for examination

of the biliary tree by endoscopic retrograde cholangiopancreatography (ERCP).

Patients are to take nothing by mouth starting the evening prior to operation. We have routinely given antibiotic coverage preoperatively, usually with a cephalosporin. Patients are asked to void just prior to entering the operating room, which eliminates the need for intraoperative bladder catheterization. Sequential compression stockings are applied either in the preoperative area or in the operating room, but in either case they are functioning prior to the induction of anesthesia to minimize the risk of deep venous thrombosis.

Operative Technique

The patient is placed on the operating table in the supine position with both arms tucked by the side. Ulnar pads are used to protect the elbows. We have found that even with rather obese patients, this positioning can be accomplished.

Once general endotracheal anesthesia has been initiated, an orogastric tube is placed and connected to suction. By decompression of the stomach, the chance of trocar injury to the stomach is lessened, and visualization of the right upper quadrant is improved. The abdomen is shaved, if necessary, around the umbilicus and the right subcostal area extending to the epigastrium. The abdomen is then prepared with a surgical preparation extending from nipple line to groin and on the right side to the midaxillary line.

The operating room is depicted in Fig. 28-1. The equipment on the primary cart includes a high-flow insufflator, carbon dioxide (CO_2) tank, camera input, light source, VCR, monitor, and an in-line printer. The secondary cart will have only a monitor connected to the primary cart monitor.

A grounding pad is placed on the patient's thigh and connected to the electrocautery. We no longer use the laser, as it was not cost-effective and offered no advantage over the cautery.

The surgeon stands on the patient's left side, as does the camera person. The assistant surgeon works from the patient's right side, as does the scrub person. European surgeons have expressed a preference for having the patient in the litho-

tomy position, with the surgeon standing between the legs. Use of a robotic arm to hold the camera—or an experienced surgeon holding the camera for him- or herself—eliminates the need for a dedicated laparoscopic camera operator.

After the insufflator tubing, the camera cord, and the light source are connected, white balance is obtained in the camera, and the irrigation tubing is connected. Pneumoperitoneum may be achieved by either an open or a closed technique. The closed method consists of making a small stab wound at the base of the umbilicus, and with gentle upward traction on the umbilicus, a Veress needle is placed into the abdomen through the incision. The Veress needle is then aspirated to ensure that the needle has not been placed in a vessel or hollow viscus. If aspiration is negative, then a drop of water is put in the needle, and the water should be sucked into the peritoneal cavity by the lower intraabdominal pressure. Many experienced laparoscopists merely attach the insufflator tubing to the Veress needle and ascertain the position of the needle in the peritoneal cavity by the low-pressure reading (usually around 3 to 5 mm Hg) on the insufflator.

The open or Hasson trocar technique is performed by making an incision in the umbilicus and dissecting down through the fascia into the peritoneal cavity using digital examination of the peritoneum to ensure that there are no underlying adhesions or intestine. A blunt-tipped trocar is then placed into the abdominal cavity and secured to the fascia by sutures or held in place by a balloon attached to the sleeve of the trocar. The obvious advantage of the open technique should be avoidance of injury to underlying structure by the Veress needle or the subsequent insertion of the umbilical trocar. However, even with the open technique, the bowel may be injured when it is intimately adhesed to the peritoneum. If sutures are used to secure the Hasson trocar, they may limit the ability of the laparoscope to have full range of motion.

Following insufflation by either technique, the trocar is placed in the umbilicus. We have not used the infraumbilical curvilinear ("smiley face") incision for two reasons. First, the shortest distance from the skin to the peritoneal cavity is through the base of the umbilicus, and there is very little adipose tissue at this point. This is important for avoiding trocar-site infection when a markedly infected gallbladder is removed. Second, cosmesis is much better when going through the umbilicus.

Obviously, when the patient has had previous abdominal surgery, the open technique may be preferred; alternatively, we have insufflated with the Veress needle placed subcostally in the right upper quadrant. A 5-mm trocar is placed in the same position, and exploration for adhesions and visual guidance of secondary trocar sites can be carried out using a 5-mm laparoscope.

The pneumoperitoneum is taken to 15 mm Hg. Higher pressures are not necessary and carry the risk of vena caval compression or hypercarbia from absorption of CO_2 across the peritoneum.

Key to avoiding injury to underlying bowel or blood vessels when the first trocar is inserted by the closed technique is to make the skin incision slightly larger than the diameter of the trocar. This allows the trocar to slide easily through the tissue, even when covered by a protective shield. If this is not done, the point of the trocar penetrates the peritoneum while the shaft hangs on the skin, allowing injury to occur as one attempts to force the trocar inward.

The umbilical port usually is the first port placed. When the closed technique is used, a vertical incision is made in the umbilicus on either side of the Veress needle. Classically, insertion of the umbilical port is described as being aimed toward the pelvis. This tends to create a "bind" in the trocar when it is then aimed cephalad toward the right upper quadrant. Our experience has led us to picture the pneumoperitoneum as a dome of gas over the viscera. We therefore aim the trocar into this dome, slightly upward toward the right upper quadrant. Insertion should be smooth and almost effortless. With this technique, injury to the aorta and the iliac vessels should not occur. Insertion should never be aimed directly posteriorly.

Once a 10-mm trocar is inserted, the insufflator tubing is connected to the side port of the trocar, and the laparoscope is inserted through the trocar sleeve. It is imperative to inspect the abdominal cavity for injury to the viscera or vessels immediately on entering the peritoneal cavity. Any blood noted in the peritoneal cavity should arouse suspicion that an injury may have occurred. This mandates irriga-

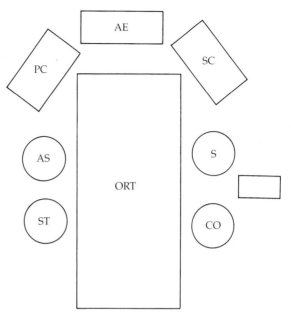

Fig. 28-1. Operating room setup. (ST, scrub technician; AS, assistant surgeon; PC, primary cart; AE, anesthesia; SC, secondary cart; S, surgeon; CO, camera operator.)

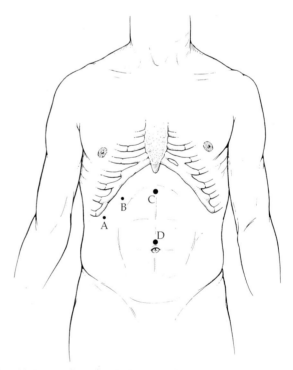

Fig. 28-2. Trocar sites. (A, 5 mm at liver edge; B, 5 mm over GB; C, 5 or 10-mm epigastric; D, 10-mm umbilicus.)

tion of the bloody area and visual inspection of all the viscera and vessels in that area.

All subsequent ports must be placed under direct visualization of the laparoscope. We place a 10-mm port in the epigastrium at the right edge of the falciform ligament (Fig. 28-2). Now that a 5-mm clip applier has been developed, a 5-mm port may be used in this area. Beginning laparoscopic surgeons may be better served by using the 10-mm port here, as the cystic duct may not be adequately ligated by a 5-mm clip, thus requiring introduction of the clip applier through the umbilicus with a 5-mm camera in the epigastric port.

The right upper quadrant ports are 5-mm in size and have been described as being placed subcostally at the midclavicular and anterior axillary lines. Realistically, the midport should be positioned directly over the gallbladder and the lateral port at the inferior edge of the liver. After all ports are placed, the patient is placed in a reverse Trendelenburg position and slightly rotated to the left so that the abdominal viscera will tend to fall away from the right upper quadrant.

A grasping forceps is placed through the lateral port to grasp the fundus of the gallbladder and push it up over the liver. This should not be done forcefully, and often one will need to remove adhesions from the gallbladder to fully retract it upward. With cystic duct obstruction, the gallbladder is markedly distended and cannot be grasped without risk of rupture. This requires decompression of the gallbladder with a needle and syringe. For thickened gallbladder walls, a laparoscopic "screw" may be placed in the fundus and used to retract the gallbladder cephalad. Toothed graspers may also be used in this setting; however, this may result in tearing of the gallbladder wall with spillage of bile and/or stones.

The middle port is used to place a grasper on the neck of the gallbladder and retract downward and slightly to the right side to open up the triangle of Calot (Fig. 28-3). Dissection of the gallbladder is accomplished using instruments placed through the epigastric port. This should be done in a stepwise and careful manner.

Initially, adhesions to the gallbladder are removed by grasping them at their insertion on the gallbladder wall and pulling inferiorly. This is done without applying electric current to avoid an arc current injury to the bowel. Blood loss in doing this is usually minimal. With the adhesions removed, dissection is begun at the neck of the gallbladder by spreading the fibroareolar tissue with the dissector and gently teasing it from the inferior edge of the gallbladder. Often, a large lymph node is present and can obscure the anatomy in this area. The cystic artery usually lies in close proximity to this node. By dissecting the tissue on the gallbladder above the node, one can identify the cystic artery and develop a plane, thus freeing the artery.

Electrocautery should not be used in this area until all structures have been identified; otherwise, thermal damage to the CBD can occur. Once the cystic duct, cystic artery, and cystic duct–gallbladder junction have been positively identified, a hook cautery may be used to complete the dissection. Small amounts of tissue are

lifted up with the hook, placed on tension, and divided with short bursts of low-wattage electrical current.

The cystic artery should be dissected up on the gallbladder, and clips applied in that area to avoid inadvertent damage to the right hepatic artery. When the dissection is complete, one should see the neck of the gallbladder dissected away from the liver with two tubular structures (cystic duct and artery) traversing Calot's triangle (Fig. 28-4).

To avoid injury to the CBD, we utilize the approach of identifying the gallbladder–cystic duct junction and dissect only enough cystic duct to allow placement of three clips. Dissection of the cystic duct down to its junction with the CBD increases the risk of injury to the CBD.

Some reports have alluded to the "cystic duct syndrome," associated with leaving a long cystic duct stump. This syndrome, however, is likely caused by the presence of a stone in a long cystic duct. Using this technique, we have not had a CBD injury at our institution in over 3,500 laparoscopic cholecystectomies. Generally, the CBD can be visualized through the visceral peritoneum as a point of reference. If stones are noted in the cystic duct, they should be milked back into the gallbladder prior to the application of clips on the distal side of the cystic duct (Fig. 28-5).

It is extremely important in dissecting the cystic duct not to retract the neck of the gallbladder superiorly, as this can tent the CBD. This can result in injury to the CBD when clips are applied to its tented portion. When dense adhesions are encountered, hydrodissection is often useful.

It is at this point in the procedure that a cholangiogram may be performed. It has been our philosophy to utilize selective intraoperative cholangiography. Indications for this include unclear anatomy, elevated liver function studies (especially bilirubin and alkaline phosphatase), a dilated cystic duct or CBD, and inability to clear the CBD by preoperative ERCP. Cholangiograms are best performed using fluoroscopic techniques. Dynamic cholangiograms are much more useful than static ones, as the anatomy can be manipulated in real time. The dye is diluted to 50% strength with normal saline, as full-strength dye can obscure small stones in the CBD.

The first step in performing cholangiography is to place a clip at the gallblad-

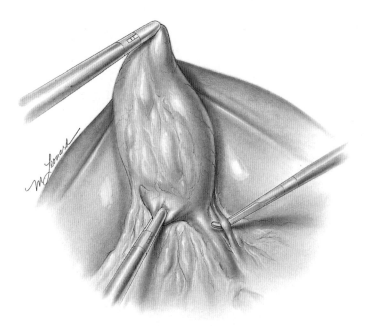

Fig. 28-3. Calot's triangle.

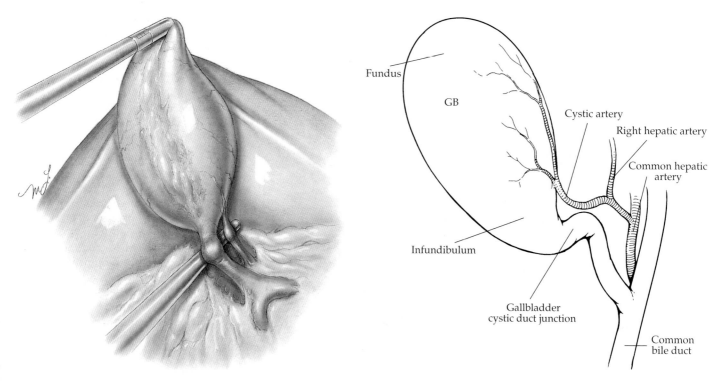

Fig. 28-4. Anatomy following dissection: the triangle of Calot.

der–cystic duct junction to prevent small stones from falling into the cystic duct. There are many good cholangiogram catheters on the market, and the surgeon should find the one with which he or she is the most comfortable. We normally use a catheter that traverses and is fixed in place by a cholangioclamp (Fig. 28-6).

The cystic duct is incised just below the clip at the gallbladder–cystic duct junction by scissors placed through the middle port. The catheter is then inserted into the ductotomy, while gently being flushed with saline. Once the catheter is placed in the cystic duct and secured, the graspers and camera are removed. It is helpful if the epigastric port and the midport are radiolucent to avoid obscuring the cholangiographic images. If this is not the case, then these trocars should be held out of the field with a towel clip. Other methods of obtaining cholangiograms include placing contrast medium directly into the gallbladder or using a 21- or 23-gauge scalp vein needle inserted directly into the CBD. If the contrast medium does not flow into the duodenum, one must assume the presence of stones. However, spasm of the ampulla may give the same picture. To relax the ampullary sphincter, glucagon, 1 mg, or cholecystokinin-op, 20 mg/kg, may be given intravenously.

Following the clipping of the cystic duct and artery, both structures are divided by scissors, and the dissection of the gallbladder from the liver bed is begun. The dissection is performed with electrocautery using either monopolar or bipolar current.

The ultrasonic scalpel is also useful for this, although it does add additional expense. The coagulation mode of the cautery is used (with a blend setting of 2) with a power setting of 30 W. The power should be at its lowest setting to accom-

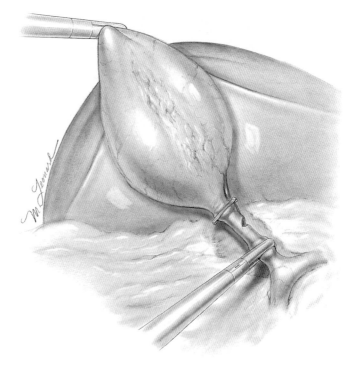

Fig. 28-5. Milking stones out of the cystic duct.

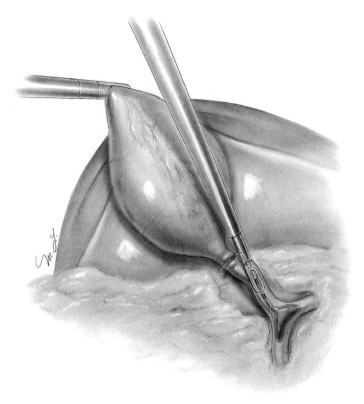

Fig. 28-6. Performance of cholangiography using a catheter placed using a cholangioclamp.

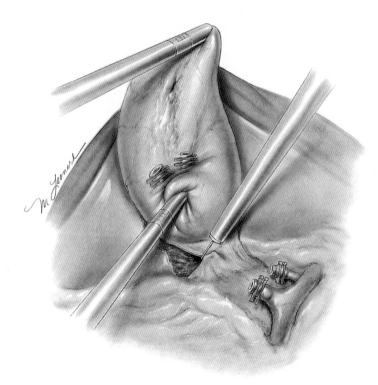

Fig. 28-7. Dissection of the gallbladder from the liver bed.

plish the dissection, for higher settings are more likely to cause an arc of current, resulting in thermal injury to surrounding tissue. Early in the history of laparoscopic cholecystectomy, a laser was used for dissection; however, we abandoned this mode after the first 100 cases in favor of electrocautery. The expense of the laser does not appear to be justified.

During dissection of the gallbladder from its bed, the expertise of the assistant surgeon is of paramount importance, as the gallbladder is manipulated from side to side to expose the plane of dissection and place it under tension (Fig. 28-7). When tears in the gallbladder occur, they may be closed by preformed loop ligatures ("endoloops") to prevent spillage of stones (Fig. 28-8). Occasionally, this ligature is also used to occlude the cystic duct, especially when it is thin or dilated and when a postoperative ERCP is anticipated. Bile leakage should be removed by copious irrigation.

Every effort must be made to retrieve stones that have fallen out of the gallbladder, for there is ample documentation that stones may be a nidus for subsequent abscess formation. Prior to completion of the dissection, the liver bed must be closely inspected for bleeding or bile leakage. It is helpful to reduce the intraabdominal pressure to a setting of 8 mm Hg to inspect for liver bed hemorrhage. Once the dissection is completed, copious irrigation of the subhepatic space is used to remove bile, blood clot, and debris, when present. The liver bed and clips are again checked.

To remove the gallbladder, the camera is placed in the epigastric port, and a heavy-toothed grasping forceps is introduced through the umbilical port and directed to the right upper quadrant. The gallbladder neck is then grasped and removed through the umbilicus. When large stones are present, the umbilical incision will need to be enlarged. When there are many small stones and the gallbladder neck has been pulled up to the abdominal wall, the gallbladder may be opened and stone forceps used to empty the gallbladder to facilitate its complete removal (Fig. 28-9).

Following removal of the gallbladder, the port site at the umbilicus is occluded, the lateral and midports are removed, and the pneumoperitoneum is evacuated by applying suction to the epigastric port. This is especially important in human immunodeficiency virus–positive patients, as it

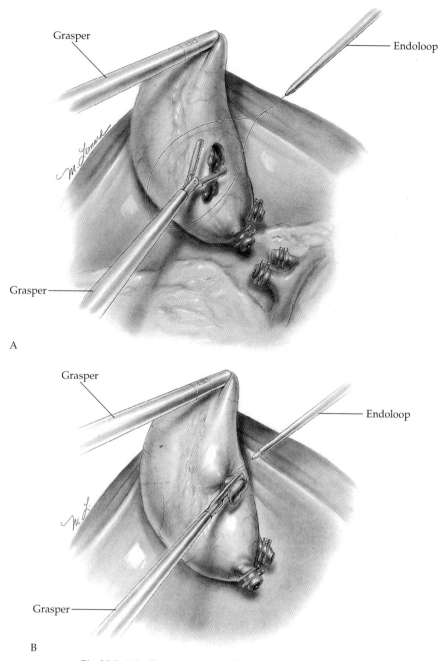

Grasper

Endoloop

Grasper

A

Grasper

Endoloop

Grasper

B

*Fig. 28-8. **A,B:** Closure of tear in gallbladder wall using preformed loop ligature.*

has been demonstrated that the flume from the pneumoperitoneum may transport live bacteria and/or virus particles. Complete evacuation of the pneumoperitoneum is important for reducing the incidence of shoulder pain due to irritation of the diaphragm.

We have not routinely used drains in cholecystectomy; however, in "dirty" cases with inordinate contamination, a drain may be placed prior to removing the gallbladder from the abdominal cavity. This is best accomplished by placing a grasper through the lateral port and into and out the epigastric port. The drain is grasped and brought out the lateral port site. (It is necessary to remove the lateral port at this point.) The drain is then positioned in the subhepatic space. The fascia at the umbilicus is closed with a no.1 long-term absorbable suture. Early experience with nonclosure of the fascia or closure with 0 short-term (less than 120 days) absorbable suture led to a significant number of hernias. The fascia at the epigastric port need not be closed, as the falciform ligament prevents herniation at that area. The skin is closed with 4-0 absorbable suture at all port sites.

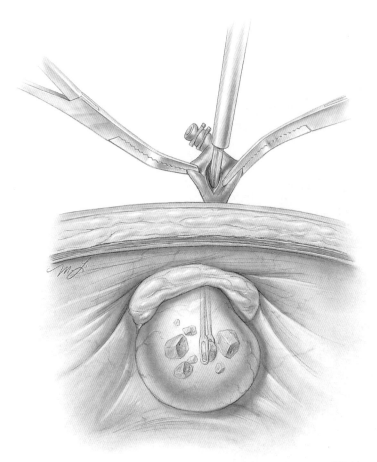

Fig. 28-9. Removing gallbladder stones through the opened infundibulum to facilitate gallbladder extraction from the abdominal cavity.

ducing the trocar too far. Insertion of the initial trocar, especially when performed in a closed fashion, has been reported to cause injury to the bowel, bladder, aorta, iliac artery, or vena cava. When a trocar injury to a major blood vessel is suspected, patients must be opened immediately without removing the trocar until the involved blood vessel is isolated. In contrast, if the small-bore Veress needle enters a viscus or blood vessel, the operation can generally be completed and patients monitored closely for signs of complications in the postoperative period.

The laparoscopic trocars may also lacerate blood vessels in the abdominal wall. Prior to removal, each trocar should be visualized from the peritoneal aspect using the laparoscope. If significant hemorrhage is seen, it can generally be controlled with cautery, intraoperative tamponade with a Foley catheter, or a through-and-through suture on each side of the trocar-insertion site.

Results

Many clinical series of laparoscopic cholecystectomy have been reported. Morbidity ranges from 1% to 9%, and CBD injuries range from 0.2% to 0.7%. Morbidity is rare after this procedure and is usually attributed to unrelated events. The conversion rates from laparoscopic to open operation in most series range from 1.8% to 7.8% and are generally greater early in a surgeon's experience with the procedure.

Conclusion

Laparoscopic management of symptomatic gallstones has rapidly become the new gold standard for therapy in the United States and throughout the world. Many patients can now undergo this operation in an ambulatory setting. Occasionally, anatomic or physiologic considerations will preclude the laparoscopic approach, and conversion to an open operation in such cases reflects sound judgment and should not be considered a complication.

Postoperative Care

A complete blood cell count is obtained approximately 2 hours postoperatively to ensure there has been no postoperative bleeding. Postoperative antibiotics are not necessary, except in cases of bile spillage. Patients may be discharged when vital signs are stable and patients are taking oral fluids, have voided, and are comfortable with oral analgesics. Overnight hospitalization is usually reserved for patients with medical problems (e.g., cardiac, pulmonary).

Instructions on discharge usually include bathing after 24 hours and removing all dressings in 48 hours. Activity and diet are unrestricted. Most patients return to normal activity within 3 to 4 days and to manual labor by 7 days. Follow-up in the office is at approximately 10 days postoperatively, and if no problems occur, patients are discharged to their primary care physician.

Complications

Many complications related to laparoscopic removal of the gallbladder are similar to those occurring during open cholecystectomy. These complications include hemorrhage, biliary duct injuries, bile leaks, retained stones, pancreatitis, wound infections, and incisional hernias. Other potential complications are pneumoperitoneum-related (gas embolism, vagal reaction, ventricular arrhythmias, hypercarbia with acidosis) and trocar-related (injuries to the abdominal wall, intraabdominal organ, or major blood vessels). The protective shield on certain trocars is not an insurance against perforation of intestine or major vessels, especially in the previously operated abdomen. Regardless of the make of trocar, one should never aim toward the spine or the location of the great vessels, and a hand is used as a brake to prevent inadvertently intro-

Suggested Reading

Baird DR, Wilson JP, Mason EM, et al. An early review of 800 laparoscopic cholecystectomies at a university-affiliated community teaching hospital. *Am Surg* 1992;58:206–210.

Barkun JS, Barkun AN, Sampalis JS, et al. Randomised controlled trial of laparoscopic versus mini-cholecystectomy. *Lancet* 1992;340:1116–1119.

Deziel DJ, Millikan KW, Economou SG, Doolas A, Ko ST, Airan MC. Complications of laparoscopic cholecystectomy: a national survey of 4,292 hospitals and an analysis of 77,604 cases. *Am J Surg* 1993;165:9–14.

DuBois F, Icard P, Berthelot G, Levard H. Coelioscopic cholecystectomy: preliminary report of 36 cases. *Ann Surg* 1990;211:60–62.

The Southern Surgeons Club. A prospective analysis of 1518 laparoscopic cholecystectomies. *N Engl J Med* 1991;324:1073–1078.

Reddick EJ, Olsen DO, Daniel JF, et al. Laparoscopic laser cholecystectomy. *Laser Med Surg News* 1989;7:38–40.

EDITOR'S COMMENT

Dr. Mason and Dr. Duncan have drawn on their extensive experience with laparoscopic cholecystectomy to summarize the appropriate perioperative considerations and describe their technique. Several points bear emphasis. The indications for cholecystectomy should not change as one becomes able to perform the operation using laparoscopic techniques. This having been said, there has been a marked increase in the frequency with which laparoscopic cholecystectomy is performed since its introduction. I hope that this represents a resetting of the threshold for performing cholecystectomy soon after symptoms begin, as asymptomatic stones, even in diabetics, should rarely be treated.

This chapter describes the typical American four-port technique, with the surgeon operating through a single port. Many valid alternative techniques exist and bear mentioning. In the French technique, the surgeon stands between the legs, with the patient in the lithotomy position and the epigastric port placed lower in the abdomen. Rather than elevation of the liver by grasping the gallbladder, the liver is retracted with an instrument placed through the lateral port. Many surgeons also use a two-handed technique, manipulating instruments placed through the middle subcostal port with the left hand while operating through the epigastric port with the right hand. When assistants are inexperienced, this technique proves particularly worthwhile. Use of this method also facilitates performance of other, more advanced procedures that require two-handed operating.

Comment must also be made regarding the performance of intraoperative cholangiography. Common to many other practicing surgeons, Dr. Mason and Dr. Duncan perform selective intraoperative cholangiography and have demonstrated that this may be practiced safely without CBD injuries. I advocate the liberal use of cholangiography and include as an indication for it the presence of cystic duct stones, as these stones predict the presence of CBD stones. More recently, I have also been using laparoscopic intracorporeal ultrasonography to image the CBD, and believe that this will be a complementary imaging technique to standard fluoroscopic cholangiography. In addition, the authors do not address the type of laparoscope that they use when performing laparoscopic cholecystectomy. I advocate the use of an angled laparoscope (30 or 45 degrees) during all cases, as the surgeon is given alternative views of the anatomy and clear visualization of the triangle of Calot is offered in patients who are obese or whose transverse colon is distended.

Regardless of how one performs laparoscopic cholecystectomy, it is imperative to perform a dissection that will prevent injury to the major biliary structures. CBD injury is the Achilles heel of the procedure and very nearly resulted in discrediting the operation. As the authors have emphasized, the critical anatomic landmark is the junction of the gallbladder with the cystic duct. I emphasize the clearance of the gallbladder neck away from its hepatic bed and view Calot's triangle for both its ventral and dorsal aspects by manipulating the infundibulum and fundus of the gallbladder to expose these areas sequentially. This allows a three-dimensional reconstruction of the anatomy as displayed on a two-dimensional video screen. When, and only when, the critical view is displayed—the fully dissected neck of the gallbladder with duct and artery entering it—are clips applied. Surgeons must constantly strive to reduce the risk of ductal injury to as close to zero as possible.

Finally, a historical note should be added. The anatomic triangle that Calot described in the 1890s has been expanded by surgical educators immemorial, including the authors of this chapter. The triangle that Calot described was bounded by the cystic duct, the cystic artery, and the gallbladder wall, thereby including very few relevant structures except for twigs from the cystic artery. What most of us refer to as Calot's triangle is the hepatocystic triangle bounded by the cystic duct, inferior gallbladder wall, and liver edge. It is this triangle that must be cleared along its upper borders in an attempt to clarify all anatomic relationships when laparoscopic cholecystectomy is performed.

N.J.S.

29

Laparoscopic Common Bile Duct Exploration

Richard L. Friedman and Edward H. Phillips

For hundreds of years, nonoperative management of patients with common bile duct (CBD) stones was the standard of practice, as most calculi pass spontaneously. However, some patients go on to develop biliary enteric fistulas or die of sepsis and hepatic failure. The early surgical treatment of biliary disease involved the creation of external or internal biliary fistulas. With the introduction of cholecystectomy in the 1880s, CBD stones were managed by either forcing them back into the gallbladder via the cystic duct or fragmenting them in the CBD, facilitating spontaneous passage.

In 1889, Thorton in the United Kingdom and Abbe in the United States presented their experiences with direct incision of the CBD to remove calculi, changing forever the treatment of patients with stone disease. In 1899, Halsted wrote that every biliary operation was an exploratory one and the type of procedure should be dictated by the operative findings. Even with this revolutionary approach to biliary disease, operative morbidity was high, and decisions were based on subjective clinical experience. It was not until Mirizzi in 1934 introduced intraoperative cholangiography that the mortality of CBD surgery was decreased. Prior to intraoperative cholangiography, a negative CBD exploration occurred in as many as 50% of patients explored; this incidence was reduced to 6%. In addition, the incidence of retained CBD calculi decreased from 25% to 11%. This substantially contributed to the decrease in morbidity and mortality, since reoperation carried with it a 30% morbidity and 5% mortality.

The next advance in operative biliary surgery was the introduction of rigid choledochoscopy in 1941 by McIver. Un-

fortunately, this technique was not widely accepted until the late 1970s. It further reduced the incidence of retained calculi to 3%. The most important advance occurred in 1974. The introduction of endoscopic retrograde cholangiopancreatography (ERCP) with endoscopic sphincterotomy (ES) changed the treatment and significance of retained stones. In experienced hands, ES has a success rate of 95% with a morbidity of 10% and a mortality of 1%. In addition, patients with cholangitis have been shown to have improved outcomes if they had ES rather than an open CBD exploration. This led to several studies comparing open CBD exploration and endoscopic stone clearance.

Neoptolemos and colleagues in 1987 and 1992, Heinerman, Ponchon, Stiegmann and their associates in 1989, and Stain and coworkers in 1991 reported trials of preoperative clearance of CBD stones prior to open cholecystectomy. All but Stain and colleagues showed reduced hospitalization, but none showed a decrease in morbidity or mortality with preoperative ES. In fact, Stain showed an increase in morbidity when preoperative ES was added to cholecystectomy, compared with cholecystectomy and open CBD exploration. Heinerman and associates' study was the only one to show a reduction in morbidity in patients undergoing ES compared with open CBD exploration, but 74% of patients having open CBD exploration had undergone concomitant transduodenal sphincterotomy.

Consequently, preoperative ES for patients suspected of harboring CBD stones did not become common practice until the introduction of laparoscopic cholecystectomy by Mouret in France in 1987 and Reddick in the United States in 1988. The

treatment of CBD stones prior to laparoscopic cholecystectomy was fairly routine. Patients underwent cholecystectomy, and cholangiography was performed when CBD stones were suspected. If stones were found, a CBD exploration was performed. However, the advent of laparoscopic cholecystectomy brought with it an aversion to convert to open surgery, which initially was the only surgical option for removing CBD stones. Consequently, preoperative ERCP became the standard for patients suspected of having choledocholithiasis, and postoperative ES was reserved for patients whose CBD stones were found either intraoperatively or postoperatively.

One of the problems with a protocol of preoperative ES is that it is difficult to predict which patients have choledocholithiasis. If strict criteria are used, many patients with CBD stones will be missed, and if liberal indications are used, most preoperative endoscopic retrograde cholangiography (ERC) examinations will be negative. In fact, all series utilizing preoperative ERC have a 40% to 70% negative rate for CBD stones. This is consistent with the negative CBD exploration rate in the era prior to intraoperative cholangiography.

Another problem with a preoperative ES protocol is the cost of the study. A single negative ERC costs approximately $3,000. This would pay for more than 15 intraoperative cholangiograms. In addition, the long-term effects of sphincterotomy in young patients with a normal-diameter CBD is unknown, but strictures and cancer induction are possible.

Now that surgeons are more experienced with laparoscopic cholecystectomy and intraoperative cholangiography, less reliance should be placed on preoperative ERCP. Surgeons should learn the various techniques of laparoscopic CBD exploration to treat patients with CBD calculi in one session and to avoid potential complications of ES. Transcystic duct exploration with balloon dilation of the cystic duct, fluoroscopic wire-basket retrieval of calculi, flexible choledochoscopy, and laparoscopic choledochotomy are all good techniques. Intraoperative ES, either antegrade or retrograde, and ampullary balloon dilation have also been employed, but are more rarely necessary and should perhaps be utilized in specialized centers for the time being. How and when to perform these techniques are the focus of this chapter.

Patient Evaluation

All patients undergoing laparoscopic cholecystectomy should have preoperative ultrasound examination of the liver, gallbladder, CBD, and pancreas. Careful analysis of the ultrasound can provide important information and may indicate the need for further studies (i.e., ERCP). Liver function tests are also important to evaluate, as well as prothrombin time and albumin level to assess liver function. About two-thirds of patients with CBD stones have elevated liver function tests, but only one-third of patients with elevated liver function tests will have CBD stones (Table 29-1). A serum amylase level should be obtained in patients with abdominal or back pain and tenderness. A baseline amylase level can be helpful when ERC or CBD exploration is anticipated. Nuclear biliary studies are not usually helpful in the diagnosis of choledocholithiasis, and tomographic intravenous cholangiography is being reevaluated. Magnetic resonance imaging has recently been shown to be an excellent method of visualizing the CBD, even the intrapancreatic portion.

The clinical presentation of choledocholithiasis can be subtle. An attack can include epigastric pain that tightens around the waist and radiates to the back, shoulder, or neck. It may be associated with nausea, vomiting, darkening of the urine, and lightening of the color of stool. Fever and rigors can occur. Often, it is difficult to differentiate between acute cholecystitis with empyema of the gallbladder with or without choledocholithiasis and cholangitis. In our experience, 18% of patients with acute cholecystitis have choledocholithiasis at the time of surgery.

Transcystic Duct Common Bile Duct Exploration

The transcystic duct technique offers an excellent approach to CBD stones, while avoiding a choledochotomy and the difficulty of suturing laparoscopically. Most transcystic duct techniques of CBD exploration involve dilation of the cystic duct with balloon dilators (preferred) or sequential graduated bougies. Biliary flexible endoscopy is our primary approach to the CBD regardless of entrance site. Nevertheless, balloon trolling of the CBD, fluoroscopy-guided wire-basket stone retrieval, ampullary balloon dilation with lavage, and transcystic endoscopy-assisted sphincterotomy are all techniques that can be employed laparoscopically via the cystic duct without the need for dilation.

Flexible biliary endoscopy with wire-basket retrieval of calculi is our preferred technique. It appears to be the safest technique because the endoscope, wire-basket manipulations, and stone capture are performed under direct vision without manipulation of the ampulla. This technique is feasible in 80% to 90% of patients. One limitation is that the endoscope cannot be passed into the proximal CBD in 90% of patients. Multiple stones, small, fragile cystic ducts, and stones proximal to the cystic duct–CBD junction usually must be dealt with by choledochotomy, ES, or ampullary balloon dilation. Larger stones (greater than 8 mm) should be dealt with via a choledochotomy but can be removed with the transcystic technique if the stones can be fragmented with a pulsed dye laser or electrohydraulic lithotripsy. These more difficult situations occur in about 10% of cases of choledocholithiasis in the United States.

Technique

The patient is positioned on the operating room table in the supine position as for laparoscopic cholecystectomy. Because any patient can have unsuspected CBD stones, trocar location is critical. The most medial subcostal trocar should always be placed in as lateral a position as possible and as close to the costal margin as possible. This facilitates insertion of the scissors for incising the cystic duct and introducing the cholangiogram catheter. It eventually provides the best angle of approach for the flexible choledochoscope (Fig. 29-1).

After dissection of the cystic duct and the cystic artery, a clip is placed on the junction of the gallbladder with the cystic duct as high as possible on the gallbladder. A cholangiocatheter, a 4-French (4-F) end-hole ureteral catheter, is inserted in the cystic duct and secured in place with a clip or cholangiocatheter clamp (Fig. 29-2), and cinefluoroscopic cholangiography is performed. Although the procedure can be performed solely with static films, we recommend digital fluoroscopy. Considerable time is saved during the cholangiogram, and this equipment greatly improves accuracy and facilitates insertion of the guidewires, catheters, and other instruments during CBD exploration.

If it is difficult to intubate the cystic duct and a better intubation angle is needed, an additional 5-mm trocar should be inserted. This can be used for direct insertion or for

Table 29-1. Incidence of Specific Liver Function Test Abnormalities and Prediction of Common Bile Duct (CBD) Stones ($n = 727$)

Abnormality	n	%	CBD Stones	%
ALP	35	5	12	34
SGOT/PT	32	4	5	16
ALP + SGOT/PT	31	4	13	42
ALP + SGOT/PT + Bilirubin	22	3	12	55
Bilirubin	19	3	4	21
Bilirubin + SGOT/PT	13	2	5	38

ALP, alkaline phosphatase; PT, prothrombin time; SGOT, aspartate transaminase.

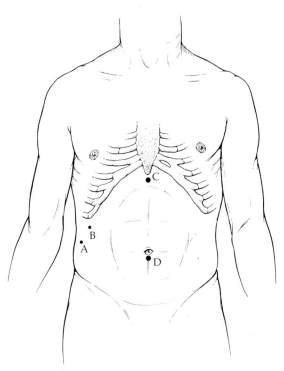

Fig. 29-1. Trocar sites and instrumentation ports for laparoscopic transcystic common bile duct exploration.

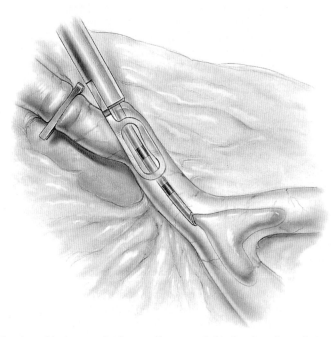

Fig. 29-2. Cholangiographic clamp used to insert and secure a cholangiocatheter in cystic duct for intraoperative cholangiogram.

a special endoscope grasper to gently guide the endoscope into the cystic duct (Fig. 29-3). When a stone or stones are seen on intraoperative cholangiography, their number, size, and location should be noted, as well as their relationship to the entrance of the cystic duct and CBD. The anatomic pattern is studied with particular attention to the entrance of the cystic duct to the CBD (Fig. 29-4).

After review of the intraoperative cholangiogram, a strategy for the treatment of choledocholithiasis should take into account the number of stones and their loca-tion. If the location of the stones and the patient's condition permit, the cystic duct should be dissected bluntly down close to its junction with the CBD. It is often neces-sary to make an incision in the larger por-tion of the cystic duct closer to the CBD so that less cystic duct requires dilation. The

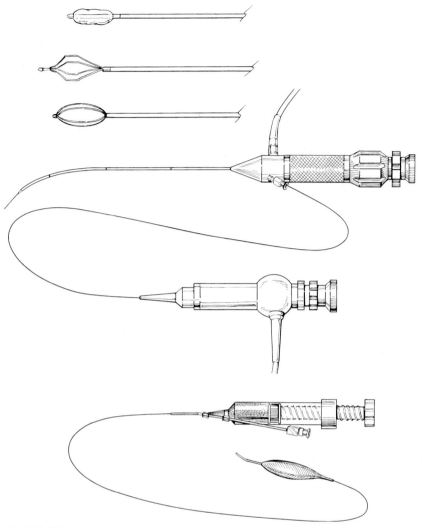

Fig. 29-3. Choledochoscope and instruments used to facilitate laparoscopic common bile duct exploration.

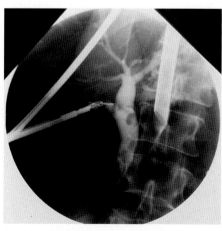

Fig. 29-4. Operative cholangiogram shows multiple common bile duct stones in a dilated duct and their relationship to the cystic duct.

location of the incision should allow an adequate length of cystic duct stump for closure with an Endoloop (Ethicon, Cincinnati, Ohio) at the end of the procedure. This maneuver increases the success of the procedure. A no.5 Phantom balloon dilating catheter (Insurg, Watertown, Massachusetts), which has a balloon that is 4 cm long and 6 mm in outer diameter, is preloaded with a 0.35-inch, 150-cm long hydrophilic guidewire (see Fig. 29-3). The assemblage is inserted via a 5-mm reducer sleeve in the trocar in the right anterior axillary line just under the costal margin.

When one is learning the technique, it is best to obtain x-ray or fluoroscopic confirmation of the guidewire location before advancing the balloon dilating catheter or

sequential bougies over the guidewire (Fig. 29-5). Two-thirds of the balloon should be inserted. The balloon is then slowly inflated with a LeVeen syringe attached to a pressure gauge. The balloon and cystic duct are observed laparoscopically while an assistant or nurse slowly inflates the balloon as the pressures are read aloud. The balloon should be inflated to the insufflation pressure recommended by the manufacturer (usually 12 atm) and held there for 3 minutes (Fig. 29-6). If the cystic duct begins to tear, inflation should stop for 1 minute before further inflation is attempted. With patience, most cystic ducts can be dilated to 7 mm, but they should never be dilated larger than the inner diameter of the CBD. When a

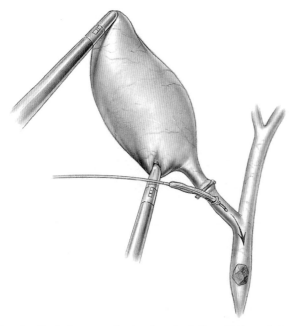

Fig. 29-5. Positioning of guidewire in preparation for advancing balloon dilating catheter for cystic duct dilation.

small CBD is being explored, care must be taken to choose the proper-diameter dilating balloon based on the intraoperative cholangiogram. The cystic duct must be dilated to the size of the largest CBD stone so that the stone entrapped in the wirebasket does not become impacted on removal. Stones larger than 9 mm must usually be fragmented with a pulsed dye laser or electrohydraulic lithotripsy, or removed via choledochotomy. After the cystic duct is dilated, the balloon catheter is deflated and withdrawn.

The endoscope can be inserted over a 150-cm-long guidewire, inserted free-hand, or gently guided with an atraumatic grasper. The working channel of some endoscopes is eccentric to their cross section, making insertion over the guidewire difficult. The endoscope should have bidirectional deflection and a working channel of at least

1.2 mm; an outer diameter of 2.7 to 3.2 mm is ideal. Smaller scopes compromise the working channel, and larger scopes are more difficult to pass. A camera should be attached to the endoscope, and the image should be projected on a monitor with an audiovisual mixer (picture in picture), or it should be projected on its own monitor. It is best and most convenient to set up a mobile cart with a monitor, a light source, camera box, video recorder, endoscope, wire baskets, balloon dilating catheters, and other instruments needed for a laparoscopic CBD exploration. This cart can function as an emergency laparoscopic cart and/or a backup cart for other laparoscopic procedures. Having all the required instruments in one place decreases frustration and delays when CBD calculi are encountered.

Once the endoscope is in the cystic duct, irrigation with warm saline should be initiated. Attention must be paid to the temperature of the irrigant, as hypothermia can occur from instillation of cold fluid. The operating surgeon manipulates the scope, inserting and torquing with the left hand while deflecting the endoscope with the right hand or the deflecting lever. Once the stone is seen, irrigation is turned off or decreased. The stone should always be entrapped closest to the scope and none should be bypassed, as they may be irrigated up into the liver. A straight no.4 wire basket (2.4 F) is preferable. The closed basket should be advanced beyond the stone,

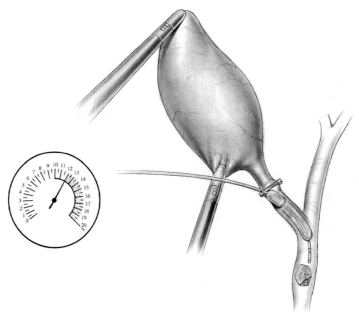

Fig. 29-6. Balloon catheter attached to LeVeen syringe during cystic duct dilation.

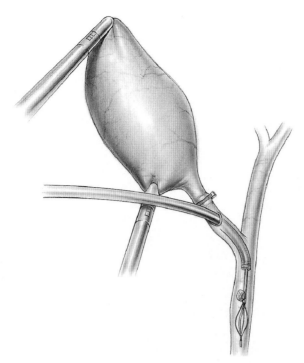

Fig. 29-7. Advancement of wire basket through choledochoscope for stone entrapment.

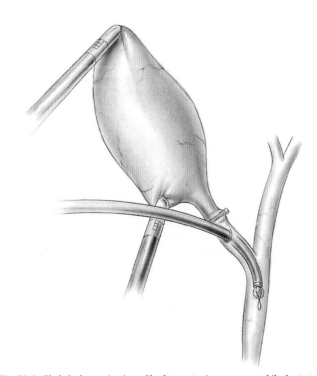

Fig. 29-8. Choledochoscopic view of basket capturing a common bile duct stone.

opened, and then pulled back to entrap it (Fig. 29-7). The basket should be gently closed, and it and stone should be pulled up lightly against the end of the endoscope so that they can be withdrawn together (Fig. 29-8). This process is repeated until all stones are removed. A completion cholangiogram is essential. At this point, a decision regarding cystic duct tube drainage may be made. Elderly or immunosuppressed patients with cholangitis should have a latex (not silicone) tube placed for postoperative decompression of the biliary system. In patients who are likely to be harboring a retained stone, a tube should be placed for postoperative cholangiography and percutaneous tube tract stone extraction, if necessary. If the

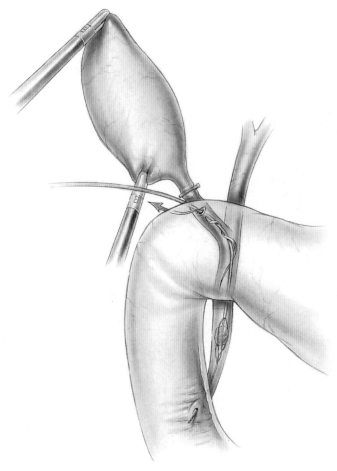

Fig. 29-9. Fluoroscopic transcystic basket retrieval of a common bile duct stone.

2. Fluoroscopic wire-basket stone retrieval requires special spiral wire baskets with flexible leaders to avoid injuring the CBD (Fig. 29-9). The basket is placed in the CBD via the cystic duct. It is advanced with fluoroscopic guidance into the distal CBD and opened. Hypaque 25% is injected through the wire-basket catheter. The basket is then pulled back until the stone is captured. The advantage of not having to dilate the cystic duct is offset by the problem of extracting the wire basket with the captured stone through the nondilated cystic duct. In our experience, this technique is not as successful as other transcystic duct techniques, and it can lead to an impacted basket and stone that require choledochotomy for removal. Nevertheless, it can be an easy and successful technique in selected patients: those with relatively few CBD calculi whose size is close to the inner diameter of the cystic duct.

3. Biliary balloon catheter stone retrieval is useful especially in cases with a dilated cystic duct. A biliary balloon catheter can be passed blindly or under fluoroscopic control via the cystic duct into the distal CBD or the duodenum. The balloon is gently inflated, and the catheter is then withdrawn, modulating the pressure on the balloon. This is often successful via choledochotomy but has the potential to pull the stone into the common hepatic duct out of reach of an endoscope, when used via the cystic duct.

Results

Results of transcystic CBD exploration are shown in Table 29-2.

Laparoscopic Transcystic Ampullary Balloon Dilation

In an effort to enhance our ability to lavage small stones and debris from the CBD when an endoscope cannot be inserted into a small, fragile cystic duct, we apply the laparoscopic technique of balloon dilation of the sphincter of Oddi (SO) via the cystic duct. Although our series is small, initial results indicate that this technique is a useful adjunct to laparoscopic CBD exploration techniques. However, it should be used when the only alternative is ES.

preexploration intraoperative cholangiogram shows a different number of CBD stones from that found on endoscopy, a tube should be placed. The cystic duct stump must be closed with Endoloops, as clips may slip off the thinned duct.

If the cystic duct cannot be dilated enough to allow insertion of an endoscope, or the cystic duct becomes transected, there are three other transcystic duct techniques that may be employed. Intraoperative fluoroscopy is crucial for these maneuvers:.

1. Glucagon, 1 mg, is administered intravenously, 3 minutes are allowed to pass, and the CBD is forcibly lavaged to flush the stones through the ampulla into the duodenum. This may work with stones 2 mm or smaller and is usually tried before cystic duct dilation.

Table 29-2. Laparoscopic Common Bile Duct Exploration Experience

Surgeon	Year	Total Cases	Transcystic Route	%	Choledochotomy Route	%	Total Successful Clearance	%	Mortality
DePaula	1994	119	107	90	12	10	108	91	1
Dion	1994	59	18	31	41	69	52	88	0
Ferzli	1994	24	13	54	11	46	24	100	0
Franklin	1995	113	2	1.8	111	98	112	99	1
Petelin	1995	173	154	89	19	11	168	97	1
Phillips	1995	162	145	90	17	10	150	93	1

Technique

When CBD stones and/or debris discovered at fluorocholangiography during laparoscopic cholecystectomy are less than 4 mm in diameter and cannot be extracted by endoscopic wire basket or lavage, laparoscopic transcystic balloon dilation of the SO can be performed. A 6-mm-diameter balloon dilating catheter (no.5 Phantom) is inserted via the right subcostal trocar over a floppy-tipped 0.035-inch hydrophilic guidewire (Fig. 29-10). The wire is advanced through the incision into the cystic duct and is gently passed under fluoroscopic control into the CBD and then the duodenum. The balloon catheter is advanced over the guidewire, through the cystic duct, and into the CBD and passed through the SO. Radiopaque markers on the balloon catheter identify its position spanning the SO. Care is taken to avoid repeated in and out manipulations through the SO. Using a LeVeen syringe, the balloon is slowly dilated under fluoroscopic view with 50% Hypaque only to the diameter of the largest stone in the CBD; it should never be dilated larger than the inner diameter of the CBD. After 3 minutes (using a pressure not greater than 12 atm), the balloon is deflated. Forceful irrigation into the cystic duct is then performed with warm saline solution, and completion cholangiogram is obtained (Fig. 29-11). The cystic duct is then ligated with an Endoloop, and a drain is placed in Morison's pouch. Placement of a cystic duct tube should be considered in cases in which percutaneous access or follow-up cholangiography may be required.

Results

Any manipulation of the ampulla of Vater can produce hyperamylasemia and/or clinical pancreatitis. In our experience, 17 (85%) of 20 patients had successful laparoscopic transcystic balloon dilation of the SO with clearance of stones from the CBD. Hyperamylasemia occurred in 15% of patients, and clinical mild pancreatitis occurred in three patients. Although this procedure appears to have a lower rate of clinical pancreatitis than endoscopic retrograde methods of SO dilation, surgeons should take this risk into consideration when applying this technique.

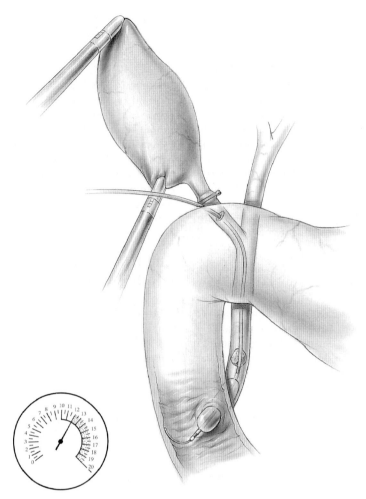

Fig. 29-10. Laparoscopic transcystic ampullary balloon dilation of the papilla.

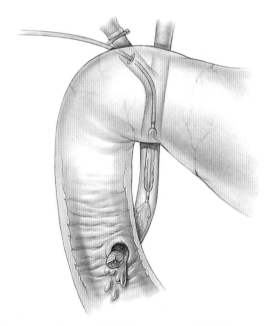

Fig. 29-11. Laparoscopic transcystic flushing of common bile duct after ampullary dilation.

Postoperative Course

Postoperatively, patients are observed for sepsis, bleeding, pancreatitis, or bile leak. These complications will usually occur within the first 24 hours. Routine postoperative laboratory tests should include a hematocrit, liver function tests, and serum amylase. If there is a question of bile leak, an ultrasound examination is the best first test; occasionally, a HIDA scan is helpful. An ERCP is sometimes needed not only to diagnose a leak but also to place a transampullary stent in association with percutaneous drainage. Reoperation will rarely be necessary.

Patients who have had a transcystic duct approach can be separated into four groups: those with suspected or unsuspected CBD stones and those under or over 60 years of age. Patients whose stones were preoperatively suspected are discharged on average 3.6 days postoperatively. Patients with unsuspected stones are discharged on average 1.7 days postoperatively. Both groups tend to return to work and regular activities on average 10 days after surgery. In contrast, between 1982 and 1988, 216 open CBD explorations were performed at Cedars-Sinai Medical Center, Los Angeles, without mortality in patients under 65 years of age and with 4.3% mortality in those over 65 years of age.

Complications

Complications with the transcystic duct stone extraction technique include perforation of the cystic or extrahepatic bile duct, cystic duct stump leak, pancreatitis, persistent cholangitis due to high intraductal pressures with lack of CBD decompression, delayed strictures due to mechanical injury or thermal injury from lithotripsy, and retained stones. All these complications can be minimized by careful attention to detail and proper patient selection. Patients with large stones greater than 8 mm, multiple stones, or proximal stones are better served by choledochotomy.

The transcystic duct approach has an 8% incidence of minor complications and a 6% incidence of major complications. Mortality is approximately 1% or less and is usually due to comorbid illness, most commonly cardiac and pulmonary. All deaths

occurred in patients over 65 years of age. Aspiration pneumonia occurred in 2% of our patients and was the cause of death in one (see Table 29-2).

By contrast, ERCP with ES has 0.5% to 1% mortality in all age groups. Because the transcystic duct technique of CBD exploration is so effective and is relatively safe, especially in patients under 65 years of age, we restrict preoperative ERC and sphincterotomy to patients over 65 years of age with significant cardiac and pulmonary disease who do not require cholecystectomy.

Laparoscopic Choledochotomy

Laparoscopic choledochotomy is an excellent approach in patients with a dilated CBD (greater than 8 mm), calculi 1 cm or larger, or multiple calculi or in those who require lithotripsy for impacted calculi. It is contraindicated in small ducts because of the risk of stricture. The advantage of choledochotomy is that calculi can easily be irrigated out of the CBD, and an endoscope can be inserted up into the intrahepatic ducts. CBD explorations, especially for solitary large stones, can be performed without a choledochoscope by milking the CBD stone into the choledochotomy. However, this technique cannot be relied on to accurately locate and/or remove all stones on a consistent basis. Therefore, we recommend use of a 10.5-F (3.3 mm) choledochoscope that can be flexed in two directions and has a 1.2-mm working channel that accommodates larger and less delicate wire baskets. Another advantage of this technique is that a T-tube is placed that decompresses the duct and provides access for cholangiography and retrieval of calculi. The disadvantages of choledochotomy are that a T-tube is required and considerable laparoscopic suturing skill is needed to close the choledochotomy.

Laparoscopic choledochotomy should not be performed without first performing an intraoperative cholangiogram. After completion of the cholangiogram and ascertainment of the exact location and number of CBD stones, a choledochotomy can be made at the point most desirable for extraction of the stones.

Technique

The procedure is performed before the gallbladder is removed so that the gall-

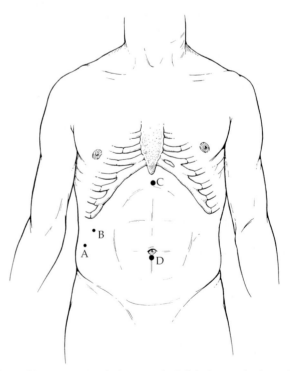

Fig. 29-12. *Trocar sites and instrumentation for laparoscopic choledochotomy. (A, large claw grasper with gallbladder; B, latex T-tube, scissors, grasper, cholangiocatheter, needle holder; C, hook coagulator, grasper, flexible scope, scissors, needle holder; D, video camera.)*

bladder can be used to elevate the liver and apply tension to the cystic duct (Fig. 29-12). The anterior wall of the CBD is bluntly dissected. Occasionally, it is necessary to aspirate bile to confirm the identity of the structure suspected to be the CBD. Intraoperative ultrasound is an additional method that can be used to identify the CBD and locate stones. The choledochotomy is placed in the anterior aspect of the CBD, preferably below the junction of the cystic duct into the CBD. This results in less chance of compromise to the lumen during closure of the choledochotomy. Two stay sutures should be placed in the CBD, and its anterior wall should be tented before an incision is made with microscissors (Fig. 29-13). The choledochotomy should be made only as long as the circumference of the largest calculus to minimize the suturing required for closure. Sometimes, the stay sutures on the edge of the choledochotomy need to be crossed alongside the endoscope, so the irrigation can distend the CBD.

The most efficient technique is to insert a choledochoscope into the CBD and irrigate with warm saline solution. The choledochoscope should be oriented so that flexion is in a vertical manner, as this assists in its passage through the choledochotomy. The CBD should be entered at a right angle, and the scope turned after entering the CBD. A biliary balloon catheter or wire basket, or both, can be used to remove calculi in most patients (Fig. 29-14). Occasionally, a three-pronged grasper or biliary lithotripsy is necessary to remove an impacted calculus.

Pulsed dye laser energy is the safest technique of lithotripsy, but electrohydraulic lithotripsy can be used safely if it is performed carefully under direct vision. After the CBD is cleared, a decision must be made regarding the need for a drainage procedure. This can be accomplished laparoscopically by performing a choledochoduodenostomy, Roux-en-Y choledochojejunostomy, or postoperative or intraoperative facilitated ES. When a drainage procedure is not needed, a latex T-tube must be inserted entirely intracorporeally to avoid carbon dioxide loss and permit easier manipulation of the tube. We frequently use a 10- to 14-F T-tube that has been tailored with a long and short end. The entire T-tube is brought into the abdominal cavity, and the long tail is allowed to extend over the top of the liver. The long

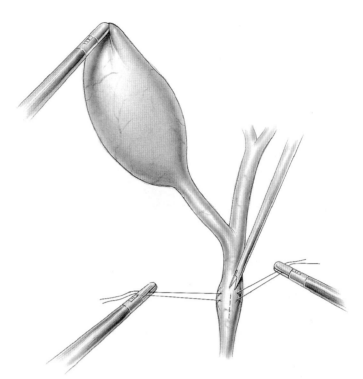

Fig. 29-13. Laparoscopic choledochotomy after placement of stay sutures.

end of the cut T-tube is introduced into the distal aspect of the CBD and the short end into the proximal end (Fig. 29-15). After the T-tube is well situated in the CBD, a pretied loop, which is very advantageous for the first suture, is placed immediately below the neck of the T-tube as the T-tube is being pushed cephalad (Fig. 29-16). This results in trapping of the T-tube and lessening of the chance of subsequent dislodgement. The next suture should be placed in the most proximal end of the choledochotomy, and the two sutures are lifted to facilitate closure of the choledochotomy. Our preference is to close the choledochotomy with interrupted sutures of Vicryl (Ethicon, Somerville, NJ) lubricated with mineral oil. The long end of the T-tube is brought through the abdominal wall, and completion cholangiography is performed. Care must be taken to ensure as close to a watertight seal as is possible without causing ischemia to this segment of the duct. It is better to have a small leak than to have an ischemic duct.

Results

Results with this technique have been excellent (see Table 29-2). Franklin and colleagues (1994) performed 111 procedures, with one retained calculus. Morbidity was 5% and mortality 1%. Surgeons who per-

form transcystic CBD exploration as the first technique in the treatment of CBD calculi perform laparoscopic choledochotomy only in the most challenging cases of choledocholithiasis (10%). This explains why the incidence of complications associated with laparoscopic choledochotomy (11% to 17%) and retained calculi (8% to 22%) is higher for these surgeons than with laparoscopic choledochotomy or even open CBD exploration as the primary method of calculi removal. Biliary drainage procedures should be performed in many of these difficult situations to reduce the incidence of retained calculi. ES or choledochoduodenostomy can be performed laparoscopically, but because drainage procedures are needed in only 1% of all patients undergoing laparoscopic cholecystectomy, converting these operations to open procedures seems appropriate, except in the hands of experienced laparoscopic surgical teams.

Laparoscopic Antegrade Transcystic Sphincterotomy

In 1993, A.L. DePaula and associates described their technique combining methods of laparoscopic CBD exploration and

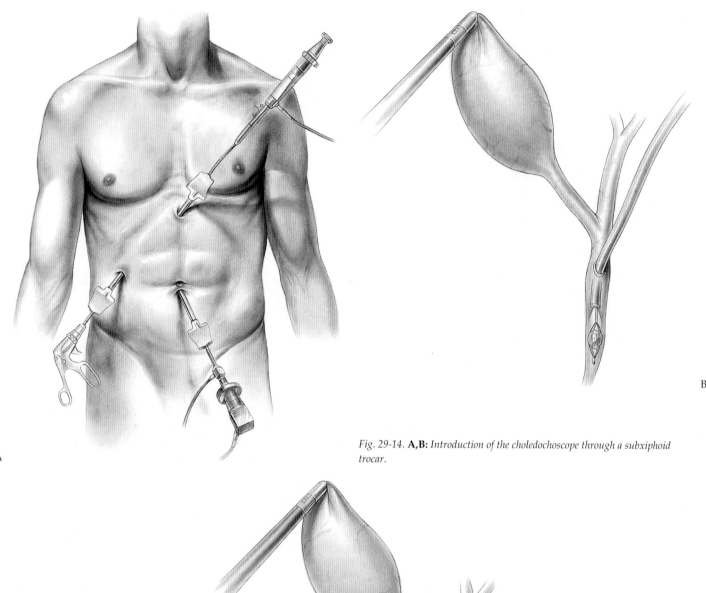

Fig. 29-14. **A,B:** *Introduction of the choledochoscope through a subxiphoid trocar.*

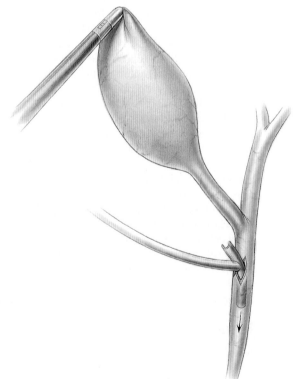

Fig. 29-15. *T-tube placed in choledochotomy after stone removal and brought out through subcostal trocar site.*

A

B

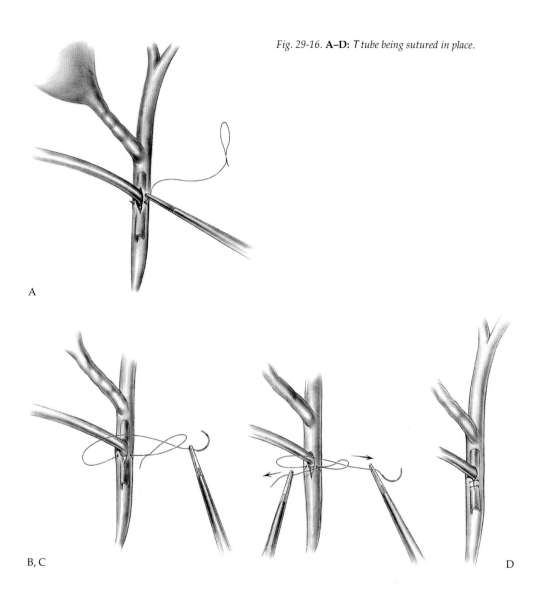

Fig. 29-16. **A–D:** *T tube being sutured in place.*

A

B, C

D

ES. According to their report, this procedure is indicated for any patient with multiple CBD stones, a CBD measuring greater than 20 mm, ampullary dyskinesia, or any evidence of impaired CBD emptying. Most who perform this procedure do it for patients with complex choledocholithiasis in whom transcystic CBD exploration and laparoscopic choledochotomy have failed to clear the CBD, which should be less than 3% of patients.

Technique

A cart should be available that contains a side-viewing duodenoscope, a selection of endoscopic sphincterotomes, guidewires, and a cautery cable compatible with the sphincterotomes. Antegrade sphincterotomy is usually performed after an at-

tempt has been made at laparoscopic CBD exploration. The transcystic or choledochotomy access to the CBD can be used for performing antegrade sphincterotomy (Fig. 29-17). The first step is to pass the sphincterotome directly into the distal CBD and across the ampulla (Fig. 29-18). Different types of endoscopic sphincterotomes are commercially available, including a 30-mm short-nose sphincterotome or a Classen-Demling–type sphincterotome designed originally for intubating the ampulla following a Billroth II gastrectomy. The sphincterotome is introduced via the right upper quadrant port. A grasping forceps is inserted through the subxiphoid sheath and then used to guide the sphincterotome into the lumen of the cystic duct or through the choledochotomy. While the sphincterotome is being manipulated into

the biliary tree, a second member of the surgical team passes a side-viewing video duodenoscope through the mouth and into the duodenum. Glucagon, 0.5 to 1.0 mg, is then administered intravenously to minimize duodenal peristalsis. The duodenoscope is positioned across from the ampulla (Fig. 29-19). As the sphincterotome passes through the ampulla, it is visualized. The surgeon withdraws and manipulates it, usually by twisting it, until the cutting wire is bowed at the 12-o'clock position (Fig. 29-20). Cautery is applied until the sphincter and overlying mucosa are divided up to the first transverse fold of the duodenum. An outpouring of bile and/or stones usually signifies a successful sphincterotomy. The CBD is then flushed copiously with saline to wash out any remaining stones or debris. The choledocho-

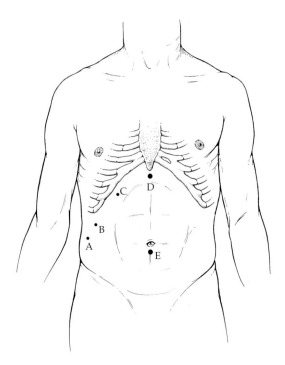

Fig. 29-17. Trocar sites and instrumentation for laparoscopic antegrade transcystic sphincterotomy. A fifth cannula (5 mm) can be inserted in the right upper quadrant for introduction of the choledochoscope, sphincterotome, and so on. (A, gallbladder grasper; B, grasper, cholangiocatheter; C, flexible scope, cautery cable, side-viewing duodenoscope; D, clip applicator, scissors, cautery hook, grasper; E, video camera.)

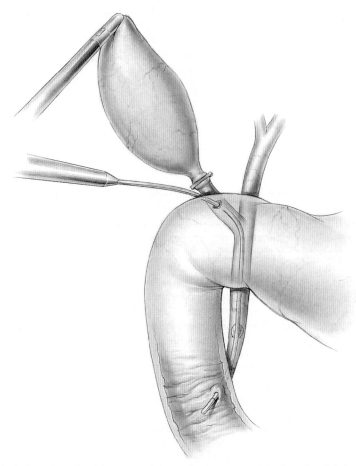

Fig. 29-18. An endoscopic sphincterotome is inserted using a suture introducer to minimize gas leakage.

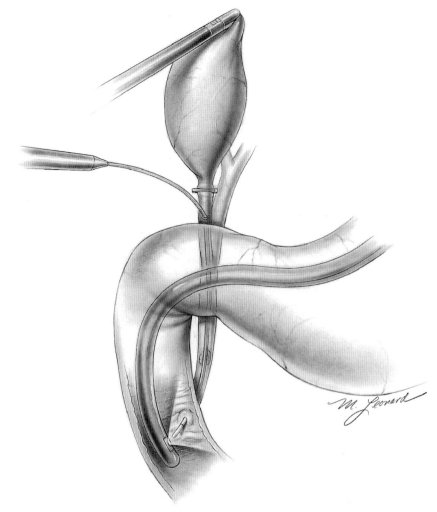

scope can then be reinserted to explore the CBD, flush the duct, and push stones out through the widened ampulla. If one or more stones are impacted in the distal CBD or ampulla, it may be difficult to pass the sphincterotome antegrade into the duodenum. In these cases, one can advance the choledochoscope as far distally as possible, maneuver a smaller guidewire through the working channel across the ampulla, and then follow the above mentioned steps. If the sphincterotomy is successful, insertion of a T-tube for postoperative biliary decompression is not necessary. Often, a small amount of bleeding is visualized from the sphincterotomy site, but it usually stops, although it occasionally requires injection of epinephrine or coagulation.

Comment

Laparoscopic antegrade sphincterotomy has a number of advantages over conventional methods of ES. First, the sphincterotome is passed quickly through the bile ducts and across the ampulla. DePaula and associates reported a mean time of 17 minutes to perform this procedure, and Zucker was able to complete antegrade sphincterotomy in just over 25 minutes (excluding time spent at attempted CBD exploration). Inadvertent cannulation of the pancreatic duct is also eliminated, and other complications associated with ERCP, such as creation of false passages, perforation of the CBD or duodenum, and the so-called "trapped basket or sphincterotome," should be dramatically reduced. In addition, patients expect complete management of all their biliary tract problems in one sitting, which this provides. However, antegrade sphincterotomy does have its disadvantages as well. Operative and anesthesia time is prolonged. Antegrade sphincterotomy does require additional equipment and experience in upper gastrointestinal endoscopy. Despite these disadvantages, laparoscopic antegrade sphincterotomy may have an increasingly important role in the surgical management of complex choledocholithiasis.

Fig. 29-19. The side-viewing duodenoscope is positioned directly opposite the ampulla so that the sphincterotome may be guided into proper position under direct vision.

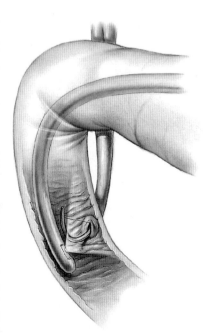

Fig. 29-20. The sphincterotome is bowed exposing the cutting wire that is maneuvered until it is at the 12-o'clock position.

Conclusion

Laparoscopic cholecystectomy has become the primary treatment for symptomatic cholelithiasis, and concomitant CBD stones are present in 10% to 15% of patients. Several approaches to their management have been described. Laparoscopic transcystic CBD exploration with choledochoscopy and stone extraction should become the primary technique because it is relatively safe, efficient, and most cost-effective for managing CBD stones in one session. If unsuccessful, it still allows other laparoscopic approaches, open choledochotomy, or postoperative ES.

Suggested Reading

Cotton PB, Lehman G, Vennes J, et al. Endoscopic sphincterotomy complications and their management: an attempt at consensus. *Gastrointest Endosc* 1991;37:383–393.

Curet MJ, Martin DE, Pitcher DT, et al. Laparoscopic antegrade sphincterotomy for complex choledocholithiasis. *Ann Surg* 1995;221:149.

DePaula AL, Hashiba K, Bafutto M, Zago R, Machado MM. Laparoscopic antegrade sphincterotomy. *Surg Laparosc Endosc* 1993;3:157–160.

Franklin ME Jr, Pharand D, Rosenthal D. Laparoscopic common bile duct exploration. *Surg Laparosc Endosc* 1994;4:119–124.

Hunter JG, Soper NJ. Laparoscopic management of bile duct stones. *Surg Clin North Am* 1992;72:1077–1097.

Petelin JB. Laparoscopic approach to common duct pathology. *Am J Surg* 1993;165:487–491.

Phillips EH. Laparoscopic transcystic ampullary balloon dilatation. In: Phillips EH, Rosenthal RJ, eds. *Operative strategies in laparoscopic surgery*. Germany: Springer-Verlag, 1995.

Phillips EH. Controversies in the management of common duct calculi. *Surg Clin North Am* 1994;74:931–951.

Phillips EH, Carroll BJ, Pearlstein AR, Daykhovsky L, Fallas MJ. Laparoscopic choledochoscopy and extraction of common bile duct stones. *World J Surg* 1993;17:22–28.

Phillips EH, Liberman M, Carroll BJ, Fallas MJ, Rosenthal RJ, Hiatt JR. Bile duct stones in the laparoscopic era: is preoperative sphincterotomy necessary? *Arch Surg* 1995;130:880–886.

Soper NJ, Brunt LM, Kerbl K. Laparoscopic general surgery. *N Engl J Med* 1994;330:409–419.

EDITOR'S COMMENT

Dr. Friedman and Dr. Phillips have an extensive experience with laparoscopic removal of CBD stones and succinctly describe the various techniques. Unfortunately, too many surgeons have relinquished the management of CBD stones to gastroenterologists by preoperative or postoperative ERCP since laparoscopic cholecystectomy has been adopted on a widespread scale. Clearly, patients with cholangitis, severe acute biliary pancreatitis, or otherwise unexplained jaundice should undergo preoperative ERCP. For most patients with relatively "soft" signs of choledocholithiasis, laparoscopic cholecystectomy with intraoperative cholangiography is an appropriate first step. Most patients will not have CBD stones and are saved the cost and morbidity of an ERCP. When stones are discovered at the time of cholangiography, numerous techniques exist for their removal using laparoscopic methods. If an individual surgeon does not feel comfortable dealing with the stones and is uncertain whether or not the local endoscopists will be able to remove the stones in the postoperative interval, one technique that will ensure the ability to remove the CBD stones postoperatively is to insert a latex tube through the cystic duct into the CBD at the time of laparoscopic cholecystectomy. This will allow postoperative cholangiography to assess whether the stones have passed spontaneously. If not, either a wire can be placed through the tube into the duodenum to guide a safe sphincterotomy, or the stones can be removed by radiologic techniques after tract maturation.

Unfortunately, there have been no well done prospective, randomized trials to guide decision making for management of CBD stones in the era of laparoscopic cholecystectomy. Until these studies are done, surgeons should learn and perfect the various techniques for laparoscopic stone removal. At present, patient and stone factors (number, size, location), as well as expertise (both surgical and endoscopic) at the local institution, determine the appropriate management of choledocholithiasis.

N.J.S

30

Laparoscopic Bile Duct Injuries

Steven M. Strasberg

Biliary injury is by far the most common serious complication of laparoscopic cholecystectomy. The incidence of biliary injury has increased since the introduction of laparoscopic cholecystectomy. Injury is largely preventable; a leading objective of the field of laparoscopic hepatobiliary surgery is to reduce the incidence of these morbid and costly injuries to an absolute minimum as soon as possible.

New Classification of Biliary Injuries

Laparoscopic biliary injuries differ from open biliary injuries in several respects. For instance, bilomas and injuries to aberrant right hepatic ducts are much more common. Older classifications focused on major bile duct injuries, and it was difficult to fit the wide spectrum of laparoscopic biliary injuries into these classifications. For this reason, a new classification of laparoscopic biliary injuries was recently introduced (Fig. 30-1). The classification includes five types: A to E. Type E injuries are subclassified into types E1 to E5. Type E injuries are identical to the Bismuth classification of major biliary injuries.

Type A: bile leak from a minor duct still in continuity with the common bile duct (CBD). These are minor lateral injuries to the biliary tract. They include bile leakage from the cystic duct or liver bed. Cystic duct leaks are usually due to improper clip application. Retained CBD stones will increase the severity of bile leakage. Bile leaks from the liver bed are most commonly caused by dissection in too deep a plane when the gallbladder is taken from the liver bed. This results in injury to a

small peripheral hepatic duct (Fig. 30-2). Type A injuries can usually be readily cured by decompression of the biliary tree by endoscopic sphincterotomy and external drainage of the biloma if one is present.

Type B: occlusion of part of the biliary tree and *type C: bile leakage from a duct not in communication with the CBD.* Aberrant right hepatic ducts are more prone to injury during laparoscopic surgery. The cystic duct joins a right hepatic duct rather than the common hepatic duct in about 2% of patients. The aberrant duct then continues on to unite with the common hepatic duct. Not surprisingly, the junction of the aberrant duct with the hepatic duct can look very much like a cystic duct–hepatic duct junction, with resultant potential for biliary injury. Type B injury occurs when an aberrant right duct is occluded, and type C when it is transected. Presentation and management of the two types of injury are different. Type B injuries may lead to cholangitis but are often asymptomatic. Type C injuries result in intraperitoneal bile collections or bile peritonitis.

Type D: lateral injury to major extrahepatic bile ducts. The CBD or common hepatic duct are the ducts that are usually lacerated in this type of injury. Like type A injuries, these are lateral injuries, and decompression by sphincterotomy may be curative. However, sometimes, type D injuries are more serious. They may progress to stricture and complete obstruction (i.e., convert to a type E injury), especially if caused by cautery.

Type E: circumferential injury of major bile ducts (Bismuth classes 1 to 5). These are circumferential injuries of major bile ducts, as described by Bismuth. Subclassification into types E1 to E4 is based on the level of

injury, while type E5 is a combined common hepatic duct and aberrant right duct injury. Type E injuries separate the hepatic parenchyma from the lower biliary tract and may be due to a stenosis or a complete occlusion with or without loss of ductal tissue. To classify the injury properly, one must state the subtype that establishes the level (E1 to E5) and whether it is a stenosis, a complete occlusion, or a complete occlusion with loss of ductal tissue. If the latter is present, then the length of tissue loss should be given (e.g., E4: 3-cm duct excised).

Most reports of ductal injuries come from tertiary centers, and these reports have focused on type E injuries. However, it is likely that type A and type D injuries are really the most common, since most of these injuries can be treated without referral to a tertiary center.

Incidence of Laparoscopic Biliary Injury

Many reports suggest that the risk of biliary injury is increased during laparoscopic cholecystectomy. These include institutional, regional, and national case series, as well as case series of laparoscopic injuries treated at referral centers. Like others, the center I am associated with has experienced a large increase in patients referred for management of biliary injuries since 1990. There are many potential errors in incidence studies of this type. To be accurate, the methodology must absolutely ensure collection of results from every laparoscopic cholecystectomy in the study population. To be representative, the population studied must be large, and it

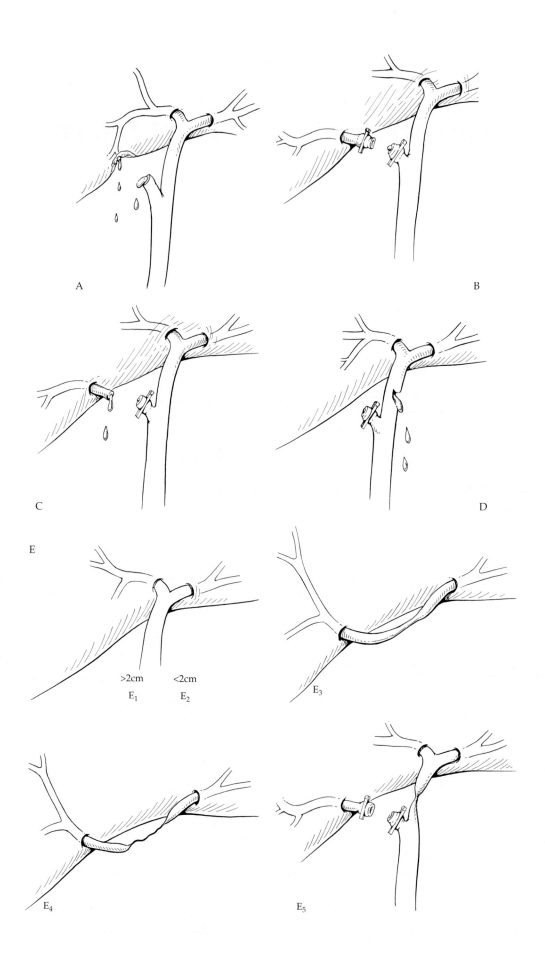

A

B

C

D

E

$>2cm$ $<2cm$

E_1 E_2

E_3

E_4

E_5

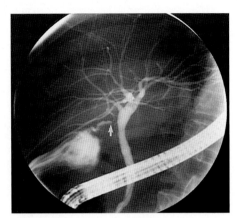

Fig. 30-2. Postoperative endoscopic retrograde cholangiogram in a patient in whom a biloma developed. Note that the injury is to a small tributary of a hepatic duct. (From Strasberg et al., 1995.)

should be regional, such as a state or a country, rather than selected institutions or surgeons. Almost all reports fail to achieve these standards. Fortunately, four good data sets exist, including statewide evaluations from New York and Connecticut, a report from the armed services, and one from Denmark. In these studies, the major bile duct injury rate was between 0.3% and 0.6%. If all types of biliary injuries are included, such as injuries to minor ducts in the liver bed, the injury rate in these reports ranges from 0.6% to 1.5%. In comparison, the major bile duct injury rate for open cholecystectomy was about 0.1%, and the total biliary injury rate was 0.15%. Therefore, laparoscopic cholecystectomy has been associated with a large and unacceptable increase in such injuries. About 500,000 cholecystectomies are performed in the United States annually, and thus one may estimate that 1,500 to 2,500 laparoscopic biliary injuries occur annually.

Etiology and Pathogenesis of Injury

There are three main risk factors for biliary injury: (a) inadequate training and experience, (b) inflammation, and (c) aberrant anatomy. Lack of training and experience were important risk factors in the early years of laparoscopic cholecystectomy. The learning curve for the operation was steep, most injuries coming within the first 30 cholecystectomies performed. Since almost all practicing surgeons have passed through this phase, injury due to these factors should be decreasing. However, inexperience in unusual or difficult situations, such as acute cholecystitis, may still be contributing to the problem.

As in open cholecystectomy, biliary injuries are more likely to occur when the procedure is difficult. Most case series of biliary injuries report acute and/or chronic inflammation, frequently with dense scarring, at the time of the laparoscopic cholecystectomy. An association between bile duct injury and surgery for acute cholecystitis was found in several series. Operative bleeding that obscures the field and fat in the portal area are also cited as possible contributing factors. Oozing of blood hampers dissection much more in laparoscopic than in open cholecystectomy, and gentle dissection in the face of inflammation is required to avoid bleeding that then obscures vision.

Aberrant anatomy is a frequent and well established danger in biliary surgery. Aberrant right hepatic ducts (see types B and C injuries above) are the most likely to be involved in ductal injury. However, other ductal anomalies can occur, including left-sided anomalies. As in the era of open cholecystectomy, surgeons must always operate as if aberrant anatomy is present.

Inexperience, local inflammation, and aberrant anatomy increase the risk of injury but are not the causes of injury. The causes of injury number only two: (a) misidentification of a duct as the cystic duct and (b) technical problems, especially the misuse of cautery. Misidentification of the CBD as the cystic duct leads to type D or type E injuries. Misidentification of an aberrant right duct as the cystic

duct causes type B and type C injuries. In a common scenario described as the classic injury, the CBD is mistaken to be the cystic duct and is clipped and divided (Fig. 30-3A). To excise the gallbladder, the surgeon must divide the bile ducts again (Fig. 30-3A), producing types E1 to E4 injuries. Such injuries are often associated with injury to the right hepatic artery. The common hepatic duct may be either clipped or divided, resulting in obstruction or bile leakage. Other injury patterns are shown in Fig. 30-3B,C. Injuries to the aberrant right duct occur in a similar manner (Fig. 30-3D,E,F). The misidentification involves the segment of the right hepatic duct between the point where the cystic duct enters it and where the right and hepatic ducts unite. This segment is thought to be the cystic duct. The misidentified segment is clipped or cut. The aberrant duct must be cut a second time at a higher level to remove the gallbladder. Variations of this injury are shown in the figure.

The direction of traction of the gallbladder may contribute to the appearance that the CBD is the cystic duct. When the pouch of Hartmann is pulled superiorly rather than laterally, the CBD and cystic bile ducts come into alignment, appearing to be a single duct (Fig. 30-4). Other contributing factors are a short cystic duct and a large stone in the pouch of Hartmann that makes retraction and display of the cystic duct difficult. Misidentification also seems to be more common when adhesive bands tether the gallbladder to the CBD.

The most common technical causes of laparoscopic ductal injury are (a) failure to securely occlude the cystic duct, (b) too deep a plane of dissection when taking the gallbladder off the liver bed, and (c) thermal injuries to the bile duct. The cystic duct is usually occluded with clips, and clip failure is more common than failure of ligatures or suture ligatures, the standard methods of securing the cystic duct during open cholecystectomy. Clip failure may result in part

Fig. 30-1. Classification of laparoscopic injuries to the biliary tract. Type A to type E injuries are illustrated. Type E injuries are subdivided according to the Bismuth classification. **A:** Type A injuries originate from small bile ducts that are entered in the liver bed or from the cystic duct. **B,C:** Type B and type C injuries almost always involve aberrant right hepatic ducts. **D,E:** Types A, C, and D injuries and some type E injuries may cause bilomas or fistulas. Type B and other type E injuries occlude the biliary tree, and bilomas do not occur. The notations >2 cm and <2 cm in type E_1 and type E_2 indicate the length of common hepatic duct remaining. (Redrawn from Strasberg et al., 1995.)

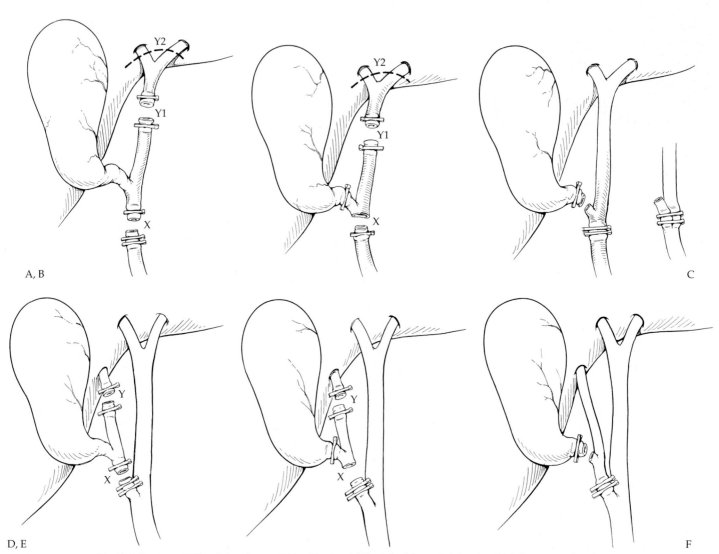

Fig. 30-3. Patterns of biliary injury due to misidentification. **A:** The "classic" type E injury in which the common duct is divided between clips at point x. The ductal system is later divided again to remove the gallbladder either at point y1, producing type E1 or type E2 injuries, or at point y2, producing type E3 or type E4 injuries. **B:** Variant of type E injury that leads to bile leakage into the operative field and thereby an increased chance of recognition before the entire injury evolves. **C:** Variant of type E injury leading to clipping but not excision of the duct. This injury also causes intraoperative bile leakage, except when cystic and common bile ducts are both occluded, as shown in the inset. **D,E,F:** Variants of injury to an aberrant right hepatic duct, producing type B or type C injuries. The injuries shown in D, E, and F correspond to the injuries shown in A, B, and C but affect the aberrant right duct. (Redrawn from Strasberg et al., 1995, with permission.)

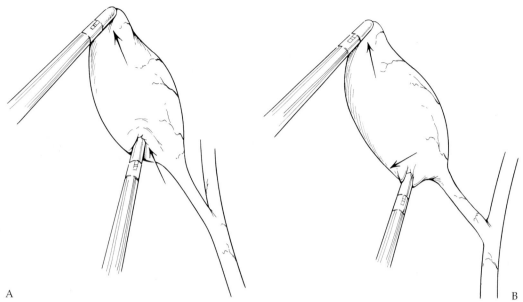

A   B

Fig. 30-4. Effect of the direction of traction on the appearance of the bile ducts. **A:** *Both graspers pulling superiorly bring the common and cystic ducts into alignment, giving the appearance of a single duct.* **B:** *When the grasper on the pouch of Hartmann is pulling laterally to the right, the cystic and common ducts appear as separate structures, and the common bile duct is less likely to be mistaken for the cystic duct and injured.*

from untreated choledocholithiasis with increased biliary pressure, but most cases occur without choledocholithiasis. Clip failure may be due to clipping a thick, rigid duct or including extraneous tissue. Clips may "scissor" during application, resulting in faulty closure. They may be loosened by

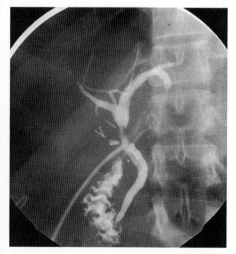

Fig. 30-5. T-tube cholangiogram in a patient 2 months after a thermal injury. The common hepatic duct (arrow) *appears shrink-wrapped over the T-tube. At the time of reconstruction, the common hepatic duct was replaced by scar. (From Strasberg et al., 1995, with permission.)*

subsequent dissection close to the clip. Using monopolar cautery to divide the cystic duct may result in delayed thermal necrosis of the cystic duct stump or bile duct. Injury to ducts in the liver bed may occur by entrance into too deep a plane when the gallbladder is excised. Removal of the gallbladder from the liver bed is usually easy in laparoscopic cholecystectomy, but may be difficult in the presence of acute or chronic inflammation or in patients with an intrahepatic gallbladder. Cautery-induced injuries are more likely to occur in the presence of severe inflammation that may lead to the use of excessively high cautery settings to control hemorrhage or to application of the cautery without being sure of the position of the duct. Misuse of cautery has led to some very serious bile duct injuries; characteristically these are type E injuries with loss of ductal tissue due to thermal necrosis (Fig. 30-5).

Prevention of Biliary Injuries

General

Laparoscopic cholecystectomy should be performed only by surgeons properly

trained and proctored in the procedure. Experience should be graded, with difficult procedures such as cholecystectomy in patients with acute cholecystitis not attempted until experience in elective laparoscopic cholecystectomy has been gained. Laparoscopic cholecystectomy is more likely to be difficult when scarring or inflammation is present, when patients are men or elderly, or when there have been repeated attacks of pain. These factors are additive. A previous attack of acute cholecystitis is also a significant contributing factor to operative difficulty. Inexperienced surgeons should be aware of these predictive factors and take appropriate steps to ensure adequate assistance in the operating room.

Avoidance of Misidentification of Ducts

Misidentification is due to a failure to conclusively identify the cystic structures before clipping or division. Injury due to misidentification can be prevented by adhering to certain principles. The cystic duct and artery are the only structures in the porta hepatis that need to be divided during a cholecystectomy. Therefore, the objective of dissection should be to conclusively identify these structures. Furthermore, only these structures need to be identified. The key phrase is "conclusive identification," and this is achieved when the dissection reaches the "critical view of safety" (Fig. 30-6). At this point, only two structures are connected to the lower end of the gallbladder, and lowest part of the gallbladder attachment to the liver bed has been freed so that the liver bed is visible. The latter is an important step that precludes the possibility of injury to an aberrant duct. It is not necessary to see the CBD. To get to the critical view, the triangle of Calot is dissected free of fat, fibrous, and areolar tissue, and the lower end of the gallbladder is dissected off the liver bed. Once the critical view is attained, cystic structures may be occluded, as they have been conclusively identified. Failure, due to any cause, to achieve the critical view of safety is an absolute indication for conversion to open cholecystectomy or possibly cholangiography to define ductal anatomy.

Several technical tips help achieve clearance of the triangle of Calot. Dissection should proceed from both dorsal and ventral aspects of the triangle. Various dissection techniques are used in combination, including pulling techniques, gentle spreading with forceps, hook cautery, and blunt dissection with a nonactivated spatula cautery tip or anchored pledgets. The pouch of Hartmann should be pulled laterally and interiorly to open the anterior-left side of Calot's triangle and to create an angle between the cystic duct and the CBD. Additionally, the posterior-right side of Calot's triangle is exposed and dissected while superior and medial traction to the gallbladder infundibulum is applied. At the start of the dissection, the gallbladder should be followed down to the presumed point of the infundibulum–cystic duct junction, and dissection should be started there and not at the presumed location of the middle of the cystic duct. Staying on or close to the gallbladder during clearance of Calot's triangle is an important principle of safe dissection. The triangle will open as structures fall away from the gallbladder, which is maintained on traction.

Routine operative cholangiography has been recommended to avoid ductal injury, but there are no good data to confirm this view. Operative cholangiograms have frequently been misinterpreted in the presence of injury. The most common problem is the failure to recognize that an injury may be present when only the lower part of the biliary tree is seen. In reality, this often means that the CBD has been cannulated and a clip placed across it so that contrast cannot flow into the hepatic ducts. Failure to fill the proximal ducts must be taken as abnormal and is a reason to convert to an open procedure. Routine operative cholangiography may limit the extent of the injury.

In my view, conclusive identification should be sought by dissection rather than cholangiography. Performance of a cholangiogram for purposes of identification means that at times a duct other than the cystic duct will be incised for the purposes of doing the cholangiogram (Fig. 30-7). While incising a small CBD or aberrant right bile duct is better than excising it, I do not believe that either option is desirable. Learning the technique of dissection to the critical view of safety avoids the need for cholangiography for ductal identification in almost all cases. When ductal identification cannot be achieved by dissection, it is my current practice to convert to an open

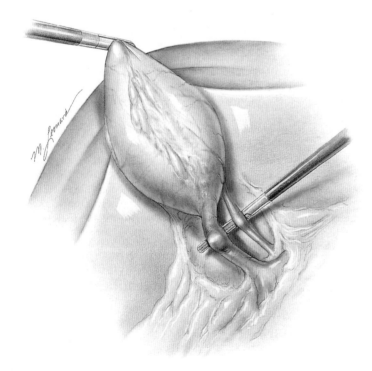

Fig. 30-6. The critical view of safety. The triangle of Calot is dissected free of all tissue except for the cystic duct and artery, and the base of the liver bed is exposed. When this view is achieved, the two structures entering the gallbladder can only be the cystic duct and artery. It is not necessary to see the common bile duct. (From Strasberg et al., 1995, with permission.)

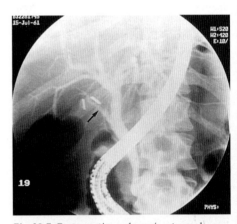

Fig. 30-7. Postoperative endoscopic retrograde cholangiogram in a patient with an aberrant right hepatic duct (arrow). Note that the intrahepatic biliary system appears normal. Clips indicate the position of the cystic duct and artery. Note how the point of union of the aberrant duct with the common hepatic duct looks like a cystic duct–common duct junction. Mistakenly doing a cholangiogram through the aberrant duct rather than identifying it by dissection would have led to a ductal injury that would have been difficult to repair because of the small size of the aberrant duct. (From Strasberg et al., 1995, with permission.)

procedure. Cholangiography can also be done through the gallbladder. For ductal identification, this technique has the advantage that no duct needs to be cannulated. There is little information on the feasibility of this method. It is theoretically limited by obstruction at the neck of the gallbladder, which frequently occurs in difficult cases. There is also the potential for flushing stones into the bile duct.

Avoidance of Technical Errors

There are several steps for avoiding technical causes of ductal injury. To occlude the cystic duct, two clips are applied to the end of the cystic duct remaining in the patient, and one is applied to the specimen end. Clips must be placed so that the tips can be seen projecting beyond the duct, free of extraneous material. Clips should not be manipulated in the subsequent dissection. Clips should not be used when the cystic duct is thickened to the point that the tips of the clips do not meet on closure. Under these circumstances, two preformed ligature loops should be applied and tightened to occlude the cystic duct.

Avoidance of ductal injury in the liver bed depends on staying in the correct plane of dissection. Use of the spatula dissector combined with irrigation to keep the field clear of blood is often helpful in difficult cases; dissection is done by a combination of pushing, cauterization, and irrigation all with one instrument. The cautery scissors also are often helpful. There is no substitute for meticulous technique and experience in this dissection.

To avoid cautery injuries, bleeding must never be controlled by blind application of clamps, clips, or cautery. Brisk bleeding that impairs visualization is an indication for converting to an open procedure. Lesser degrees of hemorrhage may be thought to be more serious than they actually are because of the magnification of laparoscopy. The operating surgeon must use judgment in such cases, as the bleeding often stops spontaneously. Direct pressure with an anchored pledget or pads of oxycellulose is often effective in stopping bleeding and rarely causes tissue damage. Cautery should not be used or used with great care in the triangle of Calot. Low cautery settings are mandatory, as higher settings may lead to arcing. Cautery should never be used to divide the cystic duct because this may lead to thermal necrosis of the cystic duct stump or adjacent CBD.

Presentation and Investigation

Except for type D and type E injuries, intraoperative identification is uncommon. Even in type E injuries, identification during the operation occurs in only 25% of cases. Injuries have been detected as a result of seeing bile or an open duct. At other times, they have been diagnosed by cholangiography or after conversion to an open procedure.

There are several modes of presentation in the postoperative period, but pain with sepsis and jaundice are the two most common. Pain with sepsis tends to occur in injury types associated with biloma—types A, C, and D—while understandably jaundice is the most common way that type E injuries present. Type B injuries (occluded aberrant right duct) may remain asymptomatic indefinitely; cholangitis and right-sided pain are the most common symptoms and may take years to appear. Patients who develop bilomas or even bile peritonitis may present only with complaints of malaise or distention or an increased requirement for analgesia; at other times bile leakage may result in fistula formation. Investigation depends on the mode of presentation. The goal is to use the least invasive and least costly route of investigation.

Pain/Sepsis or Distention/Malaise

With these presentations, the first step is to search for intraperitoneal fluid collection by ultrasound or computed tomography and to initiate appropriate antibiotic therapy if sepsis is present. When a collection is found, it is drained percutaneously to determine whether or not it is bilious. Next, biliary scintigraphy is done to ascertain whether or not the leak is continuing. If not, no further treatment is needed; if bile leakage is continuing, endoscopic retrograde cholangiography (ERC) is performed. In almost all type A injuries, endoscopic sphincterotomy combined with either an internal stent or a nasobiliary catheter controls the problem (see Fig. 30-2). Sometimes, endoscopic biliary intubation without sphincterotomy is used. Many type D injuries may be managed by these techniques also.

Jaundice

ERC is the first-line investigation. The distal duct will usually be found to be occluded or transected, with continuity to the proximal duct having been lost; often clips are seen at this point (Fig. 30-8). Next, percutaneous transhepatic cholangiography (PTC) is used to outline the proximal ducts and provide external drainage of bile. If stenotic rather than occluded ducts are found, the entire extent of injury may be diagnosed by ERC.

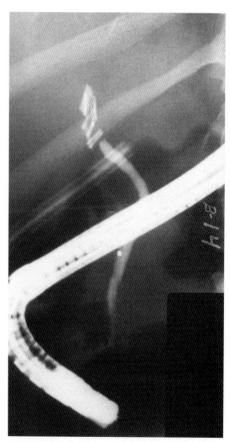

Fig. 30-8. Postoperative endoscopic retrograde cholangiogram in a patient who was noted to have bile in the operative field at the time of surgery. The surgeon placed a drain in the right upper quadrant and referred the patient for further management. Note complete occlusion of the bile duct and the position of clips at the top of the column of dye. (From Blumgart LH, Fong Y, eds. Surgery of the liver and biliary tract, 2nd ed. Churchill Livingstone, 1996.)

External Bile Fistula

External bile fistula is a less common presentation. It may occur in any type of injury. The first-line investigation is a fistulagram. Subsequent management depends on the anatomic findings.

Management of Biliary Injuries

Management of a laparoscopic biliary injury depends on the time of diagnosis and the type of injury. Successful treatment depends on the following principles:

All injured ducts must be recognized and repaired.
If reconstruction is required, it should almost always be done by hepaticojejunostomy.
Anastomoses should be of adequate caliber, mucosa to mucosa, without tension, and with good blood supply.

Injuries Recognized at Initial Operation

Intraoperative recognition of biliary injury is almost always an indication for conversion. Repair should proceed, based on the following two additional principles:

1. A repair should not be attempted if dissection or reconstructive techniques are required that are not commonly used by the primary operating team.
2. The injury should not be worsened by attempting a dissection for the purpose of making an exact diagnosis.

Types A, D, and E1 injuries require reconstructive techniques that are commonly practiced by most general surgeons. Types B, C, and E2 to E5 injuries require operative skills gained by performing high CBD resections with reconstruction, and liver resections. When these skills are not available at the time of injury, closed suction drains should be placed in the right upper quadrant, and the patient referred to an appropriate center. The best chance at repair is the first chance, and the patient's future health may be compromised by an inadequate initial repair. Type A injuries are directly repaired by suture and drainage. Type D injuries are repaired by closure of the defect using fine absorbable sutures over a T-tube. The T-tube should be brought out through a separate incision in the duct, if possible. Complete transections should be repaired with a hepaticojejunostomy Roux-en-Y anastomosis, applying the principles of anastomosis given above. Absorbable sutures only should be used in the biliary tree because nonabsorbable sutures can migrate into the lumen and become the nidus for stone formation.

Biliary Injuries Found in the Postoperative Period

Management of injuries found postoperatively depends on the type of injury, the type of initial management and its result, and the time elapsed since the initial operation or repair.

Type A injuries. The intraperitoneal bile collection is drained, and if bile leakage continues, intrabiliary pressure is reduced by endoscopic sphincterotomy with placement of a stent or a nasobiliary catheter. PTC may also be used to decompress the duct if ERC fails.

Type B injuries. These injuries may remain asymptomatic or present with pain and fever as late as 10 or more years after the initial injury. Symptomatic patients require treatment, usually hepaticojejunostomy and, more rarely, partial hepatic resection when biliary enteric anastomosis is not possible.

Type C injuries. The bile collection is drained and a biliary-enteric anastomosis is performed. If the duct is very small (i.e., less than 2 mm), then biliary-enteric anastomosis is unlikely to be successful, and ligation is preferable.

Type D injuries. Most cases should be treated by ERC and stenting. These patients should be followed closely because there is the potential for E type injuries to develop.

Type E injuries. Treatment of these injuries is quite similar to equivalent injuries occurring at open cholecystectomy. Strictures and sometimes clip occlusions may be treated primarily by nonsurgical means, including balloon dilation and stent placement either by ERC or percutaneously through the liver. There have been reports of good results using these techniques. However, these case series usually include many patients who presented with symptoms months or years after the cholecystectomy. In my experience, type E injuries that present within 1 or 2 months after cholecystectomy are rarely successfully managed in the long run by nonsurgical means, unless they are partial stenoses or are very short in length.

When patients present very early in the postoperative period (i.e., within the first 4 to 5 days), immediate repair may be undertaken. In my experience, patients are usually referred 1 week or more after cholecystectomy. In these, biliary decompression is obtained by PTC, and surgery is performed 3 months later when inflammation has subsided and the injury has evolved to its final state. The main goals of operative therapy have been stated above, namely, to obtain a tension-free, mucosa-to-mucosa anastomosis of adequate diameter of all bile ducts with a good blood supply to both ends of the anastomosis. Several series recommend preoperative placement of transhepatic tubes to aid identification of the ducts at surgery, and this is my practice (Fig. 30-9). Use of postoperative stents is controversial, and there is no evidence that they are useful if a large-caliber, mucosa-to-mucosa anastomosis has been achieved.

Hepaticojejunostomy is used in almost all cases. For types E1 and E2 injuries, my standard technique is to go above the area of scarring and perform a long side-to-side anastomosis to the extrahepatic portion of the left hepatic duct after it is lowered by dividing the hepatic plate, as described by Couinaud. This technique minimizes dissection behind the ducts and decreases the chance of devascularizing the duct at the point of anastomosis. It also permits a wide anastomosis, even when the ducts are not large, because the whole extrahepatic length of the left hepatic duct can be used. For higher and type E5 injuries, repair may require suture of several ducts (see Fig. 30-9), often after joining individual hepatic ducts. Dissection of the ducts on the right side may be particularly difficult. The ducts are found by dissection along the Glissonian plane. Often, removal of liver segment IVb will facilitate both the dissection and the anastomosis.

An adequate repair has an excellent prognosis, although patients must be followed throughout their lives. There is a progressive restenosis rate. Most recurrences are diagnosed in the first 2 years after repair, but restenosis has been described up to 15 years. The restenosis rate varies from 5% to 28%. In my opinion, modern restenosis

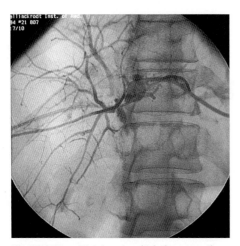

Fig. 30-9. Type E4 injury in which there were three separately transected ducts: the left hepatic duct and the right anterior and posterior ducts. Preoperative placement of percutaneous transhepatic tubes facilitated identification of anatomy at surgery. (From Blumgart LH, Fong Y, eds. Surgery of the liver and biliary tract, 2nd ed. Churchill Livingstone, 1996.)

rates should be less than 5%, using the principles enunciated above.

Restenosis and reoperation may lead to a vicious cycle of stenosis, stone formation, and liver damage. Although rarely required, liver resection and liver transplantation may be needed if repair has been inadequate.

Conclusion

Biliary injury is the most serious common complication of laparoscopic cholecystectomy. The key to this problem is prevention. Prevention requires a commitment to perform an exact dissection so that only structures that have been unequivocally and conclusively identified are divided. Diagnosis is usually made in the postoperative period; treatment depends on the type of injury.

Suggested Reading

Asbun HJ, Rossi RL, Lowell JA, Munson JL. Bile duct injury during laparoscopic cholecystec-

tomy: mechanism of injury, prevention, and management. *World J Surg* 1993;17:547–552.

Bernard HR, Hartman TW. Complications after laparoscopic cholecystectomy. *Am J Surg* 1993; 165:533–535.

Davidoff AM, Pappas TN, Murray EA, et al. Mechanisms of major biliary injury during laparoscopic cholecystectomy. *Ann Surg* 1992;215: 196–202.

Hunter JG. Avoidance of bile duct injury during laparoscopic cholecystectomy. *Am J Surg* 1991; 162:71–76.

Lillemoe KD, Pitt HA, Cameron JL. Current management of benign bile duct strictures. *Adv Surg* 1992;25:119–174.

Stewart L, Way LW. Bile duct injuries during laparoscopic cholecystectomy: factors that influence the results of treatment. *Arch Surg* 1995; 130:1123–1129.

Strasberg SM, Hertl M, Soper NJ. An analysis of the problem of biliary injury during laparoscopic cholecystectomy. *J Am Coll Surg* 1995;180: 101–125.

EDITOR'S COMMENT

Bile duct injury is the Achilles heel of laparoscopic cholecystectomy. The incidence of such injuries appears to be 5 to 10 times greater than that during open cholecystectomy. Older classification schemes for biliary injuries during cholecystectomy did not encompass all the injuries seen following laparoscopic cholecystectomy, therefore resulting in a number of new classification schemes, including that of Dr. Strasberg. The main message of this chapter is not how to *treat* biliary injuries but how to *prevent* them.

Several limitations of the laparoscopic technique must be overcome to minimize these injuries. First, as exposure of the porta hepatis is gained by cephalad retraction applied to the gallbladder, there is a natural tendency to pull the gallbladder vertically and align the cystic duct with the CBD, thereby giving the mistaken impression that the CBD is a continuation of the cystic duct. This optical illusion can be overcome by lateral traction

on the neck of the gallbladder, thereby exaggerating the angle between the cystic duct and the CBD. Second, the two-dimensional visualization of most laparoscopic systems renders spatial discrimination difficult: The surgeon must therefore view the anatomy from all sides by moving the infundibulum back and forth and assessing from both the dorsal and ventral aspects of the hepatocystic triangle. Third, most surgeons use monopolar electrocautery to obtain hemostasis and to dissect the gallbladder from its bed. When used injudiciously, cautery can cause injury to the CBD. Alternatively, too deep a plane of dissection in the gallbladder bed may be developed, unroofing peripheral bile ducts and leading to postoperative bile leakage that may be ascribed to the so-called ducts of Luschka. Fourth, the cystic duct is usually occluded by clips that may be improperly applied or that control the duct inadequately, and surgeons must be prepared to ligate the duct in the presence of a large or friable cystic duct.

Cholangiography has been hailed by some authors as the necessary step to prevent biliary injuries during laparoscopic cholecystectomy. However, misidentification of ducts prior to insertion of the catheter can result in type D biliary injuries, and bile duct injuries have been known to occur following cholangiography. It is probably true that performance of cholangiography with correct interpretation of the resulting films may limit the extent of bile duct injury if the CBD has been misidentified for the cystic duct. It thus seems wise to obtain cholangiograms liberally and certainly if there is any doubt of the anatomy. The primary means of preventing bile duct injuries, however, is meticulous dissection of the neck of the gallbladder and the junction between the gallbladder and the cystic duct. When this is done, virtually all bile duct injuries may be avoided during laparoscopic cholecystectomy, which may allow the operation to maintain its true position as a major advance in the treatment of cholelithiasis.

N.J.S.

31

Laparoscopic Management of Liver Disease

Namir Katkhouda, Eli Mavor, Donald Waldrep, and Jean Mouiel

Surgical Anatomy

Laparoscopic liver surgery requires the surgeon to have a good understanding of liver anatomy, as well as a solid knowledge of surgical techniques in open liver surgery. Fortunately, laparoscopic surgery mimics open liver surgery, and many of the fundamental principles are the same.

Descriptions of liver anatomy may be based on either morphologic or functional considerations. Morphologically, the liver consists of four lobes: right, left, quadrate, and caudate (Fig. 31-1). Morphologic lobes are divided by visible fissures. Though easily defined, these lobes do not necessarily correspond to circulatory patterns or liver function.

Surgically, we are primarily concerned with functional liver anatomy. In other words, surgical anatomy is defined by circulatory patterns. Functionally, the liver is divided into two major lobes, which may also be called hemilivers (Fig. 31-2A), as opposed to the four morphologic lobes. These hemilivers are divided by a plane starting at the medial border of the gallbladder bed and extending to the vena cava posteriorly. This division is based on portal and hepatic venous circulatory patterns. Each hemiliver can be further divided into segments, based on venous branching. The right hemiliver is subdivided into anterior and posterior segments by the right segmental fissure. The left hemiliver is subdivided into medial and lateral segments by the left segmental fissure, which is marked by the falciform ligament. Fig. 31-2B shows the segmental liver anatomy, delineating eight functionally independent segments.

Liver resections are classified as either typical or atypical, depending on whether segmental anatomy is observed. Atypical liver resection does not follow segmental anatomy. An example of atypical resection is wedge resection, which can be used in the treatment of focal liver lesions. Typical liver resection observes segmental anatomy and removes circulatory segments of liver. Typical liver resection includes all segmentectomies as well as right and left hepatectomies (removal of a hemiliver).

To avoid confusion, liver resections should be described using segmental anatomy. The term *lobectomy* should only be used in reference to classical lobectomy, which is removal of a morphologic liver lobe. For example, a left lateral segmentectomy may also be called a classical left lobectomy.

Laparoscopic Liver Surgery

Hepatic surgery has become very advanced, and its technology has been thoroughly tested. It is nevertheless important to emphasize the specialized nature of this type of surgery. For proper performance, the surgical team must have extensive ex-

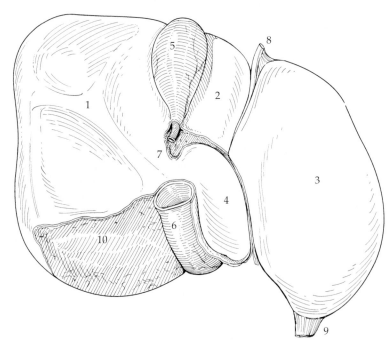

Fig. 31-1. Visceral surface of the liver showing morphologic anatomy (1, right lobe; 2, quadrate lobe; 3, left lobe; 4, caudate lobe; 5, gallbladder; 6, inferior vena cava; 7, portal vein; 8, ligamentum teres; 9, left triangular ligament; 10, right triangular ligament).

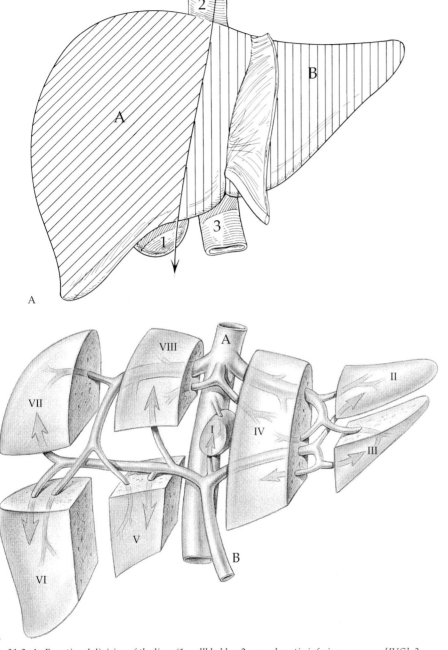

Fig. 31-2. **A:** *Functional division of the liver (1, gallbladder; 2, suprahepatic inferior vena cava [IVC]; 3, infrahepatic IVC; A, functional right lobe; B, functional left lobe).* **B:** *Vascular segmentation of the liver (A, IVC and hepatic veins; B, portal vein and segmental distribution).*

must also have access to an experimental laboratory to gain experience in laparoscopic technique. It is imperative that the surgeon get used to handling laparoscopic instruments for use in the liver and that he or she master the techniques of hemostasis and biliostasis. This can only be achieved by experimental surgery on animals.

It is very important to emphasize that the surgeon must be proficient in open hepatic surgical technique. Problems can crop up at any time during hepatic surgery, and one must be able to convert immediately for the patient's safety.

Certain specialized equipment is also required for laparoscopic liver surgery. These requirements are more important for surgery of the liver than for surgery of other abdominal organs. Unfortunately, specialized equipment, such as the neodymium:yttrium-aluminum-garnet (Nd:YAG) laser, can be very expensive. To alleviate this problem, it is essential that the various disciplines share surgical equipment.

Equipment and Instruments

In addition to the basic laparoscopic instruments, it is necessary for the operative team to have certain unique instruments that are adapted to hepatic surgery.

High-quality scopes with 0-degree, 30-degree, and 45-degree viewing ranges must be available (Karl Storz, Inc., Tuttlingen, Germany). The 30-degree scope is indispensable, as it enables observation of the blind areas of the liver not usually visible with traditional 0-degree scopes. The 30-degree scope allows visualization of the upper, posterior, and lateral regions of the liver. Moreover, the examination of tumor blood supply often requires visualization of the tumor base. This view can only be achieved with a 30-degree scope. Although it is our opinion that the 30-degree scope is not imperative in other intraabdominal laparoscopic surgeries, it is an absolute necessity in laparoscopic liver surgery.

The video camera needs to be of high quality and must have the discernment capacity needed to realize complete hemostasis and biliostasis. A powerful light source of 300-W xenon is also very important. Two video monitors are necessary to allow the surgeon and assistants comfortable view of the operation. Finally, each video screen must be at least 51 cm.

perience with the various techniques of hepatobiliary surgery.

Laparoscopic surgery is now out of its infancy and has been applied to most abdominal organs. The liver remains the last point of resistance due to its size, highly vascular nature, and a certain mystery that surrounds liver surgery. Laparoscopic liver surgery must be performed with caution and only by experienced hepatobiliary surgeons.

Prior to performing laparoscopic liver surgery, the surgeon must not only be proficient in open hepatobiliary surgery but

There is nothing specific about the trocars used for laparoscopic liver surgery. However, sufficient trocars and instrumentation must be available. Only atraumatic forceps should be used on the liver, preferably with no teeth. Forceps with large teeth are ineffective and increase the risk of hemorrhage. All forceps should be insulated and preferably rotating. The surgeon should have rotating coagulation scissors and an insulated hook on hand. Both should be insulated to the tips. For laparoscopic liver surgery, automatic clip appliers, which allow the clips to be reloaded without withdrawing the instrument, must be available. Finally, stapling devices with vascular clips will be useful for certain vascular pedicles.

The Nd:YAG laser is the instrument most highly adapted to surgery of the liver. We highly recommend it for use in laparoscopic liver surgery. Due to its capacity for greater penetration than carbon dioxide (CO_2) or argon lasers, it enables a correct cut to be carried out. The Nd:YAG laser was compared to conventional electrocautery experimentally during the excision of hepatic metastases (in rats). At the conclusion of this randomized, prospective study, the Nd:YAG laser proved to be clearly superior. When the Nd:YAG laser is not available, argon-beam coagulation can also be useful.

The ultrasonic dissector (CUSA, Valleylab, Boulder, Colorado) is another extremely valuable instrument. It enables precise dissection of the hepatic parenchyma by exploding hepatic cells using a cavitation mechanism. This exposes vasculobiliary radicles and allows a step-by-step dissection and division of these structures. The ultrasonic dissector is ideal for the resection of small, limited tumors, allowing enucleation with an adequate margin while maintaining control of pedicles.

A laparoscopic ultrasound (US) probe is also very useful, especially when coupled to Doppler. Laparoscopic US enables the surgeon to better visualize the liver while assessing for defects or hemostasis.

Another instrument that can be of great help in performing liver resection is the Harmonic Shears (LCS, Ethicon Endosurgery Inc., Cincinnati, Ohio). This instrument works on high-speed oscillations of the blades that induce cutting and hemostasis by a protein coagulation process without thermal damage. Experimen-

tal work has shown efficient sealing of biliary ducts with this device. Finally, laparoscopic argon-beam coagulating devices have recently become available that are valuable for stopping hemorrhage from raw hepatic surfaces.

Appropriate needle holders are mandatory. A wide range of models is available. Pretied endoligatures should be available, as well as finer sutures for internal suturing. These sutures should be strong and monofilament, preferably without memory. This type of monofilament ligature is also useful for extracorporeal tying with the Roeder knot. To avoid spillage of resected specimens, specimen bags must be strong and equipped with a closure system.

Tisseel fibrin sealant (Baxter Healthcare Corp. Hyland/Immuno Div., Deerfield Illinois) is indispensible for hemostasis and biliostasis after laparoscopic liver resection. It has proven its efficacy in controlling bleeding in hepatic and splenic trauma. Its ideal application is on raw hepatic surfaces to control oozing and for sealing of biliary leaks. In addition to its hemostatic effect, it has the properties of enhancing tissue healing by serving as a network for fibroblast proliferation and the creation of soft adhesions, thus promoting closure of dead spaces. Omentum may also be used to cover the raw surfaces of the liver at the end of the procedure.

Indications

Diagnostic laparoscopy is valuable in evaluating the liver for metastases that may not be detectable by conventional imaging techniques such as computed tomography (CT), magnetic resonance imaging, scintigraphy, or hepatic angiography. Small liver metastases dispersed throughout the liver may not be picked up by the usual imaging methods. However, with the laparoscope, these same metastases can frequently be seen. While CT and US can image intraparenchymal lesions, laparoscopy is more sensitive for small capsular hepatic lesions of 1 cm or less. Thus, laparoscopy makes it possible to change an indication for a curative resection into palliative surgery or to avoid unnecessary laparotomy in advanced cases. An example of such a case occurs with cancer of the pancreas. Pancreatic cancer is frequently accompanied by multiple hepatic metastases that are small and well dispersed in

the liver. Because of their size, these metastases are often not detected by conventional imaging. Laparoscopic evaluation, however, can usually pick up these metastases, altering the surgical management.

Laparoscopy can also be used to further evaluate liver masses seen by noninvasive techniques. Laparoscopy-directed biopsy of a liver mass previously detected on CT increases sensitivity and specificity over blind percutaneous biopsy. Laparoscopic US further increases the operator's ability to assess the liver parenchyma.

Diagnostic laparoscopy has also been used in the evaluation of hepatic trauma. In this capacity, laparoscopy is primarily used as a means of diagnosing injuries following blunt or penetrating trauma to the abdomen. In some cases, liver injury may be diagnosed and treated laparoscopically.

A further indication for laparoscopy is the possible resection of tumors confined to the liver (Fig. 31-3). Metastasectomy with a 2-cm margin is sufficient, and this enucleation can be performed using the laparoscope. A segmentectomy limited to one or at most two segments can also be performed laparoscopically. Finally, a classic left lobectomy (left lateral segmentectomy) is also possible, but this calls for a surgeon who possesses considerable experience. Laparoscopic liver resection should not be applied to a cirrhotic liver. The risk of hemorrhage with fatal consequences is too great.

In primary liver cancer, tumors are often very large at the time of diagnosis, and resection by laparoscopy is not a reasonable procedure. Therefore, laparoscopic resection most often concerns hepatic metastases. Laparoscopic resection may also be applied to nonmalignant tumors for which there is a formal indication, such as a hepatocytic adenoma (in women taking oral contraceptives) that has increased in size or is complicated by hemorrhage. Apart from risks of serious complications, limited resection is recommended with this type of tumor, as the histologic diagnosis is frequently uncertain.

Unroofing of liver cysts is an excellent indication for laparoscopic liver surgery. Laparoscopic unroofing is applied to either large, symptomatic, solitary cysts or polycystic liver disease. Solitary cysts presenting with intracystic hemorrhage or infection or causing pain due to their size are treated surgically. Anteriorly located polycystic liver disease can also be handled la-

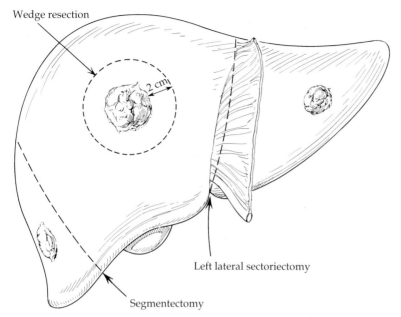

Fig. 31-3. Reasonable possibilities for laparoscopic liver resection.

Wedge resection

2 cm

Left lateral sectoriectomy

Segmentectomy

is very comfortable for the surgeon, who gets a symmetric view across the patient without unnecessary bending. It allows free use of the hands, while enabling the foot pedals to be maneuvered. The French position is also quite convenient for the assistants on each side.

Two monitors are necessary to allow all members of the surgical team a comfortable view of the surgery. These monitors are placed near the patient's head on either side of the anesthesiologist, making the whole arrangement coherent and ergonomic. The scrub nurse should be to the right of the surgeon beside the assistant, allowing him or her to pass instruments to the surgeon's right hand. In addition to the laparoscopic surgical instruments, the traditional basic instruments for open surgery must be on hand in a sterilized area, should the need for conversion arise.

paroscopically. Finally, it is possible to treat hydatid cysts using a laparoscopic technique.

Complications

The major intraoperative risks associated with laparoscopic liver surgery are hemorrhage and possible complications of CO_2 pneumoperitoneum. The usual rules of anesthesiology for hepatic surgery are followed, but it is necessary to emphasize that the anesthesiologist must be aware of the additional hazards of laparoscopic surgery, such as the complications of CO_2 pneumoperitoneum including hypoxemia, respiratory acidosis, arrhythmias, and, rarely, circulatory collapse. Additionally, vascular management by the surgeon is important in preventing CO_2 gas embolization. Measures must also be taken to ensure that there is equipment in the operating room for the rapid transfusion of blood. A sufficient supply of plasma and blood must be made readily available.

Close attention to vascular control throughout liver surgery is imperative. Bleeding that appears to be controlled at the outset can suddenly take a dramatic turn. The surgeon must be able to quickly decide to convert to open surgery in the event of sudden hemorrhage. It is likewise extremely important that the surgeon be able to use all laparoscopic methods neces-

sary for maintaining hemostasis. It is essential for every surgeon embarking on this kind of surgery to master the techniques of laparoscopic suturing with both intracorporeal and extracorporeal ligatures. As in open liver surgery, meticulous control of biliary radicles is also important. This can be achieved with clips or ligatures, as well as intracorporeal sutures.

Because of the high risk of hemorrhage, laparoscopic hepatic surgery is more technically demanding than other types of laparoscopic techniques. It is necessary to become familiar with the intraoperative use of the Nd:YAG laser, the ultrasonic scalpel, and automatic stapling devices.

Finally, another possible problem to be considered is the extraction of the excised specimen once resection has been performed. Specimen extraction is discussed in detail below (see "Maneuvers Common to All Laparoscopic Liver Surgery").

Patient Positioning and Operative Team

We recommend the "French" position for laparoscopic liver surgery. The surgeon positions him- or herself between the patient's lower extremities, which have been spread and placed into stirrups. The surgical assistants are positioned to either side of the patient (Fig. 31-4). This positioning

Approach to the Liver

If the planned intervention is more than just diagnostic laparoscopy, a minimum of four trocars will be introduced. The placement of trocars must allow enough space between them to avoid "sword fighting" with the various instruments. A trocar for the endoscope is usually introduced through the umbilicus. The graspers are introduced through a port on the patient's right side, and an instrument port is placed on the left. This triangle is converted to a rectangle by placing the fourth trocar for the palpator and irrigator/aspirator probe (Fig. 31-5A). This general scheme can be modified according to the location of the lesion and the surgeon's operating style. There is no ideal position for the trocars in this kind of surgery.

All trocars must be at least 10 mm to allow repositioning of the camera for visualization of the lesion and parenchyma from different angles. Other trocars—at most five or six—will be introduced for the use of the Nd:YAG laser or ultrasonic surgical dissector.

Adding trocar sites can affect the operative ergonomy. When the manpower is available, it is ideal to use the four-hands approach, with two surgeons operating simultaneously. One surgeon uses a grasper and the laparoscopic ultrasonic dissector, while the other surgeon manipulates scissors and clip appliers (Fig. 31-5B).

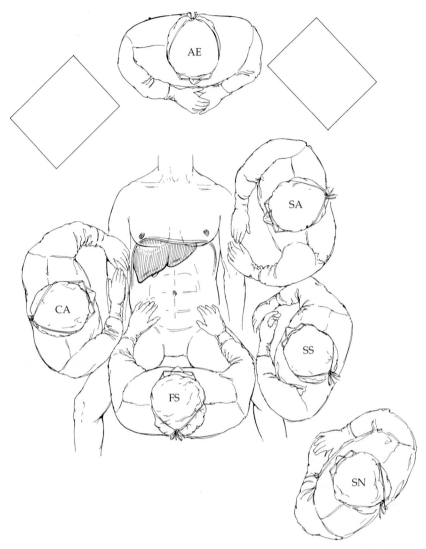

Fig. 31-4. The "French" position for laparoscopic liver surgery. (AE, anesthetist; SA, second assistant; SS, second surgeon; SN, scrub nurse; FS, first surgeon; CA, camera assistant.)

Maneuvers Common to All Laparoscopic Liver Surgery

Laparoscopic hepatic surgery, as open surgery, begins with mobilization of the liver. First, the round ligament is divided and ligated between clips. To lower the upper and posterior liver surfaces, the falciform ligament is sectioned. If a lesion in the left lobe exists, the left triangular ligament is then sectioned. In the event of a right posterior lesion, the right triangular ligament must be sectioned (Fig. 31-6). Generous liver mobilization is the key to success in this type of surgery, as it clears the area surrounding the lesion and allows direct access. In the case of a major resection, it is necessary to gain access to the inferior vena

cava and the trifurcation of the hepatic veins, particularly the left hepatic vein. A careful laparoscopic mobilization and dissection can be extremely useful if resection of the left lobe becomes necessary.

Once the liver has been mobilized, an US probe coupled to a color Doppler device can be of use in defining the anatomy and vascular connections of the lesion. This should be done prior to making an incision in Glisson's capsule. Glisson's capsule may then be incised using either a coagulating hook or the Nd:YAG laser. Next, long forceps are used to simulate finger-fracture methods. The ultrasonic dissector is helpful at this point, enabling parenchymatous pulverization while preserving vasculobiliary elements. All large-sized

vascular and biliary radicles must be clipped. When biliary ducts or major vessels are encountered, the surgeon must not hesitate to use extracorporeal ligatures with sliding Roeder knots.

At the conclusion of the operation, a possible problem to be considered is extraction of the excised specimen. There are different ways to do this, but the specimen should be placed into an extraction bag to prevent spillage of liver tissue into the abdomen. Usually, the umbilical incision must be enlarged to facilitate removal of the extraction bag. Kelly forceps may be used to morselize the specimen, but it is important to remember that the specimen should not be completely pulverized, as this will prevent later histologic examina-

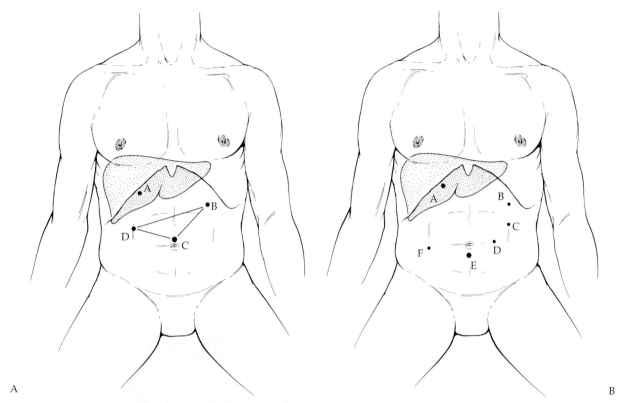

Fig. 31-5. **A:** *Trocar positioning for basic liver procedures. (A, 10 mm irrigation/suction probe; B, 10 mm right-hand surgeon; C, 10 mm umbilical scope; D, 10 mm left-hand surgeon.)* **B:** *Position of trocars and team for advanced liver procedures (four hands approach) (wedge resection, enucleation of tumors, left lateral segmentectomy). [A, irrigation/suction probe; B, clip applier (first assistant); C, scissors (first assistant); D, ultrasonic dissector (surgeon); E, camera (surgeon); F, grasper (surgeon).]*

tion of the tissue. In women requiring extraction of large specimens, a posterior colpotomy can be used. Repair of the colpotomy requires appropriate and precise reapproximation. This type of extraction does not entail any delayed complications if the repair is done correctly.

Diagnostic Laparoscopy

Diagnostic laparoscopy has several applications pertaining to liver surgery. It enables the surgeon to detect small primary tumors and metastases not detected by conventional imaging. The surgeon may also use the laparoscope to macroscopically confirm diagnoses made on preoperative assessment. Due to the magnification and precise spatial localization provided, diagnostic laparoscopy is helpful in taking directed biopsies of liver lesions. Finally, diagnostic laparoscopy may be used to as-

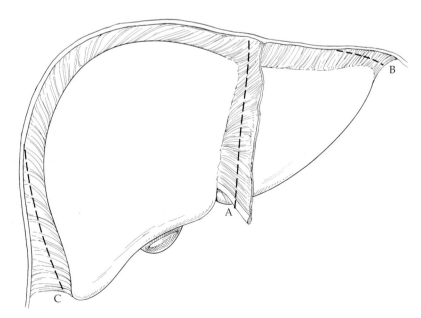

Fig. 31-6. Mobilization of the liver. **A:** *Section of the falciform ligament.* **B:** *Section of the left triangular ligament.* **C:** *Section of the right triangular ligament.*

sess liver injury following blunt or penetrating abdominal trauma.

Diagnostic laparoscopy is usually performed through a single 10-mm-trocar site placed at the umbilicus. Additional cannulas may be needed to introduce instruments to provide traction, allowing better visualization of certain abdominal regions. In some cases, mobilization of the liver may also be necessary to provide adequate access.

Laparoscopic US is an invaluable tool for the study of the liver. It permits the detection of deeper-lying metastases, as well as the definition of tumor vascular connections. Hepatic pedicles and the hilum can also be clearly seen. Thus, laparoscopic US allows biopsies to be taken without fear of causing major hemorrhage or bile leaks. Laparoscopic US precision is improved when coupled with Doppler probes.

Laparoscopic Treatment of Liver Cysts

Biliary cysts are intrahepatic lesions that usually do not communicate with the biliary tree. They are lined with bile duct–like epithelium and contain clear, serous fluid. They may be classified as either simple cysts or components of polycystic liver disease. Simple liver cysts are found in 2% to 4% of routine hepatic US evaluations. They are solitary in 50% of these patients. Polycystic liver disease is a hereditary disorder that follows an autosomal-dominant pattern and is clinically associated with progressive hepatomegaly and multiple renal cysts.

Even as cysts increase in size and number, the vast majority remain asymptomatic. In 5% to 10% of patients, however, symptoms occur as cysts enlarge and compress adjacent structures. These patients may present with abdominal discomfort, gastric or duodenal obstruction, jaundice, or even portal hypertension. Less commonly, liver cysts may become infected, bleed (intracystic hemorrhage), or rupture into the peritoneal cavity.

In the past, patients with symptomatic cysts have been treated by percutaneous aspiration alone, aspiration followed by alcohol injection, or unroofing of the cyst at open laparotomy. Although percutaneous aspiration has been popular in the recent past, its effect is usually transient. Recently, it has been shown that both solitary and multiple liver cysts can be managed laparoscopically.

Technique

The French position is used for positioning of the patient and the operating team. Four laparoscopic cannulas are introduced. Careful evaluation of the preoperative imaging studies will help guide the surgeon to sites of cyst formation and direct the exploration of the liver surface. Liver cysts, when viewed laparoscopically, appear as convex distortions on the liver surface, often possessing a characteristic bluish color.

Once the dome of the cyst is identified, it is opened with an electrocautery hook or curved scissors (Fig. 31-7A). A spurt of

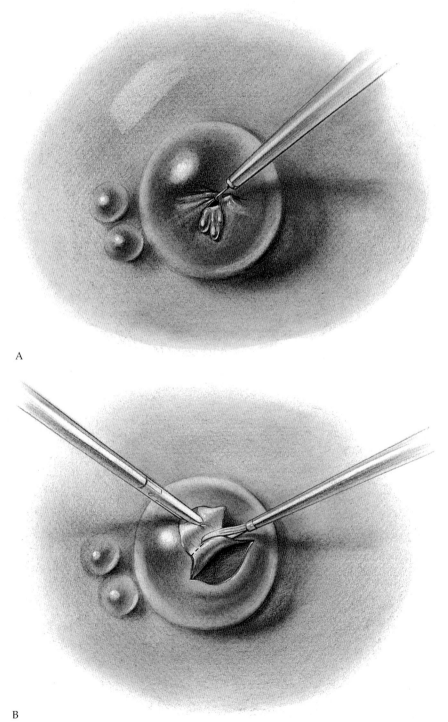

A

B

Fig. 31-7. **A:** *Opening of cyst using electrocautery hook.* **B:** *Excision of exposed cyst wall.*

serous fluid and collapse of the cyst are usually observed. This fluid should be collected with an aspiration probe and sent for bacteriologic studies. The incision over the cyst is then enlarged and the remaining fluid drained. The visible wall of the cyst is then grasped with forceps and excised using an electrocautery hook or curved scissors. This dissection is continued until the entire accessible portion of the wall is excised to a point within 2 mm of the cyst–parenchyma junction (Fig. 31-7B). A piece of the cyst wall should be sent for histologic evaluation.

Once hemostasis has been confirmed, attention can be directed toward other cystic lesions. In patients with multiple cysts, the deeper cysts may be drained through a previously opened cyst cavity, called transcystic fenestration. This process is repeated until all cysts are opened, drained, and excised. Transcystic fenestration allows laparoscopic management of multiple biliary cysts. In most patients, placement of drainage catheters is unnecessary.

From June 1989 to January 1999, we performed laparoscopic biliary transcystic fenestration in 27 patients (14 women, 13 men). The mean age was 51 years. All patients were symptomatic, experiencing epigastric pain, gastric compression, or painful hepatomegaly. All were treated in a manner similar to that outlined above. Follow-up ranged from 3 to 78 months. To date, there have been no operative complications. One patient with polycystic liver disease developed asymptomatic recurrence and underwent a reoperation.

Laparoscopic Treatment of Hydatid Cysts

Hydatid cysts are parasitic lesions of the liver that result from infestation by the tapeworm *Echinococcus granulosus*. The definitive host of this parasite is the dog. Humans, sheep, and cattle are intermediate hosts. Dogs become infected by ingesting sheep viscera containing hydatid cysts. Tapeworm scolices attach to the canine small intestine, where the worms develop into adults. Ova are later shed into the intestinal lumen and carried out with the feces. Infected feces may contaminate grass, crops, or the dog's fur. Human infection may occur by ingestion of contaminated

vegetables or even by simple contact with an infected dog.

Once ingested, the outer envelope of the ova is dissolved by gastric juices, and the liberated ova are free to penetrate the intestinal wall. Portal blood flow then carries these ova to the liver, where cyst formation occurs. Hydatid cysts occur more frequently in the right lobe of the liver. Far less commonly, ova may penetrate to the lungs, spleen, brain, and bone. Hydatid cysts usually evoke a strong inflammatory reaction within the surrounding parenchyma. Around the periphery of the cyst, fibroblasts are attracted, forming a thick capsule-like layer that often calcifies. Untreated hydatid cysts can rupture into the peritoneal cavity, resulting in anaphylactic shock or peritonitis. Cysts may also decompress into bile ducts, causing cholangitis. This may result in secondary bacterial infection of the bile ducts.

Because antihelminthic drugs are ineffective against this tapeworm, surgical excision remains the only treatment. Patients with favorably located cysts (anterior segments) may be offered total cyst excision by laparoscopy. For patients with cysts located posteriorly or near the vena cava, an unroofing technique should be used to avoid major complications due to potential venous laceration.

Technique

The principle of the laparoscopic approach to hydatid cysts is identical to that of the conventional procedure. For anteriorly located cysts, complete pericystectomy is performed without opening the hydatidoma. Careful dissection around the hydatid cyst is necessary to remove it intact. This is accomplished by creating a plane of dissection adjacent to the capsule-like cyst wall but outside the very friable hepatic parenchyma, which is often found next to the hydatidoma.

The French position is used for positioning of the patient and the operative team. Pneumoperitoneum is achieved, and four cannulas are inserted. It is important to perform an abdominal exploration to detect additional lesions that may have been missed on preoperative imaging studies. The liver is mobilized to provide access to the cyst. Occasionally, it is necessary to divide the left triangular ligament to obtain access to a lesion located in the left lobe of the liver. To facilitate hemostasis, electro-

cautery scissors are used to perform this maneuver because a moderate-sized vein usually courses through these tissues. Patients with one or more hydatid cysts often have inflammatory adhesions around the liver. If present, these adhesions should be freed using electrocautery scissors.

Total pericystectomy is used to remove anterior hydatid cysts. This technique most often applies to older, smaller cysts. When a total pericystectomy is performed, if the pericyst can be clearly delineated, it is not always necessary to inject alcohol or hypertonic saline solution into the cyst to kill the scolices and daughter cysts. Injection is avoided to prevent elevated pressure inside a cyst that is going to be entirely removed anyway.

If a posterior cyst or cysts are close to the vena cava, a different approach is preferred. The cyst is first injected with hypertonic saline to kill the parasite. After about 10 minutes, a special trocar is introduced through one of the laparoscopic cannulas, and the cystic contents are aspirated. Then, the cyst dome may be removed using the unroofing technique described in the previous section on biliary cysts.

Once the hydatid cyst is exposed, the liver capsule (Glisson's capsule) surrounding the lesion is scored with the contact-tip Nd:YAG laser set at 50 W (continuous mode). If there is persistent bleeding from smaller blood vessels, the sapphire tip can be removed and the defocused beam used for coagulation. Slow, methodical dissection is then carried out around the perimeter of the lesion. The electrocautery spatula has also proven to be useful for this portion of the procedure (Fig. 31-8A). The rounded tip of the instrument is used to bluntly dissect within the hepatic parenchyma. In contrast to other laparoscopic procedures, the electrocautery hook is rarely employed. This dissection can also be performed using the laparoscopic ultrasonic dissector, which helps to better delineate the pericyst. The magnification provided by the video laparoscope is a real advantage during hepatic dissection. It allows the surgeon to identify even the smallest vascular and biliary structures within the tissue plane. Vessels and ducts larger than 1 to 2 mm in diameter are individually ligated with surgical clips and divided with scissors (Fig. 31-8B).

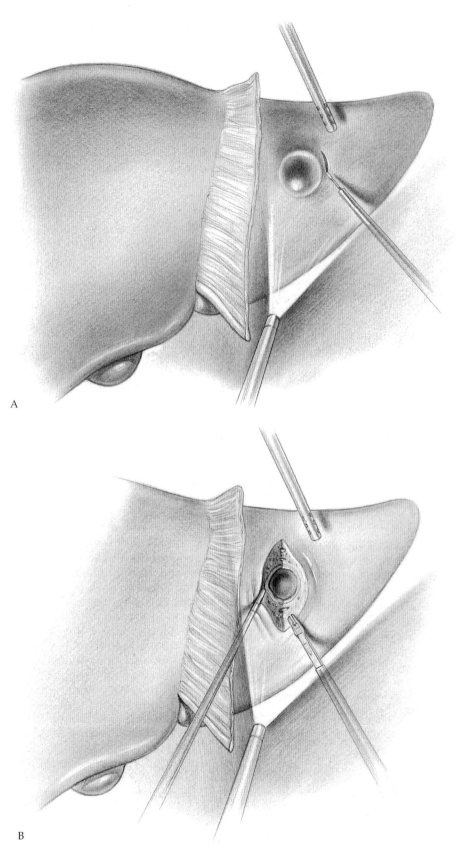

A

B

Fig. 31-8. **A:** *Scoring Glisson's capsule using the neodymium:yttrium-aluminum-garnet laser.* **B:** *Dissection around hydatidoma during total pericystectomy.*

In patients with very large hydatid cysts, numerous vascular and ductal attachments may be present. In such cases, an accurate road map is extremely helpful. Therefore, selective arteriography and cholangiography should be considered. During the procedure, if a large bile leak is suspected, the surgeon may elect to perform a cholecystectomy and obtain a cholangiogram. An alternative method is to inject methylene blue through the cholangiogram catheter and look for extravasation into the cyst cavity. On the basis of these studies, the surgeon can decide whether the ductal defect may be simply ligated with laparoscopically placed sutures or repaired over a stent (which may require open laparotomy).

Another method of providing hemostasis is the application of fibrin sealant. This material can be applied along the operative plane and is effective in controlling problematic bleeding within the liver tissue. Fibrin glue can also successfully control bile leakage from smaller transected ducts.

Following removal of the hydatid cyst from the liver, it is placed into an extraction bag in preparation for removal from the abdomen. To minimize the risk of spilling cyst contents into the peritoneal cavity, an impermeable, strong bag should be used. The bag and enclosed cyst are then removed through the umbilical fascial defect. If necessary, this opening can be gradually dilated until it is large enough to accommodate the specimen. A large Kelly clamp can be inserted through the umbilical incision and into the extraction bag and used to morselize the tissues.

After removal of the cyst, the operative site is carefully examined for bleeding or bile leakage. Once the cyst is completely removed, fibrin sealant can be injected into the remaining cyst cavity. Both edges of the cavity are then compressed with atraumatic forceps until hemostasis and biliostasis are achieved.

Closed suction drainage catheters are then placed along the liver edge under laparoscopic guidance. Such drains are routinely left in place following open liver surgery. We have decided to continue this practice with the laparoscopic approach.

Complete removal of CO_2 from the peritoneal cavity following the procedure is important, as it significantly reduces postoperative discomfort. If the umbilical fascia was dilated previously, this layer should be closed separately. Skin incisions are then closed using sutures or staples.

At present, we have performed laparoscopic hydatid cyst removal in five patients with one or more lesions. There was no mortality or identified complications. Patients were discharged from the hospital on the third postoperative day, which is dramatically sooner than patients who have undergone a similar open procedure (mean, 7 days). Postoperative imaging studies were performed on all five patients, confirming complete resolution of the cysts.

Confined Resection of Minor Neoplastic Lesions

Preliminary experience has shown that laparoscopic liver resection may have an important role in the treatment of focal liver lesions. For example, a patient with a solitary liver metastasis from adenocarcinoma of the colon can be considered for laparoscopic resection, particularly since recent data suggest that wedge resection is adequate for this type of lesion. A small metastasis located in the left lobe of the liver is an ideal example of a lesion amenable to a confined resection. This type of tumor can be safely resected using laparoscopy.

Technique

The patient is placed in stirrups, and the surgeon is located between the patient's legs. Four trocar sites are necessary. An umbilical trocar is used for the video laparoscope. The two lateral sites are used for grasping forceps and other instruments. A subxiphoid trocar is placed for the irrigator/aspirator probe. The subxiphoid site may also be used to provide access for the Nd:YAG laser and clip applier. Additional trocar sites (at most two) may be used if necessary.

Resection begins with incision of Glisson's capsule using the Nd:YAG laser 2 cm from the metastatic lesion (Fig. 31-9). Several studies have shown this to be an adequate margin. Smoke created during the incision must be intermittently suctioned through irrigation/aspiration cannula. Laser incision creates less smoke than carbonization with conventional electrocautery.

Progressive dissection more deeply into the hepatic parenchyma is then carried out

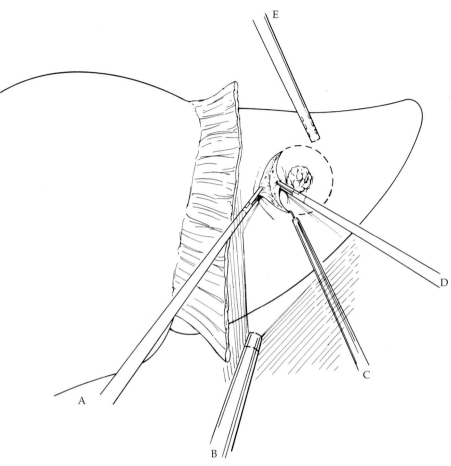

Fig. 31-9. Laparoscopic metastasectomy (with 2-cm safety margin). [**A**, atraumatic grasper (surgeon holding); **B**, camera; **C**, electrocautery hook or scissors (surgeon holding); **D**, grasper (assistant exposing); **E**, irrigation/suction.]

using the electrocautery hook or scissors with the right hand, separating the liver edges with the left-handed forceps. It is sometimes necessary to add a fifth trocar site for the insertion of the grasping forceps, so that an assistant can carefully expose the tumor. This positioning will create a groove through which a hook or coagulating scissors can pass for dissection. Fine, atraumatic forceps will allow the minute structures to be coagulated in this groove.

As larger vessels are encountered, clips must be used. We recommend using a double-clipping technique to avoid avulsion of a single clip from a vascular pedicle. The irrigator/aspirator probe must be used in the dissection groove to keep the operating field clean and dry. Maintaining a bloodless field is critical and can only be accomplished by constant rinsing of the dissection area.

Once the dissection is complete, it is necessary to insert a catheter for delivery of fib-

rin sealant. This is the last step in the resection. With a large metastasectomy, we perform cholecystectomy and routine cholangiography at the conclusion of the resection. With a smaller metastasectomy, cholangiography and drainage are not necessary.

Extraction of the resected tissue is performed in the same manner as described previously. Use of an extraction bag is important to prevent spillage. Metastases of a maximum of 5 to 8 cm can be extracted without difficulty by enlarging the umbilical incision, so that the extracted specimen is left intact.

Broader Resections: Segmentectomy and Left Lateral Segmentectomy

Liver segmentectomy can be performed laparoscopically for the treatment of liver tumors for which enucleation may be incomplete and inadequate treatment. Large lesions in the left lobe may be optimally treated by classic lobectomy, as an enucleation procedure may actually be dangerous. Because the open procedure is so much easier, laparoscopic left lobectomy (left lateral segmentectomy) should only be considered by surgeons who have extensive experience with laparoscopic surgery. Classic right lobectomy should not be attempted laparoscopically at present. Anatomic left lobectomy is discussed below, as it is a good demonstration of the principles common to laparoscopic segmentectomy and lobectomy.

Technique

Laparoscopic left lateral segmentectomy (segments II and III) follows the same rules as open surgery. The resection is preceded by a careful hepatic vascular isolation, which can be done with a little patience. The entire procedure is carried out using the four-hands technique described earlier.

The first step in the procedure is gaining control of the porta hepatis. Early control of this region allows a Pringle maneuver (clamping of the portal triad) to be applied quickly at any time during the operation. The porta hepatis is reached by opening the lesser omentum. Dissection is carried out until the region is encircled and a right angle dissector can be passed around the porta (Fig. 31-10A). This dissector is used to pass a length of umbilical tape around the vessels of the porta hepatis. This umbilical tape will be used to make a tourniquet that can be tightened, should the need arise. The ends of the umbilical tape are then exteriorized to the skin through one of the trocar sites, and a section of rubber tubing is placed over them. (A portion of a red rubber drain works well for this purpose.) Sliding the rubber tubing up the tape tightens the tourniquet and provides vascular control (Fig. 31-10B).

The falciform ligament is divided until the inferior vena cava and root of the hepatic vein are reached. Complete division of the left triangular ligament will then leave the left lobe attached only by its vascular and biliary elements. The left hepatic vein outside the liver must then be dissected out (Fig. 31-10C). A blunt right-angle dissector or a peanut dissector may be used to accomplish this. This is a tricky dissection with potentially dire consequences, and

extreme caution must be observed. If there is no left hepatic vein showing outside the liver, the dissection is not laparoscopically feasible, and the procedure should be completed via laparotomy. Once the left hepatic vein is isolated, it is ligated with 0 silk, and the suture ends are left long. This knotting should be performed intracorporeally to avoid tension that might otherwise occur with extracorporeal ligatures and could lacerate the vein.

Glisson's capsule may now be incised using the Nd:YAG laser or another electrocautery device. This incision is made parallel to the falciform ligament on its left side. The left lobe is then elevated, and this incision is continued on the visceral aspect of the liver.

A laparoscopic Kelly fracture technique is used to dissect into the liver parenchyma. This dissection may alternatively be carried out using the laparoscopic ultrasonic dissector. The ultrasonic dissector provides more precise destruction of hepatic parenchyma and better identification of

pedicles. Intraparenchymatous dissection causes the surgeon first to encounter elements of segment III. All vascular and biliary pedicles should be ligated using a double-clip technique. Double clipping prevents the accidental avulsion of a single clip from any radicle. When available, the harmonic scissors (LCS, Ethicon Endosurgery Inc., Cincinnati, Ohio) can be helpful for coagulating small vessels. Larger pedicles should be ligated using endoligatures or extracorporeal or intracorporeal sutures. Elements of segment II will become evident as the dissection progresses. These structures should be controlled in the same manner as those for segment III.

When oozing occurs on the liver surface, control can be attempted using direct compression with a small piece of cotton gauze. It is important that the liver surface be continually irrigated and suctioned to maintain a bloodless operative field so that the site of bleeding can be visualized. If oozing is persistent, the electrocautery spatula may be necessary. In our experience, use of an electrocautery spatula

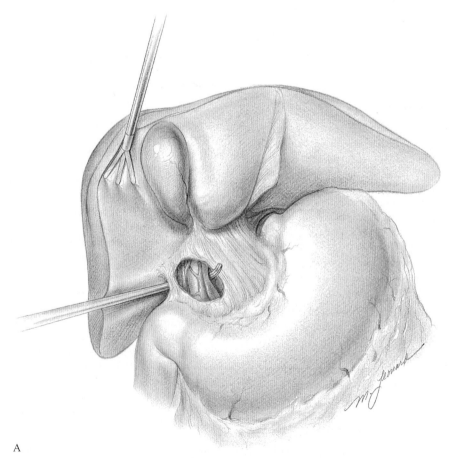

A

Fig. 31-10. **A:** *Dissection around the porta hepatis with the right-angle dissector.* (continued)

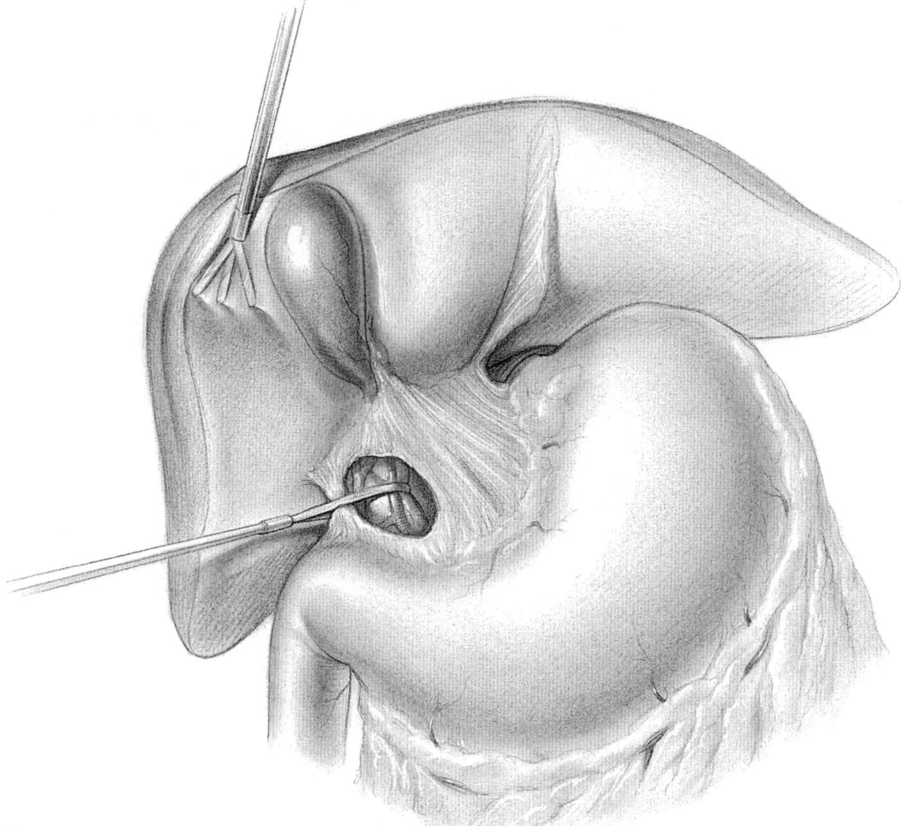

turned up to a higher setting will control most oozing. Particularly large amounts of oozing may warrant use of an argon laser.

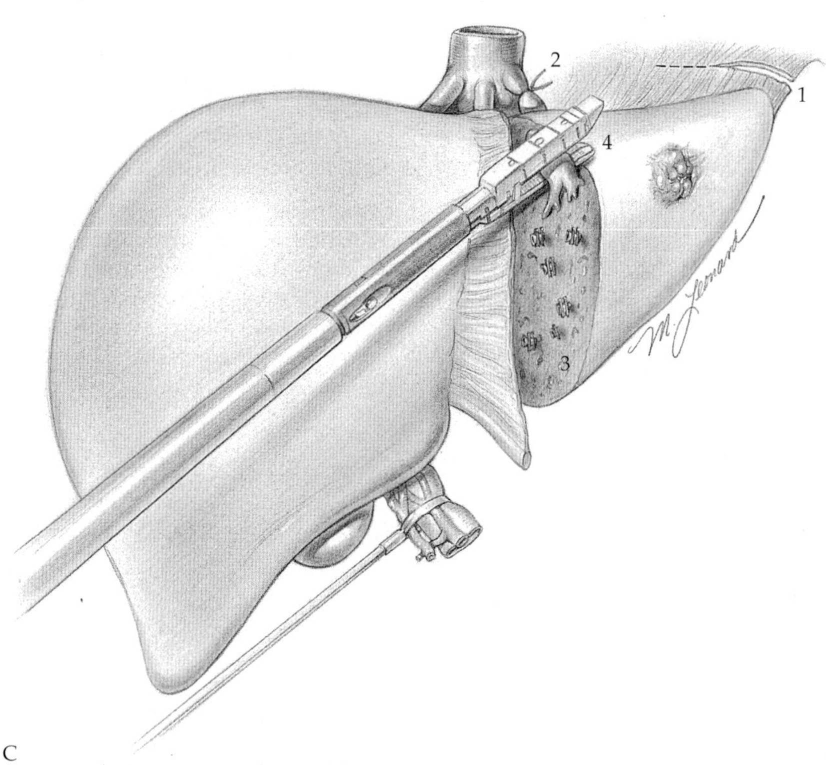

The last structure encountered during dissection of the left lateral segment is the left hepatic vein inside the liver. This vessel is not as dangerous as it may seem because the hepatic vein has been ligated earlier in the procedure. A laparoscopic linear cutting stapler with white vascular staples is then used to staple and divide the left hepatic vein. The left lateral segment's remaining attachment may now be divided using the Kelly fracture technique previously described or dissection with the flat spatula.

As with all specimens following laparoscopic resection, the lobectomy specimen must be placed into a specimen bag for extraction. Due to its size, the lobectomy specimen can only be withdrawn if it undergoes some degree of morselization or removal via a posterior colpotomy in women.

Prior to completion of the operation, the raw surface of the liver must be inspected, and hemostasis, as well as biliostasis, is completed. Cholangiographic examination after cholecystectomy is useful at this stage if significant bile leak is a concern. Remaining vascular and biliary leaks are controlled by the same means as described above. The application of fibrin sealant to raw liver surfaces is invaluable. The greater omentum can also be used to cover the raw surface of the liver at the termination of the procedure. Following left lobectomy, we recommend placing two suction drains near the edge of the wound to collect any minor persistent ooze of blood or bile and to prevent hematoma.

The same techniques for achieving hemostasis and biliostasis apply to wedge resections, as well as smaller segmental resections. For instance, resection of the anterior aspect of segment IV, resection of segment V, and resection of segment VI are all carried out in the same manner as the left lobectomy.

Prevention and Treatment of Complications

The most common intraoperative complication associated with laparoscopic liver surgery is hemorrhage. Minimal oozing may be controlled with unipolar or bipolar

Fig. 31-10. (Continued) **B:** Tourniquet around the porta hepatis using umbilical tape and a section of rubber tubing. **C:** Intrahepatic division of the left hepatic vein using the endolinear cutter with vascular staplers (1, division of left triangular ligament; 2, extrahepatic ligation of the left hepatic vein; 3, control of vascular pedicles of segments II and III; 4, division of left hepatic vein).

forceps. A coagulating spatula enables flat application of the coagulating current and can also be useful. When arterial bleeding occurs (where there is a clearly visible spurt of blood), it is necessary to grasp the artery with the atraumatic graspers and immediately apply a clip or ligature. The laparoscopic argon-beam coagulator may also help obtain surface hemostasis.

Management of venous bleeding in hepatic surgery is more complicated. Venous bleeds often entail constant oozing, and hemostasis can be extremely difficult to achieve. Panic should be avoided, as this will only make the placement of laparoscopic sutures and clips more difficult, thus delaying hemostatic control. Often appropriate, temporary tamponade will stabilize the situation and allow assessment of the venous injury. For example, a Pringle maneuver can be used to gain control in most situations, except when hemorrhage originates from a hepatic vein (Fig. 31-11). Bleeding from a small lacerated vein can generally be controlled with coagulation, a clip, or the argon laser. If the venous injury is more extensive, such as in a hepatic vein or branch of the portal vein, the surgeon should not hesitate to convert promptly to an open procedure. This will permit sufficient access to the hemorrhage and allow the operation to be completed safely. It should be stressed that conversion is not an admission of failure, but rather good surgical judgment. The safety of the patient is always the first priority.

Control of biliary leaks is generally easier to accomplish, since the biliary drainage can clearly be seen with the magnification provided by the laparoscope.

Another complication that can suddenly arise during laparoscopic liver surgery is CO_2 embolization. The gynecologic experience has shown that the risk of CO_2 embolization in laparoscopic surgery is minimal. However, this risk is much greater during surgery of organs that are well vascularized and directly linked to the inferior vena cava, such as the spleen and liver. The patient must be constantly monitored by the anesthesiologist intraoperatively. These emboli are sometimes only detected by recovery room personnel after extubation. The staff must be informed of this possible delayed complication. Precise vascular control is important in preventing CO_2 embolization. Careful handling of large vessels inside the parenchyma and avoidance of scissors injury must be stressed. Division of these vessels should only occur after coagulation or control with clips or ligatures.

The spilling of resected liver tissue (cystic debris, exfoliated tumor cells) into the abdomen can also result in complications. Appropriate handling of resected specimens to prevent this complication has been discussed in previous sections.

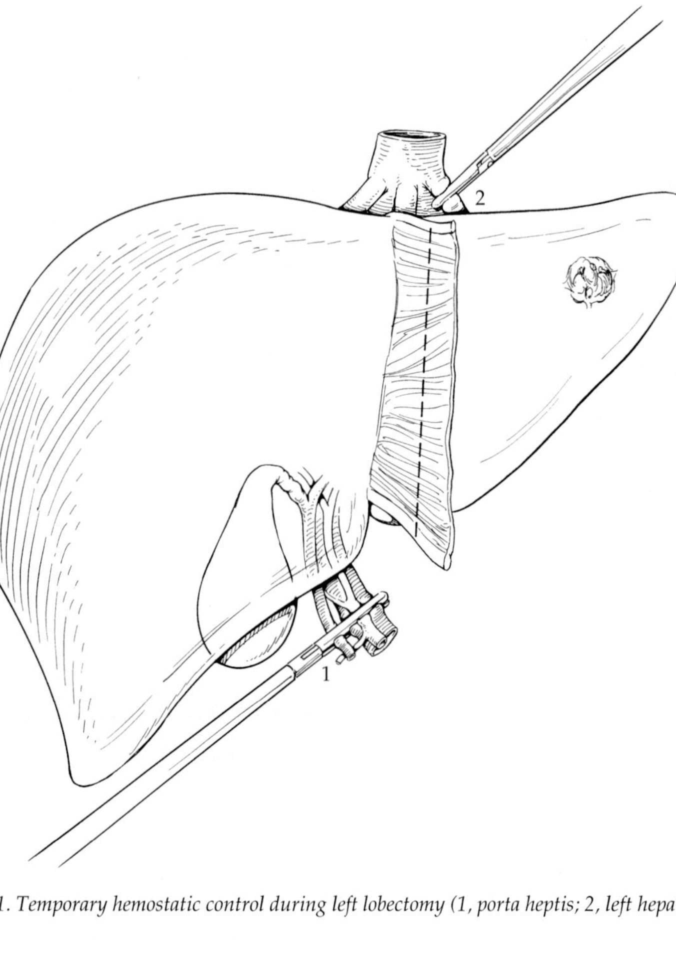

Conclusion

Diagnostic laparoscopy is a useful tool in the assessment of surgical disease of the abdomen. It is particularly helpful in evaluating widespread metastases and abdominal trauma (both blunt and penetrating), obviating laparotomy in some cases.

Laparoscopy is also an attractive alternative to open surgery for the resection of confined liver lesions. It avoids large incisions, which are painful and disabling. The efficacy of this type of surgery needs to be assessed by careful and systematic evaluation of the results, and therefore multicenter trials are required.

Laparoscopic liver surgery is technically difficult and has potentially serious complications. Therefore, it is important to approach this type of surgery with a humble attitude even when considerable hepatobiliary and laparoscopic experience and competence are available.

Suggested Reading

Barrow JL. Hydatid disease of the liver. *Am J Surg* 1978;135:597–603.

Blumgart LH, ed. *Surgery of the liver and biliary tract*, 2nd ed. New York: Churchill Livingstone, 1994.

Dixon JA. Current laser applications in general surgery. *Ann Surg* 1988;207:355–372.

Fabiani P, Katkhouda N, Iovine L, Mouiel J. Laparoscopic fenestration of biliary cysts. *Surg Laparosc Endosc* 1991;1:162–165.

Hughes K, Scheele J, Sugerbaker PH. Surgery for colorectal cancer metastatic to the liver: opti-

Fig. 31-11. Temporary hemostatic control during left lobectomy (1, porta heptis; 2, left hepatic vein).

mizing the results of treatment. *Surg Clin North Am* 1989;69:339–359.

Katkhouda N, Fabiani P, Benizri E, Mouiel J. Laser resection of a liver hydatid cyst under videolaparoscopy. *Br J Surg* 1992;79:560–561.

Katkhouda N, Hurwitz M, Gugenheim J, et al. Laparoscopic management of benign tumors and cysts of the liver. *Ann Surg* 1999 (in press).

Katkhouda N, Mouiel J. Laparoscopic applications in liver surgery. In: Zucker KA, ed. *Surgical laparoscopy update.* St. Louis, MO: Quality Medical Publishing, 1993:395–408.

Mouiel J, Katkhouda N, White S. Endolaparoscopic palliation of pancreatic cancer. *Surg Laparosc Endosc* 1992;23:241–243.

Tranberg KG, Rigotti P, Brackett KA, Bjornson HS, Fischer JE, Joffe SN. Liver resection: a comparison using the Nd-YAG laser, an ultrasonic surgical aspirator, or blunt dissection. *Am J Surg* 1986;151:368–373.

Wagner JS, Adson MA, Van Heerden JA, Adson MH, Ilstrup DM. The natural history of hepatic metastases from colorectal cancer: a comparison with resective treatment. *Ann Surg* 1984;199: 502–508.

Warshaw AL, Fernandez-del Castillo C. Laparoscopy in preoperative diagnosis and staging for gastrointestinal cancers. In: Zucker KA, ed. *Surgical laparoscopy.* St. Louis, MO: Quality Medical Publishing, 1991:101–105.

Way LW, ed. *Current surgical diagnosis and treatment*, 10th ed. East Norwalk, CT: Appleton & Lange, 1994.

Way L, Wetter A. Laparoscopic treatment of liver cysts. *Surg Endosc* 1992;6:89–90.

EDITOR'S COMMENT

Laparoscopic hepatic surgery is in its infancy. The vast majority of laparoscopic hepatic operations are currently performed for diagnostic purposes—either staging laparoscopy for hepatopancreaticobiliary malignancies or laparoscopy-guided liver biopsy. I currently perform diagnostic laparoscopy in virtually all patients with hepatopancreaticobiliary malignancy prior to consideration of laparotomy. Laparoscopy by itself is highly efficacious in demonstrating small surface metastases, and laparoscopic intracorporeal US allows assessment of the deep hepatic parenchyma. Drs. Katkhouda, Mavor, Waldrep, and Mouiel describe their extensive experience with other laparoscopic applications for hepatic surgery. It should be stressed that these operations should be performed only by those experienced in both laparoscopic and open hepatic surgery and that conversion to open operation may be required on an urgent basis. Laparoscopic hepatic surgery is obviously technology-intensive, as the argon laser, ultrasonic dissector, and Nd:YAG laser may facilitate these procedures. Thus, I have been hesitant to use pneumoperitoneum in the context of major hepatic resections due to the concern of CO_2 embolization, should an inadvertent rent in a hepatic vein develop. Therefore, I have relied on gasless laparoscopic techniques and abdominal wall–lifting devices when a potentially major liver resection is planned. Performed for the appropriate indications as described in this chapter, laparoscopic applications of hepatic surgery appear to be eminently justifiable and beneficial to patients. Certainly, these operations are for neither the faint-of-heart nor the inexperienced laparoscopist.

N.J.S.

IV

Endocrine

32

Laparoscopic Pancreatic Surgery

Michel Gagner

Anatomic Considerations

The pancreas is a soft pink gland that is approximately 15 cm long and extends from the duodenum to the splenic hilum. Proximity of the mesenteric vessels to the head of the pancreas is important during dissection. The lower part of the head has a posterior projection, the uncinate process, which surrounds the mesenteric vessels. A groove between the neck of the gland and the head cradles the gastroduodenal artery, which becomes visible after pyloric transection. The upper border of the head of the pancreas is delineated by the first portion of the duodenum, and the third and fourth portions of the duodenum are located inferiorly and to the right of the mesenteric vessels. The transverse colon and its mesentery are anterior to the pancreas. Posteriorly, the head is near the inferior vena cava, and its uncinate process lies in front of the aorta. The portal vein is also located posterior to the pancreas. The common bile duct (CBD) is posterior and transverse to the pancreatic tissue for a short distance, close to the second portion of the duodenum (Fig. 32-1).

Pancreatic Resection

Preoperative Considerations

Before pancreatic resection for cancer, a chest radiograph should be performed to identify pulmonary metastases. A computed tomography (CT) scan of the upper abdomen is performed to delineate the peripancreatic mass extension and to look for metastatic disease in the liver or peritoneal cavity. A portoscan (intravenous contrast into the mesenteric artery) may help determine whether the portal or mesenteric vein is involved. Magnetic resonance imaging may show approximately the same information and usually does not provide more information than the CT scan. The biliary tree should be delineated preoperatively to plan the operation with endoscopic retrograde cholangiopancreatography (ERCP) or percutaneous transhepatic cholangiography. Brushings and cytologic analysis of the lower CBD may be obtained as well. A cholangiogram and pancreatogram may also be obtained for anatomic delineation. During bile duct imaging, a stent may be inserted to relieve CBD obstruction. If the patient is considered to be an operative candidate, a mesenteric angiogram should be performed because mesenteric artery or vein involvement means incurability.

In deeply jaundiced and malnourished patients, preoperative bile duct decompression can improve hepatic, renal, and immunologic functions and help to sustain the patient's ability to tolerate further operative trauma. The bilirubin's response to decompression may indicate the prognosis; when there is a return to normal or near normal, the mortality rate is less than 10%.

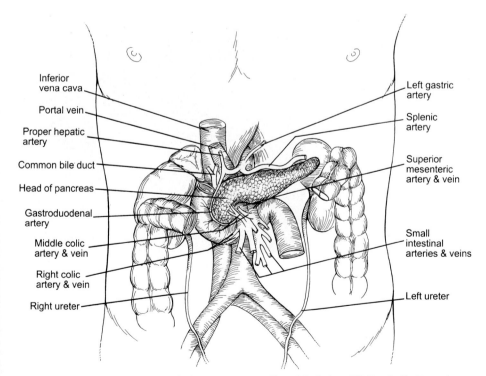

Inferior vena cava

Portal vein

Proper hepatic artery

Common bile duct

Head of pancreas

Gastroduodenal artery

Middle colic artery & vein

Right colic artery & vein

Right ureter

Left gastric artery

Splenic artery

Superior mesenteric artery & vein

Small intestinal arteries & veins

Left ureter

Fig. 32-1. Anatomy of the pancreas and adjacent structures. (From MacFadyen BV, Ponsky JL. Operative laparoscopy and thoracoscopy. *New York: Lippincott-Raven, 1996; with permission.)*

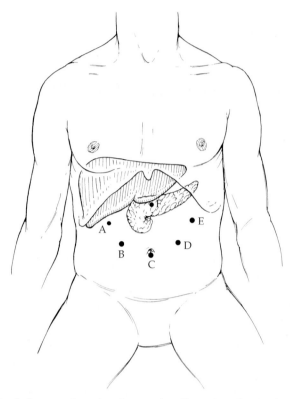

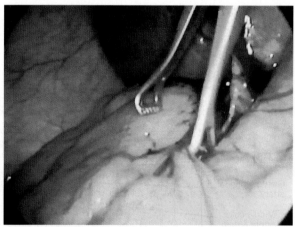

Some surgeons may prefer to perform a diagnostic laparoscopy to eliminate distant metastases and then do a second procedure (e.g., laparotomy followed by a Whipple procedure). I prefer to perform a diagnostic laparoscopy first and continue the procedure during the same anesthesia if the tumor is resectable. Warshaw and Castillo from Massachusetts General Hospital studied a series of 72 patients and found that the resectability rate was 78% when CT scan, angiography, and laparoscopy results were negative for tumor extension. Peritoneal cytology can be done but is not useful during the laparoscopy itself.

Laparoscopic staging of periampullary tumors involves the insertion of several trocars for inspection of the body and tail of the pancreas (Fig. 32-2). A window is created between the transverse colon and the greater curvature of the stomach using cautery and endoscopic clips (Fig. 32-3). A laparoscopic Kocher maneuver is performed to evaluate duodenal and vena caval involvement. Laparoscopically guided, percutaneous fine-needle aspiration or biopsy of the pancreatic lesion is usually done to confirm the diagnosis. The ligament of Treitz is inspected for mesoje-

Fig. 32-2. Trocar sites for laparoscopic staging of pancreatic malignancies or for resections. (A, 5-mm pancreatic resection; B, 10-mm exploration and resection; C, camera port; D, 12-mm exploration and resection; E, 10-mm exploration and resection; F, 5-mm resection.)

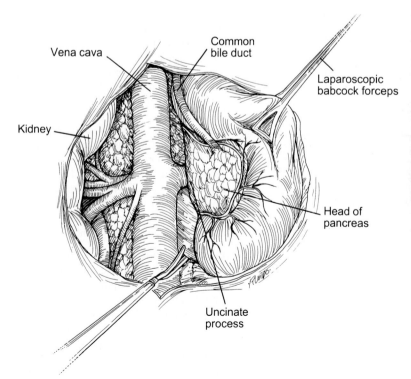

Fig. 32-3. Laparoscopic Kocher maneuver, with Babcock forceps on the second duodenum. (From MacFadyen BV, Ponsky JL. Operative laparoscopy and thoracoscopy. New York: Lippincott-Raven, 1996; with permission.)

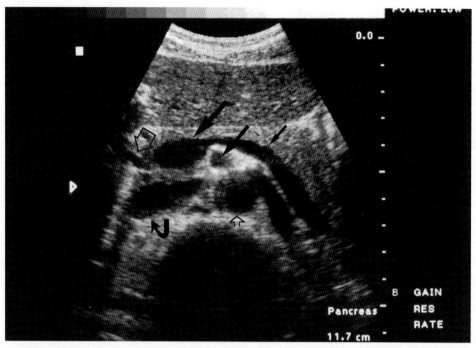

Fig. 32-4. *Portal vein as seen with laparoscopic pancreatic ultrasound (portal venous confluence, large solid arrow; superior mesenteric artery, medium solid arrow; splenic vein, small solid arrow; aorta, small open arrow; common bile duct, large open arrow; inferior vena cava, curved solid arrow). (From Staren ED. Ultrasound for the surgeon. New York: Lippincott-Raven, 1997; with permission.)*

junum involvement, and regional nodes in the paraduodenal and pericholedochal areas are sampled. A branch of the middle colic vein can be followed to the mesenteric vein with the blunt suction/irrigation probe to exclude portamesenteric vein involvement. Laparoscopic ultrasonography, with or without Doppler, can be used to evaluate vessel involvement. Using all these maneuvers, it is possible to exclude more than 90% of unresectable lesions (Fig. 32-4).

Operative Technique for Staging

The patient is kept supine in a slight reverse Trendelenburg position with both legs abducted. The surgeon stands between the legs of the patient to gain access for suturing, and assistants stand on either side of the patient (Fig. 32-5). The patient should have an indwelling Foley catheter, nasogastric tube, central venous line, and arterial line for monitoring. Carbon dioxide (CO_2) is insufflated through the umbilicus with a Veress needle using up to 15 mm Hg of pressure. A 10-mm trocar is inserted in the umbilicus, and a 30° laparoscope with a 10-mm diameter is inserted for a simple diagnostic laparoscopy.

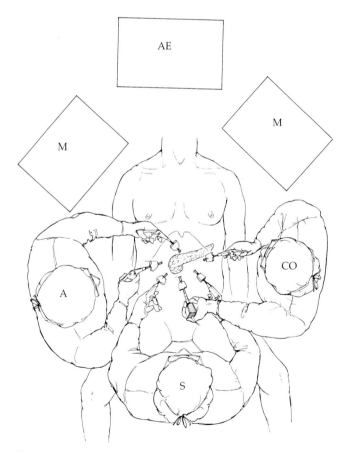

Fig. 32-5. *Operating room setup for laparoscopic pancreatic procedures. (S, surgeon; A, assistant; M, monitor; AE, anesthesia; CO, camera operator.)*

Adhesions from prior surgery may need to be released. If no obvious peritoneal or liver metastases are seen, a second 10-mm epigastric trocar and paramedian right and left trocars are inserted; these permit full evaluation of tumor extension and the possibility of resection. Through the epigastric port, a 10-mm laparoscopic Babcock forceps grasps the greater curvature the stomach. The camera is positioned in the right paramedian trocar, and the surgeon works with both hands using the umbilical and paramedian left trocars. Both instruments are used to dissect the gastrocolic ligament below the gastroepiploic vessels and enter in the lesser sac. Transverse branches from the gastroepiploic arcades are clipped, but the arcade is preserved because it supplies blood to the pylorus and antrum. Ultrasonic energy can be used for tissue dissection (i.e., ultracision). Through a 10-cm window, the body and tail of the pancreas are inspected for possible seeding (Fig. 32-6). It is also possible to inspect the upper part of the lesser sac by creating a window over the left caudate lobe and assess invasion locally. An ultrasonographic probe can be used to look for tumors behind the pancreas.

A laparoscopic Kocher maneuver is conducted by positioning the Babcock forceps on the second portion of the duodenum and lifting upward and superiorly. The dissection is carried out between the lateral border of the second and third portion of the duodenum from the transverse colon and vena cava. This maneuver frees the entire duodenal arcade, the posterior aspect of the head of the pancreas, and uncinate process. Any suspicious nodes should be biopsied with a laparoscopic biopsy forceps. When the CBD and common hepatic duct are identified (usually dilated), a cholangiogram can be performed directly on the anterior aspect of the duct using a 22-gauge metallic spinal needle percutaneously to better delineate the regional anatomy. Rarely, choledocholithiasis can be found, or tumor extension is detected on the proximal bile duct. If the gallbladder is present, it should be used for liver retraction to expose the liver hilum. The gallbladder is resected at the conclusion of the procedure.

If no diagnosis has been confirmed, my colleagues and I perform a fine-needle aspiration using a 22-gauge needle placed directly into the palpable mass or in the presumed area through the anterior head of the pancreas. This is facilitated with a Franzen aspirating syringe apparatus for cytologic sampling. Multiple passes are performed, and the aspirate is placed on the glass for microscopic examination. To complete the extensive evaluation, a branch of the middle colic vein is identified and followed until it reaches the anterior and inferior aspect of the mesenteric vein. The irrigation/suction laparoscopic probe is used with sterile saline injected in the proper plane between the pancreatic neck and the mesenteric portal vein to achieve gentle blunt dissection.

Operative Technique for Laparoscopic Whipple

The laparoscopic technique for a Whipple procedure is a modification of Longmire and Traverso; it is a pylorus-preserving pancreatoduodenectomy (Fig. 32-7). The peritoneum covering the CBD is opened anteriorly and laterally, and it is then dissected free posteromedially from the portal vein and the right hepatic artery. Using a large, curved needle, a 2-0 nylon suture is passed through the abdominal wall in the right subcostal area and passed under the bile duct to create a suspension with minimum retraction. The bile duct is transected at least 2 cm above the pancreatic border or higher above the cystic duct junction using an endoscopic linear stapler (Fig. 32-8). The first portion of the duodenum is then divided approximately 1 cm distal to the pylorus, which is easily identified by looking inferiorly for the veins of Mayo and by palpating a slight induration in the area. If there is any doubt about the anatomic landmarks, gastroscopy can be performed and the pylorus identified by transillumination. After dissection of the gastrocolic ligament is completed, gastroepiploic vessels derived from the gastroduodenal vessels are double clipped with titanium clips.

A right-angled dissector is used to dissect under the pylorus to create a window of 1 cm², which allows passage of an endoscopic linear stapler. For a 60-mm stapler, the umbilical 10-mm-diameter trocar is transformed to an 18-mm trocar by using a 10-mm-diameter plastic rod for dilation and maintenance of the tract. Reducers from 18 to 10 mm or 18 to 5 mm must be used throughout the procedure. Similarly, the duodenojejunal junction is transected as close to the proximal jejunum as possi-

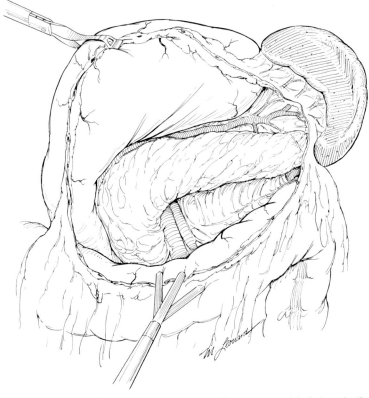

Fig. 32-6. Mobilization of the gastrocolic ligament allows exposure of the body and tail.

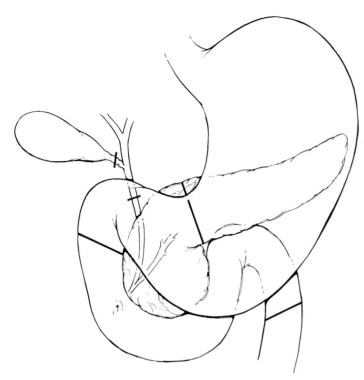

Fig. 32-7. Lines of transection for a Whipple procedure.

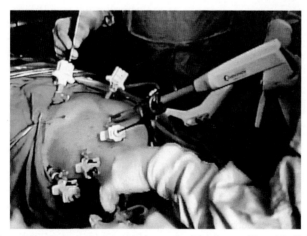

Fig. 32-8. An endoscopic stapler is used to transect the proximal duodenum. (From MacFadyen BV, Ponsky JL. Operative laparoscopy and thoracoscopy. *New York: Lippincott-Raven, 1996; with permission.)*

The uncinate process is resected from the mesenteric vessels using an endoscopic linear stapler with two cartridges 60 mm long or using the ultrasonic dissector.

The resected specimen is then inserted into a large plastic endoscopic bag with a purse string to position it in the lower quadrant of the abdomen for later extraction. After specimen insertion, closing the purse string helps to maintain all contents (potentially malignant cells or gastrointestinal secretions) within the bag.

Three anastomoses need to be created, and a good two-handed technique with fast intracorporeal knot tying is necessary. The proximal jejunal loop is prepared for this task by further mobilizing the Treitz ligament, and several vessels are taken with the hook cautery and metallic clips. The loop is passed and advanced behind the mesenteric vessels through the ligament of Treitz. The pancreas-to-jejunum anastomosis is created first because of its need for precision and delicate sutures, and it is easier to perform with the free jejunal loop. In one instance, we used a stent into the pancreatic anastomosis, a 5-French pediatric feeding tube that exits outside the jejunal loop through the right side of the abdomen. The anastomosis is created in two layers: an outer with interrupted 3-0 silk and an inner with 4-0 absorbable sutures placed with a semicurved needle, taking the duct to the antimesenteric side of the jejunum through the whole wall. Four to six interrupted sutures are positioned starting posteriorly (Fig. 32-10). Initially, we sealed the pancreatic and biliary anastomosis with fibrin glue after suturing, which was delivered by a catheter passed through the abdominal wall, but this is no longer necessary. The hepaticojejunostomy is created in a similar fashion with intracorporeal sutures starting posteriorly. No stent or T-tubes are necessary. Six to 10 sutures are placed. The distance between each of the anastomoses is approximately 10 cm. Excess proximal jejunum and staple lines are excised, and the pylorojejunostomy is created using a 3-0 absorbable, monofilament suture with a curved needle; technically, a running posterior followed by a running anterior suture is done starting superiorly. The gallbladder can be removed after sutures are placed, and the specimen is extracted through the largest trocar, which is the 18 mm in the umbilicus. The specimen is turned longitudinally and extracted.

ble with the sample stapler to the right of the mesenteric vessels. The proximal jejunum retracts in the retroperitoneum and is freed at the ligament of Treitz. After transection, the gastroduodenal artery is exposed as the antrum of the stomach is pushed toward the left upper quadrant. The artery is dissected from the pancreatic neck and more so superiorly near its origin. From the hepatic artery, it is double clipped with titanium clips and divided. In one case, a 30-mm endoscopic linear stapler with vascular staples was used. The

pancreas above the mesenteric vein and the portal vein is transected by scissors, starting on the inferior aspect and moving superiorly (Fig. 32-9). This sections the inferior and superior pancreatic vessel arcades, which are controlled with a combination of metallic clips and cautery. Alternatively, the 10-mm ultrasonic dissector can be used to transect the pancreas almost without blood loss. The pancreatic duct is easily seen because of the magnification. It is left open and can be cannulated with a 5-French pediatric feeding tube.

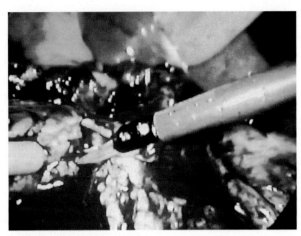

Fig. 32-9. Transection of the pancreatic neck with endoscopic scissors. (From MacFadyen BV, Ponsky JL. Operative laparoscopy and thoracoscopy. *New York: Lippincott-Raven, 1996; with permission.*)

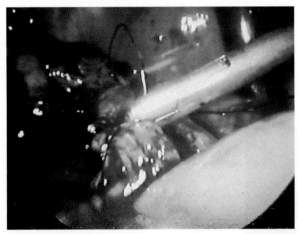

Fig. 32-10. Pancreatic jejunal anastomosis is performed using careful intracorporeal techniques. (From MacFadyen BV, Ponsky JL. Operative laparoscopy and thoracoscopy. *New York: Lippincott-Raven, 1996; with permission.*)

Jackson-Pratt drains are positioned below and above the anastomosis and passed through the trocar sites in the right subcostal and right paramedian areas. A feeding jejunostomy is inserted approximately 30 cm distal to the hepaticojejunostomy on the antimesenteric side of the jejunal loop through the left paramedian trocar site. The nasogastric tube is left in place and its position verified. All fascial wounds are closed with 2-0 absorbable sutures (Fig. 32-11).

Postoperative Care for Proximal Resections

Proximal resection results in major gastrointestinal trauma for the patient, and postoperative morbidity is high (40% to 60%). I routinely use subcutaneous somatostatin analogs (e.g., octreotide, 50 μg every 8 hours) for a minimum of 7 days to decrease the likelihood of pancreatic fistulas. Similarly, the Jackson-Pratt drains are maintained for 7 days or longer if amylase content from the drain fluid is five times greater than normal. The nasogastric tube is also maintained for 6 to 7 days, at which time a Gastrografin swallow can verify the existence of an anastomotic leak at any of the three anastomoses. If no leaks are apparent, the nasogastric tube is removed, and a liquid diet is started. Jejunostomy tube feeding is initiated on day 3 or 4 at half strength and increased progressively. Total parenteral nutrition was administered in the first patient because we did not place a jejunostomy tube.

Antibiotics (i.e., cephalosporin) are administered for 5 to 7 days. Postoperative H_2-blockers are administered intravenously to decrease the likelihood of anastomotic jejunal ulcers. To prevent deep venous thrombosis, preoperative prophylaxis is initiated by using subcutaneous heparin until the patient is fully ambulatory. Intraoperative and postoperative serum glucose levels are checked at least every 6 hours. An insulin drip may be necessary, especially during nutritional support. Pulmonary physiotherapy should be aggressive to decrease the incidence of atelectasis and pneumonia. The pancreatic stent is left in place for 6 weeks, and most patients are able to manage this on an outpatient basis. After open surgery, the average hospital stay is 20 days, and the 30-day mortality rate is 5%.

Complications of Proximal Resection

The complications encountered after proximal resection are essentially the same as those of open pylorus-preserving pancreatoduodenectomy. The most frequent complication is delay in gastric emptying, which occurs in 20% to 35% of cases in different series. Suturing between the pylorus and the jejunum should not be too tight, and the antrum-pylorus area should not be devascularized.

The most fearsome complication is pancreatic leak, which often is caused by a less than tight pancreaticojejunostomy. It is preferable to perform a mucosa-to-mucosa anastomosis rather than a dunking procedure, which invaginates the transected pancreas into a loop of jejunum. Laparoscopic suturing must be meticulous. Alternatively, a drain or stent through the anastomosis could be positioned to direct the pancreatic flow and decrease the pancreatic juice fistula. Stent placement it is more difficult to perform laparoscopically than in an open procedure because the 5-French stent has to be inserted into the jejunum loop into the anastomosis and sutured at the anastomosis for prevention of slippage.

Hemorrhage can be avoided by meticulous hemostasis during the procedure to correct possible coagulopathy. Biliary stenosis is prevented by meticulous suturing between the common hepatic duct and the antimesenteric side of the jejunal loop. Separate sutures of absorbable material should be used.

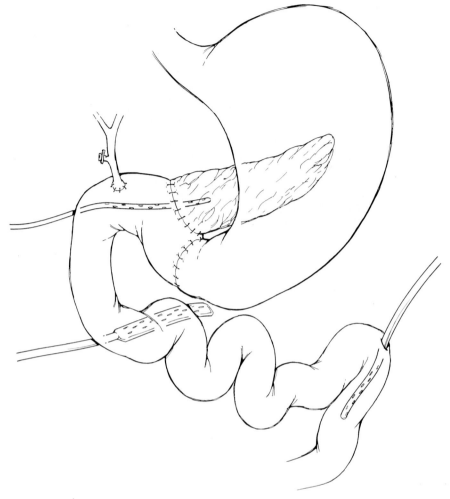

atic malignancies and are classified as serous or mucinous cystadenomas or cystadenocarcinomas, cystic papillary tumors, and mucinous ductal ectasia. They must be differentiated from pseudocysts, because treatment is different, and the prognoses vary. Pancreatic pseudocysts have no epithelial cell–lined wall, and a communication with the pancreatic duct is often seen. Pseudocysts are usually encountered after pancreatitis and tend to regress spontaneously within 6 weeks. Although true cystic tumors require resection, symptomatic pseudocysts only need drainage. The use of diagnostic laparoscopy permits classification of the cystic tumors and the possibility differentiating a pseudocyst from these tumors, excluding distant intraabdominal metastasis, and evaluating local resectability.

Preoperative Considerations

Apart from a thorough history and physical examination, the preoperative workup includes laboratory tests that may include serum levels of CA 19-9, carcinoembryonic antigen, and pancreatic enzymes and biochemical liver profile. A chest radiograph may exclude a pleural effusion associated with pseudocysts or a pancreatic-pleural fistula. Abdominal ultrasonography, CT scan of the upper abdomen, and ERCP should routinely be obtained (Fig. 32-12). If available, endogastric or endoduodenal ultrasonography is helpful for cyst wall evaluation and delineation of infiltration into

Fig. 32-11. Full reconstruction, showing the pylorojejunostomy, pancreaticojejunostomy, and the hepaticojejunostomy with drains and feeding jejunostomy.

Most postoperative complications are related to advanced age, prolonged operating room time, and increased operative blood loss. Intraabdominal sepsis occurs in fewer than 10% of patients and can be managed by antibiotic therapy with or without percutaneous drainage of abscesses. Biliary leaks are often associated with a pancreatic leak and can be managed conservatively.

Pancreatic Cyst Lesions

Pancreatic cyst lesions are diagnosed with increasing frequency because of an aggressive policy of radiologic imaging after pancreatitis or for evaluation of abdominal symptoms. Cystic tumors of the pancreas represent less than 1% of exocrine pancre-

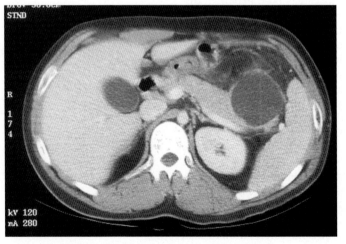

Fig. 32-12. CT image of a pancreatic pseudocyst.

adjacent organs. A preoperative mesenteric angiogram is also obtained if a resection is planned; it can delineate the superior mesenteric artery and vein and exclude vascular involvement by a cystic tumor. Cystic fluid content can be analyzed for the presence of mucin by needle aspiration under ultrasonographic guidance.

When exploration is indicated, the bowel is prepared in case the transverse colon is involved with the cystic mass and needs to be resected. A cephalosporin is given intravenously in the operating room during anesthesia induction to decrease the likelihood of wound infection from gastric organisms during the transgastric cystogastrostomy. Somatostatin (50 μg) is given subcutaneously the day before the operation to decrease pancreatic fluid secretions and decrease the likelihood of postoperative pancreatic fistula formation.

In addition to the staging procedures described previously, a laparoscopic ultrasonographic probe (10-mm, rigid or 7.5-MHz, flexible probe) can be used to locate and determine whether there is a solid component to the cystic mass. Solid tumors of the pancreas can be associated with a cystic component or a pseudocyst. Any indurated area can be biopsied with a percutaneous needle (22 gauge), and the aspirate can be sent for rapid cytologic examination.

Operative Technique for Laparoscopic Distal Pancreatectomy

Depending on the localization of the cystic tumor, resection may be performed. A distal pancreatic resection with splenic preservation is my preferred approach. After the gastrocolic space has been explored, dissection starts on the inferior edge of the pancreatic tail, which is mobilized from the splenic artery and vein. Four 10-mm trocars usually are necessary along the left paramedian and left flank areas. A right-angle forceps is useful for dissection of the transverse pancreatic vessels that must be ligated as they arise from the splenic vessels (Fig. 32-13). For visualization of the pancreatic tail, the splenic flexure of the colon and splenocolic ligament must be mobilized. Dissection in this area must be carried out with extreme care, because hemorrhage from the splenic artery or vein may necessitate large-vessel ligation. This ligation can be done safely in more than 90% of patients, because the spleen is suffi-

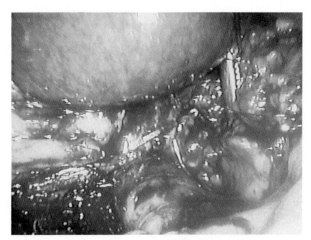

Fig. 32-13. *Dissection of the splenic artery and splenic vein with ligation of the transverse branches. (From MacFadyen BV, Ponsky JL.* Operative laparoscopy and thoracoscopy. *New York: Lippincott-Raven, 1996; with permission.)*

ciently vascularized by short gastric and gastroepiploic vessels. The posterior border of the pancreas is dissected next by dividing the retroperitoneum/pancreatic line; this plane is mostly avascular. The superior border is dissected last, and transverse vessels are often encountered.

The pancreas is transected with a 30-mm (12-mm-diameter) or 60-mm (18-mm-diameter) endoscopic linear stapler (Fig. 32-14). Conversion from an 11-mm trocar to a 12- or 18-mm trocar is necessary. This trocar must be aligned transversely with the pancreatic transection plane. The pan-

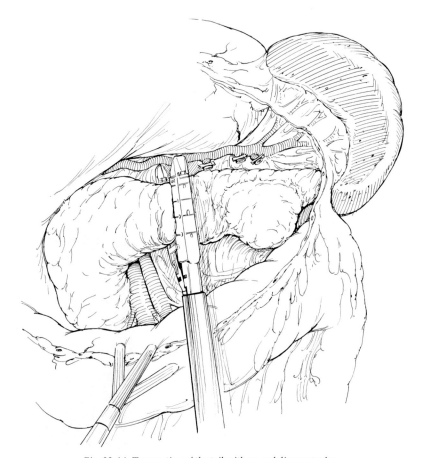

Fig. 32-14. *Transection of the tail with an endolinear stapler.*

creatic duct can be safely ligated, but application of the stapler may cause bleeding from the superior pancreatic vascular arcades, which must be ligated separately. The resected specimen is placed into a 10 × 10-cm bag and extracted by slightly enlarging the trocar incision used for the stapler. After thorough irrigation of the abdominal cavity and control of hemostasis, a Jackson-Pratt drain is left in place near the plane of resection of the pancreas.

Laparoscopic Transgastric Cystogastrostomy

Two techniques have been evaluated in our center. The first one, called laparoscopic cystogastrostomy with endoscopic guidance, is performed after diagnostic laparoscopy. Two additional trocars are placed to expose the pancreas in the retrogastric space. An intraoperative duodenoscopy is performed for endolaparoscopic creation of the cystogastrostomy with a wire that is passed through the posterior wall of the stomach. An endoprosthesis or a drain can be left in place, especially when the posterior wall of the stomach has no visible bulge. Laparoscopic control allows the surgeon to perform the anastomosis under visual guidance with sutures or fibrin glue and to manipulate the pseudocyst as necessary.

The results of this technique, which was tried in five patients, were disappointing: three conversions to open surgery were necessary because of insufficient anastomotic sealing between the posterior wall of the stomach and the anterior part of the pseudocyst, especially superiorly. In two patients, the pseudocysts collapsed after puncture and could no longer be adequately cannulated for the anastomosis. Because of these poor results, a different approach was attempted.

Transgastric Cystogastrostomy

The second technique was a transgastric cystogastrostomy, which was accomplished intraluminally with special radially expanding trocars (Innerdyne, California). This type of trocars has a balloon at the end to keep it in the stomach so an endoluminal laparoscopic procedure can be performed with two or three additional trocars. The trocars are available with a diameter of 5 or 7 mm and therefore do not allow the use of a clip applicator or stapling device. They cause small perforations in the gastric wall, which can be

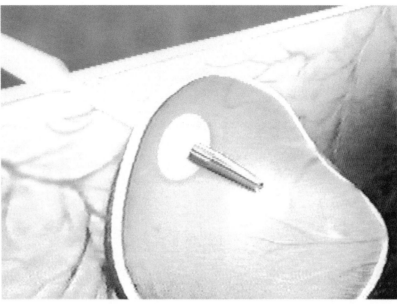

Fig. 32-15. Laparoscopic transgastric cystogastrostomy with endoluminal trocars. (From MacFadyen BV, Ponsky JL. Operative laparoscopy and thoracoscopy. New York: Lippincott-Raven, 1996; with permission.)

closed by a single 2-0 suture (silk or absorbable).

The patient is placed in a supine position, and the pneumoperitoneum is insufflated. Three trocars are introduced in the umbilical region (11 mm), left of the midline (11 mm), and on the left side (5 mm). The first endoluminal trocar is introduced in the epigastric area, above the pseudocyst through the abdominal and anterior gastric wall. After taking out the trocar, the balloon is inflated and pulled against the gastric wall for fixation (Fig. 32-15). Intraoperative gastroscopy allows placement of a nasogastric tube and insufflation of the stomach during the whole procedure. A 5-mm, 0° laparoscope is introduced to visualize the posterior aspect of the stomach. A second endoluminal trocar is placed about 8 cm lateral to the left or to the right for the laparoscopic hook or the irrigation/suction device.

The cyst is identified with the help of a long no. 16 or 18 needle, which is introduced percutaneously through the anterior gastric wall and under laparoscopic endoluminal visual control into the posterior gastric wall, where the cyst is suspected. The aspiration of cystic contents confirms the localization and avoids accidental vascular lesions. A posterior linear gastrostomy is performed with the hook over a length of 4 to 5 cm parallel to the gastric folds (Fig. 32-16). The contents of the cyst are aspirated, and the cystic cavity

is cleaned and explored. A biopsy of the cystic wall is taken to exclude a cystadenomatous tumor.

A nasogastric tube is left in the stomach, the trocar balloons are deflated, and the trocars are removed. The gastric incisions are closed with single intracorporeal 2-0 silk sutures. A no. 7 Jackson-Pratt drain is left next to the anastomosis for 24 to 48 hours.

Postoperative Considerations

After a laparoscopic distal pancreatic resection, oral intake can be started much earlier than after laparoscopic pancreatoduodenectomy, because gastrointestinal reconstruction is unnecessary. The nasogastric tube is removed on the first postoperative day, and liquids are given; intake is progressed gradually to a normal diet. The patients are mobilized progressively beginning on the first postoperative day. Somatostatin (50 μg) is given subcutaneously every 8 hours. The drain may be removed if drainage fluid does not contain amylase or is less than 30 mL per day.

After a laparoscopic cystogastrostomy, a liquid diet is given from the second postoperative day on, and the anastomosis is checked with a gastrografin swallow. If no leaks are apparent, the nasogastric tube is removed, and intake is progressed to a normal diet. We continue the somatostatin

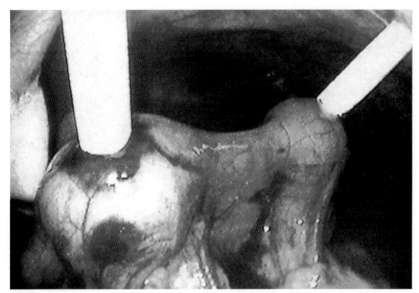

Fig. 32-16. *The linear posterior gastrostomy is made with cautery. (From MacFadyen BV, Ponsky JL.* Operative laparoscopy and thoracoscopy. *New York: Lippincott-Raven, 1996; with permission.)*

until discharge from the hospital on the third or fourth postoperative day.

Our experience with laparoscopic pancreatic surgery remains limited. We have performed four laparoscopic distal pancreatectomies and attempted the procedure in two other patients. Of those, three were performed for an islet cell tumor and one for a low-grade serous cystadenocarcinoma. The elderly man with the cystadenocarcinoma also had a left adrenalectomy for a nonfunctional adenoma and laparoscopic cholecystectomy for symptomatic gallstones during the same procedure. The operating time was 5 hours, and his hospital stay was only 7 days. The immediate postoperative course was uneventful, but he later developed a localized abscess near the pancreatic transection plane that required a percutaneous drainage on the 30th postoperative day.

For symptomatic pseudocyst, the transgastric cystogastrostomy technique was performed in six patients, and cystoduodenostomy was performed in another patient. There were no deaths and no complications. The mean size of the cysts was 16 cm (range, 6 to 20 cm); the contents were clear in 75% and necrotic in 25%. One procedure had to be converted to laparotomy because of an inability to reach the stomach caused by severe multiple small bowel adhesions. The mean operative time was 80 minutes (range, 65 to 110 minutes). Postoperative hospital stay was 4 days

(range, 3 to 10 days). On follow-up, abdominal CT scans showed complete cyst regression in 83% of patients after 3 months.

Complications after Pancreatic Resection

The complications that may occur after pancreatic resection are the same as those after open surgery. The most severe complication after pancreatic resection is a pancreatic fistula, which can often be managed by percutaneous, radiologically guided puncture and drainage but causes significantly delays in postoperative recovery. Hemorrhage can result from insufficient control of the pancreatic vessels or an injury to the spleen and may require repeat laparoscopy or a laparotomy. Complications after pseudocyst drainage include leakage of the cystogastrostomy and occlusion of the anastomotic lumen impairing emptying and regression of the cyst. If the opening is too small, infection of the cystic cavity may occur, and it can be treated with percutaneous drainage or open surgical cystogastrostomy or cystoenterostomy.

Comments on Cystic Lesions

A cystadenoma can be encountered in all parts of the pancreas, but a cystadenocarcinoma is usually located in the head of the

pancreas. Localization and CT scans cannot exclude malignancy. ERCP can show a connection of the cystic lesion with the pancreatic duct. Analysis of the cyst contents helps to differentiate pseudocysts from benign or malignant cystic tumors. Because the 5-year survival rates after resection of cystic tumors of the pancreas are 60% to 90%, the laparoscopic approach may be considered for selected patients.

The technique of endoluminal laparoscopic cystogastrostomy seems promising. The first cystogastrostomy was described by Jedlicks in 1921 and by Junes in 1932. This method was popular until 2 decades ago, when the potential risk of hemorrhage was mentioned. Studies comparing cystoduodenostomy, cystoenterostomy, and cystogastrostomy revealed similar results in the hands of experienced surgeons. The surgical principles that have been applied in open surgery for treatment of pseudocysts remain unchanged. Of the pseudocysts 6 cm or larger after 6 weeks of observation, only 15% regress spontaneously, and surgery usually is indicated. For patients with portal hypertension, this procedure is contraindicated, because collateral vessels may be injured and cause severe hemorrhage. The failure rate of open surgery is less than 10%.

The endoscopic technique alone may not be sufficient to drain the pseudocyst, and severe infections have been reported because of inadequate openings. Endoscopy has a 90% success rate, with a 15% associated severe morbidity and 4% mortality rate. The endoscopic technique may not exclude the neoplastic nature of certain cystic lesions. The laparoscopic technique may help to control bleeding from the walls during the cystogastrostomy by using hook cautery or endoluminal suturing with a two-handed technique. This technique can also bring the two walls together if they come apart during the procedure.

Infected Necrotizing Pancreatitis

When infected necrotic pancreatitis has been identified, a surgical intervention for drainage and debridement is required. The infected space may extend from the peripancreatic space to the retrogastric lesser sac area, retrocolic right and left and retromesenteric (small bowel), and perinephric right and left space. The necrotizing process occasionally extends along the psoas muscles and exits in the muscle layers of the abdominal wall or inguinal areas. The abdominal CT scan should be available for the surgeon to review while laparoscopic debridement or drainage is performed.

Operative Technique for Laparoscopic Pancreatic Necrosectomy

According to the type and location of infected necrotizing pancreatitis seen on the CT scan, three operative approaches have been designed: retrogastric-retrocolic debridement, retroperitoneal debridement, and laparoscopic transgastric pancreatic necrosectomy.

Retrogastric-Retrocolic Debridement

The retrogastric-retrocolic debridement approach is indicated for early infected fluid or severe sterile pancreatic necrosis. Because the intraperitoneal route will be used laparoscopic cholecystectomy can be performed with or without a CBD exploration if the origin of the pancreatitis is biliary. With the patient under general anesthesia, a nasogastric tube is positioned, and a Foley catheter is inserted to decompress the bladder. The whole abdominal wall is prepared. The first trocar is inserted in the umbilicus, and a pneumoperitoneum of 15 mm Hg is established. A 30°-angled laparoscope is necessary to reach all the difficult angles and to look into the lesser sac. Depending on whether the necrotic process extends along the psoas, a retrocolic approach may be used after the retrogastric approach. Two more trocars are inserted opposite to where the maximum amount of the debridement is to be performed. For a right paracolic gutter opening, a lower paramedian right trocar and an upper epigastric 10-mm trocar are inserted. The cecum is identified, and an atraumatic bowel clamp retracts the cecum medially and toward the left under some traction. A retroperitoneal opening is made with the laparoscopic curved scissors, and bulging sometimes is apparent in this area. By mobilizing the right colon and cutting its lateral peritoneal attachment, the retroperitoneal space over the right kidney and psoas is entered. The surgeon must prevent injury the right ureter. No bands are divided unless strictly identified, and the dissection is kept close to the serosa of the colon until its mesentery has been encountered. If pus and infected brown fluid are encountered, the irrigation/suction probe is used to aspirate and break the loose attachment of the pancreatic and peripancreatic debris. The right hepatic flexure often is mobilized enough to reach the second and third portion of the duodenum and the head of the pancreas. A Kocher maneuver with Babcock forceps on the duodenum from the epigastric port is performed (Fig. 32-17).

Debridement is adequately performed using a large 10-mm spoon forceps. Some of the material may be inserted into a sterile plastic bag for later retrieval (Fig. 32-18). Large sump drains are inserted from the lower right abdominal quadrant or through one of the trocar sites with an enlarged skin incision to permit easy insertion. The tip is positioned toward the upper primary focus of infection. A second or third drain may be inserted for continuous lavage of the peritoneal cavity. The left side is also drained, and the patient's position is an important factor in the success of this procedure. The table has to be tilted strongly toward the right side so that the left side is up. This helps to mobilize the sigmoid to allow entry into the left retroperitoneal space around the splenic flexure and changes the position to a reverse Trendelenburg position.

The rest of the maneuvers follow the same principles as those for a right paracolic gutter exposure, which leads to the body and tail inferior portion of the pancreas. Particular attention should be applied when dissecting the splenic flexure of the colon not to injure the inferior pole of the spleen. The lesser sac may be entered through the gastrocolic window. This retrogastric approach is performed superiorly or inferiorly (or both) to the stomach. If most of the area to be debrided is located behind the stomach in the body and tail of the pancreas, this is a good approach. At

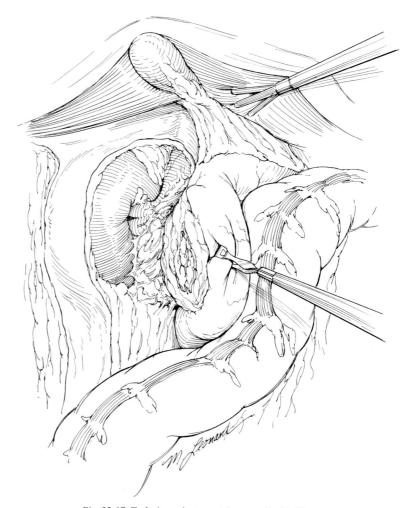

Fig. 32-17. Technique of retrogastric retrocolic debridement.

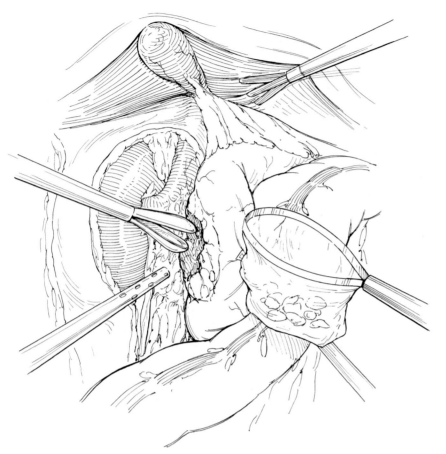

Fig. 32-18. A large cup forceps and specimen bag are needed to debride the retroperitoneum.

Retroperitoneal Debridement

Retroperitoneal debridement is advised for early pancreatic necrosis without fibrotic tissue, scarring, or thick inflammatory response, making it easy to dissect the retroperitoneal space. Edema is maximal. The patient is positioned in the lateral decubitus position, and the retroperitoneal space is entered on the left or the right, depending on where the maximum amount of disease is located. A small incision is made in the flank between the ribs and iliac crest. A finger is inserted so at least three layers of muscles are spread (i.e., external oblique, internal oblique, and transverses abdominis). The 11-mm trocar is inserted, and a 0-0 string of silk or nylon is positioned around the skin to seal the trocar. CO_2 is insufflated with a positive pressure of more than 15 mm Hg (up to 20 mm Hg if necessary). The 0° scope is used initially to push the retroperitoneal fibers and to create and delineate the work space. The right and left sides of the kidney can be used as an anatomic landmark to progress toward the head or tail of the pancreas, proceeding downward toward the psoas to drain this area. The same procedure is performed as described for debridement and drainage from the retrocolic retrogastric approach.

least three trocars are located in both the right and left paramedian areas at the level of the umbilicus. With a two-handed technique, the gastrocolic omentum is dissected. Small vessels are clipped or cauterized with monopolar dissection forceps, eventually lifting the greater curvature of the stomach. The ultrasonic dissector can be used for bloodless dissection. The irrigation/suction probe enters behind the stomach and over the body of the pancreas. The liquefied debris is aspirated, and debridement is performed after a large window has been made. Afterward, a large-bore sump drain is inserted through the window over the body and tail of the pancreas and positioned at the inferior aspect of the pancreatic tail.

The same procedure can be performed through the lesser sac over the lesser curvature of the stomach, exposing the left caudate lobe. After caudad retraction of the stomach, debridement of the superior aspect of the pancreas can be performed (Fig. 32-19).

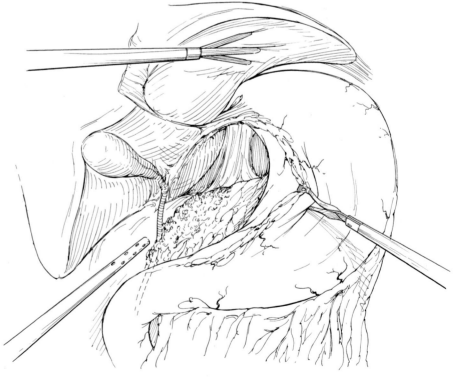

Fig. 32-19. Access to the head of the pancreas through the lesser gastric curvature.

Laparoscopic Transgastric Pancreatic Necrosectomy

The indications for laparoscopic transgastric pancreatic necrosectomy include late onset of infected pancreatic necrosis, pancreatic abscess, or infected pseudocysts (Table 32-1). Through the posterior wall of the stomach, debridement is performed with drainage into the stomach. Disease is located in the body and occasionally in the tail. If the disease is in the pancreatic head, a transduodenal approach may be applicable, but it is much more difficult to perform through the small space provided by the duodenum. Technical details were described earlier in the cystic lesions section. Debridement is performed with a 5-mm biopsy forceps, and the necrotic tissue can be left inside the stomach. A few pieces are retrieved for culturing and pathologic examination. No drains are left in the gastrostomy, but a Jackson-Pratt drain is left over the anterior gastrostomy toward the lesser sac and lesser curvature of the stomach. The endoluminal trocars are then removed by deflating the distal balloons, and with a two-handed technique, the anterior gastric wall puncture sites are closed with intracorporeal suturing technique with 2-0 silk. Planned repeat laparoscopic drainage can be performed, but the clinical

Table 32-1. Indications for Laparoscopic Pancreatic Surgery

Proximal resection
  Ampullary adenoma/adenocarcinoma
  Bile duct carcinoma
  Pancreatic adenocarcinoma
  Duodenal adenocarcinoma
  Chronic pancreatitis
  Cystic neoplasm of pancreas
  Islet cell tumor
Distal resection
  Islet cell tumors
  Cystic neoplasms
  Chronic pancreatitis
Necrosectomy
  Infected necrotizing pancreatitis
Enucleation
  Benign islet cell tumors
Cystogastrostomy
  Mature pseudocyst 6 cm, 6 weeks duration
Laparoscopic palliative procedures
  Unresectable periampullary neoplasm*
  Metastatic periampullary neoplasm*

* With more than 3 months of expected survival

status of the patient and serial CT scans can help decide when, where, and whether the procedure is needed.

Postoperative Considerations

The sites of necrotizing pancreatitis were encountered in the pancreatic head in 29% of patients, in the body and tail in 54%, and in the extending retroperitoneal spaces along the psoas and retrocolic gutters in 27%. The most frequent technique used was the retrogastric and retrocolic approach (50% of patients), followed by the transgastric approach (37%), and complete retroperitoneoscopic approach (13%). From January 1993 through September 1994, eight patients with proven infected pancreatic necrosis were operated on. The five men and three women treated had a mean age of 54 years (range, 41 to 69 years). Most patients were sick enough to be in the intensive care unit, six of them for more than 7 days, with an average hospital stay of 51 days (range, 7 to 124 days). All patients had some form of complicated preoperative and postoperative course, with five of them having respiratory failure, five with gram-negative septicemia, and two with recurrent retroperitoneal sepsis that needed reintervention. During this period, there were no fatalities. The septic process was localized in the body and tail of the pancreas in one patient, and in the second patient, it was localized in the head of the bilateral psoas extension.

It is concluded from this small but interesting experience that laparoscopic pancreatic necrosectomy with drainage is feasible and safe. The success rate after the first drainage is about 75%, although these results are preliminary. Laparoscopic reintervention was performed in one patient and was found to be extremely difficult. Laparoscopic retroperitoneoscopic and transgastric drainage has the advantage of not infecting the peritoneal cavity. This technique may be less invasive and may result in less stress in these already severely septic patients.

Because patients consumed enormous amounts of hospital resources (10 times more than other intensive care unit admissions), any decrease in their hospital stay has a significant impact on cost. By using the laparoscopic approach in treating necrotizing pancreatitis, the same goals

can be achieved as in open surgery and may be of greater benefit.

Comments on Laparoscopic Palliative Procedures for Pancreatic Cancer

Laparoscopic cholecystojejunostomy and hepaticojejunostomy have been performed with great success to palliate jaundice. Laparoscopic gastrojejunostomy can be performed alone or with biliary bypass. The laparoscopic gastric bypass sometimes is added after an endoscopic biliary prosthesis is inserted. My experience has been mostly with the use of the laparoscopic hepaticogastrostomy. Since January 1992, 19 patients (14 women, 5 men) with a mean age of 65 (range, 43 to 91 years) underwent laparoscopic hepaticogastrostomy. After transhepatic catheterization of a segment II or III bile duct, the left lobe of the liver and the lesser curvature of the stomach were perforated under fluoroscopic and laparoscopic guidance using three trocars. Anastomosis between the biliary tree and the stomach was maintained with a gastrostomy tube placed across the tract (Fig. 32-20). After 2 weeks, the tube was removed, and patency of the tract was preserved with a metallic stent.

Two-thirds of the patients had a hilar level of obstruction, and 65% of patients had unresectable cholangiocarcinoma or pancreatic adenocarcinoma determined during laparoscopic staging. One-fourth of patients palliated also had biliary obstruction from metastatic colon adenocarcinoma or gastric adenocarcinoma. The total bilirubin concentration fell from 271 to 32 (p 0.001) in less than 4 weeks. The mean hospital stay was 17 days. After a follow-up period of 47 months, the mean survival time was 7 months, with 35% of patients surviving more than 12 months. Two patients died of septicemia and pneumonia in the hospital. Early complications were cholangitis (3 patients), subcapsular hematoma (2), and gastric outlet obstruction (1). No reintervention or endoscopic procedures had to be performed. The recurrence of jaundice due to liver failure was only seen in two patients. A high level of malignant biliary obstruction can be palliated effectively with the laparoscopic method with a relatively low morbidity and mortality rate in this selected group of patients.

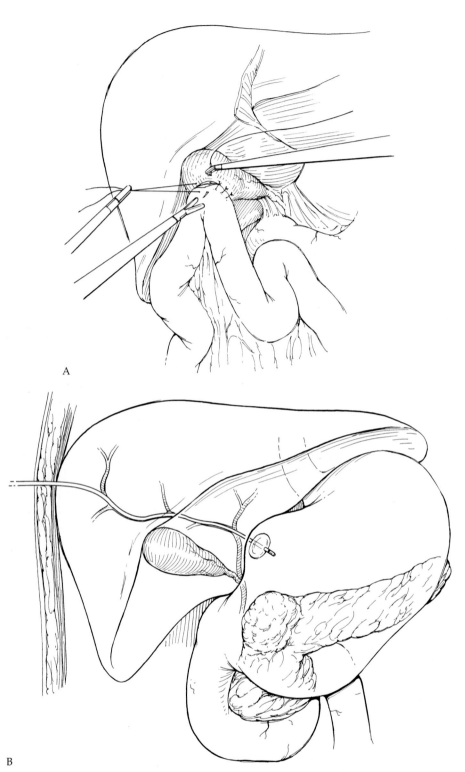

A

B

Fig. 32-20. **A:** *Laparoscopic cholecystojejunostomy.* **B:** *Hepaticojejunostomy.*

There has been resurgence of interest in splanchnicectomy (by a thoracoscopic approach) and in laparoscopic celiac ganglionectomy for chronic pancreatitis or intractable pain from pancreatic cancer. However, the results are not superior to those with an open approach with longer follow-up.

Suggested Reading

Gagner M. La pancreatectomie distale par laparoscopie pour insulinomes. Reunion des endocrinologues de l'Universite de Montreal; Hopital Sacre-Coeur, Montreal, April 5, 1993.

Gagner M. Laparoscopic transgastric cystogastrostomy for pancreatic pseudocyst. *Surg Endosc* 1994;8:239.

Gagner M, Pomp A. Laparoscopic pylorus-preserving pancreatoduodenectomy. *Surg Endosc* 1994;8:408.

Gagner M. Laparoscopic duodenopancreatectomy. In: Steichen F, Welter R, eds. *Minimally invasive surgery and technology.* St. Louis: Quality Medical Publishing, 1994:192–199.

Gagner M. Laparoscopic necrosectomy for infected necrotizing pancreatitis. In: Cuschieri A, ed. *Seminars in surgical laparoscopy,* 1995.

Litwin D, Rossi L. Laparoscopic management of pancreatic disease. In: Arregui M, ed. *Principles of laparoscopic surgery: basic and advanced techniques.* New York: Springer-Verlag, 1995: 325–331.

Shimi S, Banting S, Cuschieri A. Laparoscopy in the management of pancreatic cancer: endoscopic cholecystojejunostomy for advanced disease. *Br J Surg* 1992;79:317.

Soulez G, Gagner M, Therasse E, et al. Malignant biliary obstruction: preliminary results of palliative treatment with hepaticogastrostomy under fluoroscopic, endoscopic and laparoscopic guidance. *Radiology* 1994;192:241.

Warshaw AL, Fernandez del Castillo C. Laparoscopy in preoperative diagnosis and staging for gastrointestinal cancers. In: Zucker K, ed. *Surgical laparoscopy.* St. Louis: Quality Medical Publishing, 1991:101–104.

Way L, Leghada P, Mori T. Laparoscopic pancreatic cystogastrostomy: the first operation in the new field of intraluminal laparoscopic surgery. *Surg Endosc* 1994;8:235.

Worsey J, Ferson PF, Keenan RJ, et al. Thoraco-scopic pancreatic denervation for pain control in irresectable pancreatic cancer. *Br J Surg* 1993; 80:1051.

EDITOR'S COMMENT

This chapter on laparoscopic pancreatic surgery describes some of the most ad-vanced applications of laparoscopy cur-rently in use. The author and his colleagues have taken an aggressive leadership role in exploring the appropriate use of laparo-scopy in some of the most difficult clinical situations faced by the surgeon. Very few laparoscopic surgeons have experience with the techniques described by the au-thor and furthermore, a relatively small number of laparoscopists possess the expe-rience and skill necessary to perform lap-aroscopic pancreatic surgery.

The author provides an excellent descrip-tion of the approaches used by his team and honestly reports their experience. The lasting role of laparoscopy in the manage-ment of pancreatic disease is yet to be de-fined.

W.S.E.

33

Laparoscopic Splenectomy

Eric C. Poulin

Laparoscopic splenectomy presents the special challenges of removing a fragile and richly vascularized organ situated close to the stomach, colon, pancreas, and kidney and having to plan an extraction strategy that ensures proper histologic confirmation of the pathology while maintaining the objectives of minimal-access surgery.

Anatomic Considerations

A thorough appreciation of splenic anatomy is essential to the smooth performance of laparoscopic splenectomy, with particular focus on optimal hemostatic control and preservation of the integrity of the spleen and pancreas during the procedure (Table 33-1). Whereas most anatomy texts imply that the splenic artery is constant in its course and branches, the classic essay of Michels (1942) demonstrated that each spleen has its own peculiar pattern of terminal artery branches. Michels divided splenic artery topography into two types: distributed and magistral. He reported that the distributed type is found in 70% of dissections. By definition, the splenic trunk is short, and many long branches (6 to 12) enter over three-fourths of the medial surface of the spleen. The branches originate 3 to 13 cm from the hilum (Fig. 33-1). The magistral type, present in the remaining 30% of specimens, is characterized by the presence of a long main splenic artery that divides into short terminal branches near the hilum. In this type, the splenic branches enter over only one-fourth to a third of the medial surface of the spleen. These branches are few (three

to four) and large, originate on average 3.5 cm from the spleen, and reach the center of the organ as a compact bundle (Fig. 33-2).

The splenic branches exhibit so many variations in number, length, size, and origin that no two spleens have the same anatomy. Outside the spleen, the arteries also exhibit frequent transverse anastomoses with each other that, according to Testut (1923), arise at a 90-degree angle between the involved arteries, as with most collaterals (see Fig. 33-1). This means that the application of hemostatic clips or the embolization of coils occluding a branch of the splenic artery before such an anastomosis may fail to devascularize the corresponding splenic segment. Before it divides, the splenic trunk usually gives off a few slender branches to the tail of the pancreas. The most important of these, called the great pancreatic artery, is familiar to vascular radiologists. It is an important landmark in selective angiography of the splenic artery. Severe pancreatitis has been reported following its occlusion during embolization procedures. The number of arteries entering the spleen is not determined by its size, but the presence of notches and tubercles usually correlates well with a greater number of entering arteries.

The splenic artery in the hilum can include up to seven branches at various division levels and in various anatomic arrangements; they are the superior terminal artery, the inferior terminal artery, the medial terminal artery, the superior polar artery, the inferior polar artery, the left gastroepiploic artery, and the short gastric arteries (Fig. 33-3). Veins are usually be-

hind arteries, except at the ultimate division level, where they may be anterior or posterior. According to Lipshutz (1917), 72% of spleens have three terminal branches (superior polar and superior and inferior terminal) and 28% have two, the other remaining branches being collaterals. When the superior terminal is excessively large, the inferior terminal is rudimentary, and more blood supply often comes from the left gastroepiploic and polar vessels. Up to six short gastric arteries may arise from the fundus of the stomach,

Table 33-1. Surgical Features of Splenic Anatomy

No two spleens have the same anatomy

Two types of splenic blood supply exist: magistral and distributed

Transverse anastomosis exists between the splenic artery branches

The gastrosplenic ligament contains short gastric and gastroepiploic vessels

The lienorenal ligament contains the hilar vessels and the tail of the pancreas

Other suspensory ligaments are avascular, except in portal hypertension and myeloid metaplasia

The tail of the pancreas lies within 1 cm of the inner surface of the spleen in 73% of patients

The tail of the pancreas is in direct contact with the spleen in 30% of patients

The size of the spleen does not determine the number of entering arteries

The presence of notches and tubercles correlates with a greater number of entering arteries

If splenic artery embolization is used, it should be done distal to the great pancreatic artery

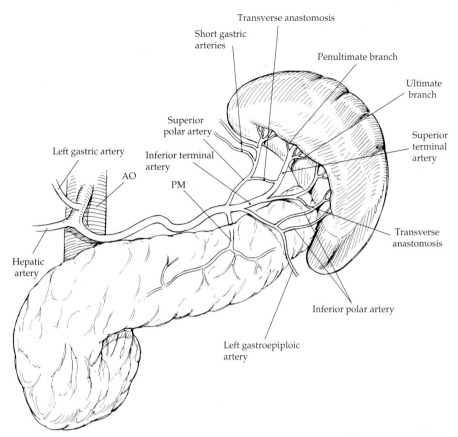

Fig. 33-1. *Distributed type of vascularization. (From Poulin and Thibault, 1993, with permission.)*

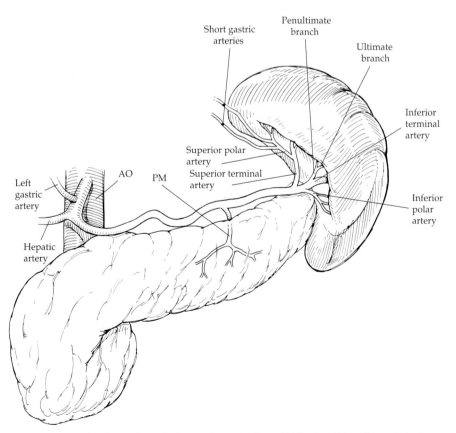

Fig. 33-2. *Magistral type of vascularization. (From Poulin and Thibault, 1993, with permission.)*

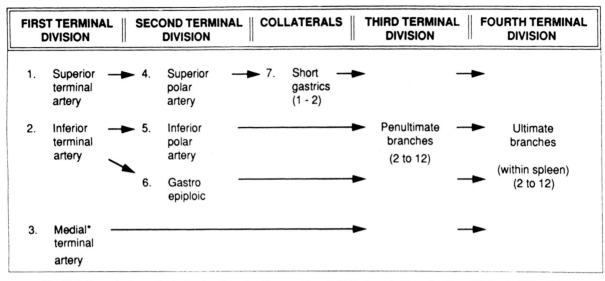

FIRST TERMINAL DIVISION	SECOND TERMINAL DIVISION	COLLATERALS	THIRD TERMINAL DIVISION	FOURTH TERMINAL DIVISION
1. Superior terminal artery →	4. Superior polar artery →	7. Short gastrics (1 - 2) →	→	
2. Inferior terminal artery →	5. Inferior polar artery	—————————→	Penultimate branches (2 to 12) →	Ultimate branches
↘	6. Gastro epiploic	—————————→	→	(within spleen) (2 to 12)
3. Medial* terminal artery	—————————————————————→		→	

Fig. 33-3. General scheme of splenic artery branches (*, present in only 20% of cases). (From Poulin and Thibault, 1993, with permission.)

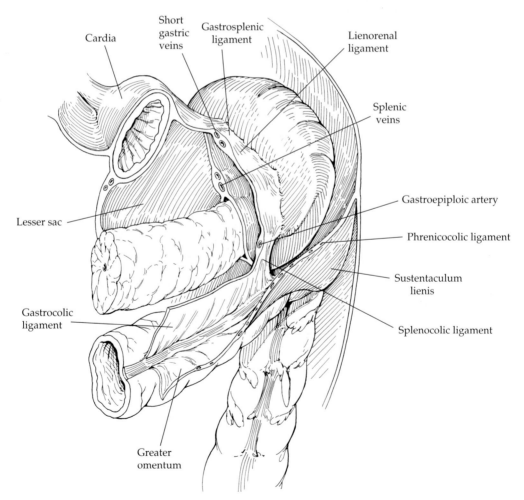

Fig. 33-4. Suspensory ligaments of the spleen. (From Poulin and Thibault, 1993, with permission.)

but usually only those (one to three) opening into the superior polar artery of the spleen need to be ligated during laparoscopic splenectomy (see Figs. 33-1 and 33-2)

Duplications of the peritoneum form the many suspensory ligaments of the spleen. On the medial side posteriorly, the lienorenal ligament contains the tail of the pancreas and the splenic vessels. Anteriorly, the gastrosplenic ligament contains the short gastric and the gastroepiploic arteries. The remaining ligaments are usually avascular, except in patients with portal hypertension or myeloid metaplasia. The longest is the phrenocolic ligament, which courses laterally from the diaphragm to the splenic flexure of the colon; its top end is called the phrenosplenic ligament. The attachment of the lower pole on the internal side is called the splenocolic ligament. Between the phrenocolic and the splenocolic ligaments, a horizontal shelf of areolar tissue is formed on which the inferior pole of the spleen rests. It is often molded into a sac that opens cranialward called the sustentaculum lienis, acting as a brassiere to the lower pole of the spleen (Fig. 33-4).

Ssoson-Jaroschewitsch (1937) found the tail of the pancreas to be in direct contact with the spleen in 30% of cadavers. Baronofsky and colleagues (1951) confirmed this finding and added that the distance was less than 1 cm in 73% of their patients.

Preoperative Patient Management

Before laparoscopic splenectomy is performed, patients undergo the same hematologic preparation as for open surgery, that is, administration of steroids, globulins, fresh frozen plasma, cryoprecipitate, or platelets when required by their hematologic disorder. Polyvalent pneumococcal vaccine is administered 2 weeks before surgery. An ultrasound examination is obtained to assess spleen size (maximum pole length), measured as the joining line between the two organ poles and divided into three categories: (a) normal spleen (less than 11 cm long), (b) moderate splenomegaly (11 to 20 cm), or (c) severe splenomegaly (greater than 20 cm). The radiologist is also asked to try to identify accessory spleens. The choice between the anterior or lateral surgical approach is of-

ten decided from determination of spleen size.

Preoperative splenic artery embolization is used as an adjuvant in some patients to reduce blood loss and makes laparoscopic splenectomy easier to perform. It involves launching 3- to 5-mm microcoils or absorbable gelatin sponge fragments in each hilar branch of the splenic artery through a 3- or 5-French cobra catheter and a coil plunger. The catheter is then pulled back 2 to 4 cm, and one or two 5- to 8-mm microcoils are launched in the main trunk of the splenic artery distal to the great pancreatic artery to avoid pancreatitis or pancreatic necrosis (double-embolization technique) (Fig. 33-5). The surgical plane of dissection is therefore situated between the proximal and distal embolization sites. The procedure is ended when it is estimated radiologically that 80% or more of the splenic tissue has been successfully embolized. Preoperative splenic artery embolization is normally not used for patients with a normal-sized spleen, but it is a useful adjunct to laparoscopic splenectomy to reduce blood loss and the conversion rate early in a surgeon's experience. Preoperative splenic embolization is also useful in the removal of larger spleens and virtually indispensable for performing partial laparoscopic splenectomy. Preoperative splenic artery embolization should be part of the armamentarium of surgeons who wish to widen the indications of laparo-

scopic splenectomy beyond the removal of normal-sized spleens.

Operative Technique

There are two principal surgical approaches to laparoscopic splenectomy: the anterior and the lateral approaches.

Anterior Approach

For the anterior approach, the patient is administered general anesthesia and placed in a modified lithotomy position to allow the surgeon to operate between the legs and the assistants to be on each side. Surgery is performed through five trocars in the upper abdomen in a steep Fowler position with left-side elevation. A 12-mm trocar is introduced through an umbilical incision, and a 10-mm laparoscope (0 or 30 degree) is connected to a video system. Two 12-mm trocars are placed in each upper quadrant, and two 5-mm trocars are inserted close to the rib margin on the left and right sides of the abdomen. Careful selection of all trocar sites is made to optimize working angles. As needed, the 12-mm ports are used to allow introduction of clip appliers, staplers, or laparoscope from a variety of angles (Fig. 33-6). Trocars can also be placed in a half circle facing the left upper quadrant. The left hepatic lobe is retracted with a grasper or retractor through the right lateral 5-mm trocar site.

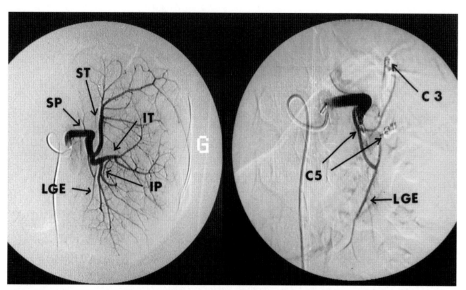

Fig. 33-5. **Left:** *An 18-cm spleen with distributed type of blood supply. Spherocytosis (SP, superior polar artery; ST, superior terminal artery; IT, inferior terminal artery; IP, inferior polar artery; LGE, left gastroepiploic artery).* **Right:** *After embolization with microspheres (not visible). The LGE is now clearly visible. (C3, 3-mm coils; C5, 5-mm coils.) (From Poulin et al., 1993, with permission.)*

While retracting the liver, the tip of the instrument should lie against the diaphragm to avoid lacerations and nuisance bleeding. The stomach is retracted medially through the left 5-mm trocar to expose the spleen after the omentum has been displaced inferiorly. Then, a fairly standard sequence is followed. First, a search is made for accessory spleens. When found, they are removed immediately, for they can be much harder to locate once the spleen is removed. The phrenocolic, splenocolic, and sustentaculum lienis are then incised near the lower pole using electrocautery and hook probe or scissors through the left 12-mm port. Some vascular adhesions, which are frequently found on the medial side of the spleen, are cauterized. The gastrocolic ligament is carefully dissected close to the spleen, and the left gastroepiploic vessels are ligated one by one with metallic clips or simply cauterized if they are small. The lower pole of the spleen is gently lifted with one grasper through a 5-mm port to expose the splenic hilum and the tail of the pancreas within the lienorenal ligament. This maneuver must be done with great care and requires constant concentration by the assistants to avoid lacerations of the spleen and troublesome bleeding. The tip of the instrument used for lifting the lower pole should therefore rest against the left lateral abdominal wall. Lifting the lower pole facilitates the individual dissection and clipping of all branches of the splenic artery and vein as close as possible to the spleen. Staying close to the spleen will decrease the likelihood of causing trauma to the tail of the pancreas.

In the anterior approach, the gastrosplenic and the lienorenal ligament and the vessels that they contain lie on top one another. Their separation is not always easily performed and requires experience with the anatomy. The operation can also differ with the type of vascular anatomy. Surgery on a spleen with a distributed type of blood supply will usually mean dissection of more blood vessels spread over a wider area of the splenic hilum, which makes individual dissection of the vessels easier. Operation on a spleen with a magistral-type blood supply will usually mean fewer vessels. The hilum will be more compact and narrow, and the dissection of each vessel will be more difficult. With the anterior approach, it is difficult to safely create a window above the tail of the pancreas to permit the application of a sta-

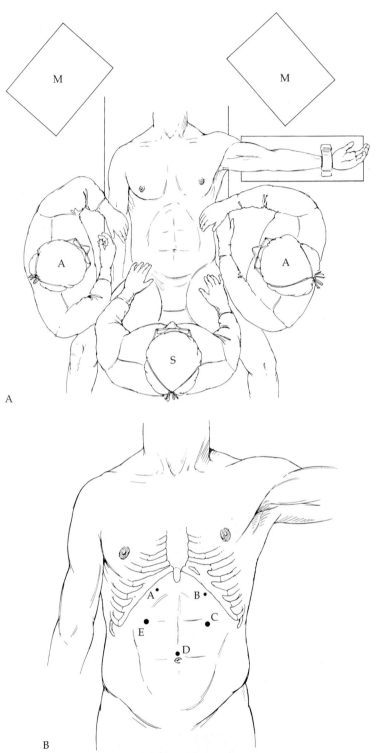

Fig. 33-6. Anterior approach. **A:** *Position of the operating team. (S, surgeon; A, assistant; M, monitor.)* **B:** *Positioning of the trocars. (A, 5-mm trocar; B, 5-mm trocar; C, 12-mm trocar; D, camera; E, 10- or 12-mm trocar.) (From Thibault C, Mamazza J, Letourneau R, Poulin E. Laparoscopic splenectomy: operative technique and preliminary report.* Surg Laparosc Endosc *1992;2:248–253; with permission.)*

pling device and to control all hilar vessels, a maneuver more easily performed using the lateral approach. Applying a stapling device across the hilum in the anterior approach is dangerous without ascertaining that the tip is free of tissue or that the tail of the pancreas has been identified and dissected away; serious hemorrhage or pancreatic trauma can result. After control of the hilar vessels, the short gastric vessels are then identified and ligated with clips or, occasionally, with a stapler. No sutures are used.

When preoperative splenic artery embolization is used, the dissection plane is situated between the sites of distal embolization of splenic artery branches and the site of proximal embolization of the splenic artery itself. Because of the segmental and terminal distribution of splenic arteries, the devascularized portions of the spleen are easily identified by a characteristic grayish color; vascularized segments retain a pinkish hue. When the organ is completely isolated, it is left in its natural cavity and hemostasis is verified.

A medium or large heavy-duty plastic home freezer bag that has been sterilized is folded and introduced into the abdominal cavity through one of the 12-mm trocars. The bag is unfolded, and the spleen is slipped inside to avoid splenosis from the manipulations necessary for extraction. Grasping forceps are used to hold the two rigid edges of the bag and effect partial closure. One should note that it is difficult to insert the spleen into the plastic bag before unfolding and opening the bag completely. Bagging the resected spleen requires patience and imagination and at first can be a frustrating experience (Fig. 33-7). The umbilical trocar is then removed, and the umbilical incision extended to 2 cm. The 10-mm jaw forceps holding the edges at the lower end of the bag inside the abdomen is pushed through the umbilical incision, and the tip of the bag is grasped and brought out of the wound. Gentle traction on the bag from outside the abdomen brings the spleen close to the peritoneal surface of the umbilical incision. It is important during this maneuver to pull out only the ridged edges of the plastic bag while keeping a finger inside. Otherwise, it is easy for the spleen to flip out of the bag, and the maneuver has to be repeated. The use of sterilized home freezer bags is the most cost-effective means of bagging and extracting the spleen. The thick freezer bags should

not be confused with other plastic bags that are thinner and prone to tearing during fragmentation and other manipulations, making them improper for extraction purposes.

A biopsy of a size suitable for pathologic identification is obtained by incising the splenic tip. Subsequently, the spleen is

fragmented with finger fracture, and the resulting blood is suctioned. The remaining stromal tissue of the spleen is then extracted through the small incision, the bag is removed, hemostasis is verified, and all trocars are removed. No drains are used. The incisions are closed with subcuticular absorbable sutures and paper strips.

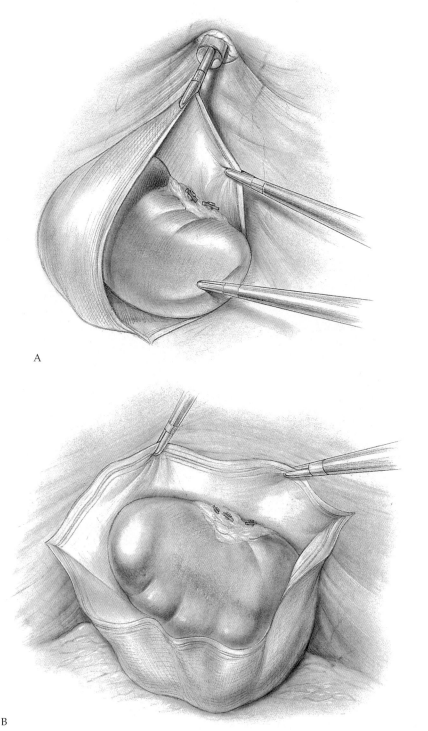

A

B

Fig. 33-7. **A–D:** *Spleen is placed in a sterile plastic freezer bag prior to extraction.* (continued)

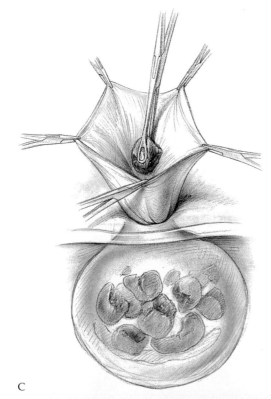

C

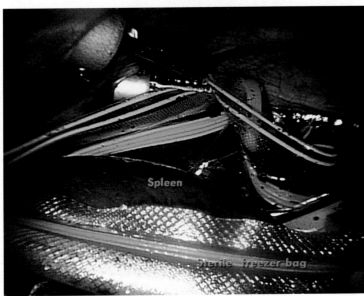

D

Fig. 33-7. (Continued)

Lateral Approach

This approach was first described for laparoscopic adrenalectomy and can be used for laparoscopic splenectomy. The patient is put in a right lateral decubitus position similar to that used for left-side posterolateral thoracotomy. The operating table is flexed, and the bolster is raised to increase the distance between the lower rib and the iliac crest. Usually, four 12-mm trocars are used around the costal margin to allow maximum flexibility for the interchange of camera, clip applier, linear stapler, and other instruments. Three trocars are located anteriorly along the rib margin, and one is located posteriorly. Enough distance between trocars is required to preserve good working angles and easy triangulation. Slightly tilting the patient backward allows more freedom to move the instruments placed along the left costal margin, especially for lifting movements. Manipulation of the instrument handles can be limited by contact with the operating table if proper patient positioning is not attained. For the same reason, it is advantageous to place the anterior or abdominal side of the patient close to the edge of the operating table (Fig. 33-8).

First, along the anterior costal margin, a Veress needle is used to create a symmetric 15-mm-Hg pneumoperitoneum, and the first trocar is inserted. The camera is inserted, and a thorough search is made for accessory spleens, which should be removed when they are found. Placement of the remaining trocars is determined by patient configuration in relation to the size of the spleen to be excised. Usually, the fourth posterior trocar cannot be inserted until the splenic flexure of the colon—or sometimes the left kidney—is mobilized. Therefore, the dissection is begun through three trocars. The splenic flexure is partially mobilized by incising the splenocolic ligament, the lower part of the phrenocolic ligament, and the sustentaculum lienis to allow access to the gastrosplenic ligament, which can be readily separated from the lienorenal ligament in this position. Gentle upward retraction of the lower pole of the spleen creates a tent-like structure, with the gastrosplenic ligament making up the left panel and the lienorenal ligament the right panel of the tent; the stomach makes up the floor of the tent. All the pertinent splenic anatomy is then readily seen in one exposure. Surgeons performing laparoscopic splenectomy through the lateral approach should always try to reproduce this maneuver to separate the gastrosplenic from the lienorenal ligament and clearly demonstrate all the noteworthy anatomic structures. The vessels contained in each ligament and the tail of the pancreas are identified and dissected (Fig. 33-9). The branches of the left gastroepiploic artery are controlled with the cautery or clips, depending on their size. The avascular portion of the gastrosplenic ligament is then incised to provide exposure of the hilar structures in the lienorenal ligament; this maneuver is facilitated by gentle elevation of the lower pole. The lateral patient position provides splenic retraction toward the left lobe of the liver by the force of gravity. The role of the assistant retracting the spleen is therefore much less critical in the lateral approach. The surgeon

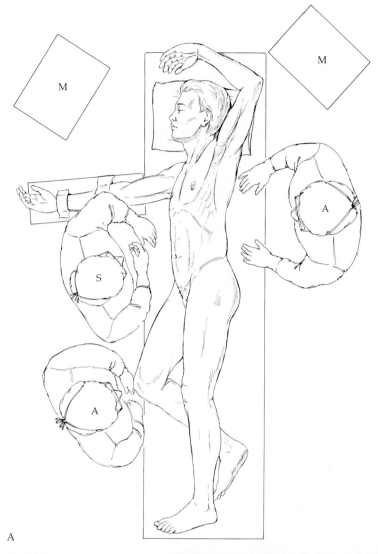

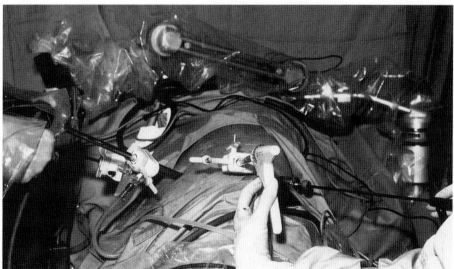

Fig. 33-8. **A:** *Patient positioning and operating room setup. (S, surgeon; A, assistant; M, monitor.)* **B:** *Lateral approach. Three 12-mm trocars are used anteriorly along the left costal margin. A fourth (5 or 12 mm) trocar is placed posterior to the iliac crest.*

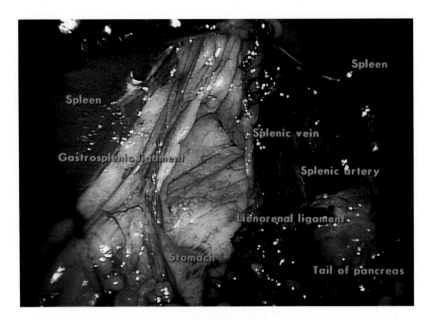

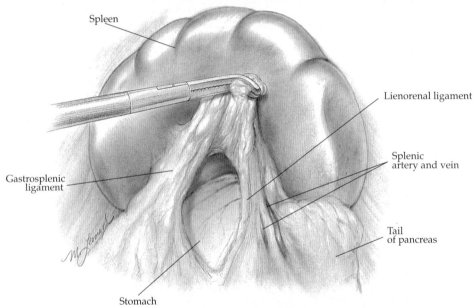

Fig. 33-9. Lateral approach—the "splenic tent." Separation of the gastrosplenic and lienorenal ligaments demonstrates all the anatomic elements as seen in the lateral approach after section of the ligaments attached to the lower pole of the spleen.

avoid pancreatic injury during control of the vessels. If a distributed type of anatomy is present with its wide hilum, the splenic branches will usually be dissected and clipped. The magistral type of anatomy lends itself to a single use of the linear stapler after the tail of the pancreas is identified and dissected away from the hilum. A window is created above the hilar pedicle in the lienorenal ligament, and all hilar structures are included within the markings of the linear stapler under direct vision (Figs. 33-9 and 33-10). The viewing angles provided by moving the camera into the various trocars make linear stapling much easier in the lateral than in the anterior approach. The dissection is continued with individual dissection and clipping of the short gastric vessels. Occasionally, these vessels can also be taken *en masse* with the linear stapler. Sutures are rarely necessary during laparoscopic splenectomy and have been used only occasionally to control a short gastric vessel too short to be clipped safely. Division of the short gastric vessels is performed while the spleen hangs by the upper portion of the phrenocolic ligament. The spleen is inserted in a plastic bag after complete mobilization, as in the anterior approach. Insertion of the spleen into the bag may be simplified by preserving the upper portion of the phrenocolic ligament. After final section of the phrenocolic ligament and diaphragmatic adhesions, extraction is performed through one of the anterior ports by the same technique used in the anterior approach. Extraction through the posterior port is made more difficult by the thickness of the muscle mass at this level and will usually require opening the incision and fulgurating bleeding muscle. After verification of hemostasis, trocar sites are closed with absorbable sutures and paper strips. No drains are used.

Extraction of Specimen

Spleens removed through the anterior approach are extracted from the umbilical trocar site after finger fragmentation in a plastic bag. It is rarely necessary to enlarge this incision to more than 2 or 3 cm. A small subcostal incision has been used as the extraction site during laparoscopic splenectomy through the anterior approach to deal better with diaphragmatic adhesions. When the lateral approach is used, extraction is more easily performed through one of the ports situated anteri-

can usually assess the geography of the hilum and have an idea of the degree of difficulty of the operation following mobilization of the inferior pole and incision of the gastrosplenic ligament. Then, the fourth trocar is placed posteriorly under direct vision, with care taken to avoid the left kidney. A 5-mm trocar can be used instead of the usual 12-mm trocar in the posterior position at the discretion of the surgeon. The trocars situated immediately anterior and posterior to the iliac crest should be positioned so that impeded

movement by the iliac crest is avoided (see Fig. 33-8).

The incision of the phrenocolic ligament is then carried toward the diaphragm. A 2-cm-wide portion of the ligament is left attached to the spleen, making a long structure from which the spleen can be manipulated with graspers. With the camera in the lower or posterior trocar site, the tail of the pancreas is dissected away from the structures of the hilum in the areolar avascular tissue of the retroperitoneum to

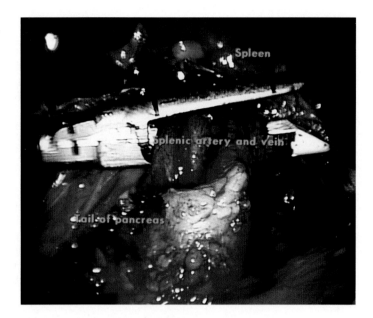

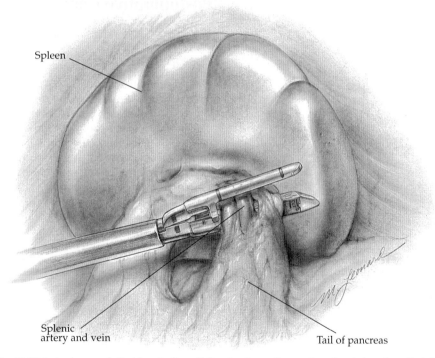

Spleen

Splenic
artery and vein

Tail of pancreas

Fig. 33-10. Lateral approach. En bloc *stapling of hilar structures after creation of a window above the tail of the pancreas.*

fragmentation in a plastic bag is not used for fear of making the histologic diagnosis difficult to obtain. Extraction of intact spleens through a small left subcostal or median incision has also been described when preserving tissue architecture is required. The various techniques of fragmentation and extraction of splenic tissue during laparoscopic splenectomy should be discussed and agreed on with the pathologists to ensure that proper pathologic diagnoses are not compromised by necrotic tissue in the case of preoperative splenic artery embolization or altered tissue architecture through finger fragmentation, especially if the diagnosis of malignancy is suspected but not proved. The choice of the appropriate extraction technique is therefore largely dependent on the type of splenic pathology or the size of the spleen.

Choice of Surgical Approach

The description by Gagner and associates (1994) of the lateral approach to laparoscopic splenectomy has been a useful addition to the armamentarium of techniques that are necessary to successfully undertake laparoscopic splenectomy for different hematologic conditions and for spleens of various sizes. This approach is especially useful for safe excision of normal or slightly enlarged spleens without prior splenic artery embolization. There are many reasons for this:

1. It allows dissection of the splenic vessels in the relatively avascular areolar tissue of the retroperitoneum, and this is an easier access than that in the anterior approach.
2. It almost eliminates inadvertent trauma from instruments usually held by assistants to lift the lower pole of the spleen, as done in the anterior approach. In the lateral approach, little force is necessary to retract the spleen. Gravity is almost all that is required, as the spleen naturally will fall toward the left lobe of the liver and out of the way, permitting identification of the vessels and the tail of the pancreas after the lower portion of the phrenocolic ligament is sectioned. Because the phrenocolic ligament is so accessible in this approach, it can be dissected early, leaving a generous portion on the splenic side that can easily be grasped to manipulate the spleen.

orly. This extraction site also requires little or no enlargement. On occasion, for a spleen longer than 20 cm, a 7.5- to 10-cm Pfannenstiel's incision is used, and the forearm is introduced in the abdomen to deliver the spleen in the pelvis for extraction in large fragments under direct vision (Fig. 33-11). The surgeon can also use this incision to hand-review the hilum videoscopically to ensure that all vascular structures have been properly identified and

controlled. The abdomen is copiously irrigated before closure. The largest spleen placed in a bag in my experience was 24 cm long, and the largest spleen removed laparoscopically was 27 cm long.

Laparoscopic splenectomy for malignant disease is performed with increasing frequency. In patients in whom lymphoma or Hodgkin's disease is suspected, preoperative splenic artery embolization or finger

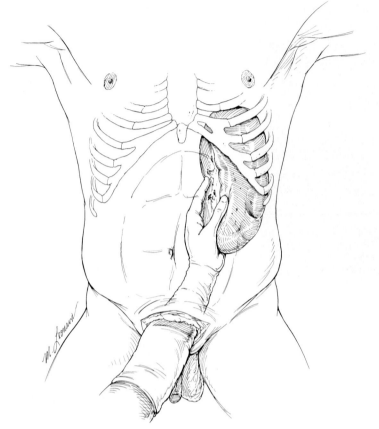

Fig. 33-11. Hand assist extraction method for laparoscopic splenectomy in massive splenomegaly. (From Poulin and Thibault, 1995, with permission.)

3. With the lateral approach, it is much easier to distinguish and separate the gastrosplenic and lienorenal ligaments to identify the anatomic structures that they contain. It is relatively easy to safely create windows through the ligaments to place clips or staples, especially above the tail of the pancreas (see Figs. 33-9 and 33-10).

4. The tail of the pancreas is more accessible to dissection, especially in its superior and posterior aspects, than in the anterior approach (Fig. 33-12).

5. When one refrains from cutting the last portion of the phrenocolic ligament at the end of the procedure, there is more room in this position to insert the spleen in a plastic bag before extraction.

All these advantages translate into a procedure that can take 30 to 60 minutes less to perform than the anterior approach.

There are some disadvantages, however:

1. The anterior approach is probably better suited to a situation in which concomitant surgery is needed, such as cholecystectomy.
2. Dealing with a large spleen is probably safer with prior splenic artery embolization and an anterior approach.
3. Performing a complete exploration for accessory spleens is possibly more difficult by the lateral approach.

The splenic hilum, gastrocolic ligament, tail of the pancreas, descending colon, and its mesentery are readily seen, but structures within the pelvis, the right side of the colon, the small bowel, and its mesentery are more difficult to evaluate. This may be more theoretical than real, as the literature states that more than 80% of accessory spleens are located in areas accessible to the lateral approach (Fig. 33-13). Moreover, in my experience so far, accessory spleens were found in 27% of patients op-

erated on with the anterior approach and in 18% with the lateral approach, which compares favorably with the 15% to 30% rate quoted in the literature on open splenectomy. A report of eight cases of recurrent hematologic disease after splenectomy successfully treated by removal of accessory spleens serves as a reminder that searching for and excising accessory spleens are essential steps in this procedure, whether access is conventional or laparoscopic.

Most patients seen for splenectomy suffer from immune thrombocytopenic purpura, and most have a normal-sized spleen; therefore, the lateral approach without prior embolization would seem to be the current technique of choice for these patients.

Postoperative Care and Surgical Complications

Postoperative Care

The postoperative care of a laparoscopic splenectomy patient is usually straightforward. The nasogastric tube is removed either in the recovery room after it is clear that the stomach has been emptied or the next morning, depending on the duration and the difficulty of the procedure. The urinary catheter is usually removed before the patient is discharged from the recovery room. Clear fluids are permitted the next day, and when this is well tolerated, the patient is allowed to move to a diet of his or her choice.

Postoperative pain medication is individualized with a view to ensuring complete patient comfort. Meperidine hydrochloride (Demerol HCl) injections can be used during the first night, followed by an oral acetaminophen/codeine preparation or acetaminophen alone. Alternatively, when the patient has no history of ulcer or dyspepsia, a 100-mg suppository of indomethacin (Indocid) is inserted before induction of anesthesia and every 12 hours for three to five doses. Then, depending on the intensity of postoperative pain, a few meperidine injections are used for the first 12 to 24 hours, followed by oral acetaminophen; this combination has produced the best results in my experience. Because of side effects of nausea, vomiting, abdominal fullness, and constipation, codeine is avoided, if possible. When indomethacin is used, prophylactic doses of

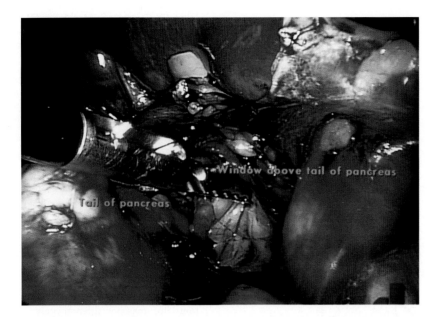

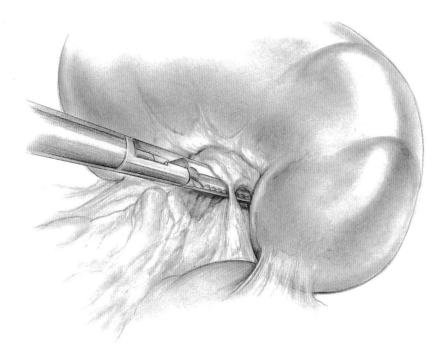

Fig. 33-12. Lateral approach. Tail of the pancreas as seen from the lateral approach in the areolar tissue of the retroperitoneum. Note the window created above the hilar vessels, making en bloc *stapling easy.*

subcutaneous heparin are avoided, especially when the platelet count is low or a platelet function abnormality is present. An oral steroid is started on the first postoperative day after an overlap intravenous injection if steroid coverage is required. Thereafter, the steroid is gradually de-

creased. Patients are advised to avoid getting the trocar wounds wet for 3 to 4 days after surgery and to keep the paper strips covering the trocar incisions for 8 to 10 days. No drains have been used so far. No limitation of physical activity is imposed, and the patient is allowed to tailor activi-

ties to his or her degree of asthenia or discomfort.

Surgical Complications

Preoperative Splenic Artery Embolization

Selective embolization of splenic artery branches demands appropriate equipment and expertise from the radiologist because many variations in arterial splenic blood supply complicate the technique. Moreover, the only embolic material used should be gelatin sponge fragments and 3- to 8-mm coils, as serious complications can occur when microspheres or gelatin powder are used. Selective embolization should also be performed distal to the great pancreatic artery to avoid causing pancreatitis. Preoperative splenic artery embolization can be performed with little morbidity and is a useful adjunct in some cases of laparoscopic splenectomy.

Laparoscopic Splenectomy

The complications of splenectomy include intraoperative and postoperative hemorrhage, left lower lobe atelectasis and pneumonia, left pleural effusion, subphrenic collection, venous thrombosis, and iatrogenic pancreatic, gastric, and colonic injury.

Success with laparoscopic splenectomy depends largely on proper preparation and avoidance of complications and technical misadventures. Recognition of anatomic elements and their arrangement is paramount. Vascular structures should be cleanly isolated and dissected from surrounding fat. Most can then be controlled safely and cost-effectively with two clips placed proximally and distally. Staplers should be used with care and should not be applied blindly. The stapler tip should be clearly seen to be free of tissue before it is closed. Otherwise, significant hemorrhage from a partial section of a major splenic branch might occur after release of the instrument. Blind application of the stapler may also result in damage to the tail of the pancreas, often lying close to the inner surface of the spleen, especially in the anterior approach.

Improper use of the cautery can cause iatrogenic injury to the stomach, colon, and pancreas. Structures close to the lower pole in the gastrocolic ligament can be approached aggressively with the cautery, but blind fulguration of fat in the hilum can result in serious bleeding. The instru-

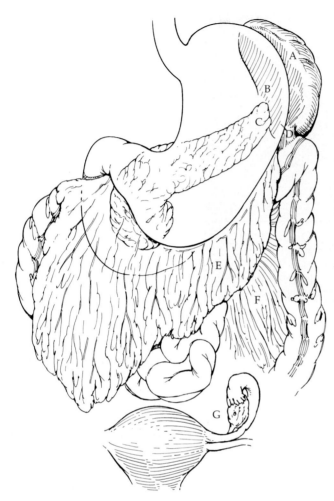

Fig. 33-13. Accessory spleens. Sites where accessory spleens are found in order of importance (A, hilar region, 54%; B, pedicle, 25%; C, tail of pancreas, 6%; D, splenocolic ligament, 2%; E, greater omentum, 12%; F, mesentery, 0.5%; G, left ovary, 0.5%). (From Curtis GH, Movitz D. The surgical significance of accessory spleens. Ann Surg 1946;123:276—298; with permission.)

Hiatt JR, Gomes AS, Machleder HI. Massive splenomegaly: superior results with a combined endovascular and operative approach. *Arch Surg* 1990;125:1363–1367.

Hilleren DJ. Embolization of the spleen for the treatment of hypersplenism and in portal hypertension. In: Kadir S, ed. *Current practice of interventional radiology: spleen.* Philadelphia: B.C. Decker, 1991:494–497.

Lipshutz B. A composite study of the coeliac axis artery. *Ann Surg* 1917;65:159–163.

Merlier O, Ribet M, Mensier E, Ronsmans N, Caulier MT. Role of accessory spleen in recurrent hematologic diseases. *Chirurgie* 1992;118:229–235.

Michels NA. The variational anatomy of the spleen and splenic artery. *Am J Anat* 1942;70:21–72.

Poulin EC, Thibault C. Laparoscopic splenectomy for massive splenomegaly: operative technique and case report. *Can J Surg* 1995;38:69–72.

Poulin EC, Thibault C. The anatomical basis for laparoscopic splenectomy. *Can J Surg* 1993;36:484–488.

Poulin EC, Mamazza J. Laparoscopic splenectomy: lessons from the learning curve. *Can J Surg* 1998;41:28–36.

Poulin EC, Thibault C, DesCôteaux JG, Côté G. Partial laparoscopic splenectomy for trauma: technique and case report. *Surg Laparosc Endosc* 1995;5:306–310.

Poulin EC, Mamazza J. Schlachta CM. Splenic artery embolization before laparoscopic splenectomy. *Surg Endosc* 1998;12:870–875.

Ssoson-Jaroschewitsch A. Zur chirurgischen Anatomie des Milzhilus. *Z Ges Anat I Abt* 1937;84:218–224.

Testut L. *Traité d'anatomie humaine*, 7th ed. Paris: Librairie Octave Doin, 1923:942–960.

ment should be activated only in proximity to the target organ to avoid arcing and spot necrosis, which may result in delayed perforation and sepsis.

The role of the assistants is also important in the prevention of complications. All instruments, including those handled by assistants, should be moved only under direct vision. Retraction of the liver and stomach and elevation of the spleen require constant concentration to avoid lacerations with subsequent hemorrhage or perforation, especially when using the anterior approach. There should be no iatrogenic trauma to the spleen during the surgery to eliminate the possibility of splenosis later on. For the same reason, if splenic trauma occurs intraoperatively or

intraabdominal fragmentation is required for extraction of a large spleen, copious irrigation should be used before closure.

Suggested Reading

Baronofsky ID, Walton W, Noble JF. Occult injury to the pancreas following splenectomy. *Surgery* 1951;29:852–856.

Fujitani RM, Johs SM, Cobb SR, Mehrenger CM, White RA, Klein SR. Preoperative splenic artery occlusion as an adjunct for high-risk splenectomy. *Am Surg* 1991;54:602–608.

Gagner M, Lacroix A, Bolte E, Pomp A. Laparoscopic adrenalectomy: the importance of a flank approach in the lateral decubitus position. *Surg Endosc* 1994;8:135–138.

EDITOR'S COMMENT

Dr. Poulin provides an excellent description of the current status of laparoscopic splenectomy with a detailed discussion of currently used surgical techniques. Several alternatives to the techniques described are currently in use but are beyond the scope of this chapter. The lateral approach—or "hanging spleen" technique—described by Dr. Poulin is being applied with increasing frequency in lieu of the anterior or anterolateral technique.

Several specific technical points warrant additional discussion. The role of splenic artery embolization remains controversial and is rarely or never used by many advanced laparoscopists. The embolization procedure adds expense and additional risks to the management of splenic disorders. There are unusual circumstances in which embolization can add safety to the performance of a laparoscopic splenectomy, but these instances are exceptional.

The majority of advanced laparoscopists utilize a four- or five-trocar technique, with the trocars positioned in a curvilinear array or L-shaped arrangement in the left upper quadrant and/or left flank. The Hasson technique is used in lieu of the Veress needle by many surgeons, and this entry site, with stay sutures placed on the fascia, is utilized for extraction of the spleen at the conclusion of the operation. Dr. Poulin describes the use of a freezer bag and warns against the risk of splenosis. Additional specimen bags are available that are extremely tough and tear-resistant. The bag may be rolled into a cigar shape and inserted via a 10- or 12-mm port site after removal of the cannula. The technique described in this chapter for positioning the spleen in the bag is appropriate. Additionally, the use of the Trendelenburg or reverse Trendelenburg position and right and left tilt of the bed may facilitate the guidance of a large spleen into an open bag by the use of gravity. The finger fracture of the spleen into four to seven large pieces usually preserves sufficient architecture for the pathologist to adequately assess the organ, regardless of the disease process for which the spleen is removed.

The risks associated with splenectomy are significant, and the laparoscopic approach is best accomplished by an experienced laparoscopic surgeon and skilled assistant. The patient should be fully informed of the risk of bleeding, injury to adjacent structures, and possible need for conversion to an open operation. The patient should also understand the risk of an undetected accessory spleen and the potential for recurrence of hematologic disorders.

W.S.E.

34

Laparoscopic Adrenalectomy

L. Michael Brunt

Since the first laparoscopic adrenalectomy was reported in 1992, the safety and efficacy of a laparoscopic approach to adrenalectomy have been demonstrated by several groups. Laparoscopic adrenalectomy has also been shown to have several advantages, compared to open adrenalectomy, including decreased pain, a shorter duration of postoperative ileus, earlier hospital discharge, and a more rapid recovery. The majority of adrenal gland tumors should be amenable to laparoscopic excision because most adrenal neoplasms are small and pathologically benign. This chapter reviews the basic principles of laparoscopic adrenal surgery, including anatomy, diagnostic considerations, indications for operation, and the technical aspects of a laparoscopic approach to adrenalectomy.

Anatomic Considerations

The adrenal glands are retroperitoneal organs located along the supermedial aspect of each kidney. The normal adrenal gland in adults weighs 4 to 6 g, measures 3 to 5 cm in length, and is 4 to 6 mm thick. The adrenal glands are comprised of a cortex and a medulla, each of which has distinct endocrine functions and separate embryologic origins. The adrenal cortex is derived from the coelomic mesoderm and is the site of synthesis and secretion of the steroid hormones: cortisol, the adrenal androgens, and aldosterone. Cortisol

secretion is regulated via a classic negative-feedback pathway involving the hypothalamic–pituitary–adrenal axis and adrenocorticotropic hormone (ACTH). The major physiologic regulator of aldosterone secretion is the renin–angiotensin–aldosterone system. The adrenal medulla is derived from cells of the neural crest and synthesizes the catecholamines, norepinephrine, and epinephrine. Catecholamines may also be synthesized in extraadrenal chromaffin tissue, most commonly in the periaortic and paravertebral regions and in the organ of Zuckerkandl.

Precise knowledge of the normal adrenal anatomy and the relationship of the adrenals to surrounding structures is essential for successful adrenalectomy, regardless of whether a laparoscopic or open technique is utilized. Each adrenal gland is embedded in Gerota's fascia and is surrounded by retroperitoneal fat. The adrenal has a fibrous capsule and is golden-yellow in color due to the high lipid content of the adrenal cortex. The right adrenal gland is somewhat pyramidal in shape and lies superior to the right kidney, whereas the left adrenal is more flattened and is in intimate contact with the medial aspect of the superior pole of the left kidney. On the right side, the adrenal gland is bordered medially by the inferior vena cava, and often a portion of the anteromedial border of the gland actually lies beneath the vena cava. The right triangular ligament of the liver crosses the anterior surface of the adrenal gland supe-

riorly, which means that the upper portion of the gland has no peritoneum covering its surface. The lower portion of the right adrenal may be overlapped or partially covered by the duodenum. Posteriorly, the right adrenal rests on the diaphragm superiorly and on the anteromedial aspect of the upper portion of the right kidney inferiorly. The left adrenal gland is bounded superiorly by the peritoneum of the posterior omental bursa, the stomach, and the superior pole of the spleen. Inferiorly, the left adrenal is covered by the pancreas and splenic vein and is closely related to the renal hilar vessels. Posteriorly, the left adrenal rests on the left crus of the diaphragm medially and the medial aspect of the left kidney laterally.

The adrenal glands are highly vascularized and derive their blood supply from numerous branches of the inferior phrenic artery, aorta, and renal arteries (Fig. 34-1). Each adrenal gland has a single, central vein, which is the key to adrenalectomy. The right adrenal vein is short (0.5 to 1 cm in length) and drains from the medial aspect of the gland directly into the posterolateral aspect of the inferior vena cava. A second right adrenal vein that enters either the vena cava or right hepatic vein is occasionally encountered. The left adrenal vein is usually 2 to 3 cm in length and exits the inferomedial aspect of the gland, where it runs obliquely to empty into the left renal vein. The inferior phrenic vein frequently joins the left adrenal vein proximal to its entry into the renal vein.

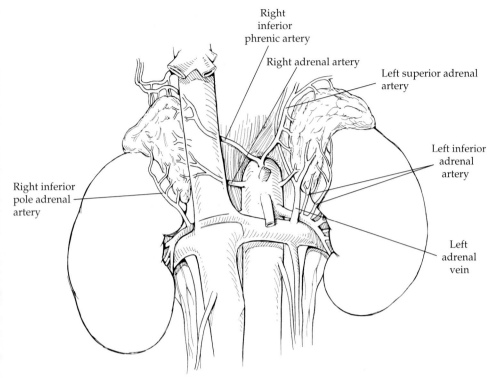

Right inferior phrenic artery

Right adrenal artery

Left superior adrenal artery

Left inferior adrenal artery

Right inferior pole adrenal artery

Left adrenal vein

Fig. 34-1. Adrenal anatomy and blood supply.

Diagnostic Considerations/Indications for Treatment

Adrenalectomy is indicated for any biochemically functional adrenal tumor and for all suspected primary adrenal malignancies. The vast majority of adrenal tumors are benign and may be considered for laparoscopic excision (Table 34-1). Suspected primary adrenal malignancies more than 5 to 6 cm in size or tumors that appear locally invasive, including adrenal cortical carcinoma and malignant pheochromocytoma, should contraindicate a laparoscopic approach because of the potential for tumor dissemination with the laparoscopic dissection and pneumoperitoneum (see "Editor's Comment"). Small, isolated adrenal metastases may be appropriate for laparoscopic surgical resection in carefully selected patients. No clear-cut size limitation has yet been defined for considering laparoscopic adrenalectomy; however, caution should be exercised in attempting a laparoscopic approach to large adrenal masses greater than 8 to 10 cm in size because of the difficulty in ma-

nipulating such masses with current laparoscopic instrumentation and the possibility of spillage of a potentially malignant tumor.

Cushing's Syndrome

Cortisol-producing adrenal cortical adenomas or carcinomas account for 15% to 20% of all cases of Cushing's syndrome. ACTH-secreting pituitary tumors comprise 60% to 70% of cases and ectopic ACTH-secreting tumors account for about 15% of cases. Occasionally, the source of

Cushing's syndrome is primary adrenal hyperplasia (pigmented micronodular adrenal hyperplasia or macronodular adrenal hyperplasia). The diagnosis of Cushing's syndrome is established by demonstration of elevated 24-hour urine-free cortisol levels or by failure to suppress plasma cortisol levels to less than 5 μg/dL after administration of 1 mg of dexamethasone. Once a diagnosis of Cushing's syndrome is made biochemically, further diagnostic tests (plasma ACTH level, high-dose dexamethasone suppression test, and radiographic imaging) may be used to determine the etiology. Patients with primary adrenal tumors usually have elevated cortisol levels, low plasma ACTH levels, and radiographic evidence of an adrenal mass on computed tomography (CT) or magnetic resonance (MR) imaging. Unilateral adrenalectomy is the treatment choice for patients with a cortisol-producing adenoma. Bilateral adrenalectomy is indicated for patients with persistent Cushing's syndrome due to either failed treatment of pituitary tumors or primary adrenal hyperplasia.

Aldosteronoma

Primary hyperaldosteronism is characterized by hypertension and spontaneous hypokalemia. The diagnosis is confirmed by demonstrating elevated plasma aldosterone levels and suppressed plasma renin activity (aldosterone-to-renin ratio greater than 30). The most common cause of primary hyperaldosteronism is an aldosterone-producing adenoma (65% of cases), and surgical excision is curative. Bilateral idiopathic adrenal hyperplasia accounts for about 30% of cases and is treated medically rather than by adrenalectomy. Dif-

Table 34-1. Indications and Contraindications for Laparoscopic Adrenalectomy

Indications	Contraindications
Aldosteronoma	Adrenocortical carcinoma
Cushing's syndrome	Malignant pheochromocytoma
Cortisol-secreting adrenal adenoma	Large benign adrenal mass
Primary adrenal hyperplasia	(>8–10 cm)
Adrenal hyperplasia after failed treatment of pituitary	Existing contraindication to
Cushing's syndrome	laparoscopic surgery
Pheochromocytoma (sporadic or familial)	
Nonfunctioning cortical adenoma (>5 cm or suspicious	
radiographic appearance)	
Adrenal metastases	

ferentiation of these two disorders is best made either radiographically with abdominal CT or MR imaging scan that shows a unilateral adrenal mass or with simultaneous bilateral adrenal vein sampling for aldosterone. Preoperatively, hypokalemia should be corrected, and the patient's blood pressure should be adequately controlled, which may be facilitated by administration of the aldosterone antagonist spironolactone (Aldactone).

Adrenal Cortical Carcinoma

Adrenal cortical carcinoma should be suspected in any patient with a large adrenal mass (greater than 6 cm) or with virilizing features. *En bloc* resection of all gross tumor with negative surgical margins at the initial operation offers the best potential for cure. Because of the difficulty in manipulating large solid masses laparoscopically and the potential for spillage of tumor with the laparoscopic dissection and pneumoperitoneum, any suspected adrenal cortical carcinoma greater than 6 cm in size should at this time be considered a contraindication to a laparoscopic approach (see Editor's Comment).

Adrenal Incidentaloma

Incidentally discovered adrenal masses are detected on approximately 0.6% of abdominal CT scans. The majority of these lesions are small, nonfunctioning cortical adenomas that do not require adrenalectomy. Patients with functional or potentially malignant lesions should undergo surgical resection. The evaluation of a patient with an incidentally discovered adrenal mass begins with a complete history and physical examination. Biochemical screening should be carried out, including 24-hour urinary cortisol measurement to exclude Cushing's syndrome and 24-hour urinary catecholamines to screen for pheochromocytoma. Evaluation for primary hyperaldosteronism is indicated if the patient is hypokalemic. Large masses greater than 5 to 6 cm in size should be removed regardless of functional status because of their malignant potential. For nonfunctioning adrenal masses, MR imaging may provide additional discrimination between benign and malignant lesions. Benign adrenal adenomas have a greater lipid content, compared to malignant lesions, and show a

loss of signal intensity on MR imaging opposed-phase gradient-echo images as compared to in-phase images. In contrast, malignant lesions do not have a high lipid content and maintain similar signal intensities on both image sequences. Fine-needle aspiration (FNA) is not useful in distinguishing benign from malignant primary adrenal tumors and should be reserved for suspected adrenal metastases. FNA should never be performed unless a pheochromocytoma has first been excluded biochemically. Patients with benign, nonfunctional tumors less than 5 cm in size should be reevaluated in 6 months, and adrenalectomy should be performed if there is any growth in the mass or evidence of biochemical function.

Pheochromocytoma

Pheochromocytoma should be suspected in any patient with hypertension and an adrenal mass. The diagnosis is made by demonstrating elevated 24-hour urinary catecholamines and metanephrines. Radiographically, pheochromocytomas can be demonstrated by CT scan, but MR imaging is more specific for this tumor because T2-weighted images typically show tumor enhancement relative to the liver. Pheochromocytomas may be removed laparoscopically, provided that they are confined to the adrenal gland and patients have been adequately prepared pharmacologically for surgery. Pheochromocytomas develop in extraadrenal sites in 10% to 15% of cases; the role of laparoscopy in the management of patients with extraadrenal tumors is presently unknown. Preoperatively, alpha-adrenergic receptor blockade with phenoxybenzamine hydrochloride (Dibenzyline) should be implemented with the goal of controlling the elevated blood pressure and other symptoms. Failure to adequately prepare patients pharmacologically may result in a severe hypertensive crisis and even sudden death intraoperatively. Beta-blockade is reserved for patients with tachyarrhythmias or predominantly epinephrine-secreting tumors.

Perioperative Patient Management

Patients with a functional adrenal mass and hypertension should have preopera-

tive control of their blood pressure and correction of any electrolyte abnormalities. Patients with a pheochromocytoma should undergo alpha-adrenergic receptor blockade, and all patients with hypercortisolism should receive stress doses of corticosteroids intravenously before and after surgery. A mechanical bowel preparation is given the day prior to surgery. Intraoperative monitoring consists of a urinary catheter in all patients and an arterial line in all hypertensive patients. A central venous catheter should be used liberally both for intravenous access and for monitoring of central venous pressure. Swan-Ganz catheterization is reserved for patients with associated cardiac disease or unstable hypertension. All patients should be typed and crossmatched for two units of packed red blood cells.

Operative Technique

The retroperitoneal location of the adrenal glands makes them surgically accessible with a variety of operative approaches—either via the abdomen or flank or through the retroperitoneum. As a result, the laparoscopic approaches to adrenalectomy have been designed to mimic their open counterparts. The most widely used approach to laparoscopic adrenalectomy is a transabdominal lateral flank approach that provides excellent exposure in the retroperitoneum by allowing gravity retraction of adjacent organs. This technique also permits examination of other intraabdominal organs, although it does not allow access to the contralateral adrenal gland. The adrenal gland may also be removed laparoscopically using an anterior transabdominal approach with the patient supine or slightly rotated. This approach provides a conventional view of abdominal anatomy and may allow access to both adrenal glands. However, operative exposure is more difficult because additional effort must be expended to maintain exposure and retraction of overlying organs including the spleen, pancreas, stomach, liver, and colon. Operative times have generally been longer with this approach than with other techniques. Finally, a retroperitoneal endoscopic approach to adrenalectomy has been reported in a small number of centers. The retroperitoneal technique allows a totally extraperitoneal approach and may have special utility in patients who have had previous abdominal surgery or require bilateral adrenalectomy. Disadvantages of the retroperitoneal endoscopic approach include the smaller working space that may complicate the removal of larger tumors, difficulties with dissecting the retroperitoneal fat, and the unfamiliarity of the anatomic relationships. The transabdominal lateral flank approach is the most commonly used technique and will be described in detail.

General Principles of Dissection

Laparoscopic adrenalectomy should follow the general principles of open adrenalectomy regardless of the approach employed. Dissection should remain extracapsular to the gland both to avoid injury to and bleeding from the friable adrenal parenchyma and to prevent fracture and spillage of tumor cells. Grasping the adrenal gland or tumor with the laparoscopic instruments should be avoided. Exposure is obtained by pushing or elevating the gland with a blunt instrument or by gently grasping the periadrenal fat. Meticulous hemostasis is essential to maintain a clear field of view and to avoid damaging adjacent structures. Isolation of the adrenal vein is accomplished early in the dissection in cases of pheochromocytoma, which reduces the release of catecholamines into the systemic circulation. The potential for hypertension due to dissection and manipulation of the tumor is reduced by early ligation of the adrenal blood supply. Small arterial branches are secured with endoscopic clips. Vascular branches may retract into the retroperitoneal fat if inadequately cauterized, and may cause troublesome or delayed hemorrhage. Finally, the gland should be removed using an impermeable entrapment sac. Morcellation of the specimen should be avoided so that pathologic examination is not compromised.

Patient Positioning and Operating Room Setup

The first key to success in this operation is proper patient positioning. Before the induction of general anesthesia, a well padded beanbag mattress is placed beneath the patient. General anesthesia is induced with the patient supine. An orogas-

tric tube and urinary catheter are inserted. Arterial and central venous pressure lines are placed, as indicated clinically. The patient is rolled into the lateral decubitus position with the side up that harbors the adrenal tumor, and secured with a combination of the beanbag mattress, safety straps, and tape. All pressure points including the axilla and hips must be well padded to prevent nerve compression injuries. The operating table is flexed at the waist to increase flank exposure (Fig. 34-2). Placement of the table in a reverse Trendelenburg position also facilitates endoscopic exposure and allows fluid and blood to drain away from the operative field.

Video monitors are positioned on each side at the head of the operating table. For both right and left adrenalectomy, the surgeon may stand to the patient's right, and the assistant should be on the opposite side. The camera operator is usually stationed on the same side as the surgeon for left adrenalectomy and opposite the surgeon for right adrenalectomy. However, these positions may be interchangeable, if necessary, according to the exposure required in any individual patient.

Initial Access and Port Placement

With the patient in the lateral decubitus position, initial access to the peritoneal cavity is most easily accomplished using a closed technique with the Veress needle. Alternatively, open insertion of a blunt-tipped cannula may be utilized, but this technique is somewhat more difficult because of the thickness of the lateral abdominal wall musculature. The first port should be inserted in the anterior axillary line two fingerbreadths below the costal margin. Subsequent ports are then placed as shown in Fig. 34-2 from the subcostal region to a point just dorsal to the posterior axillary line. All ports should be 11 mm in diameter so that there is flexibility in insertion of the laparoscope and dissecting instruments. An angled (30 or 45 degree) laparoscope is used to allow improved viewing angles. The ports are spaced at least 5 to 7 cm apart to avoid clashing of the instruments and the ports both externally and within the abdomen. Some retroperitoneal dissection is usually necessary before the most dorsal (fourth) port can be inserted. A two-handed dissection

technique is mandatory for this operation, and the surgeon must be comfortably situated relative to the ports because of the time required to complete the procedure. Once the first three ports have been inserted, the next step is to expose the retroperitoneum and adrenal gland, as described below for right and left adrenalectomy.

Right Adrenalectomy

Removal of the right adrenal gland laparoscopically is somewhat easier than removal of the left because of the shape and location of the gland; right adrenalectomy is potentially more hazardous, however, due to the anatomy of the adrenal vein and its drainage into the inferior vena cava. Adequate exposure and meticulous dissection and hemostasis are therefore critical to a successful procedure. Once access to the peritoneal cavity has been accomplished, a fan-shaped retractor is inserted through the subcostal port and is used to elevate the right lobe of the liver. The right triangular ligament is then incised from the inferior border of the liver superiorly to the diaphragm (Fig. 34-3). This maneuver allows medial rotation of the right hepatic lobe and exposes the adrenal gland and inferior vena cava. In some cases, the hepatic flexure of the colon may require mobilization, but it is not usually necessary to mobilize or retract the duodenum or kidney.

Following division of the right triangular ligament and elevation of the right hepatic lobe, the adrenal gland and tumor should be visible in the retroperitoneum superior to the kidney (Fig. 34-4). Extracapsular dissection is usually begun adjacent to the medial border of the adrenal. Using a combination of blunt dissection and either cautery scissors or an L-hook electrocautery, the medial border of the gland and the lateral border of the inferior vena cava are further delineated by dividing connective tissue fibers and small arterial branches in this area. The adrenal vein is usually visible at this point in the dissection and is isolated with the help of a 10-mm right angle dissector (Figs. 34-4 and 34-5). The vein is ligated with 9- or 11-mm endoscopic clips—two clips placed proximally and one or two clips distally. Minimal traction should be placed on the vein during dissection and clipping because of the risk of its tearing into the vena cava.

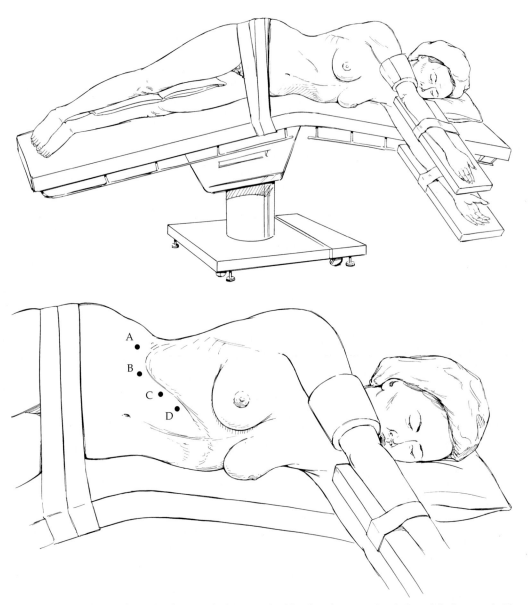

Fig. 34-2. *Patient position and port-site placement for laparoscopic right adrenalectomy using the lateral flank approach. The letters adjacent to the sites marked in the* **inset** *for port placement reflect the sequence in which the ports are generally inserted (A, 5 mm; B, 5 mm; C, 11 mm; D, 5 mm). Further details regarding positioning and port placement are given in the text.*

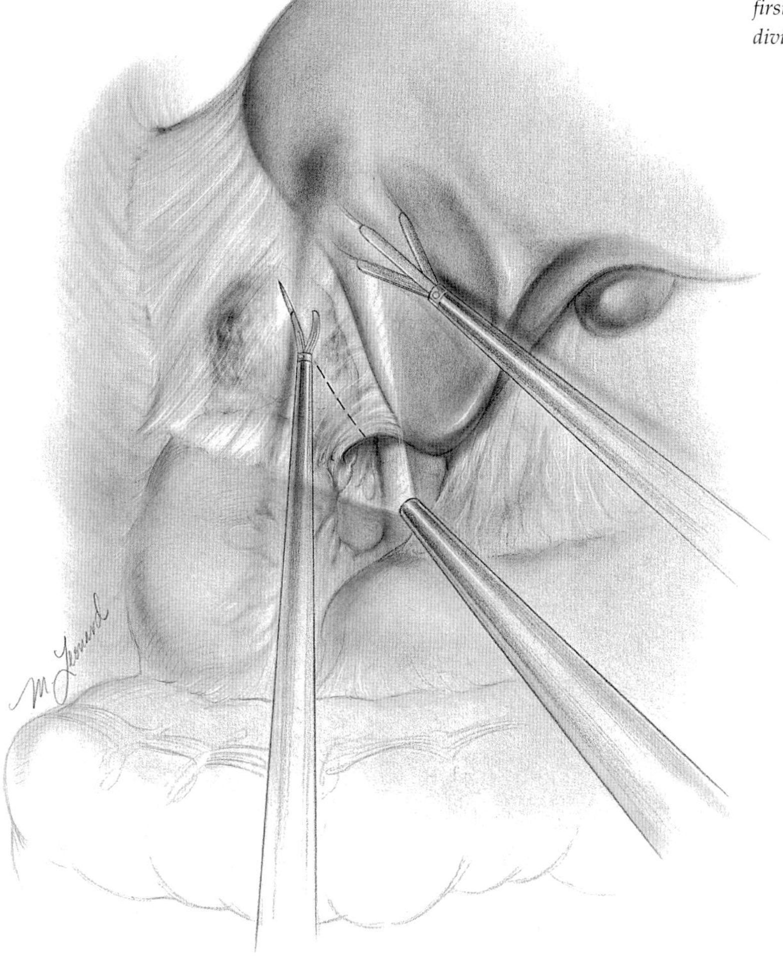

Fig. 34-3. Anatomic relationships as viewed during laparoscopic right adrenalectomy with the transabdominal lateral flank approach. The first phase in the operation entails retraction of the liver medially and division of the right triangular ligament.

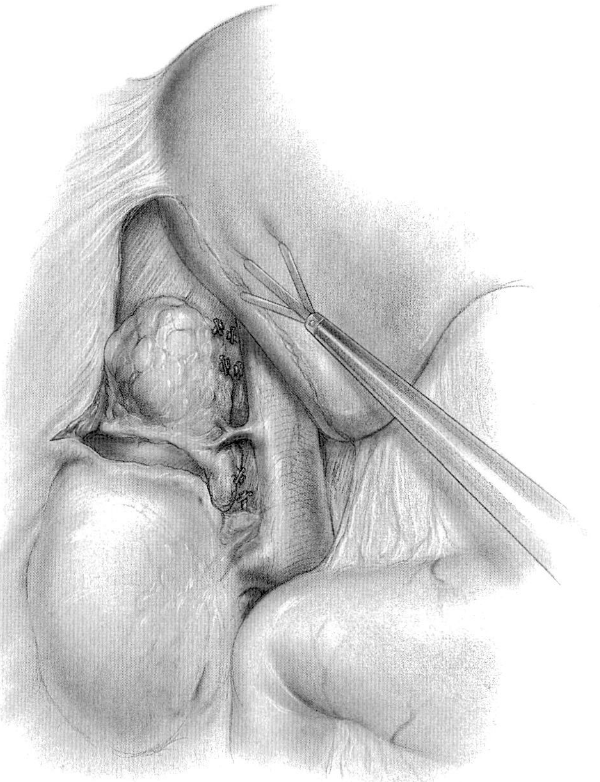

Fig. 34-4. Schematic view of the right adrenal gland as exposed laparoscopically. The triangular ligament has been divided, and the medial border of the adrenal gland has been partially dissected free, exposing the adrenal vein and inferior vena cava.

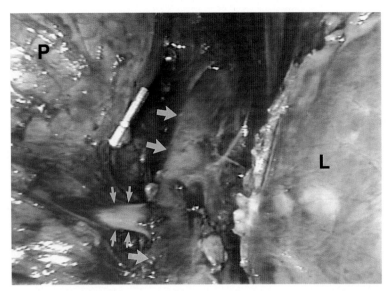

Fig. 34-5. *Endoscopic view of the right adrenal vein* (small arrows) *and inferior vena cava* (large arrows). *A 4-cm pheochromocytoma* (P) *is seen to the left, and the liver* (L) *is on the right.*

sorbable subcuticular sutures. A closed suction drain may be inserted into the retroperitoneum via one of the ports, if deemed necessary, but is not routinely indicated.

Left Adrenalectomy

Mobilization of the splenic flexure of the colon is the first step in left adrenalectomy; following this maneuver, the dorsal fourth port can be inserted. Dissection lateral to the kidney should be avoided, as this will result in medial rotation of the kidney and compromised exposure of the adrenal gland. The next step in the operation—and the key to laparoscopic left adrenalectomy—is complete division of the splenorenal ligament superiorly to the diaphragm and rotation of the spleen medially (Fig. 34-6). This maneuver allows ac-

Once the adrenal vein has been ligated, arterial branches to the adrenal inferiorly, medially (crossing posterior to the vena cava), and superiorly are sequentially isolated, clipped, and divided. A combination of techniques is used for this portion of the dissection, including blunt dissection, electrocautery, and ligation of vessels with endoscopic clips. Alternatively, an ultrasonic dissector may be used for coagulation of small vessels. Retraction on the gland is accomplished by gently pushing or elevating it and the tumor with a blunt instrument. One may also retract the gland by grasping the periadrenal fat but should avoid grasping the adrenal gland or tumor itself because the gland is friable and will bleed or the tumor may be spilled into the retroperitoneum. Finally, the lateral border of the adrenal is mobilized from the surrounding retroperitoneal fat. One should remain close to the adrenal gland throughout the dissection to avoid injury to the inferior vena cava medially, diaphragm and hepatic veins superiorly, and kidney and renal vein inferiorly. Once the specimen has been dissected free, it is placed in an impermeable entrapment sac inserted via either the subcostal or anterior axillary port site. The retroperitoneum is irrigated and inspected for hemostasis, and the specimen is removed by enlarging the port incision. Each port site greater than 5 mm in diameter is closed with a fascial suture, and the skin is closed with ab-

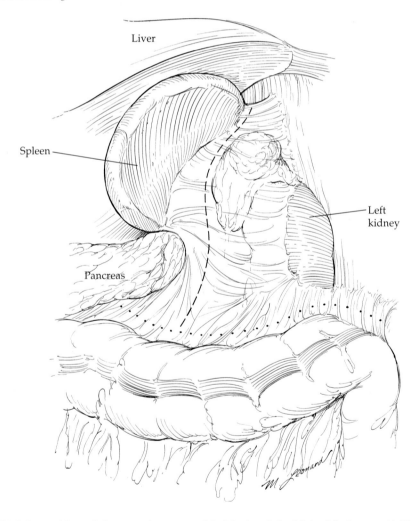

Fig. 34-6. *Sequential steps in laparoscopic exposure of the left adrenal gland (lateral flank approach). The splenic flexure of the colon is divided first* (dotted line), *followed by complete division of the splenorenal ligament* (dashed line).

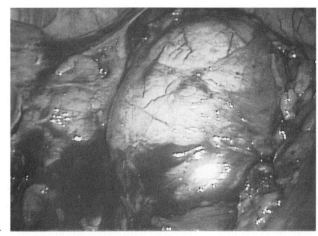
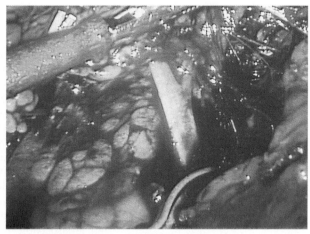

A   B

Fig. 34-7. Laparoscopic view of **(A)** *a 3.5-cm cortical adenoma of the left adrenal and* **(B)** *the left adrenal vein. The vein is usually 2 to 3 cm in length and runs an oblique course from the inferomedial aspect of the adrenal to its junction with the left renal vein.*

cess to the superior retroperitoneum and minimizes the need to retract the spleen. As the dissection continues within the retroperitoneal fat, the adrenal gland should be found closely applied to the supermedial aspect of the kidney. It is helpful to divide the connective tissue between the kidney and the tail of the pancreas to expose the inferior portion of the adrenal gland and the left adrenal vein. Retraction of the pancreas is usually not necessary, as patient positioning and mobilization of the tail of the pancreas provide adequate exposure. Locating the left adrenal gland may be difficult at first, especially in a patient with extensive retroperitoneal fat or with either a small tumor or adrenal hyperplasia. Laparoscopic ultrasonography can facilitate localization of the adrenal gland and tumor and help define the relationship of the gland to adjacent vascular structures.

Once the adrenal gland has been located, its borders should be clearly defined. In some patients, it is possible to directly approach the inferomedial border of the gland early in the operation and expose the adrenal vein (Fig. 34-7). However, if the inferior aspect of the gland is not visible, the dissection should begin superiorly and medially. One must be aware of the inferior phrenic vein, which frequently joins the adrenal vein prior to its entry into the renal vein. The dissection methods for isolation and division of the blood supply to the left adrenal gland are identical to those for the right side. The relationships of the relevant structures and the position of the laparoscopic instruments during ligation

of the left adrenal vein are illustrated schematically in Fig. 34-8. After the adrenal vein has been ligated and the inferior and medial borders of the gland have been cleared, the dissection continues laterally and superiorly. Arterial branches from the renal artery are frequently encountered along the medial and lateral

borders of the left adrenal gland. The superior pole of the kidney is usually well visualized with left adrenalectomy, and one must be careful not to damage the renal capsule because of the risk of hemorrhage. Other structures that may be injured include the renal vessels, the tail of the pancreas, the diaphragm, and the spleen.

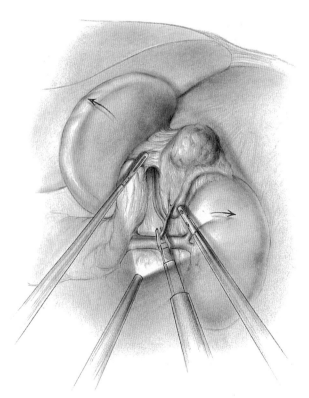

Fig. 34-8. Exposure and ligation of the left adrenal vein. The spleen has been rotated medially, and the kidney is retracted laterally. The vein is ligated at the inferomedial border of the adrenal with endoscopic clips. Note the inferior phrenic vein entering the left adrenal vein proximal to the latter's entry into the renal vein.

Bilateral Adrenalectomy

The most common indication for bilateral adrenalectomy is adrenal hyperplasia due to failed treatment of pituitary Cushing's disease. Other indications in patients with Cushing's syndrome include ectopic ACTH production that does not respond to medical treatment, primary pigmented micronodular hyperplasia, and macronodular adrenal hyperplasia. Bilateral pheochromocytomas may also be an indication for laparoscopic bilateral adrenalectomy.

With the lateral flank approach, bilateral adrenalectomy is carried out as two separate procedures with repositioning of the patient between sides. The technical aspects to the operation are identical to those described for right and left adrenalectomy. Alternatively, a retroperitoneal endoscopic approach can be used that may eliminate the need to reposition the patient.

Surgical Complications and Postoperative Care

Patients who undergo laparoscopic adrenalectomy are subject to the same potential risks as with open adrenalectomy. Bleeding is the most likely complication, and the best approach is a preventive one with a careful, meticulous dissection technique. Intraoperative hemorrhage can usually be managed laparoscopically if it comes from small retroperitoneal vessels, including the adrenal arteries or the adrenal gland. Bleeding from the adrenal veins is potentially more serious, as this may also involve the inferior vena cava on the right or the renal vein on the left. The surgeon must clearly visualize these structures before attempting to dissect around them and must be prepared to convert rapidly to an open operation in the event of major hemorrhage. In my experience with laparoscopic adrenalectomy involving 40 patients, there have been no episodes of bleeding from the adrenal veins or vena cava and no need for conversion to an open operation. Another potential site of hemorrhage is the right lobe of the liver, which may be lacerated by the retractor during right adrenalectomy. Bleeding from this area is usually self-limited and does not require any specific treatment. The operative field, however,

must be kept clear of blood to adequately visualize the dissection laparoscopically. Injuries to the liver, kidney, or bowel may also occur with insertion of the Veress needle and initial trocars into the abdomen. These risks are inherent in any laparoscopic surgical procedure, and a closed insertion technique should be avoided in any patient with extensive previous abdominal surgery or abdominal distention. Fracturing the tumor and spilling tumor cells are usually avoidable events during laparoscopic adrenalectomy if one adheres to the precautions described above. Hypertensive exacerbations may occur during laparoscopic removal of pheochromocytomas. These episodes are best controlled by adequate preoperative alpha-adrenergic receptor blockade by intravenous administration of sodium nitroprusside (Nitropress) intraoperatively and by early ligation of the adrenal vein.

After laparoscopic adrenalectomy, the vast majority of patients can be cared for in a regular nursing unit. The intensive care unit is reserved for patients with unstable hemodynamics or associated cardiopulmonary disease. Patients are started on oral liquids once they are fully awake, and the diet is advanced as tolerated. A parenteral narcotic may be required in some patients during the first 24 hours postoperatively, but most individuals are taking oral analgesics exclusively by the first postoperative day. A complete blood cell count is obtained the morning after surgery, and electrolytes are monitored as clinically indicated. Most patients can be discharged from the hospital within 48 to 72 hours of the operation. Patients are discharged to home without restrictions in physical activity and should be able to return to work within 10 to 15 days of surgery. A follow-up examination should be performed in the office 2 to 3 weeks after discharge. Wound healing problems are rarely seen postoperatively, even in patients with Cushing's syndrome.

Stress doses of a steroid should be administered intravenously in the perioperative period to patients with Cushing's syndrome and to all patients who undergo bilateral adrenalectomy. Once the patient is taking an oral diet, oral hydrocortisone therapy should be instituted at a maintenance dose of 12 to 15 mg/m² each day. Patients with Cushing's syndrome due to an adrenal cortical adenoma may require up to 2 years for the contralateral adrenal

gland to completely recover. Maintenance of hydrocortisone therapy should continue until normal function of the hypothalamic–pituitary–adrenal axis has been demonstrated with the ACTH-stimulation test. Patients who have undergone bilateral adrenalectomy also require life-long mineralocorticoid replacement with fludrocortisone acetate (Florinef Acetate), 100 μg per day. Acute adrenal insufficiency may develop postoperatively in any patient with Cushing's syndrome or following bilateral adrenalectomy for whatever cause. Acute adrenal insufficiency often presents as cardiovascular collapse with hypotension and shock, and if not recognized and treated promptly, it may be fatal. Patients may also experience abdominal pain, weakness, fever, nausea, and vomiting, and leukocytosis may develop. One must have a high index of suspicion for this diagnosis and institute prompt treatment by administration of intravenous hydrocortisone.

Patients with a pheochromocytoma may develop hypotension and require large amounts of intravenous fluids postoperatively due to intravascular volume expansion from the loss of alpha-adrenergic receptor–mediated sympathetic tone. Rebound hyperinsulinism and hypoglycemia may also develop in these patients from the loss of inhibition of insulin secretion by circulating catecholamines. Following resection of a pheochromocytoma, all patients should have urinary catecholamines measured postoperatively and then on an annual basis.

Suggested Reading

Brunt LM, Soper NJ. Laparoscopic adrenalectomy. In: Arregui ME, Fitzgibbons RJ Jr, Katkhouda N, McKernan JB, Reich H, eds. *Principles of laparoscopic surgery: basic and advanced techniques.* New York: Springer-Verlag, 1995: 366–378.

Brunt LM, Doherty GM, Norton JA, Soper NJ, Quasebarth MA, Moley JF. Laparoscopic adrenalectomy compared to open adrenalectomy for benign adrenal neoplasms. *J Am Coll Surg* 1996;183:1–10.

Gagner M, Lacroix A, Bolte E, Pomp A. Laparoscopic adrenalectomy: the importance of a flank approach in the lateral decubitus position. *Surg Endosc* 1994;8:135–138.

Mercan S, Seven R, Ozarmagan S, Tezelman S. Endoscopic retroperitoneal adrenalectomy. *Surgery* 1995;118:1071–1076.

Peplinski GR, Norton JA. The adrenal glands. In: Zinner MJ, ed. *Maingot's abdominal operations*, 10th ed. Norwalk, CT: Appleton & Lange, 1996:723–760.

Prinz RA. A comparison of laparoscopic and open adrenalectomies. *Arch Surg* 1995;130: 489–494.

Scaljon WM. Adrenal glands. In: Skandalakis JE, Gray SW, Rowe JS, eds. *Anatomical complications in general surgery*. New York: McGraw-Hill, 1983:186–198.

Takeda M, Go H, Imai T, Nishiyama T, Morishita H. Laparoscopic adrenalectomy for primary aldosteronism: report of initial ten cases. *Surgery* 1994;115:621–625.

EDITOR'S COMMENT

Dr. Brunt has provided an excellent overview of the indications, techniques, and potential complications related to laparoscopic adrenalectomy. He has described in detail only one of several approaches to this operation. Additionally, there are multiple methods of managing the vascular pedicle during a laparoscopic adrenalectomy. Suture ligature of the vessels provides an excellent method of securing hemostasis. Clips may be applied to ligate the vessel in addition to or in lieu of suture material. Ultrasonic dissection is extremely useful during a laparoscopic adrenalectomy for providing hemostasis during the dissection of the periadrenal tissue while minimizing the risk of collateral coagulation injury. The harmonic scalpel is not recommended for division of the main arterial and venous supply to the adrenal gland.

The contraindications emphasized by Dr. Brunt for a laparoscopic approach to adrenalectomy place emphasis on oncologic concerns. While a prudent approach regarding adrenal carcinoma is warranted, there currently exists no scientific foundation to exclude the application of laparoscopic techniques in the management of adrenal cancer. The uncertain potential for recurrence or trocar-site implantation should be discussed at length with the patient as a portion of the informed consent process until adequate data are available. An appropriate curative cancer procedure should not be compromised in any manner to accomplish the procedure through smaller incisions. Potential complications associated with this procedure range from minor wound problems to life-threatening bleeding and death. The potential for a fatal air embolus secondary to a major venous injury should be kept in mind as the dissection of the vascular pedicle is carried out. A plan for management of inferior vena cava or renal vein bleeding should be designed prior to the initiation of the operation. The appropriate instrumentation for vascular control and conversion to an open procedure must be readily available.

Laparoscopic adrenalectomy is an excellent operation for the appropriately selected patient, when performed by an experienced laparoscopist. Specific courses or training for the performance of laparoscopic adrenalectomy are not currently available, but advanced laparoscopic skills are necessary.

W.S.E.

V

Small Bowel, Appendix, and Colon

35

Flexible Endoscopy of the Lower Gastrointestinal Tract

Christopher J. Bruce and John A. Coller

Anatomic Considerations and Instrumentation

Flexible endoscopy of the lower gastrointestinal (GI) tract, which encompasses both flexible sigmoidoscopy and colonoscopy, is an essential tool for the surgeon in the diagnosis and management of disorders of the colon and rectum. Although colonoscopy may seem to be simply an extension of flexible sigmoidoscopy, it is in fact a considerably more complex procedure. Flexible sigmoidoscopy is performed in the office setting without the need for sedation or a complete bowel preparation. In contrast, colonoscopy is technically more demanding, is associated with increased risks, and requires supervised training and certification for competence. However, the techniques of intubation of the rectum and sigmoid are similar for both procedures, and experience in one complements the other. Whether the flexible sigmoidoscope or colonoscope is used, redundancy and acute angulations of the colon pose problems requiring manipulative skills that often disappoint even the most resourceful endoscopist. A thorough knowledge of the anatomy of the colon and an understanding of the mechanics of the flexible endoscope and its interaction with the bowel are necessary for the performance of a safe and expeditious examination.

Flexible endoscopes are available from a wide variety of vendors. Most of these instruments use similar optical devices and differ mainly in length, diameter, and maneuverability. Diameters vary from 10 to 15 mm, while flexible sigmoidoscopes range from 60 to 71 cm in length and colonoscopes are typically 115 to 180 cm long. Pediatric colonoscopes (10 mm) can prove invaluable when a tight stricture prevents access with a standard instrument, but their inferior maneuverability limits their routine use. Maneuverability has improved greatly from the prototype instruments developed in the 1960s, which provided only two-way tip deflection, compared to modern-day devices that allow a full 360-degree articulation. All endoscopes have buttons for air insufflation and aspiration, as well as a water jet directed at the distal lens to clean away debris and mucus. Various devices such as biopsy forceps, diathermy snares for polypectomy, baskets for the removal of foreign bodies, grasping forceps, laser fibers, needle injectors, and balloon dilators may be inserted through the suction/accessory channel of the scope. Colonoscopes designed with two instrument channels are available for specialized procedures, such as a difficult polypectomy or acute bleeding, but these are somewhat stiffer than the standard, smaller-diameter, single-channel scopes and have a greater potential to cause patient discomfort.

A recent advance has been the introduction of video imaging as an alternative to fiberoptics. A small charge-coupled device chip, built into the endoscope tip, transmits coded data to an image processor that converts the electronic signal to a color picture on a video monitor. The video endoscope provides brighter images with superb resolution, while maintaining flexibility and ease in handling compared to its fiberoptic counterpart.

Each segment of bowel has its own distinct endoscopic characteristics. The anal canal and distal rectum may be evaluated with a retroflexion maneuver of the flexible instrument; however, the role of anoscopy and rigid proctosigmoidoscopy should not be overlooked. The rectum is recognized by its ample lumen and prominent semicircular valves. The rectosigmoid junction is approximately 15 to 20 cm from the anal verge, and this is the first major angulation that is encountered. The sigmoid colon turns toward the left and follows the convexity of the sacrum. Effectively negotiating the sigmoid colon is key to successful colonoscopy. Different processes may limit the mobility of the sigmoid, namely, scarring from previous surgery, pelvic sepsis, or irradiation. The descending colon–sigmoid junction is commonly an acute angle, but once past this obstacle, intubating the descending colon is usually not fraught with difficulty. The typical muscular rings help in negotiating the lumen as it runs a relatively straight course before turning medially and anteriorly at the splenic flexure. Not infrequently, a bluish discoloration may be seen here, representing the spleen through the relatively thin colonic wall. A distinctive gate-like fold is commonly seen just below the splenic flexure. Once around the splenic flexure, the characteristic triangular folds of the transverse colon are seen. Advancing the scope through the transverse colon is usually uneventful, unless a deep pelvic bend or gamma-loop is present. The hepatic flexure is identified by widening of the lumen and the presence of prominent arcuate folds that do not fully encircle the lumen. The blue color of the liver can be seen through the colonic wall where the right lobe of the liver causes a flattened impression on the superior aspect of the flexure. The ascending colon is usually short and dilated with prominent arcuate folds that do not fully encircle the lumen. The ileocecal valve is pointed toward the base of the cecum, and its orifice is usually not identifiable during colonoscopy. The location of the ileocecal valve can usually be seen as an indentation of a colonic valve approximately 4 to 6 cm above the appendiceal orifice or the blind end of the cecum. The appendiceal orifice and the ileocecal valve are the most reliable landmarks for confirming the position of the tip of the scope in the cecum.

Fluoroscopy during colonoscopy is an invaluable tool in the training of young endoscopists to gain an appreciation of both normal colonic anatomy and its variations. The colon is usually fixed at the rectum, descending colon, and ascending colon, allowing the sigmoid and transverse colon to move freely on their mesenteries. The amount of movement depends on the length of colon and the elasticity of the mesenteries. The sigmoid colon may take the shape of the Greek letter α, while a redundant transverse colon occasionally conforms to a γ configuration. Both the splenic and hepatic flexures may have a reversed configuration, and these are important to recognize because a straightening maneuver converting them to a normal orientation is often required. The mobility of the cecum is variable and depends on the extent of its posterior attachments. During negotiation of these difficult formations, it is often prudent to take advantage of this mobility, rather than trying to counter it.

Only by understanding the anatomy of the colon and its variations will one appreciate the complexity of the scope–colon interaction. The ease with which intubation of the colon can be accomplished depends on the smooth integration of several independent control mechanisms. In this chapter, each of the various maneuvers, namely, tip deflection, shaft torquing, advancement/withdrawal (dithering), and insufflation/aspiration of gas, are discussed separately and then collectively applied to intubation techniques.

Indications

Flexible Sigmoidoscopy

The indications for flexible sigmoidoscopy are similar to those for rigid proctosigmoidoscopic examination, but the flexible scope has been shown to be superior in terms of the length of colon examined, diagnostic yield, and patient compliance. In contrast, examination with the rigid scope is associated with fewer complications, is less time-consuming, requires less training to perform, and is more accurate in assessing the distance of a rectal lesion from the anal verge. Furthermore, flexible instruments are more expensive and require greater maintenance. Flexible sigmoidoscopy has been found to yield pathology three times more often than rigid sigmoidoscopy. However, the length of bowel that can be examined with the flexible endoscope is often overestimated. By placing a clip marking the point at which 60 cm of the flexible sigmoidoscope was inserted and then confirming its position with a barium enema examination, Lehman and colleagues found that in only 81% of patients was the entire sigmoid colon visualized. This study emphasizes the importance of utilizing various straightening maneuvers when negotiating the sigmoid colon.

Flexible sigmoidoscopy is not a substitute for colonoscopy or radiologic evaluation of the colon when a complete assessment of the entire colonic mucosa is indicated, such as when occult blood is present or when polyps have been documented. Flexible sigmoidoscopy indications can be divided into two main groups:

Diagnostic

Polyp or cancer screening,
Evaluation of GI complaints when colonoscopy is not indicated,
Interim polyp and cancer surveillance between colonoscopic examinations,
Evaluation of questionable radiographic findings within the range of the instrument,
Confirmation of radiographic findings within the range of the instrument,
Follow-up examination in patients with inflammatory bowel disease,
Differential diagnosis of diverticular disease and malignancy,
Inspection of colonic anastomoses within the range of the instrument.

Therapeutic

Detorsion of a sigmoid volvulus,
Removal of a foreign body within the range of the instrument,
Dilation of a stricture within the range of the instrument.

It should be specifically noted that electrocautery should not be used during flexible sigmoidoscopy unless the patient has undergone a complete purgative preparation as used for colonoscopy. Explosive mixtures of methane and hydrogen may be present if the colon has not be adequately cleansed.

Colonoscopy

There is a long-standing debate about the relative merits of contrast radiography versus colonoscopy, but each examination has its benefits and limitations. The advantages of double-contrast barium enema (DCBE) include its general availability, quick completion, lower cost, and low morbidity. In diverticular disease, a DCBE is actually superior at defining the number and anatomic distribution of the diverticula. For neoplastic disease, however, one study by Saito and associates showed that DCBE alone missed almost 50% of lesions in the rectosigmoid region that were detected by endoscopy. In addition, DCBE inevitably results in considerably more radiation exposure, requires a cooperative patient, and is not without potential complications such as perforation, bleeding, or barium peritonitis. Colonoscopy demonstrates greater surface detail for determining mucosal vascular patterns in inflammatory conditions or the presence of arteriovenous malformations. In addition to imaging, colonoscopy permits the performance of other diagnostic and therapeutic maneuvers, such as biopsy of abnormal mucosa and removal of polyps and foreign bodies. Primary colonoscopy without a preceding DCBE is indicated in specific clinical situations, such as when a patient has lower GI bleeding or when an index adenoma is discovered on rigid or flexible proctosigmoidoscopy. Primary colonoscopy is also indicated for patients at high risk for the development of colon and rectal neoplasia. This group includes patients with a strong family history of colon cancer and those with long-standing inflammatory bowel disease. It is generally agreed that colonoscopy supplements but does not replace DCBE in the evaluation of most colonic disorders. Indications for colonoscopy are outlined below:

Diagnostic

Evaluation of suspected (or equivocal) abnormalities on DCBE,

Presence of a polyp on sigmoidoscopy or DCBE,

Unexplained GI bleeding, either overt or occult,

Unexplained iron deficiency anemia,

Surveillance of colonic neoplasia,

High-risk patients for colonic neoplasia (strong family history),

Follow-up evaluation after prior colonic surgery,

Evaluation and follow-up of inflammatory bowel disease,

Clinically significant diarrhea of unexplained origin,

Intraoperative colonoscopy for localization of a lesion (e.g., polyp, bleeding source).

Therapeutic

Treatment of a bleeding lesion,

Excision of colonic polyps,

Reduction of a sigmoid volvulus,

Foreign body removal,

Decompression of a dilated colon,

Balloon dilation of a stenotic lesion (e.g., anastomotic stricture),

Palliative treatment of a stenosing or bleeding neoplasm.

There are relatively few absolute contraindications to endoscopic examination of the lower GI tract. Both flexible sigmoidoscopy and colonoscopy should not be performed in patients suspected of having a perforated viscus, severe acute diverticulitis, or fulminant colitis. Relative contraindications to performing these procedures include patients that are uncooperative, have a poor or inadequate bowel preparation, or have a poor general medical condition, such as a recent myocardial infarction or pulmonary embolism. Caution should be exercised in the presence of coexisting abdominal pathology, such as hypersplenism or aortic aneurysm.

Preoperative Patient Management

The success of the procedure is not entirely dependent on the technical skills of the endoscopist. In addition to an adequate bowel preparation, the patient's understanding of the procedure is very important. Experience has shown that well informed patients who fully comprehend the implications, circumstances, and potential risks and benefits of the endoscopy show less apprehension and less anxiety during it.

Conscious sedation is generally not required for flexible sigmoidoscopy but may be advantageous in certain circumstances, including children, extremely anxious patients, or those with painful perianal disease. Although recent studies question the need for the routine use of conscious sedation for colonoscopy, most endoscopy centers still use a combination of an opiate analgesic plus a benzodiazepine administered intravenously for this procedure. The American Society for Gastrointestinal Endoscopy (ASGE) has developed guidelines for the use of monitoring devices during conscious sedation, but mechanical monitoring techniques such as pulse oximetry and continuous electrocardiography are not a substitute for an alert and competent endoscopy assistant. It is also imperative that the endoscopist have a thorough knowledge of the pharmacology, indications and contraindications, recommended dosages, duration of action, side effects, and methods of reversal for each of the drugs used.

For flexible sigmoidoscopy, one or two saline or phosphate enemas are usually satisfactory for adequate visualization. Colonoscopy, on the other hand, requires a more complete bowel-cleansing program including dietary restriction and purgation. Since colonoscopy is usually performed as an outpatient procedure in a hospital, clinic setting, or office setting, most patients undergo bowel preparation at home. However, frail, elderly, and mentally retarded patients may require hospitalization for supervised bowel preparation. The extent of preparation required depends on the clinical indication; for example, a patient who has profuse diarrhea or has undergone a subtotal colonic resection will require much less preparation than an elderly patient with chronic constipation. According to ASGE guidelines, patients with active colitis and diarrhea should not receive enemas or lavage.

The most widely used bowel preparation for colonoscopy utilizes an electrolyte solution containing primarily sodium sulfate with polyethylene glycol (PEG) as an additional osmotic agent (Colyte, GoLYTELY). Due to problems with patient compliance, another, more palatable preparation has been sought. In a prospective study, Fleet Phospho-soda was shown to be safe, effective, less expensive, and better tolerated than the standard PEG preparation. Both techniques require a no-residue or low-residue diet 24 to 48 hours prior to colonoscopy.

Practice parameters have been published by the American Society of Colon and Rectal Surgeons regarding the use of prophylactic antibiotics. In general, a prophylactic antibiotic is not routinely indicated because lower GI endoscopy carries a low risk of significant bacteremia. However, in certain high-risk individuals, such as those with a prior history of infective endocarditis or with a prosthetic heart valve, surgically created systemic pulmonary shunt, or recent (less than 1 year) insertion of a prosthetic vascular graft, broad-spectrum prophylaxis is recommended. Medications including aspirin, nonsteroidal antiinflammatory agents, anticoagulants, and iron-containing compounds should be discontinued at least 1 week prior to colonoscopy.

Technique

Colonoscopic intubation is a marvelous example of the interaction between human and machine. Some examinations are rather straightforward, while a good many require at least some manipulations of note and a sufficient number of procedures challenges the examiner to draw from his or her bag of tricks, learned by experience, to accomplish the objective. It is vital that the endoscopist have a thorough understanding of the relationship of the relatively unforgiving scope and the variably compliant colon. If the colon were an absolutely fixed structure, a totally different instrument would have to be constructed to afford optimal intubation. There would be no manipulation of the organ itself; the instrument would simply be advanced and would follow the contour of the organ. But the colon is not rigid, and it is not fixed in position. Although there are areas of the colon that are relatively fixed, the wall of the colon at these points is usually still quite compliant. Consequently, unlike intubation of other structures, such as the esophagus, the ureter, and the aorta, successful colon intubation depends in great part on appropriate manipulation of the compliant structure.

Successful intubation makes use of a number of individual maneuvers. These include tip deflection, shaft torquing, and shaft dithering. Combinations of these maneuvers are used along with gas insufflation and deflation, patient positioning, and abdominal pressure.

Tip Deflection

Clearly, it is not difficult to see how the articulating deflection tip is the essential element of the colonoscope that makes retrograde examination of the colon possible. Deflection permits the endoscopist to look around a bend or fold to see in just which direction one needs to go. Folds can be pressed against the wall so that small lesions that might otherwise stay hidden are exposed. This articulation is essential during therapeutic maneuvers to aim a snare or biopsy forceps in the proper direction.

However, it is this very characteristic, the articulating tip, that becomes what is probably the single biggest impediment to intubation. For the novice endoscopist, it is also the most likely source of injury. As the tip is deflected from straight, a gentle curve forms along the distal 10 to 12 cm of the scope. As deflection increases to beyond the 90-degree level, the radius of this curve becomes shorter, and the distribution of forces against the colon wall changes abruptly. The application of extreme deflection to both dial controls does not have the effect that one would predict. This can be observed with any scope before the procedure is started. Maximum application of the up/down dial will give a 180-degree deflection in the up direction (Fig. 35-1). Similarly, maximum application of the left/right dial will give 180 degrees to the right. One would think that maximum application of both dials would give 180-degree deflection halfway between up and right. Instead, while there is a little movement of the tip between the two quadrants, there is a much more dramatic overtightening of the deflection bend to well beyond 180 degrees. Longitudinal advancement of the scope no longer follows the tip of the scope but is instead distributed along the side of the deflection bend against the bowel wall. At a deflection of 180 degrees, which can usually be achieved with extreme application of a single deflection dial, the force to the bowel wall is over a relatively small surface area (Fig. 35-2). This can easily lead to serosal injury or frank perforation of the bowel. The operator should be aware of this situation simply by recognizing that he or she is using extreme deflection and that as the scope is advanced, the bowel under view seems to be getting farther away rather than closer. It is impossible for the scope to advance along the axis of the colon with this configuration. On occasion, extreme deflection must be used to find the lumen. But once it is found, the deflection should be eased, preferably to less than 90 degrees, before attempting further advancement of the scope.

The following generalizations relative to deflection control can be made:

1. Use the least amount of tip deflection possible.
2. Use the up/down dial for most deflection needs and resist applying both controls.
3. Release deflection when the lumen is found.

Shaft Torquing

Torquing the colonoscope shaft is an essential maneuver for effective intubation and good surface visualization during extubation. If the shaft is straight and there is a modest deflection to the scope's tip, the lumen can most easily be located by twisting or torquing against the inside surface of the bend in the colon. This torquing into the lumen is often more effective than searching for the lumen with the deflection tip.

As more scope is introduced, the response to torquing becomes more complex. If there is a simple loop in the sigmoid, an alpha loop, the effect of clockwise torquing, especially when combined with withdrawal, is to reduce the loop, accordionizing the sigmoid onto the scope without loss of intubation distance. Once reduced, this sigmoid loop will usually have a tendency to reform, particularly if counterclockwise torque is applied during scope advancement. Therefore, if a reduced redundant sigmoid loop tends to reform, it is best to advance the scope while maintaining clockwise torque. One can readily sense this tendency to reform the loop in the following way: Apply clockwise torque, and the scope will appear to advance; apply counterclockwise torque, and the scope will tend to lose ground.

On occasion, the sigmoid will have two major complete loops that are created during intubation. Nearly always, both these loops are reducible. However, in this situation, the first loop is removed by counterclockwise rotation and the second by clockwise rotation. Removing both loops is usually essential before intubation proximal to the descending colon can be accomplished. Once both loops are removed, the sigmoid is once again most likely to stay straightened by maintaining clockwise torque. This is not always compatible with the task to be accomplished at the distal end of the scope.

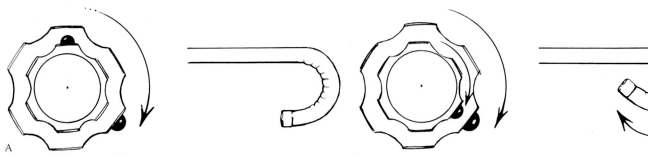

Fig. 35-1. Tip deflection. Dual coaxial control knobs determine the degree of tip deflection. **A:** *Full deflection of the up/down or the left/right controls results in approximately 180 degrees of deflection.* **B:** *Full deflection of both controls results in overdeflection.*

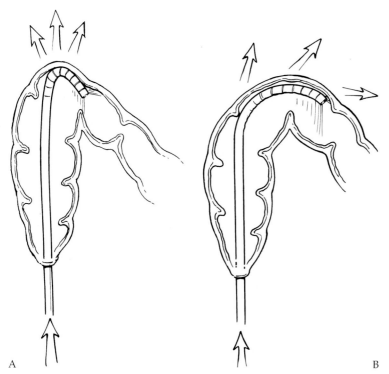

Fig. 35-2. Tip deflection. **A:** *If severe tip deflection is applied around a flexure, the bend in the deflection tip becomes the leading edge of the scope pushing against the bowel wall.* **B:** *Once the lumen is visualized, the deflection tip should be flattened to transmit advancement force in a forward direction.*

Torque also becomes very important in manipulations around the hepatic flexure. If the transverse colon is able to be held in the upper abdominal cavity (e.g., the scope takes a straight line to the hepatic flexure), clockwise torque is usually beneficial as the gently deflected tip is directed down the ascending colon. If the transverse colon is redundant, stretching down toward the pelvis, the hepatic flexure is then approached from below. By the time when the ascending colon is viewed, there is rather sharp deflection of the tip. Once again, gentle scope withdrawal along with clockwise torquing and intermittent desufflation, all combine to broaden the hepatic flexure and drop the scope down into the ascending colon and cecum.

During extubation, torquing is an extremely important manipulation for efficient examination of the colon surface. As the scope is withdrawn, the right hand is maintained on the shaft, while the left hand supports the scope head, with the thumb free to move the up/down control to make small deflections at the time. Torquing while the scope is withdrawn and readvanced 10 to 20 cm at a time affords a thorough view of the entire colon surface. This permits the colon that has

been accordionized onto the scope to be dropped off a bit at a time. If, rather than torquing, the scope is simply withdrawn while both hands of the dial controls are used, the view behind prominent folds is likely to be insufficient. In addition, if the colon is quite redundant, it will likely fly off the scope at an uncontrollable rate.

The following generalizations relative to shaft torquing can be made:

1. Clockwise torque straightens the sigmoid; counterclockwise torque promotes loop formation.
2. Torquing is more effective than tip deflection for negotiating bends and for surface examination.

Scope Advancement/Withdrawal (Dithering)

If the colon were a simple noncompliant tube without redundancy or irregularity, colonoscopic intubation would be a rather simple endeavor of advancing the scope while following the tip. Occasionally, especially if there has been a prior sigmoid resection, colonoscopy may be no more demanding than simple scope advancement.

However, straight advancement usually promotes the development of loops, stretching the colon. When progression of the scope is not impeded by severe tip deflection, the colon can be encouraged to accordionize along the length of the scope. This is most likely to occur if the scope is repeatedly advanced and withdrawn. In some areas, particularly distally, this is most effective if it is performed with small, rapid strokes, referred to as dithering the scope. Elsewhere, such as in the transverse colon, this maneuver is often performed with long, gentle strokes of 30 to 50 cm.

Gas Insufflation

Insufflation of gas is essential to effective visualization and safe performance of colonoscopy. However, insufflation should be used sparingly. Excess gas can cause distention that results in extreme discomfort and vasovagal reaction. If the examination is undertaken into the distal ileum, only a very short period of insufflation is necessary to result in a great deal of small bowel gas accumulation. Excessive intraluminal gas often works against intubation progress, particularly at a flexure or during negotiation of a loop. The distention effectively pushes the more proximal side of the loop or flexure away. The corner to be negotiated becomes more acute and consequently harder to negotiate. This is most apparent at the hepatic flexure when the deflection tip is sharply angulated into the distal ascending colon. As air is introduced, the ileocecal valve in the distance is seen to move farther away. Consequently, the endoscopist should take advantage of this while removing air during clockwise torque. The ascending colon will collapse back onto the scope, bringing the cecum into closer proximity to the end of the scope.

Patient Positioning

Although no single patient position is distinctly preferable to others, the construction of most endoscopes and the right-handedness of most physicians favor a left lateral position for the patient. Colostomy and ileostomy patients may be examined in the lateral position or supine. In patients with poor or absent abdominal wall muscle tone (e.g., paraplegia, prior dehiscence), examination in the prone position may overcome this disadvantage. An elastic abdominal binder can also provide artificial abdominal wall resistance.

Changing the position of the patient during the examination when forward advancement of the scope is difficult is often very helpful. After all, rotating the patient 90 degrees to the left is similar to torquing the scope 90 degrees to the right. Once an excessively redundant sigmoid loop has been reduced, broad pressure from just right of the umbilicus and directed toward the left iliac fossa will discourage its reformation. Likewise, in the case of a redundant transverse colon dipping deeply into the pelvis, abdominal pressure from just below the umbilicus and directed cephalad will assist entry into the ascending colon.

An alternative—and our preference—is to apply a more generalized abdominal pressure by rolling the patient into the prone position once the sigmoid has been negotiated and is felt to be reduced. This rotation is not performed unless there is a hang-up of intubation progress. Most frequently, this position change is made at the hepatic flexure. If there is no need to change patient position, the entire examination is performed in the left lateral decubitus position. If there is difficulty with entry into the ascending colon in the prone position, the patient is rotated into the right lateral decubitus position. This is frequently the last additional maneuver that one has to perform in the case of a recalcitrant hepatic flexure. It is presumed that in this position pressure from the liver may encourage the flexure to be flattened just enough to allow the scope to slip down to the ascending colon.

Many endoscopists prefer to perform much of the examination with the patient in the supine position. We find that this position is somewhat difficult for the endoscopist. If the scope is brought out between the legs, there is minimal working room between the anus and the bed for shaft manipulation. If the scope is brought out beneath the raised right leg, one is continually having to reposition the leg, unless there is an assistant to attend to this.

General Approach to the Examination

The expert colonoscopist is able to perform an expedient and thorough examination by avoiding the formation of bowel loops that interfere with intubation while utilizing loops that facilitate intubation. The experienced colonoscopist can detect from subtle cues the suggestion that a loop is starting to form: the loss of one-to-one correspondence of instrument insertion and image movement, a gradual increase in resistance to forward motion, and signs of patient discomfort. Withdrawing the scope and losing ground to gain more proximal intubation on subsequent attempts is almost always a prudent initial maneuver.

Advancement of the scope should nearly always be under direct or nearly direct vision. The slide-by technique, whereby the tip of the scope is burrowed into the colon wall, should be avoided. Although it is often necessary to have less than a totally clear view of the lumen, insertion for any distance when the endoscopist is blind to lumen orientation is strongly discouraged. One should be suspicious that one is treading on dangerous ground if the colon surface blanches and the patient experiences pain.

There is a strong tendency not to want to lose ground. During a difficult colonoscopy, one may have spent some time getting to an area that seems to have no outlet. Because of an abrupt bend, the next segment eludes identification. The endoscopist may persist in vain, searching for a way out and not wanting to give up what has already been accomplished. Instead, it is more likely that the difficulty is being accentuated by failure to ease the scope. One should never be reluctant to withdraw shaft length when progress is arrested. Often, withdrawal is the very maneuver that is needed to advance. This point cannot be overemphasized.

Although not required for most examinations, fluoroscopy is invaluable in the training of young colonoscopists and often helpful during difficult cases. Although flexible sigmoidoscopy and colonoscopy will usually be performed in the office setting, it is worthwhile observing a few examinations under fluoroscopic control to appreciate the various configurations assumed by sigmoidoscope.

Before the start of the procedure, it is important to check that the scope is working properly, that the suction line is attached and switched on, and that air insufflation and lens washing are adequate. Examination of the mucosa for abnormalities and therapeutic interventions for polyps, tumors, and so on should usually be performed when the scope is slowly withdrawn after maximum intubation.

Sedation

Without sedation, colonoscopic manipulation of the entire colon is often uncomfortable and sometimes frankly painful. Although it has clearly been shown that a modest proportion of patients can undergo colonoscopy without sedation, we prefer to initiate the examination after administration of a minimal intravenous dose of meperidine hydrochloride (Demerol) and midazolam hydrochloride (Versed). Supplementation of this base dose, if required, will be determined by the patient's sensory and physiologic reactions. We feel that the primary objective is not to avoid medication but rather to provide a safe and comfortable examination. If necessary, naloxone hydrochloride (Narcan) is used after the procedure to expedite recovery.

Examination Performance
Rectal Examination

A digital rectal examination is an essential starting point in every patient. First, it is not unusual to find significant local pathology, such as large hemorrhoids, an anal fissure, or a prostatic nodule or mass. Second, digital rectal examination allows one to gauge anal sphincter tone; poor tone will make it difficult to retain insufflated air. A tight or strictured anus may require some gentle dilation to accommodate the scope. Third, the examination mentally prepares the patient to have the instrument inserted and provides lubrication for tube insertion.

Anorectal Intubation

After lubrication of the instrument tip, but not the lens, the scope is inserted with lateral pressure and not end on. Insertion requires two hands: one to separate the buttocks and the other to hold the tip of the scope. It is helpful to have an assistant hold the control section or place it over the endoscopist's right shoulder. Due to anatomic and technical factors, it is often difficult to initially visualize the rectal ampulla. The anal canal is oriented in the direction of the umbilicus for a short distance, at which point it joins the rectal ampulla whose axis is abruptly posteriorly oriented toward the sacrum. However, the tip deflection mechanism may respond poorly at this level, since the greater portion of the deflecting system resides outside the anorectum and has nothing to work against. It is not until the bulk of the deflecting section has traversed the sphincter mechanism that the examiner starts to have control of tip deflection. Once the scope is inserted approximately 10 cm above the anal verge, tip deflection responds properly, and the middle and upper rectum can be clearly visualized. An understanding of the limitations of tip deflection when restricted by the sphincter mechanism can avoid this initial problem. Proximal intubation for the next few centimeters into the rectosigmoid and distal sigmoid colon does not generally represent a problem even to the most inexperienced, but once the rectosigmoid is reached (15 to 20 cm), the stage is set for the technique of sigmoid intubation.

With the instrument tip seated in the rectosigmoid, one takes the control section with the left hand while the right hand is positioned on the shaft. Throughout the rest of the examination, this hand placement will be the basic posture used.

Sigmoid–Descending Colon Intubation

Properly negotiating the sigmoid colon is often challenging and sets the stage for the remainder of the examination. Avoidance of bowel-loop formation not only is more comfortable for the patient but also allows a more expeditious examination of a greater length of colon with less length of scope. The three methods of intubating the sigmoid colon are intubation by elongation, looping (alpha maneuver), and accordionization (dithering/torquing). Although these are distinctly different techniques, they are not mutually exclusive solutions to the same problem. In recognizing these basic differences in technique, the operator can more deliberately and effectively control the process of intubation.

Intubation by Elongation

Intubation by elongation merely means that the scope is inserted until either the scope no longer advances or no more endoscope is available. One relies on the deflection tip to lead the way as long as a lumen is in view. This is the simplest and most perfunctory approach: no fancy maneuvers, just doing what appears obvious. Indeed, this is probably the most common approach undertaken with flexible fiber-

optic sigmoidoscopy. Most often, this technique merely stretches a redundant sigmoid until the first major angulation is encountered. If there is only a single sigmoid loop and the sigmoid–descending junction is reached, further intubation may be accomplished with clockwise torquing, shaft withdrawal, and flattening of the deflection tip (Fig. 35-3).

Intubation by Looping (Alpha Maneuver)

The relative mobility of the sigmoid colon, which is fixed proximally and distally, is best appreciated under fluoroscopy, where a loop resembling the Greek letter α is intentionally created to permit passage of the tip of the scope into the distal descending colon, followed by reduction of this loop for further advancement. The alpha loop is promoted by counterclockwise rotation of the scope while it is advanced through the sigmoid until the tip is securely within the descending colon. By encouragement of the mid- to proximal sigmoid, through counterclockwise torque, to occupy the right lower quadrant, the sigmoid–descending junction is flattened, providing a less acute angle to negotiate. Next, the loop is reduced by withdrawing the scope while maintaining clockwise rotation on the shaft (Fig. 35-4). One can assume that this reduction is working when it is observed that the image advances despite considerable scope withdrawal. Once derotation has been accomplished, the scope can be advanced toward the splenic flexure by maintaining clockwise torque during advancement of the shaft. This technique is an expeditious way to negotiate the entire sigmoid colon when only a moderate degree of redundancy is present and multiple, tightly adherent loops are absent. If several adherent loops are present, this technique is technically impossible and only serves to increase the level of discomfort for the patient. If the loop cannot be reduced on entry into the descending colon, then one should maintain the loop, traverse the splenic flexure, and attempt derotation after the scope is well into the transverse colon. No effort should be made to derotate with the deflection tip hooked around the splenic flexure.

Intubation by Accordionization (Dithering/Torquing)

This approach most consistently enables the examination of the greatest length of

colon with the least amount of scope. In contrast to the first two techniques, in which the scope is advanced up into the colon, the accordionization method should be viewed as bringing the colon down onto the scope.

This technique employs simultaneous application of both dithering and torquing. While the shaft is being advanced approximately 6 to 10 cm, a small amount of counterclockwise torque of about 45 to 60 degrees is applied. The process is reversed by applying clockwise torque and simultaneous withdrawal of the scope for the same length. This cycle is repeated in a rhythmic manner at a rate of about one cycle per second, but without net advancement of the shaft. It is useful to hold the shaft of the scope close to the anus to avoid overadvancing. Although the first few dithering/torquing cycles may appear to accomplish little, by rhythmically continuing this motion, the cumulative effect is to pleat a short segment of sigmoid colon onto the scope. As one acquires experience with this technique, it soon becomes apparent that the cyclic rhythm, amount of torque, degree of tip deflection, and shaft advancement distance are all variables that can by altered to achieve maximum effect. If this technique is successful, the descending colon can be readily intubated as far as the splenic flexure by applying clockwise torque during shaft advancement with minimal deflection of the tip. With this approach, the endoscopist is attempting to straighten the colon as he or she progresses, rather than intentionally creating a loop that has to be removed later. Several principles should be kept in mind when this technique is performed:

1. This method should be started early in the process of intubation in the rectosigmoid to minimize the deflection angle.
2. It is not always necessary to see the entire lumen, but one should avoid pushing directly into the colonic wall.
3. The endoscopist should resist the temptation to advance the scope as soon as the lumen is seen, and should continue with this process to maximize the accordionization of the entire sigmoid colon.
4. Excessive gas insufflation is a deterrent to accordionization.
5. If this technique is not successful, one can then proceed with intentional looping.

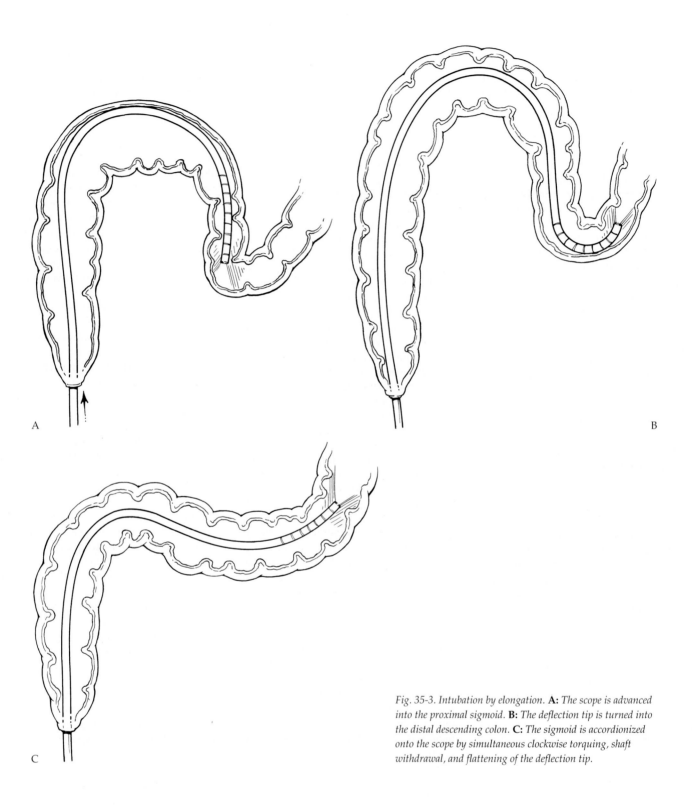

Fig. 35-3. Intubation by elongation. **A:** *The scope is advanced into the proximal sigmoid.* **B:** *The deflection tip is turned into the distal descending colon.* **C:** *The sigmoid is accordionized onto the scope by simultaneous clockwise torquing, shaft withdrawal, and flattening of the deflection tip.*

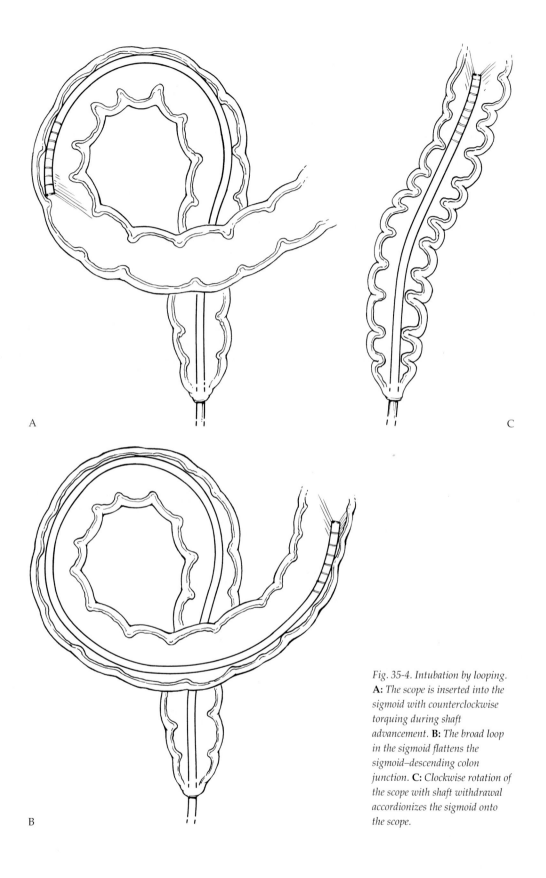

Fig. 35-4. Intubation by looping.
A: *The scope is inserted into the sigmoid with counterclockwise torquing during shaft advancement.* **B:** *The broad loop in the sigmoid flattens the sigmoid–descending colon junction.* **C:** *Clockwise rotation of the scope with shaft withdrawal accordionizes the sigmoid onto the scope.*

Splenic Flexure and Transverse Colon Intubation

If the sigmoid colon has been accordionized onto the scope and is straightened into a gentle smooth curve, negotiating the splenic flexure is usually not difficult. Even if the flexure is quite high, the deflection can be rotated into the distal transverse colon without much difficulty. It is at this point that one must remember the hazard of excess deflection bend. As soon as there is visual acquisition of the transverse colon, the degree of deflection must be eased to provide a gentle bend of less than 90 degrees. The lumen may be somewhat obscured by the outside wall, but it need not be entirely lost from view. However, in approximately 5% of individuals, there is reversal of the splenic flexure, which turns to the patient's left due to medial migration of the flexure on a false mesentery. This anomaly can cause difficulty in intubating the transverse colon and hepatic flexure. A straightening maneuver is required that involves counterclockwise rotation of the instrument shaft to convert the splenic flexure to a normal orientation. Entry into the transverse colon typically reveals a well defined triangular lumen.

Advancing the colonoscope through the transverse colon is usually uneventful. Difficulty may arise, however, if the transverse colon is redundant and assumes the configuration of the Greek letter γ. Changing the patient's position, using external pressure above the umbilicus, and/or the dithering/torquing are useful techniques when progress is impeded. In the transverse colon, dithering/torquing is often best performed with long, 30- to 50-cm strokes rather than the short strokes used in the sigmoid.

Hepatic Flexure and Ascending Colon

The hepatic flexure is recognized by widening of the lumen and a bluish discoloration of the wall superiorly where the liver is in close proximity. The lumen to the ascending colon may be readily apparent, or sharp angulation may lead one to believe that the cecum has been reached. Inability to proceed without also identifying specific cecal landmarks is nearly always evidence of incomplete intubation.

If the transverse colon can be negotiated straight across or straight down from a high splenic flexure, then intubation into the ascending colon can usually be accomplished by clockwise torquing, flattening of the deflection tip, and simultaneous gas aspiration (Fig. 35-5). These three mechanisms combine to drop the scope directly into the cecum. If the transverse colon is

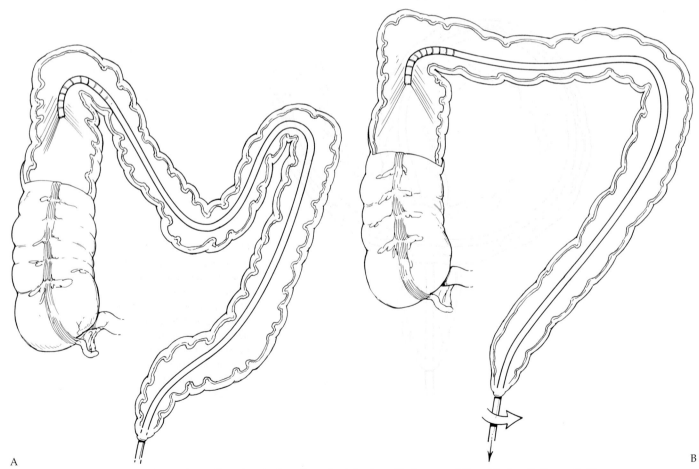

A   B

Fig. 35-5. Intubation of ascending colon. **A:** *Ascending colon is in view with sharp angulation at the hepatic flexure.* **B:** *The transverse colon is elevated into the upper abdomen during clockwise torquing and shaft withdrawal.* (continued)

excessively redundant, it may not be able to be maintained in the upper abdomen, even with abdominal pressure. In such cases, the midtransverse colon will have to be intentionally toward the pelvis, and the scope will approach the hepatic flexure from below rather than from across. Effectively, the deflection will have a 180-degree bend to negotiate. Once again, clockwise torquing, flattening deflection, and gas aspiration now combined with shaft withdrawal will be required for entry into the ascending colon. Negotiation of redundant proximal bowel is facilitated by removal of sigmoid colon loops. If the hepatic flexure is not readily passed, then the patient should be positioned onto the abdomen. For hepatic flexures that continue to defy intubation, it is most helpful to place the patient in the right lateral decubitus position.

Cecal and Distal Ileum Intubation

The most reliable landmarks for visual confirmation of reaching the cecum are the appendiceal orifice, the tenia confluence, and the ileocecal valve. Palpation of the right lower quadrant with concomitant movement of the colon endoscopically and transillumination of the abdominal wall in the right iliac fossa are less dependable signs. Fluoroscopy is most helpful, but it must be kept in mind that the cecum is not always in the right iliac fossa.

On occasion, it is important to intubate the distal ileum, especially in the evaluation of inflammatory bowel disease. The success rate for this maneuver increases with experience. The tip of the colonoscope should be partially deflected toward the ileocecal valve, which lies 5 to 7 cm proximal to the base of the cecum. By slow withdrawal of the colonoscope, the tip of the scope is pressed against the valve orifice, prying on the upper lip of the valve. With gentle air insufflation, a view of the distal ileum is apparent by the ground-glass appearance of the mucosa. Insufflation should be kept to a minimum, as small bowel gas rapidly extends proximally and is difficult to remove, leading to considerable postprocedure discomfort.

Withdrawing the Scope

Inspection of the mucosa for abnormalities is usually best performed on withdrawal of the scope. Residual debris will have been removed from the colon, and the endoscopist will already have obtained an overview of the work that has to be performed. A systematic survey of the entire colonic mucosa is mandatory, and this is more easily and completely performed on withdrawal than on insertion. Reinspection of areas behind haustra and around flexures may be required. The instrument may have to be advanced and withdrawn intermittently over varying distances to ensure that abnormalities have not been overlooked. This is best performed by keeping the right hand on the scope shaft and torquing a slightly bent deflection tip first against one fold and then the next. If a considerable length of colon has been accordionized onto the scope, it will have to be removed a small amount at a time. Steady withdrawal will result in the colon flying off the scope without adequate evaluation.

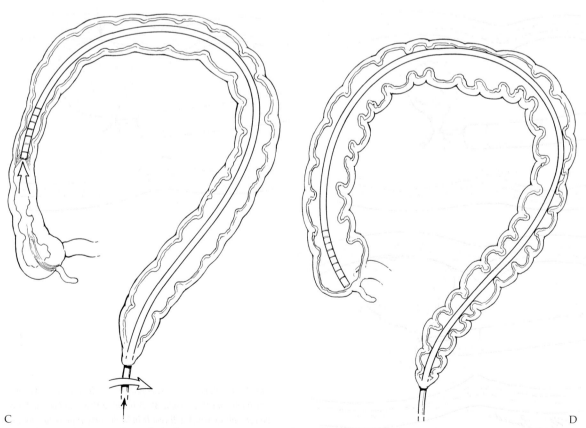

C

D

Fig. 35-5. (Continued) **C:** *Shaft advancement is accompanied by clockwise torquing, flattening of the deflection tip, and evacuation of air from the distended colon.* **D:** *Complete intubation to the cecum.*

Biopsy

Biopsy of a polyp or mass may be performed with (hot) or without (cold) the use of electrocautery. Electrocautery should only be used in patients who have undergone a complete bowel preparation to avoid the potential for explosion. All colonic biopsy catheters should be inserted under direct vision, with the tip of the scope kept centered within the lumen at all times to reduce the risk of perforation. Keeping the scope as straight as possible with minimal tip deflection will allow easier passage of the catheter.

Hot biopsy is a useful technique that destroys small polyps by coagulating the base of the lesion to provide hemostasis while preserving the tissue inside the forceps for pathologic evaluation. The tip of the polyp is grasped by the forceps and pulled into the lumen, with care taken to avoid injury to the surrounding bowel. This process is facilitated by placement of the lesion in the 5-o'clock position prior to its being grasped. Only a brief application of coagulating current is necessary to cause blanching at the base of the polyp, and with gentle traction the lesion is removed.

Snare Polypectomy

One of the most significant advances in colon surgery during the past few decades has been the development of endoscopic polypectomy. The contrast between an 8-day hospitalization for an open colotomy polypectomy and a colonoscopy polypectomy performed in less than 1 hour is dramatic.

Several disposable snares are available for polyp excision. It is our preference to use a hexagonal snare for most polyps. This configuration is most likely to hold its shape during difficult positioning or multiple excisions. For small lesions too large for hot biopsy management, a minisnare is convenient.

Prior to snare application, it is best to rotate the scope so that the polyp base is located at about 5 o'clock in the field of view.

This will ensure that the polyp stays in view while the snare loop is positioned over the polyp. In the case of a pedunculated polyp, the snare loop can be snugly tightened on the stalk under direct view. For a sessile polyp that has to be removed in a piecemeal fashion, each lobule excised can be clearly visualized.

Several techniques may be used for removing larger sessile lesions. A two-channel scope permits the endoscopist to combine both a snare and a grasper to manipulate the polyp. The snare is passed through one channel. A grasper or large biopsy forceps is placed in the second channel and passed out through the open loop of the snare. In this fashion, the recalcitrant polyp can be encouraged into the snare. On occasion, it is helpful in removing a sessile polyp to elevate it above the plane of the colon wall by injecting saline into the submucosa. This provides a greater margin between the muscularis propria and the polyp base. In addition, the greater tissue hydration makes for more efficient electrocoagulation.

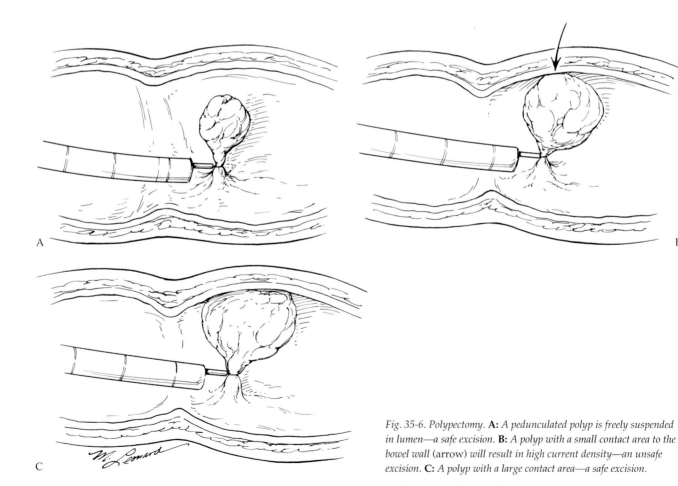

Fig. 35-6. Polypectomy. **A:** *A pedunculated polyp is freely suspended in lumen—a safe excision.* **B:** *A polyp with a small contact area to the bowel wall (arrow) will result in high current density—an unsafe excision.* **C:** *A polyp with a large contact area—a safe excision.*

Proper application of electrocautery is essential for effective and safe polypectomy. Empirically, we have found that there is no single combination of cutting and coagulation current or wattage that has to be used. A colonoscopist gradually develops confidence in his or her own electrosurgery method, and it is surprising how varied these techniques may be. The general approach that we have found effective uses short bursts of monopolar blended cutting current while squeezing on the snare. By the use of intermittent bursts, deep tissue cooling is permitted, minimizing the likelihood of a full-thickness burn. Average-size polyps are suspended within the lumen to avoid collateral injury. If the polyp is too large to avoid wall contact, then surface contact should intentionally be maximized to avoid pinpoint areas of high current density (Fig. 35-6). At no time should electrosurgery be undertaken in the absence of a thorough colon preparation.

Removal of small tissue segments with the hot biopsy forceps requires a somewhat different technique. The hot biopsy forceps presents a very small surface area and consequently results in high current density with rapid, deep injury. Consequently, the grasped tissue should be well tented into the lumen. Two or three short bursts of current are usually sufficient to provide homeostasis and tissue destruction at the base. This can be seen as the development of pallor for a couple of millimeters around the jaws. At that point, the tissue specimen is abruptly drawn back into the scope channel. If one waits for the forceps to cut through on its own, an excess amount of wall damage will result.

Blood vessel lesions, such as vascular ectasia, are best treated with a bipolar electrode. Complete destruction can be accomplished with minimal risk of full-thickness wall injury.

Malignant polyps, even if technically removable at colonoscopy, may require subsequent resection. Such lesions are unlikely to be palpable at the time of operation. Accurate localization is important, particularly if intraluminal landmarks are absent and fluoroscopic control is unavailable. We use an injection of particulate India ink applied submucosally with a sclerotherapy needle. This marker will persist indefinitely.

Complications

Complications following flexible sigmoidoscopy from eight collected series of more than 29,000 examinations between 1979 and 1988 reported no deaths, three perforations, and 10 patients with rectal bleeding. The most common problems following flexible sigmoidoscopy were syncope and persistent abdominal pain. Following colonoscopy, the reported overall complication rate is higher when therapeutic maneuvers are employed, but the mortality remains low (0 to 0.02%) in large series. The most common complications after diagnostic colonoscopy are perforation (0.16%) and bleeding (0.03%), while bleeding is more common (0.66%) than perforation (0.33%) following polypectomy.

Hemorrhage is usually from a biopsy site but may also occur from a laceration to the mucosa by the endoscope or, less commonly, from tearing of the mesentery or splenic capsule. It is usually more common after resection of a large polyp or from inadequate coagulation of the stalk. Management depends on the timing and severity of the bleed. Bleeding evident at the time of colonoscopy can usually be controlled by reapplication of the snare to the pedicle, if present, with electrocautery or by strangulation of the bleeding point for 5 to 10 minutes, if additional electrocautery is deemed unsafe. Delayed hemorrhage typically occurs 10 to 14 days later due to sloughing of the coagulum, and the majority of these bleeds are self-limited and respond to conservative management. The incidence of delayed hemorrhage is increased in patients who have a coagulopathy or take an anticoagulant or antiplatelet therapy. Repeat endoscopy with sclerotherapy or epinephrine injection, electrocautery, bipolar cautery, or heater-probe application may be necessary to control delayed hemorrhage. Rarely, angiographic techniques and/or operative intervention may be the only solution.

Perforation may be the result of excessive mechanical force or pneumatic pressure. Most perforations are located in the sigmoid colon and occur in patients with preexisting colonic disease. Perforation is diagnosed during the endoscopic procedure if intraperitoneal structures are visualized, or should be suspected if the inability to maintain insufflation is encountered. Following endoscopy, perforation is suspected on the basis of symptoms and physical findings and confirmed by the presence of free intraperitoneal air on abdominal radiographs. The management of patients with perforation depends on the timing of presentation and the clinical status of the individual. If perforation is recognized immediately, surgical intervention is warranted and usually consists of primary repair. The approach to symptomatic patients with pneumoperitoneum should also be operative, especially when it is associated with underlying colonic disease. Controversy exists in the management of asymptomatic or minimally symptomatic patients with delayed presentation and pneumoperitoneum. There are reports of successful nonoperative therapy in selected stable patients with a well prepared bowel and without peritonitis or obstruction. Management in these individuals consists of bowel rest and the administration of broad-spectrum antibiotics with careful observation for deterioration in clinical status.

Postpolypectomy coagulation syndrome or transmural burn syndrome occurs from a full-thickness thermal injury to the colon that is sealed by adjacent organs or omentum. Patients usually present with abdominal pain, fever, and leukocytosis without pneumoperitoneum 6 to 24 hours later. Care should be taken during polypectomy to avoid damaging the colonic wall opposite the lesion by minimizing contact time with the wall during application of the diathermy current. Bowel rest and broad-spectrum antibiotics with careful clinical follow-up are usually sufficient treatment for these patients.

Less frequently reported complications following colonoscopy with or without polypectomy are listed in Table 35-1. Despite these potential problems, flexible endoscopy of the lower GI tract can be undertaken with a very low morbidity. Awareness of these morbidities serves as a reminder to all endoscopists, particularly those in the learning phase, to maintain a high level of suspicion in all cases because many of these complications occur in seemingly innocuous procedures.

Table 35-1. Less Frequent Complications Following Colonoscopy With or Without Polypectomy

Oversedation (respiratory depression, hypotension)

Medical problems (myocardial infarction, arrhythmia, aspiration, pulmonary embolism)

Thrombophlebitis from intravenous injection

Pneumothorax and tension pneumothorax

Retroperitoneal pneumoperitoneum, pneumomediastinum, pneumopericardium

Pneumatosis coli

Retroperitoneal abscess

Chemical colitis

Exacerbation of an inguinal hernia

Mechanical problems (entrapped snare, incarceration of endoscope within a hernia)

Specimen labeling errors resulting in incorrect surgical resection

Loss of polyp

Bacteremia

Gaseous explosion

Vascular graft thrombosis

Appendicitis, diverticulitis

Postendoscopy distention

Colonic obstruction

Volvulus

Suggested Reading

Baillie J. *Gastrointestinal endoscopy: basic principles and practice.* Oxford: Butterworth–Heinemann, LTD, 1992.

Berk JE, ed. *Bockus gastroenterology,* 4th ed. Philadelphia: WB Saunders, 1985.

Coller JA. Technique of flexible fiberoptic sigmoidoscopy. *Surg Clin North Am* 1980;60:465–479.

Corman ML. *Colon and rectal surgery,* 3rd ed. Philadelphia: JB Lippincott Co, 1993.

Hunt RH, Waye JD, eds. *Colonoscopy: techniques, clinical practice and color atlas.* Cambridge: Chapman and Hall, Ltd., 1981.

Lehman GA, Buchner DM, Lappas JC. Anatomical extent of fiberoptic sigmoidoscopy. *Gastroenterology* 1983;84:803.

Mazier WP, Levien DH, Luchtefeld MA, Senagore AJ, eds. *Surgery of the colon, rectum, and anus.* Philadelphia: WB Saunders, 1995.

Saito Y, Slezak P, Rubio C. The diagnostic value of combining flexible sigmoidoscopy and double-contrast barium enema as a one-stage procedure. *Gastrointest Radiol* 1989,14:357–359.

Silvis SE, ed. *Therapeutic gastrointestinal endoscopy,* 2nd ed. New York: Igaku-Shoin, 1990.

The Standards Task Force. American Society of Colon and Rectal Surgeons. Practice parameters for antibiotic prophylaxis—supporting documentation. *Dis Colon Rectum* 1992;35:278–285.

Yamada T, ed. *Textbook of gastroenterology,* 2nd ed. Philadelphia: JB Lippincott Co, 1995.

EDITOR'S COMMENT

Flexible endoscopy remains a required component of surgical residency training. Many surgeons, for various reasons, fail to apply these skills in their practice of surgery. The surgeon who acquires and maintains excellent skills in flexible endoscopy possesses crucial elements in an armamentarium for the diagnosis and treatment of gastrointestinal diseases. Furthermore, the skills used in colonoscopy are similar to those necessary for the application of flexible endoscopy in other areas (e.g. bronchoscopy, choledochoscopy, esophagogastroduodenoscopy).

The authors have provided the reader with an excellent overview of flexible endoscopy of the lower GI tract while providing numerous helpful technical tips. The complications associated with diagnostic and therapeutic endoscopy must be understood by the endoscopist. Early recognition of complications such as perforation can mean the difference between a rapid repair and recovery versus life-threatening sepsis and multiple operations.

W.S.E.

36

Laparoscopic Surgery of the Small Bowel

Brett C. Sheppard and Karen E. Deveney

Anatomy

The small bowel is approximately 22 feet long. After the initial sweep of the duodenum, the jejunum begins at the ligament of Treitz and continues for approximately 40% of the proximal length of the small bowel. The transition between jejunum and ileum is not as grossly well defined as the transition from duodenum to jejunum and is somewhat arbitrary. The luminal diameter usually decreases as the small bowel proceeds distally, and the more distal segments of the small bowel are more prone to serosal tears with endoclamps, perhaps because of the thinner serosa in the ileum.

The major vascular supply for the small bowel is the superior mesenteric artery. Intestinal branches of the secondary mesenteric arteries arborize to form arcades within the mesentery. These supply the small intestine with straight end arteries. The venous drainage of the small intestine roughly parallels the arterial side and drains into the superior mesenteric vein to enter the portal vein. The lymphatic drainage of the small bowel starts within the Peyer's patches of the submucosa. These lymphoid aggregates usually are more plentiful in the ileum than in the jejunum. They may cause intussusception or perforate in patients with tuberculosis or human immunodeficiency virus (HIV)–associated coccidioidomycosis. Lymph follows along the superior mesenteric artery and ultimately flows into the cisternae chyli. The supporting mesentery of the small bowel is attached to the posterior abdominal wall. This site of attachment is usually just to the left of L-2 and drapes inferiorly toward the right sacroiliac joint. Unlike the relatively fixed mesentery of the colon, the broad-based small bowel mesentery is extremely mobile.

The unique aspects of small bowel anatomy are advantageous for the laparoscopic surgeon and pose some unique operative challenges. The ligament of Treitz is a consistent landmark and can be used to identify the duodenal-jejunal transition and provide orientation. The inferior mesenteric vein is just to the left and posterior to the ligament and can be injured inadvertently. The mobility of the mesentery facilitates mobilization. If the mesentery is not shortened from inflammatory or neoplastic processes, the small bowel is easily exteriorized for manual inspection and or anastomosis. However, the same characteristics can make operative exposure of the small bowel difficult. The convolutions of the small bowel and its mobility require frequent changes in patient positioning to optimize exposure. The absence of an easily identifiable transition from jejunum to ileum can also make orientation difficult in the distal segments. It may be difficult initially to determine whether the surgeon is running the bowel proximally or distally until the terminal ileum or ligament of Treitz is identified. The delicate nature of the small bowel cannot be overemphasized, and it requires meticulous, gentle manipulation to avoid a serosal injury or enterotomy.

Contraindications and Indications

The laparoscopic approach to surgery of the small bowel has several contraindications:

Multiply operated abdomen with dense adhesions
Positive visceral slide test results
Excessive bowel dilatation
Malignancy (e.g., adenocarcinoma, sarcoma)
Rapidly progressing peritonitis with sepsis

The indications for laparoscopic surgery of the small bowel are identical to those for open procedures and are listed in Table 36-1. The most common indication remains acute small bowel obstruction secondary to adhesions. An incarcerated hernia is the second most common cause of intestinal obstruction. Infectious diseases, particularly in recent immigrants, immunosuppressed patients, or patients infected with

Table 36-1. Indications for Surgery

Acute small bowel obstruction
Adhesions
Infectious diseases (e.g., tuberculosis, coccidioidomycosis)
Inflammatory bowel diseases
Inflammatory mesenteric disease
Hernia
Construction or take-down of ileostomy
Jejunal interposition grafts
Meckel's diverticulum, other omphalomesenteric persistence abnormalities
Malignancy (e.g., carcinoid, lymphoma)
Second-look procedures for visceral ischemia
Upper gastrointestinal hemorrhage
Evaluation of chronic abdominal pain
Evaluation of motility disorders[a]
Laparoscopically assisted intraoperative endoscopy[a]

[a] Investigative procedure.

HIV can be a cause of intestinal obstruction. Laparoscopic evaluation of chronic abdominal pain remains controversial. Several small, nonrandomized studies have had mixed outcomes. Table 36-1 indicates procedures that are investigative. For example, totally laparoscopically assisted intraoperative small bowel endoscopy has been performed in animals only. Evaluation of small bowel motility by laparoscopic electrode placement is a promising investigative clinical tool, but it has been applied in a limited number of individuals.

Laparoscopic surgery is not indicated for patients with known dense adhesions. This group of patients includes trauma patients treated with an open abdomen, patients with prior intraabdominal catastrophes or with multiple reoperations. A positive visceral slide evaluation may also be a relative contraindication to proceeding with laparoscopic surgery. Although trocars can usually be safely placed in most abdomens, excessive bowel dilatation is a relative contraindication for laparoscopic small bowel surgery. The dilated loops often obscure visualization and make safe handling difficult. Rapidly progressing sepsis is a relative contraindication, because the longer operative times may not allow for a prompt therapeutic window in patients who are acutely deteriorating. Because of the absence of conclusive clinical trials on the safety of laparoscopic oncologic resections, small bowel resection for conditions other than small carcinoids or lymphomas should be undertaken with caution.

Perioperative Management

Approximately 85% of all small bowel obstructions are caused by adhesions, hernias, or tumors. Most obstructive episodes result from adhesions. For these patients, history, examination, and a plain radiographic abdominal series are often sufficient to make a diagnosis. A chest radiograph should be done to exclude pneumonia or subdiaphragmatic air; a plain radiograph of the abdomen can appear normal in cases of closed loop obstruction. In some cases, the decision to operate may rely on clinical progression alone. In patients without prior abdominal surgery, hernia and benign or malignant neoplasms should be considered stronger possibilities. Patients with a prior history of melanoma, lung cancer, or primary gas-

trointestinal malignancy may present with small bowel obstruction as the first indication of metastatic disease. In equivocal cases, small bowel enteroclysis has been the preferred imaging study. Ultrasound may help to identify an incarcerated incisional hernia. Computed tomography (CT) scans of the abdomen have been used to evaluate the small bowel. Proponents of CT cite the ability to detect inflammatory or neoplastic disease and the ability to determine the level of obstruction as distinct advantages over other imaging modalities. The sensitivity and specificity of CT in this respect has been reported as equivalent or superior to enteroclysis studies

The visceral slide test has proved to be a useful adjunct in patients with prior abdominal operations undergoing laparoscopic evaluation for mechanical small bowel obstruction. This ultrasound evaluation can be used immediately before surgery to help determine safe trocar entry sites. With this technique, a linear-array transducer is used to maximize the scanning window aperture. A restriction of visceral slide is defined as intestinal movement of less than 1 cm in the longitudinal plane on deep inspiration. This finding indicates dense adhesions, and trocars should not be placed at these sites. This test is most accurate at the level of the umbilicus or above.

Patients undergoing evaluation for upper gastrointestinal hemorrhage require urgent resuscitation and endoscopy. In the appropriate clinical setting, a technetium pertechnetate Meckel's scan may be useful to confirm the diagnosis. We have not otherwise found nuclear medicine studies beneficial in the evaluation of upper gastrointestinal hemorrhage. Angiography in actively bleeding patients can often provide definitive localization and temporary therapy. We ask our angiographers to inject blue dye through the catheter to mark the small bowel where the hemorrhage has been localized. This staining allows laparoscopic identification of the precise small bowel segment involved, minimizes operative time, and minimizes the length of the resection required.

Operative Technique
Instrumentation

Successful laparoscopic small bowel surgery requires several critical instruments. Because more small bowel injuries

are caused by manipulation than by trocar entry, it is essential to have Glassman or similar types of endoclamps. These clamps have in common broad blades with low-profile serrations to grasp the intestine without crush injury. Noncrushing clamps should also have slightly rounded ends so that sharply angulated corners cannot cut into friable intestine. We prefer nonratcheted instruments because of the frequent need to grasp and release loops of small bowel.

Additional instruments to facilitate laparoscopic small bowel surgery are an angled laparoscope of 30° or 45° and bipolar cautery or bipolar scissors. Angled laparoscopes with 5-mm or smaller diameters may be useful for the initial phase of surgery for adhesive disease. They may also be useful as a secondary scope placed in a separate quadrant to image dense adhesions not seen well by the initially placed angled scope. The angled, 10-mm laparoscope is more than sufficient for most situations. Bipolar instrumentation is preferred to minimize the potential for thermal injury to adjacent structures or intestinal loops. If bipolar cautery is not available, monopolar energy can be used judiciously. Short-burst monopolar energy minimizes the risk of thermal energy flow through overly desiccated tissue and minimizes remote tissue injury.

Abdominal Entry and Exploration

Patients are positioned supine for small bowel procedures. The modified lithotomy (European) position tends to make these procedures more difficult. Initial trocar positions for the patient with a reoperative abdomen can be determined by the visceral slide method. If this test is not available, a site away from the prior incision is chosen. We try to avoid umbilical port entries in patients with prior midline incisions. For patients with prior lower or mid-abdominal incisions, the optimal initial trocar entry site is just to the left and below the xiphoid process or in the left upper quadrant. For patients with upper midline or transverse incisions, an initial subumbilical port is chosen. The surgeon must consider the proximity of the aortic bifurcation and iliac vessels when placing those ports.

Although safe entry into the reoperative abdomen can be accomplished with the Veress needle, liberal use of open entry (Hasson) is preferred. The use of optically clear trocars has not replaced the need for the Hasson technique.

Use of an upper abdominal or off-midline trocar entry is facilitated by placing at least one of the monitors at the foot of the bed. This monitor position allows subsequent dissection to proceed in line with the camera angle. For most procedures, one monitor positioned at the foot and another at the head of the patient provides strain-free imaging. It may be necessary to move the monitors during the procedures to provide clear fields of view and efficient dissection. A separate monitor can provide split-screen viewing if it becomes necessary to use a secondary laparoscope. After the initial port placement, the angled laparoscope is used to survey the density and pattern of adhesions. Subsequent port placements are done under direct visualization. A Maryland-type dissector and bipolar cautery are used to clear the adhesions subadjacent to the initial port to provide a wider field of view for additional port placement. Other patient-specific ports can then be placed as necessary to finish dissection. If dense adhesions prevent safe dissection, consideration should be given to placement of a second laparoscope. The port for a second laparoscope should be placed with an open technique. Use of a 5-mm laparoscope can provide the requisite visualization to safely continue the dissection.

Consideration should be given to converting to an open procedure when dense adhesions are encountered, because studies show a significantly higher reoperative rate because of inadvertent complications in laparoscopic procedures that occur in abdomens with very dense adhesions. For patients without prior abdominal procedures, our standard port placement is shown in Fig. 36-1.

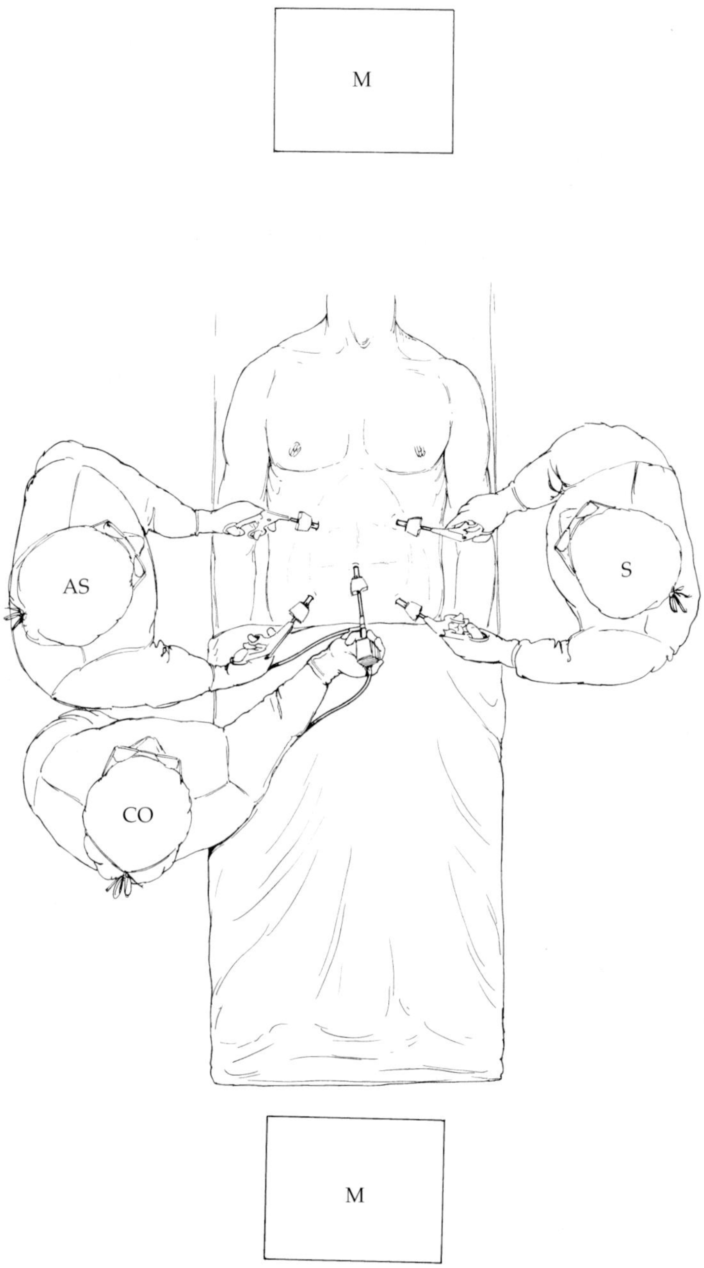

Evaluation of the small bowel is usually started near the ileocecal valve in most cases. This landmark is usually easier to identify than the ligament of Treitz. The initial part of procedure can be facilitated by positioning the patient in a Trendelenburg position with a 30° plane to the patient's left. The bowel is gently grasped and run with a two-handed technique using the Glassman endoclamp and a hand-over-hand sequence to gently grasp each successive segment. As the bowel is run proximally, the patient should be taken out of the Trendelenburg position and placed in a neutral position or a reversed

Fig. 36-1. Standard port placement for laparoscopic small bowel evaluation in patients without prior abdominal surgery. Monitors are placed at the foot and head of the bed to facilitate the axis of orientation as the procedure progresses. (CO, camera operator; AS, assistant surgeon; M, monitor; S, surgeon.)

Trendelenburg with a 30° or greater plane to the patient's right. The time spent to reposition frequently is rewarded with greater exposure and a more rapid and safer procedure. The ligament of Treitz is best identified by elevating the transverse colon and mesocolon with Glassman endoclamps, placing the patient in a reverse Trendelenburg position, and planing 30° to the right. In cases of significant adhesions or prior contamination, the inferior mesenteric vein may be closely adherent to the ligament of Treitz and prone to injury.

Applications
Small Bowel Resection

Resection of the small bowel usually can be performed through the same ports that were placed for the initial exploration of the abdomen. The technique of laparoscopic small bowel resection may be applied to a variety of purposes and pathology. Strictured or vascularly compromised small bowel segments can be identified by the laparoscope. Similarly, malignancy can be easily identified. Resection for malignancy requires adequate oncologic margins that should not be compromised to proceed with a laparoscopic procedure. These margins are thought to be 5 to 10 cm of normal bowel on the side of the lesion, with the appropriate wedge of mesentery encompassing the lymphatic drainage.

More difficult to identify may be benign lesions such as leiomyomas or Peutz-Jeghers polyps. In some cases, these can be identified more readily if endoscopic charcoal injection is done within 24 hours of surgery. Small bowel resection for upper gastrointestinal hemorrhage is greatly facilitated by injection of dye during angiography that stains the serosa and supporting mesentery of the localized segment. After the dye is injected, the angiographic catheter should be withdrawn to avoid its transection during resection.

The small bowel to be resected is grasped by Glassman endoclamps to provide tension and to stretch the mesentery to help identify vessels. The segment to be resected can also be temporarily sutured to the anterior abdominal wall. This technique facilitates the procedure and frees port sites for other instruments. Before starting the resection, transillumination of the mesentery may be necessary. We have found that the best way to provide this is by using a second 5-mm laparoscope while decreasing the intensity of illumination from the primary laparoscope and shifting its light tangentially to the mesentery.

Dissection is started by scoring the mesentery with hook cautery. After this, we use the suction/irrigator in the nondominant hand and the harmonic scissors in the dominant hand to divide the vessels and mesentery (Fig. 36-2). These instruments complement each other nicely, because the suction/irrigator can be used to provide tension for dissection and to keep the field clear. The harmonic scissors can be used for dissection and for hemostasis. If harmonic scissors are not available, the standard endoclip device can be used to individually clip vessels and divide them. Alternatively, the 30- or 60-mm gastroin-

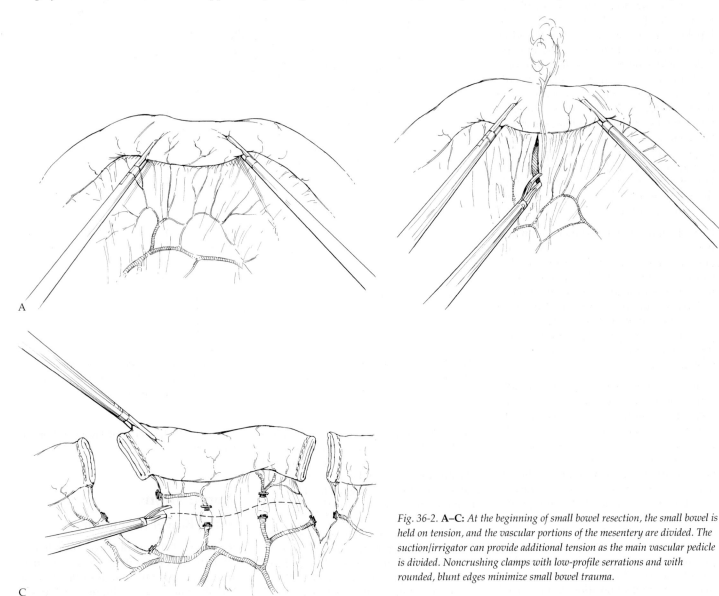

A

B

C

Fig. 36-2. **A–C:** *At the beginning of small bowel resection, the small bowel is held on tension, and the vascular portions of the mesentery are divided. The suction/irrigator can provide additional tension as the main vascular pedicle is divided. Noncrushing clamps with low-profile serrations and with rounded, blunt edges minimize small bowel trauma.*

testinal anastomosis endoscopic cutting stapler with vascular staples can be substituted. We have found that the 30-mm device is often easier to maneuver and to place accurately the 60-mm device. However, its use requires more cartridges to complete the mesenteric dissection, more instrument exchanges, and slightly more operative time.

After the division of the mesentery, the bowel is divided with a 30-mm endoscopic stapler. We routinely place the resected segment in an endo-bag before retrieval, because the bag protects the small bowel when it is harvested for free jejunal grafts and protects the wound from potential bacterial or neoplastic contamination.

Small bowel anastomosis can be performed extracorporeally through a small utility incision if there is adequate mobility of the mesentery. After exteriorization, the small bowel should be inspected to ensure that it is not twisted. An anastomosis is then performed with a standard two-layer, hand-sewn technique, and the bowel is returned to the abdominal cavity. Alternatively, a stapled functional end-to-end anastomosis can be performed extracorporeally or intracorporeally. For the stapled anastomosis, the bowel segments are aligned along their antimesenteric borders. Cautery is used to make a small stab enterotomy in the antimesenteric border of each segment of the small bowel to provide access for the endoscopic stapler blades (Fig. 36-3). The blades of the 60-mm endoscopic stapling device are then placed into each of small bowel enterotomies. This process requires slow, gentle manipulation of the small bowel over the endoscopic stapler blades. The blades cannot be forcefully thrust down the lumen of the small bowel without tearing the bowel tissue or contaminating the field. Before firing the stapler, an angled laparoscope is used to inspect the position of the endoscopic stapler and the site of anastomosis when the procedure is being performed intracorporeally. After stapling, the remaining confluent enterotomy can then be closed with sequential firing of the endoscopic stapling device transversely, or it may be hand sewn. The defect in the mesentery is then closed with interrupted, intracorporeally tied sutures of silk. Fascial defects are closed as necessary.

Stricturoplasty

Stricturoplasty has proven to be a useful procedure to preserve small bowel length in patients with Crohn's disease. Short strictures can be treated by a modification of the Heineke-Mikulicz technique for pyloroplasty, and longer strictures can be managed with a Finney-type procedure. This procedure usually can be performed through the ports used for initial exploration.

The bowel is gently grasped with Glassman-type endoclamps, and the area of stricture is identified. Unlike the previous technique of bowel resection, it is unwise to suture the small bowel to the anterior abdominal wall for traction because of the risk of sinus or fistula formation. After positioning the bowel to undergo stricturoplasty, the stricture is divided with bipolar scissors. Sutures are then placed to orient the enteroplasty and to provide traction. The procedure is completed with interrupted, intracorporeally placed sutures of 2-0 or 3-0 silk (Fig. 36-4).

Meckel's Diverticulum

Surgical therapy of Meckel's diverticula is reserved for symptomatic lesions only. Simple diverticulectomy is adequate for patients presenting with obstruction or inflammation. Segmental resection that includes adjacent peptic ulceration of the

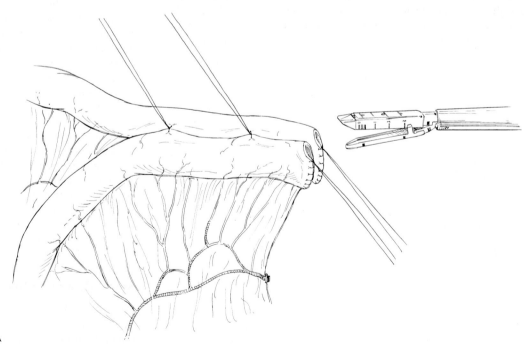

A

Fig. 36-3. **A:** *In creating a functional end-to-end anastomosis, the bowel is aligned along its antimesenteric border and approximated distally with a single stitch. Traction on this stitch can help position the stapling by providing countertension. The blades of the 30-mm gastrointestinal anastomosis endoscopic cutting stapler are gently placed in the enterotomies in the small bowel.* (continued)

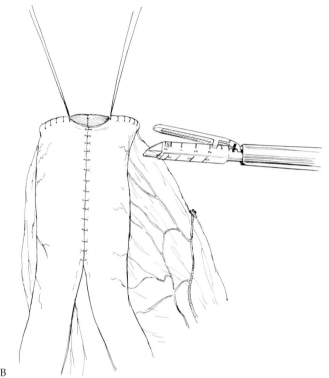

B

Fig. 36-3. (Continued) **B:** *GIA stapling of the resulting confluent enterotomy.*

viewing monitors are positioned on the patient's right side near the head and foot. A 10-mm umbilical port is placed and the abdomen inspected. Subsequent patient-specific ports are usually placed in the lower midline, right lower quadrant, and lateral to the umbilicus on the right. Only two ports plus the camera access are required for simple diverticulectomy. Segmental resection procedures usually require an additional one or two trocar sites. After exploration, the ileocecal region is identified and the small bowel run in a retrograde fashion to identify the Meckel's diverticulum. Traction is then applied near the tip of the Meckel's diverticulum with a Glassman endoclamp. The vascular supply to the diverticulum is isolated, doubly clipped, and divided. For simple diverticulectomy, the endoscopic cutting stapler is placed across the base of the diverticulum and fired after satisfactory positioning is confirmed. Depending on the width of the diverticulum base, the endoscopic stapler may need to be fired several times (Fig. 36-5).

Segmental resection is performed in a fashion similar to that for small bowel resection. The Meckel's diverticulum provides a useful traction handle and is grasped with a noncrushing clamp. After its blood supply has been ligated and the mesentery of the segment containing the Meckel's diverticulum has been divided and ligated or stapled, the segment is removed by proximal and distal firing of the endoscopic stapler. Two small stab enterotomies are then made several centimeters away from either side of the diverticular base. In a fashion analogous to that described for small bowel resection, the blades of the 60-mm endoscopic stapling device are then slipped into each enterotomy and the small bowel milked up over the tines of the blade. The stapling device is then fired and the resulting confluent enterotomies are closed with an additional transverse application of the endoscopic cutting stapler. Any mesenteric defect is subsequently closed.

Small Bowel Ischemia

Intestinal ischemia is a moderately common cause of the acute abdomen. Clinical diagnosis is often difficult, particularly in the postoperative period. Laparoscopic evaluation can potentially minimize nontherapeutic laparotomies when an ischemic bowel is suspected.

ileal mucosa is necessary in cases of a bleeding Meckel's diverticulum. Meckel's diverticulectomy can be performed with a single umbilical camera port and a solitary 5-mm port in the right lower quadrant through which the diverticulum is grasped after insufflation. This port site

can then be enlarged to a utility incision through which the surgeon can exteriorize the small bowel and perform an extracorporeal procedure. In cases that preclude this approach, such as significant adhesions or obesity, the same procedure can be accomplished intracorporeally. The

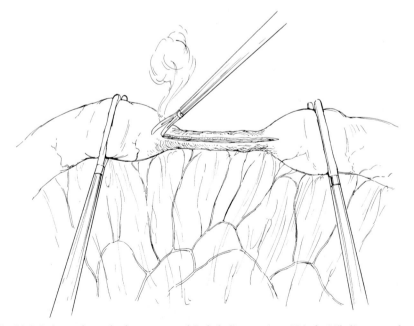

Fig. 36-4. Stricturoplasty of a short segment of Crohn's disease using a Heineke-Mikulicz enteroplasty.

Planned second-look laparoscopy after open or closed resection for ischemic bowel can be facilitated by placement of access trocars before closing. One port placed to the left and one port placed to the right of the umbilicus away from the midline incision provide initial access to begin a second-look procedure. Access site sterility can be maintained with an occlusive dressing, over which an Ioban drape is placed. Alternatively, a sterile glove can be used to cover the port site. Subsequent procedures may then be accomplished in the intensive care unit with appropriate sedation of the patient. Use of the laparoscopic Doppler may help determine small bowel viability in some cases. Laparoscopic resection within 1 cm of a normal Doppler signal from the terminal mesenteric vessels usually is sufficient to allow anastomotic healing without difficulty.

Postoperative Care and Surgical Complications

Most patients undergoing laparoscopic small bowel resection require less analgesia and ambulate sooner than patients who undergo similar open procedures. Patients may be able to aliment by the second postoperative day. Patients undergoing simple lysis of adhesions or Meckel's diverticulectomy may be discharged by postoperative day 2. Oral nutrition should await clear evidence of resolution of ileus. Principles of postoperative care should not differ from those after open procedures: patients with distended abdomens or who have no bowel tones are not ready to eat, whereas patients with good bowel tones who have a soft, nondistended abdomen are ready to begin alimentation.

Postoperative complications are similar to those experienced with open procedures. The most common of these after lysis of adhesions is an unrecognized enterotomy. This injury usually results from manipulation of the small bowel without noncrushing clamps or with excessive tension. These patients present with the classic signs of fever, tachycardia, and diminished urine output. Pain is out of proportion to that expected after a laparoscopic procedure. Abscess formation may also occur late after an anastomotic leak, even after the patient has been discharged. Although plain abdominal films may show free air or a collection of gas bubbles, a CT

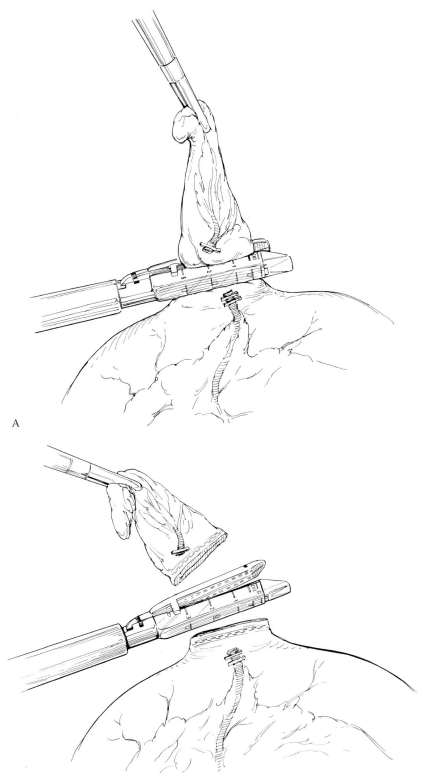

A

B

Fig. 36-5. **A,B:** *Meckel's diverticulectomy with close apposition of the gastrointestinal anastomosis endoscopic cutting stapler to the intestinal lumen.*

scan of the abdomen is frequently needed to identify possible hematoma, abscess, or phlegmon.

Postoperative bowel obstruction may also occur, as it does after open procedures. Oral contrast studies or water-soluble contrast enemas should be performed to evaluate for anastomotic obstruction or internal hernia after the CT scan has excluded other possibilities. In the absence of infectious or mechanical causes, most postoperative obstructions resolve with nonoperative therapy.

Outcomes of Laparoscopic Procedures

Anecdotal reports of laparoscopic treatment of small bowel obstruction have suggested that this procedure can be safely performed and that it may result in earlier discharge than open procedures, particularly in the geriatric age group. In larger series, patients with small bowel obstruction undergoing lysis of adhesions had an average length of hospital stay of 2.5 days, with a return to normal activity in to 4 to 17 days. Conversion rates for lysis of adhesions approximated 25% in collected series. The most common reason for conversion was the presence of dense adhesions that made dissection unsafe. The most common complication of laparoscopic lysis of adhesions is a missed enterotomy. In some series, reoperation for intestinal perforation is more common in groups treated by laparoscopy than those with open procedures. Overall, laparoscopic lysis of adhesions appears to be safe and efficacious in patients who have simple adhesive bands. Other causes of small bowel obstruction, including incarcerated hernia and malignant adhesions, are more difficult to treat laparoscopically and result in greater conversion rates.

Success rates for laparoscopic lysis of adhesions in the therapy of chronic abdominal pain range from 7% to 50%. The highest rate of success is reported in European series. Whether this success represents a distinct patient population or results from patient selection is not clear. Serious complications, such as primarily bowel perforation, are similar to those seen in laparoscopy for acute small bowel obstruction. Long-term follow-up is necessary to help determine outcomes. Laparoscopic Meckel's diverticulectomy or segmental resection appears to be safe and efficacious and results in shorter hospital stay and earlier return to normal daily activities.

The paucity of large series in regard to laparoscopic segmental bowel resection, stricturoplasty, jejunal harvest for interposition, and second-look laparoscopy make conclusions difficult. Anecdotal reports from specialized centers suggest that these procedures can be safe and result in decreased patient morbidity. They may be cost effective, but additional experience is needed to provide data for definitive conclusions.

Suggested Reading

Easter DW, Cuschieri A, Nathanson LK, Lavelle-Jones M. The utility of diagnostic laparoscopy for abdominal disorders: an audit of 120 patients. *Arch Surg* 1992;127:379–383.

Francois Y, Mouret P, Tomaoglu K, Vignal J. Postoperative adhesive peritoneal disease. *Laparosc Treat Surg Endosc* 1994;8:781–783.

Franklin ME, Dorman JP, Pharand D. Laparoscopic surgery in acute small bowel obstruction. *Surg Laparosc Endosc* 1994;4:289–296.

Freys SM, Fuchs KH, Heimbucher J, Thiede A. Laparoscopic adhesiolysis. *Surg Endosc* 1994;8: 1202–1207.

Iberti TJ, Salky BA, Onofrey D. Use of bedside laparoscopy to identify intestinal ischemia in postoperative cases of aortic reconstruction. *Surgery* 1989;105:656–689.

Kolecki RV, Golub RM, Sigel B, et al. Accuracy of viscera slide detection of abdominal wall adhesions by ultrasound. *Surg Endosc* 1994;8: 871–874.

Navez B, d'Udekem Y, Cambier E, Richir C, de Pierpont B, Guiot P. Laparoscopy for management for non-traumatic acute abdomen. *World J Surg* 1995;19:382–387.

Reissman P, Wexner SD. Laparoscopic surgery for intestinal obstruction. *Surg Endosc* 1995;9: 865–868.

Slutzki S, Halpern Z, Negri M, Kais H, Halevy A. The laparoscopic second look for ischemic bowel disease. *Surg Endosc* 1996;10:729–731.

Teitelbaum DH, Polley TZ, Obeid F. Laparoscopic diagnosis and excision of Meckel's diverticulum. *J Pediatr Surg* 1994;29-495-497.

EDITOR'S COMMENT

Many disorders affecting the small bowel are appropriate for management using laparoscopic surgery techniques. The coordinated, two-handed operative skills used in laparoscopic surgery are basic to all advanced laparoscopy. Fortunately, the ability to practice the maneuvers used in laparoscopic surgery of the small bowel is easily accomplished in inanimate and animate modes. Hand-over-hand manipulation of rope or rubber tubing in a trainer box can be worthwhile preparation for this type of surgery. The animate model adds the texture and degree of tissue friability that closely mimics human intestine.

The location of the ports used in laparoscopic surgery of the small bowel is highly variable and depends on surgeon preference and individual patient pathology. I routinely use only three ports for most small bowel procedures. These ports include the Hasson entry port and two other ports triangulated toward the quadrant containing the primary pathology. When multiple port sites are needed, I attempt to use minilaparoscopic instrumentation at those sites where deemed appropriate. The use of minilaparoscopic instrumentation and alternate energy sources, types of graspers, stapling devices, and suture material is highly variable and depends on the surgeon's experience. The chapter authors' emphasis on the importance of selecting atraumatic instrumentation warrants reinforcement. The inadvertent intestinal injury is the Achilles heel of laparoscopic surgery of the small bowel.

Diseases affecting the small bowel often increase the friability of the tissues, thereby increasing the likelihood of injury during manipulation. Patients with Crohn's disease, those with intestinal obstruction with dilated bowel, and patients on long-term steroids are examples of those at increased risk of bowel wall injury. Recognition and repair or resection at the time of operation is crucial. Ischemic intestine is also easily damaged. The ability to differentiate normal from ischemic intestine can range from being very simple to virtually impossible. The surgeon faced with determining bowel viability should readily convert to a laparoscopic assisted or an open operation if laparoscopic techniques prove inadequate to determine if ischemia exists.

W.S.E.

37

Laparoscopic Appendectomy

Jeffrey G. Tucker and Bruce J. Ramshaw

The success of laparoscopic cholecystectomy has prompted a revolution in general surgery and changed the way that surgeons approach intraabdominal pathology today. Since Kurt Semm reported the first laparoscopic appendectomy in 1983, the procedure has increasingly been utilized, and now prospective evaluations have been completed. Even though laparoscopic treatment for appendicitis has been documented to be a feasible and safe alternative to conventional methods and has enjoyed relative success to date, there remains skepticism in the surgical community with respect to its widespread implementation.

Anatomic Considerations

Appendiceal anatomy should be well known to all practicing surgeons; however, when attempting the laparoscopic approach, one does well to remember several points, since the advantage of finger dissection is removed. The only portion of the appendiceal anatomy that remains constant is the origin of the base of the appendix on the posteromedial aspect of the cecum distal to the ileocecal valve. This is due to the embryologic origin where the anterior tenia coli forms a complete outer muscular layer around the appendix. The remaining appendix is completely mobile during development, and its final position depends on the rotation of the cecum and the fixation of the retroperitoneal attachments to the side wall of the abdomen or pelvis. The blood supply is uniform, arising from the terminal ileocolic artery branches, but the mesoappendix may lie posterior to the ileum or lateral or posterior to the cecum, depending on the retroperitoneal or intraperitoneal orientation and fixation of the

appendiceal tip. When the cecum is fully rotated in its development, the appendix usually has avascular side wall attachments separate from the mesoappendix (Jackson's veil), which must be divided with care and preferably without electrocautery, given the common proximity to the iliac vessels and right ureter. Laparoscopically, these attachments will be the first bands encountered laterally as the appendiceal tip is rotated medially for mobilization, and can be best visualized with an angled lens from the umbilicus as dissection is initiated. Occasionally, when the appendix rotates anteriorly into the abdomen or pelvis, it may become adherent to the ileum or other organs. When the appendix lies adjacent to the ileum, the anterior bands to the mesentery are avascular, and electrocautery should again be avoided, if possible, since conduction along the adhesions is likely and thermal injury to the small bowel possible. Since identification of the base of the appendix and mesoappendix is paramount to a successful laparoscopic appendectomy, full mobility of the entire appendix is necessary, and thorough lysis of the above attachments becomes an important part of the initial dissection.

Diagnostic Considerations/Indications

Although appendicitis remains the most common cause of acute surgical abdomen, the diagnosis continues to pose a challenge. The history and physical examination may disclose the classic triad of fever, anorexia, and right lower quadrant pain in combination with exquisite tenderness at McBurney's point. In most patients with acute appendicitis, fever is low-grade and

rarely in excess of 37.5°C. The white blood cell (WBC) count is mildly elevated and usually demonstrates a high percentage of band cells. In patients with perforated appendicitis, high fever and WBC count, generalized peritoneal signs, and systemic signs of septic shock may become evident. Appropriate laboratory workup should include a complete blood cell count with differential, a blood chemistry profile, and urinalysis. Abdominal radiographs may be of benefit if a fecolith is demonstrated in the right lower quadrant. When early diagnostic laparoscopy is practiced, it is especially important to exclude the urinary tract as a possible source of pain or infection, since it does not lend itself to laparoscopic examination. Many patients will demonstrate microscopic hematuria when an inflammatory process exists in the right lower quadrant. Intravenous pyelogram should be considered to rule out nephrolithiasis prior to proceeding with laparoscopy. The extent of preoperative diagnostic testing varies among surgeons and different patient presentations.

Laparoscopy has proven superior as a diagnostic modality in several series. In a retrospective study of diagnostic laparoscopy in 85 consecutive cases, the authors determined that early diagnostic laparoscopy, which maintained both a sensitivity and a specificity of 100%, might have replaced expensive and less sensitive tests such as computed tomography (CT), ultrasound, or barium enema examination. The liberal use of laparoscopy is accurate for diagnosis and helpful in planning incisions when they become necessary. We commonly employ diagnostic laparoscopy in patients in good performance status with suspected appendicitis. Relative contraindications to the laparoscopic approach include cardiac instability or cardiomyopathy when pneumoperitoneum is to be employed, previous lower abdominal surgery (especially for prior inflammatory disorders), and inadequate technical support for the procedure. Laparoscopic appendectomy in the presence of intrauterine pregnancy remains to be evaluated in a prospective manner but has been demonstrated in several retrospective series to be safe when Veress needle or blind trocar placement is avoided, low-pressure pneumoperitoneum (less than 12 mm Hg) is utilized, and the procedure is performed prior to the third trimester. Nevertheless, this remains a subject of controversy, and to date many consider intrauterine pregnancy a relative contraindication to laparoscopy.

Preoperative Patient Management

Although severely septic or extremely old patients may require a more extensive preoperative workup to ensure adequate resuscitation and attention to serious medical concerns, most patients in whom the diagnosis of acute appendicitis is relatively secure require a limited time in preparation for surgery. All patients with suppurative peritonitis benefit from rehydration with balanced crystalloid solution and prompt intravenous administration of antibiotics. Although the particular agent used is the surgeon's preference, since both single- and multiple-agent therapy have enjoyed documented efficacy, it is recommended that antibiotic coverage be broad-spectrum and include adequate anaerobic activity. Antibiotics in this situation are considered to be for treatment of intraperitoneal bacterial contamination and not simply for operative prophylaxis.

Operative Technique

General endotracheal anesthesia, orogastric tube decompression, urinary bladder catheterization, and lower extremity sequential compression hose are routinely employed.

Patient Positioning

Patients may be positioned supine or in a modified lithotomy, which is our preference because it permits the operating surgeon to stand between the legs, if necessary, allowing a favorable dissecting angle if it becomes obligatory to mobilize the cecum or ascending colon extensively in case of a retrocecal appendix (Fig. 37-1). If the lithotomy position is used, it becomes important to keep the knees low so that long-instrument mobility will not be impaired later if lower abdominal trocar positions are selected. The arms are carefully padded and the fingers protected to prevent injury, and the torso must be securely strapped in anticipation of table rotation.

Trocar Placement and Initial Laparoscopic Examination

Although lifting devices have been employed with safety in laparoscopic appendectomy, we routinely employ carbon dioxide (CO_2) pneumoperitoneum because it has provided superior visualization and no complications in our experience. The umbilicus serves as the site for the initial trocar placement, where a 12-mm blunt-tipped cannula is inserted under direct vision. This facilitates rapid establishment of pneumoperitoneum, maintenance of high-flow CO_2 during the procedure, easy removal of the specimen, and insertion of an endoscopic stapling device (should it be required), as well as eliminating the need for other large trocars. A 30- or 45-degree angled laparoscope proves helpful in difficult cases but initially is not routinely used. Lower abdominal 5-mm secondary ports are used to maintain a single-surgeon operative technique and excellent cosmesis. This approach requires the availability of a high-resolution 5-mm laparoscope. All secondary trocars are placed under direct vision, and care is taken to avoid bladder or inferior epigastric vessel injury. In most patients, bilateral suprapubic trocars will prove adequate for the procedure.

Following initial inspection of the abdomen, attempts are made to localize the appendix and rule out other pathology. The small intestine, intraperitoneal colon, and pelvic structures in women are inspected. If a source other than the appendix is found to be the cause of peritonitis, appropriate surgical therapy can be undertaken, leaving the appendix *in situ*. If the appendix is retrocecal, the cecum is mobilized with graspers and scissors along the lateral peritoneal reflection. Use of electrocautery is limited, when possible, to avoid possible injury to the ureter, colon, and vascular structures in proximity. In the absence of intraperitoneal suppuration, the grossly normal-appearing appendix is removed. Some controversy exists with regard to the treatment of perforated appendicitis or localized abscess, but as long as standard surgical principles are maintained, the laparoscopic approach is feasible and safe. Nevertheless, conversion to open procedure should never be viewed as a sign of inadequate skill, but rather one of sound surgical judgment. In addition to the uniform reasons of uncontrolled bleeding, prolonged operative time, and technical inability to complete the procedure, conversion to an open procedure may become necessary in patients demonstrating a cecal mass, a necrotic appendiceal base with involvement of the cecum when tissue margins are of poor quality, or involvement of an adjacent organ (e.g., ovary, ileum) in the phlegmon or abscess. In such patients, the placement of the incision is guided by the laparoscopic examination, ensuring excellent exposure on conversion to laparotomy.

Exposure of the Appendix and Techniques of Appendectomy

Once the appendix is determined to be the cause of concern, the patient should be placed in a slight Trendelenburg position and rotated opposite the intended area of dissection. Remembering the origin of the appendix, one is advised to first identify the tenia coli on a normal-appearing cecum and then proceed inferiorly along the cecum to try to identify the appendiceal base, which is the portion of the appendix least often involved in acute appendicitis. If this proves difficult, one can follow the terminal ileum distally until the side wall attachments are encountered. These should be divided sharply, mobilizing the ileocecal junction. This will usually localize the appendiceal tip unless it is entirely retrocecal. When the appendix is found to be lying parallel to the ascending colon, one may find it helpful to retract the tenia coli medially and, utilizing an angled lens for visualization, mobilize the colon along the line of Toldt (Fig. 37-2). Once the appendiceal tip is localized, traction is necessary to allow lysis of the retroperitoneal attachments to the appendiceal body and to clarify the possible involvement of adjacent bowel. It is important not to rupture the appendix in this endeavor. When a

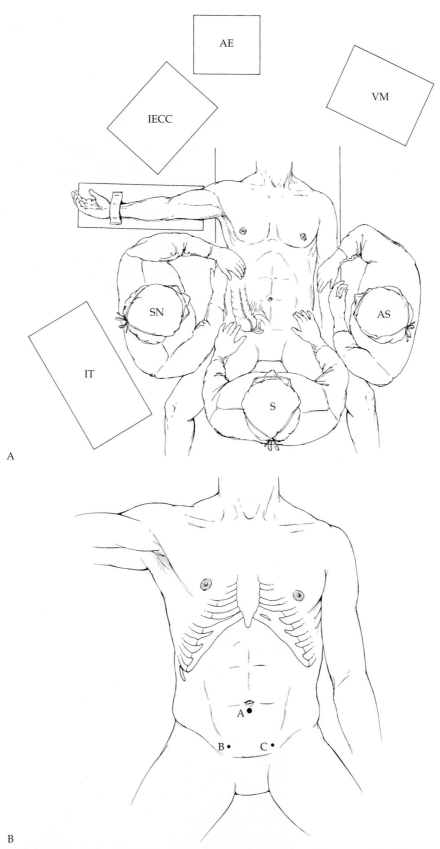

A

B

Fig. 37-1. **A:** *Suggested patient positioning for laparoscopic appendectomy. (S, surgeon; AS, assistant surgeon; SN, scrub nurse; AE, anesthesia; VM, video monitor; IECC, endoscopic instrument control console; IT, instrument table.)* **B:** *Positioning of trocars. (A, 12-mm trocar; B, 5-mm trocar; C, 5-mm trocar.)*

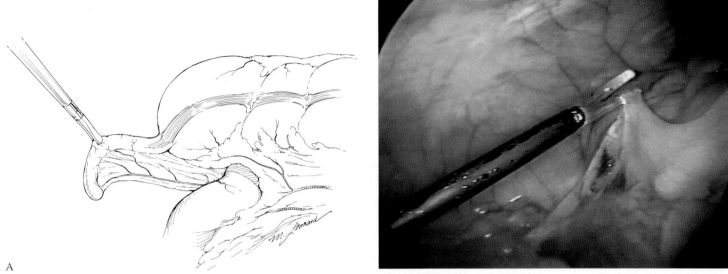

Fig. 37-2. **A,B:** *Initial mobilization of the cecum to identify a retrocecal appendix.*

moderately inflamed appendix is encountered, gentle grasping of the thickened mesoappendix with atraumatic instruments may prove adequate. However, with severe inflammation, application of a preformed loop ligature, which is not overtightened around the appendiceal tip, allows the operator to apply significant traction on the appendix without directly handling it with the instrument. Adhesiolysis surrounding the appendix proceeds laterally and superiorly along the cecal wall until the appendix can be fully rotated medially and the base fully delineated. The mesoappendix is cleared of surrounding loose adhesions and prepared for ligation. A curved dissecting grasper is utilized to create a defect in the avascular segment of the mesoappendix adjacent to the origin of the base of the appendix (Fig. 37-3). The size of the defect depends on the methods by which the appendiceal base will be ligated and divided. One may elect to divide the appendiceal base first or the mesoappendix with equal results, depending on the specific circumstances.

Established methods for securing the mesoappendix include bipolar electrocautery, ligating clips, preformed loop ligatures, and endoscopic stapling devices. We prefer stapling because the technique is rapid (offsetting instrument expense), reliable for hemostasis, independent of division of the appendiceal base, and without risks associated with electrocautery. The stapling device is inserted through the umbilicus, and the application viewed through the lower trocar (Fig. 37-4). After

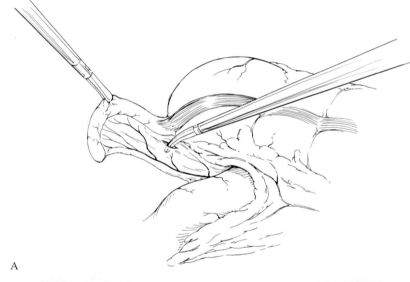

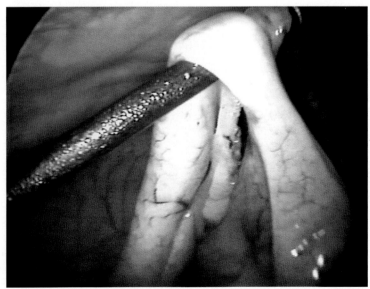

Fig. 37-3. **A,B:** *The mesoappendiceal defect is created at the appendiceal base.*

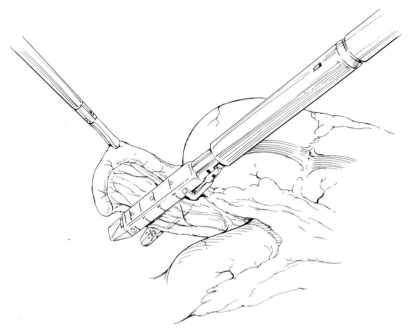

Fig. 37-4. *Diagram demonstrates the application of the endoscopic stapling device across the mesoappendix.*

the device is closed but before cutting proceeds, the entire end segment should be visualized. In general, the vascular cartridge will be used, unless the tissue is exceptionally thick, and in some cases multiple applications of the device will be necessary for complete division of the mesoappendix. The orientation of the stapler must be transverse and perpendicular to the ascending colon to prevent tangential application resulting in numerous applications of the stapler in an improper direction.

Double ligature with endoscopic loops or endoscopic stapling is an appropriate means for securing the base of the ap-

pendix. Neither single-loop ligature nor metal clips are reliable. If loop ligature is preferred, it will be necessary to first divide the mesoappendix with cautery or clips and scissors, which is at times difficult in cases of periappendiceal phlegmon. It remains paramount to divide the appendix at its origin if endoscopic stapling is employed (Fig. 37-5). If necessary, a small portion of the cecum may be excised in addition to the appendix to maintain division of healthy tissue (Figs. 37-6 and 37-7). In this case, an endoscopic gauge can be employed to test the appropriate depth of staple cartridge to be utilized. Endoscopic suturing may be used to bury the appendiceal stump if it is the surgeon's preference. If loop ligature is used, some authors advise coagulating the mucosa of the stump, but electrocautery is not to be used along a staple line, if possible, because the current may conduct along the staples, resulting in thermal injury and possible necrosis of the cecum.

Once the appendix is excised from the cecum, the specimen should be removed through a trocar or within a specimen bag to prevent contamination of the umbilicus, since the incidence of omphalitis approaches 10% in acute appendicitis when the specimen contacts the trocar wound at the umbilicus. Pneumoperitoneum is reestablished following specimen removal, and peritoneal irrigation is performed.

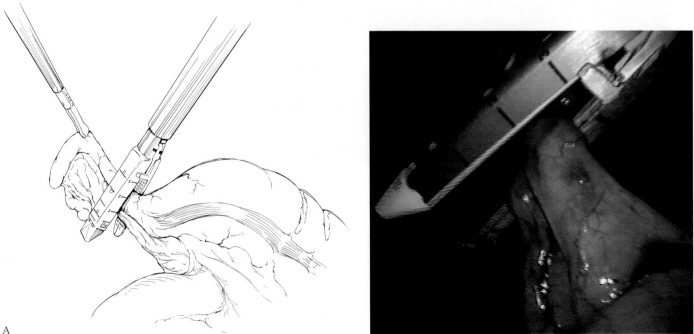

A

B

Fig. 37-5. **A,B:** *The endoscopic stapling device is applied across the appendiceal base.*

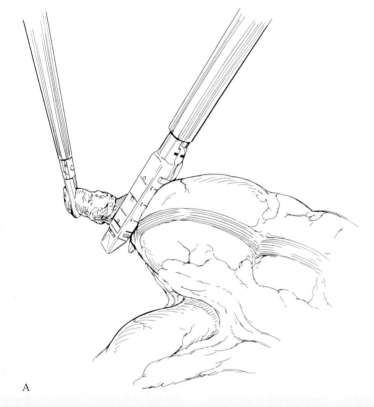

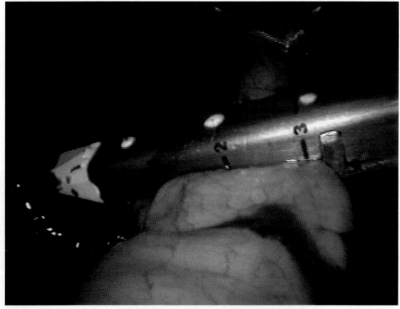

Fig. 37-6. **A,B:** *The endoscopic stapling device is applied across the anterior cecal wall.*

the pelvis and lower abdomen, and suction is employed to remove as much of the irrigant as possible. Intraperitoneal instillation of antibiotics has not been shown to be advantageous. The subdiaphragmatic spaces should be lavaged copiously and fluid evacuated as completely as possible. Manipulation of the table position facilitates adequate fluid removal.

Drain management is identical to that of traditional appendectomy. Selective drainage is beneficial in patients in whom an abscess is discovered, but not with diffuse peritonitis. Closed suction drains are preferable to Penrose or other open systems. When selected, drains are placed into the abdomen through the largest trocar in use, brought through the right lower trocar site or through a separate stab incision, and secured to the skin with suture.

The lower trocars are removed under direct vision to ensure that there is no inadvertent inferior epigastric vessel injury, and all fascial trocar defects larger than 5 mm are closed with absorbable suture, utilizing an endoscopic closure device, if necessary. All trocar sites are irrigated copiously. The fascia at the level of the umbilicus is approximated with absorbable suture, and skin incisions are loosely approximated with subdermal absorbable sutures.

Antegrade Appendectomy

Often, in patients with retrocecal appendicitis, the appendiceal tip may be found to be perforated or densely incorporated into phlegmon with the ascending colon, while the base of the appendix is free of inflammation. When it becomes cumbersome to mobilize the mesoappendix in such cases, it is wise to divide the appendix at the base and utilize this for traction while the appendix is subsequently mobilized in an antegrade fashion (Figs. 37-8 and 37-9). Care must be taken in such cases to handle the mesoappendix carefully to avoid avulsion. The endoscopic stapling device proves advantageous for this situation.

Crohn's Disease Involving the Cecum

Inflammatory bowel disease is usually appropriately treated medically, but if medical management is elected, the appendix should be left *in situ* to prevent fistulization or leaks. If resection is elected, the entire cecum and terminal ileum should be removed.

The option of withholding or limiting irrigation of the abdomen is not appropriate when laparoscopic appendectomy is performed because any containment of suppuration has been violated by pneumoperitoneum or lifting devices and the entire peritoneal cavity has been contaminated by any microorganisms present in the peritoneal fluid. After cultures are obtained, a complete peritoneal toilet is warranted. Prior to irrigation, however, it is important to regain the supine position to prevent subsequent irrigation solution from flowing to the left upper quadrant, where evacuation may prove unsatisfactory. Sterile saline (1 to 2 L) is instilled into

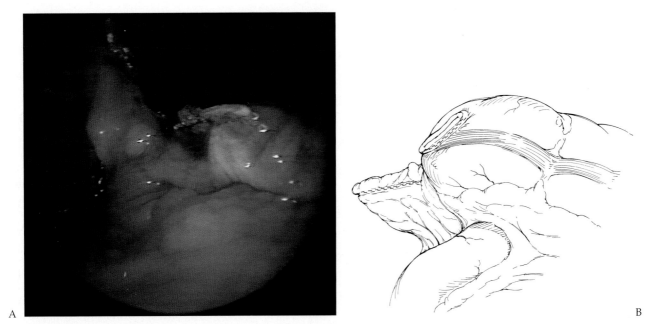

Fig. 37-7. **A,B:** *Endoscopic view of the staple line on the cecum. Note the healthy tissue surrounding the staple line, minimizing the chance for necrosis.*

Localized Perforation with Abscess

Laparoscopic treatment of such a process depends on the availability of resources and the laparoscopic expertise of the operating surgeon. Procedures range from drainage alone to laparoscopic resection of the terminal ileum and cecum. If one chooses to convert to laparotomy in these cases or to simply drain the abscess, it is not advisable to manipulate the involved structures laparo-scopically because of the likelihood of contaminating the entire peritoneal cavity.

Necrosis of the Appendiceal Base

Laparoscopic debridement of the cecum may be undertaken by experienced surgeons. Definitive laparoscopic options include tube cecostomy, limited cecal resection with endoscopic stapling, or endoscopic suture closure.

Surgical Complications and Postoperative Care

Complications are inherent to all surgical procedures, and laparoscopic appendectomy shares with open appendectomy the complications of wound infection, abscess or fistula formation, appendiceal stump necrosis, and small bowel obstruction. In addition, laparoscopic appendectomy carries the potential risks of Veress needle or trocar injury, depression of cardiac preload or exacerbation of obstructive airway disease secondary to pneumoperitoneum, and trocar-site Richter's hernia. To decrease the likelihood of these events, placement of all trocars under direct visualization, careful patient selection, and suture closure of all trocar defects larger than 5 mm are recommended.

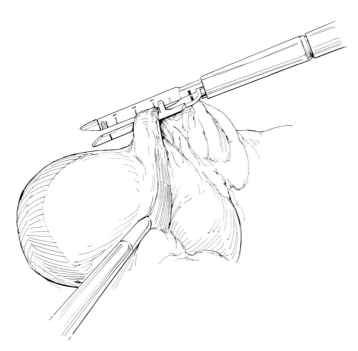

Fig. 37-8. *Antegrade appendectomy. The division of the grossly normal appendiceal base is carried out first, enabling the appendix to be placed on traction as the mesoappendix is dissected.*

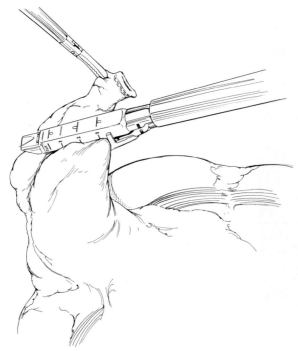

Fig. 37-9. Antegrade appendectomy. After division of the base and dissection of the appendiceal body, the thickened mesoappendix can be sequentially divided with the stapling device.

Relieving the abdomen of CO_2 as completely as possible at the operating table will prove helpful in postoperative pain control. Most patients may begin oral liquid intake when awake and alert, and oral analgesics will prove adequate in most cases. Intravenous fluids are tapered, and an oral diet is advanced with the return of peristalsis. Antibiotic administration is dictated by the severity of the disease found at the time of operation. Most patients with uncomplicated appendicitis will be satisfactorily treated with less than 24 hours of an intravenous antibiotic. In patients with perforated appendicitis, several days of broad-spectrum coverage to include anaerobes should be continued until the patient has defervesced and bowel function has resumed.

Patients who demonstrate persistent fever, leukocytosis, and ileus after 5 to 7 days of antibiotic therapy warrant ultrasound or CT to rule out pelvic abscess. Radiographically directed percutaneous catheter drainage as a definitive treatment for postappendectomy abscess (laparoscopic or open) maintains a success rate approaching 100% and should be considered as the primary therapeutic modality in such cases. Extreme circumstances of persistent pelvic abscess, interloop abscess, or early small bowel obstruction justifying reoperation are uncommon but must be managed aggressively when encountered.

Results of Laparoscopic Appendectomy

Data available from several prospective randomized trials are summarized in Table 37-1. Based on current prospective trials, several general conclusions have been drawn by experienced laparoscopic surgeons:

1. Indications for laparoscopic appendectomy should be the same as those for open appendectomy, and diagnostic laparoscopy dramatically improves the accuracy of the operative diagnosis.
2. Laparoscopic appendectomy can be safely performed in both children and adults with minimal increases in operative time, compared to open appendectomy. Perforation or abscess formation is not a strict contraindication to the laparoscopic approach, but successful endoscopic management will depend on the experience of the operating surgeon. The safety of laparoscopic appendectomy in pregnancy has yet to be demonstrated in a prospective study.
3. Wound infections are reduced with laparoscopic appendectomy and are dramatically lower when the appendix is removed via a specimen bag.
4. Hospital stays are similar for laparoscopic and open appendectomy patients, but adult patients have less pain and return to normal activities more rapidly following laparoscopic appendectomy.

Table 37-1. Results of Prospective, Randomized Trials of Laparoscopic Appendectomy

Reference	n		Operation Time (min)		Conversion Rate (%)	LOS (days)		RTNA (days)		Wound Infection (%)		Complications (%)	
	L	O	L	O		L	O	L	O	L	O	L	O
Atwood et al. (1992)	30	32	61	51	6.7	2.5	3.8	21	38	0	3	0	13
McAnena et al. (1992)	29	36	48	52	6.7	2.2	4.8	—	—	4	11	—	—
Kum et al. (1993)	52	57	43	40	0.0	3.2	4.2	17	30	0	9	0	0
Tate et al. (1994)	70	70	70	47	22	3.5	3.6	—	—	10	14	21	25
Frazee et al. (1994)	38	37	87	65	6.6	2.0	2.8	14	25	—	—	8	5

n, number of patients; LOS, length of hospital stay; RTNA, return to normal activity; L, laparoscopic appendectomy; O, open appendectomy.

Conclusion

Laparoscopic appendectomy presents a safe and effective alternative to open surgery when utilized in a competent manner, if established surgical principles are maintained. Advantages including a shortened hospital stay, reduced incidence of wound infection, and hastened convalescence justify a moderately increased operating room expense secondary to advanced instrumentation.

Suggested Reading

Attwood SE, Hill AD, Murphy PG, Thornton J, Stephens RB. A prospective randomized trial of laparoscopic versus open appendectomy. *Surgery* 1992;112:497–501.

Frazee RC, Roberts JW, Symmonds RE, et al. A prospective randomized trial comparing open versus laparoscopic appendectomy. *Ann Surg* 1994;219:725–731.

Kum CK, Ngoi SS, Goh PM, Tekant Y, Isaac JR. Randomized controlled trial comparing laparoscopic and open appendicectomy. *Br J Surg* 1993;80:1599–1600.

McAnena OJ, Austin O, O'Connell PR, Hederman WP, Gorey TF, Fitzpatrick J. Laparoscopic versus open appendicectomy: a prospective evaluation. *Br J Surg* 1992;79:818–820.

Neugebauer E, Troidl H, Kum CK, et al. The E.A.E.S. consensus development conferences on laparoscopic cholecystectomy, appendectomy, and hernia repair. Consensus statements—September 1994. The Educational Committee of the European Association for Endoscopic Surgery. *Surg Endosc* 1995;9:550–563.

Olsen JB, Myren CJ, Haahr PE. Randomized study of the value of laparoscopy before appendicectomy. *Br J Surg* 1993;80:922–923.

Talamini MA. Laparoscopic appendectomy and herniorrhaphy. *Adv Surg* 1993;26:387–396.

Tate JJ, Dawson JW, Chung SC, Lau WY, Li AK. Laparoscopic versus open appendicectomy: prospective randomised trial. *Lancet* 1993;342:633–637.

38

Laparoscopic Right Colectomy

Edward J. Brennan, Jr. and W. Peter Geis

Minimally invasive colon resection was first reported in the literature in 1991. Use of laparoscopic and laparoscopic-assisted colon resection has steadily grown over the past 5 years. Currently, 5% to 10% of colon resections are undertaken using the laparoscopic approach. These procedures have generated much controversy, with many authors questioning the advisability of performing laparoscopic colon resection, particularly in cases of malignancy. Questions regarding the adequacy of the resection have been addressed by proponents of the operation. However, reports of port-site recurrences have again raised doubts about the appropriate use of these procedures.

The majority of reported port-site tumor implantations have occurred following right colectomy. A randomized trial sponsored by the National Cancer Institute (NCI) has begun accruing patients in an attempt to define the role of laparoscopy in the treatment of colon cancer.

Despite oncologic concerns, many investigators have demonstrated that laparoscopic colectomy can be performed safely and, after a brief learning curve, in a time-efficient manner. In addition, the postoperative benefits of less pain, earlier feeding, and earlier discharge have also been shown.

Indications

Three fundamental psychomotor skills are required for the performance of laparoscopic colectomy (in order of increasing technical difficulty): (a) mobilization, (b) regional devascularization, and (c) intracorporeal anastomosis. These three skills are best learned sequentially and are demonstrated on a complexity scale delineating 13 different laparoscopic colectomy procedures (Fig. 38-1). Laparoscopic-assisted right colectomy with only mobilization performed laparoscopically prior to exteriorization is the least complex lap-

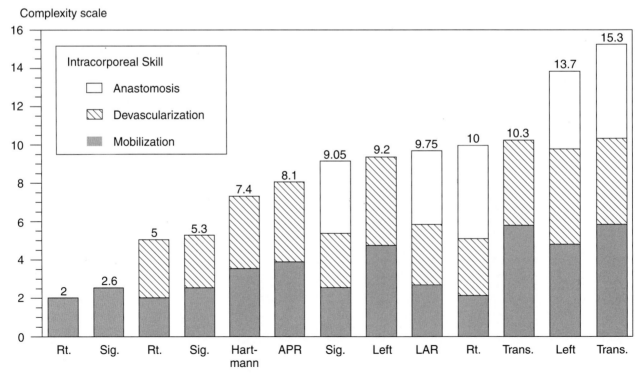

Fig. 38-1. Complexity scale. (From Geis, Coletta, Jacobs, et al., 1994, with permission.)

aroscopic colectomy procedure and is appropriate for surgeons in the early stages of their laparoscopic experience. In addition, mobilization alone prior to exteriorization of the specimen is appropriate for patients with benign diseases of the right colon, including adenomatous polyps, bleeding arteriovenous malformations, cecal volvulus, ischemia, colonic inertia, and inflammatory bowel disease. Malignancy of the right colon requires an increased level of expertise, as adherence to standard oncologic principles mandates that devascularization must be performed intracorporeally prior to exteriorization. Early vascular control has been shown to decrease intravascular spread of viable cancer cells.

Recent reports of port-site recurrence after laparoscopic colectomy have escalated the debate over the appropriate role of laparoscopy in the treatment of colon cancer. Twenty-three documented cases of port-site recurrence have been published. An NCI-sponsored randomized, prospective trial is underway to study the results of laparoscopically treated colon cancer. At this time, we recommend that the laparoscopic approach for the cure of malignancy of the colon be performed only as part of an established investigational protocol and by experienced laparoscopic surgeons.

Operative Technique

Prior to induction of anesthesia, sequential compression devices are placed on the patient's legs to increase venous return and prevent venous stasis during the operation. The patient is given a single preoperative dose of a broad-spectrum antibiotic (e.g., cefoxitin sodium [Mefoxin]) prior to the initial incision. The patient is placed on the operating room table in a modified lithotomy position. The monitors are placed at the patient's right shoulder and right knee (Fig. 38-2). The surgeon and first assistant stand on the patient's left side. The surgeon often moves to between the patient's legs while working on the hepatic flexure and transverse colon. A robotic arm can be used to hold and move the laparoscope, and it is also placed on the patient's right side and affixed to the table. The robotic arm provides a perfectly steady visual field and allows both the sur-

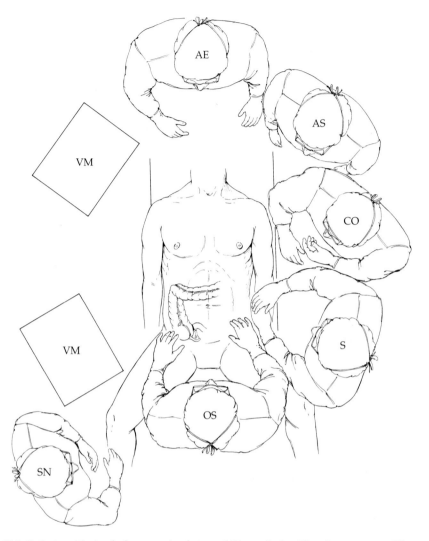

Fig. 38-2. Patient positioning for laparoscopic colectomy. (AE, anesthetist; AS, assistant surgeon; CO, camera operator; S, surgeon; OS, optional surgeon; SN, scrub nurse; VM, video monitor.)

geon and the assistant to operate with both hands.

Proper placement of laparoscopic ports can greatly increase the likelihood of a safe and efficient operation. For right colectomy, two ports are placed remote from the right colon to allow maximum radius of movement for the Babcock retractors and maximum versatility in retracting the colon in a variety of directions. These two ports are placed in the epigastrium and the left upper quadrant (or both in the left hemiabdomen). The umbilical placement of the laparoscope allows visualization of the entire abdomen and pelvis. Four or five port sites are routinely used for laparoscopic right colectomy. Additional

ports may be required for difficult anatomy or for obese patients (Fig. 38-3).

Mobilization

Gravity facilitates organ retraction. After placement of the ports and inspection of the abdomen, the patient is placed in a steep Trendelenburg position with the right side up. This position allows the mobilization to begin in the safest area—the peritoneum lateral to the cecum. With traction on the cecum and countertraction applied to the lateral peritoneum, dissection can be carried inferiorly to mobilize the distal 10 cm of the ileum (Fig. 38-4). This course of dissection crosses the right ureter, which should be identified and

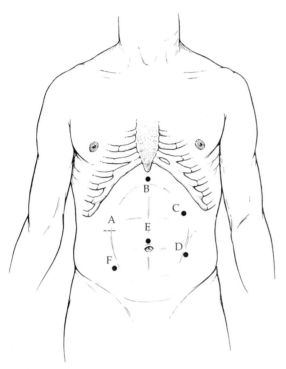

Fig. 38-3. *Location of port sites for laparoscopic right colectomy. (A, optional incision; B, 10- or 12-mm port; C, 10- or 12-mm port; D, alternate umbilical 10- or 12-mm port; E, 10- or 12-mm umbilical port; F, optional 10- or 12-mm port.)*

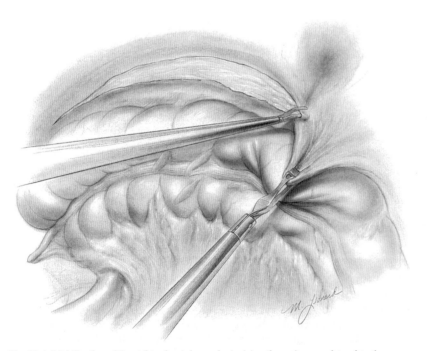

Fig. 38-4. *Mobilization of the right colon is begun by incising the peritoneum lateral to the cecum.*

protected. Mobilization is then continued cephalad along the white line of Toldt to the level of the hepatic flexure. Care is taken to divide only the peritoneum to avoid the iliac vessels and right ureter, which lie deep and medial to this plane.

Retraction of the mobilized cecum and right colon to the left permits sharp and blunt dissection of the right mesocolon from the underlying retroperitoneal structures under direct vision. An ultrasonic dissector can be used as an alternative to

cautery in an attempt to limit the lateral spread of energy to adjacent structures. This device allows the dissection to be performed with minimal blood loss. Again, the right ureter is identified as it crosses the right iliac vessels. Access to the hepatic flexure and transverse colon is established by placing the patient in the reverse Trendelenburg position with the right side up. The midtransverse colon is retracted caudad with the Babcock clamp, and the greater omentum is retracted cephalad. The gastrocolic ligament is separated from the transverse colon in the avascular plane, and the lesser sac is entered. Dissection in this avascular plane is carried from the midtransverse colon to the hepatic flexure. Endoscopic staples are used to provide hemostasis when vessels are encountered. Division of the hepatocolic ligament at the hepatic flexure completes the mobilization of the right colon and allows separation of the specimen from the underlying duodenum. The middle colic artery is identified as it arises from the superior mesenteric artery along the superior border of the third portion of the duodenum.

Grasping and manipulating the bowel in the area of the disease is to be avoided. The majority of the retraction should be performed by grasping mesentery or peritoneum. Injury to the wall of the intestine during mobilization can be repaired by seromuscular inverting sutures. If the segment injured is part of the specimen to be removed, the injured area may often be approximated with an Endoloop (Ethicon, Cincinnati, Ohio), since it will be removed shortly. The diameter and mobility of the small intestine allow easy retraction above the skin level through a dilated port site to inspect for suspected injury and to subsequently repair the injury. The small bowel is then returned to the abdominal cavity, and the procedure continues.

Devascularization

Following general mobilization, the regional blood supply to the right colon should be freely accessible from both sides of its associated mesentery. Safe intracorporeal devascularization of the right colon includes accurate visualization, traction, proximal control, and Trendelenburg position with the right side up to allow gravity to displace the small intestine. The mesentery of the ileocecal complex is grasped with a Babcock clamp and retracted directly opposite the root of the mesentery. The mesenteric peritoneum will tent up as it resists lengthening, identifying the location of the ileocolic vessel beneath the tented peritoneum. An avascular window is present on both sides of the origin of the vessel. The peritoneum is divided along the avascular space, and the vessel is isolated. A Babcock or right-angle clamp is used to control the proximal vessel during this procedure. The vessel is ligated and divided using either endoscopic clips followed by vessel transection and reinforcement of the ligature with an Endoloop, or an endoscopic stapling device with vascular staples (Fig. 38-5). The stapling device should be used when the vessel and surrounding tissue are of large enough volume to preclude safe use of endoscopic clips. Following vessel transection, proximal control is maintained by the right-angle clamp until the surgeon is convinced that no bleeding is present. If bleeding occurs, reinforcement with an Endoloop under direct vision secures the vessel. If the vessel retracts into the mesenteric areolar tissue and bleeds, an expanding hematoma is present, and we recommend immediate open abdominal exposure to gain control of the lost bleeding vessel.

Once the ileocolic vessel has been ligated and divided, a large window is present in the mesentery. Similar ligation and division of the right colic artery at its origin is easily accomplished. Access to the middle colic vessel is accomplished using the reverse Trendelenburg position, grasping the undersurface of the mesentery of the transverse colon, and retracting it cephalad and anteriorly. The origin of the middle colic vessel is identified by the tented mesenteric peritoneum. The avascular window is carefully opened on both sides of the vessels. Careful tension to avoid undue longitudinal traction on the middle colic vessel is necessary. Ligation and division of this vessel are accomplished utilizing the endoscopic clip or stapler techniques, followed by reinforcement with an Endoloop. Proximal control with a Babcock clamp is maintained until absolute hemostasis is ensured.

It is possible to ligate and divide the regional blood supply to the right colon as the first step in the operative procedure if the surgeon believes this process is of oncologic benefit. However, in this circumstance, the vessel must be isolated and carefully separated from surrounding tissue to ensure that no other structures are inadvertently included in the ligation or stapling of the proximal vessel. The structure most vulnerable to injury is the right ureter during dissection and ligation of the ileocolic vessel.

Miniincision Strategy

A miniincision in the abdominal cavity allows removal of the resected specimen. An exception to this method is abdominoperineal resection, in which the specimen may be removed through the perineum. The mini–abdominal incision may also be used for completion of devascularization and resection of the specimen and for intestinal anastomosis. Therefore, the choice of location of the mini–abdominal incision should be made based partially on whether or not both ends of the resected segment of intestine will reach above the skin level through that particular incision. Choice of location of the miniincision will therefore be affected by (a) the ability to mobilize a generous segment of proximal and distal intestine adjacent to the resected segment, (b) the surgeon's preference regarding the most acceptable cosmetic incision, and (c) the least painful and least morbid location. As a result, mini–abdominal incisions performed for extraction of the right colon will most often be right lower quadrant muscle-splitting incisions or a midline lower abdominal incision. Occasionally, however, the midtransverse colon will be limited in its mobility due to adhesions, inherent disease, and other factors, including prior operative procedures. In these circumstances, the transverse colon at the expected line of transection will not be mobile enough to reach an incision in the right lower abdomen. In these circumstances, an upper midline or muscle-splitting incision in the upper abdomen may be necessary.

The right colon is often exteriorized as a long loop of intestine. The advantage of the loop method of extraction is that it allows both segments of resected intestine to be extracted immediately adjacent to each other and without possible inadvertent torsion of one of the bowel segments beneath the abdominal wall. The disadvantage of the method is that it requires a larger incision to accommodate two limbs of intestine with its mesentery. Further, extraction of the right colon by the loop method prior to devascularization of the specimen may be associated with undue traction and injury to the vascular regional vessels, especially the middle colic vein. Care must be taken to avoid the occur-

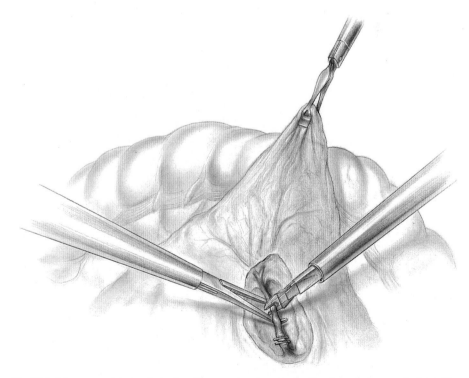

Fig. 38-5. Intracorporeal devascularization. The mesentery is grasped with a Babcock clamp and retracted to identify the vessel, which is then divided between endoscopic clips.

rence of this injury, which will result in a mesenteric hematoma or postoperative blood loss.

To avoid the disadvantages associated with the loop extraction, the right colon may be removed after first transecting the distal ileum and devascularizing the segment at vessel origins. By this method, the transected distal ileum and cecum are removed through the miniincision as a long tubular structure, with the last portion extracted being the midtransverse colon. The transverse colon is transected at the skin level, and the specimen is removed. An atraumatic clamp is affixed to the ileum proximal to the line of resection. Once the specimen has been extracted and resected, the distal ileum is carefully presented to the miniincision by the atraumatic clamp.

Anastomosis

An ileocolic anastomosis is performed at the skin level, and the anastomosis is replaced in the abdominal cavity (Fig. 38-6). The surgeon must be certain that torsion of the intestine has not occurred. It is important that the miniincision is large enough to accommodate the right colon and mesentery without risk of damage to the specimen or contamination of the miniincision wound. A variety of techniques for ileocolic anastomosis may be used: a functional end-to-end (side-to-side) stapled anastomosis, an end-to-side anastomosis utilizing the circular stapling device, or a hand-sewn end-to-end anastomosis.

Rarely, one of the two ends of transected intestine will not reach the skin miniincision because of adhesions or primary disease processes. In these circumstances, an intracorporeal sutured or stapled anastomosis is required. Again, the anastomosis may be performed using an end-to-end, end-to-side, or side-to-side technique, based on the discretion and experience of the surgeon.

Mesentery

Many surgeons believe that the mesentery must be approximated following colon resection, especially right colon resection, in which a mesenteric opening may result in herniation of the loop of small intestine through the mesenteric opening, followed by the risk of incarceration, strangulation, and bowel obstruction. Prudence dictates that the surgeon deal with the mesenteric defect in exactly the same manner as he or she does in the open approach to the colectomy procedure. It is important to close the defect completely without residual small mesenteric defects. Small defects are much more likely to result in incarceration and strangulation of the small intestine. The defect may be sutured by either an extracorporeal or an intracorporeal method.

Precautions are recommended in cases of malignancy. These include (a) early stapling across the proximal and distal segments of colon to isolate the segment, (b) early ligation of regional vascular supply, (c) avoidance of direct grasping of the colon, especially adjacent to the tumor, (d) bagging of the specimen prior to extraction, (e) allowing carbon dioxide (CO_2) to escape only through the lumina of trocars, and (f) irrigation of all ports sites and the miniincision with sterile water or dilute povidone–iodine (Betadine).

Postoperative Care

Postoperatively, the Foley catheter and nasogastric tube are removed. The hematocrit is evaluated in the recovery room, and a complete blood cell count is ob-

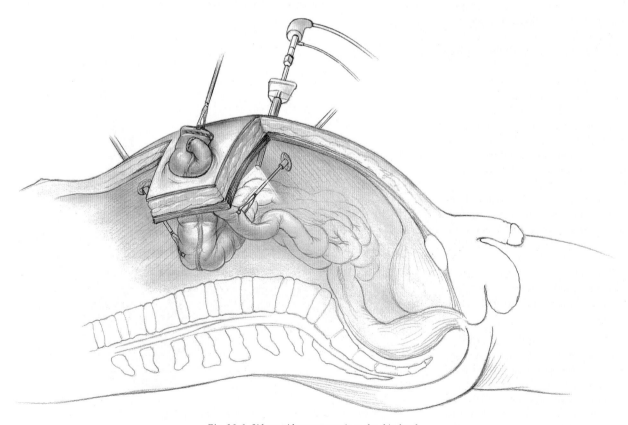

Fig. 38-6. Side-to-side anastomosis at the skin level.

tained on the first postoperative morning. One or two postoperative doses of the previously chosen intravenous antibiotic are also administered. The patient is begun on a clear-liquid diet on the morning of the first postoperative day. The diet is quickly advanced to a mechanically soft diet. In our series, patients have an average length of stay of 4.5 days, and 15% have been discharged prior to the third hospital day.

Complications

In a recent series of 327 patients who underwent laparoscopic colectomy, 15 patients required conversion to an open procedure: a conversion rate of 4.6%. Thirteen of these patients were converted for technical reasons, primarily extensive adhesions. Most conversions occurred during the early learning experience and because of assistants' inexperience in laparoscopic colectomy. Two patients were converted due to a progressive rise in CO_2 in the blood or in the end-tidal CO_2 level. There were 29 complications in this series, for a 9% complication rate. The majority of the complications were wound infections, which were all superficial and did not require prolongation of the hospital stay. Small bowel obstruction subsequently developed in six patients, and five patients underwent reoperation. Two patients had adhesive small bowel obstruction, and one had incarceration of the small bowel through a mesenteric defect that had been partially closed. There have been no port-site or abdominal-wound recurrences in our malignant cases.

Suggested Reading

Bernstein M, Wexner SD. Laparoscopic resection for colorectal cancer: a USA perspective. *Semin Laparosc Surg* 1995;2:216–223.

Geis WP, Coletta AV, Jacobs M, Plasencia G, Kim HC. Benefits of complexity scales in laparoscopic colectomy. *Int Surg* 1994;79:230–232.

Geis WP, Coletta AV, Verdeja JC, Plasencia G, Ojogho O, Jacobs M. Sequential psychomotor skills development in laparoscopic colon surgery. *Arch Surg* 1994;129:206–212.

Ramos JM, Beart RW Jr, Goes R, Ortega AE, Schlinkert RT. Role of laparoscopy in colorectal surgery: a prospective evaluation of 200 cases. *Dis Colon Rectum* 1995;38:494–501.

Wexner SD, Cohen SM. Port site metastases after laparoscopic colorectal surgery for cure of malignancy. *Br J Surg* 1995;82:295–298.

EDITOR'S COMMENT

Laparoscopic right hemicolectomy performed in a thin patient who lacks adhesions or excessive mesenteric fat can be a rapid, effective, and enjoyable operation. Conversely, the markedly obese patient or hostile abdomen can make this operation a challenge for the most skilled laparoscopic surgeon.

The authors have described their specific version of a widely used technique for laparoscopic right hemicolectomy. An alternate technique that has gained the support of a large number of general and colorectal surgeons involves the high ligation of the vasculature prior to mobilization of the colon. This technique more closely mimics the approach used by many colorectal surgeons for the open right hemicolectomy for cancer. Regardless of the sequence in which the initial steps of the colectomy are performed, the procedure is destined to fail unless healthy, well-vascularized bowel is used for the ileocolic anastamosis.

An avoidable pitfall of laparoscopic partial colectomy is to discover that the target lesion is not contained within the segment of colon that has been resected. This scenario usually occurs when the surgeon relies upon the colonoscopist's estimation of the location of the lesion. Tattoo marking of the lesion with India ink during colonscopy provides a visual landmark at laparoscopy. A barium enema will demonstrate the precise location of most lesions in need of surgical resection.

W.S.E.

39

Laparoscopic Surgery of the Left Colon

Wayne L. Ambroze, Jr.

The application of laparoscopy to biliary surgery revolutionized the treatment of cholelithiasis. The overtly apparent advantages of less pain, scaring, hospitalization, and recuperative time were incentive enough to pursue this novel technique despite early controversies regarding surgeon training and complications related to lack of experience with this new operation. This success, as expected, led to the application of laparoscopy to other surgical procedures, though often with less resounding results. Shortly after the initial favorable results for laparoscopic biliary surgery were published, case reports, followed by small series of laparoscopic-assisted colectomies, appeared in the literature. Interest in these procedures was initially high, but skepticism, which in the case of biliary surgery was dashed by the overt benefits of the technique, continued to grow, and enthusiasm for laparoscopic-assisted colectomy waned.

The reasons for the lack of acceptance of laparoscopic-assisted colectomy by a majority of surgeons are varied:

1. The procedures are technically difficult, requiring multiple changes in the visual fields as the procedure progresses, as well as requiring the dissection of large tissue planes and control of large vascular pedicles.

2. While there appear to be advantages in terms of pain, hospitalization, and recuperation for laparoscopic colectomy patients due to manipulation of the bowel, resulting in an adynamic ileus (albeit shorter in duration than for open procedures) and the need for an incision to remove the bowel, the advantages over similar open procedures are not as pronounced as for laparoscopic biliary surgery.

3. Carcinoma of the colon is the most frequent indication for colectomy in the United States. With the report of trocar-site recurrences following laparoscopic-assisted colectomy, the issue of the adequacy of this procedure as a cancer operation has been questioned.

Despite these concerns and difficulties, many surgeons at various institutions continue to perform increasing numbers of laparoscopic colectomies. They believe that the benefits of laparoscopic colectomy for properly selected patients exist and outweigh the technical difficulty for experienced laparoscopic surgeons, with no added risk to patients. Retrospective studies are being published supporting this view, and national prospective, randomized studies are underway to further address these issues.

It is my belief that laparoscopy has a significant role in bowel surgery, as is evident by the number and variety of procedures performed in my colorectal practice (Table 39-1). At the present level of experience and technology, laparoscopic surgery is not the procedure of choice for the majority of colon operations; however, it is a part of my surgical armamentarium to be applied when benefit to a patient is likely to be realized. This chapter discusses laparoscopic left colectomy with emphasis on patient selection, technique, and minimizing complications.

Indications and Preparation

To date, the indications for laparoscopic left colectomy are similar to those for open left colectomy, with the possible exception

of procedures for carcinoma. Because of issues raised regarding the adequacy of laparoscopic resection as a curative cancer operation, I perform these procedures only in the setting of an ongoing national randomized, prospective trial. In addition, the decision to perform surgery is made when it is felt that the benefit-to-risk ratio for surgery exceeds that against surgery. Though this benefit-to-risk ratio may be improved with laparoscopic bowel procedures, compared to similar open procedures, this is yet to be conclusively decided, and consequently I use the classic indications for open procedures as the initial criteria for performing any bowel surgery. When surgery is indicated based on classic criteria, I offer laparoscopic-assisted surgery to patients who I believe would benefit in terms of pain, hospitalization, return to full activity, and overall risk over similar open procedures, based on disease, comorbid conditions, prior surgery, and body habitus. For a healthy, thin patient with a villous tumor of the sigmoid colon and no prior abdominal surgery, there is a reasonable expectation that the procedure could be completed laparoscopically and that the patient would be discharged from the hospital in 3 or 4 days and be back to work in 2 to 3 weeks. These would not be reasonable expectations for an obese patient with multiple medical problems or prior abdominal surgery requiring surgery for a diverticular abscess. To the first patient, I would offer the option of laparoscopic-assisted colectomy. The second patient would not be offered laparoscopy as an option.

The most common diagnosis for which I perform laparoscopic-assisted bowel surgery is inflammatory bowel disease; however, the most common indication for

Table 39-1. Laparoscopy-assisted
Bowel Procedures Performed Between
September 1992 and December 1995

Procedure	n
Right colectomy	39
Left/sigmoid colectomy	36
Proctocolectomy/J-pouch	26
Total/subtotal colectomy	24
Stoma/bypass	23
Ileocolic resection	22
Low anterior resection	19
Abdominoperineal resection	5
Small bowel resection	5
Lysis of adhesions	5
Colotomy	2
Colostomy takedown	1

laparoscopic-assisted left colectomy in my practice is diverticulitis (Table 39-2). Contraindications to laparoscopic-assisted bowel surgery include diffuse peritonitis, severe chronic obstructive pulmonary disease, or severe congestive heart failure. With peritonitis, there is the risk that the pressure of pneumoperitoneum might spread the infection further throughout the peritoneal cavity. Carbon dioxide (CO_2) retention during prolonged pneumoperitoneum is well documented and must be considered in patients with chronic obstructive pulmonary disease whose metabolic compensatory mechanisms are already stressed. Pneumoperitoneum also decreases venous return, further decreasing cardiac output in patients with congestive heart failure.

Table 39-2. Indications for
Laparoscopy-assisted Bowel Procedures

Indication	n
Carcinoma	41
Crohn's disease	41
Polyps/polyposis	34
Ulcerative colitis	26
Diverticulitis	21
Colonic inertia	12
Anal incontinence	9
Rectovaginal fistula	8
Rectal prolapse	7
Volvulus	4
Endometriosis	2
Arteriovenous malformation	2

Preoperative preparation of the patient undergoing laparoscopic-assisted left colectomy is similar to that for the open procedure. A mechanical bowel preparation is started with a clear-liquid diet the day prior to surgery. Four liters of an oral polyethylene glycol preparation (Colyte, GoLYTELY) are given over 4 hours the day before surgery, followed by a single oral dose of metronidazole, 2 g. The patient is admitted to the hospital the morning of surgery, and intravenous fluids are started to offset the dehydrating effects of the bowel preparation. Prior to surgery, the patient is given instruction in the use of the incentive spirometer, and antithrombotic venous compression hose are placed on the patient in the preoperative holding area. Cefoxitin sodium (Mefoxin), 1 g, is given intravenously prior to the procedure. A urinary Foley catheter and a nasogastric tube are placed after the induction of general endotracheal anesthesia.

Operative Technique

Instrumentation

Laparoscopic-assisted left colectomy requires two separate sets of instruments. A sterile laparotomy set is opened and counted and is available in the room. Though rarely necessary, these instruments must be immediately available because of the possibility of urgent laparotomy for uncontrolled bleeding during laparoscopy.

For reasons of cost and efficiency, the laparoscopic instrumentation is kept to a minimum. The electronic instruments are similar to those used in most laparoscopic procedures, including a camera attached to a 10-mm-diameter 0-degree laparoscope, an air insufflator with two CO_2 canisters, and two video monitors. The entire left colectomy is performed using a total of four trocars including a 10-mm reusable Hasson trocar for the laparoscope, two 10-mm disposable trocars, and a single 12-mm disposable trocar. The 12-mm trocar with an appropriate reducer can accommodate the 5-, 10-, and 12-mm instruments, including the laparoscopic linear vascular stapler. Adjustable stability threads are used with each disposable trocar. In addition to the trocars, the only other instruments necessary for the dissection for a left colectomy are two 10-mm-diameter Babcock clamps, dissection scissors

with unipolar cautery, and a laparoscopic suction/irrigation system. A reusable vascular clip applier is kept in the operating room, but the vascular clips are not opened unless needed.

Patient Positioning

Proper patient positioning for a laparoscopic-assisted left colectomy is essential to successful completion of the procedure. Everyone participating in the operating room has access priorities to the patient and instruments, and if the room is set up inappropriately or the patient not properly positioned, interference among participants or between participants and the patient will add time and confusion to the procedure. The anesthesiologist needs access to the patient's head and upper body. Two surgeons need access to the patient's abdomen and perineum, while the sterile scrub nurse needs access to both surgeons and the instrument tables. To best accommodate these access needs, I use the room setup shown in Fig. 39-1.

The patient is placed in a modified lithotomy position with both arms extended laterally on arm boards. Arm extension helps stabilize the patient during lateral rotation of the table. The patient's legs are placed in Allen stirrups in a modified lithotomy position (Fig. 39-2). In this modified position, the legs are only minimally elevated, allowing access to the perineum but with the anterior thighs low enough not to interfere with instrument mobility when the splenic flexure of the colon is being dissected. As this portion of the dissection is often difficult, limiting the mobility of the surgeon can result in the surgeon's inability to complete the procedure without a laparotomy.

Trocar Placement

The concept of keeping the procedure uncomplicated applies to the surgical technique, as well as the instrumentation. I use a similar trocar placement with minor variations for most laparoscopic-assisted bowel procedures. For uncomplicated right colon or sigmoid colon resections, I might use only three trocars. However, if the dissection is expected to be difficult or splenic flexure or pelvic dissection is required, then four trocars are used. The Hasson trocar is placed in the umbilicus, with the 12-mm trocar placed in the right lower quadrant and 10-mm trocars placed

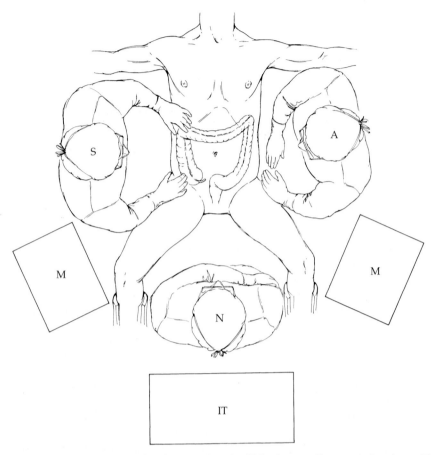

Fig. 39-1. The operating room setup for a laparoscopic-assisted left colectomy. (S, surgeon; A, assistant; N, nurse; M, monitor; IT, instrument table).

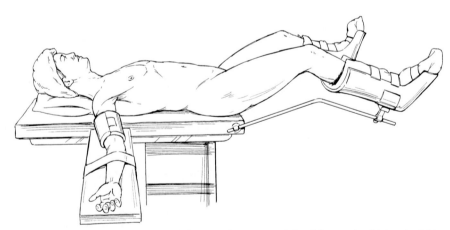

Fig. 39-2. Modified lithotomy position with the patient's arms extended and the anterior thighs raised 15 degrees from the horizontal plane.

nothing in the abdomen is found to preclude proceeding with the laparoscopic-assisted procedure, the three other trocars are placed under laparoscopic vision.

For reasons of aesthetics, I try to place the trocars in a symmetric fashion and, when possible, place the three nonumbilical trocars below the panty line. In taller patients, this may not be possible, and the trocar sites may need to be placed higher on the lower abdomen, though placing a trocar above the level of the umbilicus should not be necessary. Keeping the trocars below the umbilicus not only is more aesthetic but also should help decrease postoperative pain and improve postoperative pulmonary inspiratory effort.

Dissection

Unlike laparoscopic cholecystectomy, which requires visualization of a single field, laparoscopic bowel surgery usually requires visualization of multiple fields as the procedure progresses. For a laparoscopic-assisted left colectomy, three distinct fields are involved, each requiring repositioning of the patient and the retractors to obtain adequate visualization. The three fields include the splenic flexure (the distal transverse and proximal descending colon included), the sigmoid colon (the distal descending colon included), and the upper pelvis (the proximal rectum if indicated). The dissection of each of these fields is completed prior to repositioning and proceeding to the next field. Visualization of the region for dissection is obtained by rotating the operating table, taking advantage of gravity, as well as traction on tissue using the Babcock clamps. These maneuvers can consume a significant amount of time, which is why it is important to complete a region, including inspection for hemostasis and thoroughness of dissection with complete mobility of the bowel, before moving to the next field to avoid excessive repositioning. A common mistake for those with limited experience in laparoscopic bowel surgery is to begin dissection of one field and, if difficulty is encountered, to move to the next field with plans to return later to complete the original field. This usually results in conversion to an open laparotomy after much time is spent repositioning the patient—only for the surgeon to find that the dissection is not any easier when he or she returns to the original field. I usually begin dissection with the field that I anticipate

in the left lower quadrant and above the pubic symphysis (Fig. 39-3). I prefer an open technique to enter the abdomen. Kocher clamps are used to grasp the lateral aspects of the umbilicus, and a 1-cm incision is made at the base of the umbilicus. The peritoneum is grasped using hemostats and incised. The Hasson trocar is placed under direct vision and stabilized with two 0 Vicryl sutures to the periumbilical fascia. The peritoneal cavity is inflated with CO_2 to a maximum pressure of 15 mm Hg. The entire abdomen and pelvis are inspected with the laparoscope. If will be the most difficult. If I cannot complete the dissection laparoscopically and need to convert to an open laparotomy, I prefer to know this early on in the procedure. For a left colectomy, the splenic flexure dissection is usually the most difficult. However, if the operation is for diverticulitis with extensive inflammation, the sigmoid dissection may be difficult, and I would begin with this field. The pelvic dissection is usually easier once the sigmoid colon is mobilized.

For the splenic flexure dissection, the patient is rotated to the right and placed in a reverse Trendelenburg position. I preserve the omentum and dissect it from the left transverse colon, rather than ligating the vessels of the gastrocolic ligament. The omentum is grasped with a Babcock clamp by the assistant surgeon and pulled upward toward the liver, while the distal transverse colon is retracted caudally, with the dissection carried along the avascular plane between the omentum and colon. With the omentum free of the left transverse colon, it can be draped out of the surgical field over the stomach and right lobe of the liver, allowing access to the splenocolic ligament (Fig. 39-4). If the splenocolic ligament is not well visualized because of a high splenic flexure, being obscured by the apex of the colon, the colon can be mobilized from its left lateral peritoneal attachment first until the ligament is visualized, and can be cut using the cautery shears.

After the splenic flexure is mobilized completely, the patient is repositioned for dissection of the distal descending and sigmoid colon. With the operating table tilted to the patient's right, the patient is placed in the Trendelenburg position. The sigmoid colon is grasped with two Babcock clamps and retracted supermedially. The peritoneal reflection is transected using the cautery shears down to the intersigmoid fold. The intersigmoid fold is carefully dissected, and the left ureter, which lies under the fold as it crosses the left iliac artery, is identified (Fig. 39-5). After the left ureter is identified, the inferior mesenteric artery is isolated and transected. This is done by tilting the operating table to the patient's left, retracting the small bowel superiorly, and pulling the sigmoid colon anteriorly to the abdominal wall. This places the vessels on tension, making them easier to identify. The mesentery surrounding the base of the inferior mesen-

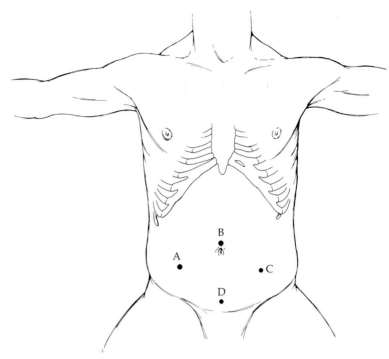

Fig. 39-3. Trocar placement for a left colectomy. A Hasson trocar in the umbilicus **(B)**, a 12-mm trocar in the right lower quadrant **(A)**, and 10-mm trocars in the suprapubic **(C)** and left lower quadrant sites **(D)**.

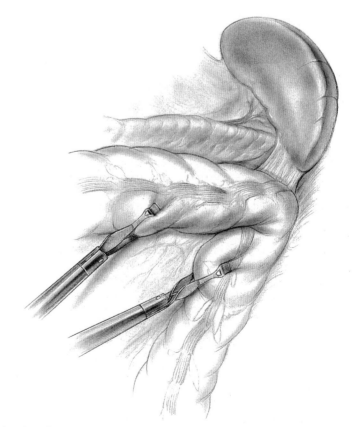

Fig. 39-4. The splenic flexure is dissected with the patient in the right-side-down Trendelenburg position. The mobilized omentum is draped over the stomach out of the surgical field, and the colon is retracted downward.

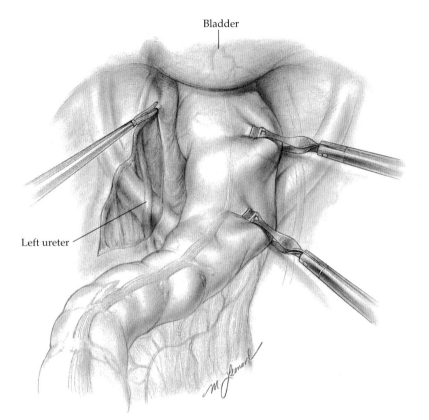

Bladder

Left ureter

Fig. 39-5. The intersigmoid fold is dissected, with the distal sigmoid colon retracted medially, exposing the underlying left ureter as it crosses the left iliac vessels.

teric artery is dissected using the cautery shears (Fig. 39-6). If the anastomosis is placed at or above the sacral promontory, depending on the indication for surgery, the superior hemorrhoidal artery is preserved and the left colic artery is transected as it comes off the inferior mesenteric artery. If the anastomosis will be below the sacral promontory, the inferior mesenteric artery is transected at its origin below the superior hemorrhoidal artery. The vessel is transected with a linear vascular stapler. The ureter is inspected to be certain that it is not incorporated in the stapler, and the device is fired. A Babcock clamp is positioned in proximity to the vessel for vascular control if the staple line is not completely hemostatic. A vascular clip or Endoloop (Ethicon, Cincinnati, Ohio) can be applied to establish hemostasis.

The third field for dissection in a laparoscopic-assisted left colectomy is the proximal pelvis. The extent of this dissection is determined by the level of the anastomosis. Some dissection of the rectum is usually helpful, even for a proximal anastomosis, to relieve the tension on the staple line. This dissection is done without lateral tilt of the table and with the patient in a steep Trendelenburg position to help keep the small bowel and mobilized sigmoid colon out of the pelvis. The rectosigmoid junction is retracted anteriorly, and the avascular plane posterior to the superior hemorrhoidal artery is dissected. If the anastomosis is below the sacral promontory, a second firing of the vascular stapler across the rectal mesentery at the level of the anastomosis is necessary. The peritoneum of the left and right perirectal gutters is dissected medial to the ureters, completing the mobilization of the intraperitoneal rectum.

Mesentery

The mesentery to the colon being resected can be managed intracorporeally or extracorporeally. For cancer, I perform an intracorporeal high (proximal) ligation of the vessels, as described previously for the inferior mesenteric artery, using a vascular stapler. For benign disease, much of the mesentery is transected extracorporeally when the bowel is brought out through a small abdominal wall incision. With the bowel exteriorized, the mesentery is taken down between Kelly clamps and suture-ligated. Often, during a left colectomy, the inferior mesenteric vessels tether the distal sigmoid colon so that it cannot be exteriorized without first transecting the vessels intracorporeally. In obese patients with a short mesentery, this can be true for the majority of the left colon. In this situation, the colon is resected, and the entire mesentery to the colon is transected intracorporeally using multiple firings of the vascular linear stapler.

Specimen Removal

Because of the size of the specimen being removed during a left colectomy, a small abdominal wall incision is necessary. A technique whereby the specimen is removed transanally through an open rectal stump has been described; however, this appears technically more difficult, and concerns exist regarding pelvic contamination with manipulation of the open rectum in the pelvis. For a left colectomy, the trocar site is extended to 4 cm in length. If the anastomosis is above the sacral promontory, the umbilical trocar site is used; if the anastomosis is below the sacral promontory, the suprapubic trocar site is used. If the umbilical site is used to remove the specimen and perform the anastomosis, a vertical incision is made, while a transverse incision is made if the suprapubic port site is used.

Anastomosis

An intracorporeal anastomosis is technically possible using either multiple applications of the linear stapler or placement of two intracorporeal purse-string sutures with use of an end-to-end circular stapling device. Both techniques are difficult and expose the abdomen to open bowel for a significant amount of time. Since a small incision is needed to remove the left colon specimen, using the same incision to perform the anastomosis is preferred. For an anastomosis above the sacral promontory, a side-to-side stapled anastomosis is performed (Fig. 39-7). For a lower anastomosis, an end-to-end double-stapled anastomosis is performed using a circular stapler. This is performed by transecting the rectum intracorporeally using two applications of the laparoscopic linear stapler. The specimen is removed through an enlarged trocar site as previously described. The proximal bowel is brought

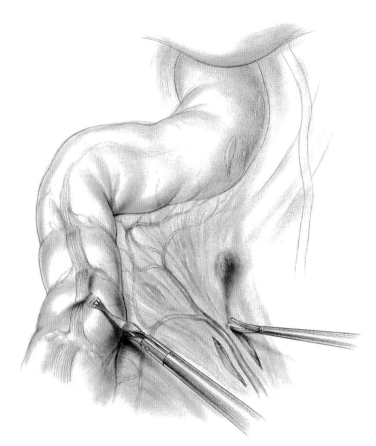

Fig. 39-6. The inferior mesenteric artery is isolated using the endoscopic shears prior to transection with the vascular stapler.

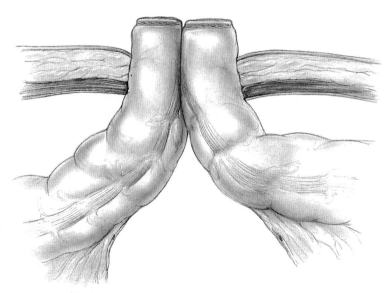

Fig. 39-7. A completed side-to-side double-stapled left colon anastomosis.

above the skin level through the same incision. A purse-string suture is placed in the proximal bowel and tightened around the anvil of the circular stapling device. The circular stapler is placed into the rectum, and the trocar is advanced through the rectal staple line. In thin patients, the anvil can be approximated to the stapling device under direct vision through the abdominal wall incision using a straight Kocher clamp to direct the shaft of the anvil. When this is not possible, the proximal bowel limb with the anvil can be placed in the abdomen and the wound closed so that pneumoperitoneum can be reestablished and the double-stapled anastomosis completed under laparoscopic vision using the Babcock clamps to grasp the anvil (Fig. 39-8). On completion of the anastomosis, the pelvis is irrigated with sterile saline, and a flexible sigmoidoscopy is performed to check for bleeding or defects in the anastomosis. Each of the abdominal wounds is closed in two layers, with a 0 Vicryl suture used in the fascia and a 4-0 Vicryl running subcuticular stitch on the skin (Fig. 39-9).

Postoperative Care and Results

The endotracheal and nasogastric tubes are removed in the operating room. The Foley catheter and venous compression hose are removed when the patient is ambulatory, usually on the first postoperative day. When active bowel sounds are noted, and if the patient has no nausea, clear liquids are started, with the diet advanced as tolerated. When the patient tolerates a regular diet, he or she can be discharged from the hospital.

In my experience with 207 laparoscopic-assisted bowel procedures, the complication rate has been 10%. This included two visceral injuries (one to the spleen and one to a ureter), both noted and treated at the initial operation. There were no perioperative deaths. The conversion rate to open laparotomy was 11%. The average time to perform a left colectomy (sigmoid colectomies included) was 130 minutes (range, 60 to 200 minutes). The estimated blood loss per procedure was 185 mL, and the average total wound length for completed procedures was 7 cm. On average, liquids were started on postoperative day 3, and the average length of stay in the hospital was 4.8 days.

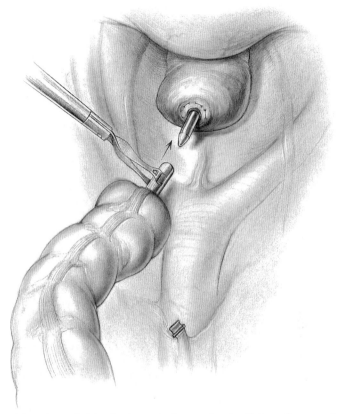

Fig. 39-8. *The rod from the anvil of the circular stapler is grasped and guided over the trocar that has been advanced through the staple line of the transected rectum.*

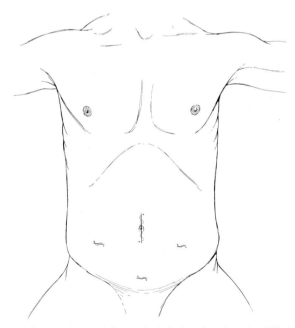

Fig. 39-9. *The abdomen following closure of all wounds, including the enlarged umbilical trocar site for a laparoscopic-assisted left colectomy.*

Suggested Reading

Ambroze WL Jr, Orangio GR, Armstrong D, Schertzer M, Lucas G. Laparoscopic surgery for colorectal neoplasms. *Semin Surg Oncol* 1994;10: 398–403.

Falk PM, Beart RW Jr, Wexner SD, et al. Laparoscopic colectomy: a critical appraisal. *Dis Colon Rectum* 1993;36:28–34.

Fine AP, Lanasa S, Gannon MP, et al. Laparoscopically assisted bowel surgery: analysis of 114 cases. *Surg Endosc* 1995;9:297.

Forde KA. Colectomy: the evolving role of laparoscopy. *Surg Endosc* 1996;10:13–14.

Liberman MA, Phillips EH, Carroll BJ, Fallas M, Rosenthal R. Laparoscopic colectomy vs. traditional colectomy for diverticulitis: outcome and costs. *Surg Endosc* 1996;10:15–18.

Liu CD, Rolandelli R, Ashley SW, Evans B, Shin M, McFadden DW. Laparoscopic surgery for inflammatory bowel disease. *Am Surg* 1995;61: 1054–1056.

Senagore AJ, Luchtefeld MA, Mackleigan JM, Mazier WP. Open colectomy versus laparoscopic colectomy: are there differences? *Ann Surg* 1993;59:549–554.

EDITOR'S COMMENT

The author of this chapter provides the reader with an excellent, detailed explanation of the patient selection process and preoperative preparation prior to laparoscopic colectomy. Additionally, the logic that guides the intraoperative decision making process is revealed. The approach taken in this chapter equips the surgeon not only with details explaining how to perform the operation but also with an understanding of why the maneuvers are performed in the manner and sequence described.

The surgeon wishing to initiate an experience with laparoscopic colectomy must first acquire an understanding of the technologies and techniques of laparoscopy. Comprehension of the physiologic effects of pneumoperitoneum is essential for appropriate patient selection. Additionally, excellent two-hand operative skills are a basic requirement for the performance of this and other advanced laparoscopic operations. Furthermore, a thorough knowledge of the disease processes affecting the left colon will guide the surgeon in the proper application of laparoscopic techniques.

Many surgeons have taken a technical approach for cancer patients that involves identification, high ligation, and division of the inferior mesenteric vessels as the initial step in this operation. Extreme caution is warranted in this approach when dissecting near the ureter as this occurs prior to extensive mobilization. I have personally found this to be a satisfactory technique with a relatively brief learning curve (in the context of extensive experience with laparoscopic bowel surgery) but have used the techniques described in this chapter more frequently. Others have chosen to restrict laparoscopic operations to those patients with benign disease. There remain many questions to be answered regarding the influence of pneumoperitoneum and laparoscopic techniques on the recurrence of cancer. Although we do not have definitive evidence that the laparoscopic approach is the preferred surgical technique for colon cancer, we likewise do not have statistical proof that condemns this operation. There are worrisome anecdotal reports regarding port site recurrences. Currently there are several large clinical trials underway that are designed to evaluate this issue. Additionally, numerous basic science laboratories are focused on defining the factors involved in tumor recurrence following laparoscopic and open operations.

The patient benefits from a laparoscopic colectomy can be significant in the properly selected patient. Unfortunately, often the patient who seems to need the minimally invasive approach most (e.g. the markedly obese patient) is a poor candidate or at high risk for conversion to the open procedure.

W.S.E.

40

Laparoscopic-assisted Abdominoperineal Resection

Claude Thibault and Heidi Nelson

Since the first description of abdomino-perineal resection (APR) by Ernest W. Miles in 1908, the technique and its indications have changed in many respects. Whereas previously advised for all rectal tumors, APR is now principally indicated for distal rectal malignancies, with lesions of the proximal and middle thirds of the rectum typically managed with anterior or low anterior resection. Even distal rectal tumors are not exclusively treated with APR due to increasing enthusiasm for sphincter-saving procedures, such as local excision and coloanal anastomosis. In addition to changes in indications, techniques have changed as well. One example of a significant change in techniques is the recent introduction of the laparoscopic approach to APR. Laparoscopic abdominal access has been applied to APR with the intent of reducing postoperative pain, ileus, and prolonged hospitalization. Whether or not laparoscopic APR offers significant advantages over open APR remains to be proven. In fact, since malignancy is the most frequent indication for APR, it must be stated up front that the application of laparoscopy for colorectal resections in the context of malignancy is a subject of considerable debate. Controversies regarding the role of laparoscopy in cancer treatment deserve special attention, and therefore this issue will be discussed below in a separate section (see "Cancer Concerns"). Meanwhile, this chapter describes indications, patient selection, and techniques of laparoscopic-assisted APR.

Indications and Patient Selection

Laparoscopy, which allows unique abdominal access, is not intended to replace conventional abdominal procedures but rather to provide alternate, perhaps less traumatic, strategies for accomplishing these well defined procedures. Due to the relatively recent introduction of laparoscopic bowel surgery, careful patient and procedure selection is required for safe and successful application of this new approach. Procedure selection begins before deciding the issue of laparoscopy, with consideration of the procedure most suited to the patient and the disease. Although APR is most often indicated for distal rectal cancer, it must be said that benign indications for APR may exist, with possibilities including severe perianal Crohn's disease, severe radiation proctitis, or complete rectal prolapse with irreversible sphincter dysfunction. In such cases, after the decision for an APR has been settled, laparoscopy may be contemplated according to patient and technical factors, as described below.

With the focus now on the most common indication for APR, distal rectal cancer, a number of alternate surgical options are available, including for both palliative and curative therapies. For palliative management of stage IV disease, where concomitant curative hepatic and primary rectal resection is not possible or reasonable, laser or cautery fulguration or colostomy placement may provide symptomatic relief. For

curative surgery, local excision and coloanal anastomosis are two alternate options available. Local excision is generally reserved for high-risk patients who have small, clinically favorable tumors, that is, those for whom the surgical risk is thought to be greater than the cancer risk. When patients are considered for local excision, it is often possible to complete the selection process prior to surgery, based on macroscopic and microscopic factors. Only if adverse findings, such as positive margins, are discovered after surgery would such patients be reconsidered for APR or perhaps coloanal anastomosis. In contrast to local excision, preoperative selection for coloanal anastomosis is typically not possible. Rather, choosing between coloanal anastomosis and APR is more often decided intraoperatively, once the adequacy of distal margins is accurately ascertained. In this regard, going into surgery, the patient has to accept the hope of a sphincter-sparing coloanal anastomosis and the possible reality of an APR and permanent stoma. Just as open surgery offers the flexibility of APR or coloanal anastomosis, determined intraoperatively, so must, and so does, the laparoscopic approach. Since it is essential to guarantee maximum flexibility with laparoscopic surgery, technical issues relevant to the handling of intraoperative transitions from sphincter-sparing resections to APR are covered in the text below.

Once the optimal surgical procedure has been determined, it has to be decided whether or not the laparoscopic approach is applicable. The choice between conventional or laparoscopic approach will depend on tumor, patient, and technical factors. As with any therapy, a favorable risk-to-benefit ratio must be maintained. Preoperative factors that would predict undue risk or marginal benefit should be thoughtfully examined. For example, the presence of a locally adherent rectal cancer would favor conventional rather than laparoscopic surgery because such a large invasive lesion may necessitate extended *en bloc* resection. Similarly, the presence of a distal obstructing lesion that produces small bowel dilatation and increased intraabdominal pressures would be difficult and risky, if approached laparoscopically.

In addition to the effects of the tumor, selection for conventional or laparoscopic surgery is also influenced by the patient's overall condition and body habitus. Obese patients are not ideal candidates for the laparoscopic approach. Especially early in the experience of a novice in laparoscopic bowel surgery, thin women with wide pelves would be preferable candidates. Similarly, patients with severe chronic obstructive pulmonary disease are probably not ideally suited for laparoscopic APR because the pneumoperitoneum and increased operative times reported for laparoscopic colorectal procedures may not be well tolerated. In general, the temptation to proceed with laparoscopic APR in patients in poor general condition or with advanced illnesses such as liver or lung disease should be resisted. Although it has been suggested that patients with compromising medical conditions fare better with laparoscopic compared to open cholecystectomy, laparoscopic APR and laparoscopic cholecystectomy are not truly comparable, and the advantages of laparoscopic over open cholecystectomy have not yet been clearly demonstrated for laparoscopic colorectal procedures. Further, patients must be capable of tolerating open APR in the event that conversion is necessary.

Finally, technical factors should be taken into consideration in the decision for laparoscopic APR. A history of previous lysis of extensive adhesions or peritonitis is a relative contraindication to laparoscopic surgery because of the risk of both inadvertent small bowel injury and undue prolongation of the operation for laparoscopic adhesiolysis. Because surgical times may be prolonged, emergency procedures for colon disease in acutely ill patients (rarely indicated for rectal cancer) are also not suitable for laparoscopic surgery.

Perioperative Management

One day prior to surgery, the bowel is mechanically prepared with a solution of polyethylene glycol followed by a nonabsorbable antibiotic regimen. A systemic antibiotic with gram-negative and anaerobic coverage is administered on call to the operating room and for three doses postoperatively. Preoperative marking of the stoma site is essential to ensure proper stomal positioning and optimal postoperative care and function. An additional benefit to preoperative stomal marking is that it allows interchange between the patient and enterostomal therapist, and this represents an opportunity to further reduce patient anxiety. Informed consent must be obtained and must include discussion specific to the uncertainties of long-term results with respect to local and systemic tumor recurrence. Additionally, patients need to understand that it may be necessary and prudent to convert to open APR for any number of reasons.

Antiembolic stockings and intermittent pneumatic compression devices are applied before the induction of anesthesia. A urinary catheter and a nasogastric tube are routinely inserted, and the patient is positioned in a modified lithotomy position (Fig. 40-1). It is important that the thighs are not flexed more than 15 to 20 degrees because this will interfere with the maneuverability of instruments positioned in the lower ports. Both arms are wrapped with wrist and elbow protectors and tucked in at the sides of the patient to avoid any tension on the shoulders or brachial plexus injury that may occur as a result of repositioning of the operating table during the procedure. The monitor can be placed on the patient's left side to give free access to the perineum, or it can be placed between the patient's legs and then moved at the time of the perineal dissection (Fig. 40-2). Two monitors, if available, one on the left and one on the right, alleviate the problem of monitor repositioning.

Operative Technique

Laparoscopic Equipment

Over the last few years, the rapid multiplication of and numerous revisions in available laparoscopic devices and instruments have rendered the selection of equipment challenging. Surgeons rapidly become accustomed to specific instruments, but just as rapidly new and improved tools become available. Updating and upgrading instruments is beneficial, but the economic impact must be considered. In general, a personal tray of standard reusable laparoscopic instruments (Figs. 40-3 and 40-4) can be supplemented by case-specific, disposable tools (Fig. 40-5).

First, for the basic equipment, a 30-degree laparoscope is preferred for its flexibility, but if one is not available, a 0-degree scope can be substituted. The 30-degree laparoscope is preferred because it provides better visualization in the pelvis and less often interferes with other instruments in the pelvis. Second, good atraumatic bowel graspers are necessary. Two basic types of bowel graspers are available: the Babcock and the "alligator." Although laparoscopic Babcock forceps are quite useful, they are not ideal for directly handling bowel because the pressure applied is localized to a small surface area. If slippage occurs, serosal tears may result. For this reason, the Babcock forceps is best applied alongside the bowel, on the mesentery, or on opposing peritoneal surface rather than directly on the bowel. Alternatively, the atraumatic or alligator bowel grasper appears to be better able to distribute pressure on a large surface area of bowel and may replace or supplement the Babcock in the standard instrument tray. Finally, sharp, preferably curved scissors that are the electrocautery-connected are essential for any instrument tray. Curved scissors allows more maneuverability, especially if the tips can be rotated (see Fig. 40-5). The ability to cauterize with scissors can save many precious minutes because this can obviate removal and reinsertion of coagulating instruments for small vessels.

Two final important details deserve mention: (a) the style of cautery connectors and (b) the length of the instruments. The most suitable cautery connectors on reusable instruments are the male-type connectors

(text continues on page 383)

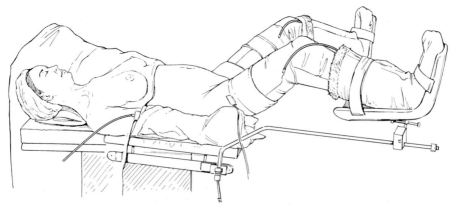

Fig. 40-1. The patient is placed in a modified lithotomy position, with hip flexion less than 20 degrees to prevent lower cannula manipulation interference.

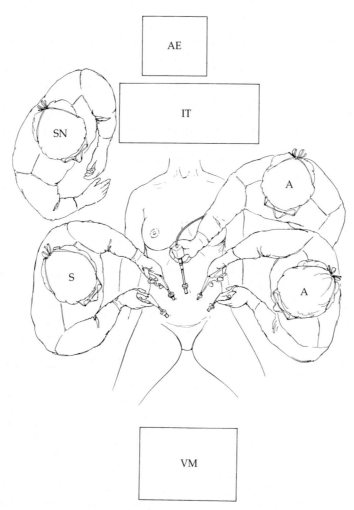

Fig. 40-2. Suggested positions for operating room personnel. The surgeon typically works on the left side of the patient for part or all of the rectal dissection. (A, assistant; AE, anesthesia; IT, instrument table; S, surgeon; SN, scrub nurse; VM, video monitor.)

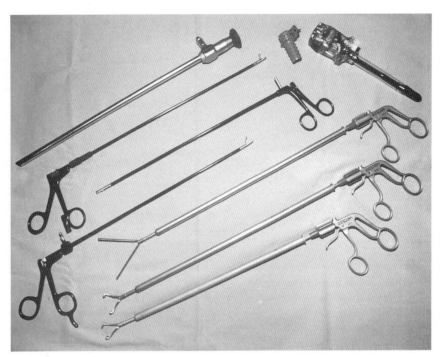

Fig. 40-3. *Suggested laparoscopic instruments for laparoscopic abdominoperineal resection. Note the 30-degree laparoscope, disposable cannulas with stability threads, and two Babcock graspers.*

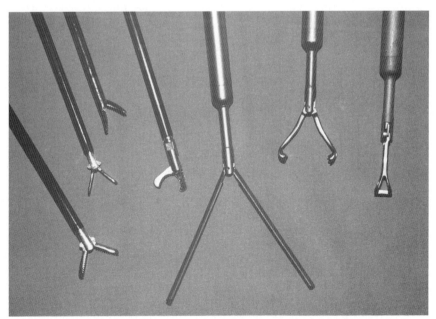

Fig. 40-4. *Each laparoscopic instrument has its own utility according to its functional end. During laparoscopic abdominoperineal resection, it may be necessary to use many different instruments because of the complexity of the procedure.*

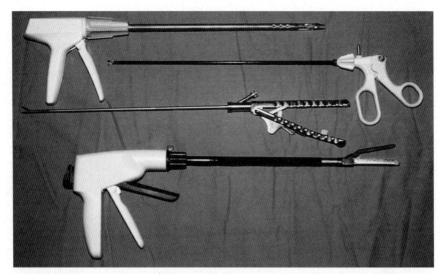

Fig. 40-5. **From top to bottom:** *The automatic clip applier is useful for dissecting the sigmoid colon mesentery. The rotating curved scissors with a connector for the cautery is almost indispensable. The laparoscopic needle holder should be mastered in the event of small or large bowel laceration. The laparoscopic linear stapler allows transection of the colon without contamination.*

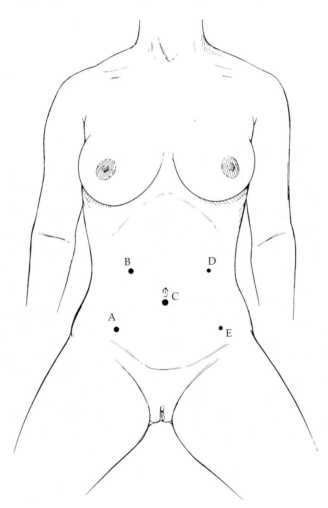

Fig. 40-6. *Suggested cannula sites. Positions can be modified according to patient body habitus. (A, 10- or 12-mm trocar; B, 10- or 12-mm trocar; C, 12-mm trocar; D, 5-, 10-, or 12-mm trocar; E, 5-, 10-, or 12-mm trocar.)*

that point upward, away from the patient. Too often, when the connector is the female type and pointing downward, the cautery cable loosens, disconnects, and must be adjusted, reattached, and secured. Optimally, all instruments should have the same type of connector to ensure compatibility. The second detail concerns instrument length. For an APR, the field of dissection may require that the ports and instruments reach all the way from the splenic flexure and diaphragm to deeply within the pelvis. Because of the diverse number of fields managed through limited ports, it is essential to have instruments that are at least 38 to 40 cm in length. Minor reach problems can be overcome by adjusting the cannulas and pushing in against the abdominal wall, but longer reaches generally result in breaks in the pneumoperitoneal seal.

Abdominal Portion

A 1-cm incision is made longitudinally just below the umbilicus. Although a circular incision may be preferred cosmetically, a longitudinal incision is easier to manage if conversion is required. A Veress needle is inserted or a cutdown performed, and then a 12- to 15-mm-Hg carbon dioxide pneumoperitoneum is achieved. A 10- or 12-mm standard or Hasson cannula is inserted, and two other trocars on the right side of the abdomen and one or two trocars on the left side are placed under direct vision (Fig. 40-6). The placement of cannulas should be individualized according to the patient's body habitus. Port positions may have to be modified to ensure adequate field reach in a tall or obese patient and to avoid cross-field interference in a thin, short-waisted patient.

Generally, on the left side, one trocar is inserted at the site marked for the colostomy. Although the technique of laparoscopic APR has been described using four trocars, the use of five ports offers more flexibility. The exclusive use of 10- or 12-mm trocars allows the introduction of all instruments in all ports and thus favors maximum versatility for camera and instrument insertion. Once the technique is well mastered, some of the 10- or 12-mm cannulas can be replaced with 5-mm ports, particularly on the left side of the abdomen. To facilitate the rectal dissection and retraction of intraperitoneal organs, other 5-mm trocars can be inserted as necessary. There are no rigid rules or limitations for the number and position of trocars, and because no patient has exactly the same anatomy, only experience will dictate optimal cannula placement.

Once the cannulas are inserted, laparoscopic exploration is undertaken, including inspection of the liver, peritoneum, and pelvic organs. The patient is then placed in Trendelenburg position, and the white line of Toldt along the sigmoid colon is incised. The sigmoid is retracted medially and caudally using Babcock clamps or atraumatic bowel graspers. The dissection is best performed with curved scissors and judicious use of cautery. Caution should be exercised when opening the peritoneal reflection. If the peritoneum is not sufficiently elevated with proper bowel traction, the iliac vessels may be positioned just beneath the peritoneal line of dissection, and inadvertent injury may occur. In the retroperitoneum, part of the dissection can be done bluntly. Cautery should always be used under direct vision to avoid inadvertent burns or electric arc that can result in necrosis and late bowel perforation. During the application of cautery, the entire length of the noninsulated, conducting tip must be visualized in the field to avoid inadvertent burn injury. Smoke can be evacuated without loss of pneumoperitoneum by periodically opening the side valve of a cannula. The left ureter should be carefully dissected and clearly visualized as in open surgery (Fig. 40-7). After the lateral adhesions of the sigmoid have been dissected, the small bowel is retracted from the pelvis. Sometimes, the distal ileum needs to be freed from the retroperitoneum at the level of the sacral promontory to facilitate retraction of small bowel loops. Following cephalad retraction of the small bowel, the right peritoneal attachments of the sigmoid are incised close to the base of the mesentery, starting distal to the sacral promontory and continuing proximal to the superior rectal artery. The superior rectal artery is usually identified by its strong pulsation and characteristic mesenteric fold. A window in the mesosigmoid just proximal to the sacral promontory and superior rectal artery usually is easily accomplished. Through this window, it is usually possible to verify the position of the left ureter.

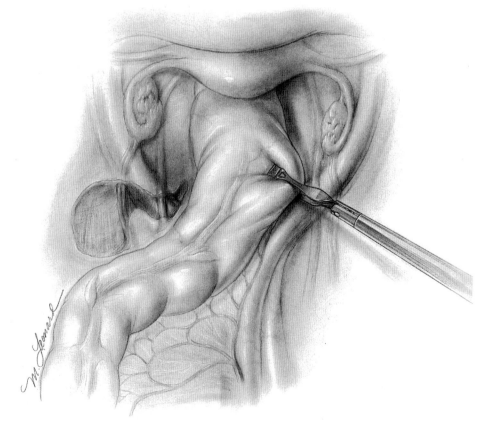

Fig. 40-7. *The left ureter should always be clearly visualized when the left and sigmoid colon is mobilized.*

The superior rectal vessels are identified, dissected, and ligated at their base with a linear stapler (Fig. 40-8), clips, or Endoloops (Ethicon, Cincinnati, Ohio). When the linear vascular stapler is used on the vascular pedicle, it is important to apply proper tension on the vessels before closing the stapler. If the pedicle is overstretched, the staples will pierce the vessels but will not accomplish proper apposition, and bleeding will ensue. Proximal vessel ligation just below the origin of the left colic artery not only ensures that oncologic principles are respected but also facilitates further dissection of the mesosigmoid, since few vessels remain to be dissected and ligated. Although high ligation proximal to the left colic artery is not required for oncologic reasons, it may facilitate reach of the proximal colon to the pelvis in the event of a coloanal anastomosis.

Once the superior rectal vessels are ligated, the rectal dissection begins posteriorly at the level of the sacral promontory distal to the window in the sigmoid mesentery (Fig. 40-9). The sigmoid colon is grasped and traction applied in a cranioventral direction using atraumatic graspers. The presacral avascular plane is entered using sharp dissection, and the posterior rectal mobilization is performed as low as possible. It may be convenient for the surgeon to perform the rectal dissection from both sides of the patient. To facilitate rectal dissection, different methods of traction on the sigmoid colon have been described. A large retention suture can be inserted through the abdominal wall into the abdominal cavity and passed around the sigmoid through its mesentery and then back through the abdominal wall to be secured outside the abdomen. Alternatively, a large vessel loop or an umbilical tape can be inserted inside the abdomen, passed around the sigmoid, and held with a laparoscopic grasper to free the assistant from continuously grasping the bowel wall with the risk of tearing and perforation. Such slings are usually not necessary, and their placement takes additional time.

Once the posterior dissection is completed to the level of the levator ani muscles, the lateral rectal dissection is accomplished using a combination of electrocautery and blunt dissection. Large vessels can be clipped. External pressure applied to the perineum by the assistant may facilitate exposure and dissection of the middle and distal thirds of the rectum. To exert lateral tension on the rectum and therefore guide the pelvic dissection, a rigid proctoscope, flexible sigmoidoscope, or a finger can be introduced into the rectum. The anterior perineal dissection is performed last, after the lateral ligaments have been freed (Fig. 40-10). The bladder and seminal vesicles in men or the uterus and vagina in women are lifted forward to dissect in the plane in front of the rectal wall, corresponding to the fascia of Denonvilliers. The dissection must be precise to avoid injury to the prostate or vagina that may result in troublesome bleeding. In women, a tenaculum-type uterine manipulator can be used to lift up the uterus and provide better exposure, but this device is usually not necessary.

After complete mobilization of the rectum has been accomplished, it is essential to determine the length of rectum distal to the inferior edge of the tumor by inserting a proctoscope into the rectum. In some cases, especially for posterior tumors, there may be sufficient length gained by rectal mobilization to accomplish a laparoscopic low anterior resection with a 2-cm distal margin. In this situation, the colorectal anastomosis can be completed using a double-staple technique. Briefly, the rectum distal to the tumor is transected with a linear stapler, and the specimen is extracted through a small left lower quadrant transverse incision. The descending colon is transected outside the abdomen, and the anvil of a circular stapler is introduced into the lumen and secured with a purse-string suture. The bowel is returned into the abdomen and the incision closed. It is also possible to transect the colon inside the abdomen both distal and proximal to the tumor using a linear stapler. If this technique is used, then a sterile plastic bag is inserted into the abdominal cavity, and the specimen placed in the bag and extracted through a left lower quadrant incision. Use of a bag has been suggested to eliminate contamination of the incision by tumor cells to reduce the risk of tumor im-

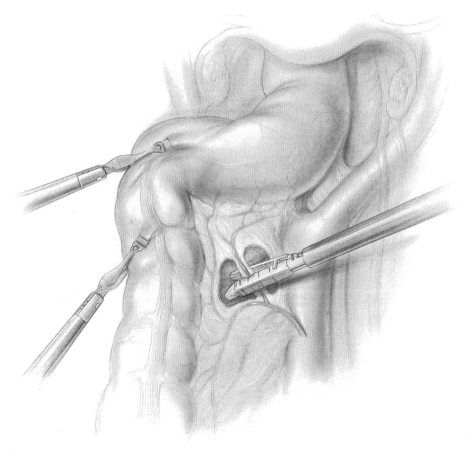

Fig. 40-8. Superior rectal vessels at their proximal extent are dissected and ligated with a linear stapler at their base to provide generous lymphadenectomy and to limit the number of vessels that have to be controlled.

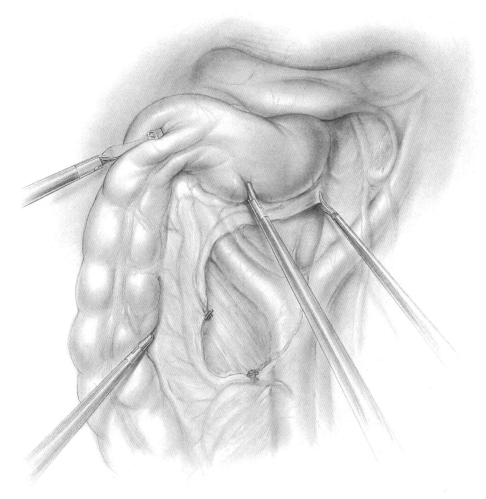

Fig. 40-9. *The rectum is dissected from the sacral promontory to the levator ani muscles in the avascular retrorectal plane.*

plantation at the wound site. As an alternative, it is probably easier to protect the abdominal wall with a plastic bag in which the bottom has been cut or with a commercially available plastic wound protector.

Once the specimen is extracted, the colorectal anastomosis is performed under laparoscopic vision in the usual fashion with a circular stapler inserted through the anus. Of note, it may be necessary to mobilize the splenic flexure for adequate reach for a tension-free anastomosis. The trocar of the stapling shaft pierces the rectal staple line and then connects with the proximal anvil, after which the stapler is closed and fired. The circular rings are inspected, and the anastomosis is tested in a saline-filled pelvis using rectal insufflation.

Sometimes, the distance between the inferior edge of the tumor and the superior part of the anorectal ring measures a scant 2 cm. This does not allow use of the linear stapler because the margin will be considerably reduced using this approach. In this case, it is still possible to proceed with a coloanal sphincter-saving procedure. Final transection of the rectum may be accomplished from the perineal side using a standard mucosectomy technique. The buttocks are retracted using two Gelpi retractors or a Lone-Star retractor, and the mucosectomy is performed using electrocautery dissection of the mucosa, starting at the dentate line. If preferred, submucosal injection of a solution of bupivacaine hydrochloride with 1:200,000 epinephrine may be employed to decrease bleeding and facilitate mucosal elevation and dissection. After the mucosa is elevated, it is grasped with Kocher clamps, and the mucosal dissection is continued proximally until the rectum is finally transected. The

proximal colon is divided with a laparoscopic stapler, which allows the specimen to be delivered through either a small wound-protected incision or the anal opening. It may be necessary to mobilize the splenic flexure to ensure adequate colon length. The proximal colon is delivered through the anal musculature and anastomosed with interrupted 3-0 resorbable sutures in a fashion typical for any hand-sewn coloanal anastomosis. A protective ileostomy is fashioned according to the surgeon's discretion and standard practice.

When the distal margin is not adequate for a proper oncologic low anterior resection or coloanal anastomosis, it is indicated to proceed with the perineal resection. The mesentery of the sigmoid colon is further dissected to isolate the bowel at a site suitable for colostomy creation. The descend-

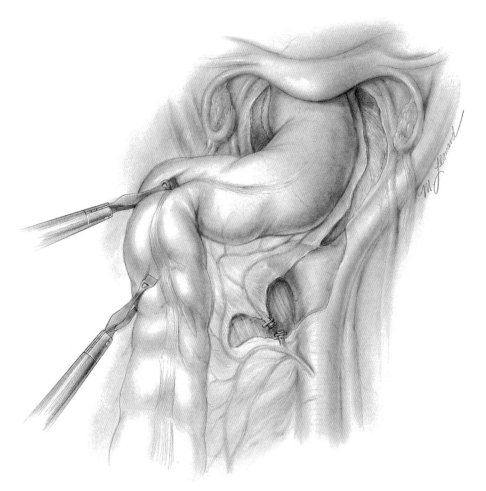

Fig. 40-10. The anterior dissection of the rectum is performed last, after the lateral stalks have been freed up.

ing colon is then transected with a laparoscopic linear stapler. The proximal bowel is further mobilized, as needed, to avoid tension on the stoma. Hemostasis is verified, and the proximal transected end of large bowel is securely grasped to be delivered later through the colostomy orifice.

Perineal Portion

The perineal dissection is performed as for conventional APR. A purse-string suture can be used to close the anus; alternatively, the perianal incision is performed first, and four clamps are applied to close the anus and serve for traction (Fig. 40-11). Dissection of the perirectal fat is carried out using electrocautery to expose the levator ani muscles and the coccygeal ligament. The anococcygeal ligament is incised with a strong scissors to penetrate into the pelvic cavity. If the pneumoperitoneum is not deflated until the perineal dissection is contiguous with the pelvic dissection, the abdominal assistant may be

able to help the perineal surgeon. For example, the abdominal surgeon can hold the rectum up and out of the way of the perineal dissection and can further guide the pelvic portion of the dissection by guiding the light and camera into the pelvis (Fig. 40-12). The levators are incised using electrocautery. This dissection is facilitated by retracting the muscles with a finger introduced into the previously created posterior defect (Fig. 40-13). The anterior dissection is performed last, and careful technique is necessary to avoid entering into the urethra in men and the vagina in women. For this part, it is helpful to deliver the proximal rectum and sigmoid colon through the posterior perineal defect. Ultimately, the entire specimen is removed through the perineal incision. Two round closed suction drains are positioned in the pelvis and externalized through lateral perineal stab wounds. The perineal wound is closed in sequential layers using absorbable suture, and the skin is

closed in a subcuticular fashion (Fig. 40-14). The drains are then clamped, pneumoperitoneum is resumed, and the orientation of the descending colon is verified to ensure that it is not twisted. The colostomy site is fashioned, and the large bowel is presented at the colostomy orifice using the laparoscopic grasper. At least a 3-cm length of colon is extracted through the skin, and the colostomy is then matured in a Brooke fashion by inverting the bowel wall so that the stoma is slightly raised above the skin. This permits better stoma face-plate application and facilitates care of the stoma by the patient. Finally, cannulas are removed under direct vision, and fascia and skin at the port sites are closed with absorbable sutures.

Conversion

At any time during laparoscopic APR, conversion to open surgery may be necessary for a number of reasons. It is important to remember that conversion itself is not a complication, even though intraoperative complications may necessitate conversion. Other reasons for conversion include difficulties with rectal mobilization, inability to recognize important anatomic structures such as the ureter, and unexpected findings such as anatomic variants or locally advanced tumors. Conversion may also be appropriate when the operation is unduly prolonged. It is suggested that time limits be set and adhered to because prolonged pelvic procedures can be complicated by pulmonary atelectasis, infection, lower extremity compartment syndrome, and pulmonary embolism from pelvic vein thrombosis. Conversion rates for laparoscopic colorectal procedures are typically between 10% and 20%. Again, when conversion is required, it should not be viewed as a failure but rather as the application of sound surgical judgment.

Intraoperative Complications

Operative complications can be roughly divided into intraoperative and postoperative categories. Because postoperative complications of laparoscopic APR are not unlike postoperative complications of open APR, only intraoperative complications will be discussed here. Further, because complications specific to the use of pneumoperitoneum are covered in a pre-

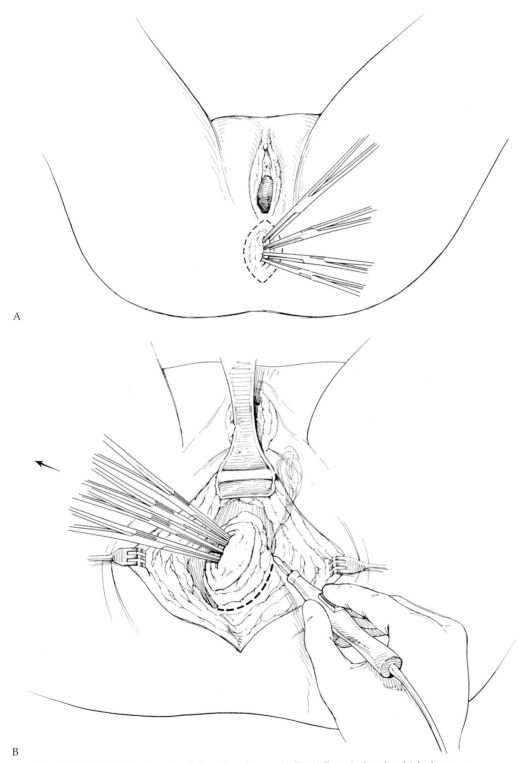

A

B

Fig. 40-11. **A,B:** *To start the perineal dissection, the anus is elliptically excised, and multiple clamps are applied to occlude the lumen and permit traction.*

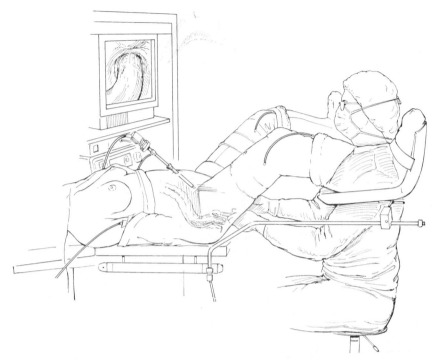

Fig. 40-12. *During the perineal dissection, the pneumoperitoneum is not released until the pelvic cavity is entered because the laparoscopic view may guide the surgeon to ensure dissection in the correct plane around the rectum.*

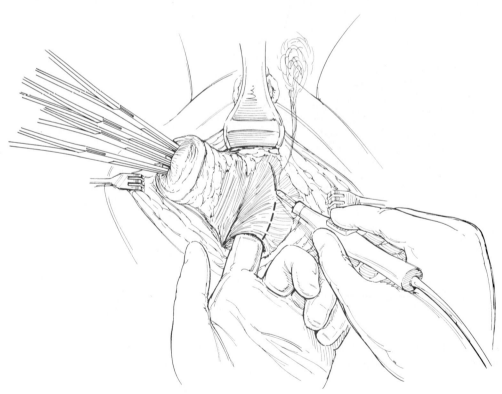

Fig. 40-13. *The levator ani muscles are retracted and dissected using a finger introduced into the posterior defect created by the incision of the anococcygeal ligament.*

vious chapter, they are not detailed here. When intraoperative injuries are considered in laparoscopic cases, two issues need be addressed: (a) what corrective action is required and (b) which approach, open or laparoscopic, is best suited to accomplish this correction. According to the severity of lesions and the laparoscopic experience of the surgeon, control of the problem may be accomplished laparoscopically or by conversion to laparotomy.

Significant bleeding may occur during dissection of the sigmoid mesentery or the lateral rectal stalks. Most often, the offending vessel can be grasped and clipped, and hemostasis can be achieved. Sometimes, a gush of blood directly blurs the lens of the camera. If this happens, the laparoscope should quickly be withdrawn, washed, and reinserted, with the assistant holding the colon in a slightly modified position so that the lens does not become soiled a second time. Sometimes, the origin of bleeding cannot be readily identified. Pressure on the area of bleeding with a grasper usually provides enough time to momentarily stop the bleeding and introduce a laparoscopic suction device. The area is washed, the blood aspirated, and control of the bleeding accomplished. Finally, whenever the laparoscopic linear stapler is used to clamp and transect large vessels, it is essential that the tip of the instrument be seen to be free of any tissue. Otherwise, closure and firing may result in troublesome partial section of a major vessel or incorporation of structures not intended for transection.

Another intraoperative complication that may have disastrous consequences in the postoperative period, if unrecognized at the time of laparoscopy, is small bowel laceration. A small serosal or even transmural perforation may be repaired laparoscopically, depending on the laparoscopic experience of the surgeon and the extent of injury. For this reason, the laparoscopic surgeon is best equipped if he or she is familiar with the technique of intracorporeal suturing. Alternatively, if laparoscopic suturing is not feasible, the bowel injury can be exteriorized and repaired through a small incision. As a final resort, conversion to an open procedure may be necessary.

Finally, ureteral injury represents another potential problem. When recognized at the

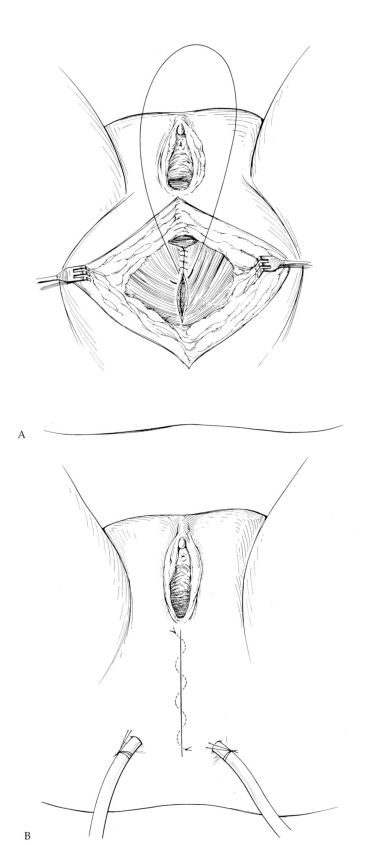

A

B

*Fig. 40-14. At completion of the perineal dissection, two round drains are inserted through lateral incisions (**A**), and the wound is closed with multiple layers of interrupted sutures (**B**).*

time of surgery, inadvertent suture ligation of the ureter can be corrected by removing the offending suture, and inserting a double-"J" ureteral stent under cystoscopic guidance. Stents should be left in place for 3 to 6 months after surgery. If a partial or complete ureteral laceration is encountered, conversion to an open procedure is warranted either to proceed with a spatulated end-to-end anastomosis with internal stenting or to perform a ureteroneocystostomy for distal ureteral injury below the iliac vessels. Because delayed recognition of ureteral injury increases the rate of nephrectomy, immediate recognition is important. If doubt exists, intraoperative administration of indigo carmine or methylene blue may help delineate a small perforation or a devitalized segment of ureter.

Postoperative Care

The nasogastric tube is removed preferably in the recovery room or the day following surgery. Ambulation is started as early as the day of surgery, especially if the operation was performed in the morning. Dietary intake is rapidly offered, usually the day after surgery, and advanced as tolerated according to hunger and bowel function. The urinary catheter is typically removed on the morning of the fifth postoperative day. Postvoid residual volumes may be helpful to identify patients with urinary retention early. The deep pelvic drains are also removed on the fifth postoperative day if the output is less than 50 mL per day. Stoma care and training are initiated early. Because many patients will be ready for dismissal before stoma teaching is complete, it is essential to have outpatient teaching opportunities available.

Cancer Concerns

The role of laparoscopic surgery in the treatment of colorectal cancer remains a subject of considerable debate. Because laparoscopic colon and rectal procedures were only introduced as recently as 1991, most reports in the literature address issues of feasibility and safety rather than long-term oncologic outcomes, such as recurrence and survival rates. Fueling these concerns and this debate are recent publications reporting trocar-site cancer recurrences following laparoscopic colon cancer surgery. Caution is advised in the widespread use of laparoscopic techniques in cases of cancer until true risks are delineated. With this in mind, two aspects of this subject deserve further discussion: (a) the technical ability to complete a proper oncologic resection and (b) the theoretical risks and concerns raised about trocar recurrences.

At a minimum, before a laparoscopic APR is embarked on, the principal features of an oncologic rectal resection should be considered, including the adequacy of distal and lateral mesorectal margins, extent of mesenteric lymphadenectomy, avoidance of intraoperative tumor contamination, and special attention to tumor extraction and wound protection. Although controlled trials will be key to determining the relative risk-to-benefit ratio for laparoscopic APR, some reports provide reassurance that at least these oncologic principles can be adhered to. With regard to margins of resection and number of lymph nodes removed, several reports have demonstrated that there are no differences between laparoscopic and open colectomy techniques and that indeed laparoscopic colectomy and APR can be performed according to accepted surgical oncologic principles.

Even if the same cancer operation can be performed laparoscopically as well as open, there remains at least a theoretical risk that the new approach alters tumor behavior through local or systemic effects. For laparoscopic colectomy, reports of trocar- and wound-site tumor implants have generated concern regarding the influence of laparoscopy on tumor cell dissemination at the time of surgery. It is postulated that laparoscopic-assisted tumor extraction techniques predispose to the risk of wound recurrence. Further, it is postulated that the presence of a pneumoperitoneum predisposes to trocar-site recurrences, specifically in cases in which viable free-floating tumor cells are present in the abdominal cavity. Because viable tumor cells can be isolated in some colon cancer patients prior to surgical manipulation, such high-risk events may occur despite the use of meticulous, "no touch," laparoscopic techniques. The focusing of tumor cell inocula at trocar sites may occur during surgery secondary to pneumoperitoneal leak or at closure when cannulas are being removed. Although these concerns have been raised for laparoscopic-assisted colectomy for colon cancer, a number of issues remain unresolved.

First, are recurrences truly different for laparoscopic versus open colon cancer resection? Second, are the same risks relevant for laparoscopic rectal cancer procedures? With regard to the first issue, controlled trials are under way. With regard to the second issue, a number of differences seem pertinent, including the fact that with laparoscopic APR or coloanal anastomosis, the rectal cancer is generally removed through the perineum or anus, respectively, as for standard open practice. Additionally, because rectal tumors are not intraperitoneal, the risk of free-floating intraperitoneal tumor cells and therefore spread secondary to pneumoperitoneal pressures would be expected to be exceedingly small. In the final analysis, the risk-to-benefit ratio of laparoscopic-assisted APR must be determined clinically, preferably in controlled trials.

Conclusion

Laparoscopic APR is an advanced-level, minimal-access procedure requiring more training, experience, and time than most other laparoscopic interventions such as appendectomy or cholecystectomy. Successful completion of laparoscopic APR requires a solid knowledge of rectal anatomy, solid experience with laparoscopic procedures, and patience. As with every new intervention, a learning curve is to be expected. Approximately 10 to 20 cases are required to achieve a modicum of comfort and reasonable operating times. Technical recommendations such as those listed in this chapter may allow avoidance of some of the common pitfalls of this procedure. Finally, long-term results of this operation when performed for malignancy are not well defined, and careful patient selection in the context of clinical research protocols is recommended.

Suggested Reading

Chindasub S, Charntaracharmnong C, Nimitvanit C, Akkaranurukul P, Santitarmmanon B.Laparoscopic abdominoperineal resection. *J Laparoendosc Surg* 1994;4:17–21.

Cirocco WC, Schwartzman A, Golub RW. Abdominal wall recurrence after laparoscopic colectomy for colon cancer. *Surgery* 1994 [Review];116:842–846.

Decanini C, Milsom JW, Bohm B, Fazio VW. Laparoscopic oncologic abdominoperineal resection. *Dis Colon Rectum* 1994;37:552–558.

Kockerling F, Gastinger I, Schneider B, Krause W, Gall FP. Laparoscopic abdominoperineal excision of the rectum with high ligation of the inferior mesenteric artery in the management of rectal carcinoma. *Endosc Surg Allied Technol* 1993;1:16–19.

Larach SW, Salomon MC, Williamson PR, Goldstein E. Laparoscopic assisted abdominoperineal resection. *Surg Laparosc Endosc* 1993;3: 115–118.

Simons AJ, Anthone GJ, Ortega AE, et al. Laparoscopic-assisted colectomy learning curve. *Dis Colon Rectum* 1995;38:600–603.

Thibault C, Nelson H. Laparoscopic proctectomy for malignant disease. In: Andrus C, Cosgrove J, Longo WE, ed. *Minimally invasive surgery: principles and outcomes.* Amsterdam: Harwood Academic Publishers, 1998.

Velez PM. Laparoscopic colonic and rectal resection. *Baillieres Clin Gastroenterol* 1993 [Review];7:867–878.

EDITOR'S COMMENT

Advanced technical skills are required to safely perform a laparoscopic APR. The possession of such skills does not provide sufficient indication for an APR to be performed using minimally invasive techniques. Drs. Thibault and Nelson have clearly described the logic used in selecting patients for various techniques. A minority of patients possessing anorectal surgical diseases requiring an APR will be suitable candidates for a laparoscopic approach.

Technical alternatives to those described by the authors include early proximal division of the sigmoid or descending colon. Early division of the proximal extent of resection may facilitate mobilization of the distal sigmoid colon and rectum and provide enhanced visualization of the mesentery and vasculature. Other authors have described an approach in which the mesenteric vessels are addressed from the right side of the colon as the initial step in the operation. A word of caution is warranted when this technique is used. The ureters are at increased risk for injury, especially in obese patients. It is advisable for the surgeon to clearly identify the vessels, as well as the ureters, prior to clipping or dividing any structures within the mesentery or retroperitoneum.

The authors have provided an excellent concise overview of the oncologic concerns with laparoscopic surgery for colorectal cancer. Many questions remain to be answered concerning the effects of pneumoperitoneum, carbon dioxide, laparoscopic techniques, and immunosuppression when laparoscopy is used for cancer surgery.

W.S.E.

41

Laparoscopic Subtotal and Total Colectomy

Dennis L. Fowler

Resection of the entire abdominal colon with or without resection of the rectum is a formidable operation. The traditional open procedure has usually required a generous midline incision and several hours to perform. It has often been associated with the need for blood transfusion and has traditionally required more than 1 week in the hospital after the procedure. Laparoscopic resection of the abdominal colon and rectum is even more technically demanding and requires a great deal of patience and laparoscopic skill. In selected patients, the length of recovery and the amount of blood loss can be significantly reduced with a laparoscopic approach. However, the procedure demands even greater attention to both anatomic and technical detail than the open procedure.

Surgical Anatomy

Several anatomic features of the colon are important in the context of resection whether open or laparoscopic. Three specific aspects of colon and rectal anatomy are particularly important during laparoscopic resection:

1. The colon has numerous attachments to other structures in the abdomen and retroperitoneum.
2. The colon has certain spatial relationships with other organs in the abdomen and retroperitoneum to which it is not actually attached.
3. As in open surgery, knowledge of the blood supply of the colon is critical to a safe resection.

The colon is attached to the right and left lateral walls of the abdominal cavity by peritoneal reflections. Beginning at the ce-

cum on the right, the ascending colon is attached by this peritoneal reflection all the way to the hepatic flexure. At the hepatic flexure and through the right transverse colon, the peritoneal reflections attach the colon to the liver and sometimes to the gallbladder and intraperitoneal duodenum. The looping portion of the transverse colon is attached to the stomach via the gastrocolic ligament. This blends into the phrenocolic ligament at the splenic flexure, which attaches the splenic flexure to the diaphragm. The spleen is also connected to the splenic flexure by the peritoneal attachment called the splenocolic ligament. The descending colon is attached to the left lateral abdominal wall by a peritoneal reflection analogous to the attachments on the ascending colon. The sigmoid colon is frequently less attached to other structures than any other segment of the colon. The rectum is completely extraperitoneal and along with the mesorectum is bounded posteriorly by the sacrum, laterally by the lateral pelvic walls, and anteriorly by the prostate and seminal vesicles in men and the vagina in women.

The cecum and its mesentery overlie the right ureter, the right gonadal vessels, and the iliopsoas muscle and fascia. Associated with the fascia are the femoral and lateral femoral cutaneous nerves. The ascending colon and mesocolon continue the intimate relationship with the ureter and gonadal vessels. The right mesocolon also overlies some of the right kidney and, most important, the retroperitoneal duodenum.

The hepatic flexure overlies the right kidney and lies inferior and posterior to the most caudal portion of the right lobe of the liver. The omentum is attached to the entire length of the transverse colon. The root

of the transverse mesocolon approaches the inferior border of the pancreas. The splenic flexure is not only close to the tail of the pancreas and to the spleen but also overlies the left kidney. The descending colon and its mesentery overlie some of the left kidney, as well as the left ureter and left gonadal vessels. Additionally, it overlies the quadratus lumborum muscle down to the medial border of the psoas major muscle. Associated within the intervening fascia are the subcostal, first lumbar, and lateral femoral cutaneous nerves.

As the descending colon becomes the sigmoid, the sigmoid colon and its mesocolon overlie the more distal segments of the ureter and gonadal vessels, as well as the left common iliac vessels near where the ureter crosses over them. The more distal portions of the sigmoid and its mesentery overlie some of the lumbar and sacral segments of the spine.

The abdominal colon receives all of its blood supply from branches of the superior mesenteric artery (SMA) and branches of the inferior mesenteric artery (IMA) (Fig. 41-1). The cecum, ascending colon, and transverse colon receive their blood supply from branches of the SMA. The terminal ileum and cecum receive blood via the ileocolic artery, while the ascending colon and hepatic flexure receive blood from the right colic artery. The middle colic artery supplies circulation to the transverse colon with communication around both flexures via the marginal artery of Drummond. This artery closely follows the colon and provides communication between all the main arterial branches to the colon. The splenic flexure, descending colon, sigmoid colon, and superior rectum receive their blood supply from branches of the IMA. The left colic

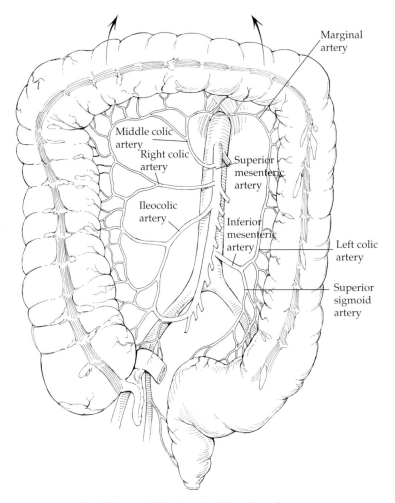

Fig. 41-1. *Arterial blood supply of the colon and rectum.*

Table 41-1. Indications for Laparoscopic Subtotal and Total Colectomy

Inflammatory bowel disease
    Chronic ulcerative colitis
    Crohn's disease
Polyposis syndromes
Colon inertia
Other benign nonemergent conditions requiring
    subtotal or total colectomy

---

artery supplies the descending colon and splenic flexure with communication via the marginal artery around to a communication with the middle colic artery. The sigmoid arteries supply most of the sigmoid, while the terminal branch of the IMA supplies the superior rectum as the superior rectal artery. Branches of the internal iliac artery supply the middle and lower rectum via the middle and inferior hemorrhoidal arteries.

Indications

Most indications for laparoscopic subtotal or total colectomy involve one of two types of disease processes: inflammatory bowel disease or polyposis syndromes (Table 41-1). Inflammatory bowel disease frequently requires removal of the entire colon, usually including the rectum. In a few patients, subtotal colectomy with ileorectal anastomosis can be utilized. Patients with

Crohn's disease will require resection by the technique described in this chapter, followed by creation of an anastomosis or stoma. Patients with chronic ulcerative colitis or polyposis syndromes may be candidates for a mucosal resection of the rectum, followed by pouch creation with an ileoanal anastomosis. Although the techniques for these latter procedures will not be included in this chapter, those patients may undergo laparoscopic resection of the abdominal colon and mobilization of the terminal ileum as described in this chapter. Patients with polyposis syndromes are often ideal candidates for laparoscopic total colectomy, and the laparoscopic approach can be used for part or all of the procedure, even if a J-pouch and pull-through procedure are contemplated.

Other patients with nonemergent conditions requiring subtotal or total colectomy may also be candidates for laparoscopic resection. However, patients with condi-

tions requiring emergent colectomy, such as ongoing lower gastrointestinal bleeding, and patients with cancer are not candidates for laparoscopic subtotal or total colectomy. In these patients, the colectomy should be performed with an open technique.

Other aspects of patients' illness may play a role in determining whether or not they should undergo a laparoscopic resection. Patients with inflammatory bowel disease may have adhesions, scarring, phlegmons, or abscesses as a result of their disease or previous surgery. Although none of these conditions is an absolute contraindication to the laparoscopic approach, any of them can make the surgical procedure much more difficult or even impossible with current technology. Colonoscopy and imaging studies such as computed tomography can provide useful information about the nature and extent of the inflammatory processes, but it may require laparoscopic visualization of the peritoneal cavity and colon before it can be determined whether or not laparoscopic resection is feasible.

Perioperative Management

Preoperative preparation of the patient for laparoscopic colon resection is no different from that for an open procedure. The patient should undergo the appropriate preoperative evaluation with colonoscopy or other imaging studies to make the diagnosis and determine the location and extent of disease. Standard bowel preparation with a purge and antibiotics are essential. Other details of patient preparation and adherence to standards of surgical care, such as using a steroid preparation in patients who are steroid-dependent, must be adhered to meticulously, just as if the patient were undergoing an open resection. All patients must have pneumatic compression boots during the operation. Particularly if pneumoperitoneum is to be used during the laparoscopy, this technique must be used to minimize the chance of postoperative deep vein thrombosis.

Operative Technique

The patient is placed in the supine position with the legs in hanging or supportive stirrups that allow the legs to be straight but abducted. Stirrups that flex the hips or knees cannot be used because elevation of the thighs interferes with movement of the laparoscopic instruments. The legs are abducted (a) to provide access to the anus for endoscopy and stapler placement and (b) to provide a position for the surgeon or assistant to stand. With this position, the surgeon can stand on either side of the patient or between the legs (Fig. 41-2). Two monitors are required, and it is preferable that they be mobile. Unlike most laparoscopic colectomy procedures, subtotal or total colectomy requires visualization of both flexures and the pelvis, and this will require pointing the laparoscope both superiorly and inferiorly. For viewing superiorly, it is best to have the monitors near the head of the bed. For dissection in the pelvis, it is better to have the monitors near the foot of the bed.

Five ports are usually sufficient for laparoscopic resection of the entire abdominal colon (Fig. 41-3). Mobilization and dissection of the colon should be completed in segments (Table 41-2). For each segment, the laparoscope is placed through the appropriate port, and then the surgeon and assistant(s) can be positioned to do that segment.

Both the port for the scope and the position of the surgeon and assistant(s) may be changed according to the segment being dissected. Although mobilization of the colon can be started with any segment of the colon, it is important to begin and complete one segment at a time so as to maintain anatomic orientation throughout the dissection.

Conceptually, the abdominal colon can be divided into four segments for mobilization and resection, and in patients requiring a total proctocolectomy, the rectum can be considered the fifth segment. The most logical point at which to begin is the cecum. Therefore, the first segment to be mobilized is the cecum and ascending colon. The second segment is the hepatic flexure and transverse colon. The third is the splenic flexure and descending colon, and the sigmoid colon is the fourth segment.

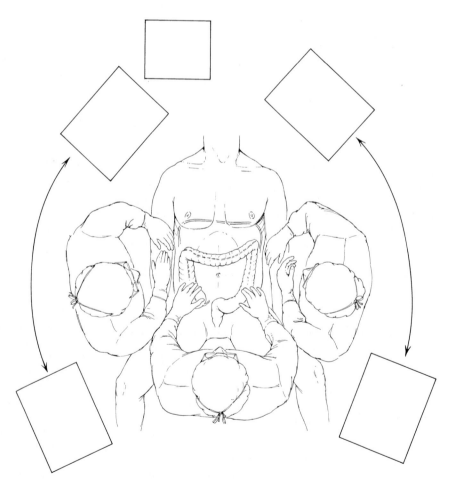

Fig. 41-2. Patient positioning and operating room setup. The surgeon, assistant, and scrub nurse may move among the three positions as necessary to perform each segment of the operation.

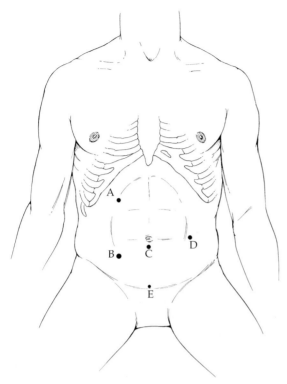

Fig. 41-3. Port sites for laparoscopic subtotal or total colectomy. (A, 5- or 10-mm port; B, 12-mm port; C, 5- or 10-mm port; D, 5- or 10-mm port; E, 5- or 10-mm port).

Table 41-2. Sequence of Segmental Dissection during Laparoscopic Subtotal and Total Colectomy

Cecum and ascending colon

Hepatic flexure and transverse colon

Splenic flexure and descending colon

Sigmoid colon

Rectum (if necessary)

Cecum and Ascending Colon

The cecum and right gutter can best be visualized by placing the laparoscope in the suprapubic midline port site (Fig. 41-4). With the scope in this port, the surgeon and assistant both stand on the patient's left side and view a monitor on the patient's right side near the head or shoulder. The cecum and ascending colon can be grasped and retracted medially and anteriorly with a grasper placed through a port on the left side of the abdomen. The lateral peritoneal reflection (white line of Toldt) can be incised with the scissors or ultrasonically activated shears (Laparosonic Coagulating Shears, Ethicon Ultracision, Inc., Smithfield, Rhode Island). This peritoneal incision is extended from the cecum to the hepatic flexure.

The ascending mesocolon is then mobilized medially with a blunt technique, although some dense attachments may need division with the scissors or shears. As this is dissected medially, it is important to visualize and preserve several retroperitoneal structures. The right ureter and gonadal vessels can be identified at the pelvic brim posterior to the cecum. Their course can be followed cephalad as the dissection progresses. The inferior pole of the right kidney is also easily identified. Equally important is identification of the retroperitoneal third and fourth portions of the duodenum. The right mesocolon must be swept away from the duodenum. If high ligation of the ileocolic vascular pedicle is critical to the procedure, the relationship between this pedicle and the duodenum must be identified prior to division of the pedicle. If the disease allows a less radical dissection of the mesentery, the duodenum should still be identified, but it may not be necessary to mobilize the mesentery away from the duodenum so extensively. In this case, the mesentery can be divided closer to the bowel.

Any of several techniques or combinations thereof can be used for division of the mesentery. Multiple factors must be considered before one is chosen. The ideal technique for dividing the mesentery would provide excellent hemostasis quickly and inexpensively. Traditional dissection of vessels followed by application of ligatures or clips can provide good hemostasis at an acceptable cost, but this approach is very time-consuming and may require too much time to do a subtotal or total colectomy. A faster technique is to divide the mesentery with the linear cutting stapler. This also provides excellent hemostasis and is acceptably quick, but this technique may require so many staple cartridges to do a subtotal colectomy that the cost would be prohibitive. A relatively newer technique involves the use of the ultrasonically activated shears. The shears can be used to divide all but the largest named vessels in the mesentery. The use of the shears avoids the need to repeatedly change instruments, and almost the entire mesenteric dissection can be done with the one instrument. The shears not only provide excellent hemostasis but also offer the quickest method of doing such an extensive mesenteric dissection, while still being less expensive than clips or staples.

The mesentery of the right colon should be divided from the terminal ileum toward the hepatic flexure (Fig. 41-5). A window can safely be made in the mesentery of the terminal ileum. Then, the ultrasonically activated shears can be used to divide the mesentery from this point to the hepatic flexure. Named vessels such as the ileocolic artery and right colic artery should be clipped or ligated. If the mesentery is divided relatively closer to the colon, only the branches of these vessels are divided, and this can be accomplished with the shears. If the mesenteric dissection is not radical, it may be possible to do the dissection with only the shears and without clips or ligatures.

Hepatic Flexure and Transverse Colon

The dissection of this segment is visualized by placing the laparoscope through the umbilical abdominal port site. Grasping devices are passed through the left midabdominal and lower midline ports. The surgeon stands to the right of

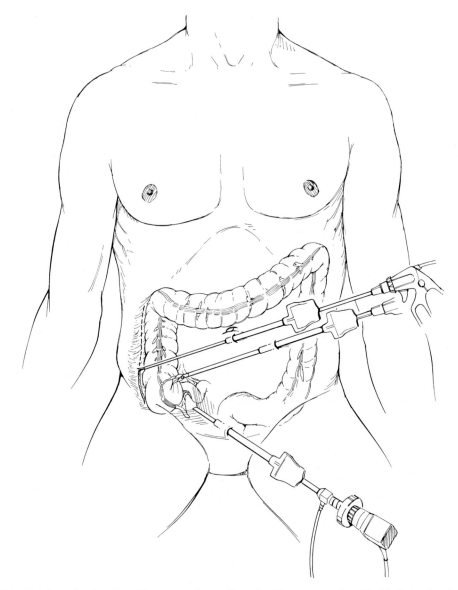

Fig. 41-4. Setup for dissection of the cecum and ascending colon. The surgeon and assistant both stand on the patient's left side.

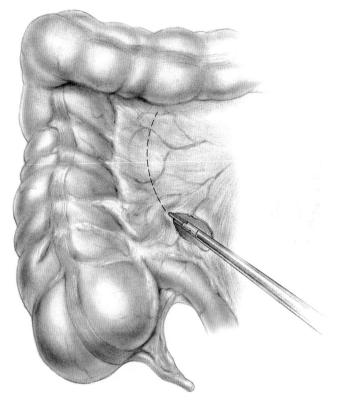

Fig. 41-5. Dividing the ascending mesocolon using the ultrasonically activated shears.

the patient and operates through the two right-sided ports (Fig. 41-6). The assistant stands between the patient's legs. The monitors must be positioned near the patient's head or shoulder on each side.

After the right mesocolon is divided, the hepatic flexure can be freed by dividing the peritoneal attachments superiorly. As this dissection is carried from right to left, the right transverse colon is mobilized away from the gallbladder and intraperitoneal duodenum. Soon, the lesser sac can be entered, and then the gastrocolic ligament can be divided from hepatic flexure to splenic flexure. Here again, this dissection is most expeditiously completed using the ultrasonically activated shears. With this technology, the dissection of the gastrocolic ligament/omentum can be done almost bloodlessly. The flexures and transverse colon are then attached only by their mesentery. The mesentery can be divided with any of the previously described techniques, but as with the previously described dissections, the ultrasonically activated shears are the preferred method of doing the dissection. The middle colic artery can be divided as proximally or distally as necessary. A high division of the middle colic artery reduces the amount of vascularity in the remainder of the wide dissection of the mesentery, but all of the mesentery can be divided with the shears, if the mesentery is divided closer to the bowel. At the time of the division of the middle colic artery, the ligament of Treitz must be identified and the proximal jejunum carefully protected.

Splenic Flexure and Descending Colon

For visualization of the splenic flexure, the scope should remain through the umbilical port. The surgeon should stand between the patient's legs, and the assistant should move around to the patient's right side. A monitor on the patient's left side near the head of the bed can be used by both surgeon and assistant. The splenic flexure is probably the most difficult part of the abdominal colon to mobilize, and it is helpful to have both the transverse colon and descending colon mobilized first. Therefore, the descending colon is mobilized prior to mobilizing the actual flexure. With the scope through the umbilical port, the right-sided abdominal ports can be used for bowel graspers to expose the

splenic flexure. These graspers can be used to retract both the distal transverse colon and the descending colon medially. Via a left-sided port, the shears or scissors can be used to divide the peritoneal reflection from the junction of the sigmoid colon up to the splenic flexure (Fig. 41-7). With traction on both the left transverse colon and the descending colon caudally and medially and with tilting of the patient into a reverse Trendelenburg position with tilt to the right, the dissection can be carried around the splenic flexure. In some patients, an angled scope may facilitate visualization superior to the splenic flexure between the splenic flexure and spleen. Here, the phrenocolic and splenocolic ligaments are divided. Once the dissection is around the splenic flexure, this incision can be connected with the previous incision made through the gastrocolic ligament.

After the splenic flexure is mobilized, the mesocolon of the splenic flexure and descending colon can be divided, just as the previous mesentery was divided. The mesentery here is relatively avascular. Beginning at the ligament of Treitz with dissection proceeding to the left, the mesentery contains only the marginal artery of Drummond all the way around to the left colic artery. Prior to division of the left colic artery or its major branches, the sigmoid colon should be mobilized.

Sigmoid Colon

For the remainder of the procedure, the laparoscope can remain through the umbilical port. The surgeon stands on the patient's right and the assistant on the patient's left. Both monitors are moved to a position near the feet. It is imperative that the patient be placed in the Trendelenburg position. The small bowel can be pulled up out of the pelvis so that it will lie in the upper abdomen. The Trendelenburg position should be sufficiently steep to allow the small bowel to stay in the upper abdomen without the use of retractors. The sigmoid colon is grasped with graspers placed through ports on the left and lower midline. The surgeon operates through the right-sided ports (Fig. 41-8). With the sigmoid retracted medially, the lateral peritoneal attachments of the sigmoid colon can be divided, allowing it and its mesocolon to be brought up into the space of the peritoneal cavity. The left ureter is easily identified in the retroperitoneum as the sigmoid mesocolon is elevated. With the sigmoid colon elevated, the sigmoid meso-

(text continues on page 400)

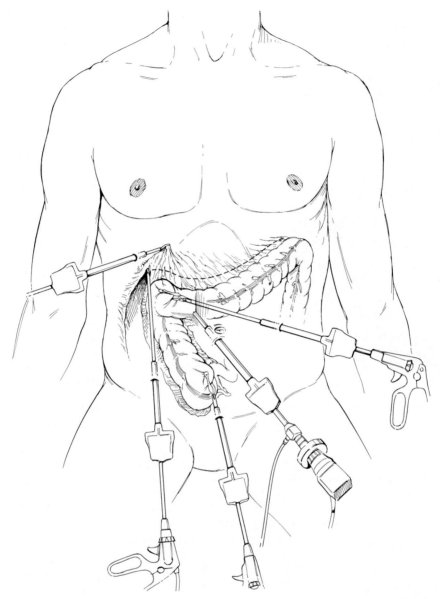

Fig. 41-6. *Setup for dissection of the hepatic flexure and transverse colon. The surgeon stands on the patient's right side, and the assistant stands between the legs.*

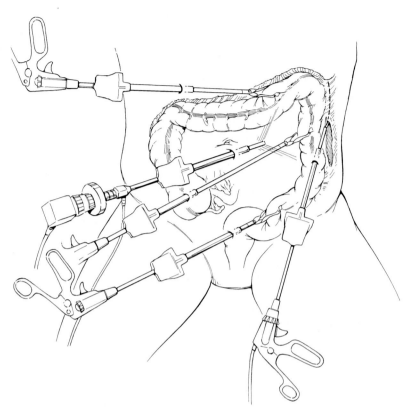

Fig. 41-7. Setup for dissection of the splenic flexure and descending colon. The surgeon stands between the legs, and the assistant stands on the patient's left side.

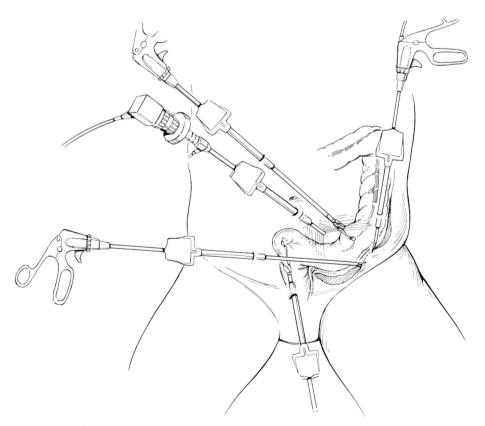

Fig. 41-8. Setup for dissection of the sigmoid colon. The surgeon stands on the patient's right side, and the assistant stands on the patient's left side.

colon is divided, beginning at the previous point of division of the mesentery of the descending colon. This mesocolic dissection is continued down into the pelvis. The sigmoid mesocolon can be taken radically by dissecting it away from the hollow of the sacrum, or it can be divided less radically with the previously described techniques, with some of the mesocolon and the presacral nerves left intact. This may be particularly important in men when preservation of sexual function is critical. Here, once again, division of the mesentery relatively close to the bowel can be done almost bloodlessly with the ultrasonically activated shears, and this spares the nerves critical to sexual function.

If the procedure does not involve proctectomy, the sigmoid mesocolon is dissected to the site chosen as the distal line of resection, usually in the distal sigmoid colon just above the rectosigmoid junction. Once the colon at the distal line of resection is circumferentially exposed, it can be divided with the linear cutting stapler. The stapler can be placed through the right lower quadrant port site. Either a 30-mm or a 60-mm stapler can be used. If the distal line of resection is deep in the pelvis, the 30-mm instrument should be used, even if two or more firings of the stapler are required. In this situation, the 60-mm stapler is so long that it divides the bowel

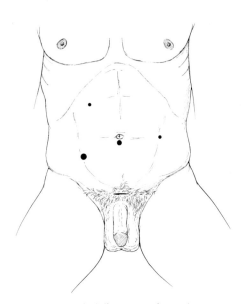

Fig. 41-9. Site of minilaparotomy for specimen removal after laparoscopic subtotal colectomy.

with a very oblique angle. The angle of division can be kept more nearly transverse using the 30-mm stapler twice.

Specimen Removal

In patients undergoing a subtotal colectomy, the specimen should be removed through a minilaparotomy. Although an extension of the umbilical wound works well, I prefer to make a 3 to 4 cm transverse incision in the pubic hair just above the symphysis pubis (Fig. 41-9). After division of the sigmoid colon at the distal line of resection, as described above, it is important to place a ratcheted clamp on the stapled end of the specimen prior to making the minilaparotomy and deflating the pneumoperitoneum. With this clamp, the end of the specimen can be passed through the minilaparotomy without having to search for the end of the specimen.

As soon as the minilaparotomy incision is made, a plastic wound protector is placed in it. The wound protector acts as a barrier against contamination of the wound with bacteria (or malignant cells in the case of malignancy). By grasping the stapled end of the distal sigmoid as it comes through the wound, the surgeon can pull the entire colon out through the minilaparotomy. When the entire colon has been exteriorized, the terminal ileum is pulled into the wound and divided, thus completing resection of the entire abdominal colon.

Anastomosis

The anastomosis can be created with the circular stapler or with laparoscopic suturing. If the stapler is to be used, the anvil of the stapler is placed into the end of the ileum extracorporeally. After division of the terminal ileum, a purse-string suture is placed in the end of the ileum using either an automated purse-string device or a hand-suturing technique. The anvil of the circular stapler is positioned in the end of the ileum through the purse-string, and the purse-string is tied. The end of the ileum holding the anvil of the stapler is dropped back into the abdominal cavity through the minilaparotomy. The wound protector is removed, the wound is closed, and the pneumoperitoneum is reestablished. Laparoscopic visualization is then used to create the anastomosis. The circular stapler (without anvil) is introduced into the rectum through the anus. The center spike of the stapler is protruded through the staple line in the distal sigmoid colon. The spike is

removed from the stapler and then removed from the abdomen through one of the ports. The anvil is then connected to the protruding shaft of the stapler, and the stapler is closed. Firing the stapler creates the anastomosis, and the stapler with attached anvil can be removed from the rectum through the anus.

If the anastomosis is to be created by suturing, the end of the terminal ileum is dropped back into the abdomen, and pneumoperitoneum is reestablished. Using laparoscopic visualization, the staple line on the rectal stump is cut off and removed through a port. The terminal ileum can then be sutured end-to-end to the distal sigmoid. A single-layer, double-layer, or even a partial running closure technique can be used, depending on the skill and preference of the surgeon.

Once completed, the anastomosis should be tested for integrity. A combination technique of visual inspection and insufflation offers the most complete evaluation of the anastomosis. The anastomosis can be carefully visualized by a flexible sigmoidoscope inserted into the rectum. This provides visual confirmation of a circumferentially intact anastomosis. At the same time, the rectum can be insufflated with carbon dioxide (CO_2) through the sigmoidoscope while the pelvis is filled with saline. Any bubbling of CO_2 through the saline, seen laparoscopically, would indicate that the anastomosis is not intact.

After the integrity of the anastomosis is confirmed, the mesenteric defect should be closed. The cut edge of the mesentery of the terminal ileum should be stapled or sutured to the presacral mesenteric edge down to the anastomosis. This closure must be complete and should prevent internal herniation and bowel obstruction. Although laparoscopic suturing works well for this, closing the defect with a hernia stapler is usually faster.

Rectum

Positioning for proctectomy is the same as that for sigmoid mobilization and resection. The surgeon remains on the patient's right and the assistant on the patient's left. The laparoscope should remain through the umbilical port. The mesosigmoid is grasped via the left midabdominal port. The mesosigmoid and rectosigmoid junction is retracted anteriorly to the right or to the left to provide exposure and traction as needed to do the dissection.

Laparoscopy provides excellent visualization for dissection of the mesosigmoid and mesorectum posteriorly. These structures can be divided using any of the techniques described above. Here again, the ultrasonically activated shears can be used very effectively to divide the mesorectum with minimal blood loss. If the dissection is to be radical, the dissection can be continued through a relatively bloodless plane in the presacral area. If there is no need for a radical dissection, the mesorectum can be divided closer to the rectum. After the posterior attachments are divided, the lateral dissection can be done on each side. By retraction of the rectum and mesorectum to the left, the attachments to the right side of the rectum, including the middle hemorrhoidal artery, can be visualized and divided. Visualization of this dissection is usually much clearer laparoscopically than it is with an open technique. A similar technique is used to retract the rectum and mesorectum to the right and divide the lateral attachments on the left. As with other aspects of the dissection, the lateral dissection of the rectum can be accomplished with scissors and clips, the ultrasonically activated shears, or even the linear cutting stapler.

The anterior dissection of the rectum is the most tedious. In women, the rectum must be dissected away from the posterior wall of the vagina. In men, the dissection plane is between the rectum and the prostate and seminal vesicles. This dissection is also better seen laparoscopically than with an open technique. Mobilization of the rectum anteriorly should be done either with sharp dissection using scissors or with the ultrasonically activated shears. The rectum is grasped and retracted superiorly while the vagina or prostatic area is pushed anteriorly. This provides tension on the plane between the two, facilitating the dissection. In most patients, some of the lateral and anterior dissection must be done to allow more of the rectum to be pulled up out of the pelvis before the posterior dissection can be completed. Therefore, some of the dissection must be done circumferentially before the most distal portion of the rectum can be dissected.

The dissection posteriorly should be carried to the tip of the coccyx. Since it is impossible for the surgeon to feel the tip of the coccyx with his fingers, he or she must rely both on the sensation of palpating the tip of the coccyx with a laparoscopic instrument and on the visual impression of the extent of the dissection. When the dissection reaches the tip of the coccyx, the remainder of the dissection can be completed through the perineal incision.

The proctocolectomy specimen will be removed through the perineal incision. However, the proximal line of resection must be divided, and the stoma must be created before the perineal part of the procedure is done. Once the anterior portion of the dissection of the rectum is completed laparoscopically, the terminal ileum should be divided with the linear cutting stapler. This concludes the laparoscopic portion of the dissection. Next, the stoma is created and the laparoscopic wounds are closed before the perineal portion of the procedure is concluded.

An ileostomy is fashioned using the same technique as in open surgery. A circle of skin is excised at the site for the stoma, and then an opening is made through the muscle layers. The stapled end of the ileum is brought through the opening after the terminal ileum is cleared of mesentery. The staple line is excised, and the ileostomy is matured. The end of the ileum can be everted and sutured using standard technique to create a Brooke ileostomy, or a pouch can be created. After completion of the stoma, the perineal incision and dissection are performed.

The perineal dissection of the rectum is an open dissection using direct visualization, and does not differ from the perineal dissection done at the time of an open proctocolectomy. The anterior dissection done laparoscopically in this case should prepare the rectum superiorly and anteriorly just as well as an open dissection, leaving only the distal rectum to be dissected through the perineal incision. Once the distal rectum is completely dissected through the perineal incision, the rectum and colon are entirely free of any attachments. The rectum and entire colon can then be brought out through this incision. Closure of the pelvic peritoneum and pelvic floor musculature can be completed using standard techniques that are not unique to a laparoscopic procedure.

Postoperative Care

Despite the minimally invasive appearance of this procedure, the patient will have undergone a very large amount of dissection. With such a large dissection, there is the potential for large fluid shifts and for bleeding from the extensive areas of dissection. The third-space loss may be large. Despite the potential for these large fluid shifts, the intestinal tract usually resumes function early after this procedure. Most patients can expect to pass gas and liquid stool within 24 to 48 hours.

Postoperative care of these patients should include routine, close monitoring of vital signs and urine output for the first 2 days after surgery or until patients are stable. However, other aspects of the recovery are usually more rapid than after an open subtotal or total colectomy. Therefore, much of the postoperative care of these patients can be accelerated. Most patients appreciate an indwelling bladder catheter during the first night after surgery, but if urine output is good, it can be removed on the first morning after surgery. Although postoperative pain is probably less severe than after a comparable open operation, patients will require parenteral narcotic administration for the first 2 days after surgery. The intensity of the pain decreases rapidly over that time, and subsequently a mild oral narcotic such as propoxyphene hydrochloride is usually sufficient. Patients should be offered clear liquids orally either the evening after surgery or the following morning. By the second morning, most patients tolerate a regular diet.

Many patients can be dismissed within 3 to 4 days after surgery. At that time, they can steadily increase their activity and diet until they completely resume normal activities. Certainly, patients with an ileoproctostomy will have numerous loose stools every day for several weeks or months, but this is no different from the situation after a similar open operation. Patients with an ileostomy will require the usual care and teaching of a stoma therapist, usually as an outpatient after an early dismissal. For working patients, most can return to work within 3 weeks after the surgery.

Complications

Complications after laparoscopic colectomy are similar to those after open colec-

Table 41-3. Complications after
Laparoscopic Subtotal and Total Colectomy

Pulmonary complications
   Atelectasis
   Pneumonia
Wound complications
   Infection
   Hernia
Deep vein thrombosis/pulmonary embolism
Bleeding
Anastomotic complications
Urinary tract complications
Small bowel obstruction
Trocar injury

tomy (Table 41-3). Pulmonary complications and wound complications seem to occur less frequently after laparoscopic colon resection. The risk of deep vein thrombosis and pulmonary embolism after a lengthy laparoscopy using a pneumoperitoneum would seem to be greater unless pneumatic compression boots are used on the legs. Bleeding, anastomotic complications, urinary tract complications, and postoperative small bowel obstruction appear to occur with a similar low incidence after either open or laparoscopic colon resection.

In addition to these complications, there is the risk of a complication specific to the laparoscopy. Most notable among these risks is bowel injury caused by Veress needle or trocar insertion. Other risks in this category are related to the pneumoperitoneum (air embolus) and the laparoscopic instrumentation (bowel perforation by grasping devices or cautery). The overall incidence of complications after laparoscopic colon resection is not different from that after open colon resection.

Suggested Reading

Harnsberger JR, Longo WE, Vernava AM. Vascular anatomy. *Semin Colon Rectum Surg* 1994;5:24–27.

Liu CD, Rolandelli R, Ashley SW, Evans B, Shin M, McFadden DW. Laparoscopic surgery for inflammatory bowel disease. *Am Surg* 1995;61:1054–1056.

Lointier PH, Lautard M, Massoni C, Ferrier C, Dapoigny M. Laparoscopically assisted subtotal colectomy. *J Laparoendosc Surg* 1993;3:439–453.

Ortega AE, Beart RW Jr, Steele GD Jr, Winchester DP, Greene FL. Laparoscopic bowel surgery registry: preliminary results. *Dis Colon Rectum* 1995;38:681–686.

Rhodes M, Stitz RW. Laparoscopic subtotal colectomy. *Semin Colon Rectum Surg* 1994;5:267–270.

EDITOR'S COMMENT

Laparoscopic subtotal and total colectomies can be some of the most tedious and time-consuming operations performed by the laparoscopic surgeon. Despite the reduced trauma to the abdominal wall compared to the laparotomy approach, the amount of intraperitoneal and retroperitoneal dissection remains significant. The trauma associated with these operations reduces the differences in the postoperative course experienced by open versus laparoscopic patients.

The author provides us with an excellent review of the surgical anatomy of the colon and reminds us of the importance of a thorough knowledge of these structures and their anatomic relations. The loss of the ability to manually palpate the retroperitoneal structures directs the surgeon to maintain a 3-dimensional mental image of the anatomy to reduce the risk of inadvertent injury. Should such a complication occur, the long-term sequelae can usually be minimized through immediate recognition and correction.

It is clearly not advisable for the surgeon to undertake this operation until experience has been gained with other bowel procedures. This is a four-quadrant procedure with each area presenting unique challenges. Appropriate port placement and patient positioning enhances the likelihood of successful completion.

W.S.E.

42

Laparoscopic Enterostomies and Closures

Gillian Q. Galloway

Progress in laparoscopic surgery has allowed surgeons to perform increasingly advanced procedures, including colon and small bowel resections. As a result, laparoscopic techniques for enterostomies have also been developed. The creation of an enterostomy laparoscopically is a relatively simple procedure and may serve as an introductory procedure for the development of skills needed to perform more advanced bowel procedures.

The most common conditions requiring the creation of an enterostomy result from obstruction, perforation, or removal of a chronically diseased colon (Table 42-1). Creation and closure of a stoma can be readily performed by laparoscopic tech-

Table 42-1. Indications for Colostomy

Most common
Palliation for nonresectable obstructing cancer
Diversion following resection of diverticular disease
Trauma
Other
Inflammatory bowel disease
Sigmoid volvulus
Toxic megacolon
Arteriovenous malformation
Abdominoperineal resection
Rectal prolapse
Fistulas
Severe endometriosis
Hirschsprung's disease
Anal atresia
Ischemic colitis
Radiation enteritis
Severe motility disorders
Constipation

Table 42-2. Benefits of Laparoscopic Enterostomy

Less pain
Shorter hospital stay
Return to work/activity sooner
Faster return of gastrointestinal function
Less incidence of ileus
Few narcotic requirements
Less scarring externally
Fewer adhesions

nique in most patients. Those patients who undergo laparoscopic enterostomy or closure have fewer problems than patients who receive open procedures (Table 42-2).

Advantages of laparoscopic techniques over standard open methods for creation or closure of a stoma include the following:

Shorter hospital stay,
Faster return to normal activity and work,
Almost immediate resumption of oral intake after surgery,
Lessened narcotic requirement,
Low incidence of ileus,
Low incidence of significant atelectasis,
Less external scarring and fewer adhesions.

Temporary stomas created laparoscopically can be reversed in just a few weeks because there is no need to wait for healing of large midline scars or softening of adhesions. Thus, use of the laparoscopic technique for the formation and closure of stomas provides patients distinct advantages, compared with conventional open techniques.

Indications for Enterostomy and Patient Selection

Laparoscopic techniques can be used to create an enterostomy to decompress the colon or small bowel and divert the fecal stream away from a resected or diseased distal segment of bowel. Laparoscopic colostomy formation is most commonly performed following colon resection or closure for injury, diverticulitis, or palliation of unresectable obstructing cancer. Other indications for laparoscopic colostomy include colonic obstruction secondary to inflammatory bowel disease, ischemia, congenital defects (Hirschsprung's disease, anal atresia), sigmoid volvulus, hemorrhage, prolapse, severe endometriosis, or radiation injury. Severe motility disorders, incontinence, and toxic megacolon are also occasional indications for laparoscopic colostomy. Many colon cancers are resectable laparoscopically, but laparoscopic resection with colostomy is currently controversial for colon cancer treatment due to the incidence of port-site implantation in several studies.

Temporary or permanent laparoscopic ileostomy can be used in the treatment of Crohn's disease and obstructing cancer or for the decompression of newly created rectal pouches (e.g., J-pouch) after total colectomy for ulcerative colitis or polyposis coli (Table 42-3).

There are few absolute contraindications to the use of laparoscopic techniques to create or close a stoma (Table 42-4). Insufflation of a "hostile abdomen" resulting from dense adhesions may be difficult

Table 42-3. Indications for Ileostomy

Crohn's disease
Obstructing cancer
Trauma with severe contamination

Table 42-5. Surgical Instruments for Laparoscopic Enterostomy

Veress needle or Hasson Trocar
Three-chip camera
30- or 50-degree angled scope
Bipolar scissor cautery
Babcock graspers
Glassmann atraumatic grasper
Harmonic Scalpel (Ethicon Endosurgery)
Endo-GIA-30 stapler (Auto Suture/USSC)
Circular anastomotic stapler
Laparoscopic needle drivers

even with the open laparoscopic (Hasson) technique. Massive adhesions also make safe assessment and mobilization of the bowel difficult. Patients with end-stage chronic obstructive pulmonary disease or other contraindications to general anesthesia are not acceptable candidates for laparoscopic enterostomy. Relative contraindications to this procedure include morbid obesity, pregnancy, dense adhesions, and bleeding disorders.

Instrumentation and Preparation

Insufflation of the abdomen with carbon dioxide (CO_2) can be obtained by Veress needle access or via an open or Hasson technique. The Hasson technique is considered safer in patients who have had previous surgery and are likely to have intraabdominal adhesions. Local anesthesia and insufflation with nitrous oxide may be used in selected patients who cannot tolerate general anesthesia or intubation. An alternative to insufflation for abdominal access is an abdominal wall–lifting device for exposure. This gasless technique allows the use of conventional open instruments.

Table 42-5 provides a list of the usual instruments used for laparoscopic enterostomy creation or closure. A three-chip camera mounted on a scope with a 30- or 45-degree visualization field is currently

considered optimal. Most instruments are 5 mm in diameter. These include Glassman atraumatic bowel graspers, Babcock graspers, bipolar cautery scissors, and monopolar dissectors. Ten- and 12-mm ports are usually used for clip appliers, the ultrasonic scalpel, and endoscopic staplers. It is possible to forgo using a 12-mm port by removing the 10-mm port and placing the 12-mm stapler directly into the abdomen.

Preoperative Considerations

The optimal location for a stoma is selected by the surgeon or an enterostomal therapist prior to performing an enterostomy. Patient education begins preoperatively, as knowledge will help allay fears and allow the patient time to mentally prepare for a significant change in body image. Location and type of enterostomy are determined by the injury or disease process being treated and plans for restoration of intestinal continuity (Table 42-6). The stoma is

placed in a location that is easily accessible, away from skin creases and belt lines. Poor stoma placement can lead to skin excoriation and predispose to cellulitis and fistula formation. Preoperative planning is especially important for stomas that will be permanent. Once the site is chosen, indelible ink is used to tattoo the skin to allow visualization following the surgical scrub.

A standard bowel preparation is begun 2 days before the procedure. Patients receive oral and intravenous antibiotics for elective cases. Preoperative patient education regarding the importance of early postoperative activity and pulmonary toilet is accomplished.

Fundamentals of Laparoscopic Enterostomy

A modified lithotomy position with padded stirrups for the prevention of nerve injury is used for closure of left-side colostomies. This position allows transanal stapler techniques. Patients may be supine for other laparoscopic stoma procedures. Deep venous thrombosis prophylaxis is begun preoperatively with sequential compression stockings or pulsatile pedal compression boots. For very short-duration procedures (less than 2 hours), patients may void preoperatively and avoid catheterization. A Foley catheter should be placed in patients who will undergo lengthy procedures or distal sigmoid and rectal dissection.

For left-side colostomy formation and takedown, the surgeon is positioned on the right side of the patient, and the camera and working ports are on the right side of the abdomen (Fig. 42-1A and B). An additional 5-mm port can be placed at the planned colostomy site to facilitate dissection of the lateral peritoneal reflection and colon mesentery when the left colon is mobilized. Adhesions that do not obstruct vision for working ports are left *in situ*. When necessary, lysis of adhesions is performed with bipolar cautery scissors. Adhesions to the anterior abdominal wall are dissected close to the peritoneum to minimize bleeding from omental vessels and avoid inadvertent enterotomy.

Table 42-4. Patient Selection for Enterostomy

Absolute Contraindications	Relative Contraindications
Hostile abdomen	Morbid obesity
Unable to tolerate general anesthesia	Significant adhesions
	Pregnancy
End-stage chronic obstructive pulmonary disease	Bleeding disorders

Table 42-6. Types of Laparoscopic Enterostomies

End colostomy with Hartmann pouch
Loop colostomy
End colostomy with mucous fistula
End-loop colostomy
Brook ileostomy
Decompressive ileostomy after ileoanal anastomotic procedure (J-pouch)

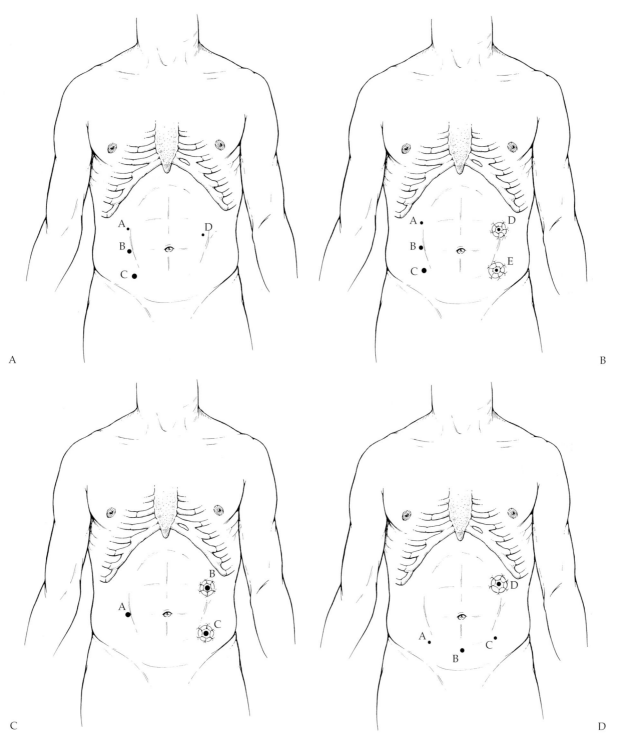

Fig. 42-1. **A:** *Laparoscopic port sites for enterostomy creation. (A, 5-mm port; B, 10-mm port; C, 12-mm port; D, 5-mm port.)* **B:** *End colostomy with mucous fistula. (A, 5-mm port; B, 10-mm port; C, 12-mm port; D, 5-mm port [colostomy]; E, 5-mm port [colostomy].)* **C:** *End colostomy with mucous fistula (alternative).* **D:** *Loop colostomy. (A, 5-mm port; B, 10-mm port; C, 5-mm port; D, 10-mm port [colostomy].)* (continued)

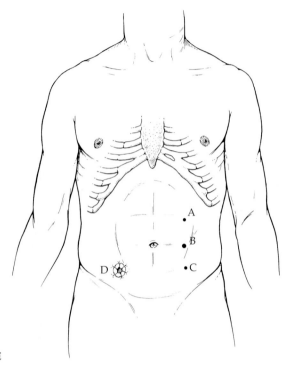

E

Fig. 42-1. (Continued) E: Ileostomy. (A, 5-mm port; B, 10-mm port; C, 5-mm port; D, ileostomy.)

Ileostomy creation and takedown is best performed from the patient's left side with ports located on the left (Fig. 42-1E).

Colostomy Technique

Skin incision sites are infiltrated with 1 to 2 mL of bupivacaine hydrochloride 0.25% with epinephrine before incisions are made. Use of local anesthesia prior to the initial incision significantly reduces postoperative discomfort, compared to infiltration at the end of the procedure. The 10-mm camera-port incision is made 4 to 6 cm lateral to the umbilicus on the contralateral side of the ostomy. Insufflation is established to 14-mm-Hg intraabdominal pressure with CO_2. A high-flow insufflator is preferred for consistent intraperitoneal pressure maintenance. Although the umbilicus has commonly been used for camera placement in laparoscopic cholecystectomy, it is not ideal for colon or small bowel procedures, as it is typically too close to the operative site and obstructs access of other instruments. It is best to place the camera away from the planned side of the procedure. For an end colostomy on the left side, the best camera placement is 4 to 6 cm to the right of the umbilicus. A mirror-image placement to the left of the um-

bilicus is used for the creation of a right-sided ileostomy (see Fig. 42-1). The camera port is placed in the midline below the umbilicus for transverse colon procedures or left upper quadrant colostomy formation or closure. The camera should be located midway between the operating surgeon's two primary ports, as this allows the best visualization and facilitates a two-handed operating technique.

A port may be placed at the proposed site of the stoma to provide increased abdominal access with no added patient morbidity (Fig. 42-2A). In addition, external division of the bowel can be accomplished through the site of the planned stoma to minimize abdominal incisions. Surgical access, visualization, and traction can be greatly facilitated by manipulation of table position. Shifting the position of the patient by tilting the table allows the use of gravity to position the bowels out of the operative field. Optimal patient positioning decreases the need for instrument retraction and lessens the incidence of organ injury.

Following camera placement into the peritoneal cavity, the abdomen is evaluated laparoscopically in a thorough, systematic fashion to assess the anatomy, determine the need to perform adhesiolysis, confirm

that no injury has occurred due to Veress needle or trocar insertion, and look for unsuspected lesions, masses, or metastases. After assessment of the feasibility of performing a colostomy, the best location for the working ports is determined visually. Probing gently with the fingers on the anterior abdominal wall helps locate the ideal spot for port placement. The 5- or 10-mm working ports are introduced safely under laparoscopic visualization.

Colostomy with Hartmann Procedure

The left colon is transected (Fig. 42-2B), and a segment is excised (if necessary), as described in Chapters 39 and 40. The distal rectum can be marked with a nonabsorbable suture for easy visualization if reanastomosis is planned. The mesentery of the proximal colon is dissected to establish adequate length for colostomy formation (Fig. 42-2C). Cautery scissors are used to incise the lateral peritoneal reflection, and the colon is bluntly dissected from adjacent tissues. The mesentery on the medial portion of the left colon is scored with the scissors. Left colic artery branches are identified by two-handed dissection technique using a suction/irrigator, scissors, or a dissector in one hand and the clip applier in the other. Larger vessels are clipped twice proximally and once distally before being transected sharply. Alternatively, an ultrasonic dissector can be used to transect the mesenteric vessels to free an appropriate length of bowel while the blood supply to the remaining bowel is carefully maintained via the left colic branches and marginal arteries. Care is taken to prevent the bowel from twisting or rotating. Babcock graspers are used to elevate the proximal end of the bowel to the anterior abdominal wall to determine the proper length of colon needed for stoma formation. Dissection of the splenic flexure may be required if a large amount of descending colon is initially resected. If the proximal stapled end can easily touch the abdominal wall at the planned site of colostomy in an insufflated abdomen, there is generally no tension once the abdomen is deflated. The ratcheted Babcock grasper is placed on the proximal bowel end to maintain proper orientation and identification from the outside after the pneumoperitoneum is evacuated.

(text continues on page 409)

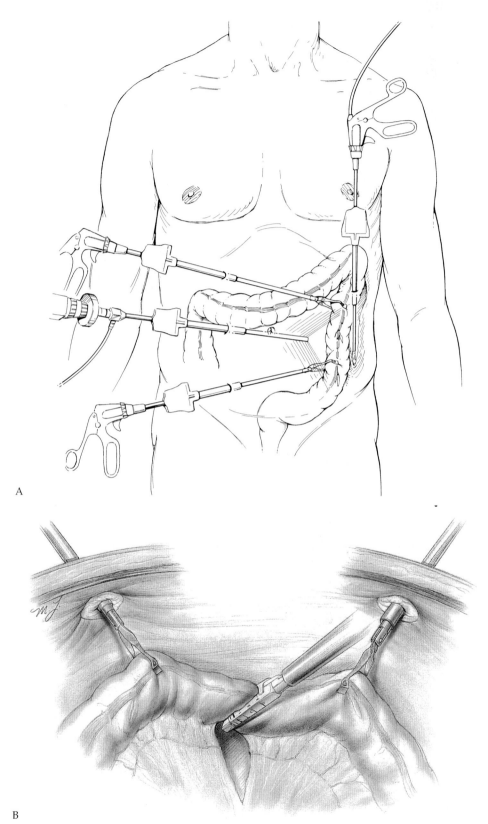

A

B

Fig. 42-2. **A:** *Exposure of sigmoid colon in preparation for resection and/or colostomy. The scope port is placed on the right side of the abdomen lateral to the umbilicus between the two working 5-mm ports. A 5-mm camera port may be used if a smaller laparoscope is available. The planned colostomy site can be used to bring in a port for bipolar cautery scissors to assist colon mobilization. The ureter must always be visualized and protected during dissection of the sigmoid colon.* **B:** *Babcock graspers retract the sigmoid colon on the antimesenteric border. The mesentery is opened, and an 30-mm endoscopic linear cutting stapler is inserted from the right lower quadrant through the mesenteric opening and perpendicular to the sigmoid colon for transection.* (continued)

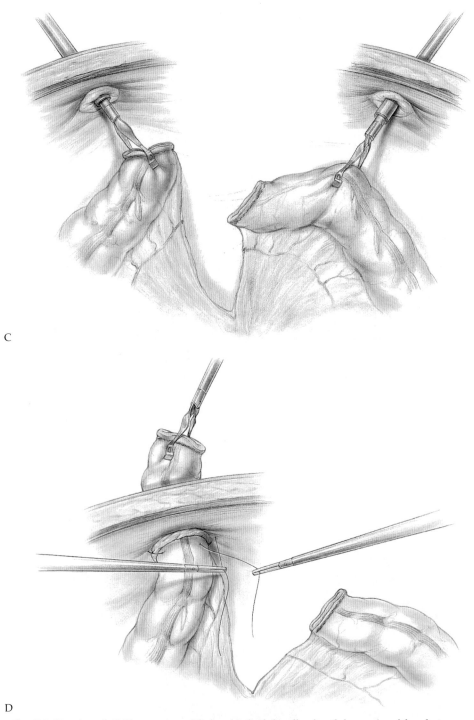

C

D

Fig. 42-2. (Continued) **C:** *The mesentery of the bowel is divided to allow length for creation of the colostomy and removal of sigmoid colon, if necessary. Adequate blood supply must be ensured to prevent necrosis of the colostomy. Three techniques can be used to mobilize the colon via mesenteric dissection (see text).* **D:** *Protruding sigmoid colon allows reinsufflation of the abdomen. Intraabdominal 3–0 Vicryl sutures are used to anchor the bowel to the peritoneum and fascia.*

A circular incision is made around the port at the previously chosen stoma location. The port is removed and the peritoneum stretched to allow two fingers to be placed into the peritoneal cavity. When a segment of bowel is to be resected, the stoma site is enlarged slightly to allow removal of the diseased bowel with subsequent formation of the colostomy. The abdomen is desufflated before the port site is opened in an attempt to prevent unnecessary extravasation of aerosolized blood, smoke, and tissue particles.

A standard Babcock grasper is used to grasp the proximal bowel end and bring it out the incision site while the laparoscopic Babcock is released (Fig. 42-3). Excess mesenteric fat is excised, and small bleeding vessels are controlled externally. Pulling the colon through the incision site creates a seal and permits reinsufflation of the peritoneal cavity, allowing evaluation of the bowel and mesentery within the peritoneal cavity to ensure proper orientation, hemostasis, and laxity. Three intracorporeal 3-0 Vicryl sutures are placed between the tenia of the bowel and the anterior abdominal wall for anchoring (see Fig. 42-2D). The peritoneal cavity is thoroughly irrigated, and the irrigant is aspirated. Larger trocar sites are closed with 0 Vicryl sutures through the anterior and posterior fascia of the rectus abdominis. Smaller ports are removed under direct vision, and the skin is approximated with 4-0 Vicryl subcuticular stitches. The

colostomy is matured, and a temporary appliance is placed.

Transverse Colostomy

Transverse loop colostomy is a useful procedure for decompressing the colon and protecting distal anastomoses or for diverting the fecal stream in an obstructing distal cancer. Less commonly, a transverse loop colostomy is performed to rest an inflamed or infected segment of distal bowel prior to resection, as in diverticular disease, while the patient receives antibiotic therapy.

Laparoscopic formation of a transverse double-barreled (loop) colostomy is fairly simple, since this portion of the colon is usually quite mobile and easily reaches the anterior abdominal wall. However, laparoscopic transverse colon resection is challenging due to the thick gastrocolic omentum and transverse colonic mesentery.

When a simple stoma for loop colostomy is created, the transverse colon is elevated with two laparoscopic Babcock graspers, which are inserted through lower quadrant ports and placed on the antimesenteric border of the transverse colon. The mesentery can be scored with scissors, if increased bowel mobility is needed. A separate port is introduced under direct laparoscopic vision at the site of the planned

colostomy. The colostomy should be placed to the right or left of midline well below the costal margin but above the umbilicus. Preoperative planning and enterostomal therapy involvement are important, as previously described.

The transverse colon is grasped with a Babcock grasper through the planned colostomy site as described for end colostomy formation. The loop of colon is pulled out to the skin surface. A bridge is placed through the mesentery of the transverse colon and left in place for several weeks to prevent retraction of the loop colostomy. Port sites are closed, and the colostomy is matured in the usual fashion.

Diverting Colostomy with Mucous Fistula

A colostomy with mucous fistula is a good way to provide complete fecal diversion when the remaining distal segment of colon is long (i.e., greater than 20 cm). This procedure can be performed with a minimally invasive technique using the planned stoma sites as working ports (see Fig. 42-1C). Only one additional incision is necessary for a camera placement port. The procedure may be made even less invasive by using a 5-mm camera with 25-degree lens.

The stoma sites are determined and marked preoperatively as previously described. Insufflation is obtained by Hasson or Veress needle technique through any of the planned port sites. Once the camera is in position, the abdomen evaluated, and the determination made that the colostomy and mucous fistula can be performed laparoscopically, the stoma sites are created in the usual fashion. The peritoneal layer is left intact, and ports are placed under direct vision. A 10-mm trocar is placed in the left upper quadrant site and a 12-mm trocar in the left lower quadrant.

The lateral peritoneal reflection is incised along the white line of Toldt using bipolar cautery scissors and blunt grasper dissection (see Fig. 42-2A). The colon is mobilized to allow adequate length for both the proximal and distal ends to reach the anterior abdominal wall. The mesentery is incised with cautery scissors perpendicular to the bowel. Mesenteric blood vessels are controlled by one of three techniques:

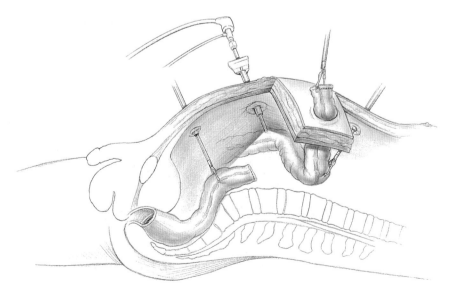

Fig. 42-3. View from the patient's left side. Any diseased segment of sigmoid colon can be resected prior to colostomy formation. Laparoscopic visualization within the abdomen ensures no twisting of bowel or undue tension.

1. Two-handed dissection with suction, grasper, or scissors in one hand and clip applier in the other hand. This technique allows serial clipping and cutting of blood vessels with good hemostasis.
2. Ultrasonic dissector transection of mesenteric vessels;
3. Serial application of an endoscopic linear cutting stapler with 30-mm vascular loads via the 12-mm trocar site.

Electrocautery and a Maryland dissector are used to cauterize small bleeding vessels. The appropriate segment of sigmoid colon is transected with one or two firings of the 30-mm laparoscopic linear cutting stapler (see Fig. 42-2B). The proximal end is grasped on the staple line with a Babcock clamp and held in position to prevent torsion. A separate Babcock clamp is inserted through the left upper quadrant 10-mm port. The intraabdominal Babcock clamp is released, and the bowel is passed through the abdominal wall after enlargement of the trocar hole in the peritoneum. The abdomen is reinsufflated, and the distal bowel staple line is grasped from the outside with the Babcock grasper. The distal bowel is brought through the abdominal wall after the peritoneal defect is enlarged. The abdomen is again reinsufflated, and the position of the proximal and distal loops is evaluated to assess for torsion or undue tension. The abdomen is thoroughly irrigated and aspirated prior to removal of the camera port. A 10-mm camera port site should have both layers of fascia approximated with 0 Vicryl suture. Skin edges are approximated with 4-0 Vicryl subcuticular suture. The end colostomy and mucous fistula stomas are matured in the usual fashion.

Laparoscopic Ileostomy

The stapled end of the transected distal ileum is elevated to the anterior abdominal wall at the previously chosen position. The technique is essentially the same as described for colostomy formation. Adequate length is obtained by scoring the mesentery with electrocautery. Preservation of adequate blood supply prevents necrosis of the stoma. Once the end of the ileum is exteriorized, the abdomen is reinsufflated and the bowel secured to the abdominal wall at three sites using intracorporeal sutures of 3-0 Vicryl. There must be no tension or twisting of the bowel.

Laparoscopic Closure of Enterostomy with Circular Stapled Anastomosis

Laparoscopically performed enterostomy can be closed soon after the initial procedure once there is adequate healing, resolution of infection, or improvement of inflammatory processes. Whereas with open enterostomy it has been common to wait 8 to 12 weeks for healing of the midline wound and maturation of adhesions, it is often possible to close a laparoscopic bowel diversion after as few as 2 to 3 weeks. The incidence of anastomotic leak does not appear to be increased by early closure.

Minimally invasive techniques can be used to close an enterostomy following an open procedure once the midline incision is adequately healed. Occasionally, adhesiolysis needs to be undertaken with bipolar cautery scissors to allow adequate exposure for reanastomosis. Closure of an end-loop colostomy or double-barreled (loop) colostomy can easily be performed as an open outpatient procedure, and laparoscopic assistance is generally unnecessary. Laparoscopic technique is most useful for ileostomy, end colostomy with Hartmann's pouch, or end colostomy with mucous fistula. The bowel anastomosis is created with external handsewn or stapled technique or internal laparoscopic suturing or stapled technique (Table 42-7). I prefer to perform an internal anastomosis using a circular end-to-end anastomosis stapler because of the relative ease, speed, and adequacy of the anastomosis with this method (Fig. 42-4). The circular stapler is useful for anastomosing the rectal pouch to the descending colon or small bowel if the distal pouch can accommodate the stapler.

The patient receives a standard mechanical bowel preparation, with intravenous and oral antibiotics preoperatively. After initiation of general anesthesia, the patient is placed in modified lithotomy position, and the abdomen is insufflated. Ports are placed as shown in Fig. 42-5. The stoma site may be used as a port site once the stoma is closed and the bowel returned to the abdomen. In addition, a 5-mm port can be used for the paraumbilical access site if a 5-mm camera is

Table 42-7. Closure of Enterostomy

Laparoscopy-assisted extracorporeal hand-sewn

Laparoscopy-assisted extracorporeal stapled

Laparoscopic dissection with circular stapled EEA anastomosis

Laparoscopic takedown with intracorporeal anastomosis

available, thereby precluding the need for a larger, 10-mm port. The mucosa of the enterostomy is sharply separated from the skin edges. Bovie cautery and scissors dissection are used to free the proximal bowel from the subcutaneous fat and fascia. Careful blunt finger dissection may be useful while a gauze sponge is used to hold the stoma. Insufflation of the abdomen and laparoscopic scissors dissection may be used to mobilize the stoma. Any remaining sutures between the bowel and peritoneum or fascia can be visualized laparoscopically and cut.

The stoma is sized for placement of the circular stapler anvil. Typically, a 28- or 31-mm stapler can be used. A 3-0 Prolene purse-string suture is placed through all layers of the stoma bowel, and the anvil is inserted and secured. The edges of the bowel must approach the center connector on the anvil circumferentially. Any loose or drifting edges create the potential for incomplete anastomosis when the stapler is fired. The bowel and the anvil are carefully relocated into the peritoneal cavity, and the fascia is closed. Alternatively, a purse-string suture may be placed in the fascia if a port is to be used at the stoma site.

The circular stapler is inserted via the anus after the appropriate diameter is determined with the sizers. The end of the rectal pouch is visualized with the laparoscope. The body of the stapler is carefully placed to prevent tearing of the muscular layers of the rectum or inadvertent puncture of the distal rectal pouch by the tip of the circular stapler. The proximal bowel is approximated to the distal pouch without tension. It may be necessary to perform more dissection of the proximal bowel to ensure adequate length for a tension-free anastomosis. Occasionally, the splenic flexure is mobilized to provide adequate length for re-

(text continues on page 414)

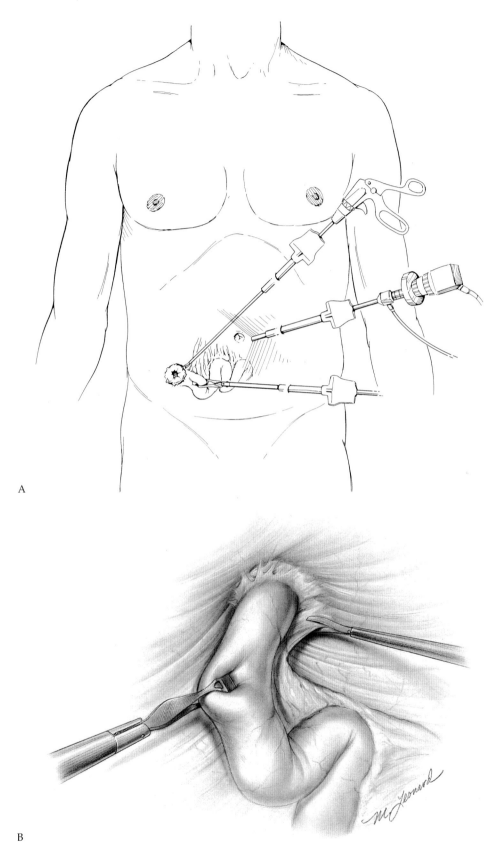

A

B

Fig. 42-4. **A:** *Laparoscopic exposure and dissection of the ileostomy.* **B:** *Cautery scissors are used to remove attachments holding the ileostomy to the anterior abdominal wall.* (continued)

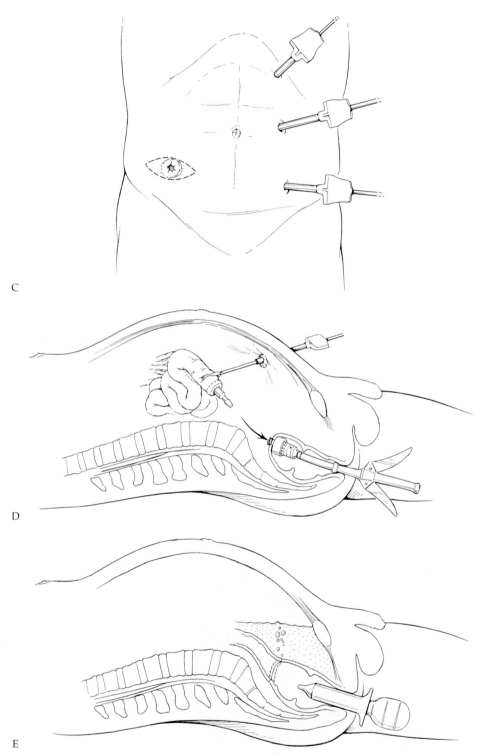

C

D

E

Fig. 42-4. (Continued) **C:** *Elliptical incision for closure of the ileostomy.* **D:** *The circular end-to-end anastomosis stapler is assembled with the assistance of a Babcock grasper.* **E:** *Saline irrigation is used to test the patency of the anastomosis.*

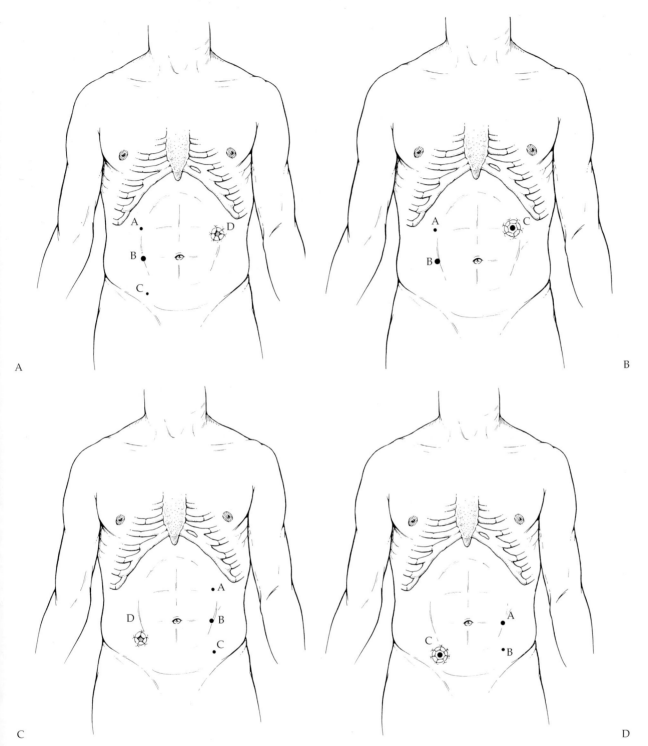

Fig. 42-5. **A:** *Laparoscopic port sites for colostomy closure. (A, 5-mm port; B, 12-mm port; C, 5-mm port; D, colostomy.)* **B:** *Alternative colostomy closure. (A, 5-mm port; B, 10-mm port; C, 11.5-mm port [colostomy].)* **C:** *Ileostomy closure. (A, 5-mm port; B, 10-mm port; C, 5-mm port; D, ileostomy.)* **D:** *Alternative ileostomy closure. (A, 10-mm port; B, 5-mm port; C, ileostomy.)*

anastomosis after colostomy formation. The tip of the circular stapler is advanced through the rectal wall away from any existing staple lines. If avoidance of staple lines is not possible, the trocar should be placed through the center of the staple line. Excess peritoneum or preperitoneal fat over the distal pouch can be dissected with cautery scissors and blunt dissection to expose the underlying muscularis. Once the trocar has protruded through the rectal wall and there is adequate exposure of muscularis for anastomosis, the proximal male appendage on the anvil is then inserted into the receiving-end trocar and snapped into place (see Fig. 42-4D). The plastic spike of the circular stapler can be removed with a Babcock grasper. A Babcock grasper or specially designed anvil grasper can be used to facilitate the connection between the two ends of the bowel, which are progressively approximated by turning the handle of the circular stapler prior to firing. The residual circular sections of bowel excised by the staple line are examined after anastomosis formation to ensure that there are two complete circles of bowel. The circular stapler is carefully withdrawn from the rectum to prevent anastomotic disruptions. The pelvis is filled with saline, and air is injected into the rectum to look for bubbles indicating an anastomotic leak (see Fig. 42-4E). Alternatively, proctosigmoidoscopy can be performed and povidone–iodine (Betadine) or methylene blue instilled in the rectum to test the anastomosis for leakage. The anastomosis is carefully examined with the laparoscope to ensure that no undue tension or twisting has occurred. The abdomen is thoroughly irrigated, and the colostomy site is inspected from the peritoneal surface with the laparoscope. Defects at the stoma site can predispose to herniation. The skin at the stoma site and the port sites are closed in the usual fashion.

Complications of Laparoscopic Enterostomies and Closures

Proper patient selection, thorough preoperative workup, and good planning can minimize the incidence of complications from laparoscopic enterostomy creation and closure. Despite careful planning, these procedures are fraught with potential complications (Table 42-8).

Problems related to insufflation include organ and vessel injury secondary to Veress needle or trocar placement. The increased intraabdominal pressure can lower cardiac output and cause hypotension, as well as pneumothorax and subcutaneous emphysema. Gas embolization is a potential life-threatening complication due to insufflation. Pressure from the CO_2 may tamponade venous bleeding and obscure potential sources of postoperative bleeding. It is appropriate to open the abdomen and control bleeding that cannot be adequately controlled laparoscopically.

The complications associated with open bowel surgery are neither increased nor reduced by laparoscopic technique. Bleeding, infection, anastomotic leakage, stricture, stoma necrosis, and bowel obstruction occur with the same frequency as in open procedures. Port-site hernias can be prevented by proper closure of both anterior and posterior layers of fascia.

Table 42-8. Complications of Laparoscopic Enterostomies

Insufflation problems
  Veress needle injury to organs/vessels
  Subcutaneous emphysema
  Hypotension
  Gas embolism
  Pneumothorax
Bleeding
Organ injury
Infection
  Cellulitis
  Abscess
Anastomotic breakdown
Anastomotic stricture
Wound hernia
Small bowel obstruction
Ischemic necrosis of the colostomy
Retraction of colostomy into abdomen
Stenosis
Prolapse

Suggested Reading

Fuhrman GM, Ota DM. Laparoscopic intestinal stomas. *Dis Colon Rectum* 1994;37:444–449.

Lyerly HK, Mault JR. Laparoscopic ileostomy and colostomy. *Dis Colon Rectum* 1994;37: 444–449.

Nyhus LM, Baker R, eds. *Mastery of surgery*, 2nd ed. Boston: Little, Brown and Company, 1992.

Sosa JL, Sleeman D, Puente I, McKenney MG, Hartmann R. Laparoscopic assisted colostomy closure after Hartmann's procedure. *Dis Colon Rectum* 1994;37:149–152.

Vernava AM III, Liebscher G, Longo WE. Laparoscopic restoration of intestinal continuity after Hartmann procedure. *Surg Laparosc Endosc* 1995;5:129–132.

Wexner SD, Cohen SM. Port site metastases after laparoscopic colorectal surgery for cure of malignancy. *Br J Surg* 1995;82:295–298.

43

Laparoscopic Surgery for Rectal Prolapse

James Knoetgen III and Garth H. Ballantyne

History

Prolapse of the rectum, or procidentia, denotes a full-thickness eversion of the rectal wall through the anal canal. This uncommon clinical entity has plagued mankind and challenged physicians since ancient times. The earliest clinical case of rectal prolapse was identified in a male mummy from Antinoe, Egypt (400 to 500 BC). A Biblical description of a disease that caused "bowels [to] fall out by reason of the sickness day by day" is testimony to the ancient history of this affliction. As surgeons' understanding of pelvic floor, colorectal, and anal anatomy improved, so did the operative procedures devised to treat rectal prolapse. Current surgical therapies employed to treat rectal prolapse are based largely on causes originally postulated by surgeons during the Renaissance period and 18th century.

Hippocrates recognized rectal prolapse as a clinical disorder and described several treatments. For the reduction of difficult cases, he advocated suspending patients by their ankles. For permanent reduction, he applied caustic potash to the rectal mucosa. The development of more sophisticated treatments awaited more precise delineations of human anatomy.

The Roman period anatomist Galen (133 to 199) provided accurate descriptions of the colon but did not focus on the anus or rectum. The understanding of colorectal and anal anatomy stagnated and regressed during most of the Middle Ages. Magnus Hundt's (1449 to 1519) *Anthropolagium,* published in 1501, contains an illustration of the small intestine leading directly to the anus without depicting a colon or rectum.

From the Renaissance period came the first detailed description of the colon, rectum, and anus. Vesalius' (1514 to 1564) *DeHumani Corpus,* published in 1543, meticulously describes colorectal and anal anatomy, including the levator ani and anal sphincter. Renaissance surgeons were able to construct etiologic theories of rectal prolapse based on these novel anatomic concepts. The 16th century surgical literature contained writings on procidentia from Mercurialis, Lowe, Riolannus, and Fabricius from Aquapendentes. Two mechanisms of prolapse proposed during this period were debility of the levator ani and relaxation and paralysis of the anal sphincter. Ambrose Pare (1510 to 1590) advocated a third theory that attributed this malady to improper functioning of the levator ani and both anal sphincters. For the first time, operative repairs were aimed at rectifying specific anatomic defects.

Morgagni (1682 to 1771) attributed rectal prolapse to a laxity of rectal suspensory ligaments and was the first to suggest rectal intussusception as the inciting mechanism. VonHaller, a noted pioneer of physiology and experimental medicine, reported rectal prolapse in humans and animals. After observing prolapse in rabbits, he was successful in producing "an antrosusception in frogs at pleasure," which constituted the first experimental model of rectal prolapse.

John Hunter (1728 to 1793) advanced the intussusception theory and wrote, "Procidentia Ani differs from introsusception as not being contained in a gut . . . and as it inverts it pushes out of the body." Two hundred years later, the advent of cinedefecography has provided radiographic evidence for the intussusception theory advanced by Morgagni, von Haller, and Hunter.

In the early 20th century, Moschowitz observed deep rectovaginal or rectovesical cul-de-sacs in prolapse patients and advocated a sliding hernia theory. By obliterating the abnormally deep pouch of Douglas, his operation prevented elevated intraabdominal pressures from driving the anterior wall of the rectum through a defect in the pelvic fascia and into the anal canal.

Twentieth century surgeons have described an array of surgical procedures aimed at correcting the anatomic defects associated with rectal prolapse. These anatomic features include diastasis of the levator ani muscles, an abnormally deep pouch of Douglas, a redundant sigmoid colon, a patulous anal sphincter, and attenuation of the rectal ligaments. More than 100 operations to correct these pathologic anatomies have been described.

The approaches for these procedures usually are transabdominal or transperineal. Perineal procedures are less invasive and can be performed under local or regional anesthesia but have poorer functional results and higher recurrence rates. Abdominal procedures are generally accepted to have superior long-term results but require general anesthesia, are potentially morbid, and have longer postoperative periods of disability. Several abdominal procedures have readily adapted to a laparoscopic approach.

The advent of laparoscopic surgery has changed the technical, but not conceptual, approach to many abdominal operations. Laparoscopic cholecystectomy has received the most attention and has clearly demonstrated reduced morbidity. Advantages of laparoscopic cholecystectomy over the open procedure include less operative trauma and therefore shortened postoperative disability. Large abdominal wall wounds are replaced by several smaller incisions that are associated with less postoperative pain and increased mobility. This approach should lead to decreased morbidity, fewer pulmonary complications, earlier return to a normal diet, and earlier discharge.

Patients who must undergo transabdominal operations for the treatment of rectal prolapse are ideal candidates for the application of laparoscopic surgery. Elderly patients who previously were deemed unfit for abdominal surgery may be candidates for laparoscopic abdominal procedures such as rectopexy and anterior resection. Operations for rectal prolapse that are approached laparoscopically include anterior resection, proctopexy, and abdominal perineal resection. Perineal rectosigmoidectomies can also be performed with laparoscopic assistance. The number of reported cases in the literature remains small for most of these procedures, and long-term follow-up is not yet available. Early published results are encouraging and justify further applications of laparoscopic approaches and randomized trials.

Surgical Options
Abdominal Procedures

More than 100 abdominal and perineal operations have been described for the surgical treatment of rectal prolapse, which suggests that no operation has yielded completely satisfactory results. Abdominal procedures include pelvic floor repair, suspension-fixation of the rectum, and resection of the rectum, sigmoid colon, or both.

Pelvic Floor Reconstruction

Reconstruction of an abnormally lax pelvic floor was first advocated by Moschowitz. Based on the concept that prolapse is a sliding hernia, Moschowitz obliterated the deep pouch of Douglas with purse-string sutures. Recurrence rates of nearly 50% encouraged Graham to modify the procedure by approximating the levator ani anterior to the rectum. Further modifications were made by several surgeons, including

Hughes, who suggested a combined abdominal and perineal pelvic floor repair. Functional results were reportedly excellent, and recurrence rates were estimated at 11%. However, these operations are complex and foreign to most surgeons and have therefore been replaced by simpler procedures with equally good functional results.

Rectopexy Procedures

Based on the notion that rectal intussusception induces a prolapse, operations were described to fix the rectum within the pelvis to prevent intussusception. Proctopexy operations were introduced in the 1950s, and the Ripstein anterior sling rectopexy remains one of the more commonly performed abdominal procedures for the treatment of rectal prolapse. Ripstein and Lanter attributed rectal prolapse to an intussusception of a loosely supported rectum and believed that associated pelvic floor defects were secondary features. The goal of their repair was to fix the rectum to the posteriorly curved sacrum to prevent abdominal pressures from being directed toward the rectum in a straight line. Bowel straightening and intussusception could therefore be avoided.

Ripstein described an operation for producing a circumferential sling of fascia lata fixed to the anterior rectum and anchored to the sacrum, which created anterior and lateral tethering of the rectum. A variety of other materials have since been used, including Teflon, polypropylene, Gore-Tex, peritoneum, and nylon strips. Complications such as obstruction and stool impaction, presumably caused by the encircling material, led surgeons to perform a partial rectal wrap, leaving the anterior surface free.

Posterior sling rectopexy (i.e., Wells procedure) is accomplished by first suturing a polyvinyl alcohol (Ivalon) sponge to the posterior surface of the rectum and then to the sacral promontory. Fixation of the rectum is ensured by a sponge-induced inflammatory fibrosis. Pelvic computed tomography has revealed rectal and pararectal thickening postoperatively. The thickened wall is believed to mechanically prevent intussusception and assist continence in patients with poor sphincter muscles by impeding the flow of stool into the lower rectum. Tissue thickening, however, does not correlate with the site of sponge placement, and similar thickening is ob-

served in most patients who undergo complete rectal mobilization.

The greatest disadvantage of this procedure is infection of the sponge, or pelvic sepsis. Pelvic sepsis can be a disastrous complication that necessitates sponge removal, although removal of the sponge does not result in prolapse recurrence. This is further evidence that rectal fixation within the presacral space is a result of rectal mobilization and subsequent postoperative scarification instead of Ivalon sponge implantation. Although the Wells procedure remains popular in the United Kingdom, the Ripstein operation is the preferred abdominal rectopexy in the United States.

Rectopexy procedures are nonresective and therefore less morbid than other abdominal operations, although a generous laparotomy is required, which is a significant determinant of postoperative disability. Rectopexy has become an ideal procedure for a laparoscopic approach. The laparoscopic rectopexy accomplishes the same anatomic goals as the open procedure without the operative trauma. The bowel lumen is not entered during a laparoscopic rectopexy, making it a more attractive procedure than other laparoscopic colorectal operations. Long-term results are not yet available, but early results are comparable to the results of open surgery and are encouraging. Further investigation is warranted.

Resection Procedures

The treatment of rectal prolapse by low anterior resection was first described by Muir in 1955 and remains a favored procedure at the Mayo Clinic. The low anterior resection has multiple advantages, including familiarity to most surgeons because of its use in carcinoma of the rectum. Resection of the redundant sigmoid and proximal rectum removes the portion of bowel where intussusception initiates, preempting rectal prolapse. Bowel function is improved with subsequently less constipation. Patients therefore experience less straining at stool, which decreases the chance of a recurrence.

Advocates of the low anterior resection think that synchronous rectopexy is obviated by postoperative fibrosis in the pelvis and between the anastomotic suture line and sacrum. Pelvic scarification lends significant posterior support to the rectum and retards the recurrence of rectal prolapse. The low end-to-end anastomosis, however, has the disadvantage of a potential leak and infection. To minimize the complications of an anastomotic leak, high anterior resections with an end-to-end anastomosis above the peritoneal reflection are favored by many surgeons.

Anterior resection is readily adapted to a laparoscopic approach. The first case report of a laparoscopic anterior resection was in a middle-aged woman institutionalized for diffuse cerebral injury with an anticipated long life span. Laparoscopic anterior resection was successfully performed without complication. The left colon and rectum can be satisfactorily mobilized, and the redundant sigmoid and proximal rectum are readily resected. Extensive posterior dissection to the coccyx promotes postoperative scarring and fixation of the remaining rectum to the sacrum. Virtually no postoperative pain or ileus are experienced, and diet can be rapidly advanced. Although the risk of an anastomotic leak and pelvic infection remains a concern, standardized results can be anticipated.

Abdominal sigmoid resection with rectopexy was initially advocated by Frykman in 1955. Many surgeons consider this procedure the standard of care for low-risk patients. The rectum is mobilized to the levator ani, but the lateral stalks and rectal blood supply are preserved. As the rectum is retracted cephalad, the tented lateral stalks are sutured to the sacral periosteum to maintain an elevated rectal configuration. Redundant anterior cul-de-sac peritoneum is excised and reconstructed. A standard sigmoid colon resection with an end-to-end colorectal anastomosis is performed.

Perineal Procedures

Although abdominal operations are associated with lower recurrence rates and improved postoperative bowel function, perineal procedures are preferred for treating elderly and debilitated patients, who are poor candidates for general anesthesia and may not tolerate a potentially morbid abdominal procedure such as a sigmoid resection. Postoperative morbidity is reduced, and the time to full recovery is considerably more rapid. The risk of presacral nerve injury, which is significant in young male patients, also is avoided in some perineal procedures. Because these

operations usually are reserved for older patients with limited life expectancies, long-term follow-up data usually are unavailable.

Thiersch Anal Encirclement

Anal encirclement was described by Thiersch in 1891. A ring of silver wire placed in the ischiorectal fat around the anus provided a mechanical obstruction that prevented prolapse of the rectum. A variety of other materials have since been used. This procedure has the advantage of requiring only local or regional anesthesia. Two small incisions anterior and posterior to the anus are created through which the encircling material is passed. Postoperative complications are common, including erosion and disruption of the material, fecal impaction, and infection. Recurrence rates are high, and skeptics argue that high-risk patients tolerate perineal rectosigmoidectomy equally well. This procedure has been abandoned by most surgeons.

Delorme Procedure

Delorme, a French army surgeon, reported in 1899 minimally invasive operative techniques for the correction of procidentia in three young men. The rectal prolapse is recreated after the induction of local or regional anesthesia. Mucosa is stripped from the prolapsed bowel, the denuded muscular wall is telescoped with interrupted longitudinal sutures, and the resulting mucosal edges are approximated. Uhlig and Sullivan modified this procedure by performing a simultaneous pelvic floor repair. The Delorme procedure is technically simple and less invasive than abdominal or large-scale perineal procedures. However, the underlying anatomic abnormalities are not corrected, and incomplete or improper mucosectomies predispose to recurrent prolapse. Recurrence rates are therefore higher than for any intraabdominal operation, but bedridden and debilitated patients tortured by rectal prolapse may benefit from this operation.

Perineal Rectosigmoidectomy

One of the major disadvantages of intraabdominal intestinal resection is the risk of anastomotic dehiscence. The risk is much lower if the procedure is performed through a perineal approach. Mikulicz in

1889 presented six cases of complicated procidentia treated by amputation of the prolapsed bowel. Satisfied with the results, he broadened the indications for perineal rectosigmoidectomy to include cases of uncomplicated rectal prolapse. This procedure was advanced by Miles in 1933 and Gabriel in 1948, and it is usually associated with Altemeier.

The operation can be performed under spinal or general anesthesia. The redundant rectum and sigmoid colon are delivered through the anus for resection, and excess peritoneum from the anterior cul-de-sac is excised. An end-to-end coloanal anastomosis is constructed between the proximal sigmoid colon and the anal canal. This operation is associated with a low morbidity and is a viable option for elderly patients. Incontinence may persist partly because of the loss of a rectal vault. The approach allows access to the pelvic floor for synchronous repair. When combined with total pelvic floor repair, there is a marked decrease in postoperative incontinence. Reported recurrence rates vary, with the highest rates from Hughes of St. Mark's Hospital and the lowest from Altemeier et al.

Patient Selection

Before evaluation for surgery, all patients must undergo colonoscopy or air contrast barium enema to completely evaluate the colon for evidence of malignancy. Tumors can serve as lead points for intussusception and prolapse. A variety of effective operative techniques are available for the treatment of rectal prolapse, and the selection of the appropriate procedure must be made after evaluating several patient factors. The patient's age, gender, comorbid conditions, bowel function, and degree of continence can significantly affect the operative course and postoperative results. These factors must therefore be considered before planning surgical intervention.

The incidence of rectal prolapse increases with age. Many patients who present with this affliction are elderly and have significant comorbid conditions. Abdominal procedures, even laparoscopic, are generally reserved for younger and more robust patients who are better able to tolerate a major operation and general anesthesia. The lower morbidity rates of perineal operations make them the preferred procedure for elderly patients deemed unfit for a major abdominal procedure and general anesthesia. The higher risk of recurrence carried by perineal procedures may be irrelevant in a patient with a limited life expectancy.

Special considerations must be made for laparoscopic procedures. Carbon dioxide (CO_2) pneumoperitoneum may elevate the serum partial pressure of CO_2. A patient with chronic obstructive pulmonary disease who retains CO_2 or a patient with cardiac arrhythmias may not tolerate this blood gas disturbance. This potential source of complications may be nullified by the advent of helium and gasless pneumoperitoneums for laparoscopic surgery.

Six times more women than men have rectal prolapse. Men who suffer from this problem often present at a younger age than women, and an abdominal procedure may be preferred in men. However, Meyers et al. found an increased incidence of sexual dysfunction in male patients treated with abdominal proctopexy compared with perineal rectosigmoidectomy. The risk of sexual dysfunction in men after posterior mobilization of the rectum is therefore significant and should be considered when deciding on an operation.

Anal manometry and electromyography are often performed preoperatively. Objective measurements of sphincter tone and pudendal nerve latency are helpful in identifying truly incontinent patients. Prolapse repair results in full recovery of pudendal nerve and internal sphincter function in approximately 60% of patients, but it is difficult to predict which patients will recover. Incontinent patients benefit from sacral rectopexy when approached abdominally or by a perineal proctectomy combined with rectopexy and posterior sphincter repair.

Constipation often accompanies rectal prolapse. Large bowel transit studies can identify patients with slow-transit constipation. Anorectal physiology tests are required in this setting to exclude outlet obstruction. If there is no evidence of outlet obstruction, patients with slow-transit constipation often respond favorably to subtotal colectomy with ileorectal anastomosis combined with sutured rectopexy. This operation is unsuitable for patients with low sphincter pressures demonstrated by anorectal manometry. Sound judgment must be used before performing a subtotal colectomy, because resections may result in impaired continence.

Laparoscopic Technique

Rectal prolapse has been successfully treated by means of the laparoscope by rectopexy, anterior resection with and without fixation, abdominal perineal resection, and perineal rectosigmoidectomy. The operations remain conceptually the same, but the technical aspects have changed.

Patient Preparation and Positioning

Patients are admitted to the hospital on the night before the operation and receive conventional bowel preparation and perioperative antibiotics. The patient is usually placed in a supine position on an electric operating room table. The patient's legs are supported by modified Lloyd-Davies stirrups that allow access to the perineum for placement of a vaginal cannula if necessary (Fig. 43-1). Laparoscopically assisted perineal rectosigmoidectomies are performed in the prone jackknife position (Fig. 43-2). The thighs are maintained as straight as possible, because flexed thighs impede the movement of the laparoscope and laparoscopic instruments. A nasogastric tube and urinary catheter are inserted in all patients, diminishing the risk of stomach and bladder injury during trocar insertion.

Trocar Placement

Between three and five trocars are used according to the surgeon's preference (Fig. 43-3). During a surgeon's early experience, a five-trocar technique should be used. As a surgeon becomes more experienced, the operation can be accomplished with just three trocars. The five-trocar technique is illustrated in Fig. 43-3. A 10-mm trocar is placed in a supraumbilical or periumbilical position for the laparoscope. A 10-mm trocar and a 12-mm trocar are placed in the right lower quadrant, and two 10-mm trocars are placed in the left lower quadrant lateral to the rectus muscle. Some surgeons suggest an optional 5-mm trocar above the umbilicus on the left side for sigmoid retraction. A suprapubic 10- to 12-mm port can also be used for retraction in unusually difficult cases.

Laparoscopic Anterior Resection

After the induction of general endotracheal anesthesia and preparation of the abdomen, the patient is dropped into a deep Trendelenburg position. A CO_2 pneumoperitoneum is established with a Veress needle in the supraumbilical site. The needle is replaced with a 10-mm trocar, and the abdomen is inspected for evidence of trocar-induced injury. The additional trocars are inserted, and the abdomen is explored for unsuspected disease.

The small bowel is pulled out of the pelvis. The sigmoid colon and rectum are grasped and retracted medially and cephalad. The course of the common iliac vessels is identified. The posterior peritoneum is elevated off of the iliac vessels and incised. The sigmoid mesentery is bluntly swept medially. The magnified video image broadcast from the laparoscope conspicuously exposes the avascular planes in the retroperitoneum.

The left ureter usually is found where it crosses the iliac vessels (Fig. 43-4) and is important to identify. A clear field of view must be maintained throughout the operation. All tissues are divided with cautery. Clots of blood are troublesome because they clog aspiration devices and because the deep color absorbs light and darkens the laparoscopic video image. Clot formation is prevented by irrigation of the operative field with heparinized saline (3000 U/1000 mL of saline) before dissection is initiated.

The rectum is mobilized off of the sacrum (Fig. 43-5). Postoperative scarring of this plane helps fix the rectum in place and hinders the recurrence of prolapse. The rectosigmoid and proximal rectum and deflected laterally. The course of the right iliac vessels is visualized. The hard sacral promontory can often be identified by "palpation" with the laparoscopic scissors.

The visceral peritoneum over the sacral promontory is incised. All vessels in the presacral space are cauterized. The mesorectum is pushed bluntly off of the sacrum. The magnification provided by the telescope facilitates the dissection. After the rectum is mobilized, the mesenteric dissection is accomplished (Fig. 43-5). The inferior mesenteric and superior hemorrhoidal vessels are preserved, ensuring an excellent blood supply for the colorectal

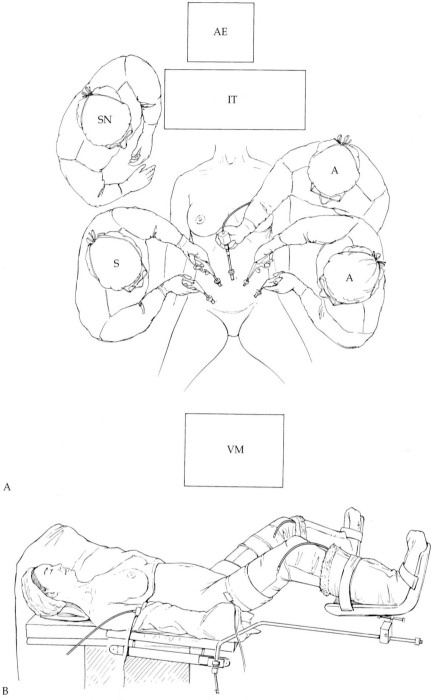

A

B

Fig. 43-1. Room setup **(A)** and patient positioning (VM, video monitor; S, surgeon; SN, scrub nurse; IT, instrument table; AE, anesthesia; A, assistant.) **(B)** for standard laparoscopic approach to rectal prolapse.

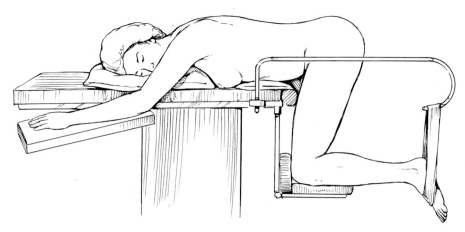

Fig. 43-2. Alternative prone, jackknife patient position for endoscopically assisted prolapse treatment procedures.

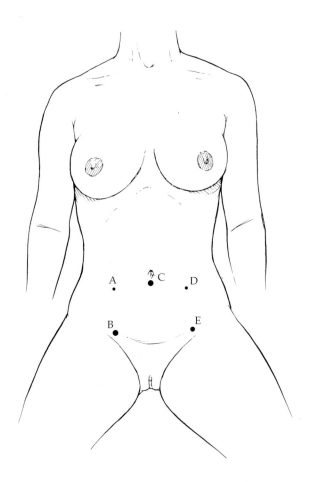

Fig. 43-3. Trocar placement for most anterior prolapse treatment (i.e., proctopexy or sigmoid resection). (A, 5-mm dissector; B, 12-mm dissector; C, camera; D, 5-mm dissector; E, 10-mm retractor.)

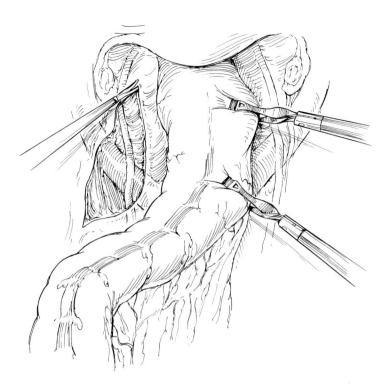

Fig. 43-4. The left ureter must be identified and protected throughout the procedure.

anastomosis. The visceral peritoneum of the mesosigmoid is incised anteriorly to the inferior mesenteric vessels. The individual sigmoid branches are sharply and bluntly separated at the base of the mesosigmoid. The vessels are divided by clipping each side twice. Transection of vessels is continued distally until the selected point of distal transection of the rectum is reached.

Exposure of the more proximal sigmoid branches becomes increasingly difficult. Space limitations within the abdomen limit the ability to lay out the mesosigmoid for inspection, and division of these branches is more easily achieved extracorporeally. It is necessary to divide enough of the sigmoid mesentery so that the distal sigmoid can be easily delivered through an incision in the left lower quadrant. Mobility of the distal sigmoid is checked by its elevation up to the abdominal wall at the planned site of incision.

The rectum is transected beyond the rectosigmoid junction in its proximal third (Fig. 43-6). The rectosigmoid junction is identified as the point of coalescence of the taeniae with formation of a complete longitudinal layer of rectal muscle. The anastomosis is positioned above the anterior peritoneal reflection because of the lower risk of anastomotic dehiscence at this level. The caudad 10-mm trocar in the right lower quadrant is replaced with a 12- or 15-mm trocar. This position allows perpendicular transection of the rectum with the laparoscopic stapling device (Fig. 43-7). The rectum is transected and divided with multiple applications of the 30-mm endoscopic staples or a single application of the 60-mm stapler. The 3.5-mm-long cartridge is used. The tips of the instrument are checked before firing.

The stapled closure of the specimen is grasped with a Babcock clamp, which is inserted through the caudad trocar in the left lower quadrant. The trocar is slid out of the abdominal wall over the shaft of a Babcock-type clamp. The trocar site is extended as a transverse incision 1.5 inches (3.8 cm) long. The distal end of the specimen is withdrawn from the abdomen through this incision, and the pneumoperitoneum is deflated.

The remaining sigmoid branches are divided between clamps and ligated. The point of proximal transection is selected. The wall of the colon at this point is

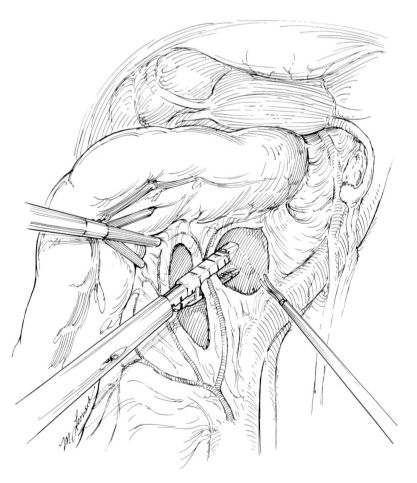

Fig. 43-5. Technique of rectosigmoid mesentery mobilization.

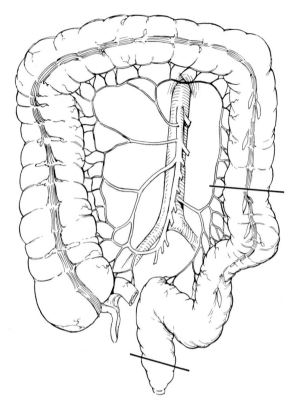

Fig. 43-6. Transection lines for sigmoid resection for treating prolapse.

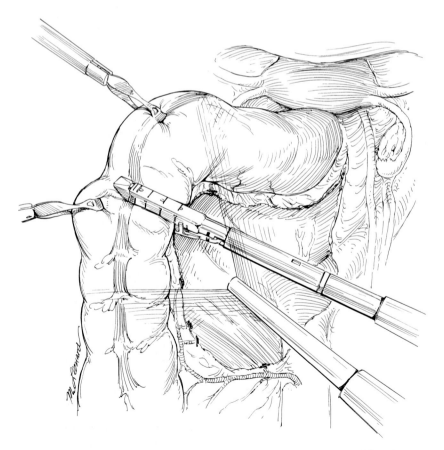

Fig. 43-7. Placement of endoscopic staples through the right lower quadrant of the colon.

cleared of mesenteric fat for a distance of 1 inch (2.5 cm). An automatic penetrating device is applied, and a crushing bowel clamp is placed on the specimen side. The colon is transected with curved Mayo scissors. The specimen is handed to a pathologist for gross inspection in the operating room.

The penetrating device is opened. The edge of the colon is grasped with three Babcock clamps. The diameter of the colon is sized. Generally, a 31-mm-diameter cartridge can be used. The low-profile anvil with modified shaft is inserted into the colon and tied into place with a purse-string suture. This end of the colon is returned to the abdomen and carefully placed into the pelvis with the point of the shaft pointing toward the rectal stump. The abdomen is liberally irrigated, and any clot in the operative field is removed. The incision is closed, and the pneumoperitoneum is recreated.

The anus is dilated to admit four fingers. The head of the circular stapling device is inserted through the anus and advanced up the rectum to the stapled closure. A suture is tied in a loop through the hole in the tip of the white trocar before the stapling device is inserted into the rectum. The white trocar is screwed through the staple line until the orange collar is visible. A grasping instrument pushes against the rectal wall as the trocar is advanced to help prevent a tear in the rectal wall.

The loop in the tip of the white trocar is held by a grasping instrument. A Babcock clamp can be used to pull the trocar out of the head of the stapling device. The white trocar is withdrawn through an anterior abdominal port site. When an older type of white trocar is used that does not have a hole in its tip, the white trocar is lassoed with a pretied endoscopic ligature. A Babcock clamp pulls the stapling trocar out of the head of the stapling device. The suture is used to pull the stapling trocar out through the 12-mm port. The Babcock clamp helps align the trocar with the axis of the trocar.

An Babcock clamp is inserted into the abdomen through the 12-mm trocar and used to grasp the modified shaft. The jaws of the Babcock clamp are locked into the groove of the shaft. It is important that the Babcock clamp be aligned perpendicularly to the long axis of the stapling device (Fig. 43-8). The shaft is inserted into the orange collar of the cartridge of the circular stapler. After docking the anvil-shaft assembly with the stapler, the taeniae of the colon are inspected to ensure that the colon is not twisted. Similarly, the mesentery of the colon is examined for evidence of a volvulus. The stapling device is screwed closed and fired. It is opened one full turn and withdrawn from the rectum. The anvil is opened, and the shaft is inspected for two intact donuts.

The pelvis is filled with warmed saline. A sigmoidoscope is advanced through the anus up to the anastomosis. The staple line is scrutinized for hemostasis, and the rectum is insufflated. The pool of water in the pelvis is observed for leakage of bubbles through the anastomosis. The saline is aspirated, and the operative field is inspected for hemostasis.

Drains can be inserted through a trocar and positioned near the anastomosis. After trocar removal, each fascial defect is closed. The placement of sutures is observed with the laparoscope. The pneumoperitoneum is deflated, the skin edges are closed, and dressings are applied.

Laparoscopic Rectopexy

Laparoscopic rectopexy techniques have been described in several articles. Patient preparation, anesthesia, and trocar placement are performed as previously described for laparoscopic anterior resection. The small bowel and sigmoid colon are pulled from the pelvis and placed in the right paracolic gutter. Retraction of bowel by the assistant may be required. After identification of the left ureter and presacral nerves, the peritoneum is incised. Starting at the root of the sigmoid mesentery, the incision is extended laterally on both sides of the rectum at the peritoneal reflection and anteriorly in the pouch of Douglas. The rectum is mobilized to the anorectal junction in the relatively avascular posterior and lateral planes. Anterior dissection is then performed between the anterior rectal wall and the vagina or the seminal vesicles and prostate. A fan retractor may be helpful with this dissection (Fig. 43-9).

If a mesh rectopexy is to be performed, a rectangle of mesh measuring approximately 10 by 12 cm is fashioned. It is inserted as a tight roll through one of the lower abdominal trocars, unraveled, and placed horizontally across the sacrum. The

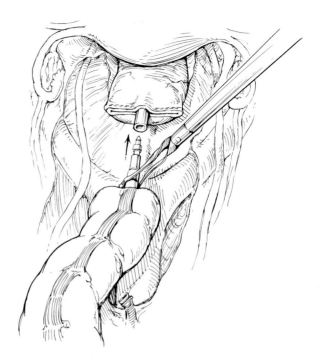

Fig. 43-8. The transrectal circular stapler is advanced and the anvil inserted under laparoscopic visualization.

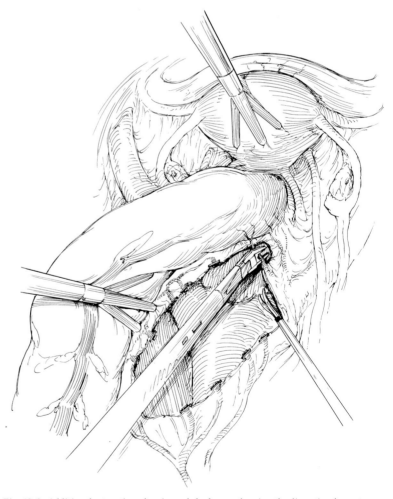

Fig. 43-9. Additional retraction often is needed when performing the dissection for rectopexy.

mesh is fixed to the sacrum in the midline using sutures, endoscopic staples, or a modified tack. A vaginal port may be employed to guarantee perpendicular placement of the fixing device into the sacrum. Fixation of the mesh is confirmed by pulling the mesh with laparoscopic forceps. The lateral limbs of the mesh are sutured or stapled to the side walls of the rectum (Fig. 43-10). Residual mesh is trimmed to achieve a partial wrap (usually three-fourths to two-thirds) of the rectum. To avoid adhesion formation to loops of small bowel, the mesh is hidden by reconstruction of the pelvic peritoneum.

Pelvic fixation of the rectum can also be accomplished with sutures. This is the required rectopexy if a synchronous sigmoid resection is planned. The procedure is conducted similarly to the mesh rectopexy. Sutures are placed from the mesorectum to presacral fascia or from the lateral ligaments to the sacral promontory (Fig. 43-11).

Laparoscopically Assisted Perineal Rectosigmoidectomy

Laparoscopically assisted perineal rectosigmoidectomy is performed in the standard fashion with laparoscopic visualization of the descending colon, sigmoid, and rectum to ensure complete mobilization. Laparoscopic mobilization or enterolysis can be performed if necessary to completely mobilize the bowel.

With the patient in the prone jackknife position, traction is applied to the rectum to reproduce the prolapse. A full-thickness circumferential incision is created through the rectal mucosa approximately 2 cm proximal to the dentate line to expose the inner tube of prolapsed bowel. The inner rectal tube is delivered through this incision while the mesentery is divided and ligated. The deep pouch of Douglas is entered, and a 0° laparoscope is inserted in each anterolateral quadrant. It is not necessary to create a pneumoperitoneum. The intraperitoneal descending colon, sigmoid, and remaining rectum are inspected. Additional dissection or lysis of adhesions can be performed laparoscopically if required. Laparoscopic instruments are removed, and the operation proceeds in the traditional fashion. Prolapsed rectosigmoid colon is resected, and a coloanal anastomosis and levatoroplasty (if desired) are constructed.

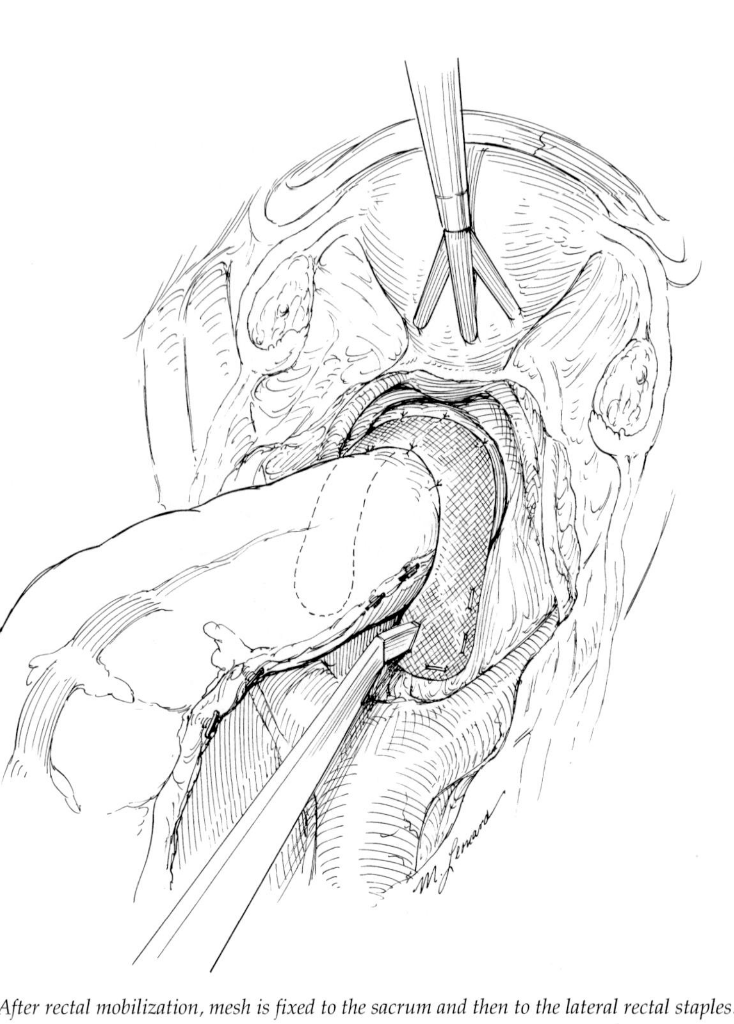

Results
Abdominal Rectopexy

Abdominal rectopexy operations are safe and effective and have therefore gained wide acceptance. Some series have demonstrated control of the prolapse in almost all patients with low morbidity and mortality rates. Functional results after rectopexy, however, are easily criticized.

The mortality rate in most series approaches 0% (Table 43-1). Recurrence rates of complete rectal prolapse for the anterior sling rectopexy are approximately 2% to 3%, with recurrence of mucosal prolapse in about 7% of operations. Mucosal prolapses do not generally require operative intervention. The Ripstein procedure is successful at restoring continence, with reported improvement ranging from 60% to 80%. This improvement may depend on the degree of preoperative sphincter impairment and the restoration of sphincter function postoperatively.

Gordon et al. polled members of the American Society of Colon and Rectal surgeons, obtaining information on 1111 patients who had received the Ripstein procedure. The overall complication rate in this report was 30%, but the rate of complications specific to the procedure was 16.5%. Critics of this operation point to the relatively high incidence of postoperative constipation and occasionally associated outlet obstruction and fecal impaction. This problem was originally attributed to a mechanical obstruction created by the sling of material. Current evidence indicates that mobilization of the rectum may result in a denervated rectum and impaired motility. The incidence of constipation after rectopexy is reduced if the procedure is combined with a colectomy. The wrap of material has also been blamed for rectal stricture formation. Most series have a 0% to 2% incidence of rectal strictures as a late complication.

Fig. 43-10. After rectal mobilization, mesh is fixed to the sacrum and then to the lateral rectal staples.

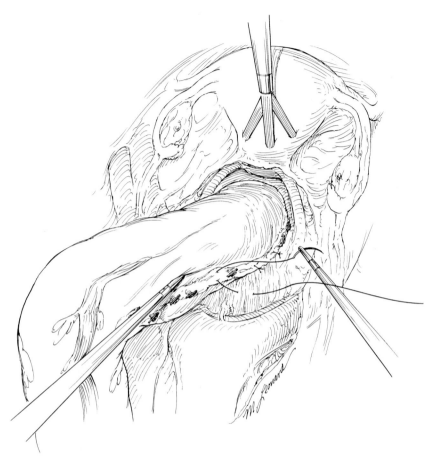

Fig. 43-11. An alternative technique for rectopexy is intracorporeal suturing with nonabsorbable sutures.

Table 43-1. Results after Anterior Sling Rectopexy (Ripstein Procedure)

Study	No. of Patients	Follow-up	Mortality (%)	Recurrences (%)	Stricture (%)
Roberts et al., 1988	135	(41 mo)[a]	1	10	2
Holmstrom et al., 1986	59	(4.5 yr)[a]	5	5	1
Leenen and Kuijpers, 1989	64	6–86 mo	0	0	
Hiltunen and Matikuinen, 1991	54	1.5–5 yr	0	2	

[a] Values in parentheses are means.

Table 43-2. Results after Posterior Sling Rectopexy (Wells Procedure)

Study	No. of Patients	Follow-up (mean)	Mortality (%)	Recurrences (%)	Sepsis (%)
McCue and Thomson, 1991	53	36.7 mo	0	0	4
Mann and Hoffman, 1988	53	6 yr	0	0	0
Rogers and Jeffrey, 1987	25	1.8 yr	0	4	0
Anderson et al., 1984	42	4.2 yr	0	2.5	2.5

The Wells posterior sling rectopexy is equally effective in preventing rectal prolapse compared with the Ripstein. Most series demonstrate improved continence postoperatively in approximately two-thirds of patients (Table 43-2). Long-term morbidity and mortality rates are acceptably low, but functional results are significant and preclude the use of this procedure by many surgeons. Marked increases in constipation after surgery is a common cause of patient dissatisfaction and is apparently multifactorial. Patients with demonstrated slow colonic transit may benefit from partial colectomy combined with rectopexy.

Strictures and fecal impaction, as seen after the Ripstein anterior sling procedure, are not observed after the Wells procedure. Division of the lateral rectal ligaments resulting in denervation and subsequent motility dysfunction of the rectum is a potential complication. However, proponents of this procedure claim that constipation postoperatively is a consequence of a preexisting tendency for constipation that is revealed after surgery and not a result of the procedure.

Infections associated with implantation of the Ivalon sponge have been estimated at approximately 2% of cases, with some series reporting pelvic abscess rates as high as 16% of cases. The increased potential for infectious complications precludes performance of a synchronous bowel resection. This complication may manifest 1 week to 6 years after surgery and necessitates sponge removal. If the septic material points toward the vagina or rectum, it may be transluminally removed through these organs.

The anterior and posterior sling rectopexies provide acceptable control of the rectal prolapse with low morbidity and mortality. Morbidities specific to each procedure include stricture formation after the Ripstein procedure and infectious complications after the implantation of an Ivalon sponge. Functional results are frequently cited causes of patient dissatisfaction with postoperative constipation and persistent incontinence. Rectopexy procedures without resection should probably be limited to patients with no evidence of constipation.

Laparoscopic Rectopexy

Rectopexy is the most frequently performed laparoscopic operation for the control of rectal prolapse. A number of series and case reports (Table 43-3). have described techniques using mesh and sutures. The sutured rectopexy takes 4 to 5 hours, and the mesh technique requires about 2 to 4 hours. The length of the procedure seems to be related to a surgeon's experience. Intraoperative complications have been limited to minor bleeding, which can be easily addressed by converting to an open procedure if necessary. One death from myocardial infarction has been reported. Two recurrences after mesh rectopexy and one after suture rectopexy have been reported. The sutured rectopexy recurrence was attributed to a concomitant enterocele observed but not repaired at the original operation, and the mesh recurrences were attributed to poor staple placement. Two cases of trocar-site hernias have been reported. One hernia was asymptomatic, and the other required reoperation and resection of incarcerated bowel.

Longer operative times, especially for relatively inexperienced surgeons, may increase potential risks. The incidence of deep venous thrombosis may increase, especially in patients in a Lloyd-Davies position with flexed legs. Some authorities have suggested performing these procedures with patients in the supine position and reserving the Lloyd-Davies positions for laparoscopic procedures requiring transanal manipulations.

Functional results are encouraging, with restoration of continence observed in 4 of 5 patients in one series. A satisfaction rate of 6 of 7 patients was demonstrated in another series. The virtual absence of postoperative abdominal pain and ileus has accelerated recovery time and mobilization. The length of hospitalization usually is 4 to 6 days.

Solomon et al. compared 21 laparoscopic rectopexies with 24 open abdominal rectopexies. Postoperative morbidity and mortality at 1 month of follow-up was 19% for the laparoscopic group and 29% for the open group. One death occurred in the open group. Mean operative time was 198 minutes for the laparoscopic operations and 130 minutes for the abdominal procedures. Length of time until a solid diet was tolerated was 2.7 days in the laparoscopic group and 5.8 days in the open group. Length of stay was 6.3 and 11.0 days, and analgesia requirements during the first 48 hours postoperatively were 42.4 and 71.5 mg of opiates, respectively.

The laparoscopic rectopexy is therefore a safe and effective option for the treatment of rectal prolapse. It is less invasive than an open rectopexy procedure with decreased postoperative disability. The indications for rectopexy may be extended to include elderly patients previously deemed unfit for an abdominal procedure.

Anterior Resection

Anterior resections have low, long-term rates of recurrence. Colon and rectal surgeons at the Mayo Clinic have favored this operation for treating rectal prolapse for 2 decades. The procedure is safe and performed frequently by surgeons for other conditions. It is therefore more familiar than prolapse procedures that have no other indications. The increased potential for infectious complications related to the colorectal anastomosis, which is absent in rectopexy procedures, is this operation's greatest disadvantage. Long-term results for laparoscopic anterior resection are not yet available.

Wolff et al. reported a series of 150 patients with mortality and morbidity rates of 0.7% and 28%, respectively (Table 43-4). These statistics compare favorably with the Lahey Clinic report on the Ripstein procedure with mortality and morbidity rates of 0.7% and 51.9%, respectively. Wolff's group experienced a 9.3% infection rate that included a 3.3% anastomotic leak rate, 3.3% wound infection rate, and a 2.6% incidence of deep abscess. Their recurrence rate of 8.9% compares favorably with the popular rectal suspension operations. The Lahey Clinic and Cleveland Clinic series had 9.6%

Table 43-3. Results after Laparoscopic Rectopexy

Study	No. of Patients	Follow-up (mo)	Mortality	Complications	Recurrences
Graf, 1995	5	10	0	0	0
Henry, 1994	5	2–10 (6)[a]	0	Incarcerated hernia in port site	0
Solomon, 1996	21	1	0	1 converted to open; 1 port site hernia	0
Kwok, 1994	1	3	0	0	0
Cuschieri, 1994	6	4–27	0	Constipation (2)	0
Schweizger, 1994	7	14–24 (19)[a]	0	0	1
Herold, 1994	19	6–18	0	Bleeding (1)	0
Kiff, 1994	37	2–10 (5)[a]	1	0	1
Munro, 1993	1	9	0	0	0
Senagore, 1993	6	12	0	Port bleed (1)	0
Cuesta, 1992	4	1–8 (4)[a]	0	0	0
Berman, 1992	1	1	0	0	0
Kockerling, 1992	4	—	0	0	0
Kusminsky, 1992	1	—	0	0	0
Darzi, 1993	7	3	0	0	0

[a] Values in parentheses are means.

Table 43-4. Results after Anterior Resection for Rectal Prolapse

Study	No. of Patients	Mortality	Recurrence	Morbidity (%)
Wolff et al., 1991	150	0.7	8.9	28
Muir, 1962	50	2	0	Frequent mucosal prolapses
Thauerkauf et al., 1970	28	3.6	3.7	7.1
Thauerkauf's review	202	2.0	3.6	Not reported
Schlinkert et al., 1985				
Low anterior resection	29[a]	0	9	76
High anterior resection	52[a]	2	11	19

[a] Incomplete patient follow-up.

and 12.2% failure rates, respectively, with the Ripstein operation. Theuerkauf et al. reported a 3.6% failure rate after anterior resection in a combined report of their series and review of the literature. Suspension procedures have the additional potential disadvantages of presacral hemorrhage and pelvic sepsis. The Lahey Clinic now proposes anterior resections as the "procedure of choice for full-thickness rectal prolapse in men . . . and probably young active women."

Low anterior resections, when compared with high anterior resections, have more infectious complications and poorer functional results. In a paper comparing these two operations, low anterior resections had a 52% rate of pelvic sepsis, and the high anterior resection rate of sepsis was 19%. Recurrence rates were similar in the two groups. Continence after low anterior resection was poorer than after high anterior resection, which was attributed to a smaller rectal vault.

Sigmoid Resection and Proctopexy

Resection with proctopexy is often used for young, healthy patients with constipation

and is an effective procedure (Table 43-5). Because the anastomosis is created at a convenient site proximal to the rectum, it is technically easier than a low anterior resection and has fewer anastomotic and infectious complications. The major advantage is the marked improvement in constipation postoperatively. A prospective study by Sayfan et al. comparing Marlex mesh rectopexy with sigmoidectomy and posterior suture rectopexy revealed significantly less postoperative constipation in the resection and rectopexy group. Morbidity, mortality, and recurrence rates were similar. Symptoms of constipation are improved in 60% to 80% of patients. Improvements in continence are reported for about 35% to 60%. Recurrence rates range from 0% to 9%.

Perineal Rectosigmoidectomy

Rectosigmoidectomy with total pelvic floor repair is a safe procedure (Table 43-6) and is often used for elderly patients with rectal prolapse. Postoperative constipation is generally not a problem and the incidence of incontinence is low. As reported by the Prasad, Altemeier, and Gopal groups, improvement in continence is much higher af-

ter synchronous pelvic floor repair. The coloanal anastomosis is associated with a low risk of dehiscence. Loss of a rectal reservoir and a resulting sense of urgency is a source of patient dissatisfaction. Many patients develop a stricture at the anastomotic site that can usually be treated by dilatation and rarely requires surgery. Hughes reported a greater than 60% recurrence rate in his series from St. Mark's hospital. Altemeier reported only three recurrences after 106 operations. These results have yet to be matched in the literature.

Suggested Reading

Altemeier WA, Culbertson WR, Schowengerdt CJ, Hurt J. Nineteen years' experience with the one stage perineal repair of rectal prolapse. *Ann Surg* 1971;173:993–1006.

Ballantyne GH. Anterior resection for rectal prolapse. In: Ballantyne GH, Leahy PF, Modlin IM, eds. *Laparoscopic surgery*. Philadelphia: WB Saunders, 1994:565–574.

Ballantyne GH. The historical evolution of anatomical concepts of rectal prolapse. *Semin Colon Rectal Surg* 1991;2:170–179.

Ballantyne GH. Laparoscopically assisted anterior resection for rectal prolapse. *Surg Laparosc Endosc* 1992;2:230–236.

Cuschieri A, Shimi SM, Vander Velpen G, et al. Laparoscopic prosthesis fixation rectopexy for complete rectal prolapse. *Br J Surg* 1994;81:138–139.

Johansen OB, Wexner SD, Daniel N, et al. Perineal rectosigmoidectomy in the elderly. *Dis Colon Rectum* 1993;36:767–772.

Kwok SP, Carey DP, Lau WY, Li AK. Laparoscopic rectopexy. *Dis Colon Rectum* 1994;37:947–948.

Meyers JO, Wong WD, Rothenberger DA, et al. Rectal prolapse in males—implications for management. *Dis Colon Rectum* 1990;33:28.

Sayfan J, Pinho M, Alexander-Williams J, Keighley MRB. Sutured posterior abdominal rectopexy with sigmoidectomy compared with Marlex rectopexy for rectal prolapse. *Br J Surg* 1990;77:143–145.

Senagore AJ, Luchtefeld MA, MacKeigan JM. Rectopexy. *J Laparoendosc Surg* 1993;3:339–343.

Wilson PD, Williams NS. Laparoscopic treatment of rectal prolapse. *Semin Laparosc Surg* 1995;2:262–267.

Wolff BG, Madoff RD, Goldberg SM. Choice of procedures for rectal prolapse. *Semin Colon Rectal Surg* 1991;2:217–226.

Table 43-5. Results after Sigmoid Resection and Rectopexy

Study	No. of Patients	Follow-up (years)	Recurrence (%)	Continence (%) WORSE	Continence (%) BETTER
Madoff et al., 1992	47	5.4 (mean)	6	23	38
Sayfan et al., 1990	13	NR	0	NR	67
Husa, 1988	48	0.6–2.5	9	33	94
Watts et al., 1985	102	0.5–30	2	1.6[a]	30[a]

NR, not reported.
[a] Sixty-one of 102 patients were interviewed.

Table 43-6. Results after Perineal Rectosigmoidectomy (Altemeier Procedure)

Study	No. of Patients	Follow-up (mo)	Mortality (%)	Morbidity (%)	Recurrence (%)
Johansen et al., 1993	20	26	5	5	0
Williams, 1992	114	(12)[a]	0	12	10
Finlay and Aitchison, 1991	17	(24)[a]	6	18	6
Ramanujam and Venkatesh, 1987	41	6–48 (20-mo mean)	0	7	5
Theuerkauf et al., 1970	13	NR	0	8	38
Altemeier et al., 1971	106	NR	0	32	2.8

NR, not reported.
[a] Values in parentheses are medians.

44

Transanal Endoscopic Microsurgery

Peter W. Smiley and Timothy W. Bax

Transanal endoscopic microsurgery (TEM) was initially described by Gerhard Buess of Tübingen, Germany. Since its introduction in 1982, TEM has been used to treat mid- and high rectal lesions ranging from small adenomas to invasive carcinomas. TEM technique allows precise dissection under direct visualization, as well as the ability to close the full-thickness rectal wall defect left by the resection. Several investigators have demonstrated that this less invasive technique for removing rectal lesions is equally effective and less morbid than conventional open surgery for selected patients. However, the technical skills needed for TEM are more demanding than those for standard laparoscopic procedures or traditional transanal techniques and require considerable training and practice before clinical practice can begin.

Indications

Any patient with a mid- or high rectal lesion is a potential candidate for TEM resection. Treatment of large sessile adenomas is often impossible with a conventional colonoscope, and patients with such lesions are ideal candidates for TEM resection. The lesion can be removed entirely using a submucosal dissection plane, and the mucosal defect can be closed primarily. These adenomas can be circumferential, and the upper limit of dissection is approximately 24 cm from the anal verge. Some controversy exists around the treatment of cancers. Full-thickness excision of the rectal wall can safely be accomplished with TEM technique. Patients who have undergone endoscopic removal of a pedunculated adenoma in which a small focus of invasive carcinoma is seen can have the base of the adenoma excised using TEM. Early, small adenocarcinomas (stage T1) can be excised using TEM, and the cure rate is probably similar to that of conventional approaches. Frail or elderly patients who might not survive a large transabdominal or abdominoperineal excision can undergo TEM resection of more advanced and larger lesions (stages T2 to T3) with less operative risk, but the long-term results may not be as good. TEM is also a useful technique in patients with documented metastatic disease who need palliative resection. Described indications are listed in Table 44-1.

Preoperative Considerations

A standard clinical workup should be obtained in all potential TEM candidates. This includes total colonoscopy and clinical staging utilizing transrectal ultrasound. This imaging modality can accurately determine the depth of invasion and the mobility of rectal lesions preoperatively. In addition, rigid sigmoidoscopy should be performed in all patients for whom the level of the lesion is in question. This will not only help the surgeon determine the suitability of TEM for individual patients but also determine the circumferential location of the lesion, which will affect positioning the patient intraoperatively. While lesions up to 90% of the circumference are resectable, high lesions (above 20 cm) are probably best treated by a transabdominal approach. A standard bowel preparation is used in all patients.

Operative Technique

Instrumentation

Currently, there are two TEM operating systems available. We have experience with the system manufactured by Richard Wolf GmbH (Knittlingen, Germany), and the following is a description of that system. The operating rectoscope is 4 cm in diameter and is available in two different lengths, 12 cm and 20 cm. A glass endpiece may be used along with manual insufflation to position the rectoscope. Once properly positioned, the rectoscope is held in place by a double ball-jointed arm attached to the operating table. A working end-piece is used for the remainder of the procedure and contains channels with sealing sleeves to allow the introduction of a telescope and operative instruments. Dr. Buess designed an angled, stereoscopic telescope for the operative surgeon to use and an optional channel for insertion of a standard laparoscope so that the rest of the operative team can follow the progress of

Table 44-1. Indications for Transanal Endoscopic Microsurgery

---

Large, sessile rectal polyps

Excision of the base of pedunculated polyps with microinvasive carcinoma

Palliative resection of metastatic rectal carcinoma

Curative resection of stage I rectal carcinoma

Epidermoidal carcinoma

Carcinoids

Strictures

Rectal ulcers

---

the procedure. Other centers having more extensive experience with standard laparoscopic imaging believe the stereoscope is not necessary to perform TEM procedures safely and effectively. We have designed an adapter that allows the use of a 10-mm, 25-degree-angled laparoscope. By using a standard angled laparoscope, the operating surgeon and the assistants all have the same field of vision and work better as a team. Eliminating the stereoscope also reduces the price of the TEM system by nearly 50%. Several specialized instruments are available from the manufacturer of the TEM system:

Long coagulation/aspiration tube, curved to avoid interference with the other instruments,

Retractable needle for injecting vasoconstrictive agents submucosally,

Needle-point cautery device for precise dissection,

Tissue graspers and scissors angled to the left or right for right-handed or left-handed use, respectively,

Needle holders bent downward for easier suturing in a confined space,

Specialized clip applier used to place small silver clips on the ends of sutures because knot tying in a 4-cm space is nearly impossible,

Single device that controls low-pressure rectal insufflation, irrigation, and suction.

A second system is manufactured by Karl Storz GmbH (Tuttlingen, Germany). This system is similar to the Wolf system but the operating rectoscopes are 3.5 × 15 cm and 2.5 × 20 cm in size. A standard insufflator and standard laparoscopic instrumentation are used. There is no stereoscopic operating scope; an angled laparoscope is used in its place.

Operating Room Setup

The circumferential position of the lesion determines the position of the patient on the operating room table. If the lesion is located on the posterior half the rectum, the patient is placed in the dorsal lithotomy position. Conversely, if the lesion is on the anterior half of the rectum, the patient is placed prone in a jackknife position with the legs separated. This allows the surgeon to look down on the lesion while working (Fig. 44-1). General or regional (spinal, epidural) anesthesia can be used. The insufflator, camera, and light source are best

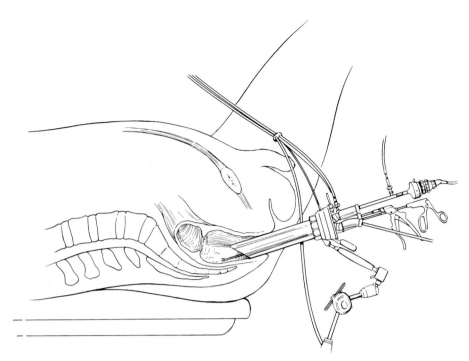

Fig. 44-1. Schematic of transanal endoscopic microsurgery system.

located lateral to the patient, with the cords and tubing draped over the thigh.

Procedure

Standard preparation and draping are used, and a perioperative dose of an antibiotic is given. After gentle digital dilation of the anal sphincters, the appropriate-length rectoscope is inserted using the accompanying obturator. Whenever possi-

ble, the shorter rectoscope should be used to make manipulation of the endoscopic instruments easier. The glass end-piece is used to position the rectoscope so that the lesion is optimally seen. Once the desired position is obtained, the rectoscope is held in place by the locking arm attached to the operating table. The working end-piece along with the sealing sleeves is then attached and the necessary tubing connected (Figs. 44-1 and 44-2).

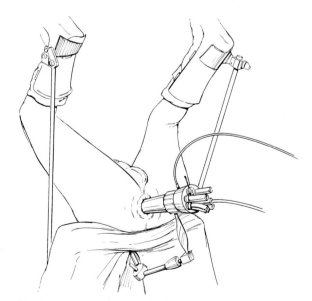

Fig. 44-2. Surgeon's view of transanal endoscopic microsurgery system in place.

The insufflator is designed to provide continuous low-level insufflation of the rectum for optimal visualization. It will adjust the inflow as the amount of suction is varied so that visualization is maintained. There is also a channel for irrigating the endoscope. (The stereoscope designed for this system has an irrigation channel built into it, but if a standard laparoscope is used, a separate scope-washing device is necessary.)

Once the lesion and the rectoscope are optimally positioned, needle-point cautery is used to mark the borders of the planned resection (Fig. 44-3). This step is vital because once the dissection is begun, the borders of the lesion are often obscured. Submucosal injection of epinephrine-containing solution is helpful in patients in whom a mucosectomy is planned. This step is slightly less helpful for full-thickness excisions. The dissection is performed using the needle-point cautery, with a tissue grasper providing gentle retraction (Fig. 44-4). For most lesions, full-thickness excision is preferred. The exceptions are high rectal lesions in which the peritoneal cavity may be entered with a full-thickness excision, and very low lesions in which anal sphincter muscles may be damaged. Once the specimen is completely excised, meticulous hemostasis is achieved using the cautery unit.

The rectal wall defect is closed with absorbable suture (Vicryl or PDS) in a transverse direction (Fig. 44-5). As a substitute for knot tying, which is very difficult in the confines of the rectoscope, a silver clip is applied to the ends of the suture (Fig. 44-6).

Postoperative Considerations

Typically, patients are fed immediately and discharged from 0 to 4 days postoperatively. Potential early and late complications are outlined in Table 44-2. Patients are warned preoperatively to expect some rectal bleeding for a few days postoperatively. Pain medications are seldom necessary.

Results

The most extensive experience with TEM is from the Tübingen group in Germany, but

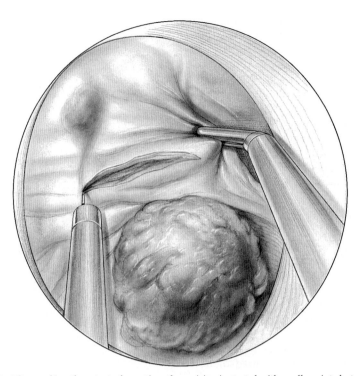

Fig. 44-3. After marking the extent of resection, the excision is started with needle-point electrocautery.

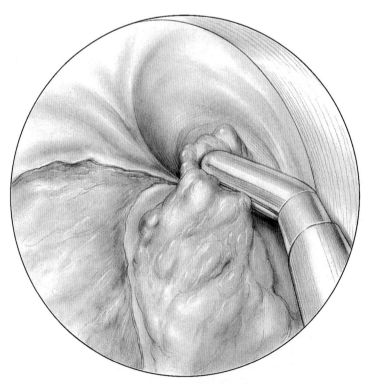

Fig. 44-4. Resection proceeds with gentle traction of the lesion.

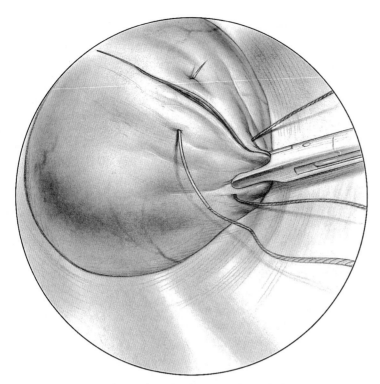

Fig. 44-5. Closure of rectal wall defect with absorbable suture.

Table 44-2. Complications of Transanal Endoscopic Microsurgery

Early
  Bleeding
  Intraperitoneal perforation
  Abscess
  Sepsis
  Suture dehiscence
  Incontinence
Late
  Incontinence
  Stricture
  Rectovaginal fistula

others have reported series of TEM as well. The results for benign lesions are good, but the results from using TEM for carcinomas are less encouraging. Results from three large series are shown in Table 44-3. The three series all represent nonrandomized patients evaluated in a retrospective fashion. In the United States, there are few centers performing this procedure. Results are being compiled in a prospective fashion by Dr. Lee Smith of Georgetown University utilizing a national registry.

Table 44-3. Results of Transanal Endoscopic Microsurgery

	Tübingen, Germany	United States	Italy
Total cases	282	154	122
Adenomas	190	82	58
Carcinomas	75	51	52
Stage T1	44	30	22
Stage T2	23	15	21
Stage T3	8	6	9
Mean blood loss (mL)	NR	68	NR
Mean operative time (min)	92	110	NR
Mean hospital stay (days)	NR	2.8	NR
Complications (%)			
Early	2.5	7.7	14.7
Late	1.8	3.9	8.3
Deaths (%)	0.7	0	0
Recurrence (%)			
Adenoma	2	11	11
Stage T1	6	10	2
Stage T2	8	40	8
Stage T3	25	67	0

NR, not reported.

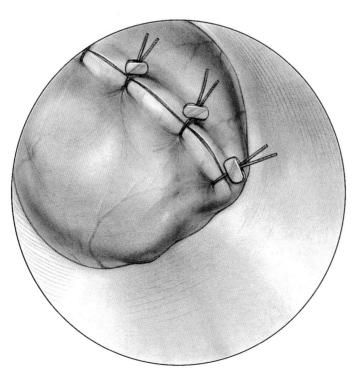

Fig. 44-6. Completed closure with a silver clip on the suture tail.

Conclusion

We believe TEM technique to be a valuable addition to colorectal surgery. Large, low-lying benign lesions can be removed with minimal morbidity and mortality, and a large transabdominal or transsacral incision can be avoided. Based on the results reported on the experience with the use of TEM for carcinomas, we believe that patients with more advanced, locally invasive carcinomas who are otherwise healthy should undergo traditional wide excision via a transabdominal or transsacral approach, until a well controlled study is done demonstrating equal effectiveness with TEM technique. Patients in need of a palliative resection for a bulky rectal tumor can also benefit from the TEM approach, but it should be made clear to them that cure is unlikely. All patients with known rectal carcinomas who are being considered for TEM should be enrolled in a study to help answer the question of the adequacy of TEM resection for cancer.

Suggested Reading

Buess G, Mentges, B, Manncke K, Starlinger M, Becker HD. Technique and results of transanal microsurgery in early rectal cancer. *Am J Surg* 1992;163:63–70.

Lirici MM, Chiavellati L, Lezoche E, et al. Transanal endoscopic microsurgery in Italy. *Endosc Surg Allied Technol* 1994;2:255–258.

Raestrup H, Manncke K, Mentges B, Buess G, Becker HD. Indications and technique for TEM (transanal endoscopic microsurgery). *Endosc Surg* 1994;2:241–246.

EDITOR'S COMMENT

Most general and colorectal surgeons at some time experience the frustration that a low anterior resection or Kraske operation are overkill, but necessary, for the removal of a benign rectal mass that is not amenable to conventional transanal techniques. The authors of this chapter have described an excellent addition to the surgeon's armamentarium for treating such lesions. The role for transanal endoscopic microsurgery (TEM) in the treatment of cancer remains undefined. The number or percentage of patients who are appropriate for TEM is relatively small. The cost of the technology needed must be considered before pursuing the acquisition of equipment and skills necessary for the performance of this operation.

The description of the procedure in this chapter sounds deceptively easy.It is worthwhile to reemphasize the point made by the authors regarding the need for excellent training and practice prior to applying these techniques in the care of patients. The complica-tions associated with a poorly performed rectal closure can lead to multiple re-operations, sepsis, and death. When properly applied by the well-trained surgeon this is a useful technique that spares the patient from unnecessary pain, recuperative time, and potential morbidity.

W.S.E.

VI
Abdominal Wall

IV

Abdominal Wall

45

Technique for Transabdominal Preperitoneal Laparoscopic Herniorrhaphy

Bruce C. Steffes

One of the leading objections to the acceptance of laparoscopic herniorrhaphy is the necessity to enter the abdominal cavity. It is argued that the need for general anesthesia, the risk of intraabdominal injury, and the late risk of small bowel obstruction outweigh the advantages of less pain, more rapid return to work, and identification of contralateral hernias. However, proper attention to technique can minimize most of these risks of the transabdominal preperitoneal (TAPP) approach. In response to these concerns, there has been an increasing interest in the totally preperitoneal (TOPP) approach, also known as the totally extraperitoneal approach, which is usually done with balloon dissecting devices. Whether this totally preperitoneal approach will prove to be safer is unknown, but the TAPP approach will always retain some of its indications and advantages. The TAPP procedure needs to be part of the laparoscopic herniorrhaphist's armamentarium for several reasons:

1. It is easier to teach the unfamiliar anatomy to surgeons learning the technique.
2. While performing the TOPP technique, peritoneal tears can occur that may be most easily handled by conversion to the TAPP technique.
3. An incarcerated hernia is more easily handled from the intraabdominal approach and allows easier confirmation of the viability of the entrapped viscera.
4. With concomitant umbilical hernia, repair of the umbilical hernia allows necessary entry to the abdominal cavity without incurring additional risk.

5. The TAPP approach allows visualization of intraabdominal viscera when there is concern about possible concomitant pathology.
6. Hernia repairs in females may be more appropriately performed intraabdominally because of the difficulty in dissecting the peritoneal hernia sac from the round ligament. This dissection is sometimes difficult from the preperitoneal approach because of the adherence of the peritoneum and often leads to tears of the peritoneum. The increased possibility of incidental pelvic pathology in women provides additional reason to use the TAPP technique.
7. Avoidance of the use of the balloon dissecting devices lowers the overall cost of the procedure. It is possible to do the TAPP procedure with reusable trocars in all three sites, thereby requiring only a disposable stapler or tacker. The TOPP procedure can be done without the balloon dissecting devices, but it usually takes significantly longer, thereby supplanting device costs with operating room costs.

Procedure

The patient is placed in a Trendelenburg position with both arms tucked to the sides. The surgeon performs most of the dissection while standing up by the contralateral shoulder. The first 10-mm trocar is placed at the umbilicus by percutaneous or open technique. Two secondary trocars (5 or 11 mm) are placed bilaterally at the level of the umbilicus on the edge of the rectus musculature. If a stapler is to be used, two 11-mm trocars usually are employed, which allows placement of the stapler from either side. If experience with the procedure allows and the surgeon is convinced that the hernia is unilateral, an 11-mm trocar is placed contralaterally and a 5-mm trocar is placed ipsilaterally. The 5-mm tackers may allow bilateral placement of 5-mm trocars, which may improve cosmesis and diminish pain and risk of trocar herniation. An angled laparoscope (30° or 45°) allows a view that is more *en face* and moves the tip of the scope more posteriorly, allowing increased space for instrument manipulation.

After visual examination of the contents of the abdomen, it is important to confirm each of the anatomic landmarks of the peritoneum, including the median, medial, and lateral umbilical folds. It is also important to identify the internal inguinal ring and be aware of where the symphysis pubis, Cooper's ligament, and iliac vessels lie beneath the peritoneum. A curvilinear incision is made that extends from the medial umbilical peritoneal fold to a point 3 or 4 cm posterolateral to the internal ring (Fig. 45-1). The incision is placed anterosuperior to any defect by about 4 or 5 cm. The peritoneum is grasped by blunt graspers placed in the contralateral port, and traction is applied medially and posteriorly. With the first nick in the peritoneum, dissection by the pressure of the carbon dioxide of the fissile areolar plane can be seen (Figs. 45-2 and 45-3). With continued traction, the peritoneum can be safely sharply incised over the lateral umbilical fold (i.e., epigastric vessels) using scissors with electrocautery. The peri-

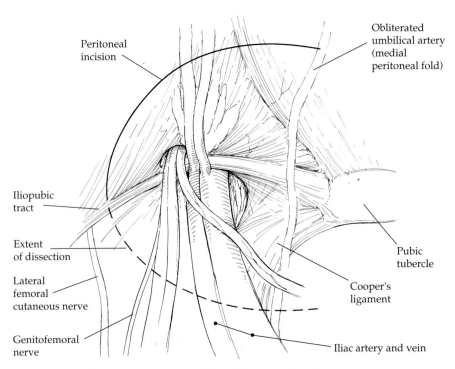

Fig. 45-1. Internal view of the peritoneal incision.

Labels: Peritoneal incision; Obliterated umbilical artery (medial peritoneal fold); Iliopubic tract; Extent of dissection; Lateral femoral cutaneous nerve; Genitofemoral nerve; Pubic tubercle; Cooper's ligament; Iliac artery and vein

toneal incision is extended into the lateral aspect of the medial umbilical fold that contains the obliterated umbilical artery. To improve visualization, the obliterated artery is sometimes carefully divided, although experience makes this maneuver increasingly less necessary. Cautery scissors are used to prevent bleeding from the small collateral vessels in this medial area. Cautery is discouraged lateral to the epigastric vessels to minimize risk of injury to the nerves. Further medial dissection is

sometimes dangerous because of the location of the bladder.

Firm countertraction provided by the contralateral grasper opens the preperitoneal space and facilitates dissection with a blunt closed grasper placed in the ipsilateral port. It is desirable to keep the fat with the peritoneum, staying directly behind the fascia and visible muscle fibers. Only occasionally is sharp dissection or cautery necessary, which carries the inherent risk of inadvertent injury to the nerves in the

area. If the normal anatomy is dissected first, the surgeon can work from the known to the unknown. For example, in the case of a indirect hernia, the area over the direct hernia site medially is dissected first, then the area lateral to the cord, and then the cord structures and the sac itself. Countertraction with the contralateral grasper is the most important factor facilitating dissection and identification of the proper planes. Retraction of the peritoneal flap should be in the direction of the middle of the pelvis away from the anterior abdominal wall. The ipsilateral grasper is used in a closed position to sweep the tissues away from the anterior wall. Approximately when the Cooper ligament first becomes visible, it is helpful to place the closed contralateral grasper into the preperitoneal space and retract the peritoneal flap with the side of the instrument in the same midpelvic direction. The ipsilateral closed grasper can then be swept along an axis parallel to Cooper's ligament from medial to lateral and usually develop this plane easily with one or two sweeps. It is important to avoid placing the grasper on the ligament to prevent injury to the fragile branches of the pudendal veins, and it likewise should not be placed much deeper than the ligament to avoid inadvertent injury to the obturator vessels and nerve laterally.

Lateral to the cord, the dissection is carried out by grasping the peritoneum or the nonvascular portion of the cord with the contralateral grasper and applying traction medially and away from the anterior musculature and the underlying iliopsoas muscle. Using the ipsilateral closed grasper, a sweeping motion from medial to lateral from the internal ring outward exposes the lateral iliopubic tract. The spermatic cord can be easily separated from the underlying iliac vessels (if mobilization of the cord is desired) (Fig. 45-4). It is during the lateral dissection and later during the securing of the mesh in this area that a full understanding the normal and variant anatomy of the genitofemoral, lateral femoral cutaneous, femoral, and ilioinguinal nerves is critical. By careful dissection and sweeping all loose tissue with the cord, the genitofemoral nerve can be preserved. The genitofemoral nerve is usually found no further than 1 cm lateral to the edge of the gonadal vessels and more commonly lies between the gonadal and the iliac vessels and exits the abdominal cavity at the internal ring. The genital

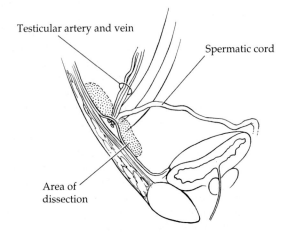

Fig. 45-2. Parasagital cut through pelvis showing area of dissection.

Labels: Testicular artery and vein; Spermatic cord; Area of dissection

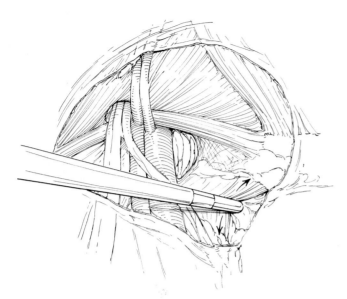

Fig. 45-3. Dissection of tissue planes.

branch sometimes parallels the iliopubic tract within the abdomen and perforates the area of Hesselbach's triangle medially. Unnecessary dissection above Cooper's ligament is discouraged to avoid injuring this variant nerve. The lateral femoral cutaneous nerve usually lies on the iliopsoas under the thin fascia and exits the abdomen beneath the iliopubic tract through the muscular lacuna about 2 cm medial to the anterior superior iliac spine. If the peritoneal incision is not carried too far laterally and if the dissection is done bluntly in the appropriate loose areolar plane, this nerve is not injured during the dissection. The normal course of the ilioinguinal nerve is to perforate the transversus and internal oblique muscles lateral to the anterior superior iliac spine, and it is not visible by laparoscopy at this location. Occasionally, a branch of the nerve is visible on the attenuated transversalis fascia laterally, paralleling the iliopubic tract and entering the internal ring from the lateral aspect. The femoral nerve is usually covered by the edge of the iliopsoas, except in a very thin individual, and is not usually vulnerable to injury at this stage in the procedure if the proper plane is maintained.

Dissection of the spermatic cord (Fig. 45-5) in the case of an indirect hernia is reserved until last. The distal sac can be handled by dissection or transection. Direct hernias and small to moderate size indirect hernias are usually dissected free (Fig. 45-6). If by reaching into the depths of the hernia sac with the ipsilateral grasper and pulling, the hernia sac can be easily everted, it can be dissected as easily, safely, and quickly as transection. Dissection of the cord is analogous to the technique used in external repairs. The peritoneum is anteromedial and is the most visible part of the cord. By grasping the peritoneum at the internal ring and applying firm countertraction up and out of the canal, the dissection grasper carefully peels the vessels and vas away. Hand-over-hand grasping of the peritoneum often is necessary to maintain sufficient tension. The characteristic appearance of the double fold of peritoneum usually is seen at the end of the sac. Occasionally, the obliterated processus vaginalis has significant substance and can be sharply divided. By grasping the end of the sac and retracting it up and into the midpelvis, the remaining structures can be bluntly dissected away until the peritoneum is adequately mobilized.

There are several options for handling the redundant peritoneum. If there is no potential for the peritoneum to cause an internal hernia, nothing is done. If the sac remains with a narrow orifice that could cause an internal hernia, it can be ligated (usually with a pretied loop ligature) or opened superiorly (which creates a new superior edge to the peritoneal flap). The sac can be everted and, after the mesh is repertionealized, fixed in a fashion similar to a diverticulopexy, but this does not offer any significant advantage and could create the potential for an internal hernia unless the sac is fixed to the parietal peritoneum along its entire length.

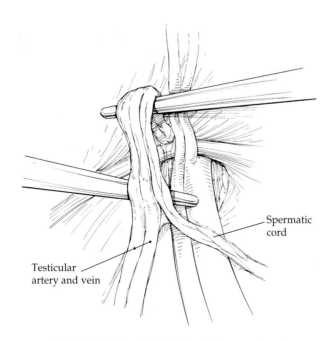

Spermatic cord

Testicular artery and vein

Fig. 45-4. Technique of mobilization of the spermatic cord.

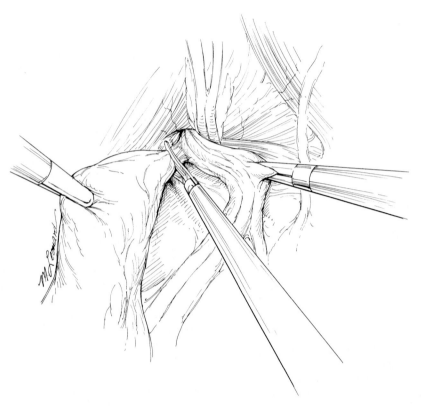

Fig. 45-5. Dissection of the spermatic cord.

Transection of the neck of the sac may be desirable in treating the large hernia, but doing so before the mobilization of the base of the sac in the preperitoneal plane and identification of the vas deferens and the vessels increases the risk of injury to those structures because of the difficulty of visualizing them as they curve around the

epigastric vessels. Transection and closure of the sac at a very high point (i.e., proximal) also causes a defect in the peritoneal flap that may make it difficult to adequately mobilize the peritoneum enough to cover the prosthetic mesh. Hernias that extend beyond the entrance into the scrotum and hernias that have scarring around the peritoneum that does not easily separate from the vas and vascular structures are best handled by transection. This approach may minimize damage to the pampiniform plexus and thereby avoid ischemic orchitis.

If transection of the sac is desirable, there are minor modifications in technique. The cord and peritoneum are pulled up out of the canal, and dissection is performed by retraction of the peritoneal sac in a direction 90° to the axis of the spermatic vessels and vas. For example, on the right side, this retraction rotates the sac counterclockwise if the retraction is toward the middle of the pelvis with the left grasper or clockwise if the retraction is away from the middle of the pelvis with the right grasper. Rotation of the peritoneal sac in the desired direction by passing the sac from grasper to grasper eventually brings the vas and vessels into view (Fig. 45-7). When the vessels and vas are freed sufficiently, careful transection of the sac (looking carefully for any visceral component) can be accomplished. The line of transection is 2 or 3 cm distal to the original neck of the sac, and the peritoneum is closed with a pretied loop ligature.

There is debate about the necessity of the mobilization of the spermatic structures to allow placement of a slit mesh compared with leaving them *in situ* and covering the area with a nonslit mesh. In our series, slit mesh is routinely used unless mobilization is likely to cause vessel injury. Placement of the slit mesh creates a new internal ring that seems desirable and, if the slit is firmly secured, prevents herniation around the cord. By firm traction of the cord medially and up into the middle of the pelvis, a window can be easily created for the placement of the "tail" of the prosthesis (Figs. 45-8 and 45-9). After this window is created, it can be enlarged by placing the graspers into the defect from both sides of the cord and applying mild force in opposing directions along the direction of the iliac vessels.

During dissection of the cord, a distinct lobule of preperitoneal fat (i.e., "lipoma"

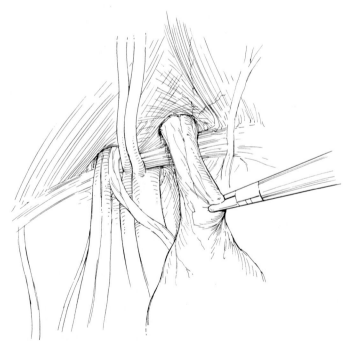

Fig. 45-6. Dissection of a direct hernia.

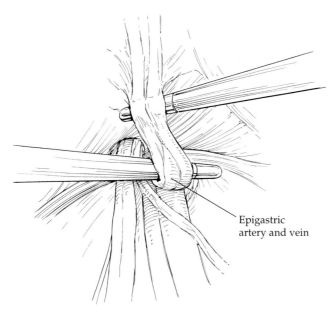

Fig. 45-7. Dissection of the epigastric vessels.

of the cord) often can be seen and is easily dissected out of the ring with traction and minimal dissection. Unless it is of sufficient size to make visualization difficult, the lipoma is usually folded back out of the way and then placed between the mesh and the peritoneum before closure of the peritoneum. If removal is desired, careful division with cautery scissors or ligation of the base with pretied loop ligature and transection is possible.

Dissection in the case of a direct hernia is usually easier. The dissection is carried out first laterally, and the cord is mobilized. With firm countertraction on the inferior flap in the direction of the midpelvis, the edge of the involved preperitoneal fat and peritoneum can usually be easily visualized. The proper plane of dissection is often marked by the double tissue fold seen anteriorly and caused by the traction and inversion of the attenuated transversalis fascia (its appearance is similar to the fold of peritoneum seen while dissecting the indirect sac but comes from the anterior direction). Careful blunt dissection can usually easily separate this plane, although sharp dissection occasionally is necessary. If the tissue is especially adherent, grasping the transversalis fascia with one grasper and the periperitoneal fat with the other allows

gentle tearing in the proper plane. Care must be taken to identify any sliding component medially to avoid injury to the bladder. The plane must be dissected in all directions sufficiently to allow easy placement of the prosthesis so that it can overlap any defect by a minimum of 2 cm.

Placement of the prosthesis behind the epigastric vessels has no effect on the efficacy of the repair. The advantage in doing so is to hold the prosthesis in position without having it fall back while it is smoothed out and stapled. It is illogical to divide the epigastric vessels unnecessarily and is recommended only if hemostasis demands; it can be safely done under that circumstance. Under the pressure of the pneumoperitoneum, the vessels bowstring and stand usually away from the muscle to some degree. A condensation of the transversalis fascia of variable density is called the *interfoveolar ligament*, which can be sharply divided to aid in the dissection. The only branch of the epigastric vessels of significance is a variable medial branch usually high in Hesselbach's triangle and extending to the falx inguinalis. It can be divided after cauterization if necessary. Sliding the closed ipsilateral blunt grasper along the top of the internal ring between the muscle and the epigastric vessels usually creates a window that is enlarged by placing the contralateral grasper into the same hole and separating the tips in opposing directions. It should large enough to allow the lateral portion of the mesh to be withdrawn without undue force and to be easily entered by the ipsilateral grasper.

We used a soft, open-weave polypropylene mesh has been used in our series because it has the best available combination of ingrowth characteristics, strength, through-visibility, and handling characteristics. The prosthesis should cover all areas of potential herniation with an overlap of any defect by a minimum of 2 to 3 cm. The average size has been remarkably consistent, with most patients served by a prosthesis 9 to 10 cm by 12 to 13 cm in the greatest dimension. Using a precut standard size and type of prosthesis that has been manufactured to these specifications has had the advantages of decreasing operative and anesthetic time and minimizing snagging of the prosthesis on the loose areolar tissue. If an 11-mm lateral trocar has been used, backloading the mesh into a 10-mm appendiceal extractor (with a 5-mm reducer) makes delivery of the mesh

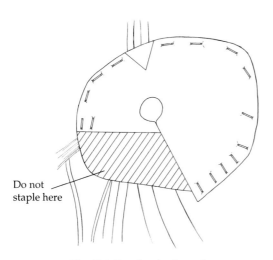

Fig. 45-8. Template for the mesh.

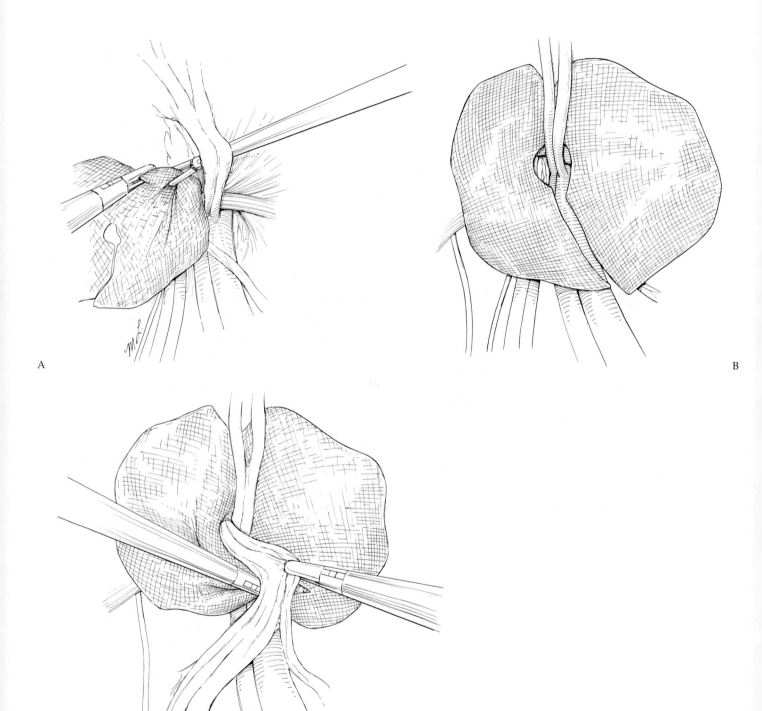

A

B

C

Fig. 45-9. **A–C:** *Placement of the mesh.*

through the valve of the trocar easier. Using the ipsilateral grasper, holding the mesh at approximately 2:00 o'clock for a right hernia or at 10:00 o'clock for a left hernia, allows the mesh to unfold with the proper orientation. It is important to keep the arm and hand in the same relative positions while advancing the mesh to prevent rotation. If the prosthesis pattern shown in Fig. 45-5 is to be used, the mesh is placed medial to the epigastric vessels and then transferred from the ipsilateral to the contralateral grasper, making sure to grasp the same spot to preserve orientation. The ipsilateral grasper then is passed behind the epigastric vessels, and the same spot is transferred back to that grasper. The mesh is pulled behind the vessels until the tail is free and the superior notch is against the epigastric vessels medially. Next, the tip of the tail is grasped by the ipsilateral grasper and the cord is held near the insertion to the internal ring by the contralateral grasper. The cord structures are pulled back out of the canal and into the midpelvis, away from the iliac vessels until the previously created window is easily visible and the tip of the tail can be laid under the cord. The prosthesis is then smoothed into place, making sure the medial inferior angle of the prosthesis is lying along Cooper's ligament. If 5-mm lateral trocars are used, the mesh must be delivered carefully and blindly through the umbilical trocar. After the mesh is within the abdomen and the laparoscope replaced, smoothing the mesh and orienting the mesh to the proper position allows identification of the proper position (10:00 or 2:00 o'clock). The mesh is then handled in an identical fashion.

The stapler is placed through the contralateral trocar. The tail of the prosthesis is stapled to the portion covering the femoral canal by precocking the stapler until the staple leg protrudes enough to snag the tail and moving it to the main portion of the patch. Only enough pressure inward is applied to the stapler to allow the other leg to snag the other side of the mesh, and the staple then is closed. This staple functions only to close the internal ring and secures mesh to mesh. Undue pressure can cause the staple to be moved laterally and injure the vein. Partial firing of the 5-mm tacker allows a similar technique, but it is important to continue the firing so that the tip of the tack is buried into the Cooper ligament or pectineus muscle. Four to six staples or tacks are placed into the mesh overlaying Cooper's ligament. These staples should be oriented at right angles to the axis of the ligament to allow better penetration of the staple legs into the ligamentous tissues. If the nature of the ligament does not allow good penetration, the staple or tack is placed just above the bony component so that it enters into the pectineus fascia. Staples are not placed too near the iliopubic tract to avoid injury to an aberrant genitofemoral nerve. Next, the mesh is smoothed out to maximum dimension laterally, and staples or tacks are placed near the edge of the mesh. Care should be taken to avoid variant nerves that may be present, and staples or tacks should not be placed below (posteriorly) the iliopubic tract to avoid injury to the femoral nerve, lateral femoral cutaneous nerve, and branches of the genitofemoral nerve. It is helpful to place the nondominant hand on the external surface of the abdominal wall to distort the muscles to create a plane at right angles to the tip of the stapler. This pressure allows equal placement of the staple legs. As a rule of thumb, no staples or tacks should be placed laterally to the ring unless the tip of the stapler is palpable. It is possible in the asthenic patient to push hard enough to entrap the ilioinguinal nerve on the other side of the internal oblique muscle or to catch the dermis, creating a dimple. It is also advisable to place the staples so that they are oriented at 90° to the axis of the iliopubic tract to avoid enclosing any nerves within the staple closure.

The medial edge of the mesh is smoothed out and stapled. As the pubic tubercle is approached, the mesh is sometimes more easily secured by placing the stapler or tacker through the ipsilateral trocar. In the event of a large direct hernia, for which the security of the mesh stapling is more critical, it is possible to place two concentric rows of staples or tacks, with the innermost being placed at or near the actual edge of the defect. It is important to watch for and avoid the variant branch of the genitofemoral inferiorly. Usually, 12 to 16 staples or tacks are used to secure the prosthesis. The peritoneum is closed by grasping the peritoneum with the ipsilateral grasper and stapling with the contralateral hand (Fig. 45-10).

Closure of the peritoneal flap is facilitated by proper placement of the original incision and by adequate dissection of the interior flap. Because of the cupped configuration formed by the pelvis and anterior abdominal wall, making the incision as cephalad as possible prevents a hanging superior flap and facilitates closure. Dissecting the posterior flap as cephalad as needed (usually about 6 cm from the internal ring) allows the peritoneum to be brought straight anteriorly without tension, even in a fully inflated abdomen. Adequate dissection of the posterior flap prevents the possibility of recurrence caused by the peritoneum being pulled through the new internal ring of mesh when the testicle goes back to its normal position.

If closing the peritoneum is difficult, lowering the intraabdominal pressure to 6 to 8 cm H_2O may allow approximation and still maintain adequate visualization and working room. Another alternative is to rotate the inferior flap laterally, using the often redundant peritoneum of the medial

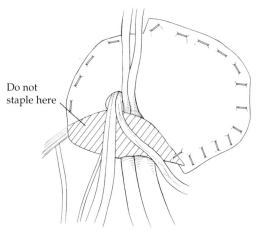

Fig. 45-10. The peritoneum is stapled and closed.

Do not staple here

umbilical fold. The technique of approximation is a point of individual preference and can be hand sewn or approximated with an automated sewing device or stapler. The technique is not as important as the security of the closure; no internal herniation should occur. If a stapler or tacker is used, partially prefiring the device until the point protrudes allows the use of the staple leg to snag the inferior flap (posterior) and carry it to the superior (anterior) edge of the peritoneum. Pressure with the other hand on the abdominal wall to distort the wall to a more vertical plane can often assist in this maneuver.

The trocars are removed, the abdominal wall defects sutured if necessary, and the skin closed with subcuticular absorbable suture. Bupivacaine is injected at the trocar sites to provide postoperative pain relief. Genital and lower abdominal wall subcu-taneous emphysema is common but absorbs rapidly. If desired, manual compression of the external genitalia to regain normal appearance may be done to avoid patient concern.

Suggested Reading

Camps J, Nguyen N, Annabali R, Fitzgibbons RJ Jr. Laparoscopic inguinal herniorrhaphy: transabdominal techniques. *Int Surg* 1995;80:18–25.

Fallas MJ, Phillips EH. Laparoscopic inguinal herniorrhaphy. *Curr Opin Gen Surg* 1994: 198–202.

Felix EL, Michas CA, Gonzalez MH Jr. Laparoscopic hernioplasty: TAPP vs TEP. *Surg Endosc* 1995;9:984–989.

Go PM. Prospective comparison studies on laparoscopic inguinal hernia repair. *Surg Endosc* 1994;8:719–720.

Nguyen N, Camps J, Filipi CJ, Fitzgibbons RJ Jr. Laparoscopic inguinal herniorrhaphy. *Ann Chir Gynaecol* 1994;83:109–116.

Phillips EH, Arregui M, Carroll BJ, et al. Incidence of complications following laparoscopic hernioplasty. *Surg Endosc* 1995;9:12–15.

Phillips EH, Rosenthal R, Fallas M, et al. Reasons for early recurrence following laparoscopic hernioplasty. *Surg Endosc* 1995;9:140–144; discussion, 144–145.

Rosser J. The anatomical basis for laparoscopic hernia repair revisited. *Surg Laparosc Endosc* 1994;4:36–44.

Seid AS, Amos E. Entrapment neuropathy in laparoscopic herniorrhaphy. *Surg Endosc* 1994;8:1050–1053.

Vogt DM, Zucker KA. The past, present and future of laparoscopic hernia repair. *Int Surg* 1994;79:280–285.

46

Laparoscopic Extraperitoneal Hernia Repair

Edward L. Felix

Interest in a laparoscopic approach to inguinal hernia repair began in 1990, shortly after the introduction of laparoscopic cholecystectomy and the rebirth of laparoscopy for general surgeons. Before this dramatic development, inguinal hernioplasty had undergone a gradual evolution over almost 100 years. In the beginning, the techniques that were developed were conventional anterior surgical approaches, such as those of E. Bassini, W. Halsted, and C. McVay. Not until the 1970s, when surgeons began to incorporate prosthetic material into their repairs to eliminate tension, was the direction of inguinal hernioplasty significantly altered. L. Nyhus, R. Stoppa, and G. Wantz applied their prosthesis to the posterior wall of the groin, developing an entirely new way of approaching the problem of inguinal hernia.

The introduction of modern laparoscopy and the development of new laparoscopic instruments and skills led surgeons to take the posterior approach to inguinal hernioplasty one step further. At first, however, they modified the posterior technique, rather than trying to duplicate the steps that had made it so successful in the first place. Because these laparoscopic surgeons failed to adequately dissect and repair the entire floor of the groin, recurrence rates of the early laparoscopic repairs were high. Once it was realized that the laparoscopic repair had to mimic the open posterior mesh repair, recurrence rates fell to less than 2%.

Initially, most laparoscopic surgeons used a transabdominal preperitoneal (TAPP) approach to reach the posterior floor of the groin. This technique was more familiar and much easier than one that required the

surgeon to laparoscopically expose the extraperitoneal space without entering the peritoneal cavity. Although the TAPP approach has been successful, a totally extraperitoneal (TEP) approach potentially offers several advantages. It might eliminate complications related to violating the peritoneal cavity to reach the extraperitoneal space, and it might reduce operative time, especially for bilateral hernia repairs.

At first, the dissection of the extraperitoneal space was difficult and sometimes confusing, but with the advent of balloon dissectors, this exposure has become quite routine. Complications related to the TAPP technique have been almost completely eliminated, operative times have been reduced, and recurrence rates kept low. There are, however, special circumstances when the TAPP approach is still preferred or when an open anterior repair will better serve the patient.

Choice of Approach

When a surgeon evaluates a patient for inguinal hernia repair, it is important that he or she be experienced in the conventional anterior approach, as well as both the TAPP and the TEP laparoscopic approaches. This allows the selection of an operation that best fits the patient's overall condition, as well as the hernia. In general, patients who are not candidates for general anesthesia should have an open anterior hernioplasty under local anesthesia. Several centers, however, have reported successful results with local or regional anesthesia for the TEP approach. Because it has been my experience that a small percentage of these patients will become anxious if carbon dioxide (CO_2) enters the

peritoneal cavity, requiring the induction of general anesthesia, I do not recommend extending the indications. Laparoscopic repair should be reserved for patients who are candidates for general anesthesia, even if a local or regional anesthetic technique is used.

An absolute contraindication to laparoscopic hernioplasty is the presence of infection. Neither the TAPP nor the TEP approach should be used in the face of local or systemic infection because of the risk of infecting the mesh.

The choice of laparoscopic approach depends on the surgeon's level of experience, the type of hernia present, and the patient's history. I favor the TEP approach for most patients because it avoids entering the peritoneal cavity. It is therefore less likely to have complications and is performed more quickly than the TAPP approach. There are, however, a few exceptions. If the patient has an incarcerated hernia, a TAPP approach is preferred. The TAPP procedure permits an accurate analysis of the contents of the hernia sac and the viability of the incarcerated structures, as well as safe and usually easy reduction of the contents. Under these circumstances, use of a balloon dissector to develop the extraperitoneal space for a TEP repair may lead to a large tear in the peritoneum or an injury to incarcerated omentum, bowel, or bladder. The TEP approach therefore should be avoided if the hernia cannot be reduced after the induction of anesthesia.

In women with abdominal pain, the etiology may be in question. If the surgeon needs to differentiate between a groin hernia and other possible causes of the patient's symptoms, such as endometriosis, the surgeon should perform a diagnostic laparoscopy and then a TAPP repair, if indicated by the findings. For women in whom the diagnosis is certain, a TEP technique is my preferred approach. The presence of a Pfannenstiel's incision is common in many of these patients because of a previous cesarean section or pelvic surgery, and this does not interfere with the TEP dissection.

Some abdominal incisions, operations, or treatments that a patient may have had previously will preclude adequate or safe dissection of the extraperitoneal space. Radical prostatectomy or pelvic irradiation will prevent the surgeon from separating the peritoneum from the abdominal wall. Balloon dissection of the extraperitoneal space may result in a large rent in the peritoneum or injury to the bladder. A lower abdominal incision crossing the rectus sheath can obstruct the safe passage of the balloon dissector. Forcing the dissector through the obstruction will tear the peritoneum and possibly injure an intraabdominal organ. A transverse incision is not a contraindication to the use of the TEP approach, but if resistance is experienced on passing of the dissector, the procedure should be converted to a TAPP approach. A lower abdominal midline incision is usually not a problem when the TEP approach is used. The dissector slides to the pubis parallel to the old incision. The midline peritoneum will separate from the abdominal wall when the balloon is inflated or can be dissected manually after the trocars are placed. If bilateral repairs are planned, however, there is a small chance that a previous midline incision may hinder the surgeon's ability to dissect the opposite side at the same sitting, and this should be discussed with the patient preoperatively.

Recurrent hernias are ideally suited for laparoscopic repair. The unobstructed view of the virgin posterior wall allows complete identification of the sites of recurrence and complete repair of the entire posterior floor. The decision as to which approach to use—the TAPP or the TEP—depends on the surgeon's expertise. The dissection of the recurrent indirect sac can be difficult using the TEP technique and requires more skill than in a primary hernioplasty. With experience, however, the difference in difficulty disappears and allows the surgeon to choose which hernioplasty he or she will use based on other factors.

Large scrotal hernias are similar to recurrent hernias in that the dissection of the indirect sac can be quite difficult via the TEP route. To avoid problems, surgeons should use the TAPP approach until they have mastered some of the special maneuvers required to deal with the long scrotal sac.

The age of a patient should influence the type of hernioplasty chosen. In general, laparoscopic hernioplasty is reserved for adults. In a few cases, a minor may be fully mature and have a truly adult-type hernia or even a recurrent hernia. Under these circumstances, the laparoscopic approach may be elected. At the other extreme are patients over 70 years of age. Some surgeons have suggested that laparoscopic repairs be limited to working younger adults. It is my experience, however, that patients of all ages benefit from the laparoscopic approach. More than 200 patients over the age of 70 years have had a successful laparoscopic hernioplasty in our center over a 5-year period. Their rapid recovery and median return to normal activity of 5 days testify to the value of laparoscopic repair for older patients. I therefore do not restrict the laparoscopic approach by age, but rather by the other criteria already discussed.

Preoperative Preparation

A full history and physical examination are essential in every patient to rule out medical problems that might preclude the laparoscopic approach or favor one laparoscopic technique over another. Before the operation, each patient should be informed of the possibility that the TEP approach might be converted to a TAPP or open repair. In addition, it is important to go over the major and minor complications that are seen with the different hernioplasties. If patients are prepared for the possible sequelae of the repair, they will be better able to deal with them. This is especially true of minor problems, such as seromas, CO_2 in the scrotum, transient neuralgia, and hematomas.

Patients should receive one dose of a prophylactic antibiotic, usually a first-generation cephalosporin, just before going into the operating room. All patients should void to completely empty their bladder immediately before the procedure to avoid the need for an indwelling catheter.

Anesthesia

For the TEP laparoscopic hernioplasty, general anesthesia is preferred for most patients. In a few instances, regional or even local anesthesia is possible with a well experienced anesthesiologist and surgeon, but they must be prepared to convert to general anesthesia if CO_2 enters the peritoneal cavity, causing the patient to become anxious. Because of the low CO_2 pressures used and the limited space present in thin or muscular patients, complete relaxation of the abdominal rectus muscles is important. Under general anesthesia, if the abdominal wall begins to regain its tone, the surgeon will become aware of it before any of the anesthesiologist's monitors become alerted. If the operative field begins to collapse, the anesthesiologist should deepen the level of relaxation to increase the available visual space.

At the end of the procedure, anesthesia should be reversed in a manner that avoids bucking on the endotracheal tube and placing a tremendous strain on the posterior floor of the groin. In our center, use of a laryngeal mask airway has markedly improved on the reversal procedure. It eliminates the endotracheal tube and its irritation. The anesthesiologist maintains control of the airway, but the postoperative sore throat and irritation are eliminated, as well as the abdominal crunches so often seen with reversal of the endotracheal anesthetic.

Operating Room and Patient Setup

The monitor and video equipment should be placed at the foot of the operating bed in the midline or slightly to the side of the hernia. The surgeon stands opposite the hernia. If there are bilateral hernias, the surgeon should start by standing opposite the larger or more complicated side and reverse sides when the second repair is begun. Usually, the scrub nurse stands on the side of the hernia and holds the camera, as well as passing instruments. The Mayo stand should be placed over the legs so that both the surgeon and the nurse can handle the instruments. It is important for both arms of the patient to be draped at the side to allow enough room for the surgeon and nurse assistant to work comfortably. The operating table can be flat or in a slight head-down position. A steep Trendelenburg position is not required.

Equipment

A unipolar scissors and a bipolar coagulator should be set up on the field, as well as two atraumatic graspers. A reusable clip applier may be used in some cases and should be available. A suction/irrigator is only used in 10% to 20% of patients and can be set up if needed. A 6- × 6-inch (15.24- × 15.24-cm) flat sheet of polypropylene mesh will be used for each hernia, as well as a single fixation device—stapler or tacker—to anchor the mesh. Endoloops (Ethicon, Cincinnati, Ohio) are used in some patients to ligate the hernia sac or close a tear in the peritoneum. I use a 0-degree scope, but a 25- or 30-degree lens will work if the surgeon is accustomed to operating with an angled scope.

I do not open a full laparotomy tray but do use Kelly and Mayo clamps to dissect the fat and muscle at the umbilicus. A no. 11 knife blade and S-retractors facilitate this dissection. A Hasson-type blunt trocar is used at the umbilicus, and two 5-mm or a 5- and a 10-mm trocar are used for the instruments. The extraperitoneal space is dissected with a balloon dissector, but this can be done bluntly without a dissector if the surgeon is experienced and so inclined.

Operative Technique

Incision

The TEP repair begins with a skin incision just below the umbilicus that extends from the midline 1 inch (2.54 cm) laterally on the side of the dominant hernia. It is important to stay off the midline to avoid entering the peritoneal cavity, where the anterior and posterior rectus sheaths merge. The side of the dominant hernia is chosen because the balloon dissector will dissect more completely on the side of the midline on which it is placed, making this dissection simpler.

After the incision is made, the fat is carefully spread with a clamp to avoid bleeding from small vessels that would obscure identification of the anterior rectus sheath. Two S-retractors are placed in the wound and used as dissectors to expose the white fibers of the fascia. The fascia is incised with a no. 11 blade and the rectus muscle exposed. The S-retractor is placed under the muscle, the muscle elevated, the posterior sheath visualized (Fig. 46-1), and the space behind the muscle dilated with a fin-

ger. At this point, the surgeon is ready to dissect the extraperitoneal space.

Balloon Dissection of the Extraperitoneal Space

The balloon dissector has simplified the dissection of the extraperitoneal space. Dissection can be done manually, without a dissector, but may be difficult and time-consuming for the inexperienced surgeon. Because the posterior rectus sheath ends at the line of Douglas, an instrument passed on top of the sheath will automatically fall into the extraperitoneal space (Fig. 46-2). The dissector is therefore placed behind the rectus muscle with its tip on the posterior rectus sheath. Aimed slightly upward, it is gently slid on top of the sheath toward the pubis until the bone is palpated with the dissector. If resistance is encountered, the dissector should not be forced into the space because it will break into the peritoneal cavity. A second attempt to pass the instrument can be tried after dilating the space with a finger and will usually be successful. If it fails, the procedure can be converted to the TAPP approach.

Once the bone is felt, the balloon portion of the dissector can be inflated. With the laparoscope in the dissector, the progress of the dissection can be followed directly on the monitor. After a maximum of 40 com-

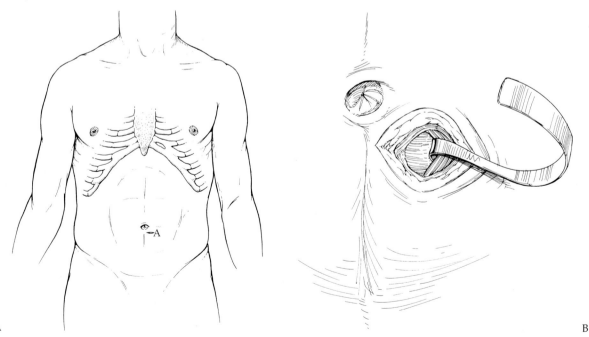

A

B

Fig. 46-1. **A:** *The initial incision is just off the midline below the umbilicus. (A, 1″ incision.)* **B:** *An S-retractor holds up the anterior rectus fascia and muscle for insertion of the balloon dissector.*

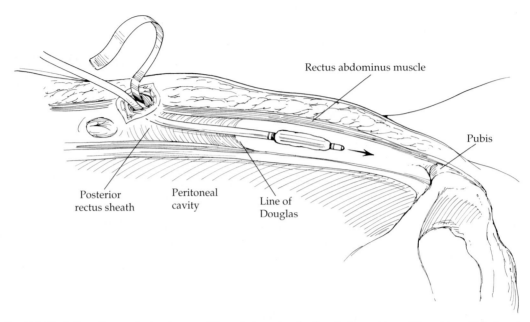

Fig. 46-2. *The balloon dissector is placed on top of the posterior rectus sheath and advanced toward the pubis until the bone is palpated.*

pressions of the bulb, the space will be adequately expanded. If the bowel is visualized during inflation of the balloon, the balloon dissection should be stopped immediately. The methods available to complete the hernioplasty laparoscopically will be discussed later (see "Intraoperative Complications"). After successful dissection of the extraperitoneal space, the balloon dissector is deflated by releasing the air valve and is then removed.

Once again, the S-retractor is placed under the rectus muscle, and the muscle is retracted upward to create a tunnel. This will ensure that when the blunt Hasson trocar is placed, it will be positioned on top of the posterior fascia and behind the muscle. Next, the Hasson trocar is positioned in the tunnel, and the extraperitoneal space is insufflated with CO_2 to a maximum of 12 mm Hg. The laparoscope is antifogged and placed in the trocar, and the dissected extraperitoneal space is examined.

The surgeon will be looking down the rectus tunnel, which opens into the dissected extraperitoneal space. If the tunnel is very short, it will not interfere with placement of the other midline trocars or with the exposure, but if it is very long, the available space will be limited and vision impaired. If the tunnel is long, a special Hasson trocar equipped with a balloon can be used to retract the posterior fascia. This opens up the exposure, facilitating the procedure.

Trocar Placement

I prefer a midline configuration for the trocars. A 10-mm Hasson trocar is placed just below the umbilicus for the camera, a 5- or 10-mm trocar in the middle, and a 5-mm trocar above the pubis. The upper instrument trocar should be as close to the subumbilical camera trocar as possible to leave space between the lowest trocar and the pubis. The inferior trocar is positioned approximately three fingerbreadths below the middle trocar, which is enough space between trocars to prevent instrument sword-fighting and still have the lowest trocar above the level of the mesh (Fig. 46-3). The penetration of both instrument trocars should be watched carefully to prevent lacerating a branch of the inferior epigastric vessel or overpenetration into the peritoneal cavity. The trocars will also need to be anchored at the skin level to prevent them from slipping in and out during instrument manipulation.

Dissection of the Posterior Floor

Dissection of the posterior aspect of the abdominal wall begins by sweeping off any tissue remaining on the pubis to expose Cooper's ligament. If a direct hernia is present, it should be completely reduced at this point. This can usually be accomplished with gentle traction on the peritoneal attachments to the defect (Fig. 46-4).

The peritoneum will peel away from the transversalis fascia, allowing the fascia to balloon into the direct hole. On a few occasions, the direct hernia will not be completely reduced by the balloon dissector, and gentle traction fails to reduce it. If this happens, the fascial defect can be incised on the superior aspect to release the incarcerated hernia. After the direct sac is reduced, it should not be ligated because the bladder may constitute the medial aspect of the sac and ligation will result in a bladder injury.

After dissection of the direct floor, the femoral area should be examined. The iliac vein will be visible just lateral to Cooper's ligament, unless there is an incarcerated femoral hernia. In this situation, the vein is under the incarcerated hernia. The surgeon must carefully reduce the hernia, taking care not to tear the small vessels present in the canal. If the hernia is stuck in the canal, an incision in the medial superior edge of the femoral ring should release the hernia (Fig. 46-5).

The dissection of the lateral floor begins with identification of the inferior epigastric vessels. The loose connective tissue and fat are swept off the posterior abdominal wall just lateral to the vessels until the peritoneum is identified (Fig. 46-6). If there is a lipoma of the cord in the canal, it will be lateral to the peritoneum and covering it. The lipoma should be pulled out of the internal ring and left in the retroperi-

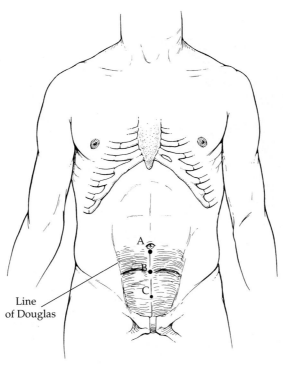

Fig. 46-3. *The second trocar is positioned at approximately the line of Douglas, and the third trocar is positioned three fingerbreadths below. (A, 10-mm Hasson (camera); B, 5 or 10 mm; C, 5 mm.)*

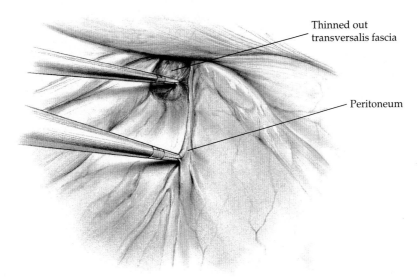

Fig. 46-4. *A direct sac is reduced by gentle traction on the peritoneum with counter traction on the transversalis fascia.*

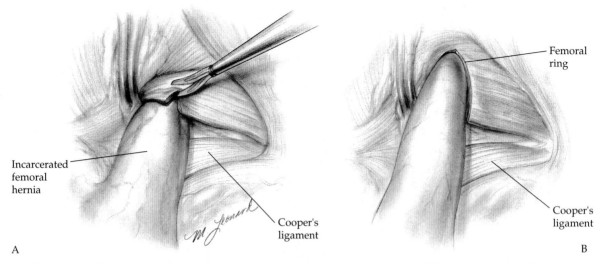

Fig. 46-5. **A,B:** *If an incarcerated femoral hernia cannot be reduced, an incision in the supermedial aspect of the ring will release the contents.*

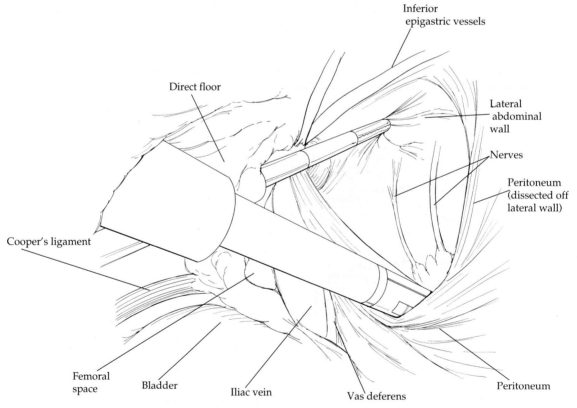

Fig. 46-6. *The dissection of the lateral floor is begun by dissecting the fat off the abdominal wall just lateral to the inferior epigastric vessels.*

toneum behind the operative field. The lateral femoral cutaneous and femoral branch of the genitofemoral nerve lie directly under the lipoma, and therefore cautery should be avoided in this part of the dissection (Fig. 46-7).

As the dissection is carried downward, the peritoneum will be identified. If there is no indirect hernia, the peritoneal edge will be found, set back from the internal ring. The edge of the peritoneum is grasped with an atraumatic grasper and lifted off the testicular vessels. It should be pulled as far cephalad as possible, so that the mesh that will be placed over the posterior floor will be covered by the peritoneum when the CO_2 is evacuated. The peritoneum must also be dissected off the vas deferens, as originally described by Stoppa in the open posterior repair, to prevent the peritoneum from lifting the mesh on the medial aspect.

If there is an indirect hernia, the peritoneal sac will be encountered anterior and lateral to the cord structures as the tissue is dissected off the lateral abdominal wall. A short or small sac can easily be delivered out of the internal ring on the anterior sur-

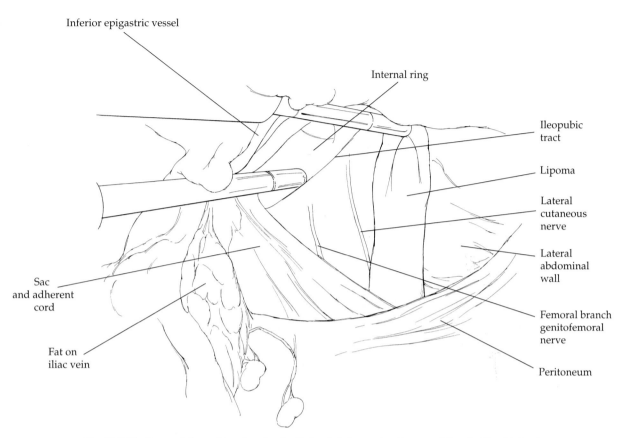

Inferior epigastric vessel

Internal ring

Ileopubic tract

Lipoma

Lateral cutaneous nerve

Lateral abdominal wall

Femoral branch genitofemoral nerve

Peritoneum

Sac and adherent cord

Fat on iliac vein

Fig. 46-7. The lipoma of the cord is reduced and pulled cephalad, exposing the nerves below the iliopubic tract.

face of the testicular vessels and vas deferens. Using a two-handed, hand-over-hand technique the entire sac can be dissected back until an adequate area is achieved for the placement of the mesh. It is essential that the peritoneum is cephalad to the inferior edge of the mesh, as described above. If the peritoneum or any of its filamentous attachments to the canal are left under the peritoneum, the door is left open for an early recurrence (Fig. 46-8).

When the indirect sac is very long, descending deep into the scrotum, the dissection of the entire sac may be difficult and traumatic. If the progress of the dissection is too slow or difficult, the superolateral edge of the peritoneum can be opened. From this point, the rest of the sac can be safely transected, if the surgeon remembers that the testicular vessels and the vas deferens are sometimes quite adherent to the under surface of the peritoneum. The vas deferens will be on the medial and the testicular vessels on the lat-

eral side. To avoid injury, both structures must be identified before the inferior peritoneal surface is cut (Fig. 46-9).

Once the proximal sac is completely separated from the distal sac, it is dissected off the cord structures and ligated with an Endoloop. An alternate technique is to circumferentially dissect the sac and pass a ligature around it. Care must be taken not to include any of the elements of the cord and to reduce the peritoneal contents before tying of the suture. In general, I believe the first technique is safer and less likely to cause complications; however, it does allow CO_2 to escape into the peritoneal cavity.

If the intraperitoneal CO_2 causes the peritoneum to balloon into the operative field, obscuring the exposure, a Veress needle or intraperitoneal trocar can be used to release the gas. Usually, however, this is unnecessary, and the surgeon only needs to dissect the peritoneum further back to hold it out of the field of vision. Some-

times, it is better to wait until the mesh is in place before ligating the indirect sac, thus leaving the peritoneal pressure in equilibrium with the extraperitoneal space. At the end of the procedure, the indirect sac and any other tears in the peritoneum must be closed to prevent an internal hernia or adhesions to the mesh. If a small hole is made in the peritoneum during dissection, it should be marked with a clip so that it can be found and completely ligated later in the procedure. If the surgeon sees quivering of the peritoneal surface during dissection, this means that CO_2 has entered the peritoneal cavity. The hole needs to be identified, clipped, and later ligated with an Endoloop.

It is important to remember that one cannot tell whether there is an indirect component to a hernia until the lateral dissection is completed. Unlike the TAPP approach, in which an indirect hernia is immediately obvious, the indirect sac cannot be identified in the TEP approach until

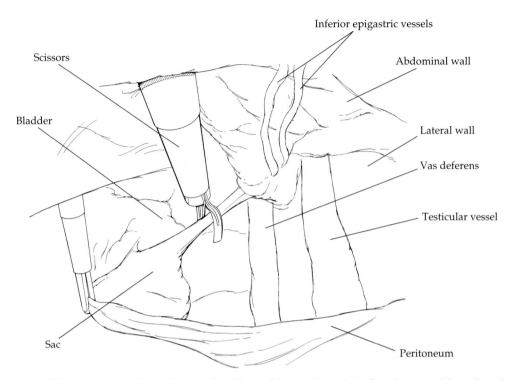

Fig. 46-8. *The peritoneal sac is dissected completely off the vas deferens and vessels to allow placement of the mesh patch.*

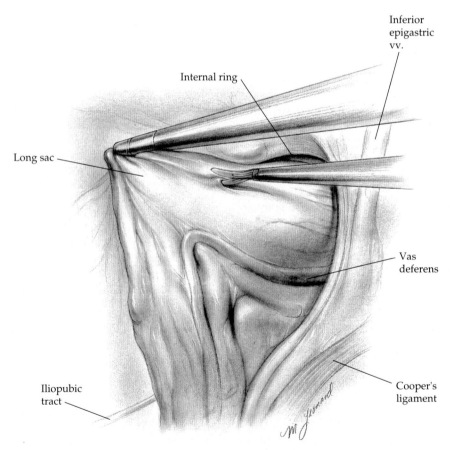

Fig. 46-9. *When the sac cannot be easily reduced, it is transected and dissected off the cord structures.*

it is dissected. The entire posterior floor needs to be dissected in every patient (Fig. 46-10). Even when there is an obvious direct or femoral hernia, up to 30% of patients will have an indirect component that must be uncovered.

Mesh

After the dissection of all three potential hernia sites, the mesh repair is begun. A 6- × 6-inch (15.24- × 15.24-cm) sheet of polypropylene is cut to fit the pelvic floor (Fig. 46-11). The medial half is cut wider than the lateral so that it drapes over Cooper's ligament when it is placed in the pelvis. The overall shape is reminiscent of a map of Australia. To differentiate the medial from the lateral side of the mesh when it is positioned laparoscopically, a stitch should be placed at the bottom of the medial side of the mesh before it is placed in the extraperitoneal space. The stitch marker will make recognition of the proper orientation of the mesh much simpler.

Placing the polypropylene mesh in the extraperitoneal space does not require any special instruments. The mesh is grasped with a 5-mm instrument and pulled into

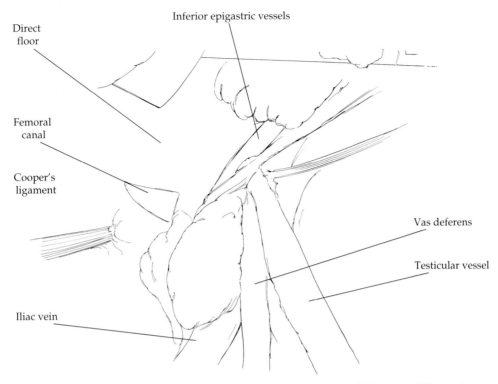

Fig. 46-10. The completed dissection of the posterior wall of the groin exposes all three potential hernia sites.

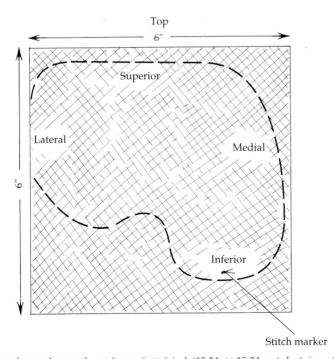

Fig. 46-11. The polypropylene mesh, cut from a 6- × 6-inch (15.24- × 15.24-cm) sheet, is made large enough to cover the entire floor of the groin.

the extraperitoneal space through the 10-mm port. If two 5-mm ports are being used in the setup, the laparoscope is removed and the mesh brought in through the camera port. The laparoscope is replaced, and the mesh is gently pushed into the pelvis with the scope. Once the mesh is fully in the extraperitoneal compartment, it is rotated using two graspers until the marking stitch is in place below Cooper's ligament. Using a two-handed technique, the smaller end of the mesh is placed over the indirect area and the larger end over the direct and femoral areas (Fig. 46-12). The mesh must cover all three potential hernia sites in every patient. When the mesh is smoothed out, it overlaps the pubic bone and crosses the midline. If the patient has bilateral hernias, the mesh from each side will overlap. It is important to examine the mesh carefully to eliminate any wrinkles or folds before it is anchored in place. It is also essential to note the location of the inferior epigastric vessels and the iliopubic

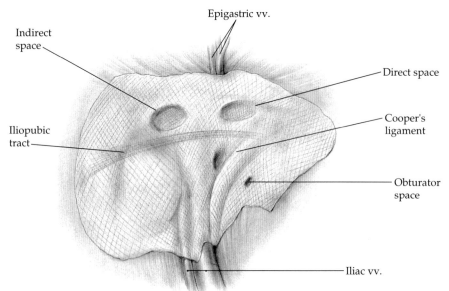

Fig. 46-12. *The polypropylene mesh covers the entire floor of the groin, with the wider half placed over Cooper's ligament.*

Anchoring the Mesh

Fixing the polypropylene mesh to the posterior abdominal wall ensures that it will be in the same position where the surgeon first placed it long after the operation. Some surgical groups have suggested that stabilizing the mesh with staples or other fixation devices is unnecessary because of the risk of nerve entrapment. This approach seems totally unreasonable because nerve injury can be avoided by the proper placement of the staples and one of the main causes of failure of laparoscopic repairs has been shown to be inadequate mesh fixation with migration of the mesh. If the surgeon understands that the nerves at risk for injury are below the iliopubic tract, injury or entrapment of the genitofemoral, lateral femoral cutaneous, or femoral nerve can be avoided by placing all mesh anchors above the iliopubic tract.

The iliopubic tract is recognized as a white fibrous band running transversely at the lower edge of the internal ring. In some patients, it is quite prominent and obvious, while in others it is subtle and barely visible. The location is confirmed by placing one hand on the abdominal wall and the other hand holding a laparoscopic grasper. The grasper is pressed against the wall, and the tip felt with the opposite hand. If the surgeon cannot feel the instrument, it is below the iliopubic tract and in an area where the nerves are at risk for injury. This same maneuver is performed when staples or fixation tacks are being placed. No anchors should be inserted into the mesh and the posterior wall unless the anchoring device can be felt with the opposite hand. In addition, using the oppo-

tract, as well as any aberrant obturator vessels, to prevent complications when the mesh is fixed to the wall.

As discussed earlier, the peritoneum and any lipomas of the cord must be well behind the inferior edge of the mesh before the mesh is fixed in place. If these elements are still under the mesh after it is properly positioned, they should be dissected back until they are comfortably superior to the mesh. In some patients, a large sac or lipoma can be placed on top of the mesh after the mesh is anchored and before the CO_2 is evacuated. Alternatively, if the mesh appears to be too large, a portion of it can be cut away with endo scissors and removed through one of the ports. This prevents the peritoneum from being lifted by the peritoneal edge when the CO_2 is released.

Occasionally, the mesh placed over the posterior floor will be too small to adequately cover it because of the unusually large size of the patient or the hernias. When this happens, a second piece of polypropylene can be added in a patchwork fashion to complete the repair. When there is a very large direct hernia, I do not hesitate to add an additional mesh running in a longitudinal direction extending well above the defect and below the pubic bone. This can also be done to add coverage to a large femoral hernia.

In a small number of patients, the testicular vessels will not lie comfortably against the pelvic floor. Instead, they seem to run across the extraperitoneal space like a

clothes line, suspending the mesh above the floor. This is more common in very thin patients or those with recurrent hernias. In these situations, to prevent a recurrence under the mesh into the internal ring, I use a double buttress repair as originally described for the TAPP hernioplasty. In this technique, a smaller 2.5- × 4-inch (6.35- × 10.16-cm) mesh with a slit in the lower third for the cord is used to secure the indirect defect. The slit is placed around the cord and reapproximated over Cooper's ligament (Fig. 46-13). A second mesh exactly like that previously described for the single-layer repair is placed over this smaller one. The second mesh prevents recurrence through the slit and completes the repair of the direct and femoral areas.

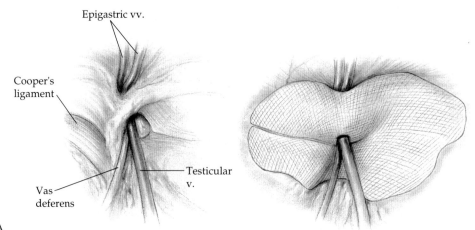

Fig. 46-13. **A,B:** *When the cord structures appear to suspend the mesh off the pelvic floor, an initial mesh is slit to accommodate the cord.*

site hand on the abdominal wall, a more perpendicular angle is created for the stapler, which improves its reliability. When pressing against the wall, however, the surgeon should not press so hard as to force the staple deeply into the wall, possibly injuring a more superficial nerve such as the ilioinguinal nerve.

The first anchors are placed through the mesh into Cooper's ligament. This stabilizes the mesh and allows the surgeon to fan the mesh out in a lateral direction, taking out any wrinkles or folds. The next staples or tacks are placed into the mesh and the transversalis fascia medial to the inferior epigastric vessels. The mesh is again smoothed out in a lateral direction, with care taken that the peritoneum and lipoma of the cord are well back of the edge of the mesh. Before the lateral fixation is completed, the mesh can be trimmed or further dissection of the sac or lipoma performed as described earlier. The lateral anchors are inserted using the bimanual technique to prevent any damage to the neural structures below the iliopubic tract (Fig. 46-14). The final mesh anchor is placed into Cooper's ligament just medial to the iliac vein. Its purpose is to remove any slack in the mesh that would otherwise allow a recurrence from under the polypropylene patch. It is mandatory to feel the pubic

bone when placing this final fixation to avoid inadvertent laceration of the iliac vessels. If aberrant obturator vessels are present coursing over the pubis, they must be avoided or serious bleeding will result.

There is no minimum number of staples or tacks that should be used to hold the mesh in place. Their purpose is not to give strength to the repair but rather to hold the mesh smoothly against the posterior wall until the body's own inflammatory response takes over in a few days. The surgeon, however, should resist placing many unnecessary anchors, especially in the lateral mesh. When the mesh is completely stabilized, the extraperitoneal space is examined for possible bleeding and, if necessary, irrigated to clear any residual blood.

Wound Closure

Closing the 10-mm trocar sites is essential to prevent the development of incisional hernias. The middle trocar is removed, and the incision closed under direct vision. Usually, a simple figure-of-eight 2-0 suture on a CT will do the job. No special closure devices are needed, as in the TAPP approach, for the lateral trocar sites. After the trocar incision is sutured, the extraperitoneal space is reinsufflated with CO_2. The position of the mesh is evaluated, and the CO_2

is slowly evacuated through the remaining 5-mm port. The peritoneum should come to rest on top of the mesh, holding it in place. If the peritoneum lifts the polypropylene patch, further manipulation can be performed using the lower port until the mesh is properly covered by the peritoneum. The 5-mm trocar is removed and closed. The camera port is closed after evacuating any CO_2 trapped in the peritoneal cavity. This can be done by holding up the abdominal wall with a clamp on the fascia and puncturing the posterior fascia and peritoneum with an intercatheter needle. The sharp needle is removed, leaving the plastic catheter to evacuate the CO_2. Once the abdominal cavity is deflated, the anterior rectus sheath is sutured closed. Bupivacaine is injected at each of the incisions to aid in early pain control.

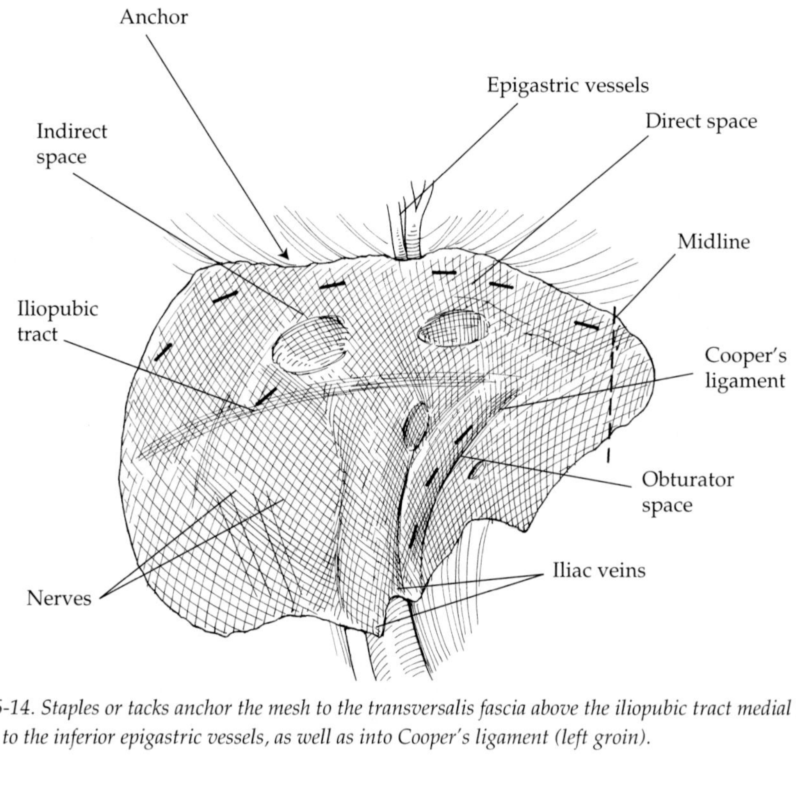

Intraoperative Complications

Three complications of balloon dissection that may cause problems for the surgeon early in the procedure are take-down of the inferior epigastric vessels, bleeding, and tearing of the peritoneum.

Any of the different-shaped balloons can lift the inferior epigastric vessels off the posterior abdominal wall, but balloons that fan out laterally are more likely to cause the problem. If the vessels are off the wall, they will interfere with further dissection. They should be ligated with clips or Endoloops or cauterized with bipolar current before further dissection of the floor.

Bleeding results when small vessels are torn from the inferior epigastrics or from the pelvic vessels. If this happens, it is only a matter of locating the bleeding site to control it with cautery or clips. Irrigation is needed if the bleeding has been brisk.

Tears in the peritoneum are the most difficult problem to handle. By avoidance of the TEP approach in patients with an incarcerated hernia, a history of pelvic irradiation, or radical prostatectomy, the incidence of significant peritoneal tears is very low. When tears do occur, the surgeon can switch to a TAPP approach or proceed with the TEP technique, making sure to close the rent at the end of the procedure. A series of Endoloops is usually sufficient and much easier than suturing a defect in the peritoneum.

Fig. 46-14. Staples or tacks anchor the mesh to the transversalis fascia above the iliopubic tract medial and lateral to the inferior epigastric vessels, as well as into Cooper's ligament (left groin).

Complications

Unfortunately, complications occur with every hernioplasty technique, but some are peculiar to the laparoscopic approach. Seromas are the most common problem but usually resolve spontaneously or with aspiration. Injuries to the femoral branch of the genitofemoral nerve, the lateral femoral cutaneous nerve, and the femoral nerve are more serious complications of the laparoscopic approach. These complications, however, can be avoided in all but rare instances if the proper techniques of anchoring the mesh are followed, staying above the iliopubic tract.

Small bowel obstruction has been reported by several authors after the TAPP approach, but only once after a TEP repair. The key to preventing this complication is the repair of all tears or holes in the peritoneum created during the operation.

Recurrence after laparoscopic hernioplasty is rare when the techniques used follow the principles outlined in this chapter. The effectiveness of the TEP repair has been demonstrated by our hernia center, as well as McKernan and Laws (1993) and others. If the surgeon, however, is not meticulous in the dissection and repair of the entire posterior floor in every patient, early recurrence of the hernia will be more common.

Bleeding during dissection of the posterior wall is usually minor and will stop spontaneously. If it does not stop, careful isolation of the bleeding point and coagulation or clipping of the individual bleeder is indicated. Mass coagulation must be avoided to prevent inadvertent injury to the cord structures or groin nerves. Severe hemorrhage can develop from dissection around the iliac vein. If bleeding develops from a tear in a small branch of the vein or the vein itself, it must be controlled promptly and CO_2 embolus prevented by compression of the bleeding site. Open exploration will be required if the surgeon cannot rapidly gain control laparoscopically.

Postoperative Care

Activity following the TEP laparoscopic repair is not restricted. Patients are told to resume all activities and work as soon as they feel able. The average return to normal activity is less than 1 week. Return to work depends on patient motivation and varies from 1 to 2 weeks. To avoid anxiety in patients, they should be forewarned about the possibility of CO_2 trapped in the scrotum, seroma formation, and discoloration of the scrotum and penis developing a few days after the operation. Wearing supportive underwear and use of antiinflammatory drugs are extremely helpful in alleviating early postoperative discomfort. If a seroma develops, usually reassurance and time are all that is needed. When patients are symptomatic or the fluid collection is large, aspiration is indicated. There does not appear to be an association between seroma formation and later development of a hydrocele, which is seen in approximately 0.5% of hernioplasties.

Results

My experience with laparoscopic approaches to inguinal hernia repair began with a TAPP technique. After performing over 500 TAPP hernia repairs, colleagues and I embarked on a study of the TEP approach. Over a 24-month period, 625 hernia repairs in 450 patients were performed, utilizing a TEP approach. With a median follow-up of 1 year, there were two recurrences. Both recurrences were the result of technical errors and became apparent within the first 6 months of follow-up. There were no deaths or other major complications such as a bowel obstruction, permanent neuralgia, bowel injury, bleeding requiring transfusion, or trocar hernia. This lack of serious complications may be due in part to the TEP technique itself and in part to previous extensive experience with a TAPP approach.

These early results are extremely encouraging. Stoppa found that recurrences after a posterior approach rarely appear after the first year of follow-up. It is our opinion that the long-term success of the TEP laparoscopic approach should mirror Stoppa's, since the TEP laparoscopic technique is based on his original repair. Continued follow-up of these patients is required to support this conclusion.

Suggested Reading

Felix EL, Michas CA, Gonzalez MH Jr. Laparoscopic hernioplasty: TAPP vs TEP. *Surg Endosc* 1995;9:984–989.

Felix EL, Michas CA, McKnight RL. Laparoscopic repair of recurrent hernias. *Surg Endosc* 1995;9:135–139.

Felix EL, Michas CA, McKnight RL. Laparoscopic herniorrhaphy: transabdominal preperitoneal floor repair. *Surg Endosc* 1994;8:100–104.

Ferzli GS, Massad A, Albert P. Extraperitoneal endoscopic inguinal hernia repair. *J Laparoendosc Surg* 1992;2:281–286.

Fitzgibbons RJ Jr, Camps J, Cornet DA, et al. Laparoscopic inguinal herniorrhaphy: results of a multicenter trial. *Ann Surg* 1995;221:3–13.

McKernan JB, Laws HL. Laparoscopic repair of inguinal hernias using a totally extraperitoneal prosthetic approach. *Surg Endosc* 1993;7:26–28.

Phillips EH, Arregui M, Carroll BJ, et al. Incidence of complications following laparoscopic hernioplasty. *Surg Endosc* 1995;9:16–21.

Stoppa RE. The treatment of complicated groin and incisional hernias. *World J Surg* 1989;13:545–554.

Tetik C, Arregui ME, Dulucq JL, et al. Complications and recurrences associated with laparoscopic repair of groin hernias: a multi-institutional retrospective analysis. *Surg Endosc* 1994;8:1316–1323.

EDITOR'S COMMENT

The laparoscopic repair of hernias has become a widely accepted option to the numerous open procedures and their myriad modifications. The author has provided insight regarding the best option for various clinical scenarios. There continue to be many surgeons who do not offer laparoscopic repairs as an option for their hernia patients. Some reasons for this include a lack of training in these techniques, poor laparoscopic skills, perceived economic disadvantages, anesthetic concerns, and personal philosophy regarding the optimal repair of hernias.

Thousands of laparoscopic hernia repairs have been reviewed and literary evidence exists that demonstrates that the laparoscopic operation can be performed with a safety profile and recurrence rate that equals or surpasses most reports of open herniorrhaphies. The experienced laparoscopist usually performs a unilateral repair in less than one hour and frequently, in less than 30 minutes. The recuperative period for the patient is usually brief and less painful than with an open approach.

Many comparisons of TAPP and TEP repairs have been presented. It is my opinion that both procedures can provide the patient with an excellent and safe repair. It is crucial to remember that the peritoneum plays no role in the strength of the repair and regardless of whether the peritoneum has been divided (TAPP) or balloon-dissected (TEP), the repair of the defect occurs at the abdominal wall. The TEP repair answers many theoretical concerns about the TAPP approach and the violation of the peritoneal cavity. Most TEP proponents consider it essential to also be facile with the TAPP repair. The development of excellent balloon dissection devices has simplified this operation and led to a marked increase in the number of surgeons who routinely perform the TEP repair.

W.S.E.

47

Laparoscopic Incisional and Ventral Hernia Repair

Michael D. Holzman and Theodore N. Pappas

The term *ventral hernia* is applied to any protrusion through the anterior abdominal wall, with the exception of those in the inguinofemoral region. Ventral hernias and diastasis recti abdominis usually appear during adulthood and are frequently associated with multiple pregnancies or obesity. Diastasis recti abdominis is related to a slow separation of the medial borders of the rectus abdominis muscles, with a diffuse bulge through the attenuated central linea alba. Though cosmetically disfiguring, diastasis recti abdominis does not lead to any complications because a true hernial sac does not exist. Spontaneous ventral/epigastric hernias are more commonly associated with incarceration and resultant pain. It is recommended that these hernias be repaired, as a risk of strangulation and necrosis exists. Another "spontaneous" anterior abdominal wall defect is a spigelian hernia: the protrusion of a peritoneal sac through a congenital or acquired defect in the spigelian fascia, the aponeurosis of the transverse abdominal muscle lying lateral to the rectus muscle. Typically, diagnosing a spigelian hernia is difficult because the defect is rarely palpable, as the external oblique muscle acts as a barrier. Recent advances in laparoscopy have made this diagnosis easier in that the defect can be visualized from the peritoneal surface.

Incisional hernias are much more common than other ventral wall hernias, resulting from an abnormal protrusion of peritoneum through a separation of the edges of a musculoaponeurotic wound. The wound may be recent or old. As with

any other true hernia, bowel obstruction, incarceration, and strangulation are possible complications, and repair is recommended in acceptable-risk patients.

Laparoscopic Ventral Herniorrhaphy

Advances in laparoscopic technique, skill, and instrumentation have lead many investigators to seek new applications in this expanding field of surgery. Though not universally accepted, inguinal herniorrhaphy by a laparoscopic approach has been widely utilized in the past several years, and at least short-term follow-up has demonstrated a low morbidity and recurrence rate. The two most commonly used techniques for laparoscopic repair of inguinal hernias are the transabdominal preperitoneal and the totally extraperitoneal approaches. Ventral and incisional hernias can be repaired via a laparoscopic approach utilizing some of the groin herniorrhaphy techniques and instrumentation. Although this technique appears straightforward and simple, advanced laparoscopic skills are mandatory to ensure a safe operation and successful outcome.

Principles

The technique used for ventral hernia repairs via the laparoscope maintains many of the same principles of the open operation. The goal is to reduce the hernia sac contents and obliterate the defect either by

approximation of the native tissue or placement of prosthetic mesh.

The laparoscopic approach utilizes prosthetic mesh to buttress the musculoaponeurotic defect. The choice of material is controversial. There are several arguments for and against each material. We routinely use polypropylene mesh (Marlex, Davol Inc., Craston, RI) because of its rapid fibrinous fixation to host tissue, its cost, and its stiffness, which facilitates its proper placement. Arguments against this material are the formation of dense adhesions and the potential complication of fistula formation from adjacent bowel. Expanded polytetrafluoroethylene (Gore-Tex, WL Gore and Associates, Phoenix, AZ) can be used for this application, but its cost-to-benefit ratio is unacceptable, and it is more difficult than polypropylene to handle in the peritoneal cavity. A composite graft with polypropylene and polyglactin (Vicryl) mesh can be applied but is more expensive and still has the potential for erosion into adjacent viscera. All prosthetic materials have some degree of adhesion formation; nonabsorbable materials may be utilized at the surgeon's discretion. The technique described uses polypropylene mesh.

The prosthetic mesh is placed intraperitoneally as a large underlay graft. This technique is not new. Large underlay grafts have been used by the French (RE Stoppa and J Rives) since the mid-1970s. The essential feature of the incisional hernioplasty is the insertion of a large prosthesis behind the abdominal muscles. The prosthesis extends far beyond the borders of the musculoaponeurotic defect and is firmly held in place by intraabdominal pressure and later by fibrinous ingrowth.

Indications

The operation is most often applied to individuals with prior celiotomies with wound complications that resulted in the development of an incisional hernia. It can easily be applied to other fascial defects, such as epigastric and spigelian hernias.

Patients with large fascial defects that involve greater than 50% of the anterior wall will pose technical difficulties in port placement to allow safe dissection and repair. Likewise, defects that extend beyond the midclavicular lines leave little room for lateral port placement, rendering this a more difficult operation from a laparoscopic approach. The cephalad and caudal extents of the hernia are less important in determination as to whether or not the patient is an acceptable candidate for laparoscopic incisional/ventral hernia repair. Obviously, prior abdominal operations are not a contraindication to a laparoscopic approach. However, patients with very dense adhesions that impair visualization or prevent safe access to the peritoneal cavity should be converted to an open repair.

The operative risk of the patient should be carefully evaluated prior to the elective repair of a ventral hernia. As with all laparoscopic procedures, there is a certain degree of stress on the cardiovascular and pulmonary systems secondary to the carbon dioxide (CO_2) pneumoperitoneum. For purposes of controlling the patient's ventilatory status with regard to CO_2 absorption, it is recommended that all patients undergo general endotracheal anesthesia. If patients have severe cardiopulmonary disease, consideration of a spinal or local anesthetic and open procedure is warranted.

Many patients with incisional hernias have experienced prior wound infections and may continue to harbor pathogenic organisms. The potential for residual infection is considered when an operative approach is selected because prosthetic material will be used with the laparoscopic approach. If infection is present, other operative techniques that avoid the use of prosthetic mesh are selected.

Preoperative Patient Management

Many patients with a large ventral hernia have poor cutaneous hygiene in skin folds below the hernial mass. Patients should shower preoperatively with germicidal soap and antifungal cream should be applied to affected skin areas. Talcum powder or corn starch may be applied to help keep the skin dry.

Aggressive pulmonary toilet should be instituted preoperatively with attempts to alleviate chronic cough, which will place unnecessary strain on the hernia repair. Pulmonary function studies are indicated in patients in whom there has been "loss of domain" of the abdominal viscera. This patient population can potentially experience ventilatory insufficiency due to the increased intraabdominal pressures created by returning the viscera into a contracted peritoneal cavity. If this entity is recognized preoperatively, some surgeons have advocated a technique of progressive pneumoperitoneum over a period of weeks to distend the abdominal wall to facilitate the return of the viscera into the abdomen. The increased intraabdominal pressure also improves diaphragmatic function but also elevates the diaphragm, to which the patients readily adjust.

A history of constipation and difficulties with urination can lead to straining and increased abdominal pressures, jeopardizing the success of the repair. These conditions should be investigated and corrected, if possible, prior to an elective herniorrhaphy.

The presence of prosthetic materials always disables the normal host defense mechanisms within the wound enough to increase the risk of infection. Parenteral antibiotics should be administered when anesthesia is induced. Since no drains are left with this procedure, continuation of antibiotics postoperatively is not necessary. A first-generation cephalosporin is the agent of choice in most cases. If a previous wound infection was present and the pathogen and sensitivities are known, a preoperative course of the specific antibiotic may be administered, because patients may silently harbor the offending organism for long periods of time.

Outpatient administration of a mechanical bowel cleansing preparation may help

during the operative procedure and will help eliminate early postoperative straining from constipation.

Operative Technique

The patient is placed on the operating table in the supine position. After induction of general anesthesia, an orogastric tube is inserted to decompress the stomach, and a urinary catheter inserted to decompress the bladder. The skin is washed and coated with a solution of providoneiodine, including both flanks.

Port Placement

Port placement may be one of the most important factors that will determine the operative success of the laparoscopic repair. For obvious reasons, it is impossible to describe the placement for every incisional and ventral hernia. A thorough understanding of the principles of port placement will allow application of the laparoscopic approach to most abdominal wall defects.

Positioning of the camera port needs special consideration. One would like to place the scope parallel to the direction in which the majority of the dissection will be performed. Working opposite the scope can be confusing and will increase the difficulty and time required for dissection and placement of the prosthetic material. Whenever possible, it is advantageous to place the scope/camera port in the midline to permit dissection and stapling from either side of the operating table. Ideally, this port is placed inferiorly so that the costal margin does not inhibit scope mobility. Avoiding previous sites of incisions permits easier access to the peritoneal cavity. The scope port needs to be placed at least 6 cm from the closest margin of the fascial defect to allow complete visualization of the defect and enough space to secure the mesh to healthy musculoaponeurotic tissue. Though the scope can be moved to other ports during dissection and mesh placement, minimizing these changes will expedite the procedure. An open placement (Hasson technique) of the scope port is utilized, since the majority of patients with anterior abdominal wall hernias have had previous abdominal operations. Once the peritoneal cavity has been entered, a finger is inserted and swept circumferentially around the anterior abdominal wall to ensure a space free of adhesions and safe access for the scope. Stay sutures are placed on either side of the fascial incision, and a blunt-tipped (Hasson type) port (12-mm diameter) is inserted and secured.

The abdominal cavity is insufflated with CO_2 to a pressure of 15 mm Hg. The scope is inserted, and the peritoneal cavity is visually explored. Though not absolutely necessary, a 30-degree scope may aid in visualization of the anterior abdominal wall and around adhesions. This scope also allows the surgeon to operate parallel to the direction of the scope.

At least 2–3 other ports will be necessary for a safe and efficient operation. On the surgeon's side, 5-mm and/or 12-mm ports are needed. These ports should be positioned so that the surgeon can comfortably operate through both ports during the dissection of adhesions and identification of the fascial defect. Ports need to be lateral enough from the fascial defect to allow room for dissection, yet not so far lateral that the range of motion of the instruments is inhibited by the operating table. Similarly, port placement in the inguinal region is inhibited by the legs and in the hypogastric region by the costal margins, making dissection of the anterior abdominal wall difficult. For this reason, the majority of operating ports are placed in the flanks at the level of the anterior axillary line for midline hernias. This location also avoids complications of vascular injuries to the epigastric vessels, which typically have been displaced laterally due to the hernia. Another matter that needs to be considered is the length of the instruments and their ability to reach the far extent of the defect during dissection and mesh placement.

Typically, the 5-mm port is placed between the scope port and the 12-mm port. This allows the greatest leeway for switching of the camera and the stapler, if necessary, during tacking of the mesh. Initial port placement for the operating instruments might be determined by what area of the abdominal wall is free of adhesions to allow safe trocar insertion. Once an instrument port is inserted, areas can be cleared for safe insertion of the other trocars. The fourth port is a 12-mm port and is typically placed opposite the 12-mm port in the contralateral flank (Fig. 47-1). Alternatively, 12-mm ports may be used at all locations to provide complete versatility with regard to placement of the stapler.

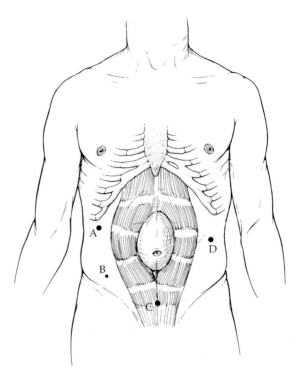

Fig. 47-1. Port placement is demonstrated for a moderate-size ventral hernia in the midline. The scope is placed via a 10- to 12-mm Hasson port inserted under direct vision, ideally in the midline. The operating ports are placed preferably in the flanks far enough away from the fascial defect to allow space for dissection, yet close enough to allow the instruments to reach the contralateral side of the hernia. A 12-mm port will be necessary on both sides of the defect to allow staple fixation of the mesh. Five-millimeter ports are added as needed to aid in dissection and mesh positioning. (A, 5/12 mm [grasper]; B, 5 mm [scissors]; C, 5/12 mm [scope]; D, 5/12 mm [grasper].)

Alternatively, a 5-mm tacker can be used instead of the 12-mm stapler, along with a 5-mm scope. This allows all secondary ports to be 5 mm. The initial port should remain 10/12 mm for safe open technique placement and to allow insertion of the mesh.

Dissection of Adhesions and Identification of Hernia

The pneumoperitoneum stretches the abdominal wall and suspends intraabdominal adhesions, facilitating the dissection and helping return the viscera to the abdomen. Using atraumatic graspers, countertraction is applied to adherent pieces of bowel and omentum. The dissection is carried out in the same plane as in open herniorrhaphy. The majority of these adhesions are filmy and avascular. Sharp dissection with scissors is initiated in the area that is both easily reached and visualized. Every attempt should be made to minimize the use of electrocautery to avoid in-

juring the adjacent bowel. Many adhesions, especially those of the omentum to the anterior abdominal wall, can be taken down with gentle blunt dissection. A Kittner dissector is placed firmly against the undersurface of the anterior abdominal wall and swept side to side, freeing these adhesions.

Extreme care is taken to maintain the plane of dissection on the peritoneal surface of the anterior abdominal wall. This technique will minimize bleeding and inadvertent injury to the adherent bowel. Though not every adhesion to the anterior abdominal wall need be taken down, at least a 2-cm and preferably a 4-cm margin of clean healthy aponeurotic tissue is cleared for placement of the prosthetic mesh. In patients with incisional hernias, the entire aspect of the previous incision should be cleared to rule out a septated or "Swiss-cheese" type of defect. Excision of the hernia sac is not routinely performed despite the potential for a slightly higher incidence of seroma formation.

Mesh Placement

Several different techniques are used by surgeons in configuring and placing the prosthetic material. One can measure the defect by placing Keith needles through the abdominal wall so that just the tip is visible on the laparoscopic view. Needles are placed on both sides of the defect in the horizontal and vertical axes, permitting accurate measurement of the defect. At least 4 cm is added in each dimension to ensure that a minimum of 2-cm overlap is available for securing of the mesh to healthy aponeurotic tissue. The greater of these two distances (vertical or horizontal) is measured, and the mesh is configured as a circle. For example, if the defect is 8 × 4 cm, 4 cm (for overlap) is added to 8 cm (the larger dimension of the defect), and a sheet of mesh is configured as a 12-cm circle. Though this leaves a greater overlap in one dimension, it simplifies positioning once in the peritoneal cavity. The center of the mesh is identified and marked with a large (1 cm) dot using a marking pen.

Prior to insertion of the mesh into the peritoneal cavity, all Keith needles are withdrawn into the abdominal musculature to ensure that inadvertent bowel perforation does not occur as the pneumoperitoneum is lost during mesh insertion. If reducers are used, they are placed on the grasper prior to grasping the mesh. This maneuver allows one to insert the mesh and reinsufflate the peritoneal cavity without having to release the mesh with the grasper. The rolled mesh is grasped and inserted into the peritoneal cavity via a 12-mm port. The pneumoperitoneum is reestablished before any adjustments are made to the mesh position. At this point, the mesh can be flattened out over the underlying omentum or bowel. A Keith needle is placed in the center of the defect to help align the mesh. This Keith needle is brought through the abdominal wall. A small bite of mesh at the previously marked center is taken, and the needle is passed back out the abdominal wall at the center of the defect. The suture is pulled firmly to raise the mesh to the abdominal wall. The mesh is properly positioned when the center is tacked by a temporary suture and the remainder is circular. This approach obviates determining the orientation of the mesh if an elliptical or odd-shaped mesh had been chosen. The other Keith needles can again be advanced until they are visualized in the peritoneal cavity.

These needles at the margins of the fascial defect should penetrate the mesh with at least a 2-cm margin (Fig. 47-2).

Using two graspers, the mesh is unfurled against the anterior abdominal wall. A hernia stapler is inserted via the 12-mm port, and staples are placed approximately 1 to 2 cm apart at the edge of the mesh, starting directly across the defect on the far side from the stapler port. It is important to ensure that the staples are placed at a right angle to the abdominal wall. This sometimes requires the surgeon to place his or her fingers on the abdominal wall over the area being secured and creating a right angle with the instrument (Fig. 47-3). This also ensures that a good bite of the aponeurotic tissue is obtained. Stapling is continued circumferentially on the far side of the mesh as long as secure staples can be applied. Eventually, the stapler is placed in the 12-mm port on the opposite side,

and the circumferential stapling of the mesh is completed. If necessary, the scope can be moved to another port and the stapler placed at that site. This is the reason for a 12-mm trocar for hernia staplers or 5-mm trocar for hernia tackers.

Alternative Techniques

Some surgeons have advocated securing each of the corners or quadrants of the mesh with sutures. These are placed using a Keith needle in a manner similar to the placement of the central suture used to position the mesh. A buttonhole incision is made in the skin at a site overlying a corner of the prosthesis. The needle is brought through the abdominal wall from this buttonhole incision; a small bite of the edge of the mesh is taken, and the needle is passed back out the abdominal wall near its entry site in the buttonhole incision. The suture is secured and the knot placed deeply in the

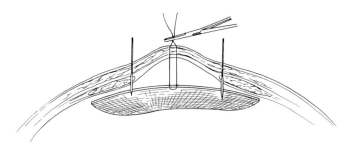

Fig. 47-2. The prosthesis is pulled up against the parietal peritoneum with a suture placed through the middle of the mesh. Keith needles on the edges of the defect allow the surgeon to assess whether the prosthesis is in place with adequate overlap for fixation.

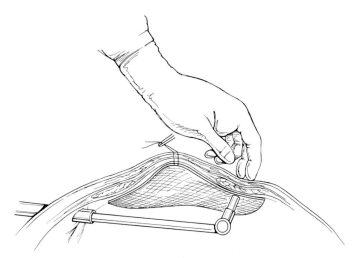

Fig. 47-3. The mesh is secured to the musculoaponeurotic tissues with the assistance of a laparoscopic hernia stapler. To ensure adequate fixation, the surgeon's hand should be placed on the anterior abdominal wall over the region of the stapler head and gently pressed downward. This will allow the staple to be seated at a right angle to the tissue and also provide a firm surface on which to seat the stapler.

buttonhole incision. These incisions are later closed with subcuticular sutures. This is repeated for all four quadrants, although some surgeons have used this technique to tack one quadrant and subsequently staple the remaining edges (Fig. 47-4).

An alternative technique is to place the suture on the mesh with long tails prior to its insertion into the peritoneal cavity. Once in place, a Grice needle can be passed into the peritoneum at the corner points, and the suture tails grasped and pulled to the anterior abdominal wall. These can be temporary, just to assist in positioning prior to stapling, or permanent if a buttonhole incision is made and two tails are pulled up at each corner within this buttonhole incision.

Another problem not infrequently encountered is a long midline incision that has several small defects with bands of fascia interspersed between them, a so-called "Swiss-cheese" type hernia. The total length of the defect may be very long with only minimal separation between the rectus muscles. These defects can be closed using the same technique described for larger single hernias, but with one or two overlapping circular pieces of prosthetic mesh. Again, this will avoid the difficulties of orienting the mesh once in the peritoneal cavity (Fig. 47-5).

Mesh Coverage

An attempt is made to drape the omentum between the mesh and the underlying bowel. If enough omentum is available, it can be tacked to the abdominal wall using the stapler. Another option is a composite graft fashioned from a nonabsorbable mesh (polypropylene) and a polyglactin absorbable mesh cut to fit and then sutured together with Vicryl suture. Other absorbable mesh materials may be used if the weave is as tight as or tighter than that of the nonabsorbable material. The nonabsorbable mesh is cut to provide a 2-cm circumferential margin on the hernia defect, and the absorbable mesh is cut with a 1-cm-larger diameter so that the former will fit completely within the dimensions of the latter (Fig. 47-6). The sutures are tied on the nonabsorbable mesh side. Knots should all be placed on the same side, as the mesh types may be indistinguishable through the laparoscope. The composite graft is then inserted into the peritoneal cavity and unfurled. It is placed over the fascial defect and secured as described above with the nonabsorbable side to the parietal peritoneum.

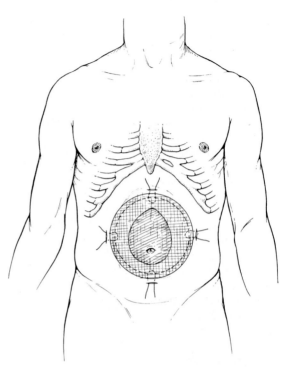

Fig. 47-4. *Buttonhole incisions are made in each quadrant of the defect at the lateral edges of the mesh. Suture is passed through these incisions: a bite from the edge of the mesh and back out the buttonhole incision. The suture is tied, securing the mesh in place.*

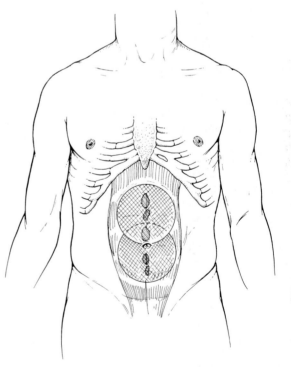

Fig. 47-5. *Multiple small fascial defects can be covered with overlapping circular pieces of mesh.*

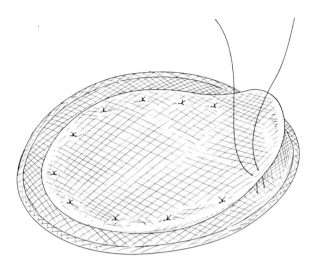

Fig. 47-6. A composite graft is created from pieces of absorbable and nonabsorbable synthetic mesh. The absorbable piece is cut at least 1 cm larger than the nonabsorbable piece. These are sutured together with absorbable sutures with the knots all on the same side. This will later help to identify the two different material surfaces. The nonabsorbable mesh is placed against the parietal peritoneum. In theory, the absorbable mesh will help diminish adhesion formation.

Closure

After the prosthetic mesh is completely secured in place, the ports are removed under direct visualization via the laparoscope. All ports larger than 5-mm require fascial closer to prevent another incisional hernia. There are several commercial devices and various techniques for port-site closure. Drains are not routinely used.

Postoperative Care

Patients are given a clear liquid diet when alert and advanced to a regular diet as tolerated. They are mobilized in the very early postoperative period and are encouraged to return to their normal activities as soon as possible. They are, however, advised to avoid unusually excessive physical effort for at least a month, until the mesh graft has been firmly incorporated. Postoperative antibiotics are not routinely necessary, and most patients can be managed on oral analgesics. Abdominal binders are not routinely used postoperatively. Binders can occasionally be applied to minimize seroma formation. Some smaller hernias are repaired on an outpatient basis, while patients with larger hernias usually spend one night in the hospital and are discharged on postoperative day 1.

Complications

Currently, there are no large published series of laparoscopic ventral or incisional herniorrhaphy. Therefore, complication rates and long-term outcomes remain unknown. Other laparoscopic procedures and conventional and laparoscopic inguinal herniorrhaphy provide the basis for the prediction of expected complication rates.

The same risks of bleeding and infection found with other minimally invasive procedures and herniorrhaphies are present when laparoscopic ventral herniorrhaphy is performed. Some surgeons have speculated that the risk of mesh infection from cutaneous pathogens is lower in the laparoscopic group due to the distance between the actual incisions and the prosthesis. This theory has yet to be proven by any clinical studies. Complications of trocar insertion are similar to those in other laparoscopic procedures. Special care should be taken to avoid the inferior epigastric vessels when the lateral ports are placed.

Complications arising from the insertion of prosthetic materials should be no different from those of an open, tension-free repair with mesh. A small but real risk exists of intestinal adhesions that could result in obstruction, strangulation, or fistula formation. This incidence in open procedures

is low, and an attempt is made to place the omentum between the intestines and the mesh.

Case reports in the literature have not discussed recurrences. Likewise, there are no published large series with follow-up from which to extrapolate some answers. Prospective, randomized studies are needed to determine the efficacy and long-term outcome of this procedure.

Suggested Reading

Barie PS, Mack CA, Thompson WA. A technique for laparoscopic repair of herniation of the anterior abdominal wall using a composite mesh prosthesis. *Am J Surg* 1995;170:62–63.

Bendavid RI, ed. *Prostheses and abdominal wall hernias.* Austin, TX: RG Landes Co, 1994.

Helfrich RB, Gianturco C. Abdominal wall hernia repair: use of the Gianturco-Helfrich-Eberbach hernia mesh. *J Laparoendosc Surg* 1995;5: 91–95.

Nyhus LM, Condon RE, eds. *Hernia,* 4th ed. Philadelphia: JB Lippincott Co, 1995.

Skandalakis JE, Gray SW, Mansberger AR, Colborn GL, Skandalakis LJ, eds. *Hernia surgical anatomy and technique.* New York: McGraw-Hill, 1993.

Wantz GE, ed. *Atlas of hernia surgery.* New York: Raven Press, 1994.

EDITOR'S COMMENT

The laparoscopic repair of ventral hernias holds great appeal when one considers the associated morbidity when using a large incision on the abdomen of most patients who are at risk for incisional hernias. Many of the comorbidities that led to the development of the incisional hernia also place the patient at an increased risk for wound infections. Infections that involve mesh prostheses is one of the most dreaded complications of hernia repair.

The authors have appropriately emphasized the importance of proper port placement. The importance of avoiding bowel injury during adhesiolysis is also worth repeating. The tips provided within the chapter regarding proper mesh placement are essential for avoiding early recurrence or incomplete coverage of the defect.

The selection of the proper prosthetic material is a difficult decision for many surgeons. Most desire tissue ingrowth yet wish to avoid adhesions between the mesh and intestines. The ability to have prosthetic materials that possess both of these characteristics while retaining optimal visibility and handling characteristics is the ideal targeted by manufacturers of these materials.

Finally, the matching of the patient to the optimal technique is the most challenging aspect of repairing ventral hernias. Rarely are these patients optimal surgical candidates and there seem to be potential negative aspects to any option chosen. The laparoscopic ventral herniorrhaphy for the proper patient can provide a safe and durable repair.

W.S.E.

VII

Chest

48

Bronchoscopy and Endoluminal Surgery

William B. Long and Allison J. Duchow

Early attempts at bronchoscopy have been described since the early 19th century. Not until incandescent lighting was available did real progress in the field occur. In the early 20th century, Chevalier Jackson founded the Philadelphia School of Bronchoesophagology, which became a general training ground for the advancement of this discipline.

In the 1980s, fiberoptic technology dramatically increased the possibilities for bronchoscopy. The flexible fiberoptic bronchoscope made the upper lobe and superior segmental bronchi accessible to biopsy, brushings, and treatment for the first time. Advances in technology derived from other endoscopy-related fields have increased the capabilities of bronchoscopy as a diagnostic and therapeutic tool.

Direct vision of the tracheobronchial tree is important for both diagnostic and therapeutic purposes. The bronchoscope allows the diagnosis of malignant and benign lesions of the tracheobronchial tree, as well as clarification of the causes of increased secretions or hemoptysis. Bronchoscopy can also be used as therapy for secretions, as well as for the removal of foreign bodies and tumors and the staunching of bleeding.

Diagnostic Bronchoscopy

Diagnostic bronchoscopy in patients with a "normal anatomic" tracheobronchial tree is quite easy, especially if the patient is under general anesthesia with mechanically controlled respirations. For sedated patients, a topical anesthetic (lidocaine hydrochloride 4%) sprayed into the hypopharynx and glottis is helpful in reducing coughing during the procedure.

Atropine sulfate (1 mg) is also helpful in reducing secretions from "salivators," which helps with airway management. The bronchoscopist should be trained to visualize every branch of the tracheobronchial tree accessible to the rigid or flexible fiberoptic bronchoscope.

Distortion of anatomy caused by pulmonary resection, radiation therapy, disease, or congenital abnormalities can make it difficult to identify anatomic structures bronchoscopically. Orientation of the bronchoscopist is facilitated by the availability of previous operative notes and imaging studies, but these are not always available.

Hemoptysis is an absolute indication for bronchoscopy to determine both its cause and its significance. Causes of endobronchial bleeding include trauma (pulmonary contusion, lobar disruption, bronchial or tracheal rupture), inflammatory diseases, infections, and neoplasms. Hemoptysis or blood in the tracheobronchial tree from trauma can be inconsequential or life-threatening. It may be the only sign of a ruptured bronchus, which is not always associated with significant air leaks. Pulmonary contusions can produce a small amount of bleeding or blood clots occluding lobar and mainstem bronchi, or they may become torrential in patients with coagulopathies.

Inflammatory diseases, infections, and neoplasms can also cause bleeding. The bronchoscopist should be prepared to identify the source of bleeding and to culture and biopsy as indicated. Granulomas or neoplasms with fresh, bright-red clots should be left alone to avoid torrential bleeding until all therapeutic resources are available to deal with the problem.

Bronchoscopic brushings and washings for cytology and culture are possible with both the rigid and the flexible fiberoptic bronchoscope. This modality has its greatest application in diagnosing segmental and subsegmental bronchial lesions and parenchymal lesions beyond the reach of a biopsy forceps. Fluoroscopy may help the bronchoscopist place the brush into bronchi distal to the peripheral lesion. Selective bronchial washing with measurement of antibody titers may help localize sites of unsuspected cancer. Earlier detection and appropriate treatment of lung cancer may improve outcomes.

Transbronchial needle biopsy via bronchoscopy is reserved for lung masses near the hilum showing no endobronchial spread (Fig. 48-1). Also available are percutaneous transthoracic needle biopsies (thin-needle aspiration) routinely performed by radiologists during computed tomography (CT) scanning. Both techniques require the skills of an experienced cytologist to interpret the aspirated specimen, and aspirates have an inherent methodologic weakness of being inconclusive 20% to 40% of the time.

Punch biopsy of endobronchial lesions is useful whenever a lesion can be reached by the bronchoscope. The bronchoscopist should be cautious and avoid biopsy of vascular lesions (e.g., arteriovenous malfunctions and carcinoids).

If the bronchoscopist suspects that an endobronchial lesion is malignant, he or she should consider its resectability based on the patient's overall health, presence of metastases, appearance of mass location on CT scan, and pulmonary function tests.

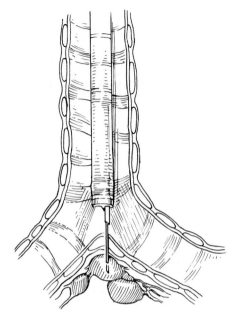

Fig. 48-1. Method of transbronchial fine-needle node biopsy.

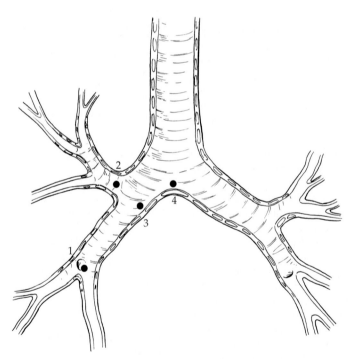

Fig. 48-2. Biopsy sites for staging an endobronchial cancer.

Endobronchial evaluation of a patient before lung resection requires a strategy for obtaining mucosal and submucosal biopsies to determine endobronchial spread (Fig. 48-2). For localized lesions of a mainstem bronchus or bronchus intermedius, which may allow a sleeve resection, the bronchoscopist should biopsy the carina of the nearest bronchus below the lesion, biopsy the lesion, and then biopsy the carina of the nearest bronchus above the lesion to determine whether endobronchial spread is present. These multiple biopsies should be done in addition to other staging procedures, such as mediastinoscopy or mediastinotomy, to determine resectability.

Therapeutic Bronchoscopy

In addition to its diagnostic uses, bronchoscopy has therapeutic functions. Among these are removal of foreign bodies, inspissated mucous, and blood clots, the control of bronchial hemorrhage, laser therapy, and stent placement.

Foreign Body Removal

Most foreign bodies aspirated into the tracheobronchial tree can be removed with the help of a bronchoscope. Foreign body aspiration should be considered in any patient with a cough, wheezing, and fever. The aspiration event may or may not have been witnessed. A chest x-ray film may show a radiopaque foreign body, lobar or lung collapse, or obstructive emphysema.

The definitive diagnosis of foreign body aspiration is made by direct visualization with a bronchoscope. Traditionally, rigid bronchoscopy has been used for retrieval. Training with this instrument is not available in the majority of training programs since the advent of the flexible bronchoscope. Flexible forceps for foreign body retrieval are now available.

Direct visualization with the bronchoscope is necessary for foreign body removal (Fig. 48-3). The forceps is passed through the operating channel of the flexible bronchoscope, and the foreign body is grasped. The scope, forceps, and foreign body are removed as a unit while the foreign body is under direct visualization at all times. Pulling the foreign body past the vocal cords can be difficult. It should be rotated to the axis of the trachea to avoid dislodgement from the forceps and subsequent damage to the vocal cords and glottis.

Radiopaque foreign bodies in the lung periphery may require both fluoroscopy and bronchoscopy. The fluoroscope is used to visualize a foreign body that may be beyond visualization with the bronchoscope. A balloon-tipped catheter (usually size 3 French [F]) can be guided fluoroscopically to the the foreign body. The balloon-tipped catheter is passed beyond the foreign body and inflated. The foreign body is then dragged into the more proximal tracheobronchial tree, where it can be grasped with forceps. The foreign body, forceps, and bronchoscope can then be brought out through the airway as a unit. This is best performed with the patient un-

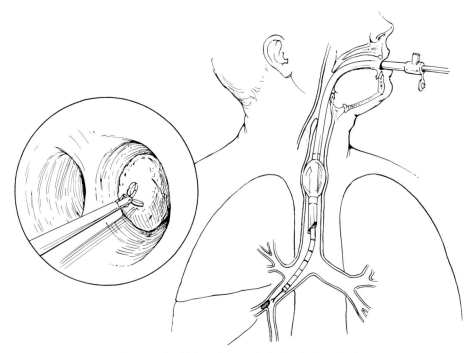

Fig. 48-3. Flexible bronchoscopy for foreign body retrieval.

der general anesthesia to allow good visualization without patient motion.

In experienced hands, these techniques have a high success rate. Removal of aspirated foreign bodies by thoracotomy should rarely be necessary.

Aspiration of Inspissated Mucus and Plugs

Patients with segmental, lobar, or pulmonary collapse may require aspiration of inspissated mucus and plugs from the tracheobronchial tree. Repeated bronchoscopy may be necessary. Flushing of involved bronchi with small amounts of normal saline has been advocated, but the bronchoscopist should be cautioned that this may push mucous plugs farther into the lung.

Control of Tracheobronchial Hemorrhage

Most pulmonary contusions cause a small amount of tracheobronchial bleeding that clears with coughing or suctioning. Hypoxemia, lobar or pulmonary collapse, or shifting segmental infiltrates should alert the physician that blood clots from pulmonary contusions may be obstructing mainstem or lobar bronchi.

Therapeutic bronchoscopy with direct visualization of the visible tracheobronchial tree enables the bronchoscopist not only to remove blood clots but also to identify the sources of bleeding. Persistent bleeding with flooding of the airways and hypoxemia may necessitate a lobectomy or pneumonectomy to save the patient's life.

Most pulmonary contusions can be managed with frequent fiberoptic aspiration bronchoscopy (sometimes every 2 hours until stable), positive end-expiratory ventilation, and correction of any coagulopathies. Should lobectomy or pneumonectomy be necessary for endobronchial bleeding, therapeutic bronchoscopy with aspiration of blood clots may be needed to clear blood from the airways of the unaffected lung despite the placement of cuffed endotracheal or bronchial tubes.

Control of Massive Hemoptysis from Trauma

Massive hemoptysis has a varying definition, ranging from several tablespoons (more than 50 mL) of blood per cough to no more than 2 cups (500 mL) of blood coughed over 24 hours. Besides trauma, the most common causes of massive hemoptysis are tuberculosis, actinomycosis, and lung carcinoma.

Regardless of etiology, a patient with massive hemoptysis needs diagnosis and treatment almost simultaneously. Small amounts of hemoptysis or aspirated blood (4 tbsp; 60 mL) can be worked up in a "routine" manner. Nonintubated patients or awake intubated patients coughing up 1 cup (250 mL) of blood or more will be frightened and hypertensive, making endobronchial bleeding worse.

The bronchoscopist should have the patient sedated, endotracheally intubated, and pharmacologically paralyzed to control the situation. An arterial catheter to monitor blood pressure may also be necessary. Continued bleeding from the endotracheal tube makes it difficult for the bronchoscopist to identify the source of bleeding.

Sometimes, the endobronchial bleeding continues vigorously despite the above measures, and the patient is in danger of drowning in blood. The bronchoscopist has several choices: (1) pushing the endotracheal tube down the mainstem bronchus opposite the source of bleeding to protect the "good" lung until thoracotomy can be performed, (2) lowering blood pressure below 100 mm Hg with afterload-reducing agents, or (3) using Gorsach's technique of placing a balloon-tipped catheter down the bronchoscope (flexible or rigid) to occlude the lobar or segmental bronchus draining the blood (Fig. 48-4).

All these endoscopic techniques for massive hemoptysis provide time for the surgeon to perform thoracotomy before the patient exsanguinates or drowns.

Laser Destruction of Endobronchial Tumors

Laser destruction via rigid or flexible bronchoscopy is most commonly used for benign endobronchial lesions, unresectable malignant lung tumors, or tracheal stenosis. Regardless of the indication, the best results are achieved in truly endobronchial lesions. When the tumor is extrinsic or below the submucosal layer, treatment is more risky (bleeding or perforation), and results are not as good.

In benign tumors, laser destruction is usually for the purpose of cure and may require repetitive treatments. Concomitant treatments, such as stent placement or dilation, are often necessary for both benign and malignant strictures. In malignant lesions, treatment is usually for purpose of

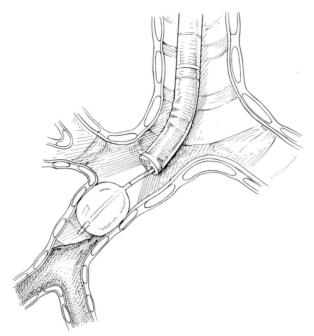

Fig. 48-4. Bronchoscopic balloon tamponade for control of acute pulmonary bleeding.

For malignant lesions, the mass is initially coagulated at low power with long pulse times, allowing more tissue destruction and hemostasis of the tumor surface. The bulk of the tumor is destroyed at higher power settings. The remnants of a destroyed tumor are removed with forceps, and final hemostasis is achieved with laser coagulation of the airway wall at lower powers. Tumor destruction should not be pursued beyond the tracheal or bronchial cartilage. This can lead to massive hemorrhage or collapse of the airway, requiring stent placement to maintain airway patency.

Usually, general anesthesia is employed. Anesthesia can be administered through a ventilating rigid bronchoscope or an endotracheal tube through which a fiberoptic bronchoscope is passed. Jet ventilation may be necessary to maintain adequate oxygen saturation in some circumstances (Fig 48-5).

More recently, the potassium titanyl phosphate (KTP) laser has been employed in pediatrics because its fibers can be passed through very small flexible bronchoscopes. The laser fiber is passed down the suction port of the bronchoscope. It can be used in a contact or noncontact manner. The laser delivers 3 to 5 W of power in a pulse or continuous mode. The KTP laser can cut, coagulate, or vaporize and is preferentially ab-

palliation and rarely cure. Cure is generally only possible in endobronchial cancers limited to the mucosa and submucosa.

Diathermic or electrocautery destruction of tumors is also an option. This was the preferred method of endobronchial ablation before the advent of laser bronchoscopy. A diathermic loop is passed through a rigid bronchoscope, and the lesion is resected by dragging the loop across or under the lesion. Debris is then removed with forceps. The lesion must be in the trachea or a mainstem bronchus to use the diathermic loop. A laser's focused beam has the advantages over electrocautery of causing less destruction to surrounding tissues and because of its flexibility reaching lesions beyond the reach of electrocautery.

Laser Types
The most commonly used laser is the neodymium:yttrium-aluminum-garnet (Nd:YAG) laser. This laser emits radiation of 1.06-μm wavelength, transmitted via a 2.5-mm diameter flexible quartz fiber coated with polytef (Teflon) and cooled by a continuous air jet. A 10-degree divergence in the beam allows its use 5 to 10 mm from the lesion being treated. The power of the Nd:YAG laser ranges from 20 to 100 W. It can be used as a pulse or continuously. Cavaliere and associates (1988) suggested a 40- to 50-W power setting with 0.7- to 1.2-second pulses for most situations. Large tu-

mors may require a longer pulse time (several seconds), with a slightly lower power.

Higher power and shorter exposure times (0.5 seconds at 70 to 80 W) may be used for benign strictures, as there is less tissue destruction adjacent to the path of the beam.

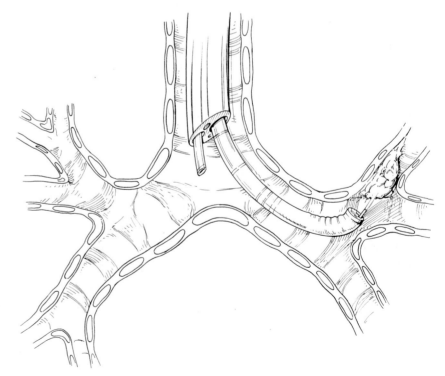

Fig. 48-5. Setup for bronchial endoscopic laser tumor ablation.

sorbed by hemoglobin. It has twice the destructive power of the carbon dioxide laser but causes less tissue necrosis than the Nd:YAG laser. It is also useful in adults with lobar and segmental bronchial lesions.

When a rigid bronchoscope is used, laser therapy is generally limited to the trachea or mainstem bronchi. Rigid bronchoscopy also allows placement of stents after tumor destruction or resection of benign strictures. The flexible bronchoscope permits access of laser therapy to the lobar and segmental bronchial orifices.

In experienced hands, laser destruction of tumor via the bronchoscope is an excellent palliative or curative procedure. Results are very good in tumors that are truly endobronchial, as well in treatment of benign stenosis. Both the complication rates and morbidity are acceptably low in well selected patients.

Stent Placement

Tracheobronchial airway stents are useful for maintaining airway patency in benign stenosis, postsurgical strictures, malignant invasion by tumor, extrinsic tumor compression of the airway, and loss of cartilaginous support (segmental tracheomalacia). Stents are often used in conjunction with dilation, debridement, or laser resection of tumor or benign strictures.

Stenting of an obstructed airway has been performed for decades. Metal stents were placed surgically in conjunction with thoracotomy in the 1950s. Montgomery introduced the silicone T-tube in 1965 for relief of subglottic stenosis. The ideal stent would be placed in a noninvasive manner and would be of an inert material that would fit snugly into the airway, hold its shape, and cause little or no inflammation that could lead to buildup of granulation tissue. A stent should also be easily tailored to different sizes and lengths of strictures and be easily replaced in the event of tumor overgrowth. Several different materials have been tried alone and in combination. Most modern stents are made of silicone (Montgomery T-tube, Integral/Heyer Schulte, Anasco, Puerto Rico, dist. V. Mueller; Harrell-Dumon, France; Dumon style stent, Bryan Corp., Woburn, MA) or a wire mesh of either stainless steel (Gianturco Roubin, Cook Inc., Bloomington, IN) or a cobalt-based alloy [Wall Stent, Schneider (USA), Inc., Boston, MA]. The advantage of silicone is that it is more eas-

ily removed and replaced, but metal stents have less chance of slipping out of position.

Traditionally, stent insertion is performed under general anesthesia. After localization of the lesion with rigid or flexible bronchoscopy, any necessary debridement or laser destruction is done. If a stent is still necessary at this point, one of several techniques is employed. For tracheal or bronchial tube stents, a rigid bronchoscope is fitted with a 36-F chest tube and placed over the scope. The stent is then fitted onto the end of the bronchoscope just proximal to the bevel and distal to the chest tube. The combined apparatus is then introduced through the vocal cords into the trachea. Once the stent is properly located, it is unloaded from the end of the bronchoscope using the chest tube as a pusher (Fig. 48-6). Positioning may be adjusted with forceps through the bronchoscope.

Tracheobronchial Y-stents are placed in a similar manner. The danger in placement of Y-stents is the possibility of folding the short limb of the Y before it reaches the right

mainstem bronchus. To avoid this, a Fogarty balloon catheter is inserted through the short limb prior to the stent's being loaded onto the bronchoscope. The catheter is guided into the right mainstem bronchus under direct vision. The balloon is inflated to fix the catheter in position. The bronchoscope and stent are then introduced into the trachea as described earlier, and the stent is pushed off into the trachea and left mainstem bronchus, while the right limb is guided into the right mainstem bronchus by the Fogarty catheter (Fig. 48-7).

A method of placement of expandable metal stents using a flexible bronchoscope and topical anesthesia has been described. Local anesthesia is achieved with a lidocaine spray, and the bronchoscope is introduced through the mouth. The lesion is identified, and the extent of the lesions is marked exteriorly with skin markers using fluoroscopic guidance. A guidewire is then placed through the operating channel of the bronchoscope past the lesion, and the bronchoscope is removed. A sheath is placed over the guidewire, and the delivery system

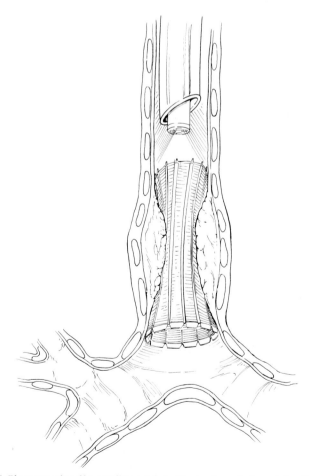

Fig. 48-6. Placement of a self-expanding metal stent for tracheomalacia or obstructing tumor.

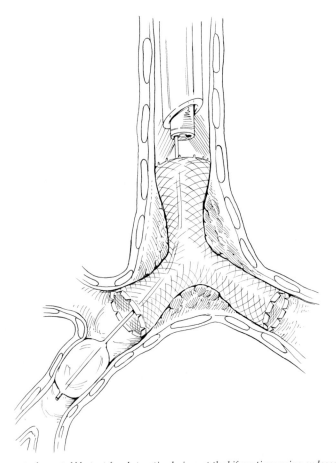

Fig. 48-7. Placement of a coated Y-stent for obstructive lesions at the bifurcations using endoscopic guidance.

with compressed stent is inserted through the sheath. Placement is confirmed by alignment of the stent with the skin markers under fluoroscopy, and the stent is released. The sheath is then removed and stent placement confirmed with bronchoscopy.

Complications

Complications of any therapeutic bronchoscopy procedures are endobronchial hemorrhage and pneumothorax. Additional complications of laser therapy include hemorrhage, pneumomediastinum, bronchial occlusion from destruction debris, and undermining of cartilaginous support of the trachea or bronchi causing airway collapse. Palliation is often the goal of endobronchial surgery in malignant, unresectable tumors. Avoiding thoracotomy is important when endobronchial surgery is considered for benign disease, especially in the elderly or other patients at high risk with thoracotomy. The complication rate is probably proportional to the skill and experience of the operator. The two most common complications of air-

way stents are obstruction and migration. In rare cases, erosion and even bleeding have occurred. Mucociliary function may be impaired with silicone stents, which may also lead to obstruction from excessive secretions. Wire stents are more often associated with exuberant granulation tissue in growth causing obstruction.

Conclusion

The use of bronchoscopy has increased over the past 20 years because of improvements in fiberoptics, laser, and stent technology. This has enabled bronchoscopists to approach problems in patients not foreseen years ago. Most bronchoscopic techniques are adjuncts to other modalities for diagnosis and treatment.

Suggested Reading

Cavaliere S, Foccoli P, Farina PL. Nd:YAG laser bronchoscope: a five-year experience with 1,396 applications in 1,000 patients. *Chest* 1988;94: 15–21.

Colt HG, Dumon JF. Airway stents: present and future. *Clin Chest Med* 1995;16:465–478.

Coolen D, Slabbynck H, Galdermans D, Van Schaardenburg C, Mortelmanns LL. Insertion of a self-expandable endotracheal metal stent using topical anesthetic and a fiberoptic bronchoscope: a comfortable way to offer palliation. *Thorax* 1994;49:87–88.

Petrou M, Kaplan D, Goldstraw P. Bronchoscopic diathermy resection and stent insertion: a cost-effective treatment for tracheobronchial obstruction. *Thorax* 1993;48:1156–1159.

Punzal PA, Myers R, Ries AL, Harrell JH 2d. Laser resection of granulation tissue secondary to transtracheal oxygen catheter. *Chest* 1992;101: 269–271.

Shah H, Garbe L, Nussbaum E, Dumon JF, Chiodera PL, Cavaliere S. Benign tumors of the tracheobronchial tree: endoscopic characteristics and role of laser destruction. *Chest* 1995;107: 1744–1751.

Sonett JR, Keenan RJ, Ferson PF, Griffith BP, Landreneau RJ. Endobronchial management of benign, malignant and lung transplantation airway stenosis. *Ann Thorac Surg* 1995;59:1417–1422.

Stanopoulos IT, Beamis JF Jr, Martinez FJ, Vergos K, Shapshay SM. Laser bronchoscopy in respiratory failure from malignant airway obstruction. *Crit Care Med* 1993;21:386–391.

Ward RF. Treatment of tracheal and endobronchial lesions with the potassium titanyl phosphate laser. *Ann Otol Rhinol Laryngol* 1992; 101:205.

EDITOR'S COMMENT

Drs. Long and Duchow effectively delineate the capabilities of flexible bronchoscopy as both a diagnostic and a therapeutic tool. Sadly, the art of rigid bronchoscopy is disappearing from surgical training programs. This is happening at the same time endoluminal bronchial stenting has become a more accepted treatment for a wide variety of problems. Fortunately, flexible bronchoscopy is becoming increasingly integrated into surgical care. This is most frequently used as a tool to provide pulmonary toilet and diagnosis of obstructive pathology in the surgical intensive care unit. In this context, bronchoscopy has become almost a routine part of resident rounds of the critically ill.

Interventional uses of bronchoscopy can only be expected to increase as optics improve, video endoscopic units replace older fiberoptic scopes, and increasingly sophisticated instrumentation is available for even the smallest of bronchoscopes.

L.L.S.

49

Thoracoscopic Resection of Pulmonary Parenchymal Lesions

Rodney J. Landreneau and Michael J. Mack

The development of minimally invasive surgical approaches in general surgery and a wide variety of other surgical disciplines has inspired thoracic surgeons to reintroduce thoracoscopy, a nearly forgotten technique, into thoracic surgical practice. Although technically simple thoracoscopic interventions aimed at accomplishing collapse therapy for pulmonary tuberculosis were originally described nearly 90 years ago, enthusiasm with this approach waned as anesthetic techniques utilized for open thoracotomy improved and effective antibiotic therapy for tuberculosis made collapse therapy unnecessary.

The development of effective video–optical camera coupling to thoracoscopic telescopes opened the realm of endosurgery to the general thoracic surgeon. As more sophisticated endosurgical instrumentation has been developed, complex video-assisted thoracic surgical procedures could be accom-

plished. These advances led to the expansion of thoracoscopy's role from a simple pleural diagnostic procedure to an intervention through which many other thoracic operations can be performed. Collectively, these thoracic surgical approaches accomplished under thoracoscopic video camera guidance have been termed *video-assisted thoracic surgery* (VATS). This chapter describes current experience with VATS for a wide variety of pulmonary parenchymal problems previously requiring open thoracotomy for diagnosis or definitive therapeutic management. Table 49-1 lists the commonly performed VATS procedures that will be detailed in this chapter.

VATS Diagnosis of Interstitial Lung Disease

Surgical biopsy is often necessary to diagnose and direct the most appropriate therapy for patients affected by diffuse interstitial parenchymal disease (Fig. 49-1). Until the advent of VATS, the standard surgical management was open lung biopsy through a limited lateral thoracotomy. Although these open surgical interventions are seldom extensive, surgical morbidity and mortality following the procedure can be substantial due to the compromised physiologic condition of these patients. These postoperative problems are often the result of significant postthoracotomy pain lead-

Table 49-1. Video-assisted Thoracic Surgical (VATS) Procedures

Pulmonary parenchymal resection
Thorascopic lung biopsy
  Interstitial lung disease
  Indeterminate pulmonary nodule
Thorascopic lung resections
  "Compromise" sublobar pulmonary
    resection for peripheral lung cancer
  VATS lobectomy

---

* With more than 3 months of expected survival

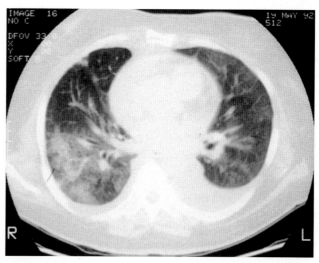

Fig. 49-1. *Pattern of interstitial pneumonia ideally suited for closed lung biopsy via video-assisted thoracic surgery. A limited lateral thoracotomy access may lead to sampling error, as the disease is heterogeneously present within the lung.*

ing to reduced respiratory effort and patient immobility.

One can intuitively assume that the operative morbidity related to surgical lung biopsy in these patients would be reduced by utilizing a VATS approach. To determine the potential benefit of a minimally invasive VATS approach to lung biopsy, we compared the diagnostic efficacy and perioperative morbidity of VATS for closed wedge resection lung biopsy against the traditional open lung biopsy procedure. This study involved the retrospective review of the records of 20 matched patient pairs undergoing elective wedge resection lung biopsy by either VATS or lung biopsy through a limited lateral thoracotomy to evaluate presumed interstitial lung disease (Ferson et al., 1993). The demographic characteristics and the degree of preoperative respiratory impairment were similar between groups. None of the patients undergoing either VATS or open biopsy required ventilatory assistance at the time of the surgical intervention. This study demonstrated that the perioperative morbidity and mortality and the postoperative length of stay were significantly less with the VATS approach to closed wedge resection biopsy compared to standard open lung biopsy. Furthermore, the diagnostic efficacy of the VATS approach was equivalent to that of open lung biopsy. Although Molin and colleagues (1994) reported a greater overall cost of hospitalization for lung biopsy with the VATS approach, our experience conflicts with their report (Hazelrigg et al., 1993). In a collaborative study, we found that although the initial operating room expenses were greater with VATS due to liberal use of disposable instrumentation, the overall cost for a VATS lung biopsy was less as a result of reduced overall length of postoperative hospital stay. Reusable instrumentation can be expected to significantly reduce operative costs in the future.

It is recognized that the preferred site of lung biopsy chosen to evaluate interstitial lung disease should be from a representative area of disease activity. Beyond the potential reductions in perioperative morbidity and overall hospital costs with VATS closed lung biopsy, the VATS approach permits virtually unrestricted visibility of the entire lung surface, which can lead to improved biopsy site selection. This is in contrast to the very restricted access to the lung achieved through the limited lateral or axillary thoracotomy approach utilized for open lung biopsy procedures.

Another potential gain for patients with interstitial lung disease resulting from the introduction of VATS closed lung biopsy is that pulmonary physicians are now tending to refer for diagnostic surgical lung biopsy earlier in the course of disease. Earlier diagnosis of inflammatory processes may result in treatment at a stage when they are more responsive to medical therapy.

VATS Closed Lung Biopsy Techniques

The techniques used for thoracoscopic closed wedge resection biopsy for interstitial lung disease are similar to those applied in thoracoscopic resection of other pulmonary parenchymal processes (i.e., wedge excision of pulmonary nodules). The general principles are described in this section.

General anesthesia is induced, and a double-lumen endotracheal tube with left endobronchial extension is introduced into the airway to accomplish selective ventilation of the contralateral lung and collapse of the ipsilateral lung during the surgical intervention. Room setup and equipment needs are the same for all thoracoscopic approaches; the patient is in the lateral decubitus position. Intercostal access is established for the thoracoscope and the resective instrumentation after ventilation to the ipsilateral lung is discontinued.

Alternatively (or occasionally in addition), a low pressure carbon dioxide (CO_2) pneumothorax can be used to displace the lung on the side being operated on. This is done by using standard laparoscopic sealed tro-

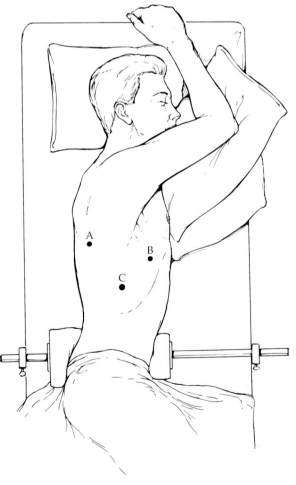

Fig. 49-2. Usual sites of intercostal access utilized to accomplish video-assisted thoracic surgical exploration and wedge resection biopsy of the lung.

cars to establish access and then connecting the port to a CO_2 insufflator. Pressure should not exceed 10 mm Hg, or mediastinal shift and cardiopulmonary compromise will result. Great care should be used with this technique, as it results in high levels of CO_2 absorption; this can be especially troublesome in patients with intrinsic pulmonary disease. Occasionally, if the double-lumen endotracheal tube is not working to collapse the lung, a brief period of positive-pressure CO_2 pneumothorax will force the residual air from the lung and achieve visualization.

The intercostal access orientation of the thoracoscope and instrumentation established should facilitate exploration of the entire thoracic cavity and identification of "target" lung pathology as determined through careful preoperative review of the chest radiograph and computed tomo-

graphic (CT) images. Generally, for diffuse interstitial pulmonary processes, intercostal access is achieved for the thoracoscope at the seventh intercostal space in the midaxillary line. Endosurgical instrumentation and the stapling device are introduced through intercostal access at the fifth or sixth interspace along the posterior axillary line and at the fourth or fifth interspace on the anterior axillary line (Fig. 49-2). This intercostal access arrangement allows ideal thoracoscopic visualization of the entire pleural space and the lung surfaces for appropriate biopsy site selection. The free edges of the lung along the fissure and along the tips of the superior or basilar segments of the lower lobe are usually easy sites for biopsy (Fig. 49-3). Similarly, the apical segments of the upper lobes or the lateral segments of the lingula and middle lobe are also readily accessible with this VATS approach. This orientation

also facilitates alignment of the endosurgical stapling device along the fissures of both the right and left lungs for the proposed sites of lobar biopsy.

In spite of the severe oxygen-dependent pulmonary parenchymal disease common in this patient group, most patients tolerate single-lung ventilation during the course of the VATS intervention. Malpositioning or mucous plugging of the double-lumen endotracheal tube is the usual cause of significant intraoperative hypoxia that may occur. The anesthesia and thoracic surgical teams must be prepared to immediately suction secretions from the ventilated "down" lung and perform bronchoscopic examination of the double-lumen tube placement to correct any potential endotracheal tube malalignment. When significant hypoxia persists despite confirmation of correct tube positioning,

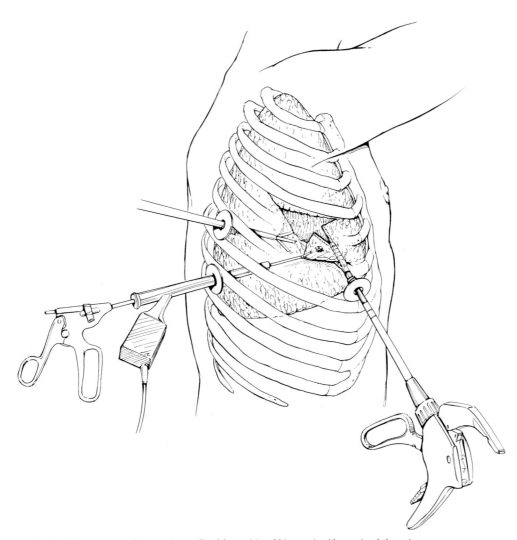

Fig. 49-3. Usual three intercostal access sites utilized for excisional biopsy via video-assisted thoracic surgery.

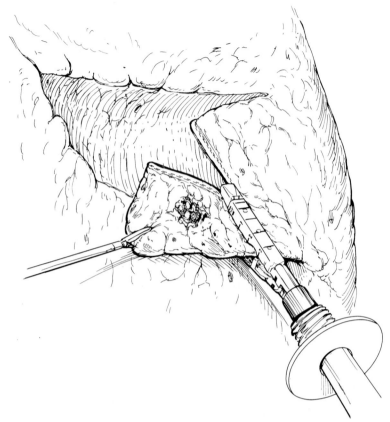

Fig. 49-4. Serial application of the endoscopic stapling device accomplishes a standard V-wedge resection of the lung. Note that the intercostal access positions of the stapling instrument and the grasping tools are reversed to expeditiously complete the stapled wedge resection.

we rely on brief periods of reexpansion of the ipsilateral collapsed lung to correct the hypoxia. Following this resuscitative maneuver, repeat isolation of the lung is accomplished to allow completion of the procedure. This latter approach will usually permit 10 to 15 minutes of operative manipulation before hypoxia recurs. If an area of lung pathology is identified along a fissure or in the lingular lobe, biopsy is accomplished by applying the endoscopic stapling device from the lateral intercostal access as the lung substance is held with a grasping forceps from the other lateral site or intercostal access (Fig. 49-4). The staple line is inspected for air leak and hemostasis. Multiple firings of the stapler may be needed to complete the excision. The pulmonary specimen is removed from the chest in a specimen retrieval bag, commercially available through a number of endosurgical companies, to avoid chest wall contamination by a potentially malignant lesion within the specimen. Alternatively, a sterile operating room latex glove can be introduced into the chest

through an intercostal access site to be used as a retrieval bag.

Following removal of the specimen, the lung is partially expanded, and the resection margin is reexamined for hemostasis and air-leak control. A singe chest tube is inserted through one of the lower intercostal access sites and positioned under thoracoscopic guidance toward an anterior apical position. The other intercostal access sites are closed primarily. The chest tube is removed when drainage is minimal and the air leak has resolved. The patient is discharged the following day.

VATS Excisional Biopsy of Indeterminate Pulmonary Nodules

Over 150,000 patients have new, indeterminate pulmonary nodules identified by chest radiography each year in the United States. Fifty percent of these patients will ultimately be found to have malignant le-

sions, of which 75% will be primary lung cancers. The most appropriate strategy for the diagnosis of such indeterminate pulmonary nodules continues to be debated. Standard radiologic assessment (chest x-ray and CT) can accurately predict the presence of malignancy in up to 60% of lesions based on their morphologic and tissue density characteristics (Fig. 49-5). Biopsy of an indeterminate lesion continues to be required, unless the lesion has remained unchanged over a 2-year period of observation or if benign calcification can be identified within the lesion.

Percutaneous transthoracic biopsy under fluoroscopic or CT guidance can diagnose malignancy in a pulmonary nodule with a reported sensitivity of more than 90%. The important limitation of percutaneous biopsy approaches is the accuracy in the determination of the true benignity of an indeterminate pulmonary lesion. A recent study by Mitruka and associates (1995) found that percutaneous biopsy techniques achieved a "specific benign" diagnosis (i.e., infectious organism identified, hamartoma, or pulmonary infarct) in fewer than 15% of patients biopsied. Unfortunately, when a nonspecific "benign" diagnosis is obtained (i.e., "benign tissue," inflammation, histiocytes, alveolar lining cells, or giant cells), many of these "benign" lesions will ultimately be found to be malignant at subsequent surgical excision. Approximately 60% of patients with

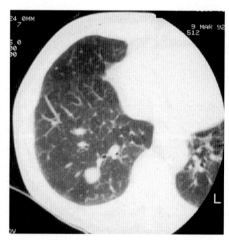

Fig. 49-5. Computed tomographic scan shows a moderate-sized pulmonary nodule within the midzone of the lung parenchyma that is not a good candidate lesion for excisional biopsy via video-assisted thoracic surgery. Percutaneous biopsy or open thoracotomy should be primarily considered to obtain a diagnosis.

a nonspecific "benign" percutaneous biopsy result in the study were found to have malignancies when surgical excision was later carried out. Actually, only 13% of patients who were physiologically fit for anesthesia and surgery were able to avoid surgery as a result of the initial percutaneous needle biopsy results. This significant limitation in affecting the clinical course of patients with indeterminate noncalcified pulmonary nodule has led many physicians to move directly to surgical excisional biopsy as the primary diagnostic modality for such lesions in patients who can withstand thoracic surgical exploration and resection.

The VATS approach offers an attractive minimally invasive surgical alternative to open thoracotomy for excisional biopsy of indeterminate pulmonary nodules. The ability to identify and accurately diagnose peripheral pulmonary nodules with thoracoscopic excisional biopsy approaches 97% (Table 49-2).

Preoperative CT localization is a useful adjunct to the thoracoscopic approach to excisional biopsy for small subpleural or deep lesions that would be difficult to locate otherwise. Localization of pulmonary nodules is supplemented with localization needle placement or methylene blue staining of the area of the lung parenchyma (Fig. 49-6). We have utilized this CT localization approach as an immediate preoperative maneuver in more than 100 patients. Dislodgement of the CT-directed needle from the lung may occur in up to 20% of cases; however, methylene blue staining of the lung in the targeted area allows successful localization and resection of a pulmonary lesion in these circumstances.

The relative accuracy, complication rate, and effect on subsequent clinical management of patients with peripheral pulmonary nodules approached with an initial VATS excisional biopsy are superior to those of an initial percutaneous biopsy approach.

Table 49-2. Candidate Lesions for Thoracoscopic Excisional Biopsy

Noncalcified, <3 cm in diameter

Indeterminate etiology after appropriate workup

Location in outer one-third of lung

Absence of endobronchial extension

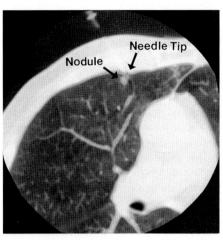

Fig. 49-6. Computed tomographic (CT) scan shows a small peripheral pulmonary nodule ideally suited for thoracoscopic resection as a primary diagnostic measure. Preoperative CT-directed needle localization of the location of lesion is a valuable adjunct to thoracoscopic excisional biopsy of such lesions.

proach. Although thoracoscopic biopsy required hospitalization, a VATS approach provides definitive diagnosis of lesions, as well as a potential therapeutic benefit through compromise nonanatomic wedge resection of peripheral lung cancers present in many patients with impaired cardiopulmonary reserve who otherwise would not have been considered for open surgical resection. A particular value of VATS excisional biopsy in this clinical setting also relates to the avoidance of open thoracotomy for the diagnosis of a pulmonary lesion that will ultimately be found to be metastatic or benign. Among patients with adequate pulmonary reserve who were found to have primary malignant lesions, immediate conversion to open thoracotomy for formal pulmonary resection can be performed. Alternatively, the thoracoscopic approach can be continued to perform a lobar resection when the pulmonary anatomy is favorable for this approach. In either circumstance, the management delay, potential complications, and added expense of percutaneous biopsy can be avoided (Table 49-3).

A percutaneous CT-directed biopsy approach is appropriate in selected instances. It is certainly a reasonable diagnostic approach for obviously unresectable pulmonary lesions, for which primary radiotherapy and/or chemotherapy are being considered. Percutaneous biopsy is also an acceptable primary diagnostic option for

Table 49-3. Advantages of VATS Wedge Resection in Management of Indeterminate Pulmonary Nodules

Minimally invasive surgical approach

Virtually 100% effective in locating and diagnosing a pulmonary lesion

No mortality and minimal morbidity

Tolerated by patients with limited cardiopulmonary reserve

Reduced postoperative hospitalization

patients with severe physiologic impairment who are not candidates for *any* surgical intervention—including VATS compromise wedge resection as primary cancer therapy. Finally, percutaneous biopsy should be considered for the diagnosis of small lesions that lie too deeply within the lung parenchyma to undergo VATS excisional biopsy. Of course, if such deep lesions have radiographic characteristics highly suggestive for carcinoma, primary surgical exploration with preexcisional "true-cut" biopsy is probably a preferred approach.

The basic techniques for VATS excisional biopsy of peripheral pulmonary lesions are similar to those used for thoracoscopic wedge resection biopsy of interstitial lung disease described earlier. Some important differences relate to the strategies for lesion localization and intercostal access for instrumentation to approach the lesion in question. Careful examination of the surface of the lung in the region of the suspected lesion identified by CT will often reveal local visceral pleural scarring or retraction. Once full atelectasis of the lung in the region of the lesion is obtained, localization can usually be achieved through effacement of the nodule against the surrounding collapsed lung. Gentle palpation of the lung in the area in question with a sponge forceps or endoscopic grasper can also identify the lesion when videoscopic inspection is less rewarding. Once the nodule has been located, strategic placement of other sites of intercostal access is critical to adequately position the endoscopic tools for wedge resection. The endoscopic stapling device can usually be positioned beneath the lung lesion when the lesion is located near an edge of the lung or when it is small (less than 2 cm in diameter) and in a subpleural location. On occasion, adjunctive use of a neodymium:yttrium-aluminum-garnet laser can allow VATS resection of deeper-seated nodules and those located on the flat surface of the lung, which are not amenable to mechanical resection with an endoscopic stapler.

VATS Pulmonary Metastasectomy

The usefulness of surgical resection of isolated pulmonary metastases from remote visceral primary malignancies is controversial as a means of improving long-term patient survival. Some investigators have reported improved survival with pulmonary metastasectomy in patients with a limited pulmonary disease burden, a favorable primary tumor histology, control of the primary tumor, and a long disease-free interval. When surgical diagnosis of potential pulmonary metastases is the objective, the VATS approach offers the obvious advantage over thoracotomy of reduced operative morbidity. When three or fewer nodules are present, thoracoscopic wedge metastasectomy is an attractive alternative (Fig. 49-7).

The fear that many surgeons have regarding the VATS approach to metastatic disease is that some foci will be missed due to restricted palpation of the lung available with these techniques. Careful examination of an adequately performed, modern CT scan of the pulmonary parenchyma makes this point moot under most circumstances. Nodules of 2 mm are consistently identified by CT scans, particularly the newer generation spiral CT scanners. Lesions of this size are usually impossible to discriminate even at the time of open thoracotomy. Lesions identified by these methods can be strategically

localized using wire needle localization techniques when a diagnosis of such lesions is important.

We find surgical excisional biopsy necessary to diagnose a minority of patients with presumed pulmonary metastases unable to be histologically confirmed by less invasive means. When surgical intervention is required, the VATS approach is an ideal means of establishing a diagnosis of such metastatic disease if it is located in the outer one-third of the lung parenchyma. Candidate lesions for pulmonary metastasectomy are similar to those described for VATS resection of indeterminate pulmonary nodules (see Table 49-2). The bottom line regarding this matter is that the intervention assumes a primarily diagnostic role if more than two or three lesions are found at thoracic exploration. The VATS approach is a valid alternative to thoracotomy for the resection of limited metastatic disease (fewer than four lesions) identified as small, peripheral nodules on CT scans. If the disease cannot be localized during VATS, conversion to an open thoracotomy may be helpful. If more extensive disease is identified, we believe that the procedure has a diagnostic intent only and minimally invasive diagnostic methods should be primarily employed.

VATS Approach to Compromise Lung Resection of Peripheral Stage I Lung Cancer

Anatomic resection by pulmonary lobectomy remains the standard of care for pa-

tients with resectable non–small cell lung cancer having adequate cardiopulmonary function. However, nonanatomic wedge resection has been reported to be a reasonable compromise surgical management plan for physiologically impaired patients with early-stage primary lung cancer. Whereas open thoracotomy has been used for nonanatomic wedge resections, we have been exploring the utility of the VATS approach to accomplish extended wedge resection as primary management of physiologically impaired patients with small peripheral non–small cell lung cancers. We caution that the thoracic surgeon should be careful to use the same anatomic criteria for VATS resection described earlier in the management of the peripheral indeterminate pulmonary nodule (see Table 49-2). Additionally, it is important to observe strict surgical oncologic principles to ensure clear surgical margins and adequate tumor staging by performing intraoperative lymph node sampling about the interlobar fissure, pulmonary hilum, and ipsilateral mediastinum. We also emphasize that specimen retrieval should be conducted with a sterile retrieval system (Fig. 49-8).

Adherence to these basic technical principles is vital for avoiding intercostal access-site recurrence, reducing the likelihood of local parenchymal recurrence, and directing appropriate adjunctive therapies for patients with more advanced-stage lung cancers. We have found that the 5-year survival of patients undergoing VATS wedge resection is equivalent to that of patients undergoing lobectomy for stage I (T1N0) peripheral lung cancer. When compared to open wedge resection, both lobectomy and VATS wedge resection demonstrate superior long-term survival results. The major drawback of primary wedge resection management of peripheral lung cancers seen by us is the local recurrence rate, which is approximately twice that seen following lobectomy for similar-stage lesions. These results parallel those reported for a randomized study conducted by the Lung Cancer Study Group (1995). Because of the local recurrence rate with wedge resection, we continue to advocate lobectomy as the primary treatment approach for good-risk patients. When wedge resection is contemplated because

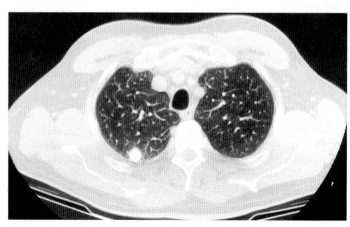

Fig. 49-7. Thoracoscopic wedge metastasectomy.

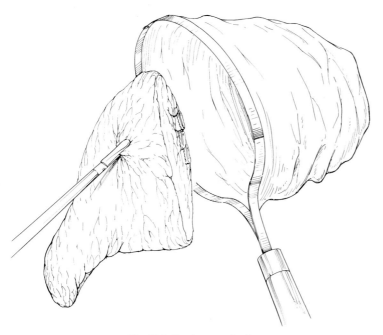

Fig. 49-8. Specimen retrieval.

thoracic surgeon is concerned about the efficacy and/or the safety of continuing the VATS approach during the operative procedure. We recommend the VATS approach to lobectomy only for patients with small, peripheral, clinical-stage I lesions without radiographic evidence of hilar or mediastinal adenopathy. Well developed pulmonary lobar fissures are also required, and the intraoperative finding of unsuspected interlobar hilar fibrosis or adenopathy would lead us to move directly to convert to an open muscle-sparing thoracotomy.

Conclusion

VATS is an important minimally invasive surgical advance in the management of pulmonary parenchymal problems previously requiring open thoracotomy for diagnosis or definitive management. However, the absolute indications for VATS in the primary management of lung cancer are yet to be firmly defined. It appears that equivalent efficacy and reduced perioperative morbidity can be achieved in many clinical circumstances when the VATS approach is appropriately chosen by thoracic surgeons experienced in these minimally invasive surgical techniques.

of a poor patient functional status, the VATS approach provides an equivalent therapeutic potential and reduced perioperative morbidity, compared to open thoracotomy approaches.

VATS Lobectomy

The use of VATS for the performance of formal resection has been investigated by our group and others (Roviaro et al., 1992; Kirby et al., 1993; Walker et al., 1993; McKenna, 1994; and Guidicelli et al., 1994). VATS approaches vary from a totally endoscopically directed procedure to the use of minithoracotomies with thoracoscopic assistance to accomplish a less invasive lobectomy without compromise of oncologic principles. Both of these minimally invasive VATS approaches are aimed at reducing the troublesome postoperative incision-related morbidity associated with standard open thoracotomy approaches to formal pulmonary resection (Fig. 49-9).

There is general agreement that adequate oncologic management of lung cancer can be achieved using VATS lobectomy approaches. Although this is assumed to be the case throughout this reported experience, Walker and associates (1993) and McKenna (1994) stated that VATS lobectomy achieved mediastinal lymph node staging and surgical resection

margins with an equivalence to those obtained with open thoracotomy approaches to lobectomy. As stated earlier, adherence to surgical oncologic principles is of paramount importance. Conversion to a standard open operative approach is most appropriate when the

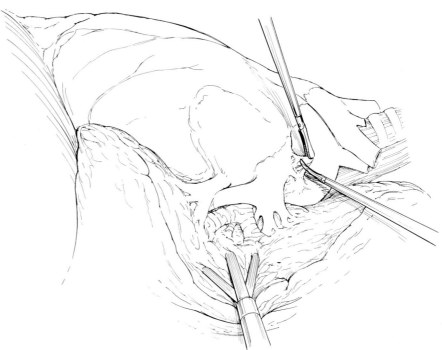

A

Fig. 49-9. **A:** *Thoracoscopic intraoperative nodal staging accompanying VATS lobectomy.* (continued)

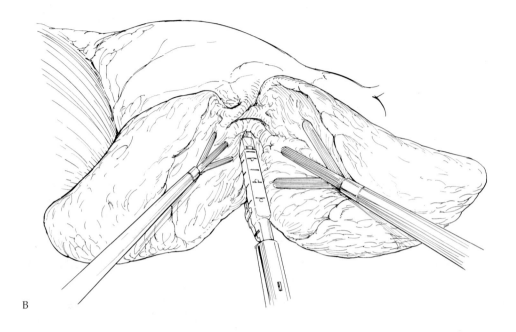

B

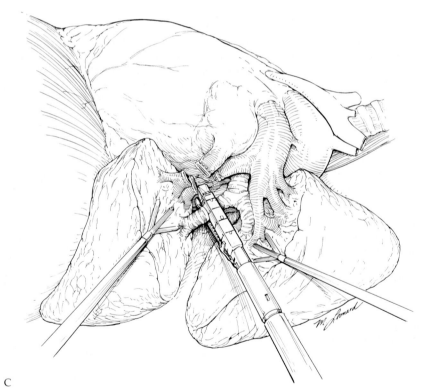

C

Fig. 49-9. (Continued) **B,C:** *Technique of thoracoscopic lobectomy.*

Suggested Reading

Calhoun P, Feldman PS, Armstrong P, et al. The clinical outcome of needle aspirations of the lung when cancer is not diagnosed. *Ann Thorac Surg* 1986;41:592–596.

Dowling RD, Ferson PF, Landreneau RJ. Thoracoscopic resection of pulmonary metastases. *Chest* 1992;102:1450–1454.

Downey RJ, McCormack P, LoCicero J III, Video-assisted Thoracic Surgery Study Group. Dissemination of malignant tumors after video-assisted thoracic surgery: a report of twenty-one cases. *J Thorac Cardiovasc Surg* 1996;111:954–960.

Errett LE, Wilson J, Chiu RC, Munro DD. Wedge resection as an alternative procedure for peripheral bronchogenic carcinoma in poor-risk patients. *J Thorac Cardiovasc Surg* 1985;90:656–661.

Ferson PF, Landreneau RJ, Dowling RD, et al. Thoracoscopic vs. open lung biopsy for the diagnosis of diffuse infiltrative lung disease. *J Thorac Cardiovasc Surg* 1993;105:194–199.

Fry WA, Siddiqui A, Pensler JM, et al. Thoracoscopic implantation of cancer with a fatal outcome. *Ann Thorac Surg* 1995;59:42–45.

Giudicelli R, Thomas P, Lonjon T, et al. Video-assisted minithoracotomy versus muscle-sparing thoracotomy for performing lobectomy. *Ann Thorac Surg* 1994;58:712–718.

Hall TS, Hutchins GM, Baker RR. A critical review of the use of open lung biopsy in the management of the oncologic patient with acute pulmonary infiltrates. *Am J Clin Oncol* 1987;10:249–252.

Hazelrigg SR, Nunchuck S, Landreneau RJ, et al. Cost analysis for thoracoscopy: thoracoscopic wedge resection. *Ann Thorac Surg* 1993;56:633–635.

Jacobaeus HC. The practical importance of thoracoscopy in surgery of the chest. *Surg Gynecol Obstet* 1922;34:289–296.

Keagy BA, Pharr WF, Bowes DE, Wilcox BR. A review of morbidity and mortality in elderly patients undergoing pulmonary resection. *Am Surg* 1984;50:213–216.

Kirby TJ, Mack MJ, Landreneau RJ, Rice TW. Initial experience with video-assisted thoracoscopic lobectomy. *Ann Thorac Surg* 1993;56:1248–1253.

Landreneau RJ, Herlan DB, Johnson JA, Boley TM, Nawarowong W, Ferson PF. Thoracoscopic neodymium:yttrium-aluminum-garnet laser-assisted pulmonary resection. *Ann Thorac Surg* 1991;52:1176–1178.

Landreneau RJ, Mack MJ, Keenan RJ, Dowling RD, Hazelrigg SR, Ferson PF. Strategic planning for video-assisted thoracic surgery "VATS." *Ann Thorac Surg* 1993;56:615–619.

Lanza LA, Natarajan G, Roth JA, Putnam JB. Long-term survival after resection of pulmonary metastases from carcinoma of the breast. *Ann Thorac Surg* 1992;54:244–248.

The Lung Cancer Study Group, Ginsberg RJ, Rubenstein LV. Randomized trial of lobectomy versus limited resection for T1N0 non-small cell lung cancer. *Ann Thorac Surg* 1995;60:615–623.

Mack MJ. Discussant: McCormack PM, Bains MS, Burt ME, et al. Role of video-assisted thoracic surgery in the treatment of pulmonary metastases: results of a prospective trial. *Ann Thorac Surg* 1996;62:213–217.

McAfee MK, Allen MS, Trastek VF, Ilstrup DM, Deschamps C, Pairolero PC. Colorectal lung metastases: results of surgical excision. *Ann Thorac Surg* 1992;53:780–786.

McCormack PM, Burt ME, Bains MS, Martini N, Rusch VM, Ginsberg RJ. Lung resection for colorectal metastases: 10-year results. *Arch Surg* 1992;127:1403–1406.

McCormack PM, Ginsberg KB, Bains MS, et al. Accuracy of lung imaging in metastases with implications for the role of thoracoscopy. *Ann Thorac Surg* 1993;56:863–866.

McKenna RJ. Lobectomy by video-assisted thoracic surgery with mediastinal node sampling for lung cancer. *J Thorac Cardiovasc Surg* 1994;107:879–882.

Mitruka S, Landreneau RJ, Mack MJ, et al. Diagnosing the indeterminate pulmonary nodule: percutaneous biopsy versus thoracoscopy. *Surgery* 1995;118:676–684.

Molin LJ, Steinberg JB, Lanza LA. VATS increases cost in patients undergoing lung biopsy for interstitial lung disease. *Ann Thorac Surg* 1994;58:1595–1598.

Plunkett MB, Peterson MS, Landreneau RJ, Ferson PF, Posner MC. CT-guided preoperative percutaneous needle localization of peripheral pulmonary nodules. *Radiology* 1992;185:274–276.

Roviaro G, Rebuffat C, Varoli F, Vergani C, Mariani C, Maciocco M. Video-endoscopic pulmonary lobectomy for cancer. *Surg Laparosc Endosc* 1992;2:244–247.

Salazar AM, Westcott JL. The role of transthoracic needle biopsy for the diagnosis and staging of lung cancer. *Clin Chest Med* 1993;14:99–110.

Shennib H, Landreneau RJ, Mack MJ. Video-assisted thoracoscopic wedge resection of T1 lung cancer in high-risk patients. *Ann Surg* 1993;218:555–560.

Sommers KE, Landreneau RJ, Fuhrman C, Hazelrigg SR, Keenan RJ, Ferson PF. The role of video-assisted thoracic surgery in the management of fungal disease. *Chest Surg Clin N Am* 1993;3:743–756.

Walker WS, Carnochan FM, Pugh, GC. Thoracoscopic pulmonary lobectomy: early operative experience and preliminary clinical results. *J Thorac Cardiovasc Surg* 1993;106:1111–1117.

EDITOR'S COMMENT

Drs. Landreneau and Mack have given a good presentation of the possibilities of thoracoscopy for advanced diagnosis and treatment of pulmonary parenchymal disease. Because of the morbidity of standard thoracotomy incisions, thoracoscopy has attained wide acceptance for diagnosing diffuse pulmonary processes (tuberculosis, chronic pneumonia, fungal infections, etc.) and for treating symptomatic pneumothorax due to blebular disease. Acceptance of the technique has been slower when pulmonary resection for suspected or known malignancy is indicated. There are three reasons for this:

1. Except for large, peripheral lesions, pulmonary masses can be difficult to locate with a thoracoscope. This makes accurate resection with margins difficult and unpredictable. The authors describe a method of preoperative methylene blue injection and hook-wire localization that has proven successful in their hands. Others have described the use of intraoperative ultrasound and even the possibility of creating new instruments that have the ability to transmit tactile feedback.

2. Performing standard resections (lobectomy) for tumors endoscopically entails some technical difficulties. When there are a well developed fissure, a well collapsed lung, and a good assistant providing exposure, a formal lobectomy is fairly straightforward. Lacking any of these elements, the procedure can be arduous and fraught with potential disaster.

3. The results of oncologic surgery performed endoscopically are unknown. There have been anecdotal reports of wound-site metastases following both thoracoscopic and laparoscopic cancer resections. What remains unknown is whether these are due to a preventable breach in technique or to a fundamental problem with minimal-access surgery for cancer. There is some evidence that positive-pressure pneumoperitoneum with insufflation of gas in laparoscopy leads to tumor cell dissemination. Obviously, this should not be an issue with thoracoscopy. Pending a final decision on the safety of this approach, it seems wise to approach such cases with caution and, if they are done, to carefully avoid overmanipulation of the tumor, to place the specimen in an impermeable bag, and not to breech any acceptable open-surgical practices.

L.L.S.

50

Thoracoscopy for Pleural Diseases

Iqbal S. Garcha

Superficial lesions of the thoracic cavity have long presented problems of diagnosis and treatment. Diseases of the pleural cavity span a wide spectrum of pathology, from incidental pleural thickening or benign masses to primary or secondary malignant processes. Traditionally, diagnosing and treating these problems required the same access as full-blown pulmonary surgery. Thoracoscopy offers a valuable tool to diagnose and sometimes treat a variety of pleural diseases without subjecting the patient to the morbidity of an open procedure.

Pleura-Based Mass

Suspicious lesions of the pleura are usually first discovered by routine chest radiography and subsequently diagnosed by computed tomography (CT) scan. Traditionally, these lesions have been biopsied by CT-guided percutaneous needle technique. Most suspicious lesions can be diagnosed successfully and safely in this way by experienced physicians. There are limitations, however. Many lesions are not accessible to percutaneous technique because of their anatomic location or their proximity to vital structures. The classic example is the pleura-based mass located in the anteroposterior window or adjacent to the diaphragm. A percutaneous approach to these lesions can be difficult and dangerous. Before thoracoscopy, these lesions required a thoracotomy for their diagnosis. Another limitation to CT-guided percutaneous biopsy is the size of the obtained specimen. Because the specimen is delivered through a fine needle, its evaluation is limited to cytologic analysis, which often is inadequate to make a defini-

tive diagnosis. Before thoracoscopy, an inadequate fine-needle specimen required thoracotomy for open biopsy.

With modern video thoracoscopic techniques, pleura-based lesions can be biopsied successfully with minimal morbidity and occasionally on an outpatient basis. All locations can be reached using thoracoscopic technique, and the size of the specimen is not limited. Although it should probably never completely replace CT-guided percutaneous technique, video thoracoscopy will continue to gain popularity as a safe, definitive biopsy method for pleura-based lesions.

Preoperative preparation of the patient for thoracoscopy is similar to that for thoracotomy. The thoracoscopic surgeon must be prepared at all times to convert to an open procedure, and for this reason, only surgeons with credentials to perform the open operation should be allowed to perform thoracoscopy. The physician first obtains a thorough history and performs a physical examination. Special attention is given to surgical risk factors, especially preexisting pulmonary disease. Single-lung ventilation is required intraoperatively, and split function pulmonary function tests should be performed if the patient has significant pulmonary disease. All other preoperative studies are routinely obtained, including the electrocardiogram and blood tests. It is not necessary to routinely type and crossmatch patients for packed cells. Each patient is instructed on the use of the incentive spirometer preoperatively and is told to plan for a 1- to 2-night stay in the hospital.

In the operating room, the patient is induced under general anesthesia and is intubated first with a standard endotracheal

tube. We routinely perform bronchoscopy for all patients in the operating room before the procedure. After bronchoscopy, the standard endotracheal tube is replaced with a double-lumen tube to allow selective lung ventilation. The patient is then placed in a lateral decubitus position with an axillary roll and with the hip extended. This is the same as for a standard posterolateral thoracotomy. For left-sided lesions, it is important to tilt the patient slightly toward the prone position, which allows the heart to fall away from the posterior chest and helps to expose the posterior mediastinal pleura. Retracting the heart thoracoscopically can be difficult and dangerous.

After positioning, the patient is prepped and draped, ensuring that access for a thoracotomy is easily available if necessary. The extent of the exposure is from the iliac crest inferiorly up to the shoulder superiorly and from the spinous processes posteriorly to the sternum anteriorly. The surgeon stands toward the patient's back with one assistant on the opposite side.

The initial approach is through a 10-mm incision at the midaxillary line, somewhere between the fifth and seventh intercostal space. This location can be adjusted according to the location of the lesion. The incision is taken down through the subcutaneous tissue and through the muscle to the rib. The dissection is then carried along the rib surface on the anterior aspect to avoid injury to the neurovascular bundle. After the parietal pleura is reached, the ipsilateral lung is deflated by clamping the appropriate side of the double-lumen endotracheal tube, and the pleural cavity is entered. Digital exploration of this tract is performed to ensure entrance into the pleural space and to ensure that the lung is free from adhesions (Fig. 50-1). A 10-mm, blunt-tipped trocar is placed through the tract. This trocar can be simple because carbon dioxide insufflation usually is unnecessary. Many devices are available, such as the U.S. Surgical Corporation's Thoracoport. Because of the rigidity of the chest wall and subsequent superfluity of positive-pressure insufflation, many argue that trocars are unnecessary. My colleagues and I agree with this argument, but we feel it is important to have one trocar at the site of the thoracoscope to protect the lens from fat and blood while going through the chest wall tract.

After the 10-mm trocar is in place, a 10-mm videoscope is placed through the trocar and into the pleural space. A 30° or 45° scope is necessary to completely evaluate the entire pleural surface (Fig. 50-2). After the scope has been inserted, the 10-mm trocar is pulled back along the scope and away from the chest wall. This allows access for a blunt instrument through the same tract (Fig. 50-3). The blunt instrument, which may be a grasper, dissector, or suction/irrigator, is used to help further deflate the lung, allowing complete exposure of the parietal pleura. In this way, all suspicious lesions of the parietal pleura can be clearly identified and localized. We use a video imaging device to produce still images of each lesion (Fig. 50-4). These images are then placed in the patient's medical record.

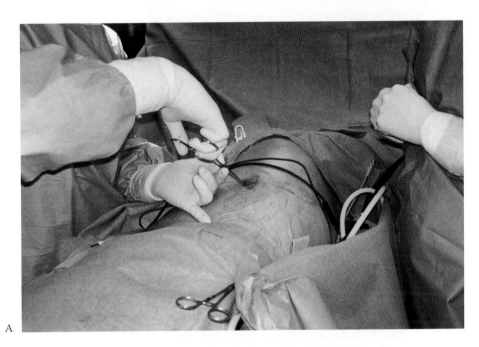

A

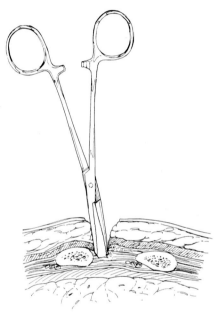

B

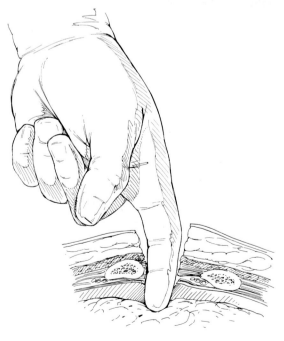

C

Fig. 50-1. **A:** Dissection is taken down over the rib into the pleural space. Proper port placement technique is essential to prevent injury to the neurovascular bundles and underlying structures. **B:** Dissection close to the superior aspect of the rib. **C:** Finger into pleural space. (From Zucker KA, ed. Surgical laparoscopy update. St. Louis: Quality Medical Publishing, 1993; with permission.)

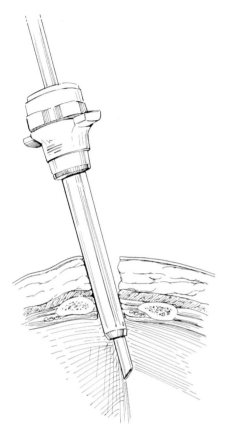

Fig. 50-2. *An angled videoscope is inserted through the 10-mm port to examine a pleural membrane.*

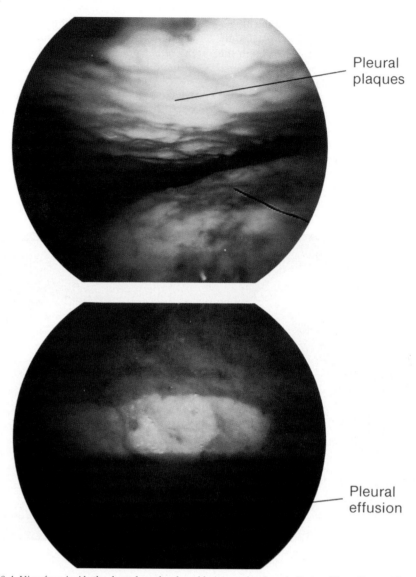

Pleural plaques

Pleural effusion

Fig. 50-4. *View from inside the chest show the pleural lesions and a pleural effusion. (From Krasna M, Flowers JL. Diagnostic thoracoscopy in a patient with a pleural mass.* Surg Laparosc Endosc *1991;1:94–97; with permission.)*

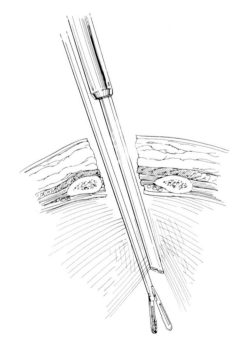

Fig. 50-3. *After the port is pulled back, an instrument can be inserted through the same incision alongside the videoscope.*

After the lesions to be biopsied have been identified and photographed, the biopsies are taken. The blunt instrument is removed and replaced with long biopsy forceps. Using these forceps under direct vision, multiple biopsies are taken of each lesion. Frozen-section analysis is routinely used to ensure adequacy of the specimens.

If a lesion cannot be reached using the biopsy forceps alone, a second port may be required. The second incision is placed to allow a 30° to 45° angle of attack at the lesion (Fig. 50-5). The exact position of this port can be facilitated by passing a long, 21-gauge needle through the chest wall and noting its location inside the chest.

This incision is 5 mm, and the dissection through the chest wall is performed bluntly under direct vision through the videoscope. A 5-mm, blunt-tipped trocar is used, and a 5-mm endoscopic scissor is inserted. Using a grasper through the 10-mm incision, the lesion is held in traction while the scissors are used to excise it from the pleural surface. Electrocautery is avoided until the specimen is removed to avoid cautery artifact that can significantly alter the histologic examination.

After all specimens have been removed and hemostasis is achieved, the entire area is irrigated before removal of the trocars. A small thoracostomy tube (24 to 28 French) is

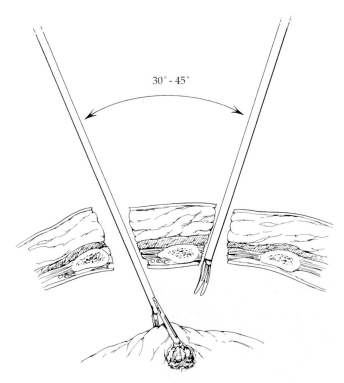

Fig. 50-5. A 30° to 45° angle of attack is optimal during biopsy of the lesion.

placed through the anterior-most incision. After all the instruments and trocars are removed, the skin and subcutaneous tissue are closed using interrupted absorbable suture. The chest tube is placed to suction.

Postoperatively, the patient is sent to the recovery room and from there to a standard floor bed. Unless the patient has a specific medical problem that requires it, an intensive care unit stay is unnecessary. In a young, healthy patient with minimal drainage form the chest tube, we frequently remove the chest tube in the recovery room. Otherwise, the chest tube is placed to a waterseal in the recovery room and removed the next morning on the floor. Diet is advanced immediately, and an incentive spirometer is used routinely. Postoperative laboratory studies are tailored to each patient's medical condition. For an otherwise healthy patient, two postoperative chest radiographs are all that is usually required.

Pleural Effusion

Determining the cause of a pleural effusion can be elusive despite analysis of thoracentesis fluid and percutaneous pleural biopsy techniques. It is estimated that the diagnostic yield of these techniques combined is only 60%. Studies have shown that, of the 40% that remain, a diagnosis can be obtained using video thoracoscopy for 85% to 90% of cases. This increased diagnostic utility probably results from the ability to completely examine and biopsy the entire parietal and visceral pleural surface through the thoracoscope. A second advantage of thoracoscopy over percutaneous techniques is the ability to provide an immediate treatment. The effusive process can be obliterated at the time of diagnosis using chemical or mechanical pleurodesis.

In the preoperative evaluation of the patient with undiagnosed pleural effusion, a meticulous search should be undertaken to locate a distant malignancy as a source for metastatic disease. If no malignancy is found, a complete metabolic workup is performed to find a reason for the effusion. Percutaneous aspiration of the fluid should be performed and the fluid sent for chemical, bacterial, and cytologic analysis. If all these steps fail to reveal the diagnosis, the patient should be prepared for diagnostic thoracoscopy. Preoperative preparation from this point on parallels that for patients with pleura-based lesions.

The patient should be initially positioned on the operating table supine with a standard endotracheal tube to allow for bronchoscopy. After diagnostic bronchoscopy is complete, a double-lumen endotracheal tube is placed, and the patient is placed in a lateral decubitus position with the affected lung side up. The patient is prepped and draped in a way to allow for a thoracotomy if necessary.

The initial incision is made in the middle to anterior axillary line at the fifth or sixth intercostal space. The dissection is taken down to the pleural membrane, taking care to stay along the superior aspect of the rib. The lung is then selectively deflated, and the pleural cavity entered using a blunt instrument. At this point, there usually is a rush of pleural fluid out of the chest. Standard suction can be used to aspirate the fluid for containment and for analysis.

After the fluid is aspirated, a 10-mm, blunt-tipped trocar is inserted. Through this port, a 10-mm videoscope is inserted. Use of 30° or 45° scope can help. A blunt-tipped instrument can be placed through the same hole to help deflate the lung and completely examine the pleural space. A second 5-mm trocar can be inserted under direct vision to facilitate the exploration if necessary. After complete exploration, any suspicious lesions are biopsied using biopsy forceps or endoscopic scissors as previously described. If no suspicious lesions are found, random biopsies of the pleural membrane are taken using endoscopic scissors and the blunt-tipped grasper (Fig. 50-6).

If a suspicious lesion or mass is found on the lung parenchyma, a wedge biopsy is performed. The technique for wedge biopsy requires a minimum of three ports, at least one of which is 12 mm in diameter. After the mass or lesion is identified, it is held in retraction with a blunt grasper or Babcock clamp. A 5-mm camera can be used to visualize the lesion through one of the 5-mm ports while the 12-mm port is used to place the endoscopic linear stapling device. While retracting on the lesion, the stapler is used to resect a wedge-shaped portion of the lung parenchyma (Fig. 50-7). Several firings of the stapler may be necessary to completely resect the lesion. After resection, the specimen is removed through the 10-mm port site. A sterile bag may be necessary to facilitate removal of the specimen.

After the diagnostic procedures are complete, a decision must be made concerning pleurodesis or pleurectomy. The preference at my institution is mechanical

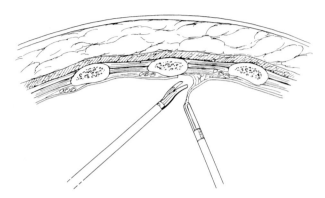

Fig. 50-6. A portion of pleural membrane is removed with endoscopic scissors for diagnostic purposes. This technique can also be used to perform a pleurectomy.

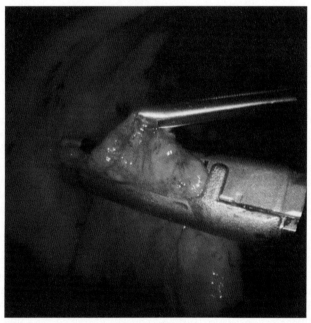

Fig. 50-7. A wedge biopsy is performed using an endoscopic linear stapling device. (From Zucker KA, ed. Surgical laparoscopy update. *St. Louis: Quality Medical Publishing, 1993; with permission.)*

pleurodesis at the time of surgery. My colleagues and I use a small piece of Prolene mesh as the mechanical device. The mesh is folded in half twice and held in the end of a long, curved sponge stick or curved Kelley clamp. The instrument is then inserted into the chest cavity. Under direct vision, the abrasive edges of the mesh are used to abrade the pleural membrane over the entire plural cavity (Fig. 50-8). Special attention is given to the apex of the chest. A complete pleu-

rodesis is confirmed by noting erythematous and swollen membrane throughout the chest.

If pleurectomy is needed to obliterate the effusion, it can be performed using the thoracoscope. Multiple portions of the pleural membrane are held in retraction by blunt graspers while the endoscopic scissors are used to cut the pleura away from the chest wall. In this way, the pleural membrane can be stripped

completely and removed. Significant bleeding can ensue, but it can be controlled with electrocautery. Chemical pleurodesis usually is unnecessary in addition to pleurectomy.

If chemical pleurodesis is to be performed, it can be done at the time of surgery. Many agents are available for chemical pleurodesis. Our preference is talc. The agent can be instilled through any or all of the port sites to obtain a complete pleurodesis. If this is to

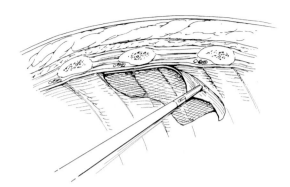

Fig. 50-8. Mechanical pleuradeses.

be performed in addition to mechanical pleurodesis, the agent should be instilled after the abrasive procedure. If it is performed instead of a mechanical pleurodesis, the agent should be instilled before closure.

After the procedure is complete, all trocars are removed and a single chest tube is inserted into the anterior-most trocar site. The wounds are closed in layers and the chest tube secured. The patient is typically extubated in the operating room, and a chest radiograph is obtained in the recovery room. After recovery, the patient is sent to the floor unless cardiac or respiratory disease necessitates an intensive care unit stay. Chest tubes can usually be removed on the first or second postoperative day, unless further chemical pleurodesis is required. If the lung parenchyma was violated during surgery, as with a wedge biopsy, care must be taken that there is no air leak before removing the chest tube.

Fibrothorax

Intervention for fibrothorax is indicated to re-expand a trapped lung. Causes include unresolved hemothorax, unresolved empyema, and solidified pleural effusion. Timing of surgical intervention can be controversial; however, after conservative measures have failed, early intervention can reduce morbidity by decreasing the risk for pneumonia in the entrapped lung. Conservative measures such as percutaneous aspiration are notoriously ineffective because they fail to deal with the thick peel surrounding the lung. In the past, definitive therapy required thoracotomy, but thoracoscopy has been successful in decorticating even difficult fibrothoraces and allowing shorter hospital stays and decreased morbidity.

The preoperative evaluation of the patient with fibrothorax is aimed at determining the cause and exhausting conservative measures. A retained hemothorax in a trauma patient is rarely amenable to percutaneous techniques, whereas a parapneumonic effusion can sometimes be treated successfully with thoracentesis. The diagnosis is usually obvious on a plain chest radiograph, but if the cause is uncertain, a CT scan may be helpful.

After the decision is made to intervene operatively, the patient is prepared for surgery. Bronchoscopy is performed through a standard oral endotracheal tube while the patient is supine. Full cultures are taken by bronchoalveolar lavage. Once complete, the endotracheal tube is replaced with a double-lumen tube, and the patient is placed in a lateral decubitus position with the affected lung up. The chest is prepped and draped to provide adequate access for a thoracotomy if necessary.

After adequate positioning, the initial incision is made in the middle to anterior axillary line at the sixth or seventh intercostal space. The dissection is taken down to the pleural membrane, taking care to stay directly alongside the superior aspect of the rib. The lung is then deflated by clamping the appropriate limb of the double-lumen tube. The pleural cavity is entered using a blunt instrument. A finger is then inserted to lyse any surrounding adhesions. Once clear, a 10-mm, blunt-tipped trocar is inserted through the chest wall.

After the trocar is in place, a 10-mm videoscope is inserted into the cavity. In most cases, the cavity is filled with fibrinous exudate that prevents collapse of the lung and obscures vision. The trocar is then pulled back along the shaft of the videoscope to al-

low placement of a suction/irrigation device through the same incision. Using this as a blunt instrument, the fibrothorax is broken up and separated from the lung. After the cavity is opened further, a second incision is made lateral to the first. Dissection is carried over the rib into the pleural space under direct vision. The suction/irrigator can then be placed through this incision to further lyse the fibrothorax. For particularly difficult cases, a Yankauer suction tip can be inserted through the incision to provide a more rigid, angled instrument to break up the fibrous material. Multiple incisions may be required for evacuation, but complete removal of the peel can usually be accomplished with only three incisions. After the lung is decorticated, a pleurectomy or chemical pleurodesis can be performed. My colleagues and I prefer to perform a talc pleurodesis.

After the procedure is complete, one or two large-bore chest tubes are inserted through the anterior-most incisions. The wounds are closed in multiple layers, and the chest tube or tubes are secured in place (Fig. 50-9). The patient is extubated in the

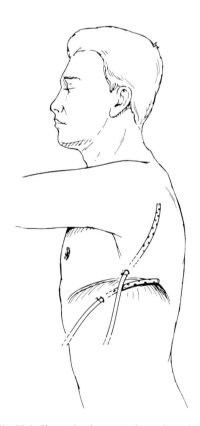

Fig. 50-9. Chest tube placement after endoscopic empyema drainage.

operating room when possible and transferred to the recovery room, where the chest tubes are placed to suction. The recovered patient is transferred to the floor unless a specific problem necessitates a stay in the intensive care unit.

Postoperative management concentrates on chest tube management. Antibiotics are used only for infectious fibrothorax and are targeted to the intraoperative culture results. The chest tubes are removed sequentially when the drainage is sufficiently low. Serial chest radiographs are usually unnecessary except to confirm complete expansion of the lung. Early ambulation is often possible and can help reduce pulmonary morbidity. If an infectious process was diagnosed at surgery by Gram stain or culture results, the chest tubes are left as empyema catheters. If not, the tubes can be removed early.

Empyema

Empyema usually develops as a result of the extension of infection from a contiguous structure. The etiologic factors and therapy have undergone a series of changes during the last 60 years. The development and availability of antibiotics has reduced the incidence of empyema due to streptococcal and pneumococcal pleuropulmonary infections. Most empyemas result from necrotizing anaerobic infections of the lung and from postoperative complications after pulmonary and esophageal resections. Regardless of the cause, definitive treatment cannot be accomplished without adequate drainage. Initial drainage can be accomplished with tube thoracostomy, but this is often unsuccessful, and subsequent surgery is required.

Preoperative evaluation is aimed chiefly at determining the cause and exhausting all conservative measures. After the decision is made to proceed with surgery, standard preoperative testing is performed.

At the time of surgery, the patient is initially placed supine to allow for diagnostic bronchoscopy through a standard oral endotracheal tube. After bronchoscopy, including bronchoalveolar lavage, is complete, the endotracheal tube is replaced with a double-lumen tube. The patient is then placed in a lateral decubitus position with the affected lung side up. The chest is prepped and draped in a fashion to allow access for a thoracotomy if necessary.

The initial incision is made in the middle to anterior axillary line. The dissection is carried to the pleural membrane, taking care to stay along the superior aspect of the rib. The pleural cavity is entered using a blunt instrument after the appropriate lung is deflated. A 10-mm port is then inserted into the chest, followed by the 10-mm videoscope. One or two more ports are placed laterally to allow access for a suction/irrigation device and a blunt grasper. Using these two instruments, the fibrous material is removed, and the adhesions are lysed. After the cavity is completely cleaned, a pleurectomy or pleurodesis can be performed.

After completion of the procedure, one or two chest tubes are inserted through the anterior-most incisions. The wounds are closed in layers, and the chest tubes are secured. The patient is extubated and sent to the floor after recovery. An intensive care unit stay is typically unnecessary.

The chest tubes are allowed to drain the cavity while continuing intravenous antibiotics. The tubes are removed when drainage is sufficiently low and the infectious process is under control. Serial chest radiographs are usually unnecessary except to ensure full expansion of the lung. Early ambulation can be accomplished by placing the tubes to a waterseal. This allows continued drainage while freeing the patient to leave the room.

Suggested Reading

Garcha I, Conn J. Outpatient thoracoscopy: a case report and discussion. *Am Surg* 1995;61: 229–230.

Jacobeus HC. The practical importance of thoracoscopy in surgery of the chest. *Surg Gynecol Obstet* 1922;34:289.

Landreneau RJ, Mack MJ, Hazelrigg SR, et al. Video-assisted thoracic surgery: basic technical concepts and intercostal approach strategies. *Ann Thorac Surg* 1992;54:800–807.

Menzies R, Charbonneau M. Thoracoscopy for the diagnosis of pleural disease. *Ann Intern Med* 1991;114:271–276.

Webb WR, Ozmen V, Moulder PV, Shabahang B, Breaux J. Iodized talc pleurodesis for the treatment of pleural effusions. *J Thorac Cardiovasc Surg* 1992;103:881–885.

Zucker KA, ed. *Surgical laparoscopy update.* St. Louis: Quality Medical Publishing, 1993.

EDITOR'S COMMENT

Diagnostic thoracoscopy for diseases of the pleural space has been described since 1910. The first therapeutic use of thoracoscopy was by Jacobaeus in 1992. Video enhancement and improved thoracoscopic tools, including angled and flexible laparoscopes, curved instruments, and stapling devices, engendered a new awareness of the potential for this modality in the 1980s. Although more invasive than image-guided biopsy, thoracoscopy remains a highly accurate and sensitive diagnostic tool. It offers all the advantages of open surgery for exposure, visualization, and ability to obtain large pathology specimens while avoiding the high degree of morbidity of a thoracotomy incision. The success of diagnostic thoracoscopy has led to it being applied to a wider spectrum of pulmonary conditions than pleural lesion assessment. Thoracoscopy is being used for treatment of empyema, spontaneous pneumothorax, and malignant pleural effusions and for evaluation and treatment of penetrating trauma of the chest wall, including diaphragmatic injuries. Thoracoscopy is an invaluable diagnostic and therapeutic tool for the diagnosis and treatment of problems of the pleural space.

L.L.S.

51

Thoracoscopic Esophageal Procedures

Jeffrey H. Peters, Luigi Bonavina, and Jeffrey A. Hagen

Minimally invasive approaches are increasingly being employed in the treatment of esophageal diseases. Laparoscopic Nissen fundoplication, myotomy of the lower esophageal sphincter (LES) and esophageal body, epiphrenic diverticulectomy, resection of esophageal leiomyomas or duplication cysts, and thoracoscopic esophagectomy have all been described. Many of these procedures can be performed through either the abdomen or chest. While the ideal approach has yet to be determined for many of these procedures, the thoracoscopic route is advantageous in many settings.

Of the thoracoscopic esophageal procedures described, only myotomy of the LES is performed with any frequency. While amenable to minimally invasive techniques, epiphrenic diverticula and esophageal leiomyomas are rarely encountered. Thoracoscopic esophagectomy for both benign and malignant disease remains highly controversial. Nearly all studies investigating the role of thoracoscopy in esophagectomy have demonstrated morbidity and mortality equal to or greater than that of traditional open procedures. At present, thoracoscopic antireflux procedures remain beyond the capabilities of safe and effective minimally invasive surgery.

Esophageal Motility Disorders

Esophageal motility disorders constitute the most common indications for a thoracoscopic approach to esophageal disease. Commonly encountered motility disorders of the body of the esophagus and LES

are shown in Table 51-1. Surgical treatment of these disorders is based on the ablation of motor activity via myotomy of the circular and longitudinal muscle layers of the LES and esophageal body. Achalasia is the primary indication for an LES my-

Table 51-1. Characteristics of the Primary Esophageal Motility Disorders on Standard Manometry

ACHALASIA

Incomplete lower esophageal sphincter (LES) relaxation (<75% relaxation)

Aperistalsis in the esophageal body

Elevated LES pressure >26 mm Hg

Increased intraesophageal baseline pressures relative to gastric baseline

DIFFUSE ESOPHAGEAL SPASM

Simultaneous (peristaltic contractions) (>20% of wet swallows)

Repetitive and multipeaked contractions

Spontaneous contractions

Intermittent normal peristalsis

Contractions may be of increased amplitude and duration

NUTCRACKER ESOPHAGUS

Mean peristaltic amplitude in the distal esophagus >180 mm Hg

Normal peristaltic sequence

HYPERTENSIVE LOWER ESOPHAGEAL SPHINCTER

Elevated LES pressure >26 mm Hg

Normal LES relaxation

Normal peristalsis in the esophageal body

NONSPECIFIC ESOPHAGEAL MOTILITY DISORDERS

Decreased or absent amplitude of esophageal peristalsis

Increased number of nontransmitted contractions

Abnormal wave forms

Normal mean LES pressure and relaxation

otomy. Patients with dysphagia and motor disorders of the esophageal body, characterized by segmental or generalized simultaneous contractions, may benefit from a long esophageal myotomy. These disorders include diffuse and segmental esophageal spasm, vigorous achalasia, and nonspecific motility disorders associated with a mid- or epiphrenic esophageal diverticulum.

Achalasia

Diagnosis and Indications

Achalasia is the best known primary motility disorder of the esophagus. It is a disease of unknown etiology occurring in 6 per 100,000 population. Patients typically present with progressive dysphagia for both solids and liquids, regurgitation, and occasionally chest pain. The diagnosis is confirmed on the basis of classic manometric features including failure of the LES to relax on deglutition, an aperistaltic esophageal body, hypertension of the LES, and elevation of intraluminal esophageal pressure. The combination of a noncompliant, nonrelaxing LES followed by peristaltic failure of the esophageal body results in esophageal retention of swallowed food and saliva and ultimately in dilatation of the esophageal body. With time, this results in the typical radiographic appearance of a dilated esophagus with tapering, beak-like narrowing of the distal end.

Selection of Approach

The goal of the treatment of achalasia is relief of the functional outflow obstruction secondary to the loss of the ability of the LES to relax fully. Successful treatment requires attention to the balance between relief of esophageal outflow obstruction imposed by the LES and the loss of LES competency. If this balance is not achieved, relief of dysphagia will be replaced by the experience of heartburn.

Four important principles govern the performance of a surgical myotomy of the LES:

1. Minimal dissection of the cardia,
2. Adequate distal myotomy to reduce outflow resistance,
3. Prevention of postoperative reflux,
4. Prevention of healing proximation of the myotomized muscle.

The development of a reflux-induced stricture due to the loss of LES competency after a myotomy is a serious problem that usually necessitates esophagectomy.

If simultaneous esophageal contractions are associated with the LES abnormality, the so-called vigorous achalasia, then the myotomy should extend over the distance of the motility abnormality as mapped by the preoperative motility study. Failure to do this will result in continuing dysphagia and a dissatisfied patient. Use of a fundoplication after a myotomy to prevent reflux has been debated. A balance must be obtained between relieving the outflow resistance responsible for achalasia and allowing free reflux through an incompetent LES. Some surgeons have chosen to perform a meticulous myotomy without an antireflux procedure, carefully limiting the extent of the dissection and distal myotomy in an effort to minimize postoperative reflux, while others have combined the myotomy with a partial or complete fundoplication. Recent studies have shown that when an antireflux procedure is added to the myotomy, it should be a partial fundoplication. A 360-degree fundoplication is associated with progressive retention of swallowed food, regurgitation, and aspiration to a degree that exceeds patients' preoperative symptoms.

Perioperative Management

Because of long-standing dysphagia, weight loss, and difficulty in tolerating oral fluids, patients with functional foregut disorders require special consideration prior to and during induction of anesthesia. Dehydration, chronic aspiration, and a dilated esophagus full of debris

make anesthetic induction hazardous for the unaware. Admission to the hospital for 24 to 48 hours prior to surgery may be required to allow intravenous hydration and pulmonary physiotherapy. Patients with achalasia should be limited to clear liquids for 48 hours prior to anesthetic induction. In the presence of a massively dilated and tortuous esophagus, lavage of the esophageal lumen via an endoscope or nasogastric tube may be required. The anesthesiologist should be cognizant of the high risk of aspiration.

Thoracoscopic Myotomy of the Lower Esophageal Sphincter

Our initial experience with minimally invasive esophageal myotomy is based on the following principles:

1. A thoracoscopic rather than a laparoscopic approach;
2. Minimal dissection of the esophagus and esophageal hiatus to preserve the normal anatomic antireflux mechanisms;
3. Precise control of the distal extent of the myotomy, limiting it to the anatomic gastroesophageal (GE) junction;
4. Definition of the GE junction via an intraluminal flexible endoscope.

The procedure is performed with the patient in the right lateral decubitus position. A double-lumen endotracheal tube is used to allow selective ventilation of the right lung.

A four-port technique is employed in addition to a small (2.5 cm) incision along the left costal margin for placement of retracting instruments (Fig. 51-1). A 10-mm port

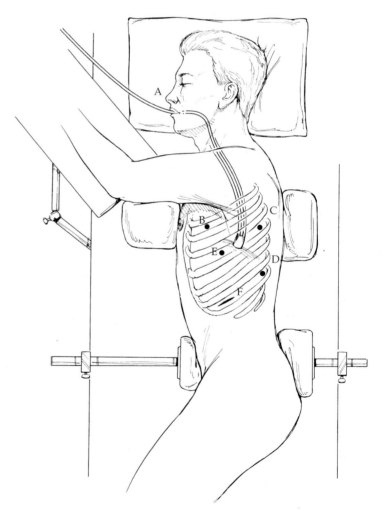

Fig. 51-1. Patient and surgeon positioning for thoracoscopic esophageal myotomy and trocar placement. Four 10-mm thoracoports and a single 4-cm incision are used. (A, endoscope; B, 10-mm port [scissors]; C, 10-mm port [camera]; D, 10-mm port [grasper]; E, 10-mm port [grasper]; F, incision.)

is placed posterior to the scapula in the fourth intercostal space and used for the camera. Meticulous hemostasis is important when the trocar holes are created. Bleeding from the trocar site is common and very troublesome during the procedure, particularly for the camera port. Air is allowed to enter the thorax, and the left lung is slowly deflated, with some assistance from the shaft of the telescope. A second 10-mm port is placed high and anterior in the second to third intercostal space at the anterior axillary line. A Babcock clamp is placed through this port and utilized as a lung retractor following dissection of the inferior pulmonary ligament. The right-handed surgeon's port is placed at the midaxillary line in the sixth to seventh intercostal space. The position should be such that the electrocautery hook placed through the right-handed trocar is directly above the esophagus and not approaching it from an angle. Placing this trocar too high can result in difficulty in performing the myotomy near the GE junction. The left-handed surgeon's trocar is placed low, inferior, and posterior, above the diaphragm in the ninth to tenth intercostal space. Finally, a 4-cm incision is made along the left costal margin directly above the esophagus for placement of three instruments: a fan retractor to displace the diaphragm inferiorly, a long vein retractor to retract the crura superiorly, and a suction/irrigation device. With selective ventilation of the right lung, it is not necessary to insufflate the left hemithorax. One advantage of thoracoscopy is that airtight ports are not necessary, allowing small incisions and the placement of standard instruments. We have found that angled-viewing laparoscopes/thoracoscopes are preferable to 0-degree scopes.

Proper retraction and exposure of the esophagus and hiatus are critical to the dissection and require some attention at the outset. The diaphragm should be forcefully displaced inferiorly via the large fan retractor, completely exposing the esophageal hiatus (Fig. 51-2). Identification and dissection of the esophagus are aided by the concomitant use of an endoscope within the esophageal lumen, allowing displacement of the esophagus to the left. In patients with achalasia, the esophagus is often dilated and easily seen. The mediastinal pleura overlying the terminal esophagus is divided sharply with scissors, and the inferior pulmonary liga-

ment divided is for 2 to 3 cm (Fig. 51-3). A Babcock clamp placed through the high anterior port is used to retract the left lower lobe and left lung toward the superior thorax.

The dissection is consciously kept to a minimum, preserving normal hiatal structures. The crural arch is dissected just as the esophagus passes beneath, allowing placement of a long vein retractor underneath the arch and retraction of the crura away from the esophagus (Fig. 51-4). The gastric serosa usually becomes evident and is recognized by its more distinct, white color. No attempt is made to mobilize any portion of the stomach, only to visualize the GE junction.

The myotomy is begun 2 to 3 cm above the GE junction and performed with an L-hook electrocautery probe (Fig. 51-5). Magnification by the telescope usually allows clear visualization of the longitudinal and circu-

lar muscle fibers. The vagus nerves are also easily seen, and care must be used to avoid injuring them during dissection. Insufflation via an intraluminal flexible endoscope allows the mucosa to pouch out between the cut ends of the muscle, clearly outlining the myotomized segment. In addition, the endoscope within the lumen of the esophagus can be used to help prevent mucosal injury by applying suction, collapsing the mucosa prior to using the electrocautery. Once the esophageal mucosa is clearly identified, the myotomy is carried distally with an electrocautery probe or scissors. The inferior extent of the myotomy is carefully judged using the endoscope. The myotomy is ended when it has reached the endoscopic GE junction, and the functional obstruction commonly associated with achalasia is alleviated.

At completion of the procedure, the dependent portion of the left chest is filled with water, and air is insufflated via the

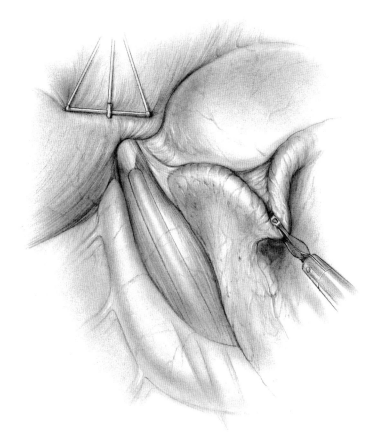

Fig. 51-2. Thoracoscopic esophageal myotomy illustrating the exposure obtained with video-assisted technology. This allows the traditional myotomy of the lower esophageal sphincter or body to be done without a thoracotomy. The diaphragm is forcefully retracted toward the patient's abdomen with a fan-shaped retractor inserted through a small incision along the left costal border. The left lower lung is retracted superiorly and anteriorly by a Babcock clamp placed in a high anterior port.

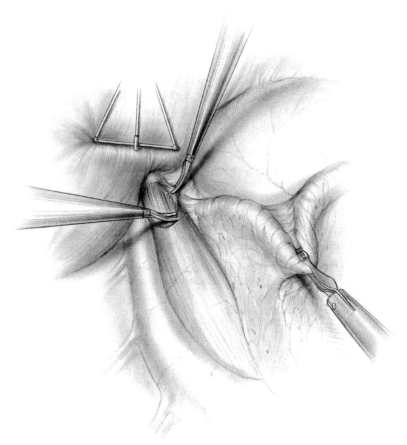

Fig. 51-3. *Videoscopic view of the initial dissection for myotomy of the lower esophageal sphincter. The pleura overlying the lower esophagus is incised, and the dissection continued by dissecting the crura of the diaphragm at the gastroesophageal junction.*

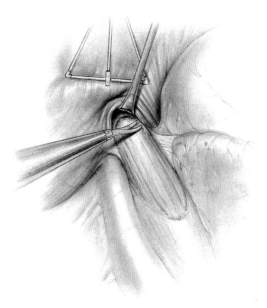

Fig. 51-4. *Initial dissection is continued by dissecting the crura of the diaphragm at the gastroesophageal junction.*

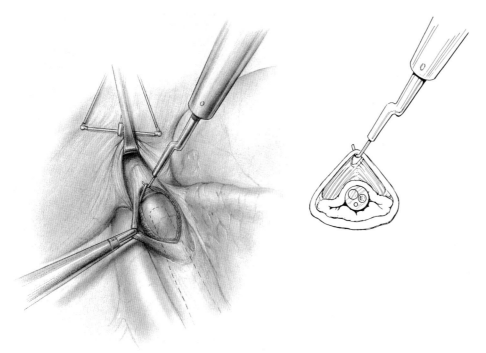

Fig. 51-5. *The myotomy is begun 2 to 3 cm above the gastroesophageal (GE) junction and carried out with an* L*-hook electrocautery instrument. Note the intraluminal endoscope as an aid in defining the GE junction. The* **inset** *demonstrates collapse of the mucosa as suction is applied via the endoscope just prior to the application of electrocautery.*

endoscope to check for esophageal mucosal integrity (Fig. 51-6). A small-caliber chest tube is placed and the left lung reinflated under direct vision. All trocars are removed and the wounds closed in a two-layer fashion.

A nasogastric tube is not necessary; its placement may be potentially hazardous following myotomy. A video contrast esophagram is performed the day following surgery, and if it is acceptable, the patient allowed liquids. Hospital stay in the absence of comorbid disease is generally 3 to 4 days.

Diffuse Esophageal Spasm

Diagnosis and Indications

Diffuse esophageal spasm (DES) is less common than achalasia, occurring about five times less frequently. It is characterized clinically by substernal chest pain and/or dysphagia. It differs from classic achalasia in that it is primarily a disease of the esophageal body, produces a lesser degree of dysphagia, causes more chest pain, and has less effect on the patient's general condition. Chest pain is typically substernal and may radiate into the back or up into the neck. The pain is often provoked by eating but may occur spontaneously. Dysphagia associated with DES tends to be less prominent than in patients with achalasia, and often occurs simultaneously with episodes of chest pain. The diagnosis of DES is confirmed on the basis of motility findings of simultaneous, high-amplitude, aperistaltic contractions in the body of the esophagus. Relaxation of the LES is normal. Radiographically, DES is evident in approximately 50% of patients, appearing as segmental spasm, pseudodiverticulosis, or rarely a corkscrew esophagus. A hiatal hernia or epiphrenic diverticulum may also be present.

The decision to operate on patients with DES is made based on the severity of their symptoms, their dietary and lifestyle adjustments as a result of the disease, and their nutritional status. The driving force should be the severity of a patient's swallowing disability. The symptom of chest pain alone is generally not an indication for esophageal myotomy, as the results in this setting have been disappointing.

Perioperative Management

In patients selected for myotomy of the esophageal body, preoperative manometry is essential to confirm the diagnosis and determine the proximal extent of the myotomy. Most surgeons extend the myotomy distally across the LES to reduce the outflow resistance to the aperistaltic

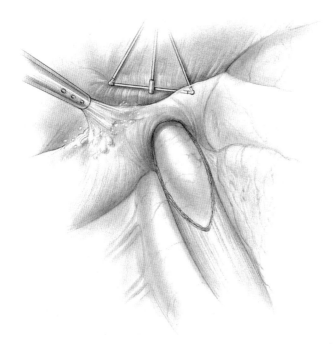

Fig. 51-6. *Following completion of the myotomy, the lower chest and esophagus are irrigated with water. The integrity of the esophageal mucosa is checked by insufflating air via the intraluminal endoscope.*

esophagus resulting from complete myotomy. Consequently, some form of antireflux protection may be added to avoid GE reflux. If symptoms suggestive of reflux are present preoperatively, particularly in patients with a concomitant hiatal hernia, 24-hour pH monitoring should be performed to confirm its presence.

Thoracoscopic Long Esophageal Myotomy

The technique of long esophageal myotomy is similar to that of myotomy limited to the LES, with the exception of the need for complete retraction of the lung to allow extension of the myotomy. In an open procedure, lung retraction is not a problem. Thoracoscopically, however, lung retraction can be difficult. Proper positioning of the patient is critical to allowing lung retraction. A prone position would be the ideal, allowing the left lung to fall forward away from the esophagus and facilitating exposure. Because of the possibility of open thoracotomy, we have been reluctant to place patients in a completely prone position, which would undoubtedly make posterolateral thoracotomy more difficult. For this reason, we prefer to place the patient in the right lateral decubitus position and then roll him

or her 45 degrees further toward prone. A bean bag and tape are used to secure the patient. The table is rolled the remaining 45 degrees so that the patient ends up nearly prone. Should thoracotomy be necessary, the table can be rolled to the lateral position and thoracotomy performed without difficulty. Prone positioning is the key element allowing simple retraction of the left lung and thus long myotomy.

Port placement and the initial dissection are identical to those of an LES myotomy. With suitable lung retraction, the myotomy is performed through all muscle layers, extending distally to the endoscopic GE junction and proximally on the esophagus over the distance of the manometric abnormality (Fig. 51-7). The muscle layer is dissected from the mucosa laterally for a distance of 1 cm. Care is taken to divide all minute muscle bands, particularly in the area of the GE junction.

Diverticula of the Esophageal Body
Diagnosis and Indications

Esophageal diverticula are not common lesions. They occur frequently enough, however, that most surgeons will en-

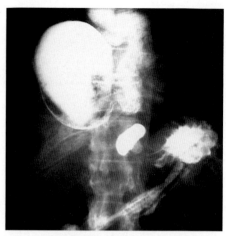

Fig. 51-8. Radiographic appearance of large epiphrenic diverticulum in a patient with achalasia.

counter several during their careers. These outpouchings of the esophageal wall have been classified based on histology, pathophysiology, and their location. Histologically, both true diverticula, containing all layers of the esophageal wall, and false diverticula, containing mucosa only, are recognized.

Epiphrenic, or lower esophageal, diverticula are generally of the pulsion type and tend to occur in the elderly. Although pulsion diverticula can develop at any level of the esophagus, they have a predilection for the distal 10 cm (Fig. 51-8). They are much less frequent than Zenker's diverticula and have a 2:1 male-to-female predominance. Most patients have mild symptoms or are asymptomatic. The predominant symptoms are dysphagia, regurgitation, or those of the underlying foregut disorder. Complications include aspiration, pneumonia, and rarely squamous carcinoma.

Physiologic evaluation of esophageal and foregut function cannot be overemphasized. Many lower esophageal diverticula are associated with motility disorders and/or GE reflux and hiatal hernia. An underlying functional or mechanical obstruction can usually be identified. Debas found that most are single and many are associated with a hiatal hernia. He also pointed out that associated manometric abnormalities of the lower esophagus such as achalasia or DES are common.

Selection of Approach

Complete treatment commonly requires not only excision of diverticula but also esophageal myotomy and/or considera-

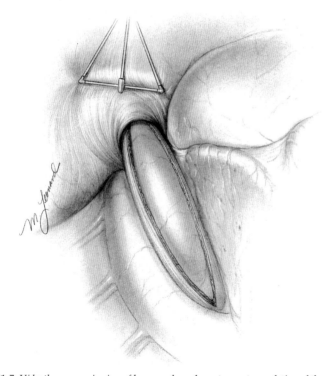

Fig. 51-7. Videothoracoscopic view of long esophageal myotomy at completion of the myotomy.

tion of other underlying disorders. Whether a diverticulum should be surgically resected or suspended depends on its size and proximity to the vertebral body. When diverticula are associated with esophageal motility disorders, esophageal myotomy from the distal extent of the diverticula to the stomach is indicated; otherwise, one can expect a high incidence of suture-line rupture due to the same intraluminal pressure that initially gave rise to diverticula. If a diverticulum is suspended to the prevertebral fascia of the thoracic vertebra, a myotomy is begun at its neck and extended across the LES. If a diverticulum is excised by dividing the neck, the muscle is closed over the excision site, and a myotomy is performed on the opposite esophageal wall, starting at the level of diverticulum. When a large diverticulum is associated with a hiatal hernia, it is excised, a myotomy is performed if there is an associated esophageal motility abnormality, and the hernia is repaired because of the high incidence of postoperative reflux when this is omitted.

Thoracoscopic Resection of Epiphrenic Diverticula

Although lower esophageal diverticula are approached in the open setting via a left posterolateral thoracotomy, most have been approached thoracoscopically via the right chest. This is because the majority of epiphrenic diverticula develop from the right side of the esophagus and are adherent to the right pleura and/or diaphragm. The ideal approach remains unknown. Treatment of an associated motor disorder via esophageal myotomy and/or repair of a hiatal hernia and fundoplication may be difficult from the right chest and require a second access through the left chest or abdomen.

A double-lumen endotracheal tube is used to allow left lung retraction. The patient is placed in the left lateral decubitus position. Four trocars are placed analogously to those described for myotomy of the LES (Fig. 51-9). Dissection is begun by taking down the inferior pulmonary ligament and freeing the right lower lobe to the level of the inferior pulmonary vein. The right lung is then retracted into the upper chest via a Babcock clamp placed into one of the anterosuperior ports. The pleura overlying the esophagus is incised, and the right lateral aspect of the esopha-

gus is dissected for a distance of 8 to 10 cm (Fig. 51-10). Usually, the diverticular sac will become evident and can be carefully dissected from its inflammatory attachments (Fig. 51-11). Meticulous dissection of the diverticular sac, which consists of mucosa only, is required to prevent injury and spillage. A Babcock clamp may be placed on the sac and gentle traction used to facilitate dissection of the diverticular neck. Analogously to the left-sided approach for esophageal myotomy, we do not hesitate to create a 4-cm incision superiorly in the tenth to eleventh interspace, through which additional instruments, a fan retractor for diaphragmatic retraction, and a suction/irrigation device may be placed. Once completely dissected, the diverticulum is excised in the presence of a large (50 to 60 French) intraesophageal bougie or, alternatively, with an endoscope in the esophageal lu-

men. Endoscopic visualization is helpful for checking the placement of the stapler after closure of the jaws, as well as for inspecting the integrity of the suture line after the diverticulum is resected. An endoscopic linear stapler is used, generally introduced via one of the more cephalad ports (Fig. 51-12). Orienting the stapler parallel to the longitudinal axis of the esophagus can be difficult. If this is unsatisfactory, a video-assisted approach can be utilized by extending the previously placed incision and inserting a hand for esophageal retraction and orientation of the stapler. The muscle layer is generally closed over the mucosal suture line with interrupted sutures of 4-0 polypropylene (Fig. 51-13). We prefer extracorporeal knot-tying techniques. Appropriate secondary procedures for achalasia or hiatal hernia and GE reflux are added, depending on the preoperative physiology. Stan-

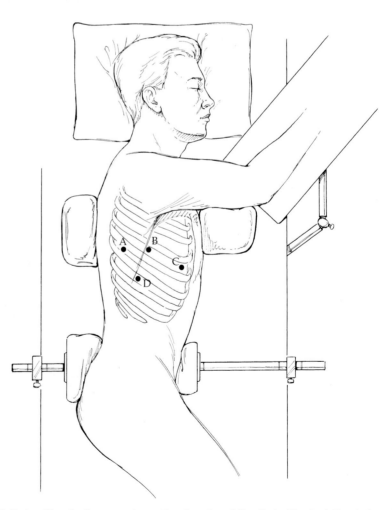

Fig. 51-9. Port positions for thoracoscopic resection of esophageal diverticula. (Proximal diverticulum: A, 10 mm; B, 10 mm; C, 10 mm; D, camera port. Resection of diverticulum: A, 10 mm; B, 10 mm; C, camera port; D, Endo GIA stapler.)

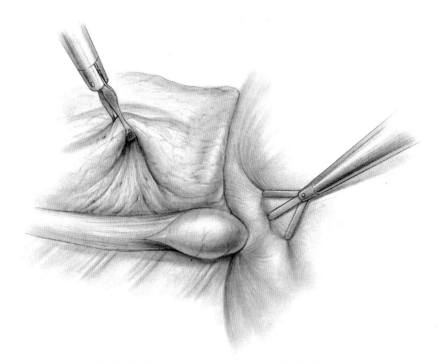

Fig. 51-10. Thoracoscopic view of an epiphrenic diverticulum.

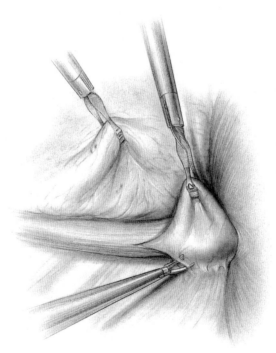

Fig. 51-11. Dissection of an epiphrenic diverticulum through a right thoracoscopic approach. The camera is positioned between the two operating instruments.

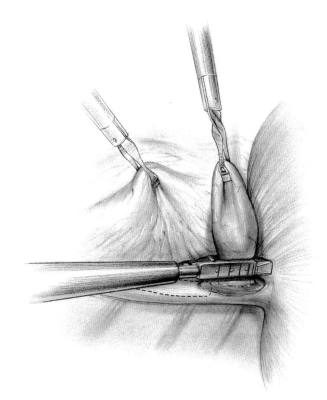

Fig. 51-12. The camera is moved to allow the endoscopic stapler to be applied to the neck of the diverticulum. Inset: Position of ports and instruments.

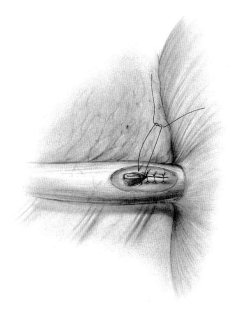

Fig. 51-13. Following diverticulectomy, the muscle edges are approximated with interrupted sutures.

dard chest tube drainage is placed, and the wounds are closed. Video esophagography is performed at postoperative day 1 to 2 to assess both the functional result

and the mucosal integrity prior to feeding.

Leiomyoma of the Esophagus
Diagnosis and Indications

Leiomyomas represent two-thirds of benign tumors of the esophagus, although still uncommon. They are more common in men than in women, with an average age at presentation of 38 years. Because they originate in smooth muscle, 90% are located in the lower two-thirds of the esophagus. They are usually solitary, but multiple tumors are found on occasion. They vary greatly in size and shape. Tumors as small as 1 cm in diameter and as large as 10 lbs (4.54 kg) have been removed.

Typically, leiomyomas are oval in shape. During their growth, they remain intramural, with the bulk of their mass protruding toward the outer wall of the esophagus. The overlying mucosa is freely movable and normal in appearance. Neither their size nor their loca-

tion correlate with the degree of symptoms. Dysphagia and pain are the most common complaints and occur more frequently together than separately. Bleeding directly related to the tumor is rare. Thus, when hematemesis or melena occurs in a patient with an esophageal leiomyoma, other causes should be investigated.

A barium swallow examination is the most useful method to demonstrate a leiomyoma of the esophagus. In profile, the tumor appears as a smooth, semilunar or crescent-shaped filling defect that moves with swallowing, is sharply demarcated, and is covered and surrounded by normal mucosa. Esophagoscopy should be performed to exclude the reported observation of a coexistence with carcinoma. The freely movable mass that bulges into the lumen should not be biopsied because of an increased chance of mucosal perforation at the time of surgical enucleation.

Despite their slow growth and limited potential for malignant degeneration, leiomyomas should be removed surgically unless there are specific contraindications. The majority can be removed by simple enucleation. If the mucosa is inadvertently entered during removal, the defect can be repaired primarily. Following removal, the outer esophageal wall should be reconstructed by closure of the muscle layer. The location of the lesion and the extent of surgery required will dictate the approach. Lesions of the proximal and middle esophagus require a right-sided approach, whereas distal esophageal lesions can be approached via the left side. The mortality of enucleation is less than 2%, and success in relieving dysphagia is universal. Large lesions or those involving the GE junction may require esophageal resection.

Thoracoscopic Resection of Esophageal Leiomyoma

Most leiomyomas should be approached from the right chest. The surgeon stands on the patient's right side and the assistant on the left. Trocar placement in general is similar to that described for myotomy and diverticular resection, with the exception that the camera position is modified, depending on the location of the lesion (Fig. 51-14). If the tumor is located in the upper part of the esophagus, the camera is positioned in the seventh or eighth intercostal space distal to the lesion. If the tumor is located in the distal esophagus the camera is placed in the fourth intercostal space just anterior or just posterior to the tip of the scapula. We prefer a 30-degree angled video telescope. Two operating ports are placed one to two interspaces below the camera: one low in the paraspinal area and one high in the mid- to anterior axillary line. We prefer 10-mm ports because they do not limit the choice of instruments. The final port is placed in the seventh to eighth interspace in the midaxillary line and is used to place a Babcock clamp to retract the lung into the superior thorax. Once the operative field is exposed and the tumor identified, the mediastinal pleura overlying the tumor is opened and the longitudinal muscle layer overlying the tumor incised (Fig. 51-15). This is best done using a combination of an electrocautery hook and scissors. A 4 × 4 gauze sponge may be introduced into the chest cavity to blot the field during esophageal dissection. Circumferential dissection of the esophagus is not necessary, unless the lesion is very large or left-sided, in which case it will be difficult and consideration should be given to converting to an open technique.

Once the tumor is identified, it should be grasped with forceps or a traction suture to allow retraction during dissection. The tumor is pulled away from the underlying muscle and mucosa as it is carefully dissected and teased away (Fig. 51-16). Care must be taken not to unduly traumatize the vagal trunks and the overlying muscle that will be reapproximated following removal of the tumor (Fig. 51-17). Gentle dissection usually allows removal of the tumor without injuring the underlying mucosa, unless a biopsy has been obtained prior to surgery. Intraoperative endoscopy is a useful adjunct, as it allows inflation of the esophagus and visual surveillance of the mucosal integrity. If the mucosa is violated, it may be repaired with fine interrupted suture and the longitudinal muscle closed over the suture line.

Following removal of the tumor, a nasogastric tube is carefully passed into the stomach, the pleural cavity is irrigated, and the trocar wounds are closed. A 28- to 32-French chest tube is left for drainage,

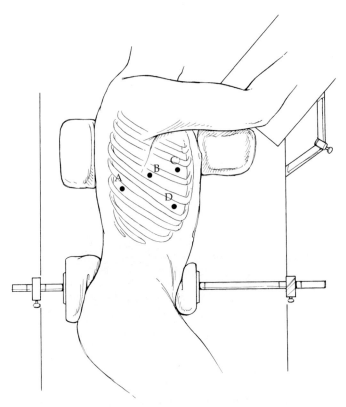

Fig. 51-14. Port positioning for dissection of esophageal leiomyoma. The position of the ports will vary, depending on the location of the tumor. (A, 10 mm; B, 10 mm; C, 10 mm; D, 10 mm.)

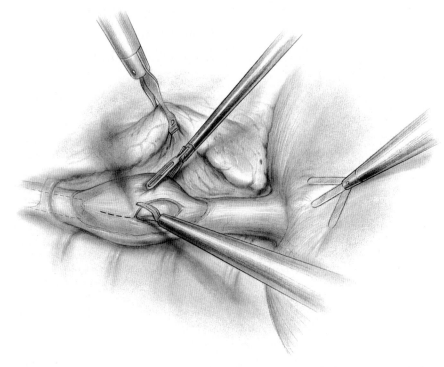

Fig. 51-15. Videoscopic dissection of an esophageal leiomyoma via a right thoracoscopic approach.

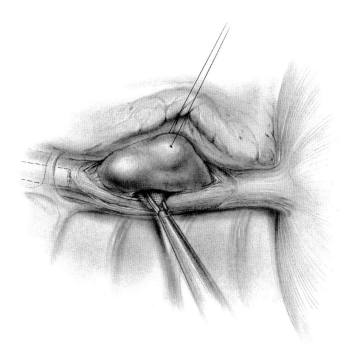

Fig. 51-16. Enucleation of a leiomyoma. A transfixing stitch is placed on the tumor to provide countertraction during its removal.

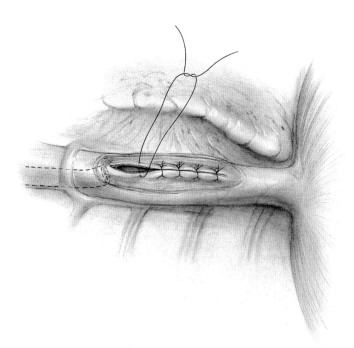

Fig. 51-17. After the leiomyoma is excised, the muscular wall is closed with interrupted sutures.

and a video esophagram is performed on postoperative day 1.

Cysts and Duplications of the Esophagus
Diagnosis and Indications

Esophageal cysts are the second most common benign lesion of the esophageal wall, occurring five times less frequently than leiomyomas of the esophagus. They represent embryonic rests and are located within the wall of the esophagus, usually in a submucosal position. A cyst may be lined with ciliated columnar (respiratory type) or stratified squamous epithelium. They are more common in the upper middle and upper thoracic esophagus and may be indistinguishable from leiomyomas on upper GI radiography. The treatment of these lesions is similar to that of esophageal leiomyomas. The cyst is asymptomatic in one-third of the patients, usually found incidentally. The other two-thirds complain of nonspecific symptoms such as dyspepsia, chest pain, or, more rarely, dysphagia. Extramucosal cysts can be complicated by intracystic hemorrhage, perforation, or infection. Malignant degeneration has also been reported.

A round or oval, regular mass in the posterior mediastinum on a routine chest film should suggest this diagnosis. Barium swallow examination shows a smooth compression of the esophageal lumen, and endoscopy confirms that the mucosa is normal. As in the case of leiomyoma, it is always advisable to avoid biopsy of the submucosal mass. Endoscopic ultrasonography is the diagnostic test of choice. Paraesophageal cysts may have ultrasonographic and computed tomographic features similar to those of leiomyoma, and a definitive diagnosis can be made only after examination of the surgical specimen.

Esophageal duplications are less common abnormalities and consist of a tubular structure composed of muscular and submucosal layers with a stratified squamous epithelial lining. The duplication may extend for a portion or the entire length of the esophagus. Esophageal duplications are commonly associated with other congenital anomalies, particularly those of vertebrae. As with simple esophageal cysts, they are treated by surgical enucleation. Because of their close association to the esophageal mucosa, long segment duplications may be difficult to remove thoracoscopically.

Thoracoscopic Resection of Paraesophageal Cysts

The operation can be performed through the right or the left chest, depending on the site of the mass. The approach is similar to that described for leiomyoma. Care must be taken to identify and preserve the vagus nerves. When the cyst is located in the esophageal wall, the muscle layer of the esophagus should be carefully dissected and closed with sutures after removal of the cyst. This is important to avoid an area of weakness in the esophageal wall leading to formation of a pseudodiverticulum. The cyst may be closely adherent to the underlying esophageal mucosa, and care must be used to avoid mucosal injury. Mucosal integrity may be checked by insufflation of air or injection of methylene blue via an intraluminal endoscope at completion of the procedure.

Postoperative Care

Following uneventful thoracoscopy, most patients may return to a step-down unit or surgical ward, although patients with comorbid disease occasionally require a 24- to 48-hour stay in the intensive care unit. Chest tubes are generally removed the day following surgery. Video barium esophagrams are obtained on postoperative day 1 or 2 to assess the functional and anatomic outcome of the procedure. Liquids are begun following the radiographic study, and patients are progressed rapidly to soft solids if dysphagia has been relieved.

Suggested Reading

Bardini R, Segalin A, Roul A, Pavanello M, Peracchia A. Videothoracoscopic enucleation of esophageal leiomyoma. *Ann Thorac Surg* 1992; 54:576–577.

Csendes A, Braghetto I, Henriquez A, Cortes C. Late results of a prospective randomised study comparing forceful dilatation and oesophagomyotomy in patients with achalasia. *Gut* 1989;30:299–304.

Debas HA, Payne WS, Cameron AJ, Carlson HC. Physiopathology of lower esophageal diveticulum and its implications for treatment. *Surg Gynecol Obstet* 1980;151:593–600.

Eckardt VF, Aignherr C, Bernhard G. Predictors of outcome in patients with achalasia treated by pneumatic dilation. *Gastroenterology* 1992;103: 1732–1738.

Ellis FH Jr. Oesophagomyotomy for achalasia: a 22-year experience. *Br J Surg* 1993;80:882–885.

Pellegrini C, Wetter LA, Patti M, et al. Thoracoscopic esophagomyotomy: initial experience with a new approach for the treatment of achalasia. *Ann Surg* 1992;216:291–299.

Shimi SM, Nathanson LK, Cuschieri A. Thoracoscopic long oesophageal myotomy for nutcracker oesophagus: initial experience of a new surgical approach. *Br J Surg* 1992;79: 533–536.

Topart P, Deschamps C, Taillefer R, Duranceau A. Long-term effect of total fundoplication on the myotomized esophagus. *Ann Thorac Surg* 1992;54:1046–1052.

EDITOR'S COMMENT

Minimally invasive esophageal surgery has become somewhat synonymous with laparoscopic esophageal surgery. This is due in large part to the inherent advantages of the transabdominal approach and, to a lesser extent, to the fact this is the approach most familiar to the current generation of endoscopic surgery practitioners.

Drs. Peters, Bonavina, and Hagen, who practice at centers noted for transthoracic esophageal surgery, remind us that many diseases of the esophagus can be well treated by a thoracoscopic approach. This chapter nicely describes the techniques for performing myotomies and benign tumor resections of the esophagus, both of which are ideal indications for a thoracoscopic approach. We agree with the authors' assessment that thoracoscopic Belsey fundoplications are difficult and probably not needed, as laparoscopic alternatives exist for partial and total fundoplications and even Collis gastroplasty. I would disagree, however, with the authors' assessment that thoracoscopy has little place in the area of esophageal resections. It is true that several studies have shown little or no improvement in morbidity or hospital stay. On the other hand, avoidance of thoracotomy incisions dramatically improves the quality of life and return to normal activity after hospital discharge for the majority of patients. In addition, the true utility of laparoscopic and thoracoscopic procedures is impossible to assess, based on small case series (e.g., with thoracoscopic esophagectomy), which typically include "learning curve" cases. Recent surgical history has shown that with experience good laparoscopic practitioners tend to decrease operative times and morbidity to a level consistent with traditional open surgery. Whether or not thoracoscopic esophagectomy for esophageal cancer is a sound oncologic procedure remains unknown. On the other hand, surgeons need to keep an open mind about thoracoscopic esophageal resection, as this procedure offers hope of a significant improvement in the quality of life for these unfortunate patients.

L.L.S.

52

Thoracoscopy for Mediastinal, Pericardial, and Cardiac Diseases

Michael J. Mack and Rodney J. Landreneau

Since the introduction of video thoracoscopy in 1990, a broader role has developed for the endoscopic approach in the management of all intrathoracic diseases. This includes applications in mediastinal, pericardial, and, more recently, cardiac diseases. In many mediastinal diseases, including posterior neurogenic tumors, as well as in esophageal surgery and cancer staging, video-assisted thoracic surgery (VATS) has been widely accepted. For other diseases, such as thymectomy for myasthenia gravis, the procedure remains unproven and therefore investigational at this stage.

The role of thoracoscopy in diseases of the pericardium has become fairly well defined, and an accepted role has been standardized for VATS. Recently, a large amount of enthusiasm has developed for cardiac applications of VATS, which will be discussed near the end of this chapter. The approach of VATS for cardiac disease is in its infancy, and we expect in the years to come a much more expanded role in coronary artery disease, as well as valvular and congenital heart disease. This chapter discusses the mediastinal, pericardial, and cardiac applications of VATS.

Mediastinal Applications of VATS

Traditionally, the mediastinum has been divided into three compartments: posterior, middle, and anterior. This is a particularly useful division for the discussion of diseases appropriate to each compartment (Table 52-1). Diseases of the posterior mediastinum are primarily benign tumors of

neurogenic origin. Tumors arise from either the sympathetic chain or the intercostal nerve and usually present as radicular pain or an abnormal chest x-ray.

Indications

Indications for surgical intervention in posterior mediastinal masses include the presence of symptoms and the potential for malignancy. Anytime an anterior approach is contemplated for a posterior mediastinal mass, computed tomography (CT) or preferably magnetic resonance (MR) imaging should be performed to rule out a dumbbell extension through the vertebral foramen into the spinal canal. If tumor extension does exist through the foramen, it does not rule out a minimally invasive approach. However, prior knowl-

Table 52-1. Mediastinal Lesions Accessible via Thoracoscopy

Posterior mediastinum
  Neurogenic tumors
  Enteric cyst
Middle mediastinum
  Pericardial cyst
  Bronchogenic cyst
  Lymphoma
  Thyroid/parathyroid adenoma
  Metastatic disease
Anterior mediastinum
  Lymphoma
  Adenopathy
  Thymoma
  Teratodermoid
  Metastatic cancer
  Hemangioma
  Lipoma

edge of this extension is necessary because a posterior approach is necessary for removal of the intraspinal component of the tumor. Enteric cysts are also occasionaly identified in the posterior mediastinum and should be removed.

Operative Technique

Posterior neurogenic tumors lend themselves particularly well to thoracoscopic extirpation. The procedure is performed in the standard manner of most thoracoscopic procedures, that is, with the patient in the lateral decubitus position under general endotracheal anesthesia with a double-lumen tube to effect ipsilateral lung collapse (Fig. 52-1). Three trocars are generally used as illustrated in Fig. 52-2. The particular level at which the trocars are placed varies depending on the level of involvement. Posterior neurogenic tumors at the levels of the T1-2 interspace to the T12-L1 interspace in either right or left chest cavity can be approached by the thoracoscopic technique. Frequently, rotation of the patient anteriorly can help drop the lung out of the operative field, obviating retraction and enhancing exposure.

The procedure is performed by incision of the parietal pleura overlying the mass and by sharp dissection to begin mobilizing the tumor. Care is taken to ascertain that the vascular supply, usually from intercostal vessels, is ligated with endoscopic clips (Fig. 52-3). The tumor is totally mobilized and excised. If any concern of malignancy exists, placement in an endoscopic bag is mandatory so that seeding of the chest wall does not occur. Meticulous hemostasis should be obtained. If the operative

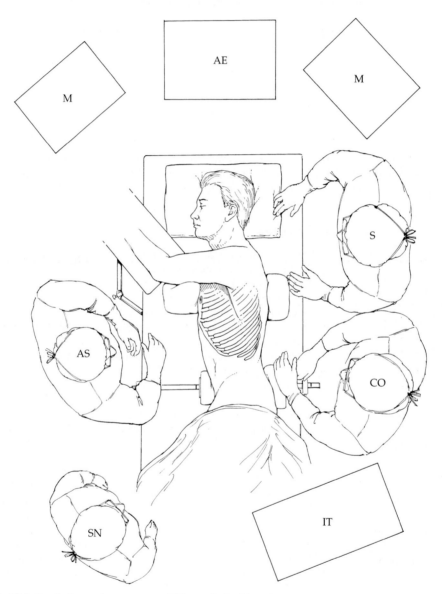

Fig. 52-1. Standard operating room setup. (AE, anesthesia; AS, assistant surgeon; M, monitor; S, surgeon; CO, camera operator; IT, instrument table; SN, scrub nurse.)

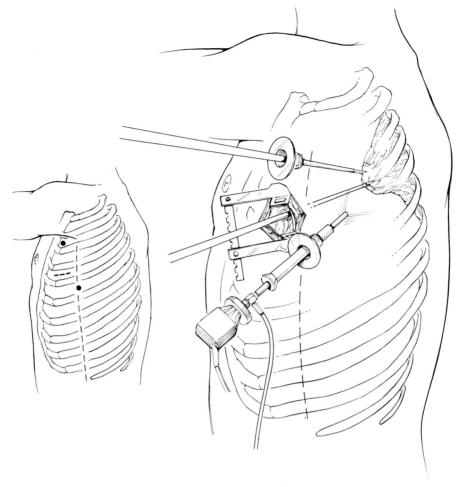

Fig. 52-2. Video-assisted thoracic surgery approach for posterior neurogenic tumors.

field is dry and no inadvertent lung injury has occurred, chest tube placement is not necessary. The lung is simply reexpanded under direct visualization, and the trocar sites are closed with a subcuticular suture.

Enteric cysts are excised in the same manner as neurogenic tumors. These masses are derived embryologically from the foregut and occasionally are very adherent to the esophagus. They can also be closely adherent or even connected to the spinal meninges. Care should be taken during dissection of these lesions to prevent injury to the esophagus or dura.

Middle-mediastinal Applications of VATS

Masses in the middle mediastinum are primarily cystic and usually benign. Cysts are usually of bronchogenic or pericardial origin and usually present as asymptomatic masses. Occasionally, when cysts become

large enough, they can cause symptoms by compression of adjacent viscera, as well as causing dysphagia, coughing, and other symptoms.

Indications

Indications for surgery include the presence of symptoms or concern regarding malignancy. Although virtually all middle-mediastinal cysts are benign, most end up being removed for diagnosis. When intervention is necessary on the basis of symptoms, simple needle aspiration of the cyst fluid is frequently sufficient. If aspiration is not successful or if the cyst recurs, then thoracoscopy is the optimal approach for excision.

Operative Technique

The general technique as described for posterior mediastinal masses is used (see Fig. 52-2). Dissection is usually started without aspiration of the cyst because dissection is easier thus. However, it often becomes necessary during the most posterior

part of the dissection to aspirate the cyst to facilitate manipulation and have a better view. Total extirpation of the cyst is performed when possible. However, if the posterior wall of the cyst is particularly adherent to the trachea or adjacent viscera, total excision is not absolutely mandatory, and the cyst wall left in place can be obliterated with electrocautery. Again, a chest tube is not often necessary after this procedure.

Pericardial cysts are usually located on the right side of the mediastinum in the cardiophrenic angle. Although they may communicate with the pericardium, they present no particular challenge for excision.

Anterior-mediastinal Applications of VATS

Thoracoscopy also has a role in the diagnosis and management of anterior-mediastinal masses. Frequently, masses in this area are malignant, and accurate

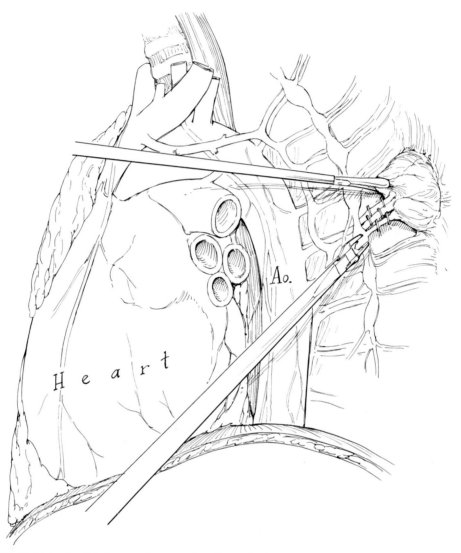

Fig. 52-3. *Ligation of the intercostal artery, vein, and nerve during resection of a posterior neurogenic tumor.*

staging and biopsy are important. When the differential diagnosis is thymoma versus lymphoma, significant amounts of tissue are usually needed to obtain an accurate diagnosis. This is particularly true of lymphoma, for which the definitive diagnosis of a particular type or subtype is obtained only by biologic tumor markers. Needle aspiration biopsy is usually inadequate in obtaining sufficient tissue to differentiate between lymphoma and thymoma, and surgical intervention is necessary.

Indications

For adenopathy in the right peritracheal or subazygous areas, cervical mediastinal ex-

ploration continues to be the preferred method for surgical approach. However, for masses in the anterior mediastinum, which previously would have been approached by a second left interspace mediastinotomy (Chamberlain procedure), we now operate through left thoracoscopy. The advantage of this approach is better access to the anterior mediastinum, with wider exposure and visualization of target tissue (Fig. 52-4). In addition, the smaller, more lateral thoracoscopy incisions are less morbid than an more anterior incision with resection of the costal cartilage. In addition, if radiation therapy is indicated, the thoracoscopy incisions are not in the field of radiation, as the Chamberlain incision would be. After appropriate preoper-

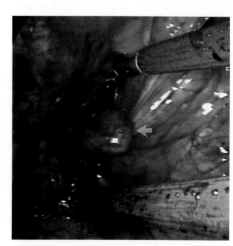

Fig. 52-4. *Video-assisted thoracic surgical removal of a large left paratracheal lymph node* (arrow).

ative workup, usually consisting of CT and/or MR imaging, the thoracoscopic approach is indicated.

Operative Technique

Just as posterior-mediastinal masses are approached from the anterior aspect, masses in the anterior mediastinum are approached from the more posterior aspect (Fig. 52-5). From a distance, this approach allows a more panoramic view of the operative field, as well as more room for maneuvering instrumentation. The target area previously identified by preoperative CT scan is identified intraoperatively. The mediastinal pleura is divided, and by careful dissection the abnormal tissue is biopsied. If concern exists regarding accurate identification of the target tissue, needle aspiration may first be performed under direct visualization to ensure that a vascular structure is not being biopsied. Again, if concern regarding malignancy exists, the suspect tissue should be placed in an endoscopic bag for extraction through the chest wall. When hemostasis has been obtained, the lung is reexpanded. A chest tube is usually not necessary for this procedure, unless inadvertent lung injury has occurred.

VATS Thymectomy

We have developed significant experience using VATS for thymectomy for both stage I thymoma and myasthenia gravis and have recently published the results from thymectomy for myasthenia gravis in 33 patients (Mack et al., 1996). Outcomes using the VATS approach have been equivalent to results from surgical resection by the more standard transternal, transcervical, or combined transcervical and transternal approaches. We feel that an equivalent operation can be performed by the endoscopic approach with less pain and better cosmesis, without jeopardizing the remission rate for the disease. As with any surgical intervention in myasthenia gravis, the earlier in the disease course that the thymectomy is performed, the better the response rate will be. Younger female patients with thymic hyperplasia appear to respond better to thymectomy than patients without these preoperative variables.

Indications

Indications for the endoscopic approach to thymoma include stage I disease that is limited to the thymus gland itself. If invasion by thymic tumor into adjacent structures occurs, then an open approach should be performed. If this is not appreciated on preoperative CT scan, thoracoscopy can make the determination, and if it is found that an anterior mediastinal mass is a thymoma that has invaded contiguous structures, then conversion to a median sternotomy should occur.

Operative Technique

No particular preoperative preparation is necessary in patients with myasthenia gravis undergoing thymectomy. They are admitted to the hospital the morning of surgery. If they are taking steroids prior to surgery, perioperative steroid coverage is increased and continued. VATS thymectomy can be performed through either the right or the left thoracic cavity. Although our initial experience involved only the left chest, we have more recently developed experience with the right thoracoscopic approach. We are developing a predilection for the right-sided approach because of the greater room for maneuverability of telescope and instruments and the better definition of the recesses around the superior vena cava and innominate vein obtainable through the right chest. Sometimes, the gland is markedly asymmetric, in which case one would choose the side on which the thymus is most prominent. Of 33 thymectomies to date, 22 have been performed through the left chest and 11 through the right chest.

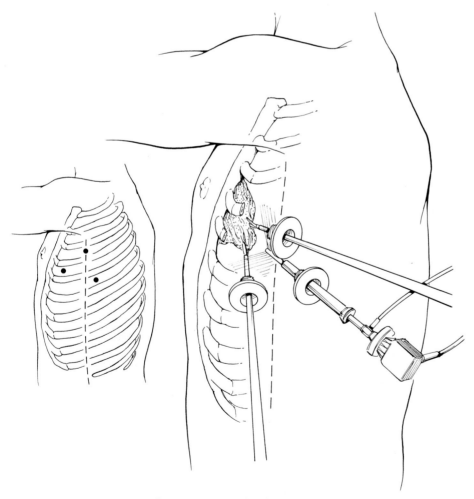

Fig. 52-5. Thoracoscopic approach to the anterior mediastinum.

The patient is positioned with the opera-tive side, elevated 30 degrees from hori-zontal. Three or four trocar sites are placed in the mid- and anterior axillary line in the third and fourth interspaces (Fig. 52-6). Once the chest cavity is en-tered and the lung is collapsed, the phrenic nerve is identified. Dissection is usually begun at the inferior aspect of the thymus gland, anterior to the phrenic nerve along the pericardium (Fig. 52-7). The mediastinal pleura is divided using a combination of sharp and blunt dissec-tion. This plane is continued cephalad until the mediastinal pleura is divided along the total length of the phrenic nerve. The thymus gland is then dis-sected off the pericardium, and the medi-astinal pleura is divided in the retroster-nal area. The thymus gland is mobilized anteriorly away from the sternum. Blunt dissection usually works well here. At this point, a plane is developed along

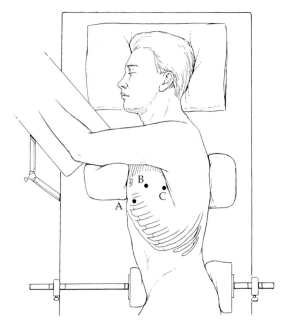

Fig. 52-6. Trocar sites for video-assisted thoracic surgery thymectomy through the left chest.

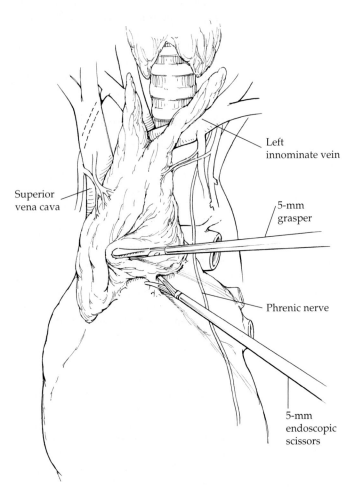

Fig. 52-7. Video-assisted thoracic surgery thymectomy is begun by dissection at the inferior pole of the gland just anterior to the phrenic nerve.

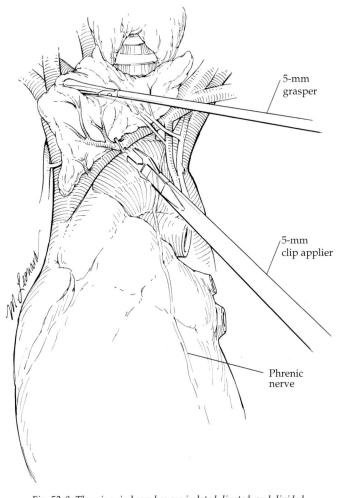

Fig. 52-8. Thymic vein branches are isolated, ligated, and divided.

the contralateral pleura. This plane is easily identified, and as long as the dissection is continued along the pleura, the contralateral phrenic nerve can be avoided. The arterial supply enters the upper poles of the thymus gland from the internal mammary artery. These branches are divided after appropriate endoscopic clips are placed. Next, dissection is continued on the posterior aspect of the gland until the main thymic vein, which drains into the innominate vein, has been identified. Once this vein has been located and carefully dissected free, it can be ligated or clipped and divided (Fig. 52-8). Finally, dissection is carried cephalad to the innominate vein and into the neck, where the uppermost poles of the thymus gland are. The fibrous attachments of the superior horns of the thymus gland to the inferior portion of the thyroid gland can be easily identified, and a complete extracapsular resection of the thymus gland can be assured.

Because of the concern of ectopic thymus tissue, all anterior mediastinal tissue is removed with the dissection (Fig. 52-9). Once the thymus gland has been removed through one of the slightly enlarged anterior sites, hemostasis is obtained. A chest tube is not usually necessary. For

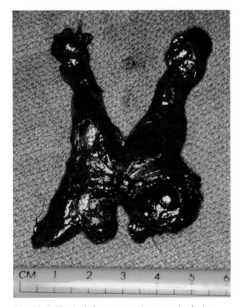

Fig. 52-9. Typical thymus specimen excised via video-assisted thoracic surgery with extracapsular dissection.

postoperative management, a stay in an intensive care unit is usually not necessary, and discharge is usually 1 or 2 days postoperatively.

VATS Staging of Malignancy

Staging of the mediastinum for spread of lung cancer is problematic. Some thoracic surgeons feel that preoperative staging by mediastinoscopy is mandatory prior to any lung resection, while other thoracic surgeons feel that mediastinoscopy is necessary only if lymph nodes larger than 1 cm in diameter exist on preoperative CT scan. If the thoracic surgeon feels that staging is necessary either as a routine or because of an abnormal CT scan, thoracoscopy has a role. Thoracoscopy has not replaced cervical mediastinal exploration, which is still the preferred method for staging of the right peritracheal lymph nodes. However, we have added a video channel to our standard mediastinoscope, and therefore term this procedure *video mediastinoscopy*. The addition of video offers better illumination and magnification of the peritracheal area, allowing safer assessment and biopsy of mediastinal lymph nodes. In addition, we feel that more accurate staging may be possible by being able to access subcarinal lymph nodes (level 7) and lymph nodes along the right mainstem bronchus (level 10). More accurate delineation of extranodal versus intranodal involvement with tumor may also be possible.

For left-sided tumors, left thoracoscopy has replaced anterior mediastinotomy (Chamberlain procedure) for staging of lung cancer. Better access and visualization of lymph node levels 5 and 6, including the aortopulmonary window, is possible by the left thoracoscopic approach. We feel that left thoracoscopy is better cosmetically and allows more effective staging by improved visualization of a wider area of the mediastinum. In addition, level 8 lymph nodes in the inferior pulmonary ligament can be accessed, which is not possible with the Chamberlain procedure. The additional benefit of being able to preoperatively stage the pleura is another reason why we feel that left thoracoscopy is preferable to the

Chamberlain approach for staging of left-sided cancers.

Pericardial Applications of VAT

Indications

Diseases of the pericardium are particularly well approached by thoracoscopy. Current indications for the use of thoracoscopy are limited to benign effusive pericardial disease. Since benign effusive disease carries a significant recurrence rate when managed by needle or catheter aspiration or a subxiphoid pericardial window, a limited anterior thoracotomy has been the standard approach. This has been replaced in our practice by thoracoscopy. The ability to perform a wide pericardial resection in a minimally invasive manner allows effective management of benign pericardial diseases. On the other hand, we prefer to manage malignant pericardial effusive disease with catheter aspiration and instillation of a sclerosing agent or by a subxiphoid pericardiectomy, which can be performed under local anesthesia. We feel that the requirements for general anesthesia and a double-lumen endotracheal tube are too invasive for patients with end-stage malignancy who are frequently debilitated at the time of presentation with malignant effusion. Since the recurrence rate with subxiphoid pericardiectomy is relatively low (15% to 20%), this is usually sufficient palliation for these end-stage patients. In a manner similar to that of cervical mediastinal exploration, we have used a video mediastinoscope to perform a subxiphoid pericardiectomy. With this technique, we can excise a wider swatch of pericardium under local anesthesia than with the standard subxiphoid approach.

In addition to its effectiveness in benign effusive disease, thoracoscopic pericardiectomy has proved useful in three patients with delayed tamponade after cardiac surgery and in two orthotopic cardiac transplant patients in whom a delayed tamponade presented because small donor hearts only partially filled large pericardial spaces. Repeated needle pericardiocentesis was only temporarily effective in relieving the problem in both patients. A thoracoscopic left pericardial window permanently relieved this pericardial space problem.

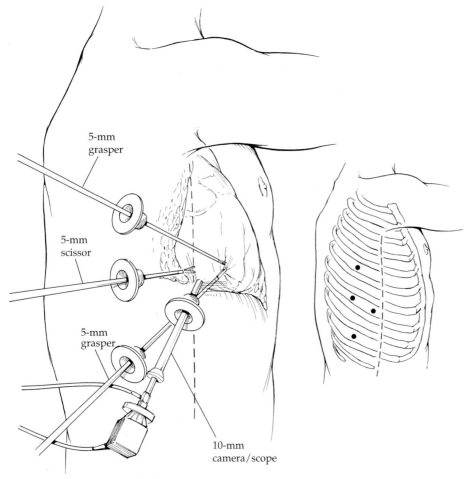

Fig. 52-10. Trocar placement for thoracoscopic pericardiectomy through the right chest.

Operative Technique

The technique of thoracoscopic pericardiectomy is quite straightforward. The pericardiectomy can be performed by either the right or the left thoracic approach. As we gain more experience, it is becoming our habit to perform this more commonly through the right thoracic cavity, since the distended pericardium on the left side frequently does not allow adequate visualization and easy maneuvering of instrumentation. The greater excursion of instrumentation allowed through the right chest significantly facilitates the procedure. Trocars are placed as shown in Fig. 52-10.

The lung is retracted cephalad and away from the operative field. If a distended pericardium is difficult to grasp, needle aspiration of the pericardial fluid can be done under direct vision. An incision is made in the pericardium, and the remaining pericardial fluid is drained. An exten-

sive pericardiectomy is performed both anterior and posterior to the phrenic nerve, with preservation of a bridge of pericardium beneath the nerve (Fig. 52-11).

At completion of the pericardiectomy, a 28-French chest tube is placed adjacent to the pericardium and left in place until the drainage is less than 150 mL in a 24-hour period. Of course, noneffusive pericardial disease is not always appropriately managed by the thoracoscopic approach. However, the bread-and-butter (fibrinous) pericarditis that occurs with uremic disease can still be managed thoracoscopically, even though there is not a large effusive component. In constrictive pericarditis, a median sternotomy with cardiopulmonary bypass is the preferable approach, thoracoscopy having no role.

As further experience is gained, most benign effusive pericardial disease can be optimally approached and managed by

the VATS approach as surgeons become increasingly comfortable with this minimally invasive approach.

Cardiac Applications of VATS

Cardiac surgery has been the last surgical subspecialty to adapt minimally invasive surgical techniques. Because of the technical complexity of procedures and the necessity for circulatory support during the operative period on the target organ system, adaptation of minimally invasive techniques has lagged. As the invasive nature of most surgical procedures continues to diminish, attention is being turned to cardiac surgery in an attempt to develop a minimally invasive approach to many procedures, including coronary artery bypass grafting (CABG).

Many simple cardiac procedures have been performed thoracoscopically, including permanent pacemaker lead placement for the few patients for whom the transvenous system is not appropriate. In addition, placement of pericardial patches for implantable defibrillators has been successful by either the thoracoscopic or the laparoscopic approach, with patches being placed on the underside of the diaphragm. These techniques have largely been supplanted by the successful transvenous systems and remain of case-report interest only. Laboratory experimentation is addressing both the maze procedure for atrial fibrillation and transmyocardial laser revascularization of the left ventricle. Neither of these procedures has reached the clinical stage yet.

Significant experience has developed in many centers with thoracoscopic patent ductus arteriosus ligation. Reports of large experiences have shown the procedure to be done safely and effectively by the thoracoscopic approach. Benefits compared with the open technique, however, are still difficult to fully define and delineate. In addition, vascular rings have been able to be divided by the thoracoscopic approach.

Minimally Invasive Coronary Artery Bypass

The main area of focus has been CABG and, secondarily, valve repair and replacement, as well as repair of intracardiac defects. The

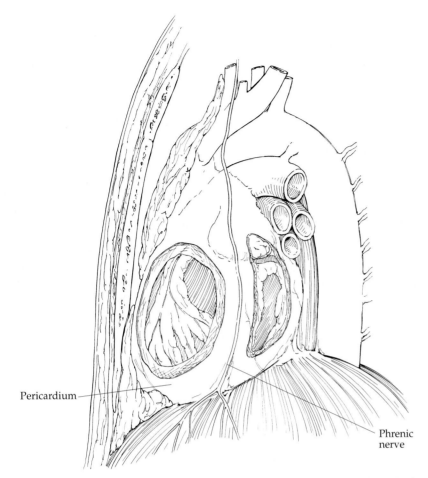

Pericardium

Phrenic nerve

Fig. 52-11. Pericardial resection both anterior and posterior to the phrenic nerve during video-assisted thoracic surgery.

minimally invasive focus has been in three areas: (1) method of access, (2) necessity for and type of circulatory support, and (3) minimalization of aortic manipulation.

Many variations of the standard median sternotomy have been developed for minimal-access cardiac surgery. These include a ministernotomy, in which the lower one-third of the sternum is divided and divided vertically and then horizontally into the third or fourth intercostal space on one or both sides. The internal mammary artery (IMA) is then harvested under direct vision, and the anastomosis of the left IMA to the left anterior descending artery and/or the right IMA to the right coronary artery is performed without cardiopulmonary bypass. An alternative approach has been the anterior minithoracotomy. This procedure has been called "keyhole" and "trap door" cardiac surgery, and more recently minimally invasive direct-vision coronary artery bypass (MIDCAB).

The basis of all these procedures is that the IMA can be harvested along its full length by the thoracoscopic approach, and the anastomosis can be performed either on or off bypass through a 6-cm anterior thoracotomy with resection of the fourth or fifth cartilage. The anastomosis is done under direct vision or eventually by video imaging techniques. Alternatively, the IMA can be harvested directly through the incision by retraction of the higher ribs. By this approach, the IMA can be harvested up to one or two interspaces above the fourth intercostal space. However, this technique leaves side branches unligated, and therefore the possibility of steal through side branches exists. Another alternative access for MIDCAB is a muscle-sparing lateral thoracotomy, which is helpful in some procedures for bypass grafting to the obtuse marginal branch of the circumflex coronary artery, especially in patients requiring repeat CABG in whom patent grafts are present. Finally, a totally endo-

scopic approach has been attempted. There has been minimal success with this approach at present because of the difficulty of performing a totally endoscopic vascular anastomosis. By this approach, the patient is placed on a femoral cardiopulmonary bypass system, and an "endovascular clamp" is placed through the femoral artery. This endovascular clamp is a balloon catheter that is placed transfemorally into the ascending aorta and inflated, occluding the aorta. Myocardial protection is then delivered into the aortic root through the catheter. The IMA harvest and anastomosis are performed endoscopically on the arrested heart. Alternatively, numerous retraction devices for providing exposure have been developed, as well as wall-motion stabilizers for stabilizing local wall areas of the beating heart while the anastomosis is performed.

Perhaps an equally important method of making cardiac surgery less traumatizing for patients, in addition to minimalization of the method of access, is minimalization of cardiopulmonary bypass. Extensive experience exists with open sternotomy for "off pump" CABG (OPCAB). During this procedure, initially described by F. Benetti, a median sternotomy is performed and the heart rate slowed pharmacologically. Vessel loops are placed around the coronary artery for occlusion, and the anastomosis is performed under direct vision on a beating heart. Alternatively, cardiopulmonary bypass can be used by the femorofemoral approach, and numerous modifications, including heparin bonding of cardiopulmonary bypass circuits, are used to minimize the inflammatory response associated with cardiopulmonary bypass. Alternative circulatory support methods, including percutaneously placed ventricular assist devices, are being examined experimentally.

Indications for MIDCAB

Optimal candidates for this procedure include patients with single-vessel disease of the proximal left anterior descending coronary artery (LAD). Lesions not approachable by percutaneous transluminal coronary angioplasty (PTCA) because of their length or located proximal to the first septal branch in the LAD are appropriate candidates. In addition, recurrent lesions following previous PTCA and/or stent placement represent good candidates for this procedure. We have experience with seven patients who have had previous CABG and have isolated disease in the LAD and patent grafts present in other vessels.

MIDCAB: Operative Technique

Our present procedure for selected patients with single-vessel coronary artery disease primarily of the LAD is a hybrid procedure in which thoracoscopic harvesting of the IMA is performed and then the anastomosis completed under direct vision on a beating heart without cardiopulmonary bypass.

In this procedure, the IMA is thoracoscopically harvested along its full length (Fig. 52-12). We feel that this is an important part of the procedure because all side branches are divided to prevent steal after the conduit has been placed to the coronary artery. The anastomosis is then performed off bypass through an anterior minithoracotomy after the fourth costal cartilage has been resected (Fig. 52-13). We have experience with 33 patients at present. The left IMA was placed to the LAD in 29 patients and to the diagonal artery in one patient; the right IMA was placed to the right coronary artery in three patients. The average time for harvest of the IMA was 48 minutes, and the ischemic time in which the anastomosis is performed averaged 12.5 minutes. The average total operating time was just over 2 hours, and the average hospital stay 2.4 days. We feel that although this procedure is a less invasive approach for patients with single-vessel disease, it is an intermediate-step procedure, performed partially open and partially endoscopically. As surgical expertise and technologic development continue, this will evolve to a totally endoscopic approach.

Conclusion

It has now been 5 years since the introduction of video thoracoscopy into thoracic surgery. Although the indications for pleural and lung diseases are fairly well defined, the role of thoracoscopy in mediastinal, pericardial, and cardiac diseases is less well defined and continues to evolve. Thoracoscopy is appropriate for resection of posterior-mediastinal tumors and for the rare occasion in which mediastinal cysts should be removed. Diag-

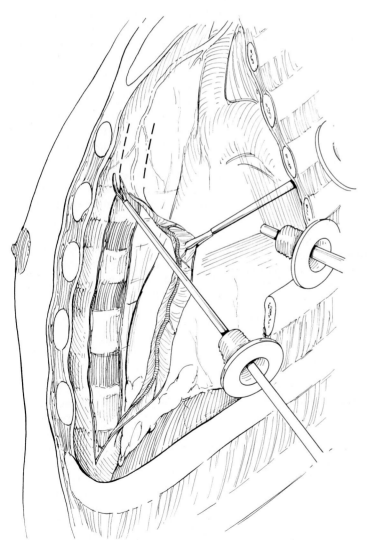

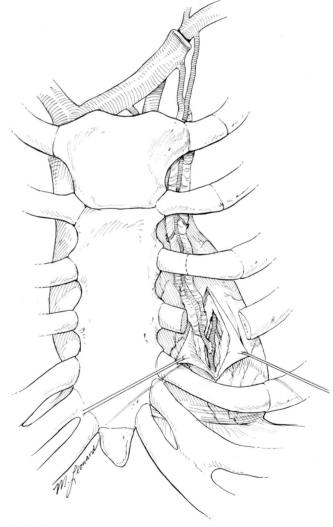

Fig. 52-12. Video-assisted thoracic surgical harvest of the left internal mammary artery.

Fig. 52-13. Anastomosis between the left internal mammary artery and the left anterior descending artery is performed under direct vision on a beating heart.

nostic biopsy of anterior-mediastinal masses is optimally approached by thoracoscopy because needle biopsy is often is insufficient in providing an accurate tissue diagnosis.

Thymectomy for myasthenia gravis has been performed by this approach with an efficacy equal to that of the more traditional open approaches, but in a cosmetically more acceptable manner. There is also a role for thoracoscopy in the staging of left-sided lung cancers.

Benign effusive pericardial disease is appropriately managed by thoracoscopy. However, malignant pericardial effusion, in which life expectancy is severely limited, is more appropriately managed by a less invasive approach.

Much excitement now exists concerning potential cardiac applications of endoscopic surgery. MIDCAB, one of these procedures currently being performed, is minimally invasive CABG, in which the left IMA is anastomosed to the LAD off bypass through an anterior minithoracotomy. Significant challenges exist, but evolution of minimal-access techniques is occurring at a very rapid rate.

Suggested Reading

Acuff TE, Landreneau RJ, Griffith BP, Mack, MJ. Minimally invasive coronary artery bypass grafting. *Ann Thorac Surg* 1996;61:135–137.

Hazelrigg SR, Mack MJ, Landreneau RJ. Video-assisted thoracic surgery for mediastinal disease. *Chest Surg Clin N Am* 1993;3:249–262.

Hazelrigg SR, Mack MJ, Landreneau RJ, Acuff TE, Seifert P, Auer JE. Thoracoscopic pericardiectomy for effusive pericardial disease. *Ann Thorac Surg* 1993;56:792–795.

Landreneau RJ, Hazelrigg SR, Mack MJ, et al. Strategic planning for video-assisted thoracic surgery "VATS." *Ann Thorac Surg* 1993;56:615–619.

Mack MJ, Landreneau RJ, Yim AP, Hazelrigg SR, Scruggs GR. Results of VATS thymectomy in patients with myasthenia gravis. *J Thorac Cardiovasc Surg* 1996;112:1352–1360.

Riquet M, Mouroux J, Pons F, et al. Videothoracoscopic excision of thoracic neurogenic tumors. *Ann Thorac Surg* 1995;60:943–946.

Stevens JH, Burdon TA, Peters WS, et al. Port-access coronary artery bypass grafting: a proposed surgical method. *J Thorac Cardiovasc Surg* 1996;111:567–573.

EDITOR'S COMMENT

Mediastinal lesions, while usually benign and seldom needing treatment, still benefit from accurate tissue diagnosis. In the past, surgical diagnosis was associated with highly morbid incisions and was considered an option of last resort. The ability to do surgical biopsy and excisions using minimally invasive techniques opens the door to earlier, more acceptable intervention. This is cost-effective. In addition, it bypasses attempts at percutaneous biopsy and reliance on imaging techniques, which have been shown to be less accurate as diagnostic tools and certainly not therapeutic modalities.

Thymectomy for myasthenia gravis is a case in point. This surgery has been shown to be highly effective in certain patient groups but is seldom used because the morbidity and cosmetic results of the traditional surgical approach in these same populations are considered unacceptable.

When the thoracoscopic approach becomes more generally available, perhaps more patients will be offered and accept this treatment alternative.

Attention should be paid to Drs. Mack and Landreneau's comments in several instances on the ease of access via the right chest for thoracoscopic procedures. I have also found that the majority of endoscopic mediastinal surgeries are best approached from the right chest, leaving the left approach for treatment of pericardial diseases.

Great care and skill are needed for thoracoscopic mediastinal surgery. Complications are potentially severe and include nerve injuries (recurrent laryngeal, vagus, and phrenic nerves) and vascular injuries (azygos vein, innominate vein, pulmonary hilar vessels, and aorta). There is also the potential for esophageal injuries, tracheal injury, and chylothorax following undiagnosed injury to the thoracic duct. Thoracoscopic mediastinal surgery should only be performed by surgeons totally familiar with the anatomy of the mediastinum, well versed in advanced endoscopic techniques, and able to convert to the open approach if complications arise.

Mastery of the thoracoscopic approach to the mediastinum for tumor staging and treatment of benign disease can be accomplished and provides definite patient benefits. It is the first step toward the performance of more complex procedures, such as thymectomy for thymoma, thoracoscopic esophageal resections, and even the major cardiac procedures outlined by the authors.

L.L.S

VIII

Miscellaneous

53

Minimally Invasive Vascular Surgery

Robert W. Thompson and Brian G. Rubin

For many years, physicians caring for patients with vascular disease have held a strong interest in minimally invasive treatment approaches. This is best exemplified by the widespread use of percutaneous transluminal balloon angioplasty, indwelling vascular stents, and the recent development of intraluminally placed endovascular stent–graft devices. Unlike other areas of general surgery, where laparoscopy has been applied to nearly every major intraabdominal operation, abdominal vascular procedures have been considered the least amenable to this additional form of minimally invasive technology. This derives from the perception that laparoscopy provides an insufficient degree of exposure and control of the aorta for prosthetic grafting due to difficulty in rapidly dissecting retroperitoneal tissues, controlling diseased arteries through laparoscopic ports, and timely creation of vascular anastomoses by intracavitary suture techniques. An additional concern has been the risk of sudden major hemorrhage from arterial or venous sources, an uncontrollable event under laparoscopic conditions. Nonetheless, in the past few years, experimental studies and early case reports attest to a growing interest in laparoscopic-assisted aortic reconstruction.

As experience has been gained in overcoming both authentic obstacles and perceived limitations of laparoscopy for operations on the intraabdominal vasculature, it has become clear that these techniques will likely provide feasible and beneficial applications for patients with vascular disease. Increasing familiarity with laparoscopic technology has also enabled vascular surgeons to extend its use to other vascular disorders, such as lower extremity venous insufficiency. The development, early clinical applications, and future prospects for laparoscopic treatment of arterial and venous disease are reviewed in this chapter.

Laparoscopic Surgery of the Abdominal Aorta

Prosthetic graft reconstruction of the abdominal aorta is commonly performed by conventional open operations for both occlusive atherosclerosis and aneurysm disease with a low morbidity and mortality in most centers. These procedures typically involve wide exposure of the aorta from the level of the left renal vein to the aortic bifurcation, a dissection that can lead to considerable third-space fluid shifts, prolonged ileus, pulmonary dysfunction, cardiovascular compromise, and wound-related morbidity. Use of the left retroperitoneal approach to the aorta, reintroduced in the 1980s, was initially thought to reduce these effects, compared to more traditional transperitoneal approaches. However, several prospective clinical trials have now demonstrated no significant difference between these two methods. Because patients with degenerative disease of the aorta often harbor significant coexisting medical problems, they frequently present increased risks for a major intraabdominal operation. A less invasive technique for aortic reconstruction might thereby be attractive and beneficial for this patient population.

Trends toward minimally invasive vascular surgery have largely focused on percutaneous transluminal approaches to arterial lesions, including balloon dilation angioplasty, catheter-directed atherectomy, placement of intravascular stents and, most recently, use of endovascular stent–graft devices. For aortoiliac occlusive disease, satisfactory long-term results have been demonstrated with balloon angioplasty of favorable lesions, such that this may often be the treatment of choice for selected patients. Despite these encouraging results, major obstacles remain to the widespread use of transluminal procedures for those with diffuse aortoiliac occlusive disease or aortic aneurysm. For example, even the recently introduced use of endoluminally placed stent–graft devices for aneurysms requires a disease-free segment of infrarenal aorta at least 2 to 3 cm in length, as well as a distal aorta of normal diameter. This pattern of disease is unfortunately found in a minority of patients with abdominal aortic aneurysm. Because endoluminal techniques for aortobifemoral bypass are still unresolved, patients with aneurysm disease extending into the common iliac arteries are also not eligible for the current generation of devices. Although these difficulties limit the use of transluminal approaches for the majority of patients, they are problems for which alternative, minimally invasive techniques, such as those using laparoscopy, might yet prove feasible. Whereas laparoscopy cannot be used for aortic operations in the same manner as it is commonly employed for biliary and gastrointestinal procedures, early experience suggests that the anticipated problems are neither insurmountable nor unobtainable.

Conventional (Open) Techniques and Potential Pitfalls of Laparoscopy

Abdominal aortic reconstruction is employed for occlusive atherosclerosis or aneurysms affecting the infrarenal aorta and iliac arteries. Because these disorders present unique problems for adaptation to laparoscopic surgery, methods currently used in conventional aortic operations are discussed below in relation to the potential pitfalls to be expected using a laparoscopic approach.

Whether a vertical midline or left flank incision is chosen, the proximal infrarenal aorta is isolated just beyond the level of the crossing left renal vein. When the midline (transperitoneal) approach is used, this involves separating the peritoneal attachments of the duodenum anterior to the aorta just beyond the ligament of Treitz, whereas the left retroperitoneal approach avoids this requirement. Retroperitoneal periaortic fat and lymphatic structures are divided to expose and achieve the proper plane of dissection on the aorta. Although it is not always necessary to completely encircle the aorta, its lateral aspects must be sufficiently exposed to permit secure clamping across the entire aortic wall. From the midline approach, this requires dissection along the sides of the aorta to the vertebral bodies of the spine. Although it is uncommon (approximately 5% of the population), the presence of a retroaortic left renal vein may provide considerable challenge if it is inadvertently injured during dissection in this region. The left renal vein may also bleed extensively if injured directly or through avulsion of its gonadal, lumbar, or adrenal vein branches during retraction. This consideration is especially important when approaching the aorta from its left lateral aspect. With the degree of exposure achieved by these maneuvers, the proximal aortic clamp will typically be placed just below the renal arteries.

For occlusive disease the distal aortic clamp is usually placed at the level of the inferior mesenteric artery, providing an isolated aortic segment approximately 2 to 3 cm in length with which to construct the proximal graft anastomosis. The prosthetic graft may be placed in either end-to-end or end-to-side fashion on the aorta, a choice largely dependent on the operating surgeon's preference. The frequency of calcific atherosclerosis requires sufficient exposure of the distal aorta to assess the local extent of disease in this region in order to select the optimal site for aortic clamp placement. It is essential that clamp occlusion of the aorta provides reliable control against hemorrhage, inadvertent aortic injury, and dislodgement of thromboembolic material. The instrumentation used to clamp the aorta must therefore be unequivocally dependable to avert serious complications.

Once the aorta is opened, bleeding from patent collateral vessels may obscure the operative field, making construction of the anastomosis difficult. During open operations, these vessels are often identified prior to aortotomy and controlled with small clamps, hemoclips, or ligatures. Because the inferior mesenteric artery must often be preserved to maintain satisfactory colonic blood flow, it is not typically ligated during operations for occlusive disease. If back-bleeding from this vessel occurs after aortotomy, it too must be seperately controlled with an additional clamp. When an end-to-side graft anastomosis is performed, atherosclerotic debris is debrided or irrigated from the aorta at the anastomotic site to avert distal atheroembolism on restoration of antegrade flow. The diseased aortic wall may also be difficult to suture with accuracy, as it may fragment with excessive manipulation. Continuous anastomoses rather than interrupted sutures are most often used because this technique provides better hemostasis of the suture line by keeping the continuous suture taught during its construction. These operations are typically performed in the presence of systemic anticoagulation, and thus bleeding from suture holes in the prosthetic material is commonly encountered on completion of the anastomosis regardless of the graft material chosen. This usually presents only a temporary problem, responding well to topical hemostatic agents. On the other hand, bleeding between the aortic wall and the graft material indicates a gap in the anastomosis that must be repaired by additional (interrupted) sutures, often used with small pledgets of prosthetic material to more evenly distribute the tension.

Once the proximal anastomosis is complete, the limbs of the bifurcation graft are passed through retroperitoneal tunnels to each groin. These tunnels must be placed underneath each ureter to avoid either compression and urinary obstruction or graft–ureteral erosion. The ends of the graft are then sewn to the common femoral arteries in end-to-side fashion, after which all clamps are removed and distal flow is restored through the new prosthetic bypass graft. The abdominal portion of the graft is excluded from contact with the gastrointestinal tract by reapproximation of the posterior peritoneal membrane overlying the aorta. This step is not necessary when the retroperitoneal approach is used, as the peritoneal lining is not opened.

Similar considerations are used in reconstruction for abdominal aortic aneurysms. In this circumstance, the enlarged aorta may present added difficulty in exposing the most proximal infrarenal aorta, if it obscures the adjacent retroperitoneal structures. When approached from the midline, the neck of the aneurysm often lies behind the anterior bulge of the aneurysm wall, making it difficult to access for sufficient exposure. Downward manual traction on the aneurysm (toward the feet) can facilitate this aspect of the dissection, if necessary. Notably, the neck of the aneurysm is often more easily and more rapidly exposed when approached through the left retroperitoneum. However, as with occlusive disease, this approach will make it difficult to identify and occlude any right-sided lumbar vessels or accessory renal arteries that are readily exposed through the midline approach.

Distal arterial control for aneurysms is most often obtained by clamping the iliac arteries rather than the aorta. The right iliac artery may be more difficult to control from the left retroperitoneal approach than it is with the patient supine. It is often easiest to use an intraluminal balloon occlusion device for this vessel, placed from within the open aorta, rather than to control it prior to opening of the aneurysm. Although the inferior mesenteric artery is usually already occluded in patients with aneurysms, if it is patent, use of an end-to-end proximal anastomosis may require that it be preserved by reimplantation into the graft. Similar concerns apply to aberrant renal arteries supplying significant proportions of functional renal mass.

One of the unique features of aneurysms is the large amount of atherosclerotic debris and laminated mural thrombus that must be removed from the aneurysmal sac. Evacuation of the thrombus often leads to brisk bleeding from lumbar collaterals entering the posterior aortic wall. These are rapidly oversewn from within the opened aorta before construction of the prosthetic repair begins.

Finally, in contrast to operations for occlusive disease, aortic reconstructions for aneurysms are always performed with an end-to-end proximal anastomosis. The graft must be placed high enough to prevent aneurysmal degeneration of the anastomotic region or the proximal aorta, and there is often little room to clamp and create the anastomosis in the 1- to 2-cm neck of the aneurysm available below the renal arteries. The frequency of diseased aortic tissue in the neck of the aneurysm also allows no tolerance for technical mistakes, as the anastomosis cannot be redone or placed higher without considerable hazards. Although aortobifemoral grafts are most commonly used when treating occlusive disease, prosthetic grafts placed to repair aortic aneurysms do not often need to be placed beyond the distal aorta (aortic tube grafts) or the common iliac artery bifurcation (aortobiiliac grafts). Thus, operations for aneurysm disease do not frequently entail the problems associated with groin incisions that exist for aortobifemoral bypasses.

Based on this discussion, it is apparent that unique considerations must be given to the potential use of laparoscopy in the treatment of occlusive and aneurysmal aortic disease. The problems inherent in applying laparoscopy to aortic reconstruction and the potential solutions that are emerging to overcome them are summarized in Table 53-1 and the following sections.

Emerging Use of Laparoscopy in Aortic Reconstruction

Experimental Studies

To begin investigating various techniques by which laparoscopy might be applied to aortic surgery, we conducted experimental studies of aortofemoral bypass in a porcine model. Early in the development of these methods, we found that the use of pneumoperitoneum adds considerable difficulty to the procedure. Thus, use of suction to control even relatively small amounts of bleeding resulted in repeated loss of intraperitoneal pressure and obliteration of the immediate operative field. Combined with the small field of dissection in the retroperitoneum and the tendency of the surrounding tissues to collapse on loss of the pneumoperitoneum, these problems required constant reexposure of the structures of interest. With the need to dissect around major blood vessels that might be easily injured, and recognition that these problems could be disastrous during stages of the operation in which anastomoses were created and tested, the problems associated with pneumoperitoneum led us to abandon this approach. In contrast, we found that gasless laparoscopy permitted more stable exposure of the aorta and uninterrupted dissection of retroperitoneal structures, even when suction was required to control bleeding.

One of the principal purposes of our experimental work has been to compare different techniques for transperitoneal and retroperitoneal approaches to laparoscopic aortic reconstruction. As it is now performed, the transperitoneal approach employs four ports that are placed as shown in Fig. 53-1. With the animal in a supine position, the abdominal wall is retracted manually, and a Veress needle is blindly inserted into the lower abdomen, directed away from the aortic bifurcation. The abdominal cavity is then insufflated with carbon dioxide to a pressure of 15 mm Hg. After a video laparoscope is inserted through the initial port, the remaining ports are placed under laparoscopic vision. One 10-mm port is placed in the right flank for bowel retraction, and two additional 10-mm working ports are placed in the left flank. After these ports are secured, the pneumoperitoneum is evacuated. Through a 2-cm lower midline incision over the aortic bifurcation, an external lifting device is used to maintain the working space. Steep (30 to 60 degrees) Trendelenburg positioning is necessary to help retract the small bowel anterior to the liver to provide adequate exposure of the infrarenal aorta. A fan retractor is used to further retract the bowel while the retroperitoneum overlying the aorta is incised. With standard laparoscopic instruments under video observation, the infrarenal aorta is dissected along each of its lateral borders to the level of the spine and longitudinally from the level of the left renal vein to the aortic bifurcation. Retraction of the

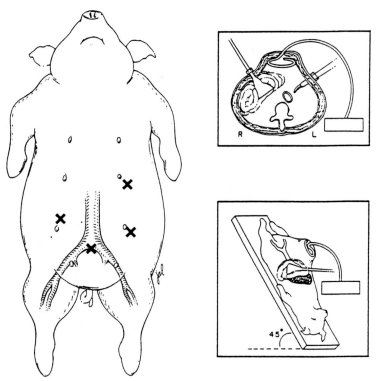

Fig. 53-1. Transperitoneal approach to laparoscopic-assisted aortofemoral bypass in the porcine model. (From Jones et al., 1996, with permission.)

After laparoscopic-assisted aortic exposure, femoral incisions are made, and each common femoral artery is exposed at the level of the inguinal ligament. Regardless of the initial approach used to expose the aorta, a 6-mm polytetrafluoroethylene (PTFE) graft (Gore-Tex, W.L. Gore, Inc., Flagstaff, AZ) is tunneled through the pelvic retroperitoneum from the femoral incision to the aortic bifurcation under laparoscopic guidance (Fig. 53-3). A 10-mm, 30-degree laparoscope (Olympus, Lenexa, KA) is used to illuminate and image the femoral dissection from the abdomen and to visualize intraabdominal passage of the graft. Retraction of the retroperitoneum under the inguinal ligament is facilitated by use of a sterile laryngoscope from the femoral incision while the graft is introduced by a blunt, 5-mm laparoscopic cherry dissector (Ethicon Endosurgery, Cincinnati, OH). Once the graft is in place, any kinking or twisting is easily detected by video imaging and corrected. The external lifting device is then removed from the central incision over the aortic bifurcation, and this incision is extended to 4 cm in length. Exposure of the anastomotic site

aorta with an umbilical tape facilitates circumferential exposure, allowing lumbar vessels and the inferior mesenteric artery to be clipped and divided under optimal visualization.

For the retroperitoneal approach, we place the animal in a right lateral decubitus position at about 45- to 60-degrees rotation (Fig. 53-2). An expandable balloon (General Surgical Innovations, Portola Valley, CA) is introduced through a 2-cm incision in the left flank. It is serially inflated with saline solution to a total volume of 600 mL to create an extraperitoneal working space. After balloon expansion, the external lifting device is inserted to maintain the space, and two 10-mm working ports are placed in the left flank for introduction of laparoscopic dissecting instruments. A separate port is created for introduction of the laparoscope. In the approach to the abdominal aorta through a plane anterior to the left kidney, the intact peritoneal sac is used to facilitate retraction of the small bowel to the right. The infrarenal aorta is then dissected circumferentially, and the lumbar vessels and inferior mesenteric artery are clipped and divided.

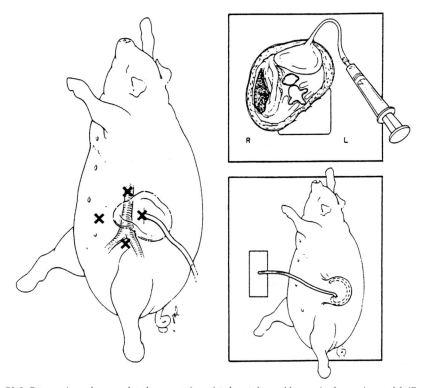

Fig. 53-2. Retroperitoneal approach to laparoscopic-assisted aortofemoral bypass in the porcine model. (From Jones et al., 1996, with permission.)

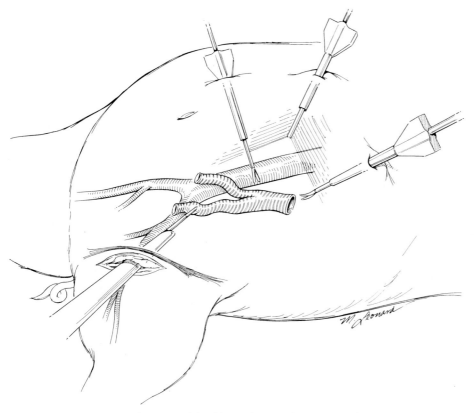

Fig. 53-3. Laparoscopic-assisted exposure of the abdominal aorta and retroperitoneal passage of the graft limb during aortofemoral bypass in the porcine model.

on the aorta is maintained by a small self-retaining retractor and gauze packing (Fig. 53-4).

Creation of the proximal aortic–graft anastomosis is performed similarly for both the transperitoneal and retroperitoneal approaches. The proximal and distal portions of the aorta are temporarily occluded either with standard vascular clamps inserted through separate ports or by large endoscopic clips. Using standard vascular instruments through the 4-cm incision overlying the aorta, an anterior aortotomy (1 cm in length) is created, followed by construction of an end-to-side anastomosis using continuous suture technique. After the anastomosis is complete, the proximal aortic clamp (or clip) is removed, the graft is flushed with heparinized saline, and a clamp is replaced on the graft just beyond the proximal anastomosis. After complete hemostasis of the proximal suture line is achieved, end-to-side femoral anastomoses are completed by conventional hand-sewn techniques. All clamps are then removed to restore distal perfusion through the aortofemoral graft.

In our initial study using this porcine model, we successfully completed unilateral aortofemoral bypass grafts in 10 animals. Five were performed with the transperi-toneal approach and five with the retroperi-toneal approach. Overall operative times (161 to 192 minutes) and aortic-clamp times (27 to 28 minutes) were indistinguishable between the two approaches. However, complications of the laparoscopic technique, principally related to the creation of the pneumoperitoneum and retraction of the small bowel, were only observed in the transperitoneal group. Thus, perforation of a distended urinary bladder occurred in one animal during initial insertion of the Veress needle, and in another animal the small bowel slipped from the fan retractor and was inadvertently cauterized. While each of these problems may have been avoidable, they serve to illustrate some of the potential hazards of the transperitoneal approach, which are overcome by performing the procedure through the retroperitoneal route.

Several additional lessons have been learned through our initial experience. For example, it is clear that "pure" endocavi-tary suturing is too difficult and time-consuming for aortic reconstruction, whereas an open technique uses instrumentation and techniques familiar to all vascular surgeons. Excellent visualization of the proximal anastomosis is achieved by a combination of direct inspection through the small abdominal-wall incision and video-guided visualization through the laparoscope (see Fig. 53-4). Indeed, the laparoscope allows even better visualization than open techniques alone because it can be used to view

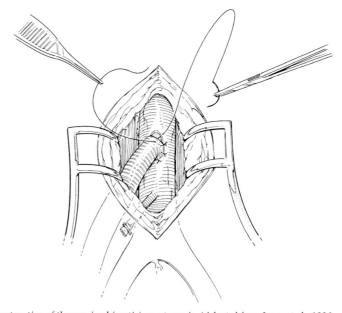

Fig. 53-4. Construction of the proximal (aortic) anastomosis. (Adapted from Jones et al., 1996; redrawn to illustrate intracavitary and extracavitary techniques for the first assistant.)

the anastomotic site from different angles and with magnification. Despite these advantages, we have nonetheless encountered difficulties in properly performing continuous suture anastomoses with instruments placed solely through laparoscopic ports, at least with the currently available instruments. This is in part due to the importance of the first assistant in "following" the suture to maintain tension during a continuous anastomosis. Thus, the assistant may either hold the suture close to the anastomotic site using metal instruments placed through laparoscopic ports (intracavitary assistance), or hold the suture straight up through the principal wound with the fingertips alone (extracavitary assistance) (see Fig. 53-4). Because polypropylene-based suture materials are prone to fracture and late failure if handled with metal instruments, we prefer the extracavitary assistance technique if these materials are to be used for vascular anastomoses. The more flexible PTFE sutures (Gore-Tex) are therefore preferred if the surgeon wishes the assistant to use port-based instruments and an intracavitary technique to follow the continuous suture line.

Other investigators have also explored the application of laparoscopy to aortic reconstruction with or without the use of pneumoperitoneum. For example, Dion and associates (1993 to 1995) reported experimental animal studies in which they used a left retroperitoneal approach and an expandable balloon similar to that described above. In 19 piglets, they were able to successfully dissect the aorta from the left renal vein to the aortic bifurcation under standard laparoscopic conditions and pneumoperitoneum. A total of five ports was used during the procedure (Fig. 53-5). After evacuation of the pneumoperitoneum and insertion of an abdominal wall–lifting device for gasless laparoscopy, complete aortobifemoral bypass was performed in four of these animals. In this circumstance, the aorta was clamped with a unique laparoscopic vascular clamp, and an end-to-end anastomosis was created. Although not specifically stated in their report, it appears that this was performed using intracavitary suture techniques. After the graft limbs were tunneled through the retroperitoneum, the femoral anastomoses were completed in conventional fashion. In their hands, the entire procedure was typically performed in less than 4 hours, with aortic-clamp times of 60 to 80 minutes to complete the proximal anastomosis.

In another porcine model, Chen and associates (1995) developed a technique for aortic reconstruction in which laparoscopy under pneumoperitoneum was also used during the initial dissection of the aorta. Twelve animals were approached through a transperitoneal route using a 10- to 12-mm infraumbilical midline incision. A silicone "fish" similar to those often used dur-

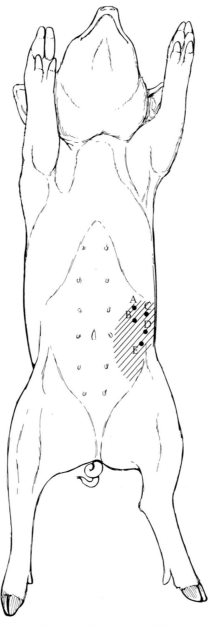

Fig. 53-5. Placement of ports for aortobifemoral bypass in the porcine model. (A, proximal aortic cross clamp port; B, Laparolift and laparoscope port; C, needle holder; D, inflatable balloon and grasper; E, grasper port; shaded section is the area lifted.) (From Dion et al., 1995, with permission.)

ing closure of the abdomen in open operations was inserted through this incision, and the peritoneal cavity was expanded by air insufflation. Six 11-mm trocars were then inserted under laparoscopic visualization. Using the silicone fish to retract the bowel, along with Trendelenburg and right lateral decubitus positioning, complete dissection of the aorta was conducted under pneumoperitoneum. After the aortic neck was sufficiently exposed, three additional trocars (11 mm) were inserted for dissection of the iliac arteries. All of the trocars were then removed, and a 10-cm midline laparotomy was performed. Standard aortic and iliac clamps were inserted through the previous trocar sites, and the proximal aortic–graft anastomosis was readily performed with conventional (hand-sewn) techniques using traditional instrumentation. The authors also found these techniques applicable to humans in a cadaver study conducted prior to clinical implementation.

Clinical Applications and Future Prospects

Several published reports have demonstrated the safe and effective application of laparoscopic techniques to aortoiliac vascular disease. The first of these was a single case report by Dion and coworkers (1993) in Québec, Canada, describing the use of laparoscopy to assist in performance of a prosthetic aortobifemoral bypass. The procedure employed seven 10-mm ports, two of which were used for the laparoscopic camera. Under pneumoperitoneum, retrograde dissection of the aorta from the bifurcation up to the left renal vein was visualized through a camera port placed in the midline 7 cm above the symphysis pubis. The inferior mesenteric artery in this patient was already thrombosed, and it was therefore ligated and divided to enhance aortic exposure. Retroperitoneal tunnels for passage of the graft limbs to the femoral arteries were created under visualization through a second camera port, placed in an upper paramedian position. These tunnels were placed beneath the ureters, largely facilitated by finger dissection from the femoral (groin) incisions. Following evacuation of the pneumoperitoneum, an 8-cm periumbilical incision was created. The aorta was clamped with a side-biting Satinsky clamp, and an end-to-side anastomosis to the graft was created with conventional suture techniques. The procedure was successfully completed by bilateral graft–femoral artery anastomoses in standard fashion.

Interestingly, in this patient, Dion and associates considered the presence of severe coronary arteriosclerosis and refusal to undergo an extraanatomic bypass as indications for a laparoscopic-assisted procedure. In most circumstances, a patient at high risk for a prolonged procedure under general anesthesia would not be considered an optimal candidate for this new surgical approach. Although any additional time required to perform the procedure with laparoscopy was not reported, the patient apparently had no cardiopulmonary complications and was ambulatory on the second postoperative day. Neither the duration of hospitalization nor return to usual levels of activity were discussed in this re-

port. The same group has recently reported an additional four patients undergoing laparoscopic-assisted aortobifemoral bypass with equally good results.

It is appropriate to reemphasize that vascular surgeons have several technical options by which to achieve lower extremity revascularization without the risk of prolonged general anesthesia, and consequently most high-risk patients need not undergo operations of this magnitude. Given that the use of laparoscopy does not avoid the need for general anesthesia in aortic reconstruction and indeed is more likely to result in a longer operative time than conventional open procedures, laparoscopic-assisted aortoiliac or aortofemoral reconstruction should not be considered a low-risk option for patients with severe cardiopulmonary disease. Investigators beginning to per-

form these procedures will do well to recognize that longer operative times and anesthetic exposure will be required than would be achieved by standard techniques for aortic reconstruction.

The most comprehensive clinical study of laparoscopic-assisted arterial reconstruction has been reported by Berens and Herde (1995) from Tucson, Arizona. After examining various methods for using laparoscopy in the laboratory, these authors described four cases of laparoscopic-assisted arterial reconstruction for occlusive disease. The procedures employed included two iliofemoral bypasses, one aortobifemoral bypass, and one aortoiliac endarterectomy. All were performed under gasless laparoscopic assistance with the Laparolift system (Origin Medsystems, Inc., Menlo Park, CA) for maintaining the working space (Fig. 53-6).

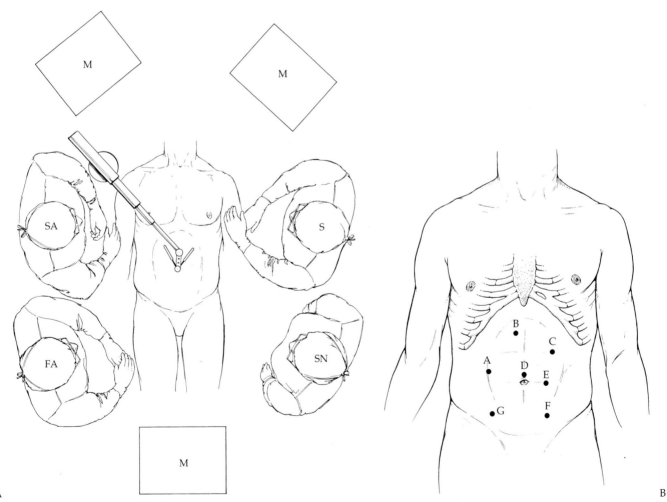

A   B

Fig. 53-6. **A:** Operating room setup and the Laparolift device used for laparoscopic-assisted aortoiliac reconstruction. (FA, first assistant; SA, second assistant; M, monitor; S, surgeon; SN, scrub nurse.) **B:** Port placement. (A, 15-mm port; B, camera port; C, 15-mm port; D, Laparolift; E, 15-mm port; F, 15-mm port; G, 15-mm port.) (From Berens and Herde, 1995, with permission.)

Five to seven laparoscopic ports (0.5 to 1.5 cm) were used in each patient, along with a 4-cm incision, and all anastomoses were performed with conventional vascular instruments and hand-sewn, end-to-side techniques. Notably, 5 to 7 hours of operating time were required to complete these operations. The patients undergoing iliac procedures were ambulatory within 24 hours and tolerating a regular diet prior to discharge on the second day, whereas those undergoing aortic procedures were ambulatory and tolerating food after 48 hours, with discharge on the third day. All of these patients resumed normal daily activities within 1 week, certainly a more rapid recovery than that following open operations. This important report emphasizes the use of gasless laparoscopy using a mechanical-arm lifting device, and it delineates the operating room setup and physical considerations required to embark on this approach.

In particular, the authors noted the use of the body mass index (BMI) (weight in kilograms divided by height in meters squared) to estimate the presence of technically limiting obesity. Based on their early experience and that of others, they recommend that laparoscopic aortic procedures be restricted to patients with a BMI less than 30.

Finally, Chen and colleagues pioneered the use of laparoscopy in the treatment of abdominal aortic aneurysms. They performed an aneurysm repair in a patient with a 6-cm infrarenal abdominal aortic aneurysm using laparoscopy under pneumoperitoneum during dissection of the aneurysm neck and the iliac vessels (Fig. 53-7). After evacuation of the pneumoperitoneum, a 10-cm minilaparotomy was made, and a prosthetic tube graft repair was performed in conventional fashion. The authors noted that this procedure took

approximately 4 hours, or about twice as long as comparable operations performed in an open fashion.

In considering the risks of laparoscopy in patients with aortic disease, Chen and colleagues noted that their patient's pulmonary artery diastolic pressure (PAD) was elevated from 10 mm Hg to around 25 mm Hg during use of the pneumoperitoneum, after which the PAD returned to the high teens on evacuation. Although there were no significant hemodynamic effects attributed to these changes based on monitored cardiac output, many patients with significant cardiac disease might not tolerate these changes. Their patient remained intubated for 1 day, did not resume a regular diet until postoperative day 4, and was not discharged until day 6. This postoperative course, similar to that of patients currently undergoing

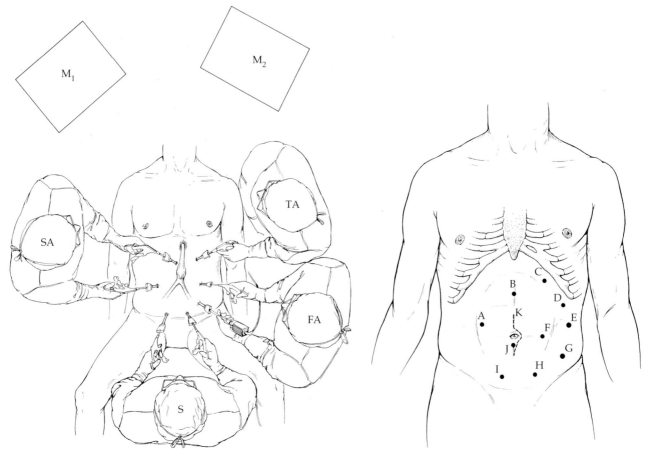

Fig. 53-7. **A:** *Operating room set-up for laparoscopic-assisted repair of an abdominal aortic aneurysm. (S, surgeon; FA, first assistant; SA, second assistant; TA, third assistant; M₁, monitor/light source/insufflator/VCR/Digivideo system; M₂, monitor/suction irrigator.)* **B:** *Port placement. (A, bowel retractor; B, bowel retractor; C, retractor; D, suction irrigator; E, camera port; F, dissector; G, camera port; H, dissector; I, dissector; J, dissector; K, incison.) (From Chen et al., 1995, with permission.)*

aneurysm repair by conventional methods, indicates that the benefits of laparoscopy for this procedure will need to be unequivocally demonstrated before it can be generally recommended. It is also notable that in their early experience Chen and associates found that a 2- to 3-cm-long disease-free segment of infrarenal aorta was necessary to allow laparoscopic-assisted aneurysm repair. This anatomic feature is not common in patients with aneurysm disease, thereby limiting applicability of this approach. Furthermore, patients with this favorable pattern of disease will also be candidates for the current generation of endovascular stent–graft devices, for which the postoperative recovery period is decidedly shorter. If it is found that this anatomic restriction persists even with more experience, applications of laparoscopy to abdominal aortic aneurysm disease will ultimately need to offer substantial advantages over endovascular treatments. At the least, it will need to be demonstrated that laparoscopy provides a therapeutic alternative with lower costs and recovery time than open operations for those patients who cannot undergo transluminal procedures.

Regarding the potential role of laparoscopic-assisted procedures for the treatment of aortic disease in the future, several as yet untested possibilities appear likely. One of these is that laparoscopic visualization and exposure of the aorta may be of additional benefit in vascular reconstructions that are otherwise based solely on an endoluminal approach. Because aortic stent–graft devices must be reliably secured in the proximal infrarenal aorta, it may be useful to use laparoscopic exposure to help secure the proximal anastomosis, such as by laparoscopically placing a supplementary ligature around the aorta at the level of the stent. Although this prospect has not yet been examined as an adjunct to the development of endoluminal stent–graft devices, it is conceptually similar to the use of previously reported "sutureless" graft materials. Indeed, the use of prostheses with a rigid ring at the proximal end might also provide another method by which to conduct laparoscopic-assisted aortic grafting without the need for conventional sewn anastomosis or endoluminal intervention.

A second possibility that may enhance the performance of aortic reconstruction under laparoscopic visualization is the use of new vascular stapling instrumentation not only to occlude the distal segment of the vessel (as in current use) but also to rapidly construct vascular anastomoses. Such devices have been shown to provide effective approximation of vascular tissues in microsurgery, and development of similar techniques for larger vessels can be expected. As various investigators continue to explore these problems over the next few years, both increasing experience and technical advances are likely to expand the use of laparoscopy in aortic surgery. These developments will undoubtedly present new challenges and opportunities for the current generation of vascular surgeons.

Endoscopic Venous Surgery

Advances in minimally invasive venous surgery have centered on new techniques for subfascial perforator ligation and saphenous vein harvesting. Subfascial perforator ligation is typically performed in selected patients who present with ulceration due to lower extremity venous insufficiency. Saphenous vein harvesting is done to provide conduits for coronary or peripheral vascular bypass grafts.

Subfascial Perforator Ligation for Lower Extremity Venous Insufficiency

Chronic lower extremity venous disease is due to either venous obstruction or valvular reflux. Valvular reflux with retrograde venous flow is the predominant problem among patients with chronic venous complaints. Therefore, venous surgery is performed primarily for treatment of refluxive venous disorders, manifested clinically as varicose veins or venous ulcers.

The formation of a venous ulcer results from transmission of high venous pressure to the skin and subcutaneous tissues around the area of the malleoli at the level of the ankle. Venous ulceration can be caused by superficial, perforator, or deep venous disease alone, or any combination thereof. Venous ulcers are preceded by hyperpigmentation, reflecting deposition of hemosiderin in the affected tissues. Heavy compression stockings are effective in preventing the formation of venous ulcers; however, they are difficult to don and re-move and are hot and often unsightly, resulting in poor patient compliance. An alternative in selected patients is to interrupt flow through incompetent perforating veins that allow abnormally directed flow from the deep venous system toward the skin. This is usually done in conjunction with elimination of superficial vein segments that demonstrate retrograde flow during preoperative evaluations. Recent clinical series suggest that elimination of superficial venous reflux can reduce or eliminate deep venous valvular dysfunction, resulting in improved or normalized deep venous system hemodynamics.

Advances in the technique of noninvasive imaging of venous abnormalities have contributed greatly to the renewed interest and success of contemporary venous surgery. Preoperative testing includes an evaluation of both the deep and superficial veins of the leg. In our institution, venous duplex imaging and venous reflux mapping using the rapid cuff deflation technique described by P. van Bemmelen are standard, although ascending and descending venography is used in other centers. Briefly, the van Bemmelen technique uses a duplex scanner and a rapidly deflatable blood pressure cuff. The duplex scanner images and records the magnitude, direction, and duration of venous flow in a venous segment immediately above the deflating cuff. A normal vein valve allows retrograde flow only briefly, typically 0.1 second. Abnormal valves have retrograde flow for several seconds. Our vascular laboratory uses a limit of 0.5 seconds of retrograde flow as the upper limit of normal. Attention is paid to documenting luminal patency and valvular function in the deep, perforating, and superficial veins of the leg. Perforating veins are abnormal if deep to superficial flow can be demonstrated, or if the vein diameter exceeds 4 mm. With detailed knowledge of the sites of valvular abnormality, surgery can be individualized and tailored to address the refluxing segments in each patient.

Perforating veins are so named because they penetrate the superficial fascial investment of the leg. Often erroneously conceptualized as simply connecting the superficial and deep venous systems, many perforating veins drain the skin and subcutaneous tissues directly into the deep venous system without any intervening connection to the superficial veins. Below the knee, some perforators connect the posterior arch vein with the deep venous system. Thus, stripping the long saphenous vein alone does not eliminate the possibility that high deep venous system pressure will continue to be directly transmitted to the skin through incompetent perforating veins. Only perforator ligation, an operation specifically designed to identify and divide the veins traversing the fascia of the leg, can serve this function. When necessary, surgical removal of portions of the superficial venous system responsible for reflux can also be combined with perforator vein ligation in patients without significant deep venous system abnormalities to permanently cure venous ulceration.

Open perforator ligation for patients with venous ulceration, referred to as the Linton procedure, is an operation characterized by frequent ulcer nonhealing and invariable problems with incisional complications. The standard open technique of subfascial perforator ligation is to raise a flap of skin, subcutaneous tissue, and muscle fascia through an incision over the medial or posterior calf and ankle. Frequently, this incision goes directly through the venous ulcer. Because of protracted problems with incisional nonhealing, this procedure has been largely abandoned. The poor clinical results from published series were due to the inability to specifically identify the venous segments that contribute to ulcer formation in any given patient. Thus, the ability to noninvasively map venous problems sparked a renewed interest in applying subfascial perforator ligation in appropriate patients, if the incisional problems could be overcome.

To avoid wound healing problems, surgeons investigated whether the perforating veins in the subfascial location could be reached from a remote incision through unaffected skin. This surgery has been called subfascial endoscopic perforator surgery (SEPS). The explosion in minimally invasive surgical products and application of techniques has now made SEPS a reality. The earliest series used a rigid bronchoscope as the viewing device, which was inserted subfascially into the posterior superficial compartment of the lower leg through a medial incision a few inches below the knee. This technique is still used in Europe and in selected American centers. Our technique is conceptually identical but takes advantage of the equipment used in standard laparoscopic surgery, together with a new balloon dissector for creating a large subfascial working space.

As detailed in Fig. 53-8, a transverse skin incision is made medially below the knee, and the fascia of the posterior superficial compartment of the lower leg is identified. A purse-string suture is placed in the fascia large enough to allow a 1- to 2-cm incision to be made in the middle of the purse-string. A blunt obturator with attached balloon is passed through a 10-mm port and is blindly tunneled posterior to the tibia. The peel-away balloon is inflated with 200 to 300 mL of saline to enlarge the potential space. The balloon and obturator are then removed, and the fascial purse-string is tied down. In addition, we prefer to place a second purse-string suture around the port at the level of the skin to prevent loss of gas from the working space. A pneumatic tourniquet is inflated around the lower thigh to superarterial pressure. Gas is insufflated into the subfascial working space. A 10-mm laparoscope is inserted and the working space examined. Typically, a few strands of fat accompany the perforating veins, which traverse from the muscle forming the floor of the working space to the fascia forming the ceiling of the working space. Under laparoscopic visualization, a second port is introduced into the working space, usually placed a few centimeters distal and posterior to the initial port. Blunt dissection cleans the remaining strands of fat from the perforating veins, which are then doubly clipped and divided. The process is continued down to the level of the medial malleolus. Usually, three to seven large perforating veins are identified and divided. Other surgeons have extended this technique, including a fasciotomy that allows identification of paratibial perforating veins. These paratibial veins contribute to the formation of venous ulcers located along the anterior ankle area. The ports are removed, and the tourniquet is deflated. Typical operating time is less than 1 hour, with tourniquet times of less than 30 minutes. After perforator ligation is completed, ablation of refluxing superficial venous segments is addressed. After completion of the procedure, the patient is placed into external elastic support wraps or hosiery. We have admitted patients the day of surgery and kept them overnight with legs wrapped and elevated after the procedure. The following morning, they are instructed to begin ambulation and are discharged home. The current medical-economic environment encourages shortening the length of stay, and several sur-

geons have reported discharging patients on the day of the procedure. Most surgeons also agree on the use of perioperative subcutaneous heparin as prophylaxis against the formation of deep vein thrombosis.

Careful cadaver dissections have identified hundreds of perforating veins in each lower leg, most less than 2 mm in diameter, that are not seen during laparoscopic perforator ligation. Presumably, the creation of a large subfascial working space disrupts many of these tiny perforating vessels and may contribute to the efficacy of the surgery. Early results of a multicenter SEPS trial demonstrated 88% healing of previously intractable ulcers. Complication rates were low. Intermediate term followup has shown that predictors of poor outcome after SEPS include venous outflow obstruction, large ulcer size, and multilevel deep vein reflux. An even less invasive treatment option for patients with a small number of incompetent perforators is a percutaneous miniincision approach described by L. Queral and F. Criado.

Endoscopic Saphenous Vein Harvesting

If SEPS is in its infancy in North America, then endoscopic saphenous vein harvesting is still in the embryonic stage. Saphenous vein conduits are used predominantly by vascular and cardiac surgeons, and major complications of full-length incisions over the length of the saphenous vein occur in about 2% of patients. Vascular surgeons using saphenous vein for *in situ* bypass grafting have tried to overcome these incisional problems by using long valvulotomes for valve lysis followed by short incisions directly over arteriovenous fistulas. However, for patients who need long saphenous segments transplanted elsewhere for use as an autograft or for reversed saphenous vein grafts in the leg, these techniques are not applicable. It is particularly the large patient population undergoing coronary artery bypass grafting using saphenous vein that drives the interest in endoscopic saphenous vein harvesting.

The procedure as currently practiced is endoscopically assisted rather than truly endoscopic, with initial incisions spaced roughly 30 cm apart over the course of the greater saphenous vein. The initial dissec-

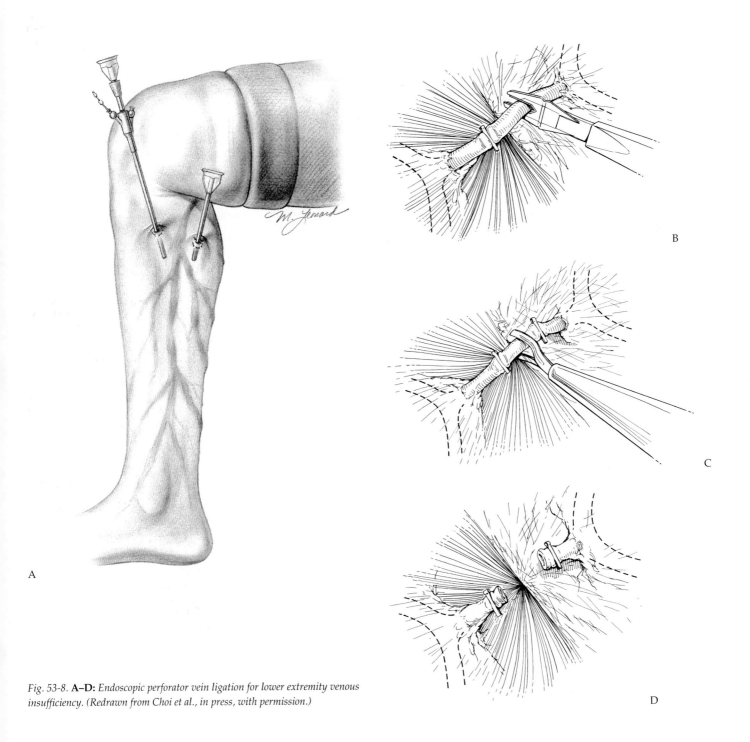

Fig. 53-8. **A–D:** *Endoscopic perforator vein ligation for lower extremity venous insufficiency. (Redrawn from Choi et al., in press, with permission.)*

A

B

C

D

tion is carried along the anterior surface of the vein as far as possible using standard instruments; then a long endoscopic retractor that accommodates a 30-degree endoscope is inserted. One group has reported using a long balloon dissector in a preliminary series of cadaver experiments to expose a length of the anterior vein surface. The dissection then continues along the vein surface with visualization through the endoscope using endoscopic instruments, with attention next directed to dissecting the side and posterior vein walls from the surrounding fat. Large side branches are clipped, while smaller branches are controlled with bipolar cautery. Because the same vantage point is used for introduction of both the endoscope and the working instruments, the vein dissection is coaxial rather than based on triangulation as typically performed for endoscopic procedures. The incisions are not closed until completion of the cardiac or vascular procedure so that the subcutaneous tunnel can be inspected to ensure hemostasis. The largest patient series from a single institution comes from Emory University in a report on experience with 30 patients undergoing endoscopic-assisted saphenous vein harvest. The investigators identified one patient who developed a limited segment of wound necrosis, and one patient who developed a bulla over the harvest tunnel. Both these problems were attributed to conduction of cautery through the endoscopic retractor to the overlying skin. Use of bipolar cautery appears to have resolved these problems, with no complications reported for the last 15 patients. Mean length of time to harvest saphenous vein was 1.25 hours. As experience accumulates, the role of endoscopic-assisted vein harvesting will become more clearly defined, and the optimal techniques for performing the surgery safely and rapidly will be clarified.

Suggested Reading

Ahn SS, Seeger JM, eds. Endovascular surgery. *Surg Clin North Am* 1992;72.

Berens ES, Herde JR. Laparoscopic vascular surgery: four case reports. *J Vasc Surg* 1995;22:73–79.

Chen MH, Murphy EA, Halpern V, Faust GR, Cosgrove JM, Cohen JR. Laparoscopic-assisted abdominal aortic aneurysm repair. *Surg Endosc* 1995;9:905–907.

Choi ET, Rubin BG, Thompson RW. Minimally invasive vascular surgery. In: Jones DB, Wu JS, Soper NJ, eds. Laparoscopic surgery: principles and procedures. St. Louis, MO: Quality Medical Publishing, Inc., 1997:412–432.

Cordts PR, Rubin BG. Noninvasive evaluation of chronic lower-extremity venous insufficiency. In: Callow AD, Ernst CB, eds. *Vascular surgery: theory and practice*. Stamford, CT: Appleton & Lange, 1995:375–378.

Dion YM, Chin AK, Thompson TA. Experimental laparoscopic aortobifemoral bypass. *Surg Endosc* 1995;9:894–897.

Dion YM, Katkhouda N, Rouleau C, Aucoin A. Laparoscopy-assisted aortobifemoral bypass. *Surg Laparosc Endosc* 1993;3:425–429.

Dion YM, Rouleau C, Aucoin A. Laparoscopy-assisted aortobifemoral bypass. *Surg Endosc* 1994;8(abst):438.

Dulucq JL. Laparoscopic iliofemoral bypass. *Surg Endosc* 1994;8(abst):438.

Gloviczki P, Bergan J, Menawat S, et al. Safety, feasibility, and early efficacy of subfascial endoscopic perforator surgery: a preliminary report from the North American Registry. *J Vasc Surg* 1997;25:94–105.

Horvath KD, Gray D, Benton L, Hill J, Swanstrom LL. Operative outcomes of minimally invasive saphenous vein harvest. *Amer J Surg* 1998;175:391–395.

Isner JM, Rosenfield K. Redefining the treatment of peripheral artery disease: role of percutaneous revascularization. *Circulation* 1993;88:1534–1557.

Jones DB, Thompson RW, Soper NJ, Olin JM, Rubin BG. Development and comparison of transperitoneal and retroperitoneal approaches to laparoscopic-assisted aortofemoral bypass in a porcine model. *J Vasc Surg* 1996;23:466–471.

Jordan WD Jr, Voellinger DC, Schroeder PT, McDowell HA. Video-assisted saphenous vein harvest: the evolution of a new technique. *J Vasc Surg* 1997;26:405–414.

Jugenheimer M, Junginger T. Endoscopic subfascial sectioning of incompetent perforating veins in treatment of primary varicosis. *World J Surg* 1992;16:971–975.

Lumsden AB, Eaves FF III. Subcutaneous, video-assisted saphenous vein harvest. *Perspect Vasc Surg* 1994;7:43–55.

Oz MC, Ashton RC Jr, Oz M, et al. Replacement of the abdominal aorta with a sutureless intraluminal ringed prosthesis. *Am J Surg* 1989;158:121–126.

Palmaz JC, Richter GM, Noeldge G, et al. Intraluminal stents in atherosclerotic iliac artery stenosis: preliminary report of a multicenter study. *Radiology* 1988;168:727–731.

Parodi JC, Palmaz JC, Barone HD. Transfemoral intraluminal graft implantation for abdominal aortic aneurysms. *Ann Vasc Surg* 1991;5:491–499.

Queral L, Criado F. Miniincisional ligation of incompetent perforating veins of the legs. *J Vasc Surg* 1997;25:437–441.

Rhodes J, Gloviczki P, Canton L, Rooke T, Lewis B, Lindsey J. Factors affecting clinical outcome following endoscopic perforator vein ablation. *Am J Surg* 1998;176:162–167.

Robbins MR, Hutchinson SA, Helmer SD. Endoscopic saphenous vein harvest in infrainguinal bypass surgery. *Amer J Surg* 1998;176:586–590.

Sicard GA, Reilly JM, Rubin BG, et al. Transabdominal versus retroperitoneal incision for abdominal aortic surgery: report of a prospective randomized trial. *J Vasc Surg* 1995;21:174–183.

Thompson RW, Anderson CB. Aortoiliac occlusive disease. In: Callow AD, Ernst CB, eds. *Vascular surgery: theory and practice*. Stamford, CT: Appleton & Lange, 1995:605–645.

54

Port-Access Cardiac Surgery: State of the Art

John H. Stevens, Mario F. Pompili, James T. Fann, and Tom A. Burdon

Minimal access endoscopic techniques have only recently been applied to the treatment and diagnosis of diseases of the chest. The geometry of the bony thorax and outcomes of applications limited to those on the periphery of the lung dampened initial enthusiasm for this approach. Subsequently, the significant benefit for patients became apparent. As the technology has improved, more thoracic surgeons and thoracic surgical procedures became amenable to minimal access techniques.

In the late 1930s, Gibbon initiated a series of pioneering experiments in an attempt to develop an extracorporeal circuit to allow temporary support of cardiopulmonary function. This culminated in 1954, when he performed the first open heart procedure using total cardiopulmonary bypass to repair an atrial septal defect. Work by Gibbon and others propagated the field of cardiac surgery. During the past 40 years, there have been dramatic advances in the safety and effectiveness of cardiopulmonary bypass and myocardial preservation. Cardiopulmonary bypass enables the surgeon to work in still and bloodless fields while maintaining systemic circulatory support. With a quiet and bloodless operative field, the heart may be manipulated fully so that complete coronary revascularization can be performed. The chambers of the heart can be opened and appropriate intracardiac palliative or corrective operations carried out.

Just as the development of cardiopulmonary bypass and myocardial preservation was essential for the development of

cardiac surgery in the 1950s, so too was the development of a system that allows the same degree of systemic circulatory support and myocardial protection to enable creation of a minimally invasive approach to cardiac surgery. During the past 4 to 5 years, a system of endovascular cardiopulmonary bypass has been developed that provides state of the art extracorporeal support and myocardial preservation to be carried out through entirely endovascular means. With the platform of a nonbeating heart, a protected patient, and still and bloodless field, cardiac diseases can be treated effectively with the minimal access techniques.

There are two fundamentally different techniques for performing minimal access cardiac surgery. Minimally invasive direct-vision coronary artery bypass (MIDCAB) grafting is a technique that was developed by several surgeons, including Benneti, Calafiore, and Subramanian. The procedure entails performing a minithoracotomy over the anterior fourth intercostal space and under direct vision, mobilizing a short segment of the internal mammary artery, and then performing an internal mammary to left anterior descending coronary artery anastomosis on a beating heart. This technique has the advantage of simplicity and avoiding the negative side effects of cardiopulmonary bypass. It is restricted to vessels on the anterior surface of the heart, because significant rotation or manipulation of the heart is not hemodynamically tolerated. A physical restraint of the portion of the coronary vessel to be bypassed must occur to increase the precision of a microvascular anastomosis on a moving tar-

get. A number of methods have been developed to accomplish this, including stay sutures, a suction device, and a compressing device much like the foot plate of a sewing machine. We believe the MIDCAB provides a nice springboard for discussion and evaluation of less invasive cardiac surgical techniques; however, it is severely limited in the scope of cardiac surgery that can be performed. Without the aid of cardiopulmonary bypass, MIDCAB is essentially relegated to single-vessel coronary artery bypass grafting to the left anterior descending artery. In the modern era of sophisticated and effective interventional cardiology techniques, this represents approximately 2% to 3% of all coronary artery bypass operations.

To extend minimal access surgery to the full spectrum of cardiac surgery, we adopted the same enabling technology that allows open chest surgery to be carried out, namely cardiopulmonary bypass (Figs. 54-1 and 54-2). Because of the unique characteristics of this approach, including combined endoscopic and direct visualization, and the use of cardiopulmonary bypass, we call these procedures *port-access procedures.*

Indications and Diagnostic Considerations

Port-access technology is applicable to patients who do not have severe aortoiliac occlusive disease, because the endovascular cardiopulmonary bypass system is introduced through the femoral artery

(text continues on page 528)

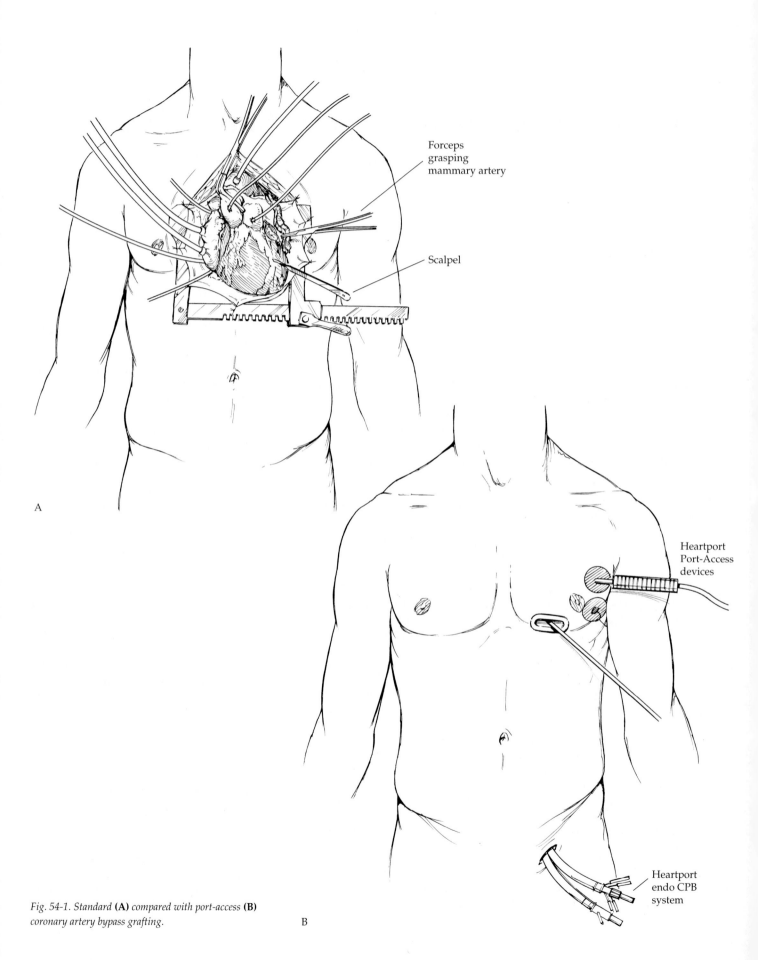

Forceps
grasping
mammary artery

Scalpel

Heartport
Port-Access
devices

Heartport
endo CPB
system

A

Fig. 54-1. Standard **(A)** *compared with port-access* **(B)**
coronary artery bypass grafting.

B

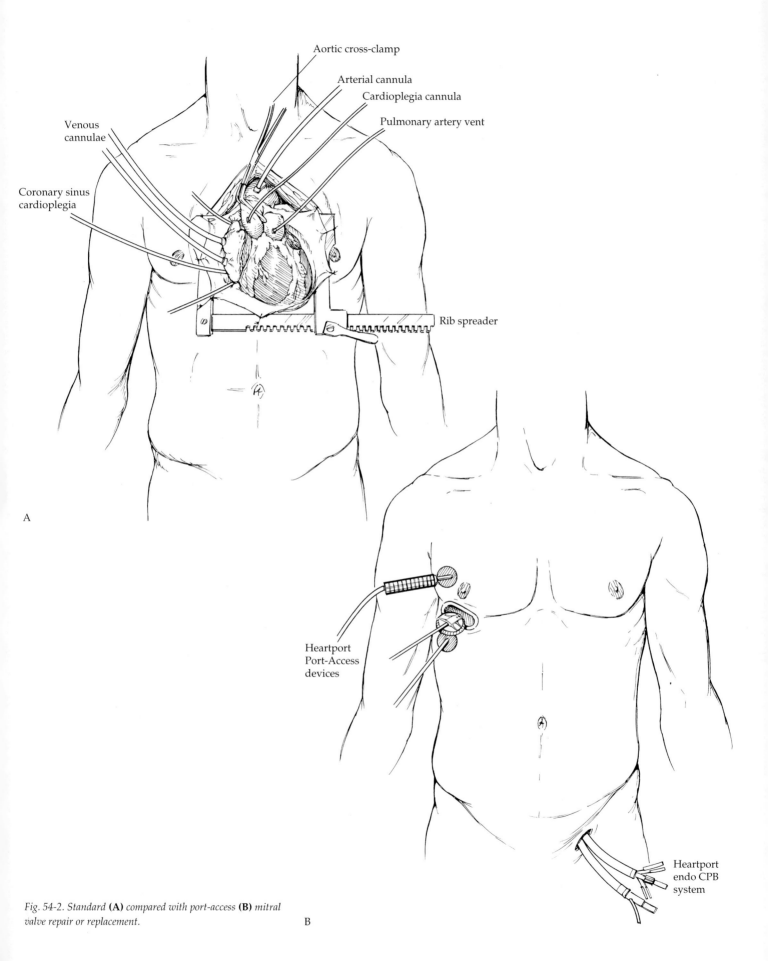

Aortic cross-clamp

Arterial cannula

Cardioplegia cannula

Pulmonary artery vent

Venous cannulae

Coronary sinus cardioplegia

Rib spreader

A

Heartport Port-Access devices

Heartport endo CPB system

Fig. 54-2. Standard **(A)** *compared with port-access* **(B)** *mitral valve repair or replacement.*

B

(Fig. 54-3). Prior major thoracic surgery, severe pleuritis, or inflammatory disease of the pleural cavity are contraindications for port-access intervention. We have performed only single-vessel coronary artery bypass grafts. Application is limited by a Food and Drug Administration protocol and by our desire to ease cautiously into this new arena of technology. However, based on the early clinical experience and our experimental and cadaveric experience, we think that multivessel bypass grafting is eminently feasible and that most patients should be candidates for port-access coronary artery bypass grafting in the near future. For patients who are candidates for mitral valve reconstruction or replacement, the only primary contraindications are peripheral vascular disease or severe inflammatory or postoperative scarring in the right pleural cavity. Prior mitral valve replacements through a median sternotomy are not a contraindication and seem to be more safely approached with this alternative strategy.

Surgical Technique
Coronary Artery Bypass Grafting

After the induction of anesthesia, a double-lumen endotracheal tube is inserted, and appropriate hemodynamic monitoring lines are placed. The patient is positioned in a modified supine position with the left and right arms elevated over the head of the patient and supported by an arm support. The left chest is raised slightly with a pillow behind the left shoulder to allow free access anteriorly and to the lateral chest. Standard skin preparation is performed for any coronary artery bypass grafting from the chin to the toes, and routine draping is carried out.

The fourth costal cartilages are palpated by identifying the manubrial sternal junction (the adjacent rib is the second) and counting inferiorly to the fourth intercostal space. An incision is made directly over the fourth costal cartilage, a 4-cm incision is carried out over this cartilage, and subperichondrial resection of the costal cartilage is performed. Single-lung ventilation is initiated. The posterior pericardium is incised with a scalpel, and the internal mammary artery is identified at this point. A pedicle of approximately 15 cm, including the internal mammary vein and artery, is then mobilized approximately 1 cm distally in either direction. Three 5- to 10-mm intercostal incisions are made in the left lateral thoracic wall, beginning in the fifth intercostal space in the middle to posterior axillary line. A thoracoscope is inserted (we most commonly use an articulating thoracoscope, the distal view 360 Welch Allen); initial inspection is carried out, and two thoracic ports are inserted, one in the fourth intercostal space in the anterior axillary line and a second in the sixth or seventh intercostal space in the middle to anterior axillary line.

The thoracoscope is inserted to the most inferior port, some gentle pericardial retraction is carried out through the anterior mediastinal incision previously made, and the thoracoscopic mobilization of the internal mammary artery is carried out (Fig. 54-4). Mobilization of the internal mammary artery is completed up to the level of the first inner space and distally to the level of the bifurcation of the internal mammary artery to the musculophrenic branches. Specially designed instruments are used for this purpose, including an angled DeBakey-type forceps and electrocautery probe that encompasses a very small electrocautery tip, constant suction, and fingertip irrigation. The femoral artery and vein are then surgically exposed. The patient is systemically heparinized, and

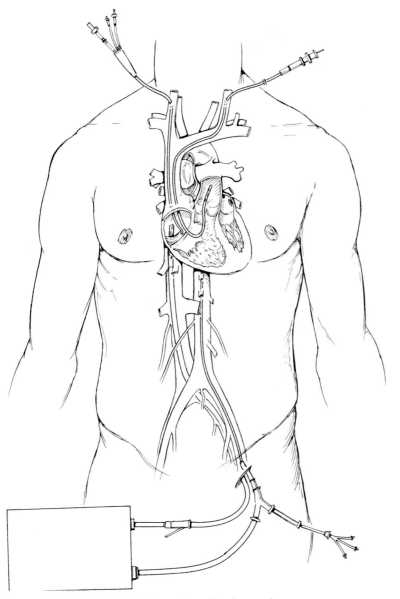

Fig. 54-3. Endovascular cardiopulmonary bypass.

the distal and internal mammary arteries are ligated distally, occluded with a temporary occluding device proximally, and divided distally. The internal mammary artery flow is checked, and the distal end is prepared for anastomosis. The endovascular pulmonary bypass system is inserted (Fig. 54-5).

Fluoroscopy and echocardiography are used to confirm appropriate positioning. Cardiopulmonary bypass is initiated, the ascending aorta is occluded with the endoaortic clamp, and cardioplegia is delivered. After satisfactory cardiac arrest has been achieved, the appropriate coronary vessel is dissected free, the arteriotomy is made, and anastomosis is carried out using a running continuous polypropylene suture. The anastomosis is completed using primarily direct vision with surgical loupes (Fig. 54-6). The temporary occluding device on the internal mammary artery is removed, and hemostasis is checked. The endoaortic clamp balloon is deflated, and spontaneous cardiac activity typically resumes. The thoracoscope is reinserted into the pleural cavity to confirm appropriate lie and position of the internal mammary artery pedicle and to secure hemostasis throughout the chest. A chest drain is inserted through one of the thoracic port sites, and routine skin closure is carried out.

Mitral Valve Replacement

For mitral valve replacement, the patient is placed in a modified left decubitus position. The right arm is gently positioned posteriorly, and the right chest is slightly elevated on the pillow. The fourth intercostal space is identified and marked with indelible ink. Routine skin preparation is carried out, and the patient is draped. A 5- to 8-cm incision is made in the fourth intercostal space between the middle and posterior axillary lines. Single-lung ventilation is initiated, and a specially designed retractor is inserted to facilitate retraction and displacement of all soft tissue without any mechanical force on the ribs (Fig. 54-7). An additional 10-mm port is created in the sixth intercostal space in the midaxillary line for insertion of the articulating thoracoscope. The pericardium is opened longitudinally approximately 3 cm anterior to the phrenic nerve pedicle. Pericardial stay sutures are placed. The sutures are passed externally through intercostal

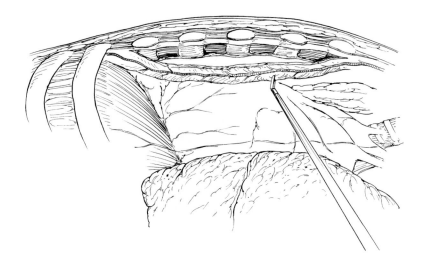

Fig. 54-4. Thoracoscopic mobilization of the internal mammary artery.

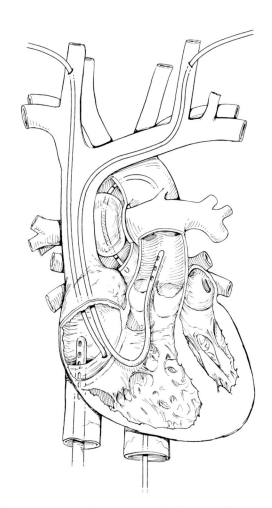

Fig. 54-5. Endovascular cardiopulmonary bypass equipment includes an endoaortic clamp, endocoronary sinus catheter, endopulmonary vent, and endovenous drainage.

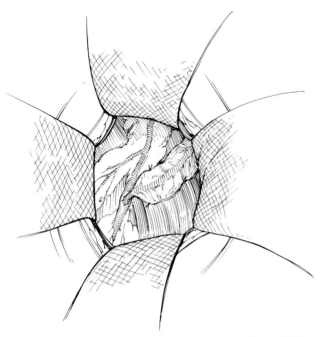

Fig. 54-6. Anastomosis of the internal mammary artery to a coronary artery. Even with limited access with an arrested heart is superb.

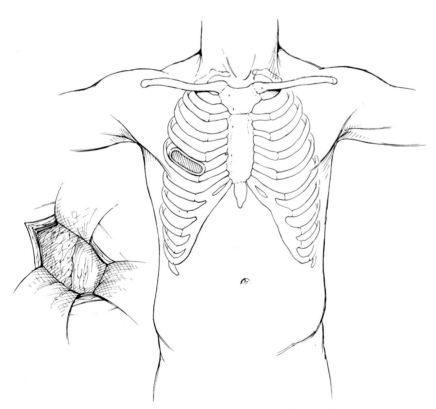

Fig. 54-7. Right chest fourth intercostal space incision (6 × 2 cm).

spaces and secured under tension. The right femoral artery and vein are exposed, and the patient is systemically heparinized and cannulated for initiation of endovascular cardiopulmonary bypass. Cardiopulmonary bypass is instituted, the endoaortic clamp is inflated, and cardioplegia is delivered (Fig. 54-6).

The left atrium is opened just posterior to the interatrial groove from the right superior pulmonary vein to the level of the right inferior pulmonary vein. The port-access left atrial retractor system then is inserted through the working port (Fig. 54-8). A 5-mm port is inserted in the second intercostal space on the right side. A retractor handle is inserted, and the retractor is assembled. Retraction of the left atrium is accomplished, and the interior aspect of the left atrium is inspected. If necessary, a sump suction device is placed in the well of the left atrium through the inferior aspect of the primary working port. The thoracoscope is positioned into view, and using a combination of thoracoscopic vision and direct vision with surgical loupes, the valve is inspected.

Standard surgical technique is used to determine suitability of reconstruction or replacement of the valve. After that determination is made, the appropriate repair is carried out. The following is a description of a port-access mitral valve replacement. Typically, the anterior leaflet is excised using port-access forceps and a long scalpel. An articulating valve-sizing device is then placed through the working port to determine the appropriate size of the prosthesis (Fig. 54-9). A series of sutures are placed in a horizontal mattress fashion using 36-inch, double-armed, 3-0 braided polyester sutures. If the tissue is friable, Teflon pledges are recommended. A series of the sutures are placed through the working port with thoracoscopic assistance and sequentially placed externally (Fig. 54-10). After all sutures have been placed appropriately, the needles are passed through the sewing ring of the prosthetic valve. The prosthetic valve is seated into place in the valve annulus (Figs. 54-11 and 54-12). All the needles are removed, and the sutures are tied extracorporeally using a single hand throw. Five to six throws are placed for securing each suture. Each knot is passed with a port-access knot pusher, which allows excellent tactile feedback and precise positioning of the knots (Fig. 54-13). All the excess suture material

(text continues on page 533)

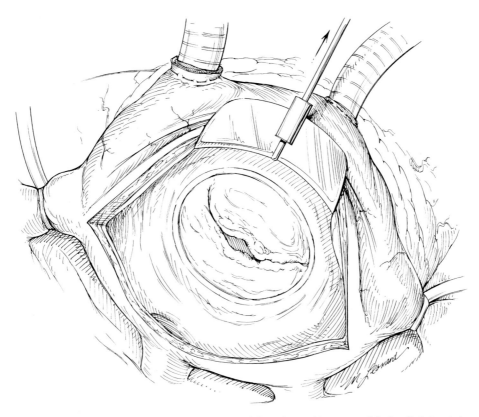

Fig. 54-8. *The left atrial retractor system blade is inserted through a working port, and the handle is inserted anteriorly through a 5-mm port. The retractor then is assembled.*

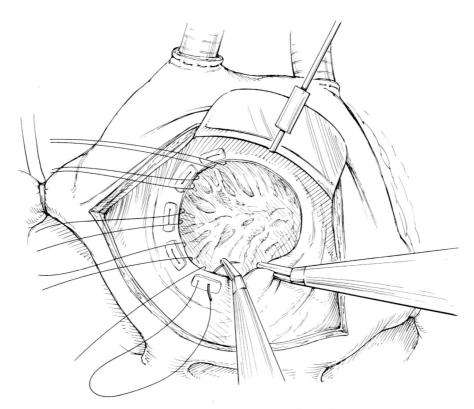

Fig. 54-9. *Valve sutures are placed into the annulus.*

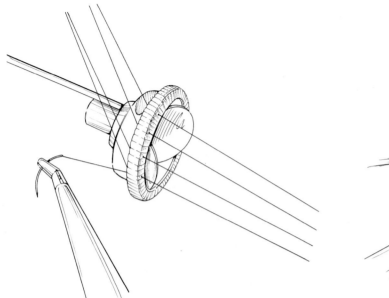

Fig. 54-10. *Sutures are placed* ex vivo *into the valve sewing ring.*

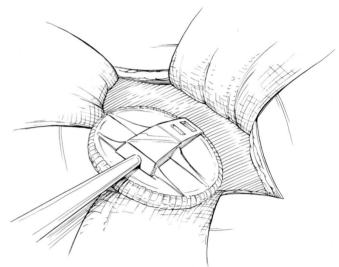

Fig. 54-11. *To press the valve into the chest, it must be oriented sideways.*

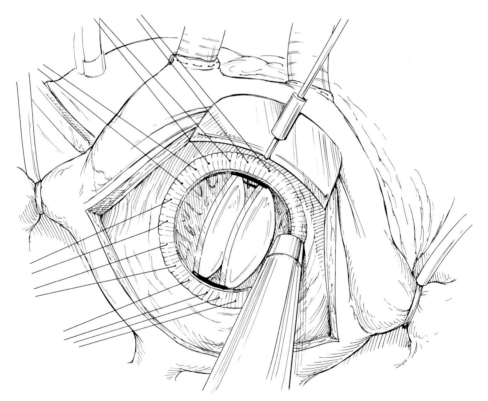

Fig. 54-12. *The valve is seated onto the mitral valve annulus.*

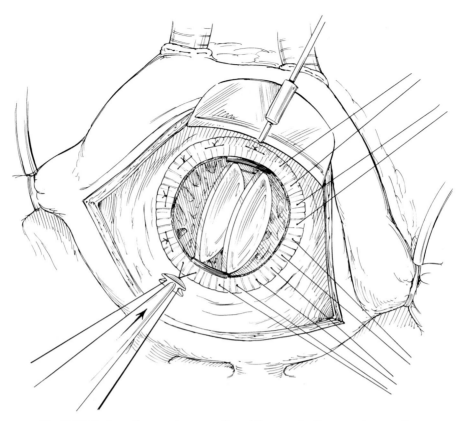

Fig. 54-13. Knots are thrown extracorporeally and then passed with a passer to secure them.

is trimmed, and the valve is tested for unhindered leaflet motion.

The left atriotomy is then closed with a running continuous suture of 3-0 polypropylene. Before complete closure of the atrium, a 10-French, soft Silastic catheter is placed across the valve to render it incompetent. Blood is returned to the patient, and cardiac venting is discontinued. The patient is placed in a slightly more left lateral decubitus position to fill the apex of the heart with blood, and vigorous Valsalva maneuvers are carried out with the left lung to displace any residual air that may lie in the pulmonary veins. Vigorous de-airing maneuvers are continued as the atrium is closed. The catheter that renders the valve incompetent is then removed. Suction is applied to the endoaortic root vent, and the endoaortic balloon is deflated. Spontaneous cardiac activity typically resumes; if not, internal defibrillation is carried out through the working port. Ventricular pacing wires are placed in all cases, as are atrial pacing wires, if deemed appropriate. The patient

is weaned from cardiopulmonary bypass in a routine fashion. Hemostasis is verified, and skin closure is routine.

Postoperative Care

For many patients, extubation may be carried out in the operating room before transfer to the intensive care unit. For others, a period of rewarming is essential in the intensive care unit. Routine cardiac postoperative care is initiated. With appropriate analgesia, most patients have minimal disturbances of their respiratory mechanics. They are able to resume ambulation rapidly in anticipation of an early discharge.

There are several real and potential complications of port-access coronary artery bypass grafting. A serious complication is injury of the internal mammary artery during harvest, rendering it unusable. Because this revascularization conduit has outstanding long-term patency rates, careful and meticulous dissection is essential. By

initiating the dissection through the anterior working port and completing it with thoracoscopic assistance, the internal artery pedicle can be mobilized with ease. If the internal mammary artery is not mobilized to the first intercostal space, it is theoretically plausible that large intercostal vessels may facilitate a steal phenomenon, thereby diminishing the coronary artery flow. Complete mobilization with thoracoscopic guidance is highly recommended. Because of the change in surgical perspective, the internal mammary artery pedicle can easily be twisted or rotated. To avoid this complication, we routinely inspect the graft through two different intercostal ports after the completion of the anastomosis to ensure a comfortable position for the internal mammary artery pedicle. We have had cases of inadequate hemostasis caused by overzealous use of electrocautery and underuse of hemostatic clips or displacement of clips. It is also important to revisit the site of dissection on the chest wall after the heparin has been reversed to ensure hemostasis.

For mitral valve reconstruction or replacement, inadvertent placement of the left atrial incision could cause right atrial entry and compromise the venous return to the cardiopulmonary bypass circuit. We have suggested the incision lie in continuity with the superior and inferior pulmonary veins to minimize this potential. Because of the enhanced magnification and the improved surgical view over the routine open surgical perspective, suture placement has become an important component to the learning curve. We have had the tendency to place our sutures further away from the annulus because of the magnified surgical perspective. Because we appreciate the high quality of the surgical exposure, we are more able to accurately place our sutures. As a consequence of errant suture placement, we had a case of permanent complete heat block. Knot securing after placing the throws is essential to minimize the risk of dehiscence of the valve or perivalvular leak. This is the most significant difference between open and port-access mitral valve surgery. It requires careful attention to both suture arms and precise visualization of the thoracoscope to ensure a secure position of the knots. A concern that we initially had was that cardiac de-airing would be difficult because of our inability to directly manipulate the heart. It appears in this early experience though

that our de-airing strategy has been very effective, but further experience is required.

Conclusions

Minimal access cardiac surgery is in its infancy. Procedure and device development will undergo significant maturation in the coming years. Looking forward, a few issues seem to be of paramount importance. The learning curve appears to be quite steep for these techniques. The similarities to a traditional open procedure are many, and the surgeon comfort and patient safety therefore are acceptable. We have strongly recommended intensive training before the initiation of these procedures, which might have obviated many of the learning curve issues.

This technology seems to hold tremendous promise for the advancement of cardiac surgery in terms of increased patient comfort, decreased patient morbidity, and a more rapid return to full and gainful activity. At the same time, modern techniques of cardiopulmonary bypass and myocardial preservation can be applied for optimal patient safety and surgical efficacy. Without doubt, much more experience and knowledge must be gained to fully appreciate these potential benefits.

Suggested Reading

Acuff TE, Landreneau RJ, Griffith BP, Mack MJ. Minimally invasive coronary artery bypass grafting. *Ann Thorac Surg* 1996;61:135–137.

Calafiore AM, DiGiammarco G, Teodorei G, et al. Left anterior descending coronary artery grafting via left anterior small thoracotomy without cardiopulmonary bypass. *Ann Thorac Surg* 1996;61:1658.

Pompili MF, Stevens JH, Burdon TA, et al. Port-access mitral valve replacement in dogs. *J Thorac Cardiovasc Surg* 1996;112:1268–1274.

Schwartz DS, Ribakove GH, Grossi EA, et al. Minimally invasive cardiopulmonary bypass with cardioplegic arrest: a closed chest technique with equivalent myocardial protection. *J Thorac Cardiovasc Surg* 1996;111:556–566.

Schwartz DS, Ribakove GH, Grossi EA, et al. Minimally invasive mitral valve replacement: port-access technique, feasibility and myocardial functional preservation. *J Thorac Cardiovasc Surg* 1997;113:1022–1030.

Stevens JH, Burdon TA, Peters WS, et al. Port-access coronary artery bypass grafting: a proposed surgical method. *J Thorac Cardiovasc Surg* 1996;111:567–573.

Stevens JH, Burdon TA, Siegel LC, et al. Port-access coronary artery bypass with cardioplegic arrest: acute and chronic canine studies. *Ann Thorac Surg* 1996;62:435–440.

55

Gynecologic Laparoscopy

Geoffrey W. Cundiff and John T. Soper

Laparoscopy has been an inherent part of gynecologic practice in the United States since the early 1970s. Although initially used for diagnostic purposes, tubal sterilization introduced operative techniques early in the evolution of gynecologic laparoscopy. These techniques were subsequently applied to treating infertility and ectopic pregnancy. As laparoscopic techniques evolved, they became applicable to more complex procedures, including urogynecologic and oncologic applications. Through this evolution, gynecologists have contributed significantly to the techniques and technologies that comprise modern operative laparoscopy.

Anatomic Considerations

Only anatomy pertinent to the performance of gynecologic laparoscopic procedures is discussed in this chapter. Figure 55-1 depicts the gynecologic organs as viewed through the laparoscope, with the uterus anteflexed toward the pubis. The uterus is between the bladder (anterior) and the rectosigmoid (posterior). The parietal peritoneum is applied directly to the uterus, fallopian tubes, and ovaries, with little intervening adventitia. It reflects anteriorly over the bladder, forming the anterior cul-de-sac, and posteriorly over the upper vagina on to the rectosigmoid, forming the posterior cul-de-sac. The vesicovaginal and rectovaginal spaces are po-

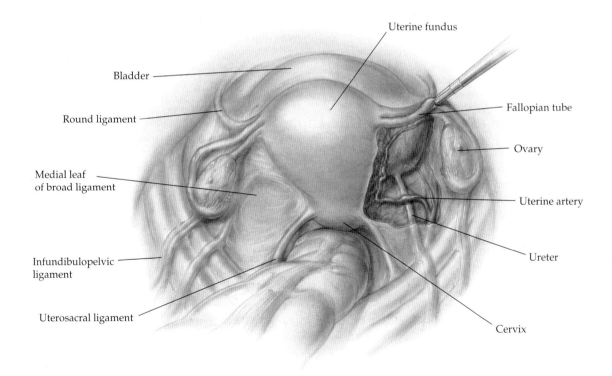

Fig. 55-1. Laparoscopic pelvic anatomy. The uterus is anteflexed toward the pubis. The parietal peritoneum is applied directly to the uterus, fallopian tubes, and ovaries and reflects over the bladder anteriorly, forming the anterior cul-de-sac, and over the upper vaginal and the rectosigmoid posteriorly, forming the posterior cul-de-sac. Lateral reflections of the visceral peritoneum applied to the adnexa and round ligaments form the broad ligaments on either side.

tential spaces that exist within loose areolar tissues along the endopelvic fascial planes.

Lateral reflections of the visceral peritoneum applied to the adnexa and round ligaments form the broad ligaments on either side. The round ligaments are condensations of perivascular fascia within the broad ligaments that pass anterolaterally from the anterior uterine cornu to exit the pelvis through the internal iliac rings. Samson's artery, an anastomotic vessel arising from the uterine vasculature, accompanies the round ligament. This must be controlled when the round ligament is divided.

The anterior leaf of the broad ligament is the flat expanse of peritoneum covering the round ligament and extending to the bladder. The middle leaf of the broad ligament is the triangular portion of peritoneum bounded by the round ligament anteriorly, the tube and infundibulopelvic ligament medially, and the pelvic sidewall laterally. When the anterior and middle leaves of the broad ligament are opened, the underlying loose areolar tissue can be easily dissected to expose the pelvic sidewall and retroperitoneal structures. The medial leaf of the broad ligament extends posteriorly to the fallopian tube, ovary, and infundibulopelvic ligament. In Fig. 55-1, the peritoneum of the medial leaf of the right broad ligament has been removed to illustrate relationships of the ureter, infundibulopelvic ligament, and uterine artery. The ureter is loosely adherent to the medial leaf of the broad ligament throughout its course in the pelvis and can be readily visualized laparoscopically through the normal peritoneum. The posterior boundary of the medial leaf is formed by the uterosacral ligaments, which extend from the cervix in a posterior and lateral direction to the rectum, inserting into the sacrum as the posterior rectal pillars.

The dominant uterine blood supply is from the uterine arteries that are anterior branches of the hypogastric (internal iliac) arteries. Each uterine artery rises and courses anteromedially, crossing anterior to the ureter approximately 2 cm lateral to the cervix. The uterine artery divides into ascending branches, which supply the uterine fundus and anastomose with vessels from the mesosalpinx, and descending cervicovaginal branches. The uterine veins coalesce and descend as a plexus that drains into the hypogastric vein.

The vascular adventitia of the uterine vessels condenses to form the cardinal ligament, which transverses laterally and provides major lateral support to the uterine cervix. The ureter passes posterior to the uterine artery through the cardinal ligament within the ureteric tunnel.

The ovarian blood supply descends into the pelvis within the infundibulopelvic ligament. The ovarian arteries are direct branches from the aorta. The right ovarian vein drains into the inferior vena cava, and the left ovarian vein drains into the left renal vein. The ovarian artery continues medially, forming the arcade of the mesosalpinx and terminates in anastomoses with ascending branches of the uterine artery adjacent to the uterine cornu. The ovaries are supported medially by the utero-ovarian ligaments.

The ureter must be isolated and visualized at all times during pelvic laparoscopic procedures. The ureter enters the pelvis at approximately the level of the bifurcation of the common iliac artery, in proximity to the infundibulopelvic ligament. The pelvic ureter courses anteriorly and medially in a shallow arc, applied loosely to the medial leaf of the broad ligament. It enters the ureteric tunnel under the uterine artery as previously described. The most common sites of injury to the ureter during pelvic surgery are at the level of the uterine artery and uterosacral ligament, followed by the level of the infundibulopelvic ligament.

Diagnostic Laparoscopy
Background and Indications

Diagnostic laparoscopy remains one of the most prevalent surgical procedures in gynecologic practice. The longevity of the technique can be attributed to the high-quality visualization of the pelvic and abdominal viscera with a minimally invasive but safe surgical approach. These are ideal qualities for a diagnostic modality. Recognition of the value of diagnostic laparoscopy rapidly led to its application to all aspects of gynecology. Common indications include evaluation of acute peritoneal signs, unexplained infertility, chronic pelvic pain, and second-look surgery after debulking of ovarian cancer. Diagnostic laparoscopy remains the first step performed in all operative laparoscopy.

The differential diagnosis of a reproductive-age women who presents with acute onset of pelvic pain and peritoneal signs is extensive, including ruptured ovarian cyst, torted adnexa, ectopic pregnancy, and pelvic inflammatory disease. These conditions require expedient diagnosis and treatment. Diagnostic laparoscopy provides a relatively safe and minimally invasive approach to this quandary. The access to the peritoneal cavity achieved for diagnostic laparoscopy facilitates surgical intervention for any discovered pathology.

Pelvic abnormalities have been demonstrated in 30% to 40% of women with infertility. Direct visualization of the abdomen and pelvis with laparoscopy provides information regarding adhesions, tubal distortion, clubbing of the fimbriated end, and evidence of ovulation. Common findings include adhesions from prior salpingitis, endometriosis, and anatomic abnormalities. Even 25% of infertile patients with negative radiographic findings have abnormalities. Findings at laparoscopy are valuable in planning future therapy, but it is best performed after the completion of noninvasive infertility tests.

Perhaps the most common indication for diagnostic laparoscopy is chronic pelvic pain, prompting approximately 40% of all gynecologic laparoscopies. Approximately 60% to 70% of diagnostic laparoscopies performed for chronic pelvic pain have abnormal findings. Endometriosis, pelvic adhesions, chronic pelvic inflammatory disease, and ovarian cysts are the most common findings in these patients, with endometriosis and adhesions comprising most of the positive findings. Operative management of pelvic abnormalities can be challenging and should be anticipated when planning diagnostic laparoscopy. For example, although a biopsy of a peritoneal implant to make the diagnosis of endometriosis is straightforward, vaporization of pelvic endometriosis requires electrocautery or laser energy and a surgeon with experience in using these modalities. Approximately, 65% to 80% of women with positive findings at laparoscopy have clinical improvement after operative management.

Technique

Although diagnostic laparoscopy is not unique to gynecology, several technical aspects are unique to the specialty. A significant proportion of the pathology within the pelvis occurs in the cul-de-sac, which can be difficult to visualize with the limited retraction afforded by laparoscopy. The uterine manipulator permits the uterus to be retracted without an intraperitoneal instrument. All of the many uterine manipulators available have a probe that traverses the cervical os and an anchoring mechanism. Although most require an assistant to elevate the instrument, some use weights to maintain the uterus in an anteflexed position.

Chromotubation is another important aspect of gynecologic diagnostic laparoscopy. Dilute methylene blue solution is infused into the uterine cavity and tubal lumen to evaluate tubal patency. Many of the available uterine manipulators provide a channel for chromotubation. Patency of the tubes is determined by detecting the spill of the dye from the fimbriated ends of the tubes. Chromotubation also has therapeutic benefit, because pregnancy rates immediately after chromotubation are significantly improved.

Gynecologic diagnostic laparoscopy begins with placement of the uterine manipulator. The patient is prepped and draped for vaginal surgery, and a Foley catheter is placed. A weighted or open-sided bivalve speculum is placed in the vagina, providing visualization of the cervical os. A single-tooth tenaculum placed on the anterior cervical portio simplifies placement of the uterine manipulator. A bimanual examination and sounding of the uterine cavity before placement of the uterine manipulator minimizes the chance of uterine perforation. After the manipulator is secured in place, the patient is draped for laparoscopy, including a drape over the vagina and handle of the uterine manipulator.

There are nearly as many techniques for achieving a pneumoperitoneum and placing trocars as there are surgeons. Generally, an umbilical port provides the best visualization of the pelvis with the least risk to the patient. A standard 10-mm telescope gives excellent visualization. Smaller-diameter telescopes (2 to 5 mm) have been used for diagnostic laparoscopy. Aside from decreasing patient discomfort, they offer the opportunity for laparoscopy to be performed outside of a traditional operating room setting. They have also been used through a Tenckhoff catheter for repeated diagnostic laparoscopy in chronic pain patients. The small-diameter telescopes have

a smaller focal length and transmit light less efficiently. These characteristics make a panoramic view of the pelvis unfeasible with the small telescopes.

Depending on the findings, a midline sheath may be sufficient to provide instrumentation for manipulation of the pelvic viscera. If extensive pathology is encountered, two paramedian sheaths may be required. Several important landmarks on the anterior abdominal wall should be identified before placement of paramedian trocars. The urachus can be identified running superiorly in the midline from the symphysis pubis. The obliterated umbilical arteries lie lateral to the urachus. They are good markers for the inferior epigastric arteries, which are often not visible through the parietal peritoneum but are 1 to 2 cm lateral to the umbilical arteries. Knowledge of their course is important when placing paramedian trocars.

A systematic approach to surveying the abdomen and pelvis is the best method to ensure pathology is not overlooked. Before the patient is placed in a Trendelenburg position, the upper abdomen and diaphragm should be visualized. After placing the patient in a deep Trendelenburg position, the pelvic organs are inspected. The anterior cul-de-sac is visualized first. The uterus is then elevated, allowing evaluation of the uterine fundus and posterior aspect of the uterus. This also gives an excellent view of the fallopian tubes (Fig. 55-1). Placing a blunt probe in the ovarian fossa permits the ovary to be elevated laterally and fully inspected. The posterior cul-de-sac is then surveyed. The sigmoid colon is followed out of the cul-de-sac. Chromotubation is performed last so that dye does not obscure pelvic structures. If the reason for evaluation is chronic pelvic pain, a thorough inspection of the small bowel and appendix should be undertaken and requires two paramedian ports. The survey should be completed before any operative procedures, because they may compromise the view of the viscera.

Laparoscopic Tubal Sterilization

Background and Indications

Permanent but reversible interruption of the oviducts to prevent pregnancy has been a surgical goal since the 19th century.

By the early 1970s, 95% of tubal sterilization in the United States was performed using monopolar high-frequency coagulation through a laparoscopic approach. This breadth of experience with sterilization by monopolar high-frequency coagulation demonstrated an unacceptable rate of tubal recanalization and a significant number of inadvertent electrical injuries. Efforts to find a safer method of tubal coagulation led to the development of bipolar high-frequency current coagulation that minimized the path of electrical current and decreased thermal spread. Semm developed the endocoagulator that uses heat without current to achieve coagulation. Investigators also sought noncoagulation techniques of laparoscopic tubal sterilization, including techniques using suture ligation and Silastic rings. Other gynecologists used clips in an attempt to improve the reversibility of laparoscopic sterilization. The use of clips is associated with a higher success rate at reanastomosis but also with a higher failure rate of the initial procedure.

Sterilization is a misnomer, because there is a failure rate associated with all sterilization techniques. Large studies have reported failure rates ranging from 2.2 to 12 cases per 1000 procedures. A rate of 4 failures per 1000 procedures is probably a good estimate for all tubal sterilization methods. This failure rate should be discussed with the patient preoperatively and should be part of the informed consent. Because the failure rates differ among different sterilization techniques, the specific method failure rate also should be discussed and documented. Failure rates are lower for puerperal and postabortion tubal sterilization procedures, demonstrating that at least a portion of the failures result from early pregnancies existing at the time of the sterilization procedure. Scheduling procedures during the follicular phase of the menstrual cycle and requiring a negative pregnancy test result the morning of surgery can decrease these luteal phase failures.

Studies of patient satisfaction after tubal sterilization have shown a surprisingly high degree of regret, and a significant portion of patients seek tubal reversal. The success rates for tubal reanastomosis also differ for the various sterilization methods. This finding may have implications in the choice of the sterilization technique used for a given patient.

Technique

Most of the laparoscopic tubal sterilization techniques are easily performed with two sheaths: an umbilical sheath for the telescope and a midline 5-mm sheath for instrumentation. Alternative sheath placement can be used. A single-puncture technique requires a laparoscope with an operating port and longer instruments that can reach the pelvis through the operating port. Most of the specialized instruments for clip or Silastic ring application are available in the longer lengths.

A variety of anesthetic techniques are appropriate for laparoscopic tubal sterilization, including general, regional, and local anesthesia. Local anesthesia is perhaps most appropriate for the single-puncture technique, and the simplicity of this approach has made it popular for sterilization programs in Third World settings. The mean operating time using this approach is 10 minutes. Nevertheless, general anesthesia is used most often in the United States.

Bipolar high-frequency coagulation is the most commonly used technique for laparoscopic tubal sterilization. It lends itself well to the single-puncture approach. After entry to the peritoneal cavity, the pelvic viscera are inspected by elevating the uterine manipulator. Before performing tubal sterilization, each tube must be identified. A Kleppinger bipolar forceps is introduced through the operating port, and the fallopian tube is grasped approximately 3 cm from the uterus. It is important to grasp the tube perpendicular to its axis so that the forceps jaws completely encompass the tube (Fig. 55-2). After ensuring that the forceps and tube are free of all other viscera, current is applied until the ohm meter demonstrates infinite resistance across the clamped tissue. The Kleppinger forceps are removed and replaced approximately 1 cm proximal to the initial site, and current is reapplied. A total of three sites should be coagulated on each tube. Care should be used while manipulating the forceps, because they get hot enough to cause burns to abdominal viscera after coagulation. Studies of the failure rates for bipolar tubal sterilization range from 4 to 7 per 1000 patients. The failure rate increases to 50 per 1000 using only a single-burn technique. The improved efficacy of multiple burn sites comes at the cost of increased tubal damage. Consequently, the efficacy of reversal of bipolar sterilization techniques is low.

Semm described a technique for laparoscopic tubal sterilization using an endocoagulator. The technique is similar to that described using bipolar current with several exceptions. The fallopian tube is coagulated at a single site and is then transected. He reports pregnancy rates of 2 cases per 1000 patients using this technique, but other investigators found no benefit to tubal transection and observed a higher failure rate and an increased incidence of hemorrhage.

Some gynecologists prefer to reproduce the open ligation techniques of sterilization rather than use coagulation. Many techniques using a pretied Roeder loop have been described. The use of this technique for fimbriectomy should be discouraged, because the failure rate approaches 10%. Ligation and resection of the midportion of the tube provides a surgical result similar to the Pomeroy technique and can be expected to have a similar failure rate of 5 per 1000 patients. In his open technique, Pomeroy advocated using absorbable catgut suture, which is rapidly absorbed and permits separation of the tubal ends. This may minimize the chance of fistula recanalization. The technique requires multiple ports, because the tube must be elevated through one port while the loop is put in place through another.

Yoon developed the Falope-Ring applicator that ligates a loop of the midportion of the tube with a Silastic band. It is considerably easier to place than a suture loop. A small Silastic ring is stretched open onto the end of the applicator mechanism. A narrow portion of tube is then grasped by atraumatic grasping forceps and elevated into the mechanism. The Silastic band is released onto the tubal segment, where it returns to its normal radius, constricting and occluding the tubal segment. The main advantage of the Falope-Ring applicator is the relative simplicity of the technique. It is adaptable to a single-puncture approach using local anesthesia. The most common complications are bleeding from torn mesosalpinx and incomplete tubal occlusion caused by improper placement. The reported failure rates range from 1 to 38 failures per 1000 procedures. The higher rates are caused by improper ring placement, and a failure rate of 6 per 1000 is probably a good estimate. The technique sacrifices 2 to 3 cm of tube because the oc-

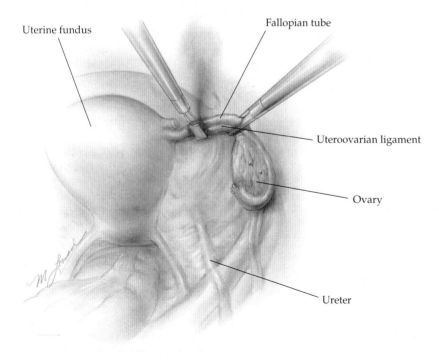

Fig. 55-2. Laparoscopic tubal coagulation by biolar electrocautery. The fallopian tube is grasped approximately 3 cm from the uterus with a Kleppinger bipolar forceps, and current is applied until the ohm meter demonstrates infinite resistance across the clamped tissue.

cluded portion undergoes necrosis, and this may be too much tissue to permit successful subsequent tubal reanastomosis.

Clips were developed for tubal sterilization in an attempt to improve the reversibility of the procedure. Hemostatic Tantalum clips were tried initially, but the metal clip had too much spring action and partially released the occlusion of the tube. Hulka introduced a clip constructed from plastic with a gold-plated stainless steel spring and an applicator for use with a laparoscopic approach. Other clips were subsequently introduced, including the Bleier clip. Regardless of the clip used, it is placed across the narrowest portion of the tube perpendicular to the tube axis. Application is not difficult provided the tube has a normal contour and is narrow. The tubal lumen must not be squeezed out of the clip as the hinge closes. This result is facilitated by maintaining tension on the tube with an atraumatic grasper during clip placement. Even with excellent technique, the failure rate of clips exceeds 6 per 1000 procedures (Hulka) and has been reported as high as 86 per 1000 procedures.

Laparoscopic Management of Ectopic Pregnancy
Background and Indications

Although the salpingectomy is definitive surgical management of a tubal ectopic pregnancy, it hinders future fertility by removing an oviduct. In an effort to preserve future fertility, more conservative surgical approaches were sought such as the salpingotomy, in which an incision on the antimesenteric aspect of the tube allowed extraction of the gestational tissue with preservation of the tube. Both techniques have been integrated into laparoscopic surgery. Experience has demonstrated that hemostasis without primary closure of the tubal incision provides similar tubal patency and decreases postoperative adhesion formation. Healing by secondary intention eliminates the need for laparoscopic suturing, greatly simplifying the procedure.

The laparoscopic approach is rapidly becoming the standard of care in surgical management of an unruptured ectopic pregnancy. It provides a minimally invasive diagnostic capability combined with a variety of therapeutic options. Advantages of the laparoscopic approach include a brief postoperative recovery with decreased hospitalization and an associated decrease in expense. In addition to these savings, the laparoscopic approach probably decreases the severity of postoperative adhesion formation and provides improved cosmesis.

Conservative therapy gained new meaning with the introduction of pharmacologic approaches to treating ectopic pregnancies. Methotrexate was introduced by Tanaka in 1982 and has been successful in approximately 90% of properly chosen patients. The American College of Obstetricians and Gynecologists recommends methotrexate for patients who desire future fertility and have an ectopic mass less than 3 cm in diameter, with a β-human chorionic gonadotropin level of less than 15,000 mIU/mL and no evidence of fetal heart tones on ultrasonography. Patients should be compliant, without hepatic, renal, or peptic ulcer disease. The College also recommends that the integrity of the tubal mucosa and the absence of active bleeding should be confirmed laparoscopically.

Conservative surgery is recommended for patients with an ectopic pregnancy who desire future fertility and are not candidates for pharmacologic therapy. An exception is made for most cornual and isthmic ectopic pregnancies. Two-thirds of ampullary ectopic pregnancies grow within the tubal lumen, whereas isthmic and cornual ectopics usually have an extraluminal implantation. With an extraluminal implantation, salpingotomy predisposes the patient to scarring and narrowing of the tubal lumen. Segmental salpingectomy has the advantage of removing the abnormal portion of the tube while preserving the proximal and distal segments for subsequent reanastomosis. Patients who do not desire future fertility are best served by a salpingectomy combined with occlusion or resection of the contralateral tube.

Persistence of viable trophoblastic tissue in the tube after intravenous methotrexate is equivalent to that after conservative surgical therapy, approaching 5%. Similarly, tubal patency is restored in approximately 80% of patients treated with pharmacologic or surgical conservative therapy. This leads to an intrauterine pregnancy rate of 75% after salpingotomy, compared with 44% after salpingectomy. The risk of recurrent ectopic pregnancy after salpingotomy is 10% to 20%, with equal prevalence in the operated and contralateral tube.

Technique

Even for a patient who is thought to be a candidate for conservative surgical therapy, access to the peritoneal cavity is essential before determining the most appropriate procedure. Linear salpingotomy is appropriate for the patient with an identified ampullary ectopic with intact mucosa in the absence of active bleeding (Fig. 55-3). The linear incision is made on the antimesenteric aspect of the tube using sharp dissection, monopolar electrocautery, laser, a harmonic scalpel, or an endocoagulator. The products of conception and blood clot are teased from the tubal lumen using forceps, suction, or hydrodissection. Irrigation with an isotonic solution facilitates identification of any sites of hemorrhage that can be controlled by point or bipolar forceps. Some surgeons inject the mesosalpinx beneath the conceptus with dilute vasopressin, but this technique may result in hypertension. If hemorrhage persists, the vessels in the mesosalpinx that serve the tube can be coagulated or ligated. The tubal incision is allowed to close by secondary intention.

A salpingectomy is the operation of choice for patients who do not desire future fertility. Although the linear salpingotomy is feasible for patients with small isthmic ectopics, these patients usually are better served by a salpingectomy. Salpingectomy can also be used in patients with tubal rupture provided they are hemodynamically

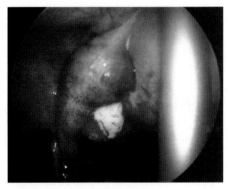

Fig. 55-3. An ampullary ectopic pregnancy of the left tube with intact mucosa.

stable. In patients who desire future fertility, a midsegment salpingectomy preserves tubal segments for subsequent reanastomosis. The midsegment resection is accomplished by coagulation on either side of the conceptus with bipolar forceps. The desiccated tissue is then cut with scissors, which permits the bipolar forceps to be placed on the mesosalpinx beneath the conceptus. After this tissue is desiccated, the abnormal segment of tube can be resected with the products of conception in place. In patients who do not desire future fertility, the involved segment and the distal portion of tube are removed. The mesosalpinx beneath the distal segment of tube can be resected using cautery followed by scissors. The tube itself can be excised in the same fashion, or it can be ligated and cut using pretied suture loops with a Roeder knot.

Depending on the size of the resected tissue, removal can be accomplished through a larger laparoscopic port (<10 mm) or through a colpotomy. A claw or large spoon forceps can be used for removal. Several commercially available devices to simplify tissue removal are safe and effective. Morcellation allows removal of larger specimens through an abdominal port. Colpotomy permits removal of the tissue specimen intact. The colpotomy can be made by incising the vaginal wall in the cul-de-sac transversely between the uterosacral ligaments. A sponge stick should be placed in the posterior vaginal fornix to place the vaginal wall on tension and facilitate cutting. Dipping the sponge stick in methylene blue before placement helps gauge the depth of the colpotomy incision because it provides visual contrast to the vaginal wall. Monopolar electrocautery is useful for this incision as it decreases hemorrhage. After the incision is made, a long clamp placed through the incision from the vagina retrieves the specimen from the cul-de-sac and removes it. The colpotomy is easiest to close from a vaginal approach using interrupted stitches.

Infertility Surgery

In treating infertility, the reproductive endocrinologist of the 1960s had limited therapeutic options consisting primarily of surgical intervention. Ovulation induction with clomiphene citrate or gonadotropins was newly available and was not widely used. Assisted reproductive technologies (ART), such as *in vitro* fertilization, were nonexistent. Reconstructive pelvic surgery therefore played an important role in the management of the infertile patient, including adhesiolysis, tubal reconstruction, myomectomies, and uterine reconstruction. Reconstructive surgery of the pelvic organs was performed by laparotomy using large reactive sutures. The introduction of microsurgical techniques by surgeons such as Gomel and Winston significantly improved reproductive outcomes for reconstructive surgery and were well accepted by the late 1970s. Reproductive outcomes were also influenced by the widespread adoption of diagnostic laparoscopy during the same period. Diagnostic laparoscopy modified the infertile population coming to surgery, because it detected less severe pelvic pathology than discovered by pelvic examination or hysterosalpingogram.

As operative skills improved, reconstructive pelvic surgery was increasingly attempted by a laparoscopic approach. Perceived advantages of the laparoscopic approach are a decrease in postoperative adhesions and shortened recovery, which permits outpatient management and provides cost savings.

During the past decade, the improving efficacy of ART has increased the use of these techniques in treating infertility. The American Fertility Society/Society for Assisted Reproductive Technology registry reported a delivery rate per *in vitro* fertilization retrieval of 17% in 1992; many centers have significantly better rates. Cumulative fertility rates for four cycles have been reported as high as 75%. The delivery rate falls dramatically with increasing age.

In a parallel trend, reproductive surgery has seen tremendous advances, largely through the application of laparoscopic approaches. Defining the appropriate role of ART and laparoscopic surgery is an ongoing effort that is best determined on the basis of individual patients. The use of a laparoscopic approach does have logical limits. For example, it has been proven that a myomectomy is technically feasible through a laparoscopic approach. However, the time required for morcellation and closure of the myoma bed using laparoscopic suturing techniques makes the laparoscopic approach unwarranted for large myomas that merit surgery. Similarly, efforts at tubal reanastomosis by a laparoscopic technique doubles the operating time and provides a patency rate of approximately 40%, significantly lower than the 60% rate achievable with open microsurgical techniques.

Laparoscopic surgery has proven invaluable in the diagnosis and treatment of peritubal adhesions. Adhesions impair fertility by distorting the normal tubo-ovarian relationships or by interfering with ovum pickup. Laparoscopic salpingo-ovariolysis has a subsequent intrauterine pregnancy rate of 62% and an ectopic rate of 5%. Patients with extensive or thick vascular adhesions have a much poorer prognosis after surgery and are better served by ART. Any patient who has failed to conceive within a year of surgery should also be directed to ART. Animal studies suggest that *de novo* adhesion formation is decreased by the laparoscopic approach, but definitive human studies are lacking. There is good evidence, however, that the rate of *de novo* adhesions is the same using laser or electrocautery for adhesiolysis.

Peritubal adhesions from prior salpingitis are often encountered in conjunction with fimbrial adhesions or phimosis. Laparoscopic fimbrioplasty has been reported to have pregnancy rates similar to microsurgical techniques, approaching 60% with an ectopic rate between 5% and 14%. True fimbrial agglutination requires more extensive surgery, including salpingostomy with eversion to create neofimbria. The subsequent pregnancy rate falls dramatically to between 17% and 4% and is inversely related to the extent of tubal distortion and degree of adnexal adhesions. Laparoscopic salpingostomies seem comparable to those performed by laparotomy. Factors that influence success include the diameter of the hydrosalpinx, fimbrial appearance after eversion, presence of adhesions, and rugal pattern on hysterosalpingography. Conceptions usually occur within the first year after surgery. Based on this information, it seems logical to offer laparoscopic tubal reconstruction to young patients with mild to moderate tubal disease and send those with more severe disease directly to ART. Younger patients benefit from reconstructive surgery because, if successful, it permits multiple future pregnancies. Multiple-site tubal occlusion mandates ART rather than surgical correction. Similarly, patients who have not conceived within 1 year should also be directed to ART.

Laparoscopic Approach to Endometriosis

Background and Indications

Some investigators estimate that up to 40% of infertile patients have endometriosis. Endometriosis is the heterotropic presence and growth of endometrial glands and stroma. Although there are several theories, the pathophysiology of endometriosis has not been definitively characterized. Typical symptoms associated with endometriosis are pelvic pain, dysmenorrhea, and infertility, but presentations are rarely typical, and a given patient may suffer from one or all of these symptoms. Moreover, the severity of symptoms is often inversely related to the severity of disease. Although there are physical findings suggestive of endometriosis, histologic confirmation is essential to making a diagnosis. Laparoscopy is useful for establishing the diagnosis and the extent of disease, and laparoscopically guided biopsy is recommended before making treatment decisions. Use of the American Fertility Society classification of endometriosis is recommended in staging endometriosis, because it is valuable in estimating prognosis.

The treatment of endometriosis can be surgical, medical, or a combination of both. Multiple variables influence the choice of therapy, including, age, reproductive desires, symptoms, and the extent and location of disease. Medical therapy is hormonally based and is based on clinical observations that endometriosis regresses during pregnancy and at menopause. Numerous sex steroids, used alone or in combinations, have been used to achieve amenorrhea by producing a pseudopregnancy or pseudomenopausal state. Commonly used medications include Danazol, gonadotropin-releasing hormone (GnRH) agonists, medroxyprogesterone, and oral contraceptives. Optimal regression occurs in patients with endometriomas less than 2 cm in diameter.

Rather than causing regression, the goal of surgical therapy is the removal of endometriosis. Surgical therapy is required for patients with ruptured endometriomas or symptomatic involvement of nongenital viscera. This includes conservative and definitive operations. The goal of conservative surgery is resection of all endometrial implants with restoration of normal

pelvic anatomy. Provided these surgical goals can be accomplished by a laparoscopic approach, fertility rates are comparable to surgery performed by laparotomy. The main advantage of the laparoscopic approach is that the patient can be treated at the time of diagnosis. Definitive surgery refers to castration with removal of the uterus, ovaries, and all foci of endometriosis. There is a role for laparoscopic resection with vaginal hysterectomy in patients with mild disease, but most definitive surgery is performed by laparotomy.

Medical and surgical therapies have implications for future fertility, and the patient's reproductive desires should be the foundation of management. Similarly, when infertility is the primary concern, the severity of disease has implications for treatment. For women with mild endometriosis and no other cause of infertility, the rate of conception without treatment is 65% to 75%. Multiple studies have demonstrated that this rate is not improved by medical therapy or conservative surgical therapy. The endometriosis is probably not the cause of infertility in these patients but rather is an associated finding. Conversely, the pregnancy rates for moderate and severe endometriosis managed conservatively are estimated at 25% and 0%, respectively, but these rates may be improved by therapy in selected patients.

Infertile women with moderate to severe endometriosis and associated adhesions, tubal obstruction, or endometriomas more than 1 cm in diameter appear to benefit from conservative surgical management. Conception rates for women appropriately treated with conservative surgery range from 50% to 60% for moderate endometriosis and 30% to 40% for severe disease. Preoperative treatment with Danazol or GnRH agonists for 6 to 12 weeks may simplify resection but does not improve fertility by itself. Similarly, postoperative medical management does not improve fertility rates. This suggests that the benefit of surgery in these patients is release of adhesions and restoration of normal anatomy rather than resection of the endometriosis. Consequently, infertile women with severe adhesions or tubal obstruction not amenable to surgical resection may be best served by ART in lieu of extensive pelvic surgery.

Pelvic pain from endometriosis mandates a different treatment algorithm. The diagnosed recurrence rate of treated endometriosis at 5 years is one case per three

patients, and this estimate is probably low because many women do not undergo a second-look laparoscopy. Medical therapy is rarely curative and cannot be used indefinitely because of the metabolic implications of a pseudomenopausal state. These two facts have important implications in treating women who suffer pelvic pain and have no plans for future childbearing. Mild to moderate disease may respond favorably to a course of medical therapy or may resolve after ablation at the time of diagnostic laparoscopy. Severe or recurrent disease should be treated with definitive surgery.

Women with pelvic pain who desire future childbearing should be offered medical therapy for mild disease less than 1 cm in diameter. If these patients have more severe disease or recurrence, they may be candidates for a presacral neurectomy, in which the sensory innervation of the uterus is ablated as it travels with the sympathetic nerves in the presacral area. Uterosacral nerve ablation has also been advocated for patients with central pain. For severe disease in women who desire future childbearing, a combination of conservative surgical therapy and medical therapy is often the best approach.

Technique

The surgical techniques used for endometriosis are similar to those used for invasive cancer. Like invasive cancer, endometriosis infiltrates tissues, causing fibrosis that prevents cleavage of normal surgical planes. Dissections can be tedious and demand excellent surgical technique. The goals of surgery are ablation or removal of all visible implants and lysis of all adhesions to restore normal anatomic relationships. Peritoneum close to the lateral surface of the ovary should be preserved if possible to minimize adhesion formation. Superficial peritoneal implants are vaporized or ablated using laser or electrocautery. Deeper endometrial implants should be excised. An elliptic incision is made through the normal peritoneum surrounding the endometrial implant. The peritoneum is then undermined using hydrodissection, sharp dissection, and electrocautery or laser energy as needed. Care is warranted during excision of implants that impinge on the bladder, ureters, or bowel. In these locations, use of the laser is preferred because there is less thermal spread than electrocautery. Hydrodissection can be used to separate the peritoneal surface from adherent bowel or adnexa.

In severe endometriosis, pelvic wall dissection may offer the greatest safety to the urinary tract. Careful identification of normal anatomy is essential to prevent damage to the urinary tract or bowel. The ureter enters the pelvis at the bifurcation of the common iliac artery and usually descends into the pelvis just superior to the hypogastric artery. The left ureter passes behind the sigmoid colon just superior to the pelvic brim, and the sigmoid colon may obscure its view. As the ureter travels further into the pelvis, it creates the posterior aspect of the ovarian fossa and then passes beneath the uterine artery and disappears from view as it passes into the bladder.

Presacral neurectomy requires opening of the retroperitoneal space over the sacrum to provide access to the afferent sensory nerve fibers before they enter the 11th and 12th thoracic segments. This requires lateral retraction of the sigmoid colon, which is best accomplished with a laparoscopic port in the left paramedian region. Special care must be taken while opening the retroperitoneum to avoid damaging the ureters or branches of the middle sacral artery. The sensory nerves can be ablated with laser or electrocautery. The technical requirements of the laparoscopic presacral neurectomy have led some surgeons to favor the laparoscopic uterosacral nerve ablation. This is accomplished by ablating the medial aspect of the uterosacral ligament inferior to its insertion into the posterior aspect of the uterus. The risk of ureteral damage increases as ablation is carried laterally.

There are several approaches to minimizing postoperative adhesions. Fine, nonreactive sutures should be used in reapproximating peritoneal surfaces. Frequent irrigation using a isotonic solution with heparin also helps to decrease postoperative adhesions. Some surgeons perform an anterior uterine suspension at the completion of surgery to minimize adhesion formation between the adnexa and raw cul-de-sac surfaces.

Laparoscopically Assisted Vaginal Hysterectomy

Background and Indications

Vaginal and abdominal hysterectomies have been performed since the 19th cen-

tury, but abdominal hysterectomy remained an extremely morbid procedure that was rarely performed until principles of sterile technique, ligature of vascular pedicles, and basic anesthesia were widely applied in the late 19th and early 20th century. Even with the advancements, vaginal hysterectomy was more frequently performed than the abdominal hysterectomy until the mid-20th century. Improvements in anesthetic techniques, antibiotics, and blood transfusion services, in addition to changing indications for hysterectomy, resulted in a relative increase in the number of abdominal hysterectomies. The advantages of vaginal hysterectomy include shorter hospital stays and less morbidity than with abdominal hysterectomy.

Reich described the first laparoscopically assisted vaginal hysterectomy (LAVH) in 1989. During the next 7 years, many anecdotal reports of LAVH described various techniques and instrumentation, and only recently have results of relatively large series of patients undergoing the procedure been reported. LAVH was widely embraced by gynecologists before the procedure was subjected to critical analysis in the literature. The use of laparoscopy along with the vaginal removal of the uterus seems to yield many of the benefits of an abdominal approach, including the ability to lyse adhesions and visualize the upper abdomen without the morbidity of an abdominal incision, and preserves the advantages of decreased morbidity and shortened hospital stay of the vaginal approach. The purported benefits of LAVH are presented in Table 55-1.

A variety of disease processes are amenable to treatment by hysterectomy. It is beyond the scope of this chapter to discuss the pathophysiology for each of these, but it is important that the surgeon be thoroughly familiar with the disease processes that may constitute indications for LAVH and have a thorough knowledge of the therapeutic options. It is inappropriate to use LAVH when a simple vaginal hysterectomy is indicated. In a randomized trial comparing vaginal hysterectomy (with or without removal of the adnexa) with LAVH, Stovall et al. were unable to demonstrate any advantage for LAVH in terms of decreased morbidity, but they documented increased cost and length of procedure for patients undergoing LAVH. The major advantage for the use of LAVH appears to be the potential to

convert hysterectomies that may otherwise be performed by laparotomy into vaginal hysterectomies. Table 55-2 has a partial listing of cervicouterine and adnexal diseases that may be approached with this technique.

A normal uterus is often removed in conjunction with removal of adnexal disease, particularly in women who do not desire to retain fertility or who are perimenopausal. Conversely, elective removal of normal fallopian tubes and ovaries is often performed in conjunction with hysterectomy in perimenopausal women. In general, the lifetime risk of developing ovarian carcinoma in a retained ovary is approximately 1.5% at age 40 and increases threefold in women with a family history of ovarian cancer, but rare families may have a much higher risk for ovarian cancer. This risk and the subsequent risk of surgery for benign adnexal disease must be weighed against the risks of surgical castration of the patient and need for

Table 55-1. Comparison of LAVH with Vaginal or Abdominal Hysterectomy

LAVH versus vaginal hysterectomy
  Superior visualization of abdominal
    contents
  Reliable removal of adnexae
  Can surgically approach adhesions,
    endometriosis, adnexal pathology
  Higher cost
LAVH versus abdominal hysterectomy
  Abdominal incision avoided
  Reduced ileus
  Reduced infectious morbidity
  Concomitant repair of vaginal relaxation
  Reduced hospital stay and convalescence

LAVH, laparoscopically assisted vaginal hysterectomy.

Table 55-2. Partial Listing of Indications for Laparoscopically Assisted Vaginal Hysterectomy

Refractory dysfunctional uterine bleeding
Adenomyosis
Uterine leiomyomas
Chronic pelvic inflammatory disease
Endometriosis
Refractory cervical dysplasia
Endometrial adenomatous hyperplasia
Benign adnexal masses and ovarian neoplasms

estrogen replacement therapy in premenopausal women.

Relative contraindications for LAVH include invasive cervical or endometrial carcinoma, cases in which extended hysterectomy or more comprehensive surgical staging is indicated, and pelvic masses that are suspected to be ovarian cancer, because intraoperative rupture of an early ovarian malignancy may adversely affect survival. Patients with ovarian cancer confined to the pelvis require comprehensive surgical staging, and those with obvious advanced intraabdominal malignancy require extended debulking procedures.

Several types of LAVH techniques have been recorded, ranging in scope from using laparoscopy to confirm the feasibility of vaginal hysterectomy through procedures that use laparoscopic ligation of all vascular pedicles and ligaments, development of the bladder flap, and entry into the vagina, leaving only removal of the uterus for the vaginal portion of the procedure. Some have recommended performing a laparoscopically assisted subtotal hysterectomy that leaves the cervix intact. In our opinion, the later procedure is rarely indicated, because most patients who are candidates for this procedure can be managed conservatively, without hysterectomy.

We teach and use a modified LAVH technique. Laparoscopic dissection is used to lyse adhesions, control the round ligaments, open the pelvic side walls, control the infundibulopelvic ligament or utero-ovarian ligaments and tubes, and partially develop the bladder flap. The procedure is then converted to a standard vaginal hysterectomy, with ligation of the uterosacral ligaments, cardinal ligaments, and uterine vessels and closure of the vaginal cuff performed vaginally. We believe that this is the safest technique to learn for physicians who do not have advanced laparoscopic skills. It avoids the potential for ureteral injury when endoscopic staplers or electric cautery are used for laparoscopic control of the uterine vessels.

Technique

Patients receive mechanical bowel preparation with clear liquids and laxatives for 1 or 2 days before surgery. All patients receive perioperative prophylactic antibiotics, preferably a first-generation cephalosporin, and receive thromboem-bolic prophylaxis consisting of minidose heparin or intermittent calf compression. The patient is positioned in a modified lithotomy position using candycane stirrups with the hips flexed 30 to 40 degrees. The arms are tucked at the patient's side. The vagina and perineum are sterilely prepped and draped but excluded from the abdominal field. A Foley catheter and uterine manipulator are placed. Two lateral video monitors are used so that the surgeon and assistant have an unobstructed view of the operation. Alternatively, a single monitor can be placed at the foot of the operating table.

Peritoneal access is performed with a 10-mm sheath placed infraumbilically using closed (direct insertion of a Verres needle) or open (Hasson trocar) techniques. Carbon dioxide is insufflated with a high-flow insufflator at pressures less than 15 mm Hg. The laparoscope is inserted, and the upper abdominal contents are visualized. The patient is placed in a 20- to 30-degree Trendelenburg position for visualization of the pelvic structures.

Additional sheaths are placed under laparoscopic guidance with transabdominal illumination and avoidance of the major vessels. Two 5-mm sheaths are placed approximately 3 to 4 cm medial to and slightly above the level of the anterior superior iliac crest. The inferior epigastric vessels should be visualized during placement of these sheaths. A 12-mm sheath is usually placed in the suprapubic location if endoscopic staplers or clips are to be used. If additional exposure is required or a large uterus is encountered, the 12-mm trocar may be placed above or below the umbilicus, or additional sheaths may be placed at these sites. If these placements are used, the sheaths should be placed just off of the midline to avoid interference between the instruments and laparoscope.

The bowel is manipulated out of the pelvis with atraumatic forceps and blunt probe. Adhesions are taken down sharply with endoscopic scissors. Electrocautery is not used on adhesions involving the bowel. The course of each pelvic ureter should be visualized through the medial leaf of the broad ligament, and its relative position should be verified during each portion of the procedure.

The uterus is placed on lateral traction. The round ligament on each side is ele-vated and divided using monopolar cautery with endoscopic scissors or divided after bipolar cautery with the Kleppinger forceps. The principles of traction and countertraction are used throughout the procedure. Although one physician can serve as the primary surgeon and the other as the camera operator and assistant, it is often easier for the two to alternate functions and serve as the primary surgeon for procedures on opposites side of the pelvis.

The peritoneum of the broad ligament is opened lateral to the fallopian tube and infundibulopelvic ligament (Fig. 55-4A). Medial traction on the utero-ovarian ligament or ovary using atraumatic graspers and the use of endoscopic scissors with monopolar cautery expedite the dissection. The peritoneal incision can be extended lateral to the ovarian vessels above the level of pelvic brim if salpingo-oophorectomy is to be performed. The loose areolar tissue within the broad ligament and the pelvic sidewall are opened using blunt dissection. Occasional small perforators can be controlled with electrocautery. The ureter remains attached to the medial leaf of the broad ligament.

When salpingo-oophorectomy is performed, a window is created with endoscopic scissors above the level of the ureter in the medial leaf of the broad ligament (Fig. 55-4B). This extends from the infundibulopelvic ligament to approximately the uterine vessels. Electrocautery may be required for control of bleeding from small vessels. Ligation of the infundibulopelvic ligament can be performed with the endoscopic stapler with the vascular staples, placed through the 12-mm suprapubic port (Fig. 55-4C). By closing the stapler and gently lifting the infundibulopelvic ligament before firing the stapler, the surgeon can ensure that the tips of the stapler are free and that the pedicle is isolated away from the ureter.

Alternatively, the infundibulopelvic ligament can be electrodesiccated with bipolar cautery and divided with endoscopic scissors (Fig. 55-4D). Care must be taken to ensure that the ureter is at least 2 to 3 cm from the point of cautery. Additional verification of hemostasis can be obtained by grasping the infundibulopelvic ligament through an open Endoloop (Ethicon, Cincinnati, Ohio) as it is being divided (Fig. 55-4E). The Endoloop is then secured around the proximal pedicle (Fig. 55-42F).

(text continues on page 546)

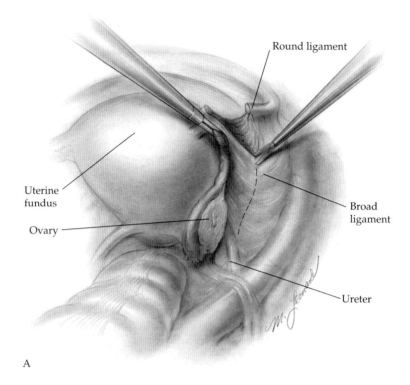

A

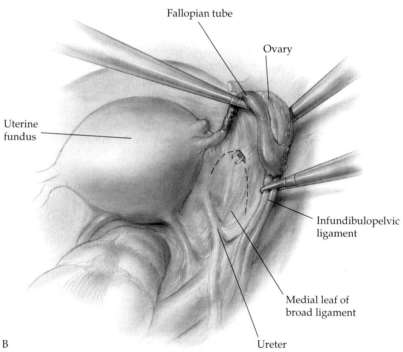

B

*Fig. 55-4. Laparoscopically assisted vaginal hysterectomy. **A:** The peritoneum of the broad ligament is opened lateral to the fallopian tube and infundibulopelvic ligament. **B:** A window is created in the medial leaf of the broad ligament above the level of the ureter with endoscopic scissors. (continued)*

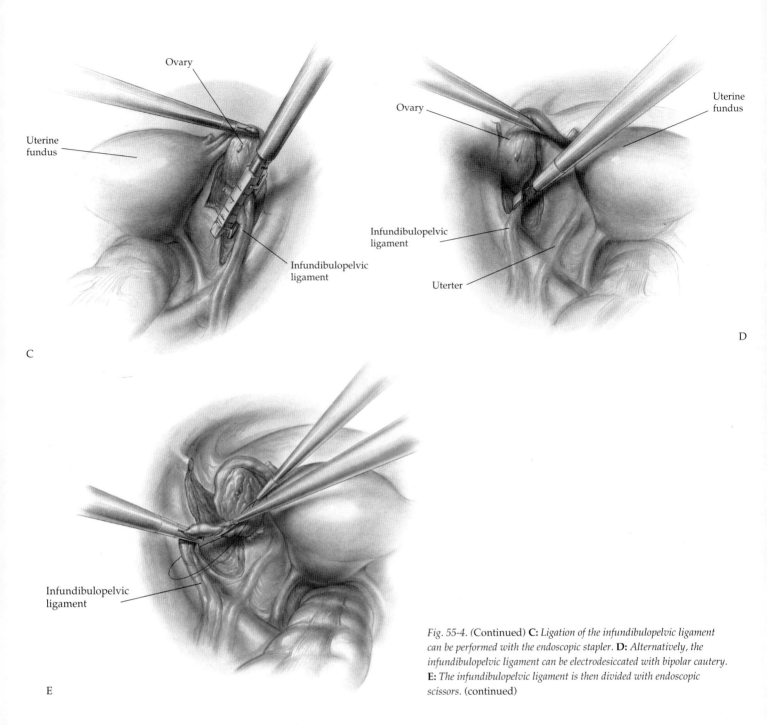

C

D

E

Fig. 55-4. (Continued) **C:** *Ligation of the infundibulopelvic ligament can be performed with the endoscopic stapler.* **D:** *Alternatively, the infundibulopelvic ligament can be electrodesiccated with bipolar cautery.* **E:** *The infundibulopelvic ligament is then divided with endoscopic scissors.* (continued)

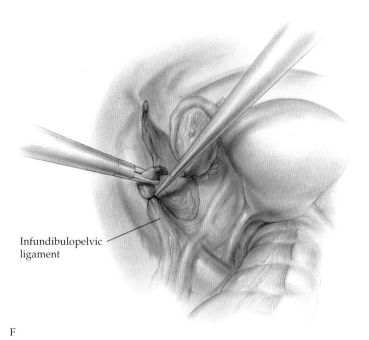

Infundibulopelvic
ligament

F

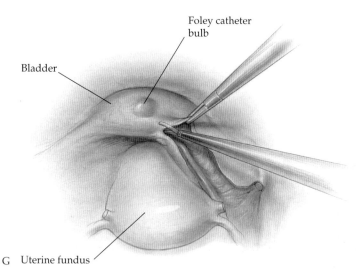

Foley catheter
bulb

Bladder

G   Uterine fundus

Fig. 55-4. (Continued) F: Hemostasis can be ensured by ligating the infundibulopelvic ligament with a pretied Roeder loop as it is divided. The Endoloop (Ethicon, Cincinnati, Ohio) is then secured around the proximal pedicle. G: The bladder flap is developed by opening the peritoneal reflection of the anterior leaf of the broad ligament using sharp dissection while the bladder is reflected anteriorly with atraumatic forceps.

Alternatively, the isolated infundibulopelvic ligament can be ligated using free suture with extracorporeal knots.

If the adnexa are to be preserved, the endoscopic stapler with the vascular staples can be used to divide the utero-ovarian ligament and tube, excluding the round ligament. This tissue can also be divided after bipolar electrodesiccation with Kleppinger forceps. If the window has been created in the medial leaf of the broad ligament above the level of the ureter, the

ureter is less likely to be damaged at this location than during division of the infundibulopelvic ligament.

The peritoneum and loose areolar tissues of the anterior leaf of the broad ligament and anterior peritoneal reflection of the uterus are opened with the endoscopic scissors. The bladder is reflected anteriorly with atraumatic forceps, and the bladder flap is partially developed with sharp dissection (Fig. 55-4G). Extensive mobilization of the bladder is not required, because

this will be completed during the vaginal phase of the procedure. The uterus should be elevated and the uterine fundus directed toward the posterior pelvis during dissection of the bladder flap. When a large uterus is being removed, electrodesiccation of the ascending branches of the uterine artery above the level of the ureter may expedite hemostasis during vaginal hysterectomy.

The instruments are removed from the sheaths, and the patient repositioned in lithotomy position with the hips flexed more than 45 degrees. The uterine manipulator is removed. Vaginal hysterectomy is completed using standard technique, and the vaginal cuff is closed. After completion of the hysterectomy, the peritoneal cavity is insufflated and the laparoscope reinserted to inspect all pedicles and raw surfaces for hemostasis. The operative field should be copiously lavaged with normal saline and intraabdominal pressure dropped to between 6 and 8 mm Hg to ensure that hemostasis is complete. The large fascial defects caused by the 10- to 12-mm trocars should be closed to prevent hernia formation using direct suture techniques or one of many laparoscopic instruments that have been developed for this purpose. Skin incisions are closed with fine, subcuticular sutures of absorbable material.

Results and Complications

The various techniques of LAVH are so new that some recent standard texts of gynecology do not describe them. Many of the reports in the literature consist only of small numbers of patients. LAVH is feasible in most patients. In some studies, performance of LAVH results in a shortened hospital stay and convalescence compared with abdominal hysterectomy. In most series, the major morbidity rate is low. Most surgeons report that the length of the procedure became shorter during the study interval as the surgeons became familiar with the technique. However, bleeding and significant injuries to the genitourinary and gastrointestinal systems have been reported after this procedure. LAVH cannot be considered a minor procedure. A randomized trial is comparing laparoscopically assisted vaginal hysterectomy with standard abdominal hysterectomy techniques to determine whether there is any advantage to LAVH.

Laparoscopic Approach to an Adnexal Mass

As newer diagnostic and laparoscopic techniques have evolved, the traditional approaches to an adnexal mass have undergone a substantial reevaluation. Until recently, the standard of care entailed ovarian cystectomy or oophorectomy by means of laparotomy for any adnexal mass larger than 7 to 8 cm discovered in a premenopausal woman or any adnexal enlargement in a postmenopausal woman. The aggressive approach to adnexal masses was a reflection of the limited means for preoperative diagnosis of an ovarian or tubal malignancy. Advances in diagnostic techniques have allowed more precise characterization of an adnexal mass as benign or malignant, and advances in laparoscopic techniques have increased the number of options for surgical management of benign adnexal masses. Laparotomy for surgical debulking and staging of ovarian carcinoma is the standard of care.

The trend toward increasing use of laparoscopic approaches to surgery for adnexal masses has raised concerns about the chances of inadvertently operating on a malignancy without proper preparation and the potential for a worsened prognosis because of tumor spill in these cases. Before considering techniques for laparoscopic adnexal surgery, it is important to consider the following questions:

1. What is the accuracy of preoperative discrimination between benign and malignant adnexal masses?
2. How reliably can ovarian malignancy be identified visually during laparoscopic surgery?
3. Is there any adverse prognostic effect if an ovarian cancer is ruptured intraoperatively?

The risks that an ovarian neoplasm is malignant increases with age from about 13% in premenopausal women to 45% in postmenopausal women. Although a clinical pelvic examination can give important information about an adnexal mass, transvaginal sonography with or without Doppler flow studies is the most frequently used radiographic test for distinguishing benign from malignant adnexal masses. In premenopausal and postmenopausal women, the incidence of ma-

lignancy approaches 40% to 60% when masses are larger than 10 cm in diameter. Regardless of size, a simple anechoic cystic mass has a less than 1% chance of being malignant. However, the entire cyst must be evaluated before this characterization can be made, which may be difficult for larger tumors. An increasing number of internal septations or increasing thickness of internal septations beyond 1 to 3 mm also increases the risk of malignancy. Solid components or clearly identified papillary excrescences increase the risk of malignancy to between 70% and 93%.

Malignant tumors are characterized by an increased flow in the vascular supply of the tumor. Doppler flow studies have suggested that a reduced pulsatility index has high sensitivity and specificity for identification of malignancy beyond the conventional ultrasound characteristics of an adnexal mass. In all studies, however, negative predictive value was substantially better than the positive predictive value, reassuring the clinician that she is not operating on a malignancy.

Serum CA 125 antigen levels have been evaluated preoperatively in women with adnexal masses. Studies report a high sensitivity (>80%) and specificity (>80%) in postmenopausal women when a threshold value of 35 IU/mL was used to discriminate between benign and malignant masses. Several studies have suggested that the use of transvaginal ultrasonography in combination with serum CA 125 values increases the accuracy for discrimination between benign and malignant masses when compared with the use of either modality alone. Clinical, sonographic, and tumor marker characteristics suggesting benign pelvic masses are detailed in Table 55-3.

Several studies have attempted to address the visual identification of an ovarian malignancy at the time of open or laparoscopic surgery for adnexal masses. Most series have been predominantly composed of premenopausal woman. Characteristics suggesting malignancy have consisted of obvious extraovarian metastasis or the presence of surface papillations or excrescences. Approximately two-thirds of the early ovarian cancers encountered in these series were diagnosed by visual appearance at the time of surgery.

The possibility of an adverse prognostic effect caused by intraoperative tumor

Table 55-3. Preoperative Criteria Suggesting a

Diameter <7–8 cm
Unilateral lesion
No evidence of ascites
Ultrasound characteristics
Unilocular, simple cyst
Rare, thin septa
Low flow and pulsatility index
Serum CA 125 <35 IU/mL

rupture must be considered. Patients undergoing laparoscopic removal of an adnexal cystic mass often require drainage of the mass or morcellation so that the entire mass can be removed through a laparoscopic trocar. Because of frequent tumor invasion into the cyst wall and adhesions to surrounding structures, malignant ovarian cysts are more prone to intraoperative rupture than benign ovarian tumors. Although there has been significant theoretical concern that intraoperative rupture of an otherwise intact ovarian malignancy might worsen the prognosis, many large series have failed to confirm this. Nevertheless, intraoperative rupture of an ovarian malignancy confined to a cyst increases the surgical stage (IA to IC) and may result in an individual patient receiving adjuvant chemotherapy or other postoperative treatment that would not have been administered if the tumor had been removed intact. Techniques used to avoid free intraperitoneal rupture of cystic masses are discussed in the following sections.

Laparoscopically Directed Cyst Aspiration or Fenestration

Small cysts of the ovaries have occasionally been managed through laparoscopically directed needle aspiration or by removing a 1- to 3-cm^2 portion of the cyst wall to allow internal drainage of the cyst contents. In most cases, these are small, simple cysts of the ovaries and often represent functional cysts related to ovarian function. This usually represents meddlesome surgery and is not recommended if pathology is suspected. Symptomatic functional cysts managed by drainage and fenestration recur in as many as one-third of cases, and occasional ovarian malignancies have been reported that developed less than 6 months after a drainage or fenestration procedure.

Laparoscopic Cystectomy

In laparoscopic cystectomy, similar to open techniques for cystectomy, the ovarian cortex overlying the cyst is incised with endoscopic scissors and using electrocautery for hemostasis. The cyst is decompressed using a spinal needle, grasped with an atraumatic grasper, and twisted to avulse the cyst from the ovarian stroma. Use of endoscopic scissors facilitates the sharp dissection, with electrocautery used for hemostasis. No sutures are required to close the defect in the ovarian capsule if hemostasis is adequate. Cystectomy is usually appropriate only for simple cysts encountered in premenopausal women and is technically difficult in cysts of more than 8 to 10 cm in diameter.

Laparoscopic Oophorectomy and Salpingo-oophorectomy

Complete salpingo-oophorectomy is preferred management of an ovarian mass in a perimenopausal or postmenopausal woman. It often is combined with laparoscopically assisted vaginal hysterectomy, as previously outlined. In these cases, the adnexal mass is usually removed trans-

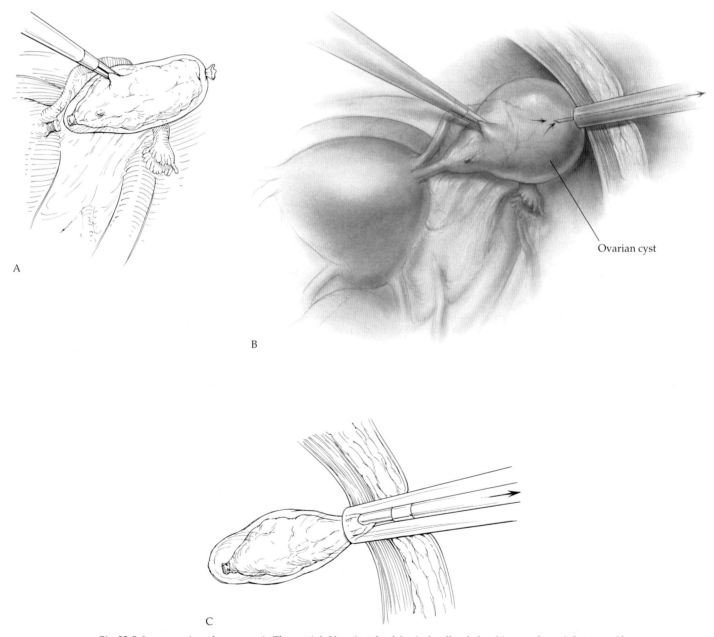

Fig. 55-5. *Laparoscopic oophorectomy.* **A:** *The cyst is held against the abdominal wall and placed in an endoscopic bag to avoid spilling intracystic fluid.* **B:** *Decompression of a large, simple ovarian cyst using laparoscopically directed needle placement into the cyst.* **C:** *After significant decompression, the cyst can be manipulated into an endoscopic bag and drainage completed before removing the deflated cyst through the 12-mm trocar.*

vaginally after completion of the vaginal hysterectomy. Alternatively, the infundibulopelvic ligament, fallopian tube, and utero-ovarian ligament pedicles can be controlled and severed; posterior colpotomy is performed; and the mass is delivered into the posterior cul-de-sac as described for an ectopic pregnancy. The vaginal operator can grasp the mass through the posterior colpotomy, drain or morcellate the mass transvaginally, and remove the mass before performing hysterectomy. This allows prompt gross inspection of the contents of the mass and frozen section if malignancy is suspected.

Performance of laparoscopic salpingo-oophorectomy is technically similar to management of the adnexae during laparoscopically assisted vaginal hysterectomy (Fig. 55-4A–F). The location of the pelvic ureter should be confirmed by transperitoneal inspection of the medial leaf of the broad ligament. The middle leaf of the broad ligament posterior to the round ligament is opened using the endoscopic scissors and electrocautery. The pararectal spaces are partially developed to allow visualization of the ureter and isolation of the infundibulopelvic ligament from the ureter. A window is created in the medial leaf of the broad ligament, and the infundibulopelvic ligament is controlled with electrodesiccation or endoscopic stapling techniques. The remaining medial leaf of the broad ligament is incised distally toward the vagina and above the level of the ureter. In patients who have undergone prior hysterectomy, the utero-ovarian ligament and fallopian tube are often densely adherent to the vaginal cuff in the vicinity of the old uterine artery pedicle. These adhesions should be taken down sharply, using electrocautery for hemostasis. The surgeon must visualize the ureter during all steps of this portion of the procedure and avoid using the endoscopic staplers in the area adjacent to the vaginal angle, because the distal ureter can easily be damaged as it courses beneath the uterine artery in its ureteric tunnel.

Figure 55-5 illustrates decompression of a large, simple ovarian cyst using laparoscopically directed needle placement into the cyst. The cyst is held against the abdominal wall to avoid spilling the intracystic fluid. After significant decompression, the cyst can be manipulated into an endoscopic bag (Fig. 55-5B) and drainage

completed before removing the deflated cyst through the 12-mm trocar.

When the residual ovarian mass cannot pass easily through the trocar, the trocar should be removed and the neck of the plastic bag opened at the skin level. Using the laparoscope to directly view the intraabdominal bag and its contents, the ovarian mass can be morcellated within the plastic bag so that there is no spill of tumor contents into the peritoneal cavity. Occasionally, the fascial incision needs to be enlarged slightly using sharp or blunt techniques to allow complete removal of the mass. When the mass and bag have been removed, the suprapubic sheath can be replaced.

After removal of an adnexal mass, the abdomen and pelvis should be copiously irrigated with normal saline. Theoretically, this reduces the chance of implantation if malignant cells were spilled intraperitoneally and reduces the risk of chemical peritonitis from intraperitoneal spill of dermoid cyst contents. The pelvic ureter should be carefully inspected and identified after completion of the procedure. If there is any difficulty in identifying the ureter, the patient should be given intravenous indigo carmine or methylene blue, and cystoscopy should be performed to confirm bilateral ureteral patency.

Results and Complications

Most series have indicated that more than 80% of adnexal masses in premenopausal and postmenopausal women that are not suspected to be malignant on preoperative evaluation can be successfully managed using the laparoscopic approach. In these women, incidence of malignancy is extremely low (<1%), and risk of complications are comparable to laparotomy. A laparoscopic approach to an adnexal mass should begin with a thorough peritoneal exploration and assessment of the mass for features of malignancy. If there is no evidence of extant peritoneal metastasis, ascites, or surface excrescences, peritoneal washings should be obtained before manipulating the adnexal mass, unless it is an obviously benign paraovarian cyst or hydrosalpinx. Washings can be discarded if the mass is confirmed to be benign. After the mass is removed, it should be carefully inspected for visible evidence of malignancy, and frozen sections should be liberally obtained if there is any question about the diagnosis. The current standard of care

mandates an immediate laparotomy for debulking and comprehensive surgical staging if malignancy is encountered. The surgeon should always be prepared for this eventuality if she is using the laparoscopic approaches on patients with adnexal masses.

Laparoscopic Procedures for Incontinence and Prolapse

Retropubic Urethropexy

Background and Indications

Advances in endoscopic instrumentation coupled with more technically capable and confident surgeons have dramatically increased the employment of laparoscopic techniques in the fields of gynecology and urogynecology. Many of the commonly used urogynecologic procedures employ a vaginal approach, but several procedures are conventionally performed through a laparotomy and are therefore amenable to a laparoscopic approach. Retropubic urethropexy, culdoplasty, and abdominal sacral colpopexy have been developed into laparoscopic procedures.

Retropubic urethropexy, originally described by Marshall, Marchetti, and Krantz in 1949, corrects the urethral hypermobility associated with genuine stress incontinence by suturing the urethrovesical junction to the symphysis pubis. Burch modified the retropubic urethropexy by using the paravaginal fascia to elevate the urethrovesical junction and fixing it bilaterally to Cooper's ligament instead of the symphysis pubis. Later studies demonstrated that retropubic urethropexy by either of these approaches has an 85% to 90% cure rate and has excellent longevity in correcting genuine stress incontinence.

The literature on laparoscopic retropubic urethropexy is not extensive and is composed primarily of retrospective descriptive reports of surgical techniques with poorly defined criteria for success and short follow-up. Most of the reports share an intraperitoneal approach in which access to the retropubic space is gained by cutting through the parietal peritoneum and pushing the bladder downward while dissecting into the space of Retzius. Reported advantages of the laparoscopic approach include easy access to the space of

Retzius, better visibility in the operative field, and minimal intraoperative blood loss. Shortened hospital stay, recovery time, and time to return of normal voiding are frequently touted benefits. Nevertheless, the operative time for the laparoscopic retropubic urethropexy remains a drawback to the procedure, as does the difficulty in mastering the technique.

The steep learning curve has led to the development of new techniques and equipment to simplify the procedure. Because the laparoscopic suturing is the most demanding portion of the procedure, it has been a major focus of modifications. For example, some laparoscopists recommend use of extracorporeal slip knots to elevate the bladder neck. Others advocate elevating the urethrovesical junction with a strip of surgical mesh anchored to the urethrovesical junction and Cooper's ligaments using surgical staples. These are significantly different procedures than the classic open retropubic urethropexy, and assuming that they have cure rates similar to the well-established cure rates for open procedures is not justified. The longevity of these modifications is suspect, but until well-designed prospective studies are done, the true benefit of these modifications remains unclear.

Approximately 15% of women undergoing a retropubic urethropexy subsequently develop enteroceles. With the intraperitoneal laparoscopic approach, a prophylactic culdoplasty is easily performed after urethropexy. The Halban or Moschcowitz technique can be used, and each is greatly facilitated by commercially available suturing devices.

Technique

The technique uses four trocar sites: a 10-mm umbilical incision for the laparoscope, two 5-mm paramedian trocars lateral to the inferior epigastric vessels, and a midline suprapubic 10-mm trocar. The suprapubic space is reached by incising the peritoneum well above the symphysis so that the peritoneum above the incision does not fall into the laparoscopic view and hinder the surgery. The bladder is filled with 400 mL of sterile saline to make it identifiable. The symphysis and retropubic space are cleaned of fat and areolar tissue using blunt and sharp dissection. The white strands of Cooper's ligament can be identified at the superior border of the symphysis (Fig. 55-6). Attention is then directed toward cleaning the vaginal fascia. The bladder is emptied, and with two fingers in the vagina and gentle traction on the Foley catheter, the vesicle neck is easily identified and the vaginal fascia laid bare by blunt dissection. A long, permanent-type suture on a curved needle is passed through the 10-mm sheath. Two sutures are taken on each side. Each suture is tied as it is placed while elevating the vaginal fornix with a vaginal finger. Sutures are tied using an extracorporeal technique and are placed with a knot pusher.

Surgical Management of Vaginal Vault Prolapse

Background and Indications

The incidence of pelvic organ prolapse is not well established, but the factors leading to it are. Anything that compromises the ligamentous or muscular support of the pelvic organs can result in prolapse, including neurologic and ligamentous damage during childbirth, chronic increases in intraabdominal pressures, and estrogen deprivation. Vaginal vault prolapse is a relatively rare complication of hysterectomy, with an estimated incidence of 4% to 5%. Prophylactic surgical techniques using the uterosacral and cardinal ligaments at the time of hysterectomy can help to prevent subsequent vault prolapse but are often insufficient for treating complete vault eversion in which the uterosacral and cardinal ligaments are attenuated. Colpopexy to another pelvic structure is an alternative approach. Many pelvic structures have been used for colpopexy, but those commonly used today are the sacrum, the sacrospinous ligament, and the fascia overlying the iliococcygeus muscle.

In 1962, Lane described an abdominal approach to repair vaginal vault prolapse by attaching the vaginal vault to the sacrum using an intervening tissue bridge. Tunneling of the bridge into a retroperitoneal location prevents visceral complications and promotes scarring. Subsequent modifications of the abdominal sacral colpopexy focused on the point of attachment to the sacrum and the material used for the intervening bridge. Different surgeons advocate the use of rectus fascia, fascia lata, Dacron, Marlex, or Gore-Tex for the intervening bridge. The artificial grafts offer greater strength and longevity, although at the risk of rejection. The surgeon's choice of repair of vaginal vault prolapse should be based on what defects are present and personal experience.

Technique

A laparoscopic sacral colpopexy requires careful retroperitoneal dissection over the sacrum and laparoscopic suturing techniques using a curved needle. The operation proceeds exactly as described for an open abdomen. The vagina is elevated by a vaginal probe. Dissection of the bladder off the cuff is sometimes required to provide 3 to 4 cm of vaginal apex for placement of sutures. Two straps of synthetic material, 2 to 3 cm wide and 12 cm long, are carried into the pelvis. One strap is sutured to the posterior vaginal cuff, and the other is sutured to the anterior vaginal vault. Permanent suture on a curved needle is used to take the six to eight circumferential sutures that anchor the straps to

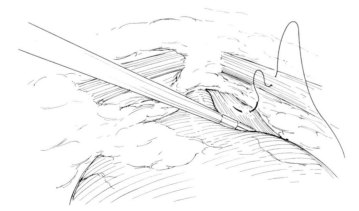

Fig. 55-6. Laparoscopic retropubic urethropexy placement. With two fingers in the vagina and gentle traction on the Foley catheter, a long, permanent suture on a curved needle is passed through the 10-mm sheath. Two sutures are taken on each side, and each suture is tied as it is placed while elevating the vaginal fornix with a vaginal finger. Sutures are tied using an extracorporeal technique and are placed with a knot pusher.

the vault. At least six extracorporeal knots are tied for each suture. The peritoneum overlying the sacral promontory is gently lifted from the underlying areolar tissue and bone and incised downward to the vagina. The sigmoid colon must be reflected laterally, and great care is taken to avoid the vessels of the sigmoid mesentery and ureters. Using careful hydrodissection and blunt dissection, the periosteum is cleaned from the promontory to the level of the third sacral vertebra (S-3). The straps are brought up to the sacral periosteum and, under appropriate tension, are anchored to the periosteum with permanent sutures. The excess fabric is trimmed from the strap, and the peritoneum is closed over the strap. If a retropubic urethropexy is to be performed, it is done after colpopexy.

Laparoscopically Assisted Management of Gynecologic Malignancies

Malignancies of the cervix, uterus, ovaries, and fallopian tubes often require surgery as part of initial treatment. In addition to removing the primary site of malignancy, surgical staging is often performed to help direct postoperative and adjuvant therapy. Surgical reassessment has been applied to patients with advanced ovarian malignancies after completion of primary chemotherapy in an attempt to assess response of intraperitoneal disease. The current standard of practice is for these procedures to be performed by open laparotomy. Table 55-4 includes the components of surgical management of cervical, endometrial, and ovarian or tubal malignancies. Because various components of these procedures have been performed laparoscopically, several small series have reported results for patients undergoing laparoscopically assisted management of gynecologic malignancies.

Table 55-4. Surgical Management of Selected Gynecologic Malignancies

Uterine cancer
  Peritoneal exploration
  Washings for cytology
  Simple hysterectomy and bilateral salpingo-oophorectomy
  Bilateral pelvic and periaortic lymphadenectomy
Cervical cancer
  Early stage (Ib/IIa)
    Radical hysterectomy
    Bilateral pelvic and periaortic lymphadenectomy
  Advanced stage
    Peritoneal exploration
    Bilateral common iliac and periaortic lymphadenectomy
Ovarian cancer
  Early stage (confined to pelvis)
    Peritoneal exploration
    Peritoneal cytology
    Biopsy suspicious lesions or multiple random peritoneal biopsies
    Intracolic omentectomy
    Simple hysterectomy and bilateral salpingo-oophorectomy
    Bilateral pelvic and periaortic lymphadenectomy
  Reassessment (second-look) procedure
    Peritoneal exploration
    Peritoneal cytology
    Biopsy of suspicious lesions or multiple random peritoneal biopsies
    Omental biopsies
    Multiple pelvic biopsies
    Bilateral pelvic and periaortic lymphadenectomy

Because gynecologic malignancies can potentially involve peritoneal structures and retroperitoneal lymph nodes, the biggest obstacle to performance of complete management of gynecologic malignancies has been development of safe approaches to the periaortic lymph nodes. Several small series have been composed of patients with gynecologic malignancies undergoing pelvic and periaortic lymphadenectomy. The Gynecological Oncology Group is conducting a series of studies in a cooperative group setting to determine the feasibility, safety, and cost of this approach. These studies are strictly controlled and require a comprehensive program intended to orient and evaluate gynecologic oncologists in performing standardized laparoscopic staging procedures before surgeons are allowed to enter patients in clinical trials. Until these prospective trials are completed, laparoscopic management of most patients with gynecologic malignancies must be considered experimental.

Suggested Reading

American College of Obstetricians and Gynecologists. Technical bulletin no. 150. Ectopic pregnancy: American College of Obstetricians and Gynecologists, Washington, DC, March 1990.

Benadiva CA, Kligman I, Davis O, Rosenwaks Z. In vitro fertilization versus tubal surgery: is pelvic reconstructive surgery obsolete? *Fertil Steril* 1995;6:1051–1061.

Dorsey JH, Cundiff G. Laparoscopic procedures for incontinence and prolapse. *Curr Opin Obstet Gynecol* 1994;6:223–230.

Howard FM. The role of laparoscopy in chronic pelvic pain: promise and pitfalls. *Obstet Gynecol Surv* 1993;6:357–387.

Martin DC. Laparoscopic treatment of endometriosis. *Clin Obstet Gynecol* 1991;2:452–459.

Soper JT. Laparoscopic-assisted vaginal hysterectomy with or without removal of the adnexae. In: Pappas T, et al, eds. *Atlas of laparoscopy*. Philadelphia: Current Medicine, 1996.

Steege JF. Laparoscopic approach to the adnexal randomized mass. *Clin Obstet Gynecol* 1994;2: 392–405.

Summitt RL Jr, Stovall TG, Lipscomb GH, Ling FW. Randomized comparison of laparoscopically assisted vaginal hysterectomy with standard vaginal hysterectomy in an outpatient setting. *Obstet Gynecol* 1992;80:895–901.

56

Laparoscopy in Urology

Todd D. Cohen and Glenn M. Preminger

Since the introduction of the first urologic endoscopes in the late 1800s, urologic endoscopic surgery has evolved into the primary method of treating intraluminal diseases of the genitourinary tract. Over the past 20 years, the development of percutaneous surgical techniques and improvements in optical systems have permitted the movement of endoscopic surgery into the upper urinary tracts (ureter and kidney). The next logical progression in urologic endoscopy was the expansion of these techniques to include extraluminal procedures. Since the first staging laparoscopic pelvic lymphadenectomy was performed 5 years ago, nearly every open urologic procedure has been performed or attempted laparoscopically in patients or in laboratory studies. Although many of these procedures are technically challenging, further improvements in laparoscopic equipment and techniques should allow laparoscopic surgery to replace several of the more conventional open urologic procedures.

Anatomic Considerations

Unlike most organs that are accessible laparoscopically to the general surgeon, the organs of the genitourinary system lie within the retroperitoneum or the extraperitoneal space. This is an important distinction, in that one must carefully consider appropriate access to these organs when developing an operative strategy. The retroperitoneum can be entered either directly or transperitoneally. The choice of the appropriate approach depends on the operation to be performed, the patient's body habitus, and the skill and ability of the surgeon. Most urologic laparoscopic procedures can be accomplished trans-

peritoneally. Direct access to the retroperitoneal or extraperitoneal spaces requires the creation of a working space, since there is no analogous cavity to the peritoneal space in these areas. Although these spaces can be created through the use of dissecting balloons, discussion of these procedures is beyond the scope of this review.

Performing successful laparoscopic surgery of the genitourinary tract requires complete knowledge of retroperitoneal and pelvic anatomy. The kidneys, adrenal glands, and ureters lie in the retroperitoneum. The presence of the liver causes the right kidney to be lower than the left; however, the right adrenal gland lies more cephalad and medial than the left gland. Both the kidneys and the adrenal glands are enveloped by a fascial sheath, Gerota's fascia. Surgery of the adrenal glands and a more detailed discussion of their anatomy is presented in Chapter 36.

A layer of perirenal fat lies between Gerota's fascia and the capsule of the kidney. The vascular pedicle enters in the midportion of the kidney. From anterior to posterior, the renal vein is the most anterior structure, followed by the renal artery and ureter, respectively. The left renal vein usually receives the main branch of the left adrenal vein, the left gonadal vein, and one or more lumbar veins. These are important considerations during any renal procedure. Supernumerary renal arteries may be present in approximately 25% of patients.

The ureters run lateral to the vertebral column along the anterior surface of the psoas muscle. They enter the true pelvis anterior to the bifurcation of the iliac artery, traverse medially, and penetrate

the base of the bladder. The ureters derive their blood supply from the renal artery, aorta, common iliac artery, and internal iliac artery, respectively, as they travel caudally. Care must be maintained when the ureter is mobilized, as stripping of the thin fascial covering off the ureteric surface may lead to segmental devascularization and stricture formation.

The pelvic organs and vasculature are separated from the peritoneal cavity by a reflection of peritoneum. This thickened layer often obscures the anatomy, making identification of important structures and dissection more difficult. The external iliac artery can often be identified through this layer, as one sees its pulsations along the lateral pelvic side wall. The external iliac vein lies inferior to the artery and often has branches emerging posteriorly and laterally that are easily avulsed. A large venous branch is generally found at the level of the inferior pelvic wall. The internal iliac arteries and veins supply branches to the pelvic viscera. These branches should be reviewed in detail prior to initiation of any pelvic surgery. In the collapsed state, the bladder rests posterior to the pubic symphysis, separated from the bone by a fat-filled space, the space of Retzius. In men, the bladder is separated from the rectum by a thin layer of fat and an atretic reflection of peritoneum known as Denonvillier's fascia. The prostate is also found posterior to the pubic symphysis and is held securely in position by reflections of the endopelvic fascia constituting the puboprostatic ligaments. In women, the bladder is separated from the rectum by the reproductive organs.

The urachus can serve as an important anatomic landmark in pelvic laparoscopic surgery. This structure courses in the midline along the anterior abdominal wall between the peritoneum and the transversalis fascia from the umbilicus to its insertion at the dome of the bladder.

The spermatic cord can be identified from inside the peritoneal cavity as it traverses through the internal inguinal ring. The vas deferens joins the cord at this point after crossing anterior to the iliac vessels. The gonadal artery and vein are covered with a layer of peritoneum but can usually be followed along the posterior abdominal wall.

Urologic Operative Procedures

Urologic laparoscopic procedures can be divided into three distinct categories: ablative, reconstructive, and diagnostic. Ablative procedures are by far the most commonly performed in adults, while diagnostic studies are done more routinely in children. Reconstructive procedures are the most technically challenging and require advanced laparoscopic skills. As techniques and instrumentation improve, many reconstructive urologic procedures will likely become more commonplace.

Ablative Urologic Laparoscopic Procedures

Laparoscopic Pelvic Lymphadenectomy

Indications
Pelvic lymphadenectomy is the most frequently performed application of urologic laparoscopic surgery in adults. This procedure may be an important part of the staging of prostate and bladder cancer. Currently, none of the available imaging modalities, including computed tomography, magnetic resonance imaging, ultrasound, and lymphangiography, is sufficiently sensitive, specific, or practical as a replacement for lymphadenectomy in determining appropriate therapy for these two malignancies. It remains controversial whether or not certain combinations of tumor size, grade, and serum values of prostate-specific antigen (PSA) define subgroups of patients with prostate cancer who are at a low enough risk for lymph node metastasis that lymphadenectomy may be omitted. Clinical data suggest that

patients with a PSA level less than 10 ng/mL and a Gleason score less than 7 have only a 2% risk of metastases to the pelvic lymph nodes. It is this group of patients who likely will not require staging lymphadenectomy. Similarly, whether or not all patients with invasive bladder cancer or, alternatively, just those with positive lymph nodes should receive preoperative neoadjuvant chemotherapy is being investigated. This chapter will not deal with these evolving treatment strategies. More important, laparoscopic pelvic lymphadenectomy occupies a central role in the evaluation and treatment of these two major genitourinary malignancies and is emerging as an alternative to standard open lymphadenectomy.

At present, pelvic lymphadenectomy is indicated for prostate cancer when positive pathology for cancer would alter the treatment strategy. In contrast, pelvic lymphadenectomy should be performed in all patients with invasive bladder cancer, except when known metastatic disease is present and the procedure would not add any additional information. Contraindications to laparoscopic pelvic lymphadenectomy include the presence of multiple pelvic adhesions (from prior surgery, peritonitis, or pelvic inflammatory disease), coagulopathy, pregnancy, and severe obesity.

Patient Preparation
Preoperatively, patients should undergo the same evaluation process as that for open surgery, including history, physical examination, routine laboratory studies, and electrocardiogram (when indicated). A complete bowel preparation with an osmotic cathartic and oral antibiotics (erythromycin with neomycin) are strongly recommended. Additionally, a povidone–iodine enema should be performed immediately preoperatively.

Operative Technique
Pneumoperitoneum is established via either a cutdown technique or a Veress needle at an umbilical or infraumbilical location. An 11-mm trocar for the endoscope and camera is inserted through this site. The remaining trocars may be placed in a standard diamond fashion: a 10-mm trocar inserted in the midline 6 cm above the pubic symphysis and right and left 5- or 10-mm trocars inserted at the level of the anterosuperior iliac crest, lateral to the course of the inferior epigastric blood vessels,

within the rectus abdominis muscles. Variations of the described diamond-shaped trocar pattern include additional lateral trocars in either more cephalad or caudal locations such that the overall trocar pattern may be more of a box or rectangular shape. Generally, the right-sided dissection is performed first. Adhesions of the sigmoid colon must be taken down before the left side can be dissected. The patient is rotated with the side undergoing dissection tilted 15 to 20 degrees upward.

The intraperitoneal laparoscopic view of common pelvic structures differs from that seen in open surgery performed in the perivesical space from an extraperitoneal approach. The peritoneal surface of the bladder is in the midline, with the urachus extending from the dome of the bladder to the umbilicus. The medial umbilical ligament courses in an anteroposterior plane between the lateral wall of the bladder and the internal inguinal ring.

The dissection is begun by grasping the peritoneum along the medial umbilical ligament (Fig. 56-1). The peritoneum is incised *lateral* to the medial umbilical ligament by sharp dissection or with electrocautery or laser. This incision provides entry into the obturator and iliac space. The peritoneal incision is extended cephalad, and the vas deferens comes into view, crossing horizontally. This anatomy is a key finding for purposes of orientation. The ureter and the internal iliac artery and vein are located just cephalad and deep (dorsal) to the vas deferens at this level. Dissection cephalad to the vas deferens risks injury to these structures.

A modified dissection technique removes the external iliac lymph nodes along the anteromedial edges of the external iliac artery and external iliac vein and the obturator nodes. This dissection corresponds to the usual open lymphadenectomy performed for prostate cancer. The lateral border of the specimen is developed by traction-countertraction and blunt and sharp dissection, cleaning off the anteromedial edge of the external iliac artery. The specimen is similarly freed from the external iliac vein. After medial retraction of the specimen, the dissection proceeds inferiorly toward the pubic bone. Frequently, an accessory obturator vein enters the inferomedial aspect of the external iliac vein.

At this point, the external iliac nodes are attached only to the obturator lymph node

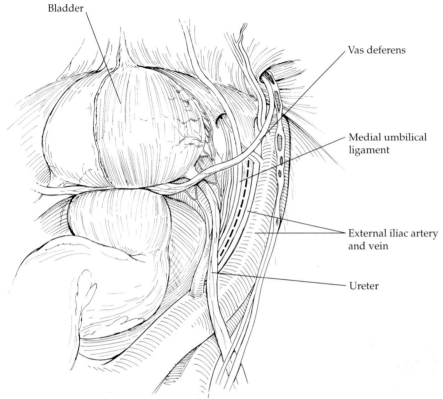

Fig. 56-1. Anatomy of the pelvic side wall on the right side. The vas deferens emerges from the internal inguinal ring, courses cephalad, and crosses anterior to the medial umbilical ligament and ureter. The line of incision should be immediately lateral to the medial umbilical ligament (as shown). This incision ensures access to the obturator fossa and facilitates visualization of the surrounding anatomy.

chain. Only blunt dissection is utilized until the obturator nerve is identified. The obturator vein and artery often lie deep to the nerve. The obturator chain of nodes is freed from the neurovascular structures. The node package is clipped inferiorly near the pubic bone and superiorly near the bifurcation of the iliac vessels to complete the dissection.

The left side is rolled 15 to 20 degrees upward, and the left-sided dissection is performed in the same sequence as the right-sided dissection. For patients with bladder cancer, the lateral limit of the dissection should be extended to the genitofemoral nerve, which courses lateral to the external iliac artery. After all dissection is completed and the specimen is removed, the pelvis is irrigated with saline and checked for hemostasis. Finally, the trocars are removed under direct vision, the pneumoperitoneum is evacuated, and the trocar sites are closed.

Laparoscopic Nephrectomy

Indications

Laparoscopic nephrectomy was initially performed to remove benign lesions of the kidney. Small, noninflamed kidneys secondary to end-stage renal failure or from renal artery stenosis are most suitable for laparoscopic "simple" nephrectomy. Kidneys associated with chronic inflammatory processes, such as chronic pyelonephritis or xanthogranulomatous pyelonephritis, are the most technically difficult laparoscopic nephrectomies to perform. Recently, the indications for laparoscopic nephrectomy have been expanded to include radical nephrectomy for small renal cell carcinomas (less than 6 cm), nephro-ureterectomy for urothelial tumors, and partial nephrectomy for benign conditions. However, further investigations are warranted to assess the safety, efficacy, and cost-effectiveness of laparoscopic nephrectomy for malignant renal lesions.

Patient Preparation

Patient preparation for laparoscopic renal procedures are similar to those for pelvic lymphadenectomy and include a full mechanical bowel preparation, as well as placement of a nasogastric tube and Foley catheter. If ureteral surgery is to be performed, a 7-French (7-F), 11.5-mm occlusion balloon catheter can be placed over a guidewire and the balloon inflated within the renal pelvis. A catheter within the ureter aides in identification of the ureter and adds stability during the ureteral dissection.

Operative Techniques

Transperitoneal Approach. Laparoscopic nephrectomy can be performed in either a supine or lateral position. While supine insufflation with subsequent repositioning of the patient to a lateral decubitus position may be the safest mode of trocar placement, this technique is often cumbersome. We have found that lateral insufflation is relatively easy to perform and offers the advantage of allowing the bowel to be passively reflected.

Veress needle or an open technique is used to create the pneumoperitoneum at the level of the umbilicus in the midclavicular line. Once insufflation has been completed, three trocars are placed: a 10-mm trocar approximately two fingerbreadths below the costal margin in the midclavicular line, a 10-mm midclavicular trocar even with the umbilicus, and a 12-mm midclavicular trocar that is infraumbilical. After these trocars have been placed, the laparoscope is positioned through the superior trocar as the surgeon works through the two inferior ports.

Prior to placement of the two remaining 10-mm trocars, adhesions are taken down from the abdominal wall, and the colon is mobilized off the abdominal side wall along the line of Toldt, allowing it to fall medially. The dissection is carried up to and around the splenic or hepatic flexure.

Once the colon has been mobilized and the retroperitoneum exposed, the two remaining 10-mm trocars are placed in the anterior axillary line: one subcostal and one at the level of the umbilicus. While the surgeon continues to work through the two midclavicular-line trocars, the assistant uses the two anterior axillary-line ports for retraction. The renal hilum (Fig. 56-2) is carefully dissected out using a combination of sharp and blunt dissection (Fig. 56-3). The renal hilum may be stretched by retracting the kidney laterally. Titanium clips (9 or 11 mm) are used to secure the renal artery, and a vascular endoscopic linear cutting stapler is used to secure and transect the renal vein. The endoscopic stapler can also be used to ligate and divide the renal artery. The artery should be ligated initially to allow the kidney to decompress before the renal vein is transected (Fig. 56-4).

Alternatively, one may begin dissection of the kidney by first identifying the ureter or gonadal vein. The ureter is readily identified as it crosses the iliac artery anterior to its bifurcation, and can be followed proximally. The gonadal vein is also easily identified as it courses along the psoas muscle and guides one to the renal vein on the left and to the proximity of the vein on the right. These maneuvers may aid in localization of the renal hilum.

Once the renal hilum has been secured, the remaining ureter is dissected free from surrounding tissue. Before the ureter is clipped, the balloon occlusion catheter and guidewire are removed. The ureter is clipped and divided and may be used as a handle to continue the dissection of the kidney. A locking grasper placed through the upper anterior axillary-line port is used to secure the ureter.

The kidney, with Gerota's fascia intact, is dissected free from surrounding fibrous tissue. A plane is easily developed bluntly between the posterior aspect of the kidney and the underlying psoas muscle. Lateral attachments are best divided using cautery. The adrenal gland may be spared, except when tumor appears to directly involve the gland or a large, upper-pole renal tumor is present. The surgeon dissects the adrenal gland off the superior pole of the kidney after entering the avascular plane between these two structures.

After the kidney is placed on the liver, an entrapment sack may be inserted through the lower 12-mm midclavicular-line port. The entrapment sack is opened using trocars placed through the lower and umbilical midclavicular-line ports and the lower anterior axillary-line port. After the kidney is placed into the entrapment sack, the drawstrings are closed, and the patient is placed back in a supine position. The drawstrings are pulled through the 12-mm um-

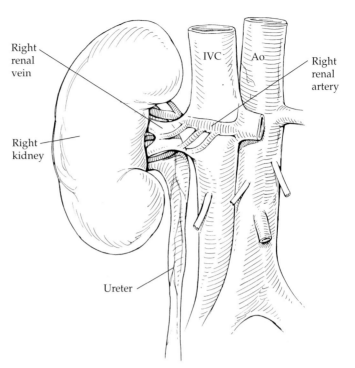

Fig. 56-2. Renal hilar anatomy. The renal vein is the most anterior structure. The renal artery is generally located posterior and slightly superior to the vein. The renal pelvis lies most posteriorly.

bilical port, and the neck of the sack is delivered. One may either morcellate the kidney using an electrical device, ring forceps, or Kelly clamp, or perform digital morcellation. However, if the kidney is being removed because of a malignant lesion, the umbilical incision may be widened to allow intact renal removal within the entrapment sack, thereby allowing adequate histologic staging of the kidney.

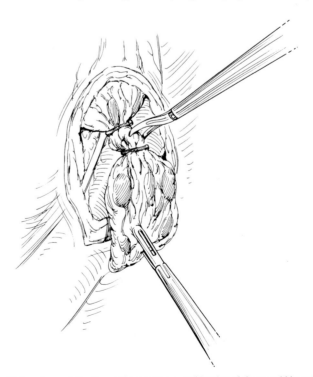

Fig. 56-3. The renal hilum is carefully dissected out using a combination of sharp and blunt dissection. Clips (9 or 11 mm) are used to secure the renal artery.

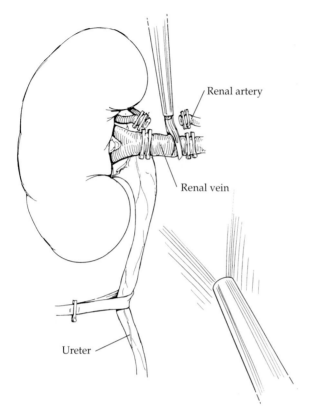

Fig. 56-4. *The artery should be ligated initially, allowing the kidney to decompress before transecting the renal vein.*

Following removal of the kidney, the clamped renal artery and vein and the dissection site should be thoroughly inspected for any evidence of bleeding. The colon may be reapproximated to the body side wall with a hernia stapler. Trocars are removed in the standard fashion after adequate inspection. The fascia of the 10- and 12-mm trocar sites should be closed with 2-0 suture.

Retroperitoneal Approach. Alternatively, the kidney may be approached via the retroperitoneum using various techniques of retroperitoneal insufflation. A Veress needle may be inserted directly into the retroperitoneal space through a location 1 to 2 cm superior to the anterosuperior iliac spine in the midaxillary line, and insufflation initiated. Once the retroperitoneum has been insufflated to approximately 18 mm Hg, a 10-mm trocar is placed into the retroperitoneal space and the laparoscope inserted to assess proper positioning. Additional techniques of lateral insufflation include making a small incision over the tip of the twelfth rib to get into the retroperitoneal space. Once correct position is confirmed, a balloon dilating device can be inserted into either the retroperitoneum or Gerota's space after Gerota's fascia is incised.

We have constructed a retroperitoneal dilating balloon using a 16-F red rubber Robinson catheter, a finger from a sterile surgeon's glove, and umbilical tape. The glove finger is secured to the end of the catheter with the umbilical tape. Alternatively, commercially available balloon dissectors are available, but most are not specifically designed for retroperitoneal dissection. We prefer balloon inflation with 1 to 2 L of sterile normal saline. Once the retroperitoneum has been insufflated/dissected with the aid of the retroperitoneal balloon, a Hasson trocar is placed through the initial incision and a laparoscope positioned to assess the completeness of retroperitoneal dissection. Working trocars are then placed under direct vision. The retroperitoneal approach has the main advantage of avoiding injuries to the abdominal organs and vasculature and approaching the renal hilum from behind, allowing initial access to the renal artery.

Laparoscopic Renal Cyst Decortication

The approach to renal cyst decortication is similar to that of laparoscopic nephrec-

tomy (either transperitoneal or retroperitoneal). Preoperatively, an open-ended ureteral catheter is positioned within the renal pelvis. The kidney is isolated as described for laparoscopic simple nephrectomy; however, the renal hilum is left undisturbed. Gerota's fascia is entered and dissected off the kidney in the vicinity of the renal cyst. The exophytic portion of the cyst wall is resected using the coagulating scissors (Fig. 56-5). The cyst cavity is inspected, and any suspicious areas are biopsied. The edges of the resected cyst wall and the bed of the cyst are then coagulated/fulgurated using either the laparoscopic argon beam coagulator or standard electrocautery. We prefer using the argon beam coagulator, as one can rapidly "spray" the edges and base of the cyst to ensure appropriate fulguration. Indigo carmine or methylene blue is injected retrograde through the ureteral catheter to determine whether a communication exists between the normal intrarenal collecting system and the base of the cyst. If blue dye is seen to come from the cyst base, the area is oversewn with absorbable suture. Perinephric fat can be procured from surrounding tissues, laid in the cyst bed, and secured to the edges of the cyst with absorbable suture. A drain is brought in through one of the ports and placed in the vicinity of the cyst. It is secured to the skin and left in position for approximately 7 days.

Laparoscopic Varicocelectomy

Indications
The appropriateness of laparoscopic varix ligation continues to be a source of controversy in the urologic community. As with many new procedures, just because we *can* perform a particular procedure, the question remains whether the procedure *should* be performed. Laparoscopic varix ligation has certain advantages; these include magnification of the spermatic cord, allowing improved identification of the veins and venous ligation; high retroperitoneal access; limited morbidity, especially for bilateral varix ligations; excellent cosmetic results; and a rapid return to work. However, some have criticized laparoscopic varicocelectomy because the spermatic vessels are approached transabdominally, with an increased potential for intraabdominal complications. In contrast, an

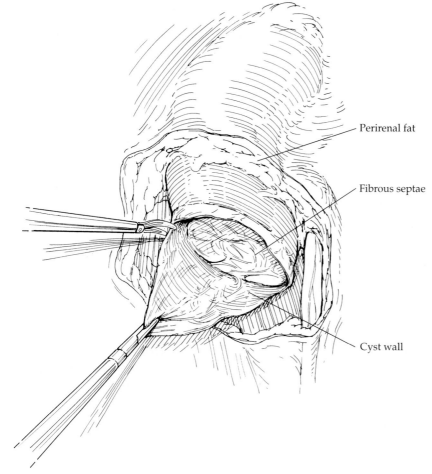

Perirenal fat

Fibrous septae

Cyst wall

Fig. 56-5. The cyst wall is resected revealing underlying fibrous septa. The cauterizing scissors help prevent bleeding from the edge of the cyst.

open inguinal varix ligation is performed through an extraperitoneal approach.

Moreover, laparoscopic varix ligation requires general anesthesia, whereas the open inguinal approach is generally performed under local anesthesia. Similarly, varix ligation can be performed by radiography-assisted vein embolization with minimal morbidity and comparable results to either an open or laparoscopic approach. Currently, many urologists believe that laparoscopic varix ligation should be reserved for patients with bilateral varices who would otherwise require a more extensive open or interventional radiologic procedure.

Indications for laparoscopic varix ligation are identical to those of standard open varicocelectomy or radiographically performed spermatic vein embolization; they include testicular pain, testicular atrophy, or a clinical varicocele associated with infertility.

Patient Preparation

Preoperative preparation is quite similar to standard pelvic laparoscopic procedures, but a laxative bowel preparation is not routinely performed because true pelvic exposure is not necessary.

Operative Technique

Transperitoneal Approach.
Following induction of general anesthesia, a Foley catheter is inserted to decompress the bladder. Standard abdominal insufflation and access are obtained with either a Veress needle or Hasson cannula. The primary 10-mm laparoscopic port is placed in an umbilical or subumbilical location. A secondary 10-mm trocar, which will accept a laparoscopic clip applier, is placed in the midline approximately two fingerbreadths above the pubic symphysis. For left-sided varix ligation, a 5-mm trocar is positioned on the right side midway be-

tween the anterosuperior iliac crest and the umbilicus. A second 5-mm trocar can be placed on the left side for access to the right spermatic vessels if bilateral varix ligation is planned.

The patient is placed in the Trendelenburg position with the right side down to help expose the left spermatic vessels. The vessels are traced from the internal ring, and the posterior peritoneal membrane is incised with laparoscopic scissors to the level where the vas deferens joins the spermatic vessels. The spermatic vessels are mobilized from surrounding tissue using mostly blunt dissection. Care should be taken to identify the spermatic artery prior to clipping the spermatic veins.

To assist in identifying the testicular artery, papaverine hydrochloride or lidocaine hydrochloride may be dripped onto the spermatic vessels, and pulsations of the artery can often be seen with laparoscopic magnification. Moreover, a laparoscopic Doppler probe (Meadox/SurgiMed, Oakland, NJ) may be used to assist in identifying arterial flow.

Once the testicular artery has been identified, the spermatic veins are clipped and divided to permit complete exposure of all spermatic vessels. Use of electrocautery should be limited during varix ligation to reduce the chance of testicular artery or vasal injury.

Dissection of the spermatic vessels may lead to carbon dioxide (CO_2) tracking through the internal ring into the scrotum. If the scrotum has been prepared into the field, it can be palpated prior to completion of the procedure, and the CO_2 can be compressed back into the peritoneal cavity prior to removal of the abdominal trocars.

Following complete ligation of the spermatic veins on the left side (or on the right if bilateral), the intraabdominal pressure should be reduced to 5 to 7 mm Hg and the dissection sites inspected for potential bleeding. The 5-mm trocar(s) are removed under direct vision. After complete desufflation of the CO_2 from the abdominal cavity, the laparoscope is removed from the 10-mm site under direct vision, with observation for possible bleeding. The 10-mm trocar sites are closed in the standard fashion with fascial sutures. The 5-mm site(s) are closed with subcuticular suture and Steri-strips.

Extraperitoneal Approach. Some investigators have recently described a "retroperitoneal" approach to laparoscopic varix ligation that would eliminate the drawbacks of a transabdominal approach. Planned insufflation of the preperitoneal space is performed to develop an extraperitoneal cavity. The cavity can be further dissected with the aid of a dilating balloon. A similar extraperitoneal approach has been described for pelvic lymph node dissection and extraperitoneal hernia repair.

Laparoscopic Pelvic Lymphocelectomy

Indications

Small asymptomatic collections of lymphatic fluid commonly occur following pelvic surgery such as renal transplantation or open pelvic lymphadenectomy. Larger collections occasionally produce a symptomatic lymphocele, which may cause obstruction of the transplant ureter, venous stasis secondary to extrinsic compression of the iliac veins draining the ipsilateral lower extremity, or a sensation of tightness and fullness in the transplant wound. Lymphoceles occur primarily from leakage of the lymphatics along the external iliac vein and to a lesser extent from the divided lymphatics in the renal hilum of the transplant allograft. Lymphoceles are most often located between the lower pole of the allograft and the side of the bladder. The degree of objective findings may not correlate with the size of the lymphocele. A relatively small lymphocele with a thick, fibrous rim may severely compress the iliac veins and produce marked lymphedema.

A variety of therapeutic approaches to lymphocele drainage have been utilized over the years. External drainage with a short incision and placement of a drain has an undesirably high risk of wound infection in transplant recipients. This procedure is limited to drainage of infected lymphoceles. Percutaneous needle aspiration under ultrasound guidance is the most common initial procedure to establish the diagnosis of lymphocele and exclude urine leak. Complete percutaneous aspiration can be therapeutic as well as diagnostic. However, lymphocele recurrence is the rule following aspiration alone. Repeated needle aspirations are possible but have a diminishing likelihood of effecting definitive therapy and an increased risk of introducing infection. Prolonged, closed percutaneous tube drainage of lymphoceles for 3 to 6 weeks has a fairly high success rate. However, patients dislike external drainage and must be fastidious in wound care to prevent infection. Open surgical drainage of the lymphocele into the peritoneal cavity represents definitive treatment yet is attendant with significant patient morbidity.

Laparoscopic internal lymphocele drainage is an example of an ideal laparoscopic procedure. The indications for intervention and the technical details of the procedure result in identical outcomes to those provided by a standard open surgical approach, yet with significantly less morbidity for the patient.

Patient Preparation

Preoperative preparation is similar to that for other pelvic laparoscopic procedures (lymph node dissection, hernia repair, etc.). A ureteral stent may be placed in transplant patients to aid in identification of the transplant ureter to avoid ureteral injury.

Operative Technique

A pneumoperitoneum is created with a Veress needle or an open Hasson technique, and CO_2 insufflation is accomplished in the standard fashion. The endoscope is placed through a 10- or 11-mm trocar at an umbilical or infraumbilical site. Working ports are established with 5- or 10-mm trocars in the right and left lower quadrants. The lymphocele should be easily recognized as a bluish cystic mass bulging inward toward the peritoneum. The renal parenchyma, renal hilar vessels, renal pelvis, and ureter all must be avoided when the lymphocele is opened. If any doubt remains regarding the site of the actual lymphocele, the cystic collection may be aspirated under direct vision with a needle passed through a working port.

A generous opening is made in the lymphocele wall using either sharp dissection, electrocautery, or laser incision (Fig. 56-6). The edge of the lymphocele defect is then cauterized to help prevent recollection of lymphatic fluid. The opening should be wide-mouthed to promote lymphatic drainage from the lymphocele into the free peritoneal cavity. Typically, the transplant ureter is located against the inferomedial wall of the lymphocele. Thus, dissection in this region should be avoided. All fluid is

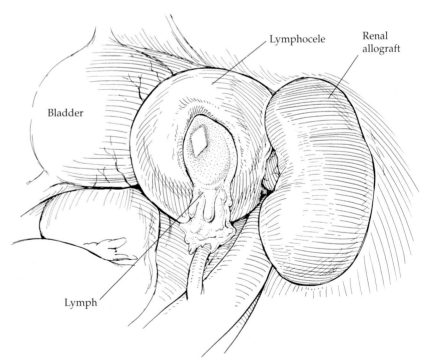

Fig. 56-6. The lymphocele typically lies between the bladder and the renal allograft. It is obvious how this collection may obstruct the transplanted ureter. A wide opening should be made in the lymphocele. The edges of the defect should either be cauterized or marsupialized to prevent resealing of the lymphocele.

aspirated, and the endoscope is passed directly into the lymphocele cavity. Loculations within the lymphocele should be broken by blunt or sharp dissection. A dependent portion of omentum may be placed into the lymphocele across the opening to prevent closure and reaccumulation of lymphatic fluid and discourage bowel from entering the cavity. The omentum may be secured in position with staples, clips, or sutures.

Reconstructive Urologic Laparoscopic Procedures

Laparoscopic Bladder Neck Suspension

Indications

Genuine stress urinary incontinence is a common condition primarily affecting postmenopausal women. The primary defect is a generalized weakness of the pelvic floor musculature resulting in the inability to support the bladder neck and urethra. With increased abdominal pressure (e.g., from coughing, sneezing, or laughing), the bladder neck and urethra descend, creating a funneling effect that allows urine leakage. Normally, the bladder neck is well supported and descent does not occur.

Laparoscopic bladder neck suspension is indicated in patients with genuine stress incontinence for whom surgical repair is the treatment of choice. Preoperative evaluation of these patients includes a thorough pelvic examination, urodynamic testing, and often radiographic studies. Patients with concomitant cystocele, primary urge incontinence, or intrinsic sphincter deficiency are not candidates for bladder neck suspension. These diagnoses will become evident with appropriate preoperative studies.

Patient Preparation

Prior to surgery, patients should be instructed in self-catheterization, since a significant percentage of patients will experience temporary urinary retention following surgery. A mechanical bowel preparation is recommended the evening before the operation, and a povidone–iodine enema should be performed immediately before surgery.

Operative Technique

The patient is positioned in such a way to allow access to the abdomen and the vagina. A lithotomy position best serves this purpose, but a frog-legged position may be used. Pneumoperitoneum is established by Veress needle or open technique at an umbilical or infraumbilical position. An 11-mm trocar is placed at this point. Two additional 11-mm trocars are placed on the left side of the abdomen: one just medial to the anterosuperior iliac spine and the second at the level of the umbilicus in the midclavicular line. One 11-mm trocar is placed on the right medial to the anterosuperior iliac spine. The left medial umbilical ligament defines the lateral border of the dissection. The initial incision is made anteriorly at the level of the pubis from the left medial umbilical ligament and extended medially across the midline. The urachus may be divided to permit improved exposure. The periosteum of the pubis is identified and the space of Retzius entered. This space is opened widely, and the bladder neck is identified by placing light traction on the Foley catheter. The tissue obscuring the pubic symphysis is cleared. Cooper's ligament is identified. This maneuver is often difficult and can be facilitated by careful blunt dissection along the pubic bone. Two fingers are then placed into the vaginal vault, and the endopelvic fascia on either side of the bladder neck and urethra is identified by removal of the tissue surrounding these areas.

To begin suture placement on the right side, the surgeon places two fingers in the vagina and retracts the bladder neck to the patient's left. The anterior aspect of the bladder neck is only minimally elevated so that the space between the endocervical fascia and the pubis may be maintained (Fig. 56-7). The suture is introduced into the operative field. The suture material should be nonabsorbable and monofilament. The needle is passed through the endocervical fascia exactly at the level of the bladder neck. The needle is then placed into the pubic bone at the corresponding level so as not to greatly distort the anatomy. The suture is knotted extracorporeally while the assistant elevates the vaginal wall against the pubis to remove tension. Only one suture per side is required if placed in the appropriate position. The identical procedure is performed on the patient's left side.

Once both sutures have been placed, many surgeons recommend cystoscopic examination to be certain that the suture has not been inadvertently passed into the bladder. The operative field is irrigated and hemostasis confirmed. Closing the peritoneal defect is not necessary. The working ports are removed under direct vision, and the sites are inspected for bleeding. The pneumoperitoneum is released, and the fascial defects are closed as described previously.

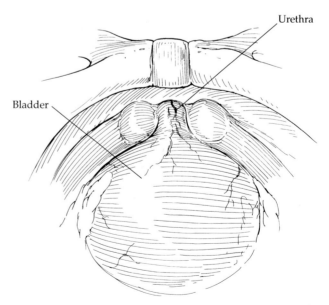

Fig. 56-7. Two fingers are placed into the vagina, and the bladder neck is gently elevated so as not to obliterate the space between it and the pubic symphysis. The sutures will be placed on either side of the bladder neck and anchored to the endocervical fascia and the periosteum of the pubis.

Postoperatively, a Foley catheter is left in place until the patient is fully mobile. The patient should begin self-catheterization every 4 to 6 hours immediately on discharge until residual urine volumes fall below 125 mL.

Laparoscopic Dismembered Pyeloplasty

Indications

Ureteropelvic junction (UPJ) obstruction is a form of obstructive uropathy that can be either congenital or acquired. The acquired form generally results from excessive fibrosis as a result of previous kidney surgery or other retroperitoneal surgical procedures (e.g., open pyelolithotomy or ureterolithotomy). In the congenital form of UPJ obstruction, collagen is found to replace the normal smooth muscle in the wall of the UPJ. This area is adynamic, thereby increasing the chance of obstructed urine flow. As increased pressures are required to overcome the obstruction and empty the renal pelvis, stretching of the renal capsule occurs and flank pain ensues. In addition, stasis of urine within the renal pelvis may occur, potentiating infection and/or calculus formation.

The workup for this condition includes an intravenous urogram (IVU), which characteristically demonstrates delay in contrast excretion, pelvocaliectasis, and nonvisualization of the ipsilateral ureter. A furosemide renal scan should confirm the presence of obstruction and indicate the relative function of the kidney; renal function of less than 10% may be an indication for nephrectomy. A retrograde pyelogram is strongly recommended to determine whether other areas of obstruction are present more distally in the ureter. The retrograde study is usually performed at the time of definitive repair to avoid another anesthetic.

Patient Preparation

Patient preparation is identical to that for the previously described laparoscopic approaches to the kidney.

Operative Technique

An internal ureteral stent is placed prior to the procedure. The patient is placed in either a supine or lateral position with the affected side elevated. Pneumoperitoneum is obtained at the level of the umbilicus by either Veress needle or open Hasson technique. Once the pneumoperitoneum is obtained, the kidney is exposed in an identical fashion to that described for laparoscopic nephrectomy. The ureter is carefully dissected free from the surrounding tissues inferiorly for a distance of approximately 8 to 10 cm. The renal pelvis is then dissected circumferentially, and the site of the UPJ obstruction is identified. The ureter is then divided at a distance of approximately 1.5 to 2 cm from the UPJ obstruction, or until normal-appearing ureter is identified. The previously placed ureteral stent is identified at this point, and care is taken to avoid cutting the stent. The stenotic area is excised sharply with coagulating scissors. We have found that articulating laparoscopic scissors facilitate excision of the UPJ and spatulation of the proximal ureter. If the renal pelvis is large and redundant, it may be tapered with a running, absorbable suture or interrupted sutures. The ureter and the renal pelvis are spatulated such that the most dependent portion of the pelvis funnels down into the ureter (Fig. 56-8). The anastomosis is begun by placing absorbable, stay sutures at the apices of the ureter to corresponding areas in the renal pelvis, juxtaposing the intended suture lines. These are not tied, as they will be used to spread out the areas to be sutured. The end of the ureteral stent is placed in the renal pelvis. The anastomosis is started on one side. The reanastomosis is most expeditiously accomplished with the aid of an automated suturing device loaded with absorbable suture (Endostitch, US Surgical, Inc., Norwalk, CT). Each suture is individually tied. When the initial side is completed, the stay sutures are brought under the anastomosis, bringing the other side into better view. The second side is completed in an identical fashion. Once the anastomosis has been completed, a drain is placed through one of the working ports and laid near the suture line. The end of the drain is fixed to the skin. The trocars are removed under direct vision, and after evacuation of the pneumoperitoneum, the trocar sites are closed.

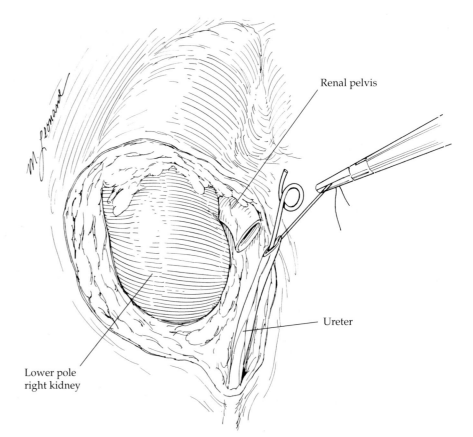

Renal pelvis

Ureter

Lower pole right kidney

Fig. 56-8. The renal pelvis has been tapered and spatulated such that the anastomosis can be performed at the most dependent portion of the new junction. The ureter is spatulated opposite that of the pelvis to facilitate suturing. The ureteral stent is repositioned within the renal pelvis prior to completion of the anastomosis.

Postoperatively, the drain is left in place for approximately 2 to 3 days. The stent should be removed in 4 to 6 weeks. Three months following the surgery, an IVU is performed to evaluate the integrity and patency of the anastomosis.

Postoperative Management

Postoperative management of urologic laparoscopic procedures is similar to that following other laparoscopic abdominal operations. Briefly, parenteral analgesics are used to control pain at the trocar sites until the patient tolerates oral medications. Ketorolac tromethamine (Toradol) may be readily substituted for narcotics if preferred by the surgeon. The Foley catheter is removed when the patient is fully awake. Discharge from the hospital may occur when the patient tolerates oral intake, ambulates well, and requires only oral analgesics.

Complications

The overall complication rate for laparoscopic surgery is less than 4% in the hands of skilled surgeons, and the mortality rate is lower than 1%. Most complications are those common to general, urologic, and gynecologic laparoscopic surgery and are discussed in detail elsewhere. Complications specific to urologic laparoscopic surgery include urine leaks and fistulas, hydroceles, and lymphoceles.

In any laparoscopic procedure that may involve purposeful or accidental entry into the renal collecting system, a ureteral catheter or stent must be placed. In cyst decortication, indigo carmine or methylene blue can be injected through the previously placed catheter to determine whether or not the collecting system has been violated. If a communication with the collecting system is identified, repair of the defect can be performed, and a drain may be left in place in proximity to the cyst. At the termination of the procedure, the catheter should be exchanged for an internal ureteral stent to facilitate healing of the defect.

Urine leaks may also be detected in the postoperative period. In these situations, an internal ureteral stent should be placed to allow the urine to pass preferentially through and around the stent. If a stent is already in place, a percutaneous nephrostomy tube should be placed to divert the urine flow. Subsequent studies, including IVU or antegrade nephrostogram, will determine whether or not the leak has healed.

Hydrocele formation is an uncommon complication of extraperitoneal lymph node dissection, occurring secondary to the accumulation of irrigation fluid in the dependent scrotum. The fluid tracks along the spermatic cord and will generally be resorbed within 10 to 14 days. Fluid reabsorption will be facilitated by scrotal elevation to allow fluid to return to the abdomen. If resolution does not occur, the fluid may be aspirated or drained under a local anesthetic.

Lymphoceles may also complicate pelvic lymphadenectomy. These lymphatic collections are best prevented through careful cauterization and ligation of lymphatic channels during the procedure. The symptoms of pelvic lymphocele are the result of obstruction of the ipsilateral ureter or compression of the pelvic vessels. The lymphocele may result in ipsilateral flank pain and/or leg edema. Radiographic studies will likely reveal some degree of hydronephrosis and the presence of a pelvic fluid collection. Lymphoceles are best managed with radiographically guided placement of a drain. Aspiration alone usually results in the reaccumulation of fluid. If closed drainage does not resolve the lymphocele, open surgery or laparoscopic procedures may be warranted.

Suggested Reading

Gerber GS, Rukstalis DB, Levine LA, Chodak GW. Current and future roles of laparoscopic surgery in urology. *Urology* 1993;41:5–9.

Gill IS, Clayman RV, McDougall EM. Advances in urological laparoscopy. *J Urol* 1995;154: 1275–1294.

Gill IS, Kavoussi LR, Clayman RV, et al. Complications of laparoscopic nephrectomy in 185 patients: a multi-institutional review. *J Urol* 1995;154:479–483.

Sagalowsky AI, Preminger GM. *Basic urologic laparoscopy.* New York: Futura Publishing, 1993.

Wolf JS Jr, Stoller ML. The physiology of laparoscopy: basic principles, complications and other considerations. *J Urol* 1994;152:294–302.

EDITOR'S COMMENT

The majority of urologists do not use laparoscopy or apply these techniques very rarely. Conversely, there are a few institutions where a urologist or group of urologists perform the majority of their operations using laparoscopic techniques. This disparity is largely due to the lack of a high-volume, relatively easy, routine procedure that is amenable to laparoscopic techniques. Therefore, the urologist who wishes to perform many operations by laparoscopy must possess exceptional skills or commit a tremendous amount of time in the laboratory to develop these skills.

Most urologic laparoscopic procedures require a surgeon who is skilled with suturing and two-hand operation techniques. The patient benefits derived from a successfully completed laparoscopic urology operation are similar to those seen with general surgical patients.

A rapidly growing trend in the United States is to harvest the kidney laparoscopically for transplantation in living related-donor cases. This new application of laparoscopy has prompted many urologists, in hospitals where transplantation is performed, to acquire advanced skills in laparoscopy.

W.S.E.

57

Surgical Endoscopy in the Pediatric Patient

Thom E. Lobe

Pediatric surgical endoscopy encompasses a broad spectrum of practice, including rigid and flexible endoscopy of the airway, thorax, abdomen, gastrointestinal tract, and genitourinary tract. Some special considerations that are common to all pediatric endoscopic procedures are necessary to effectively manage pediatric surgical endoscopic problems.

Although the average child is smaller than the average adult, most pediatric surgeons also treat adolescents who are physically as large or larger than many adults. Pediatric surgeons must be familiar with the entire spectrum of available endoscopes, from ultra-small to standard adult-sized instruments, to effectively treat patients weighing between 2 and 100 kg.

Flexible scopes that can be used for pediatric work are available from less than 1 mm in diameter to adult-sized (13-mm) instruments. The tip of the ultra-small scopes usually cannot be manipulated in multiple directions as it can on larger endoscopes, thereby restricting their usefulness. Flexible endoscopes are used for the airway and for the gastrointestinal and genitourinary tracts. The smallest of these endoscopes can be passed, often through endotracheal tubes, into the distal airway of even preterm infants. Flexible endoscopes as small as 2 mm in diameter also can have one or more working channels that can be used to aspirate or irrigate fluid or used to pass instruments for biopsy, dilatation (Fig. 57-1), or tissue ablation.

Pediatric surgeons also should be familiar with rigid telescopes, which range in size from less than 2 to 10 mm in diameter and which come in viewing angles ranging from 0 to 75 degrees. Newer telescopes use single optical fibers and smaller, more nu-

merous light bundles to deliver more intense light and have a wider viewing angle than the older Hopkins rod and lens scopes. These are often marketed as instruments for "minilaparoscopy" or "office laparoscopy" using a Verres needle introducer sheath. Whether these telescopes will prove useful in pediatric endoscopy remains to be seen.

Modern surgical endoscopy is aided by the use of video systems to monitor and record the procedure. Video monitoring allows all those involved with a procedure to be able to see the procedure as it is being performed. This is especially important for airway endoscopy, in which the surgeon and the anesthesiologist need to work cooperatively to complete any procedure that may in part compromise the airway.

Because of the wide variety of endoscopes used by the pediatric surgeon, it is helpful to have access to a video camera that can be readily adapted to all of the endoscopes used. Most video cameras can be obtained with a C-mount adapter so they can be used with any flexible or rigid endoscope. It is more economical for the pediatric surgeon to use this type of camera than it is to purchase telescopes with the camera mounted on them, even though the image may be better with such a mounted camera-telescope unit.

The weight of the camera becomes more of an issue with pediatric endoscopy than it is with adult work. The lighter the camera, the better, particularly when the camera is mounted to the smallest of the telescopes. As an example, when a heavy camera is mounted to a 2-mm Hopkins rod lens telescope, it tends to bend the scope, decreasing the light delivery and creating a crescentic shadow along the periphery of the

image, which is therefore distorted and decreased.

Another important factor with pediatric work is the mode of light delivery and the light sensitivity of the camera. The smaller pediatric telescopes tend to deliver less light. In some situations, this limits the resolution of the image. The most powerful light available should be used for pediatric work. It is better to have a camera coupler (i.e., the electronic interface, usually a box, that connects the camera to the video system and translates what the camera sees into an image on the monitor) that allows adjustment of the light sensitivity. With this capability, the gain on the system can be adjusted so that the image appears brighter. Although this decreases the resolution and makes the image appear more grainy, it allows the surgeon to see optimally in relatively low-light situations.

In many video systems, the light intensity is automatically regulated. Although this is desirable in adult endoscopic surgery, it is a problem for pediatric intracavitary work. Thoracoscopy and laparoscopy in children occur in a relatively small, confined space. There is barely enough room for all of the necessary instruments. This can result in light reflecting off of the instruments in the foreground. When this happens with a servoregulated light delivery system, the light is automatically decreased to eliminate the glare, lowering the amount of light in the operative field, which may make it difficult to see well enough to complete the surgery. To avoid this phenomenon, it is better to bypass or override the automatic mode and to place the system on manual control.

Another difference between adults and children is in the anesthetic management

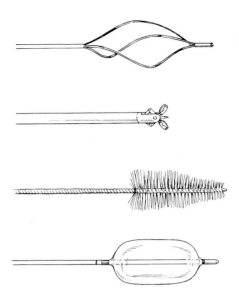

Fig. 57-1. A sample of small instruments that can be passed through 2.2-mm flexible endoscopes.

during endoscopic surgery. Many of the procedures that can be carried out under local anesthesia in adults are better performed under general anesthesia in children. Although some procedures can be performed with intravenous sedation (e.g., diagnostic upper gastrointestinal endoscopy, some cases of flexible bronchoscopy), most flexible endoscopy in children is better performed with the child asleep. This is true of the more advanced laparoscopic and thoracoscopic procedures. With older adolescents, the tolerance for a local anesthetic depends on the maturity of the individual. Minilaparoscopy or office laparoscopy, which is in vogue in adult surgery and can be performed under conscious sedation, is likely to be less applicable to all except the older, more mature adolescents.

For anesthetic techniques used in thoracoscopy, adult work is easier because the adult airway is better suited to the use of double-lumen endotracheal tubes. When isolation of a lung is desired in the smaller child, my colleagues and I prefer selective intubation with a cuffed endotracheal tube or placement of a balloon catheter as a bronchial blocker. The latter maneuver is much easier to perform than it sounds. When lung isolation is required, the patient is placed under deep inhalation anesthesia in preparation for intubation. An appropriately sized balloon embolectomy is inserted into the trachea, immediately followed by placement of a cuffed endo-

tracheal tube. A flexible bronchoscope is then inserted into the lumen of the endotracheal tube, and the deflated Fogarty balloon is manipulated into the bronchus to be blocked. Once in place, the balloon is inflated just enough to occlude the opening to the bronchus (Fig. 57-2). The anesthesiologist can adjust the pressure in the balloon as necessary to allow the lung to deflate and stay deflated during the thoracoscopy. Other than the previously mentioned reservations and some size constraints, most of the other concerns of pediatric endoscopic surgeons are similar to the concerns of those who treat adults.

Historical Review

Credit for the earliest attempts to convince pediatric surgeons that laparoscopy is important must be given to Gans. In the middle to late 1970s, Gans worked with the Stortz Company of Tutgarten, Germany, to design suitable laparoscopic instruments for surgery on infants and small children. Refinements in video technology

and the development of better and smaller endoscopic instruments, including endoscopic surgical staplers and devices for delivering various forms of thermal energy (i.e., laser, monopolar, bipolar, and the harmonic scalpel), permitted development of more advanced endoscopic procedures for children.

Instrumentation

The Hopkins rod lens telescopes revolutionized all of pediatric endoscopy (Fig. 57-3). These instruments range in size from 2 to 10 mm in diameter and are used most often in 0- or 30-degree lens configurations. The 0-degree scopes are used most frequently because they cause less disorientation and because they are the easiest to use for the novice, The 30-degree lenses are most useful in instances such as cystoscopy, endoscopic suturing, and specific procedures such as those performed in the right upper quadrant (e.g., Nissen fundoplication). The newer endoscopes, which are smaller than 2 mm in diameter, deliver

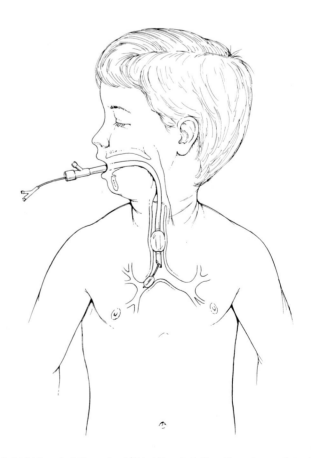

Fig. 57-2. Right lung isolation using inflated Fogarty balloon through an endotracheal tube.

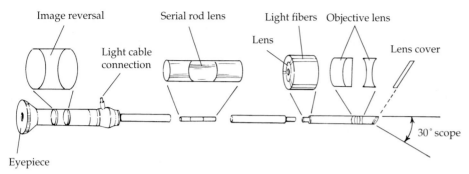

Fig. 57-3. *The Hopkins rod lens telescope and its components.*

sufficient light and have good enough optics that they can be used in selected cases in pediatrics such as screening children with chronic abdominal pain for pathology in the pelvis and lower abdomen.

Laparoscopy in infants and children requires smaller trocar and cannula sets and more delicate instrumentation. The standard lens has become a 3- to 5-mm reusable cannula for most procedures. For neonates, some instruments are 2 mm or smaller. After the small cannulae are inserted, they should be sutured to the skin to prevent traction on the cannula or instrument from dislodging them.

The smaller instruments for endoscopic surgery include smaller diameters (3 to 5 mm) and shorter shafts on instruments to accommodate the needs of the thoracic and pediatric surgeons. These shorter instruments are most effective when used with shorter cannulae. Delicate sets of 1.7- to 2.7-mm instruments are available from several manufacturers. Standard laparoscopic instrumentation is usable as well, but larger clamps and staplers should be avoided except in procedures for which they are essential.

Laparoscopic Technique

Laparoscopy in infants and children must be performed under general anesthesia, usually with endotracheal intubation. Preoperative prophylactic antibiotics are recommended to prevent trocar site infections, and they should always be used for prophylactic coverage in children with indwelling ventriculoperitoneal shuts.

The stomach and bladder are emptied immediately before the procedure. The stomach can be emptied with a suction catheter,

and in most instances, the bladder can be emptied sufficiently with use of the Credé maneuver.

The abdominal wall of the child, which is thin and elastic, presents two access problems. First, it is much easier to introduce a needle or trocar into the subcutaneous space and think that it is in the peritoneal cavity when it is not. Second, it is potentially easier to injure abdominal viscera during secondary trocar introduction because of the small size of the abdominal cavity. These problems can be easily avoided with experience and care.

Although the Veress needle technique can be used to establish a pneumoperitoneum, the open technique is probably safer. First, each trocar site is infiltrated with a 50:50 mixture of 1% lidocaine and 0.25% bupivacaine with 1:100,000 epinephrine. The lidocaine is short acting, the bupivacaine provides postoperative analgesia, and the

epinephrine makes the local effect last longer. I then make a stab wound in the skin of the inferior rim of the umbilicus. The length of the incision should approximate the diameter of the cannula to be introduced. I find it helpful to place the fascial closing suture before I introduce the cannula. This allows for easy closure of this wound at the end of the case. To introduce the umbilical cannula, I elevate the abdominal wall by grasping it on either side of the umbilicus (Fig. 57-4). I then insert the telescope to ensure that the tip of the cannula is free in the peritoneal cavity before I begin insufflation with carbon dioxide (CO_2).

The total volume of gas introduced into the abdomen of a child varies with the patient's size. It is preferable to ignore the volume and to use pressure limits controlled by a pressure-regulated automatic insufflator. For newborns and small infants, the maximum pressure is 6 to 8 mm Hg. For children, most procedures can be accomplished using pressures of 8 to 10 mm Hg. Older children and adolescents tolerate pressures of 10 to 12 mm Hg.

Insertion of the secondary trocars can be dangerous. The tip must be kept in sight during introduction, and the abdomen must be elevated instead of relying on insufflation to keep the abdominal wall away from the viscera. My colleagues and I advocate lifting the abdominal wall medial to the insertion point of the trocar and taking care to insert the trocar at 90 degrees to the abdominal wall rather than

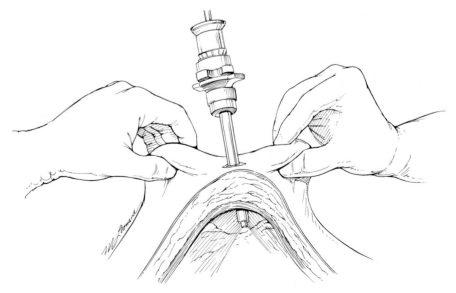

Fig. 57-4. *The abdominal wall is elevated while a needle and trocar are inserted.*

obliquely through it. This prevents the thin, flexible abdominal wall from allowing the tip of the trocar to contact with any important structures.

Postoperatively, the fascia at all trocar sites should be sutured. Because of the thinness of the abdominal wall, the possibility of a trocar site hernia is more likely in children. We therefore close the fascia and the skin with interrupted absorbable sutures. A Steri-Strip or transparent occlusive dressing is applied to each trocar site.

Patients who undergo operative endoscopic procedures (as opposed to diagnostic procedures) are placed on postoperative metaclopromide to prevent nausea.

Children have fewer complaints of postoperative shoulder pain than do adults. We have not made it our routine to leave suction catheters in the peritoneal cavity for several hours to evacuate all the CO_2 gas, as has been occasionally described in adults. Postoperative analgesic requirements are variable and should be titrated depending on the child.

A wide variety of laparoscopic procedures can be accomplished in infants and children (Table 57-1). Details of the more common procedures are provided in the following section.

Table 57-1. Laparoscopic Procedures in Infants and Children

Exploration for contralateral inguinal hernia

Exploration for nonpalpable testes

Exploration for chronic abdominal pain

Exploration and biopsy or node sampling for cancer

Exploration for intersex

Exploration and cholangiogram for biliary atresia

Ladd's procedure for malrotation (not for midgut volvulus)

Appendectomy

Cholecystectomy

Pyloromyotomy for pyloric stenosis

Fundoplication for gastroesophageal reflux

Esophagomyotomy for achalasia

Splenectomy

Nephrectomy

Oophorectomy

Resection of Meckel's diverticulum

Pull-through for hirschsprung's disease

Laparoscopic Treatment of Appendicitis

One of the best applications of laparoscopy to pediatrics is in the treatment of appendicitis. Most of the arguments against approaching this disease laparoscopically are by those unfamiliar with laparoscopic techniques. The collected data from several series of adults and some children suggest that there are no major differences in the results of appendectomy between open and laparoscopic techniques.

Varlet et al. carried out a retrospective review of 403 children with appendicitis, one-half of whom underwent a laparoscopic appendectomy. Although operative complications occasionally occurred with the laparoscopic approach, there were many more postoperative complications from open appendectomy (10.8% versus 1.5%; $p<0.0001$). The complications that occurred after open appendectomy included wound abscesses, intraperitoneal infections, and bowel obstructions.

The nature of postoperative complications appears to differ between open and laparoscopic appendectomy in most reported series. Open appendectomy is associated with more wound-related infections than intraperitoneal abscesses; the converse is true with the laparoscopic approach.

The alleged advantages of laparoscopic appendectomy over an open procedure include a better cosmetic result—particularly in young female patients—and an earlier return to full activity. Appendectomy in the obese child may be easier to perform using the laparoscopic approach.

After laparoscopic appendectomy for acute uncomplicated appendicitis, patients are discharged between 6 and 36 hours postoperatively and are allowed to return to unrestricted activity as soon as they are comfortable, usually within 72 hours. In cases of ruptured appendix, the advantages of laparoscopic appendectomy are not as great. Some claim that the involved tissues are better inspected and that the pus is more easily and directly drained when using the laparoscopic approach, but this is not established. For the young adult who would like to "return to normal as soon as possible," the laparoscopic technique does offer the opportunity to treat the disease efficiently and, af-

ter antibiotic therapy is completed, to return the patient to normal levels of activity without the restriction imposed after surgery.

One approach is to perform laparoscopy in patients who clinically appear to have appendicitis uncomplicated by rupture or abscess formation. If laparoscopic appendectomy is begun and a ruptured appendix is discovered, the surgeon could complete the appendectomy laparoscopically or convert to an open incision, unless there are anatomic contraindications to doing so.

The initial approach to laparoscopic appendectomy requires emptying the stomach and bladder. Although not essential, an indwelling urinary catheter during the procedure may be helpful. The patient is placed supine in the Trendelenburg position for most of the procedure and can be rotated toward the surgeon to allow the small bowel to fall out of the line of sight of the cecum and appendix (Fig. 57-5). A CO_2 pneumoperitoneum is established as described previously using a 5- or 10-mm laparoscope introduced through the umbilicus into the peritoneal cavity. My colleagues and I generally use a 5-mm laparoscope for patients younger than 10 to 12 years of age and a 10-mm laparoscope for older children.

On inspection of the peritoneal cavity, it is usually immediately obvious whether there is pathology in the right lower quadrant. Occasionally, cloudy fluid is seen in the pelvis. Two additional cannulae can be used to complete the operation; their size and location depends on the technique. It is preferable to place symmetric cannulae in the right and left lower quadrants below the "bikini line," lateral to the epigastric vessels on either side. One 5-mm cannula and one 10- or 12-mm cannula appear adequate. To ensure ample room for proper instrument placement and function, the larger cannula is inserted in the left lower quadrant (Fig. 57-6).

A ratcheted tissue grasper is placed through the right lower quadrant port to grasp and stabilize the tip or body of the appendix, and a dissector is placed through the left lower quadrant port. With these instruments, the tissues are mobilized so the tip of the appendix can be secured. A closed grasper is helpful as a blunt dissector in a manner similar to the use of blunt finger dissection in open

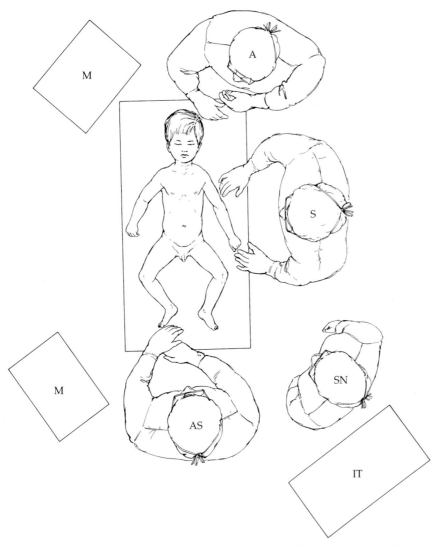

Fig. 57-5. Surgical setup for laparoscopic appendectomy. (A, anesthetist; AS, assistant surgeon; IT, instrument table; M, monitor; S, surgeon; SN, scrub nurse.)

and cannula are reinserted, the surgical site is inspected for hemostasis, and the area irrigated as necessary.

In cases of ruptured or gangrenous appendicitis, the surgeon must take care to watch for friable segments of the appendiceal wall through which a fecalith may extrude. A lost fecalith in the peritoneal cavity usually forms a nidus for abscess formation requiring subsequent intervention. In the case of an abscess, a Luken's trap is attached to the end of the suction device to obtain material for culture. At the end of the procedure, copious irrigation of the peritoneal cavity with saline and an antibiotic-containing solution is carried out.

If an abscess is drained and the abdomen is irrigated after laparoscopic appendectomy, the patient is placed in a reverse Trendelenburg position at the end of the procedure to allow the irrigation fluid to run into the pelvis, where it can be meticulously aspirated. Similarly, in cases of upper abdominal procedures during which irrigation is used, the patient is placed in the Trendelenburg position at the end of the procedure and may even be rotated to the right or to the left in a semidecubitus position so that the fluid becomes dependent, and it can be completely aspirated.

These maneuvers are important to prevent subsequent loculated abscesses from irrigation fluid. Occasionally, with retrocecal appendicitis or when the tip of the appendix is markedly inflamed and involved in an inflammatory mass, retrograde removal of the appendix is indicated. This usually is achieved by making an opening in the mesoappendix near the normal base and inserting a linear stapler through this window to divide the appendix. The surgeon can also simply divide the appendix with a laser or with endoscopic shears approximately 1 to 1.5 cm from the base of the cecum. The free ends are secured with pretied Roeder loops before grasping the resected end of the appendix and dissecting the remainder of the appendix and its mesentery free.

Patients who have a preoperative diagnosis of ruptured appendicitis are best treated with antibiotics through a percutaneously placed central line. The average hospital stay is 3 days, at which time most patients are ambulating and eating. Intravenous antibiotics should be continued at home until the patient is afebrile for 48

cases. This technique enables the separation of inflammatory adhesions and fluid loculations.

Some adhesions occasionally require sharp dissection. Bipolar scissors enable careful division of the adhesions while cauterizing any blood vessels to minimize bleeding. After the appendix is mobilized and its junction with the base of the cecum can be clearly identified, the mesoappendix and the appendix are divided. The mesoappendix can be ligated using extracorporeally tied sutures and the appendix looped with three or four nonabsorbable Roeder loops (Fig. 57-7). Endoscopic shears can be used without cautery to divide the appendix between the loops, with two of the loops remaining on the appendiceal stump. Because cautery can melt

and disengage the loops, electrical energy should not be used at this point.

With the appendix free, it is extracted through the left lower quadrant 12-mm cannula so that the inflamed or contaminated tissue never touches the cannula tract. If the inflamed appendix is so thick that it cannot be removed through the cannula, a tissue sac or pouch can be inserted through the larger cannula. The appendix is placed within it, and the sac is withdrawn into the cannula to its point of resistance. The cannula should be withdrawn completely so the neck of the sac or condom-like pouch is outside the abdominal wall. The sac usually has enough lubrication from tissue fluids that it can easily slip out through the incision. After the sac is removed, the left lower quadrant trocar

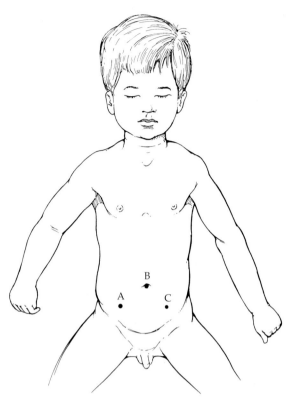

Fig. 57-6. Camera port and symmetric cannulas in right and left lower quadrants. (A, 5 mm; B, 10 mm; C, 10 mm.)

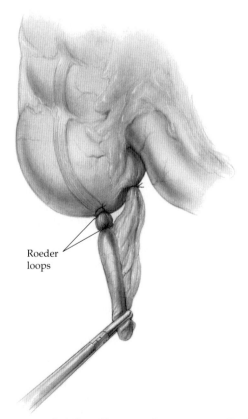

Roeder loops

Fig. 57-7. A vessel in the mesoappendix is ligated by means of an extracorporeally placed knot while the appendix is looped with three nonabsorbable Roeder loops.

hours and has a normal white blood cell count with a normal differential blood cell count. Patients are then placed on oral antibiotics, usually sulfamethoxazole-trimethoprim, for another 1 to 2 weeks and are admitted approximately 6 weeks after treatment began for an elective laparoscopic appendectomy performed as day surgery.

The laparoscopic approach is also indicated in cases of abdominal pain when the diagnosis is unclear. A recommended strategy is to perform an appendectomy and then search for other possible causes of the symptoms. It is much easier to explore the abdomen with the laparoscope than through the conventional right lower quadrant incision. In little girls, the ovaries and tubes can be atraumatically manipulated and inspected. The bowel can be inspected in its entirety, looking for a Meckel's diverticulum or other pathology, and the upper abdomen can be evaluated for cholecystitis or abscess formation.

After a laparoscopic procedure has been completed, the cannulae are removed and the wounds closed as described previously. Patients with ruptured appendicitis remain on antibiotics and nasogastric suction, as is our routine for open ruptured appendicitis. Patients with acute simple appendicitis are allowed a regular diet and normal activity as tolerated, and they are discharged on the day of surgery or as soon thereafter as possible. Because there is no significant abdominal muscle incision, patients may return to unrestricted activities immediately on discharge. They usually remain uncomfortable for a few days and then return to their normal routines.

Cholecystectomy and Common Duct Exploration

Cholecystectomy

The technique and results of laparoscopic cholecystectomy in children are similar to those for adult patients. Common indications for pediatric cholecystectomy and common duct exploration are described in Table 57-2.

The operating room setup and patient positioning is illustrated in Fig. 57-8. The surgeon is positioned to the patient's left. The scrub nurse stands next to the surgeon. The first assistant is across from the surgeon, and the camera operator stands next to the surgeon or at the foot of the table.

Cholelithiasis
    Symptomatic
    Idiopathic
    Secondary to hematogenous diseases
    Asymptomatic
        Immunosuppression
        Juvenile diabetes
        Incidental during laparoscopic
            splenectomy for hematogenous diseases
Cholecystitis
Common duct stones
    Documented (by imaging)
    Suspected (by presentation)

Some surgeons prefer to stand between the patient's legs or at the foot of the table to perform the operation.

A four-cannula technique is preferred (Fig. 57-9). The 5- or 10-mm cannula is placed in the umbilicus for insertion of the laparoscope as described earlier. Careful inspection of the liver and gallbladder is necessary to determine optimal insertion sites of the three operating cannulae, which are 3 mm for an infant or 5 mm for an older child. The anterior axillary line cannula is placed next. A grasper is inserted through this cannula, the fundus of the gallbladder is grasped, and the fundus is pushed over the anterior edge of the liver. This cannula site may be altered, depending on the position of the gallbladder. It may need to be more inferior and lateral on the abdomen in the smaller child.

The second operating cannula is placed in the midclavicular line. Another grasper is positioned through this cannula, and the gallbladder is grasped at the junction of the body and neck. When this instrument is directed in a caudad and lateral direction, it exposes the structures in the triangle of Calot. As with the anterior axillary port, it may be necessary to adjust the position of this cannula for smaller patients. It is sometimes desirable to reverse the roles of the graspers in the anterior axillary and midclavicular cannulae when retracting the gallbladder. Ratcheted instruments help to diminish the discomfort of the assistant.

The final cannula is placed in the subxiphoid position to the right of the falciform ligament in larger patients and to its left in smaller patients. The instruments in this cannula must intersect the cystic duct at a 60- or 90-degree angle. The dissector can be passed below the falciform ligament, or the cannula can be passed through the falciform ligament to provide better exposure.

Adhesions about the gallbladder are dissected free, and the cystic artery is separated from the cystic duct. The surgeon must ensure that the cystic artery, cystic duct, and right hepatic artery are clearly identified before any structure is divided. The cystic artery is ligated with sutures or clips and then is divided with shears between the ligatures. The cystic duct is separated from the surrounding structures by blunt dissection. Sutures or clips are then placed on the distal cystic duct in preparation for the cholangiogram.

Cholangiography can be performed by any one of several methods. Commercial catheters can be passed through one of the cannulae. Unfortunately, this results in a loss of exposure, because one of the graspers must be removed. An 8- or 12-inch long, 14-gauge intravenous cannula or the outer sheath of a Veress needle can be placed directly through the abdominal wall just below the edge of the liver, between the anterior axillary and midclavicular cannulae. Using curved endoscopic shears, a small opening is made in the exposed cystic duct, and the cholangiogram catheter is advanced into its lumen through the needle. A clip or suture is placed around the catheter to secure it in the duct. Alternatively, a cholangiogram catheter with a balloon at the tip can be used to secure the catheter in place. After

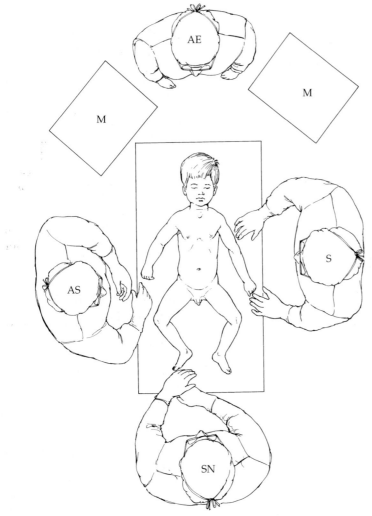

Fig. 57-8. Surgical setup for laparoscopic cholecystectomy. (AE, anesthetist; AS, assistant surgeon; M, monitor; S, surgeon; SN, scrub nurse.)

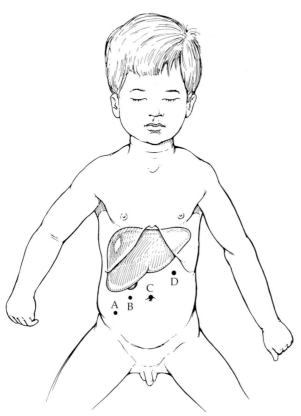

Fig. 57-9. Four-cannula placement for cholecystectomy. (A, 3 or 5 mm; B, 3 or 5 mm; C, camera 5 or 10 mm; D, 5 mm.)

the cholangiogram is obtained, the catheter and ligature are removed. Clips or sutures are reapplied, and the duct is divided. This cannulation should be accomplished well away from the junction of the common bile duct (CBD) and the cystic duct.

Common Bile Duct Stones

Some patients have known CBD stones. In these cases, a laparoscopic CBD exploration can be performed by making an incision in the cystic duct, dilating the duct with balloon dilators, and inserting a flexible endoscope into the bile duct. For a pediatric "choledochoscope," we have found it convenient to use a pediatric cystoscope. This allows for good visualization and provides access for irrigation and instrumentation (e.g., passage of a stone basket). A second camera can be attached to the choledochoscope so that the surgeon can see intraductal and extraductal anatomy simultaneously. After the endoscope is removed from the duct, the cystic duct stump can be ligated in the standard fashion.

After the cystic duct is ligated and divided, the gallbladder can be dissected free from

the liver using a combination of ultrasonic dissection or electrosurgery and blunt dissection. When the dissection reaches a point at which only the peritoneum attaches the gallbladder to the liver, the ligated cystic artery and duct are carefully inspected, and the gallbladder bed is examined for bleeding. If this is not done before division of the last peritoneal attachments, it is difficult to regain exposure. The intraabdominal pressure should be lowered to less than 8 mm Hg to check for venous bleeding that might be tamponaded at higher pressures. The peritoneal attachments are divided completely, and the gallbladder is removed through the umbilical cannula site after switching the laparoscope to the uppermost cannula. When large stones are present, the gallbladder may be opened, the stones crushed or removed with a large clamp, and all debris removed.

Results

Holcomb et al. reviewed their experience with 26 laparoscopic cholecystectomies in children. Five patients presented with acute cholecystitis. The surgeons per-

formed cholangiography in every instance. Their review suggests that laparoscopic cholecystectomy in children is safe and as cost effective as that procedure performed in adults.

Most published series have described treatment of symptomatic cholelithiasis in children with sickle cell disease. These patients, who often have recurrent abdominal pain, should also undergo appendectomy. Of interest is the finding of pathology (scarring or inflammation) in 50% of the appendices removed from these children. Complications of laparoscopic cholecystectomies in children are unusual but include hemorrhage from the liver bed, bile leaks, retained stones, common duct injury, infections, and problems related to the underlying disease of these often very ill children.

Laparoscopic Approach to Undescended Testicles

Background and Indications

Laparoscopy for nonpalpable cryptorchid testes is a well-accepted approach. Many patients with bilateral cryptorchidism or with a unilateral nonpalpable testis may benefit from laparoscopic diagnosis and treatment.

For unilateral disease, the differential diagnoses include undescended testis and testicular atrophy. At laparoscopy, the surgeon can visualize the testicle in the inguinal canal or abdomen. In cases of testicular atrophy, the testicular vessels and vas deferens are seen, but they end blindly just at the internal inguinal ring. This observation, coupled with the fact that there is no palpable tissue in the inguinal canal or scrotum, indicates that testicular atrophy has occurred, probably because of an intrauterine torsion. Laparotomy or other treatment is not required in this type of case. For bilateral disease, the surgeon can determine whether the testes are present and where they lie.

Technique

CO_2 pneumoperitoneum is established by the standard process, and an appropriately sized 3- or 5-mm umbilical cannula is placed for passage of a 2- or 5-mm laparoscope (Figs. 57-10 and 57-11). Simple inspection of both internal inguinal rings provides the required information in most cases.

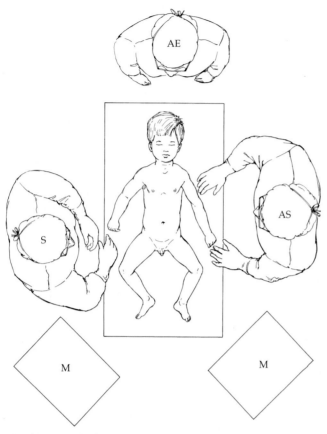

Fig. 57-10. Operating room setup for the laparoscopic approach for nonpalpable cryptorchid testes. (AE, anesthetist; AS, assistant surgeon; M, monitor; S, surgeon.)

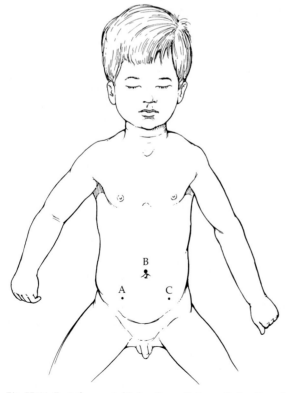

Fig. 57-11. Port placement. (A, 3 or 5 mm; B, 5 mm; C, 3 or 5 mm.)

In the treatment of the high intraabdominal testis, one option is to perform high ligation and division of the spermatic vessels to mobilize the testis and allow it to be moved to the internal inguinal ring. The testis is then secured in this position with a clip or sutures for subsequent orchiopexy, which is done several weeks or months later. This technique requires that the patient be placed in a Trendelenburg position and rotated laterally away from the cryptorchid side. The testicle and its pedicle are identified, and a small incision is made over the proximal spermatic vessels, just enough to isolate them from surrounding structures. They are divided between surgical clips, are suture ligated, or are divided with the laser, depending on the preference and experience of the surgeon. The testicle can be left in place, or the peritoneum can be incised toward the pelvis sufficiently to displace the testicle to the internal inguinal ring. After several weeks to months have passed, sufficient vascular collateralization occurs that a Fowler-Stephens type of orchiopexy can be performed safely by the inguinal or laparoscopic approach. Although the long-term results of this technique are unknown, it causes minimal disruption of the collateral vascular supply, and this approach therefore is appealing. Unfortunately, the available experimental data suggest that, although the testis is viable after spermatic vessel ligation, its endocrine and reproductive capacity may be impaired. However, neither Jordan and Winslow nor Guar et al. found evidence of testicular loss or acute testicular atrophy in their experience.

After simple inspection or relocation of the testis, the cannulae are removed and the wounds closed as described earlier. Some surgeons advocate removing an atrophic testicular remnant from the scrotum when it is found. This can be done laparoscopically. If a hernia is not present, an inguinal incision is then no longer necessary.

Based on their experience with 126 patients, Perovic and Janic concluded that laparoscopy is the most satisfactory method for the diagnosis of nonpalpable testes when carried out by an experienced endoscopist.

Brock et al. assessed 58 children with nonpalpable testes using this technique. Two of the children underwent a laparoscopic orchiectomy, and 26 underwent a standard single staged orchiopexy (11), a staged open procedure (3), or a laparoscopic-assisted staged procedure (12). Attenuated vessels were noted in 26 patients, inguinal exploration showed a viable testis in 6 patients, and a testicular remnant only in 20 patients. Four of the patients had blind-ending vessels. In their experience, the use of the potassium titanyl phosphate (KTP) laser has made the laparoscopic two-stage procedure easy.

Fundoplication for Gastroesophageal Reflux

Background and Indications

The laparoscopic approach to gastroesophageal reflux is routinely performed in many centers. The indications for performing a laparoscopic antireflux procedure for gastroesophageal reflux in children are primarily related to pulmonary problems from the eflux or severe esophagitis the same as those for open operations. The theoretical advantages of the laparoscopic approach are related to the absence of an abdominal incision and a more rapid recovery. Particularly in obese patients, a larger incision is more likely to develop wound complications. In the debilitated child, particularly one with severe mental retardation or those who cannot follow instructions, a full abdominal incision may also impair pulmonary function and dispose the patient to atelectasis or pneumonia.

The choice of operation depends on the surgeon's preference and on the patient's disease. When the patient is neurologically impaired and requires access for feeding, a 360-degree wrap is preferred. When the patient is not neurologically impaired, a 180-degree anterior wrap or a 270-degree posterior wrap are better options because of their low rates of gas bloat and dysphagia. All of these procedures can be performed laparoscopically.

Technique

The operating room setup is the same as for laparoscopic fundoplication. Five 5-mm cannulae are placed into the abdomen: one for viewing with the telescope, one for retracting the liver, two for tissue manipulation, and one for suturing (Fig. 57-12). The operation is identical to that performed by laparotomy. The liver is retracted away from the esophageal hiatus, the esophagus is mobilized, the diaphragmatic crura are approximated with sutures, the short gastric vessels are di-

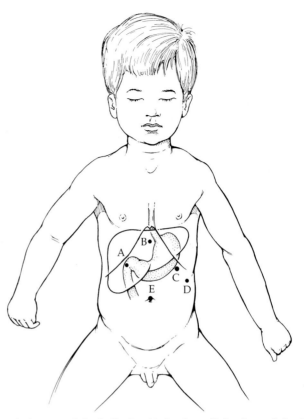

Fig. 57-12. Five ports for laparoscopic fundoplication. (A, 3 or 5 mm; B, 3 or 5 mm; C, 5 or 10 mm; D, 3 or 5 mm; E, 5 or 10 mm.)

vided, wrap is sutured into position, and a gastrostomy is placed if thought to be necessary.

Patients are best prepared by emptying the colon of gas and feces before the operation. Otherwise, the gas-distended colon is in the way, making the procedure difficult or impossible. My colleagues and I find that an osmotic cathartic is effective for this purpose.

Under general endotracheal anesthesia, the bladder is catheterized or emptied by means of the Credé maneuver, and a nasogastric tube is passed. Larger children can be placed in the lithotomy position so that the camera operator can stand between the legs and out of the way. Infants and small children are positioned in a "frog-leg" position. Using sterile technique, a CO_2 pneumoperitoneum is established and maintained, and a 5- or 10-mm, 0 or 30-degree laparoscope is passed through an umbilical cannula. A 5-mm cannula is placed below the right costal margin in the midclavicular line, and another is placed in the epigastrium. A 5- or 10-mm cannula is placed in the left midclavicular line below

the costal margin, and a 5-mm cannula is located in the left anterior axillary line below the costal margin. The liver is retracted through the epigastric cannula in small infants to expose the esophageal hiatus. Although the cannula itself is sufficient to hold the liver out of the way in smaller patients, a grasper used as a retractor is necessary in larger patients. It may be easier in larger patients to insert this grasper through the right lateral cannula and to use the epigastric cannula for dissection and suturing. The grasper can be used to grab the diaphragm anterior to the hiatus and keep the liver from flopping in the line of sight. Rarely, for large floppy livers, an additional grasper can be inserted through the patient's left side, and the two graspers together can act as a supporting structure to keep the liver out of the way of the surgery. The short gastric vessels are divided as necessary if the wrap is otherwise too tight. If, before sutures are placed, the wrap cannot stay in place without holding it, the short gastric vessels should be divided. We find it easiest to use a bipolar dissector or harmonic scalpel to isolate and divide these vessels.

The esophagus, with as large a bougie in place as it can accommodate, is mobilized and retracted using dissecting instruments passed through the right and left lateral cannulae. A short segment (approximately 6 inches) of umbilical tape is then passed behind the esophagus. The exposed diaphragmatic crura are approximated to close the hiatus using interrupted 2-0 silk sutures that have been lubricated with mineral oil. If needed, the Endo-Stitch device (USSC, Norwalk, CT) can be used to place the sutures. After exposure is obtained, it is easier to insert the sutures if the bougie is removed from the esophagus. Extracorporeal knots are the easiest for securely tying under tension. For the 360-degree and the 270-degree wraps, the stomach is passed behind the esophagus (with the bougie in position), from the patient's left to right. With the stomach held in position using an instrument passed through the right midclavicular line cannula, a suture is used to "snag" the stomach and to complete the first (distal-most) suture of the wrap. This maneuver saves having to put in another cannula. The 3- to 5-cm wrap is then secured into place using interrupted 2-0 silk sutures, as for an open procedure (Fig. 57-13). The esophageal bougie and the cannulae are then removed. These children often need a gastronomy tube placed for feeding and medications.

For placement of the gastrostomy tube, the laparoscope is used to determine the optimal position of the gastrostomy, grasping the correct spot on the anterior gastric wall, and T-fasteners are used to secure the stomach to the anterior abdominal wall. The Seldinger technique is then used to place a gastrostomy tube or a gastrostomy button over a wire while watching the procedure with the laparoscope.

Patients are fed liquids on the evening of their operation, and a full diet (orally or by tube) on the first postoperative day. They usually are discharged between 36 and 48 hours after surgery, at which time they can return to unrestricted activities. Representative data (±1 SD) are presented in Table 57-3.

Complications specifically related to laparoscopy trocar sites included a leak in a patient with a ventriculoperitoneal shunt and malposition of a wrap. All other complications in both groups are representative of those described in other series of fundoplications (e.g., small bowel obstruc-

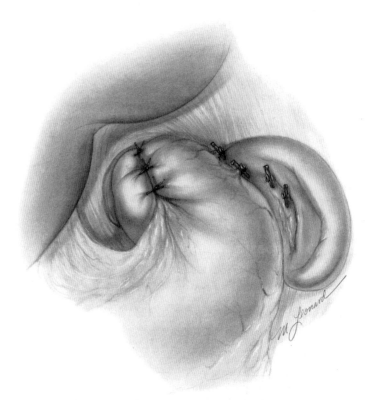

Fig. 57-13. Completed laparoscopic Nissen fundoplication.

Table 57-3. Comparison of Laparoscopic and Open Fundoplication for Gastrointestinal Reflux in Children

Characteristic	Neurologically Impaired Patients (n = 143)		Neurologically normal patients (n = 69)		All patients (n = 211)[a]	
	LAP	OPEN	LAP	OPEN	LAP	OPEN
Operating time (hr)	2.2 ± 0.9	1.8 ± 0.8	2.3 ± 0.6	1.9 ± 0.7	2.2 ± 0.8	1.8 ± 0.8[c]
Days[b]	4.6 ± 3.2	8.4 ± 6.8	3.0 ± 3.7	7.2 ± 6.3[c]	3.8 ± 3.5	8.1 ± 6.7[d]
Early complications (%)	20	41.4	16.7	5.3	18.5	30.3
Late complications (%)	13.3	42.2[d]	0	31.6[c]	7.4	38.9[d]

[a] Patient numbers are derived for three procedures: Nissen (25 laparascopic, 180 open), Thal (0 laparoscopic, 5 open), and Toupet (2 larascopic, 0 open), for a total of 27 laparoscopic and 185 open procedures.
[b] Postoperative days in the hospital.
[c] P<0.05.
[d] P<0.01.

tions, wound infections). Overall, the laparoscopic approach results in a longer operative time but shorter hospitalization and fewer late complications. Neurologically normal children had fewer early complications compared with the neurologically impaired group (5 of 69 versus 56 of 143; p<0.001).

We concluded that laparoscopic antireflux procedures are a safe alternative to open procedures. Because of the shorter

hospitalization and fewer late complications associated with the laparoscopic technique, this approach appears to be superior.

Thompson et al. reported their experience with laparoscopic fundoplication in 25 children, whose mean weight was 8 kg. Their mean operative time was 114 minutes, which included gastrostomy placement in 20 of the patients. Nineteen of the patients are alive without recurrent gastroesophageal reflux at a mean follow-up of 1 year. Perioperative complications in their experience were unusual and mild when they occurred. Six of their patients died late of their underlying disease, but none of the deaths was attributable to the laparoscopic procedure.

In France, Longis et al. had a similar experience with 30 pediatric fundoplications. Twenty-four patients underwent a Nissen-Rossetti procedure, and six underwent a Toupet fundoplication. They found only some minor complications in three of their patients. These included dysphagia in one child, a slipped wrap that did not cause problems in one patient, and recurrent episodes of gastrointestinal hemorrhage in one patient.

Laparoscopic Exploration of Inguinal Herniorrhaphy

Infants and children with unilateral symptomatic inguinal hernias can undergo safe and accurate exploration of the contralateral groin using techniques. The patients usually receive general anesthesia using endotracheal intubation. The stomach is emptied with a suction catheter, and the bladder is emptied by a Credé maneuver. The symptomatic side is explored in the normal open fashion, and the hernia sac is dissected free from the cord structures and divided. A 4-mm laparoscopic cannula is passed into the peritoneal cavity through the hernia sac and is secured in position with a 2-0 silk suture to prevent it from slipping. The abdomen is then insufflated with CO_2 to a pressure of 8 to 10 mm Hg. A 70-degree telescope (the size used for bronchoscopy) is passed into the peritoneal cavity through the cannula, and the peritoneal aspect of the contralateral internal inguinal ring is inspected. In the normal male patient, the surgeon can see the vas deferens and spermatic vessels pass through the ring and determine that there is no hernia defect. Hernias are obvious. When no hernia is found, the CO_2 is evacuated, and the ipsilateral hernia repair is completed. When a contralateral hernia is discovered, it is repaired in the normal (open) fashion after completing the repair of the symptomatic side.

Fuenfer et al. modified the technique of contralateral groin exploration. They insufflate the abdomen through the hernia sac on the symptomatic side and then pass a 1.2-mm laparoscope through a 14-gauge catheter in line with the contralateral internal inguinal ring. Using this approach, they believe that they have fewer errors in their assessment of the anatomy

Holcomb et al. studied 195 children who underwent laparoscopy before hernia repair. Eighty-six patients had a unilateral hernia with a contralateral patent processus vaginalis, and 109 had only a unilateral hernia. After anesthesia, it was suspected on prelaparoscopic clinical examination that 55 patients had a contralateral patent processus vaginalis. During laparoscopy, it was found that 31 (56%) had patent processus vaginalis, and 24 (44%) did not. Of the 140 patients believed to have a contralateral patent processus vaginalis on prelaparoscopic clinical examination, 60 (43%) did, and 80 (57%) did not. Insufflation alone was not diagnostic of contralateral patent processus vaginalis; of the 195 patients undergoing laparoscopy, insufflation resulted in a positive finding on the known side in only 129 (66%) and on the contralateral side in 23 (27%) of the 86 patients found to have a contralateral patent processus vaginalis. There were no complications related to the laparoscopy or the hernia repair in their experience. Similar results were found for 150 patients reported by Grossman et al.

Laparoscopic Splenectomy

Background and Indications

Another procedure that shows promise in children is laparoscopic splenectomy. These procedures usually are performed on patients with hematologic disorders. Patients are prepared as described earlier for a fundoplication, and they are vaccinated preoperatively with the appropriate polyvalent vaccines against pneumococcal disease and *Haemophilus influenzae.*

Technique

A 5- or 10-mm laparoscope, depending on the size of the patient, is placed through an umbilical cannula. A steep reversed Trendelenburg position is required, and the patient is slightly rotated, with the left side elevated. Two cannulae are placed first: one 12 mm in the midclavicular line and one 5 mm in the midclavicular line at or below the level of the umbilicus. The child is moved to the right lateral decubitus position, and two 5-mm cannulae are placed in the anterior axillary line, one below the costal margin and one between the umbilicus and the iliac crest (Fig. 57-14).

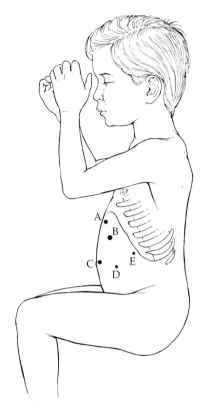

Fig. 57-14. Port placement for laparoscopic splenectomy. (A, 5 or 10 mm; B, 12 mm; C, 5 or 10 mm; D, 5 mm; E, 5 mm.)

Initially, the greater curvature of the stomach is grasped gently with an atraumatic grasper and the gastrosplenic ligament retracted to expose the short gastric vessels. The short gastric vessels are then divided using the harmonic scalpel or the bipolar electrocautery dissectors passed through the midclavicular cannula.

As the dissection progresses, it is helpful to rotate the patient from the lateral decubitus position to allow the intestines to fall out of the way. Using instruments passed through the lateral cannulae, the spleen is elevated, and the splenic artery and vein at the hilum just beyond the tail of the pancreas are identified, using gentle dissection with a curved or right-angle dissector. The splenic hilum is then isolated and the vasculature divided with an endoscopic linear stapler inserted through the 12-mm cannula used to divide both vessels simultaneously. The vascular stapler device provides excellent hemostasis and diminishes operative time significantly.

After the major splenic vessels have been divided, there are often some ligamentous attachments that should be carefully divided using Metzenbaum-type scissors. At this point, the spleen is completely mobilized and freed in the peritoneal cavity. A LapSac (Cook Urological, Spencer, IN) is then inserted through the 12-mm cannula. The sac is unfurled, and the three tabs at the mouth of the sac are held open while the spleen is placed in the sac. The neck of the sac is drawn up into a 10-mm cannula. When the entire neck is in the cannula, it should be withdrawn until the neck of the sac is exteriorized. The neck of the sac is opened and a mechanical or automated tissue morcellator placed within the pouch. The organ can then be morcellated until it is small enough that the entire pouch and any residual tissue can be withdrawn through the trocar site. The trocar and cannula are then reinserted, and the pneumoperitoneum is reestablished to ensure hemostasis.

Depending on the indication for a splenectomy, a search should be made for accessory spleens. If any are identified, they are removed. After it is established that there are no accessory spleens and that there is good hemostasis, the cannulae are removed and the incisions closed.

Rothenberg has reported on a similar technique, but uses the harmonic scalpel for most of the dissection and division of vascular structures to save on time and cost of the procedure. Hicks et al. reported their experience with laparoscopic splenectomy in 11 children compared with 10 recent cases of open splenectomy. Their technique used endoscopic clips and Roeder knots and did not require the use of linear staplers or tissue morcellators. The operative time for their laparoscopic procedure was 147 minutes, compared with 112 minutes for the open procedure. The estimated blood loss for the laparoscopic procedure was less. The patients undergoing a laparoscopic splenectomy spent an average of 3.6 days in the hospital after their procedure, compared with 5.3 days for the open

group. There were no complications in the laparoscopic group.

Data on 14 laparoscopic splenectomies from the University of Tennessee were compared with data on 47 open pediatric splenectomies (Table 57-4). Two (14%) of the 14 laparoscopic patients developed complications. One patient with Evan's syndrome developed pneumonia requiring antibiotics. A second patient required conversion to an open procedure because of poorly controlled hemorrhage from a short gastric vessel. Twelve (25%) of the open splenectomy patients developed complications: atelectasis (3), fever (4), wound infection (2), pneumonia (1), laryngospasm (1), and pancreatitis (1). The data show a trend toward a 1-day reduction in hospital stay with laparoscopic splenectomy ($p<0.02$). Operative time was 83% longer for the laparoscopic approach ($p<0.001$), and operative costs were almost $3000 greater ($p<0.001$). Total hospital costs were also greater for the laparoscopic procedures ($p<0.1$), primarily reflecting a more than $3000 difference for splenectomy alone ($p<0.02$).

Laparoscopic splenectomy is a safe but more expensive alternative to open splenectomy, primarily because of the use of disposable instruments. Benefits of the laparoscopic approach include a shorter hospital stay and a subjective improvement in cosmetic results. Disadvantages include increased operative time and cost. A larger series is needed to determine the significance of the difference in complication rates between the two approaches.

Pull-through Procedure for Hirschsprung's Disease

A modification of the Soave procedure for Hirschsprung's disease can be easily performed in newborns and infants for whom the diagnosis has been made on clinical grounds and supported with a contrast en-

ema and a suction rectal biopsy showing the absence of ganglion cells and hypertrophy of the nerve fibers. A colostomy is unnecessary in these patients.

Patients under general anesthesia are placed supine at the end of a shortened operating table and are prepped circumferentially from the nipples down. Three 3- or 5-mm cannulae are placed: one in the right upper quadrant in the midclavicular line below the costal margin (for the telescope) and one lateral to each rectus muscle at or above the level of the umbilicus. A bladder catheter is inserted, and the lower abdomen is inspected. By placing several towels underneath the patient's buttocks, a Trendelenburg position can be established. The colon is grasped, and the transition zone is identified. The mesentery is opened by blunt dissection, and the retrorectal space is dissected free. Mesocolic vessels distal to the transition zone are divided between sutures or with bipolar electrocautery. These vessels can be divided as high as necessary. The endoscopic instruments are removed at this time, and the abdomen is deflated.

Attention is then turned to the anus where, with the legs elevated over the patient's abdomen, the rectum is everted with sutures. After infiltrating the submucosa with 1:200,000 epinephrine solution, a circumferential incision is made where the infiltration was carried out in the anal mucosa at the dentate line, and a mucosal tube is dissected from its muscular cuff. After a short 1- to 2-cm dissection, the posterior rectal space is entered by dividing the muscular cuff posteriorly and extending this incision circumferentially around the colon, which is then further dissected until the transition zone has been brought down through the anus. This muscular cuff can be made quite short, until the procedure may be more similar to a Swenson procedure anastomosis than it is to that of a Soave procedure. All of the dissection is di-

Table 57-4. Comparison of Open and Laparoscopic Splenectomy Performed Alone or in Combination with Other Procedures

Procedure	No. of Patients	Age (yr)	Hospital Stay (d)	Operating Room Time (min)	Operating Time (min)	Total Cost ($)	Operating Cost ($)
Open							
Alone	28	6.5	3.6	116	81	4081	1026
Combined	19	7.4	3.7	185	140	7501	1583
Laparoscopic							
Alone	10	6.5	2.7	229	187	7233	4183
Combined	4	5.0	2.2	252	202	6445	4128

rectly on the wall of the colon in a fashion similar to the mobilization of the rectum in a posterosagittal anorectoplasty performed for imperforate anus. After a full-thickness biopsy confirms the presence of ganglion cells, any posterior muscular cuff is completely divided in the midline posteriorly, and a full-thickness anastomosis is carried out in quadrants using interrupted 4-0 absorbable sutures, which are cut to allow the anastomosis to retract into the anus.

These patients are fed the day of surgery and can be discharged the following morning. Dilation of these patients begins at 2 weeks after surgery and is continued as required.

At the University of Louisville, my colleagues and I have performed 20 such procedures and have encountered only two problems. One patient's initial radiographs suggested a transition zone in the sigmoid colon. At operation, multiple biopsies of the colon were performed, but no ganglion cells were seen. Ultimately, an ileal-anal pull-through operation was required. This patient was in the hospital for nearly 2 months for the control of diarrhea but is now thriving and has three to four normal stools each day. Because of this experience, we do not believe that it is best to perform this laparoscopic procedure on known cases of total-colon Hirschsprung's disease. One other patient underwent a laparoscopic pull-through at 2 weeks of age and had some initial difficulty. After a brief period, the patient developed a distal bowel obstruction. A contrast study showed the problem to be at the level of the anastomosis, and a sphincterotomy was performed. This patient subsequently did well. One patient with Down syndrome and congenital heart disease died several months after surgery of sudden infant death syndrome after apparently good results (e.g., normal stooling pattern, weight gain). All other patients are doing well, and have normal stooling patterns. The average hospitalization after surgery is 1.5 days.

Laparoscopy for Cancer in Children

One of the more useful functions of minimal access surgery is the diagnosis and staging of pediatric cancer.

Liver Biopsy

Background and Indications. Liver biopsy may be required for evaluation of a primary liver tumor or metastatic disease. Percutaneous needle biopsy is the simplest method to obtain liver tissue for the diagnosis. However, equivocal ultrasound or computed tomography (CT)–guided biopsies or impairment of coagulation may mandate biopsy under direct vision. Laparoscopic-assisted biopsy is an alternative to open biopsy and has several advantages over an open procedure. The color, size, structure, and consistency of the liver can be evaluated. The presence of local or diffuse hepatic processes like tumors, cysts, hemangiomas, abscesses, or miliary infections are noticed before the biopsy is taken. In the case of focal lesions, the biopsy instrument can be directed to the desired area. Direct observation prevents penetration of vascular or other easily harmed targets. Hemorrhage or bile leakage after the biopsy can be identified immediately and treated with electrocoagulation, microfibrillar collagen, fibrin glue, or sutures. A better view of the entire liver and its relation to the abdominal organs also is obtained.

Technique. One laparoscope is placed through an umbilical cannula. The abdominal contents and the liver are inspected. Core biopsies can be taken using Tru-Cut needle (Travenol Division, Valencia, CA) placed percutaneously under direct guidance of the laparoscope. An alternative method is to insert two additional cannula: one in the anterior axillary line on the right below the coastal margin and the other below the xiphoid and to the right of the falciform ligament. The size of the cannula is determined by the size of the required biopsy. In most instances, a 5-mm cannula is sufficient for obtaining adequate tissue. Surface lesions can be biopsied using a cup biopsy forceps. The biopsy is taken first, and then hemostasis is established. This sequence avoids tissue destruction and allows the pathologist to better interpret the histology. Wedge resections can be performed using laparoscopic suturing technique, and the specimen can be excised using a scalpel blade or laser. An alternative to suturing the liver is to use an endoscopic stapler to excise the wedge biopsy. This technique is useful for lesions on the edge of the liver.

Lesions situated deep in the liver parenchyma can be detected by an endoscopic ultrasound probe that can be inserted through an abdominal cannula and that is available from several manufacturers. A Tru-Cut needle can be directed by the ultrasound probe to the deep lesion, and core biopsies can be taken (Fig. 57-15). After the specimen is removed and

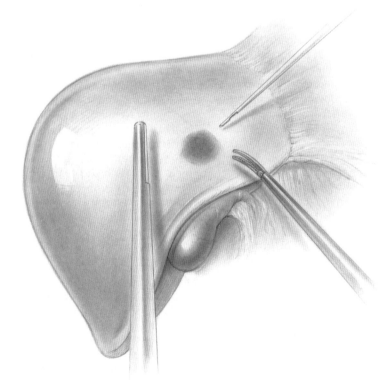

Fig. 57-15. Tru-Cut needle directed by an ultrasound probe for core biopsy of a deep lesion.

hemostasis is achieved in the biopsy bed, the cannulae are removed under direct view, and the wounds are closed.

Tumor Staging

Background and Indications. Laparoscopic examination of the abdomen in children with intraabdominal malignant disease can provide on the spread and resectability of the tumor information when the results of noninvasive modalities are equivocal. Laparoscopy is superior to CT for staging and evaluating neoplasms that seed by peritoneal spread and for the evaluation of unexplained ascites. Second-look operations to assess the response to chemotherapy in patients with neuroblastoma, germ cell tumors, or non-Hodgkin's lymphomas can be performed laparoscopically. Liver, lymph nodes, and residual tumor biopsies also can be obtained. When indicated, splenectomy also can be carried out laparoscopically.

Staging laparotomy in Hodgkin's disease is performed to direct therapy and, especially in children, to avoid unnecessary irradiation or intensive chemotherapy. Staging laparotomy includes splenectomy, wedge and needle biopsies of both lobes of the liver, biopsy of at least seven node groups, biopsy of any other suspicious lymph nodes, and an iliac crest bone marrow biopsy. In female children who receive radiotherapy to the lower abdomen and pelvis, oophoropexy is usually done. Abdominal exploration by laparotomy or laparoscopy alters the clinical staging in about 30% to 40% of children. For most, the stages are upgraded, predominantly from stages 1 or 2 to stage 3 or 4. Laparoscopy can minimize postoperative pulmonary complications and intraabdominal adhesions, and it can result in a shorter delay before definitive therapy can be started.

Technique. After the pneumoperitoneum is established, appropriate-sized cannulae are introduced, and the abdominal cavity is inspected. For difficult to reach places, such as the dome of the liver or under the diaphragm, the laparoscope can be changed from a 0- to a 30-degree or 70-degree scope to provide a better view. When biopsy is necessary, it can be carried out percutaneously under direct laparoscopic observation, using biopsy forceps or by free excision.

There are various types of biopsy instruments. The instrument to be used should be tailored to the type of specimen needed. When it is important not to crush the tissue, as in case of lymphadenectomy for cancer staging, "spoon" forceps are preferred. Laser or electrocautery can destroy the tissue and interfere with the histologic examination; therefore, the tissue is first taken by a biopsy device, and hemostasis is established later. Specimens can and should be removed in various types of endoscopic bags as to avoid spillage of malignant tissue and contact with the cannula tract. Large specimens such as a spleen or kidney can be removed from such a bag piecemeal using a ring forceps or automatic morcellator. Although histology can be identified accurately in these chunks of tissue, gross morphology and identification of surgical margins can be difficult to interpret. If tissue margins are important, the surgeon can perform marginal biopsies or mark the different areas of the specimen with India ink before morcellating the tissue. A final alternative is to make a muscle-splitting counterincision to remove the specimen intact.

Endoscopic Treatment of Idiopathic Hypertrophic Pyloric Stenosis

Background and Indications

Many surgeons consider a discussion of the endoscopic treatment of pyloric stenosis ludicrous. This is a disorder for which the conventional surgical treatment is simple, elegant, inexpensive, and associated with few complications. Conventional wisdom suggests that for a new and highly technical procedure to be warranted, it must provide some advantage to the patient. Proponents of laparoscopic pyloromyotomy suggest that the cosmetic result is better than with conventional surgery. Others refute this argument and perform the pyloromyotomy through an umbilical incision that leaves no scar.

Laparoscopic pyloromyotomy is simple, cost effective, and at worst another acceptable alternative. Whether it is a better procedure is difficult to say for certain. The studies that have been performed do not show any great advantage over the conventional approach. The diagnosis and preoperative management of pyloric stenosis is straightforward and is not different when laparoscopy is considered as an option.

Technique

With the patient under general anesthesia, the stomach and bladder are decompressed, and the abdomen is prepped as usual with infiltration of local anesthesia at the instrument insertion sites. The initial cannula is inserted through the umbilicus. This is for the telescope and need only be large enough to accept the scope (2 to 5 mm). The abdomen is insufflated, and two other instruments are inserted without cannulae directly through stab wounds. An atraumatic grasper is placed through the stab wound in the left upper quadrant. This is used to grab the stomach and expose the pylorus. A retractable knife blade (a round-ended arthroscopy knife is suitable for this purpose) is then inserted through a right upper quadrant stab wound, and the longitudinal incision is made along the pyloric mass and extended slightly onto the stomach proximally. The knife is then removed, and a laparoscopic pyloric spreader is inserted through the same right upper quadrant stab wound. The incision in the pyloric mass is carefully spread open until the two halves of the pyloric tumor move independently (Fig. 57-16). Care is taken not to make a hole in the mucosa. After the pyloromyotomy is completed, the instruments are removed. The umbilical incision may require a suture; the others can be dressed with a simple bandage without suture. The procedure takes 10 to 20 minutes to complete.

Postoperative care is the same as after conventional surgery. Proponents of the laparoscopic approach reason that, because there is no "tugging" on the pylorus to get it out of a wound, there is less postoperative ileus and the patients can be fed more quickly. A typical protocol is to feed the patients one ounce of standard formula or breast milk within 2 to 4 hours of completing surgery. If they tolerate this, they can have 2 ounces 2 hours later and then are fed *ad libitum* in 3 more hours. Using this schedule, patients are up to full feedings approximately 7 hours after surgery.

In his first few cases, Alain encountered a couple of mucosal tears. Since then, there have been few complications from the laparoscopic procedure that is performed in several centers around the world. Thompson et al. have shown that the laparoscopic approach in their hands is more cost effective than the conventional approach.

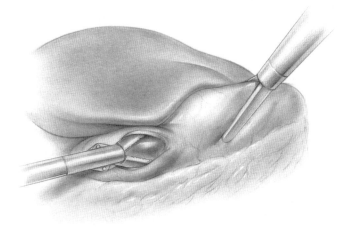

Fig. 57-16. *The pyloric tumor is being spread during laparoscopic pyloromyotomy.*

Thoracoscopy

Background and Indications

Rodgers initiated pediatric thoracoscopy in the United States in the 1970s. He and his colleagues used rigid endoscopic equipment under local anesthesia to diagnose malignancy and other disorders in infants and children. Despite several reports of success, the technique did not catch on until after laparoscopic cholecystectomy became widely accepted. The availability of lightweight, high-resolution video cameras and better endoscopic instruments made more complex endoscopic procedures more appealing, and the results justified the renewed interest.

The endoscopic linear stapler made quick, efficient endoscopic segmental lung biopsy possible. As the stapler became readily available, surgeons learned to cut and sew tissues in the chest, and as better devices for tissue extraction were developed, many complex procedures that before could only be carried out by means of thoracotomy could be performed through minor stab wounds in the chest wall. Thoracoscopy appears to cause less pain, allow the patient to go home more quickly, and make it so that the patient returns to unrestricted activity sooner than after thoracotomy.

Thoracoscopy is performed by pediatric surgeons with greater frequency than laparoscopy. In a survey of Pediatric Oncology Group surgeons, endoscopic procedures performed for cancer included 192 thoracoscopic procedures compared with 103 laparoscopic procedures. Even though most of the thoracoscopic procedures were simple biopsies, the shorter hospitalization

(which translates into dollar savings) has already made an impact on pediatric surgical practice. The increased patient comfort is dramatic. Most thoracoscopic patients are discharged within 24 to 48 hours, and more than one-half do not require chest tubes. This is not the case when thoracotomy is required. Pediatric thoracoscopic procedures are listed in Table 57-5.

The only contraindications to thoracoscopy are the inability to tolerate general anesthesia, complete pleural symphysis, and severe pulmonary insufficiency that obviates single-lens ventilation. Patients selected for thoracoscopy do not require any special preparation. It is safer to perform thoracoscopy in infants and children under general anesthesia. Plans should be made to perform a selective intubation with a double-lumen endotracheal tube in larger patients and selective intubation with a cuffed endotracheal tube or a bronchial blocker in younger patients.

Thorough patient positioning is essential. We use gravity as much as possible to allow the collapsed lung to fall out of the field of vision. Accordingly, if the lesion is in the apex, the patient should be in a reversed Trendelenburg position. If the lesion is at the base of the lung, the patient should be in the Trendelenburg position. If the lesion is anterior, the patient should be rotated 30 to 45 degrees posteriorly from the full lateral position, and if the lesion is posterior, the patient should be rotated anteriorly 30 to 45 degrees.

When the patient is prepped and draped, the anesthesiologist should allow the lung to deflate if he has not already done so. The

surgeon then is ready to make the first incision. The location of the incision depends on the procedure to be performed. As with laparoscopy, it is useful to infiltrate the trocar sites with a local anesthetic consisting of one-half 0.25% bupivacaine with 1:100,000 epinephrine and one-half 1% lidocaine to provide a short- and long-lasting analgesic effect. When the suspected lesion is in the upper chest, then we insert the telescope in the midaxillary line in a lower interspace (taking care not to put the instrument through the diaphragm). When the lesion is in the lower chest, we insert the telescope in the upper chest. This allows for the best and broadest field of vision possible in the small thorax.

The chest is entered directly with blunt dissection as though inserting a chest tube. After the initial access is achieved and the thoracoscope is inserted, the surgeon can tell if the selective intubation is effective. We often speed up the deflation of the lung by insufflating the chest with CO_2 gas at a pressure of 4 to 10 mm Hg. Although this maneuver is used initially to save time, it may be necessary to continue the insufflation if the lung remains inflated and interferes with the procedure.

If CO_2 insufflation is unnecessary, special trocars are not needed for instrument insertion but instead can be inserted directly through the small incisions in the intercostal spaces of the thin chest wall. If insufflation is necessary, standard laparoscopic cannulae must be used.

After the procedure is completed, hemostasis must be ensured. When the stapler is used to resect lung tissue, the chest tube is not routinely left in place unless the patient is on mechanical ventilation or ventilation is likely because of pulmonary insufficiency. In these instances, patients are more likely to develop a delayed pneumothorax from an air leak at the staple line and require insertion of a chest tube.

As long as the visceral pleura remains intact, it is unnecessary to leave indwelling chest tubes in patients who undergo simple biopsies. However, we routinely insert a noncollapsible suction catheter into a trocar site during wound closing. The anesthesiologist should inflate the lung several times with sustained positive pressure in an attempt to evacuate all the gas from the chest. Even with this maneuver, a small postoperative pneumothorax may occur. When this occurs in an asymptomatic patient, a repeat radiograph is obtained 6 hours later. If the pneumothorax is stable or no longer present, the patient can be discharged from the hospital. When chest tubes are inserted, they are placed in a trocar site and removed when there is no longer any air leak present (usually 6 to 12 hours).

Caution should be emphasized when considering resection and biopsy for cancer. Tumor implants have been reported to occur in trocar sites in patients with metastatic osteosarcoma. The surgeon should always extract these specimens carefully and not drag them through the muscle, subcutaneous tissue, and skin of the chest wall without first placing them into a protective sheath.

Some surgeons infuse long-acting local anesthetics into the pleural space through an indwelling catheter to improve postoperative analgesia. Most patients, however, require only oral analgesics after thoracoscopy and do not require these catheters. After thoracoscopy, patients are allowed free access to food and they are encouraged to ambulate as soon as they are awake and steady on their feet.

Three relatively innovations in pediatric thoracoscopy appear to be useful: the automatic tissue morcellator, the harmonic scalpel, and endoscopic ultrasound. The automatic tissue morcellator can be used on lung and tumor tissue to facilitate extraction of large specimens. The specimen is first placed into a LapSac (Cook Urological, Spencer, IN), the open end of which is exteriorized by drawing it through a trocar

site. The working end of the morcellator is then inserted into the sac, and the tissue is cut into 0.5- to 1.0-cm pieces of tissue that the pathologist can easily interpret. When the tissue is too large to extract through a standard trocar site but too small to justify using the morcellator, an alternative is to enlarge one of the intercostal incisions and extract the sac through the incision.

The harmonic scalpel (Ultracision, Smithfield, RI) can be inserted through a 5-mm port and oscillates at a frequency of 55,000 vibrations per second. With such rapid oscillations, the backside of the device's tip coagulates vessels up to several millimeters in diameter. The device serves as an outstanding dissection tool with relatively bloodless dissections. Because the harmonic scalpel does not conduct electrical energy like conventional electrocautery, there is no risk of inducing cardiac fibrillation when working around the mediastinum.

The latest new device is endoscopic ultrasound. This diagnostic ultrasound device is 10 mm in diameter and comes with a variety of suitable probe configurations. This device can image lesions in the parenchyma of the collapsed lung and is useful to define the vascular anatomy near points of dissection. This later use tends to minimize any hemorrhage and certainly indicates where major structures are relative to the proposed dissection. Endoscopic ultrasound has also been used to detect metastatic lesions that were not seen on chest CT images or plain chest films, suggesting that the device may play an important role in thoracoscopy for cancer.

The experience with thoracoscopy in pediatric surgical practices is quite good. Several clinical conditions lend themselves exceptionally well to the thoracoscopic approach.

Techniques

Loculated Pleural Effusion and Empyema.
In the past, children with loculated pleural effusions were admitted to the hospital and underwent repeated thoracenteses with or without the introduction of antibiotics, or they had a tube thoracostomy for drainage. As the patient failed to improve, repeated attempts at drainage were usually performed. If the child developed restriction of the lung, decortication was performed by means of thoracotomy.

The modern approach is different. The patient who first presents with fluid in the chest may undergo a thoracentesis. If the thoracentesis does not completely drain the chest, thoracoscopy is considered. Alternatively, a CT scan may be performed to determine whether loculations exist in the chest. When loculated fluid is suspected, the physician should proceed immediately to thoracoscopy under anesthesia rather than inserting a chest tube.

The surgeon first enters the fluid-filled space and bluntly enlarges the space with the end of the thoracoscope or with the tip of the finger through the trocar site. With insufflation, sufficient room is obtained to insert a second trocar for placement of a blunt instrument. With this instrument or the end of a suction catheter, all of the loculations are broken up, and fluid is evacuated. The lung is completely freed, and a chest tube is inserted in the site that was used for the telescope.

In the case of an empyema, we insert a blunt instrument such as a ring forceps through a small incision in the intercostal space to evacuate the exudate. After the exudate is removed and the cavity is irrigated, the chest tube is inserted to expand the lung. The chest tube usually stays in for 2 to 10 days, after which the process is usually resolved sufficiently well for the chest tube to be removed and for the patient to be discharged home on oral antibiotics. Thoracoscopy allows patients to spend less than one-half the time in the hospital than they used to with an open approach.

Pneumothorax.
Spontaneous pneumothoraces caused by bleb rupture or occurring in patients with cystic fibrosis can be managed with thoracoscopic approaches. Some surgeons advocate thoracoscopy with the initial episode. Under these circumstances, if a leaking bled is found, a tissue stapler can be used to staple off the segment with the bleb. A chest tube may not be required. If a single bleb is not obvious, there may be some bullae that can be shrunken down using an argon beam coagulator or laser to seal the lung tissue.

Pleurodesis may be required in some instances. Tetracycline is less readily used today than it was in the past. The most effective agent for pleurodesis is dry, sterilized USP talc. Blown through a cannula into the chest, the talc coats the pleura and creates an intense inflammatory reaction. An indwelling chest is left tube for approximately 48 hours after instilling the talc into the pleural space. These patients usually have a low-grade fever for 1 or 2 days. Analgesics may be required because of some discomfort from the inflammatory reaction. In patients with cystic fibrosis who may be candidates for lung transplant, talc pleurodesis is contraindicated because it obviates future resection of the lung.

Diagnosis and Staging of Cancer

The condition that lends itself best to thoracoscopic intervention is cancer. Mediastinal masses can be excised or biopsied. Intraparenchymal lesions also can be easily identified and biopsied. Children with cancer rarely require lung resection.

Thoracoscopic exploration of the chest with limited biopsy is the most commonly performed procedure. These patients typically present with one or two lesions identified on their diagnostic images and are best served by using thoracoscopy to identify the lesions. A tissue stapler is used for resection, or other techniques are used for biopsy of the localized lesions.

Biopsies for diffuse disease in immunosuppressed patients may be better performed through a small anterolateral incision. In these cases, the lingula can be brought up into the wound, and the stapler can be applied. This is a 15- or 20-minute operation and is much better suited for ill patients with diffuse disease.

For some patients with patchy disease, video-assisted thoracic surgery can be useful. The thoracoscope is introduced into the chest. The area of suspicion is readily seen, and a lung clamp can be passed through an incision in the intercostal space to grasp the lung and withdraw it through the incision for biopsy using a linear stapler. This combined use of open and closed technique obviates the need for a large thoracic incision, which may be painful.

Lung Biopsy. Primary intrapulmonary malignancy is rare in children, but the lungs are a common site of metastasis in childhood. Hematogenous spread appears in the lung parenchyma, and lymphogenous spread usually appears in the mediastinum. The most common pediatric malignancy with early pulmonary metastasis is Wilms' tumor. Other tumors that metastasized to the lung are bone and soft tissue sarcomas, thyroid and hepatic tu-

mors, melanoma, teratocarcinoma, and retinoblastoma. Neuroblastoma metastasizes more commonly to the pleural and mediastinal nodes. Metastatic lesions and granulomas from fungal infections usually resemble each other so closely that it is impossible to distinguish between them without a tissue biopsy. Adequate tissue may be needed to differentiate infectious processes from metastasis, especially in the immune suppressed child.

Open lung biopsy in immune suppressed patients with diffuse pulmonary disease is reported to have mortality rates of 11% to 22%. Thoracoscopy-guided biopsy in children was first reported by Rodgers in 1976. Biopsies of pulmonary tissue or the chest wall can be taken under direct vision. Lung tissue division can be accomplished with an endoscopic stapler that leaves six airtight rows of staples and cuts between the middle two rows. This device must be inserted through a 12-mm incision and requires 5 to 6 cm of working room in the pleural space. The size of the stapler makes it unsuitable for children much younger than 2 years of age. The neodymium:yttrium-aluminum-garnet (Nd:YAG) laser can be used for dissection or cutting and tends to seal the surface of the lung because of the resultant coagulative necrosis. The fiber can be placed through a cannula or placed in a position that allows dissection. The resulting segment of lung can be removed through one of the larger cannulae or placed into a tissue sac to minimize any risk of trocar site implantation of tumor during tissue extraction. Frozen section should be performed to assess the specimen. Hemostasis is achieved by electrocautery, clips, argon beam coagulator, or laser.

Rodgers reported diagnostic accuracy of 92% for evaluation of intrathoracic tumors, and 100% accuracy in the diagnosis of pulmonary parenchymal disease. There was no procedure-related mortality. Reported complications have been minor and occurred in a small percentage of patients and they include pneumothorax, hemorrhage, and conversion to open biopsy. In a series of 131 thoracoscopies reviewed by the Pediatric Oncology Group, 18 (13.7%) had to be converted to open procedures mainly for failure to gain safe access or unresectability. Non–life-threatening complications occurred in 9.2% of the thoracoscopies, and there were no deaths related to the procedure.

Mediastinal Lesions. Mediastinal masses in infancy and childhood are frequently discovered incidentally, and approximately 40% of these primary mediastinal masses are malignant. The anatomic location of the mass within the mediastinum often suggests the origin of the lesion. Neurogenic tumors such as neuroblastoma or ganglioneuroblastoma arise in the posterior mediastinum. Lymphatic tumors, such as Hodgkin's and non-Hodgkin's lymphomas, malignant thymoma, and lymphosarcoma are usually located in the anterior and middle mediastinum, but germ cell tumors such as teratoma occur most often in the anterior mediastinum.

In addition to primary mediastinal tumors, distant malignant disease can metastasize by lymphogenous routes to the lymphoid tissue of the mediastinum. Every mediastinal mass should be evaluated promptly to distinguish a malignant processes from benign masses such as a bronchogenic cyst, esophageal duplication, or thymic hyperplasia.

Diagnostic evaluations usually include posteroanterior and lateral chest radiographs. Calcification in an anterior mass suggests germ cell tumor, but calcification in a posterior mass suggests neuroblastoma. Chest and abdominal CT or magnetic resonance (MR) imaging are done to assess the origin and extent of any tumor found. MR imaging is better for evaluating posterior masses when intraspinal extension of the tumor forming a "dumbbell" lesion is suspected. This information can be obtained from MR imaging without the risks of myelography. After imaging, tissue biopsy may be still needed to differentiate malignancy from benign or infectious diseases. Reevaluation of the tumor after treatment may require a tissue sample.

Thoracoscopic biopsy of mediastinal masses and lymph nodes in pediatric patients was reported by Rodgers in 1981. Most mediastinal lesions could be biopsied using this technique with diagnostic accuracy of 88%. The approach to the biopsy is determined based on the diagnostic imaging. The patient is positioned in a way that allows the lung to fall dependently after its deflation, allowing for maximum visualization of the part of the mediastinum to be explored.

The approach to the pleural space is as described earlier for thoracoscopic lung biopsy. A 5- or 10-mm cannula is inserted at the fourth or fifth intercostal place in the midclavicular line. Another 5-mm cannula is inserted under direct vision in a place that allows manipulation of the biopsy site. The hemithorax and mediastinal structures are inspected, and the lesion to be biopsied is identified. Additional areas of tumor involvement are searched for. The relation of the lesion to the great vessels is established by inspection or by using endoscopic ultrasound. Biopsies can be taken using forceps, scissors, bipolar electrocautery, harmonic scalpel, or laser to excise the tissue. Sufficient tissue should be obtained for histopathologic diagnosis, biologic markers, and genetic evaluation of the tumor. A frozen section should be done to confirm that adequate tissue was biopsied.

In the absence of pleural adhesions, most of the mediastinal lesions are easily visualized. In the superior mediastinum, peritracheal masses or superior hilar lesions can be easily identified. Although early reports suggested that difficulty may be encountered in assessing areas of the pulmonary hilum posteriorly, adjacent to the inferior pulmonary ligament and inferior pulmonary vein, modern instruments and techniques allow even this area to be adequately inspected.

When thoracoscopy fails to establish the diagnosis of mediastinal pathology, thoracotomy is indicated to better evaluate the suspected lesion. Such may be the case when a suspected lymph node or mass is seen on the diagnostic images but is not identified using thoracoscopy alone.

Intrathoracic Cysts
Cystic lesions in the chest readily lend themselves to thoracoscopic exploration and excision. Bronchopulmonary foregut malformations can be excised when indicated using standard thoracoscopy techniques. Pulmonary sequestrations, collapsed cystic adenomatoid malformations, and enteric duplications also are managed this way.

Patent Ductus Arteriosus
Several surgeons have used thoracoscopy to ligate a patent ductus arteriosus. This procedure can be performed in even the tinniest of infants using 2.7-mm pediatric instruments. Although it can be argued that the risk of morbidity from a small in-

cision in the chest is low, the incision will grow with the child and may cause problems in the future. The optics of today's telescopes and video cameras are so good that a physician can easily see the structures for careful dissection and the ductus arteriosus can be clipped or ligated (Fig. 57-17).

In France, Laborde has performed more than 450 thoracoscopic procedures to occlude the patent ductus arteriosus. His technique uses three ports: one for the thoracoscope, one for a lung retractor, and the remaining one for a right-angled hook electrocautery device and clip applier. He used the hook cautery on low power to dissect the ductus free of its surrounding tissues. After the ductus is free, he applies two endoscopic clips to occlude the lumen. He has encountered few complications and no deaths. When complications did occur, they were minor ones, the nature of which were inherent to ductal ligation performed by any technique.

Trauma
Another application for thoracoscopy that we have found useful is in our evaluation of trauma. Some patients have had chest tubes placed in the trauma resuscitation room and have continued hemorrhage. Insertion of a telescope through the chest tube site may clarify whether there is bleeding from the pulmonary parenchyma that can be stapled off to stop the hemorrhage or there is a more significant vascular injury that requires thoracotomy for repair. We also evaluate for the possibility of diaphragmatic injuries through this approach.

There are many more procedures being performed today on children. Some surgeons are skilled enough to be able to perform pulmonary lobectomy for infection or for congenital malformations, and others have excised mediastinal tumors using thoracoscopic approaches. Although thoracoscopy may be better suited for the older child, it is safe even in the smallest

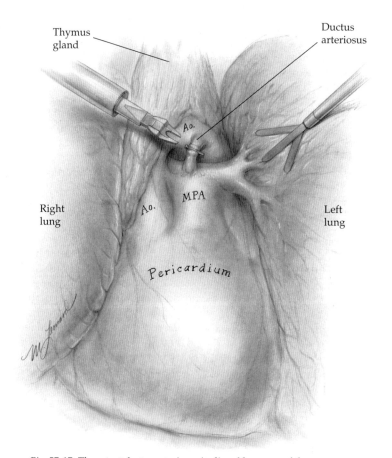

Fig. 57-17. The patent ductus arteriosus is clipped by means of thoracoscopy.

infants when used by skilled surgeons experienced in the technique.

Complications of Minimal Access Surgery in Children

We reviewed the complications associated with laparoscopy and thoracoscopy early in our experience with 636 children between the ages of 1 month and 19 years. Thoracoscopy was performed in 62 children. Conversion to thoracotomy occurred in 8 children (13%) because of an inability to localize the lesion (3), unresectability (2), inadequate tissue sample (1), unsafe access (1), and hypoxemia (1). Complications occurred in 3 children (5%). One child with an unresectable mediastinal tumor had an inadvertent esophagotomy. Two ventilator-dependent children developed a tension pneumothorax after lung resection and required chest tubes.

Laparoscopy was performed on 574 children with conversion to laparotomy occurring in 15 children (2.6%) for technical reasons (10) and intraoperative complications (5). The complication rate of laparoscopy was 2% (12 of 574). Several technical errors occurred early in our experience, including hemorrhage during appendectomy (2), cholecystectomy (1), and splenectomy (1); malpositioned Nissen fundoplication (1); esophagotomy during a fundoplication (1); and gastric volvulus after gastrostomy and Nissen because of improper gastrostomy tube position (1). Two children developed a hernia at the umbilical trocar site that had been used for contralateral inguinal exploration, and three children developed cellulitis when a gastrostomy tube was brought out through a trocar site. Other complications not specific to minimal access surgery included pelvic abscess after appendectomy (5); small bowel obstruction after jejunostomy catheter placement (1) and combined cholecystectomy and appendectomy (1); enterocolitis (1) and severe hyponatremia (1) after pull-through for Hirschsprung's disease; and pneumonia after splenectomy (1).

The overall complication rate was 4% (25 of 626), and there were no deaths. Based on this experience, we found that the initial use of endoscopic surgery was associated with technical errors that decreased with experience. We recommend routine placement of a thoracostomy tube in children after thoracoscopy if they require postoperative ventilator support; using the open hernia sac to place a 70-degree telescope for contralateral inguinal exploration; and not using a trocar site for gastrostomy tube placement. With experience, endoscopic surgery can be safely used in children for a wide variety of diseases with minimal morbidity and mortality.

Conclusions

The surgeon must be cognizant of the extensive applications of endoscopic surgery in the pediatric patient. The ability to provide surgical care in association with outpatient or short-stay appears to be cost effective and appropriate state of the art medical care. As the array of surgical instruments continues to evolve, new and innovative endoscopic procedures will become increasingly available.

Suggested Reading

Alexander J, Hull M. Abdominal pain after laparoscopy: the value of a gas drain. *Br J Obstet Gynaecol* 1987;94:267.

Altman AJ, Schwartz AD. *Diagnosis of cancer in childhood*, 2nd ed. Philadelphia: WB Saunders, 1983.

Barth RA, Jeggrey RB, Moss AA, et al. A comparison study of computed tomography and laparoscopy in the staging of abdominal neoplasms. *Dig Dis Sci* 1981;26:253–256.

Bloom D, Ayers J, McGuire E. The role of laparoscopy in the management of nonpalpable testes. *J Urol (Paris)* 1988;94:465–470.

Brock JW, Holcomb GW, Morgan WM. The use of laparoscopy in the management of the nonpalpable testis. *J Laparoendosc Surg* 1996;6:35–39.

Bufo A, Chen M, Lobe T, et al. Laparoscopic fundoplication in children: a superior technique! *J Pediatr Surg* 1996;1:71–76.

Castilho L, Ferreira U. Laparoscopy in adults and children with nonpalpable testes. *Andrologia* 1987;29:539–543.

Chen M, Schropp K, Lobe T. Complications of minimal access surgery (MAS) in children. *J Pediatr Surg* 1996;6:233–237.

Davidoff A, Branum G, Murray E, et al. The technique of laparoscopic cholecystectomy in children. *Ann Surg* 1992;215:186–191.

Diamond DA, Caldamone AA. The value of laparoscopy for 106 impalpable testes relative to clinical presentation. *J Urol* 1992;148:632–634.

Fuenfer M, Pitts R, Georgeson K. Laparoscopic exploration of the contralateral groin in children: an improved technique. *J Laparoendosc Surg* 1996;6:1–4.

Gans S, Berci G. Advances in endoscopy of infants and children. *J Pediatr Surg* 1971;6:199–233.

Gans SL. A new look at pediatric endoscopy. *Postgrad Med* 1977;61:91–100.

Garibyan H. Use of laparoscopy for the localization of impalpable testes. *Neth J Surg* 1987;39:68–71.

Grossman P, Wolf S, Hopkins J, et al. The efficacy of laparoscopic examination of the internal inguinal ring in children. *J Pediatr Surg* 1995;30:214–217; discussion, 217–218.

Guar D, Agarwal D, Purohit K, et al. Laparoscopic orchiopexy for the intra-abdominal testis. *J Urol* 1995;153:479–481.

Heiss KF, Shandling B. Laparoscopy for the impalpable testes: experience with 53 testes. *J Pediatr Surg* 1992;27:175–178.

Hicks B, Thompson W, Rogers Z, et al. Laparoscopic splenectomy in childhood hematologic disorders. *J Laparoendosc Surg* 1996;6:31–34.

Holcomb GR, Sharp K, Neblett WR, et al. Laparoscopic cholecystectomy in infants and children: modifications and cost analysis. *J Pediatr Surg* 1994;29:900–904.

Holcomb GR, Brock JR, Morgan WR. Laparoscopic evaluation for a contralateral patent processus vaginalis. *J Pediatr Surg* 1994;29:970–973; discussion, 974.

Huang E, Kelly RJ, Fonkalstrud E, et al. Effects of simulated Fowler-Stephens orchiopexy on testicular structure and function in rats. *Am Surg* 1992;58:153–157.

Janu P, Roger D, Lobe T. A comparison of laparoscopic and traditional open splenectomy in childhood. *J Pediatr Surg* 1996;31:109–114.

Jordan G, Winslow B. Laparoscopic single stage and staged orchiopexy. *J Urol* 1994;152:1249–1252.

Lobe TE. The applications of laparoscopy and lasers in pediatric surgery. *Surg Annu* 1993;1:175–191.

Lobe TE, Blucher D, Rao BN, et al. Evaluation of the role of minimal access surgery for childhood cancer: preliminary experience of the pediatric oncology group. Submitted.

Longis B, Grousseau D, Alain J, et al. Laparoscopic fundoplication in children: our first 30 cases. *J Laparoendosc Surg* 1996;6:21–29.

Moir C, Donohue J, van Heerden J. Laparoscopic cholecystectomy in children: initial experience and recommendations. *J Pediatr Surg* 1992;27:1066.

Newman KD, Marmon LM, Attorri R, Evans S. Laparoscopic cholecystectomy in pediatric patients. *J Pediatr Surg* 1991;26:1184–1185.

Plotzker ED, Rushton HG, Belman AB, Skoog SJ. Laparoscopy for nonpalpable testes in childhood: is inguinal exploration also necessary when vas and vessels exit the inguinal ring? *J Urol* 1992;148:635–638.

Rhodes M, Rudd M, O'Rourke N, et al. Laparoscopic splenectomy and lymph node sampling for hematologic disorders. *Ann Surg* 1995;222:43–46.

Rodgers BM, Moazam F, Talbert JL. Thoracoscopy in children. *Ann Surg* 1978;189:176.

Rodgers BM, Talbert JL. Thoracoscopy for diagnosis of intrathoracic lesions in children. *J Pediatr Surg* 1976;11:703.

Rodgers BM, Ryckman FC, Moazam F, et al. Thoracoscopy for intrathoracic tumors. *Ann Thorac Surg* 1981;31:414.

Rothenberg S. Laparoscopic splenectomy using the harmonic scalpel. *J Laparoendosc Surg* 1996;6: 61–63.

Saenz NC, Schnitzer JJ, Eraklis AE, et al. Posterior mediastinal masses. *J Pediatr Surg* 1993;28: 172–176.

Schropp KP, Lobe TE. Tissue extraction. In: Lobe TE, Schropp KP, eds. *Pediatric laparoscopy and thoracoscopy.* Philadelphia: WB Saunders, 1994:52.

Thompson W, Hicks B, Guzzetta JP. Laparo-scopic Nissen fundoplication in the infant. *J Laparoendosc Surg* 1996;6:5–7.

Thompson EI. Hodgkin's disease. In: Gernbach PJ, Vietti TJ, eds. *Clinical pediatric oncology,* 4th ed. St. Louis: Mosby–Year Book, 1991:355.

Varlet F, Tardieu D, Limonne B, et al. Laparoscopic versus open appendectomy in children—comparative study of 403 cases. *Eur Pediatr Surg* 1994;4: 333–337.

Ware RE, Kinney TR, Casey JR, Pappas TN, Meyers WC. Laparoscopic cholecystectomy in young patients with sickle hemoglobinopathies. *J Pediatr* 1992;120:58–61.

58

Minimally Invasive Plastic Surgery

Robert D. Rehnke and Eric R. Van Buskirk

The inclusion of this chapter in a text on surgical technique aimed at general surgeons may at first seem odd. However, it represents a process that has come full circle. Minimally invasive plastic surgery, or endoscopic plastic surgery, has evolved from the knowledge and experience gained in minimally invasive general surgery. In fact, many of the young plastic surgeons involved in the spread of endoscopy to plastic surgery were general surgery residents during the late 1980s and took their enthusiasm for this technology to their new specialty. The growth of endoscopic plastic surgery brought with it many new challenges. For example, the development of an endoscopic optical cavity, provided so naturally by the peritoneal cavity in laparoscopy, is a major obstacle for subcutaneous endoscopy. Once the cavity has been created, it must be maintained. In some instances, as in laparoscopy, this is done with gas insufflation, but in the majority of cases, subcutaneous endoscopy is performed with hand-held retractors.

This chapter presents the major endoscopic plastic surgery procedures, which will serve as practical examples of the differences between laparoscopy and subcutaneous endoscopy. We hope this will be important and useful information to general surgeons interested in expanding minimally invasive general surgery beyond the confines of the peritoneal cavity.

One of the first articles in the plastic surgery literature was by Teimourian and Kroll in 1984, who described subcutaneous endoscopy in suction lipectomy. They applied endoscopic technology to visualize the subdermal vasculature but did not incorporate it into their operative procedure. Nicanor Isse and Luis Vasconez presented

pioneering work in endoscopic plastic surgery in 1992. Foad Nahai, John Bostwick, Felmont Eaves, and others have also contributed greatly to the development of endoscopic applications in aesthetic and reconstructive plastic surgery. Jules Verne's statement, "What one man can conceive, another man can achieve," exemplifies the building and development from previous accomplishments that carries on to this day in endoscopic surgery.

Endoscopic Cavities

The creation of subcutaneous cavities to allow endoscopic views of internal anatomy and space in which to operate instruments is the fundamental first step in soft tissue endoscopy. Space must exist to allow illumination of a surgical horizon, which gives the surgeon an anatomic reference point. Once the pertinent anatomy has been identified, there must be sufficient room to insert instruments to perform the surgical procedure. Once established, the space must be maintained with hand-held retractors or gas insufflation. Procedures are often performed through one or two incisions in an effort to optimize the aesthetic impact. These aesthetic concerns place a premium on space in accessing the endoscopic cavity and support the selection of scopes, retractors, and instruments that are low-profile and multifunctional. Many minimally invasive plastic surgery procedures are accomplished in relatively small spaces as compared to the thoracic and peritoneal cavities. These smaller spaces require performing the procedure with scopes and instrumentation smaller than the standard 5- and 10-mm equipment.

Once the endoscopic cavity has been created, the surgeon must identify the anatomic boundaries of the proposed dissection. A proper perspective is maintained by combining the internal endoscopic view with the external view of the scope in relation to external anatomic landmarks. When possible, a second external-view camera can be used and shown on a monitor adjacent to the endoscopic monitor. This helps the surgeon synthesize a combined internal and external picture of the surgical field—in the same fashion that an automobile driver combines the view ahead with information from the rearview mirror. This total endoscopic picture is facilitated by periodic zooming in and out with the endoscope to place an up-close and magnified view of the operative site in perspective with the total endoscopic cavity. This endoscopic strategy helps in converting from the familiar open anatomy to the new endoscopic perspective.

Endoscopic Instruments and Fascial Cleft Balloon Dissection

All surgeons are familiar with the importance of being in the "right plane" while performing an open dissection. This is even more important in subcutaneous endoscopy. Straying from the proper plane leads to bleeding that stains the tissues and makes it difficult to identify endoscopic anatomic landmarks. The right plane is what anatomists refer to as a fascial cleft. These clefts are avascular planes between two parallel sheets of fascia that are traversed at regular anatomic locations by neurovascular perforators. Fascial clefts are potential spaces that exist throughout the body between opposing layers of fascia. These clefts can be turned into true endoscopic spaces with blunt dissection (Fig. 58-1). Balloon dissectors have proven to be the ideal instrument for performing fascial cleft dissections of endoscopic cavities. The dissectors consist of deflated balloons of varying sizes and configurations that are rolled up tightly into introducers. The device can be bluntly inserted into a fascial cleft once one has been identified through open dissection of the endoscopic port site. Once in place, the balloon is inflated with saline to perform a blunt dissection and expand the fascial cleft into an endoscopic cavity (Fig. 58-2). Unlike other methods of blunt dissection, balloon dissectors have large blunt surfaces that do not stray from the right plane of dissection. In addition, because the balloon expands in the plane of least resistance, it respects the integrity of neurovascular perforators, and anatomic lines of fascial fusion are preserved. Inadvertent destruction of anatomic landmarks during the rapid creation of an endoscopic cavity is rare, and bleeding is minimized. Finally, balloon dissection is accomplished with great speed and ease, compared to other means of endoscopic soft tissue dissection.

Once the subcutaneous endoscopic cavity is created, specialized retractors and instruments are required to perform the desired procedure. Depending on the procedure and size of the endoscopic cavity, telescopes can range in size from 4 to 10 mm and from 0 to 30 degrees. Most subcutaneous endoscopy is gasless and makes use of hand-held retractors to which the telescope is mounted. Since the scope, retractor, and dissecting instruments often all go through the same small port, space is limited. In addition, these ports are frequently in the axillary, suprapubic, or similarly confined regions. For this reason, specialized telescopes that make a 90-degree bend or that have the eyepiece and camera coupler moved out of the plane of the port are extremely useful (Fig. 58-3). This allows increased room at the port site for manipulation of instruments. Once again, for similar reasons, graspers and scissors with in-line handles, as opposed to the pistol-grip variety used in laparoscopy, optimize instrument maneuvering without interference. Whenever possible, instruments that combine functions (i.e., suction, irrigation, cautery) increase the ease and speed of the procedure (Fig. 58-4). This limits the amount of sword-fighting between instruments and prevents wasting time for insertion and removal.

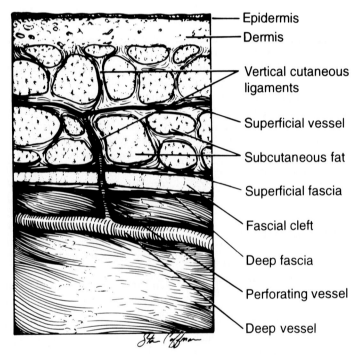

Fig. 58-1. Typical subcutaneous cross-section illustrating a superficial fascial cleft.

Epidermis
Dermis
Vertical cutaneous ligaments
Superficial vessel
Subcutaneous fat
Superficial fascia
Fascial cleft
Deep fascia
Perforating vessel
Deep vessel

Expansion of fascial cleft with balloon dissector

Insertion of endoscope in optical cavity

A   B

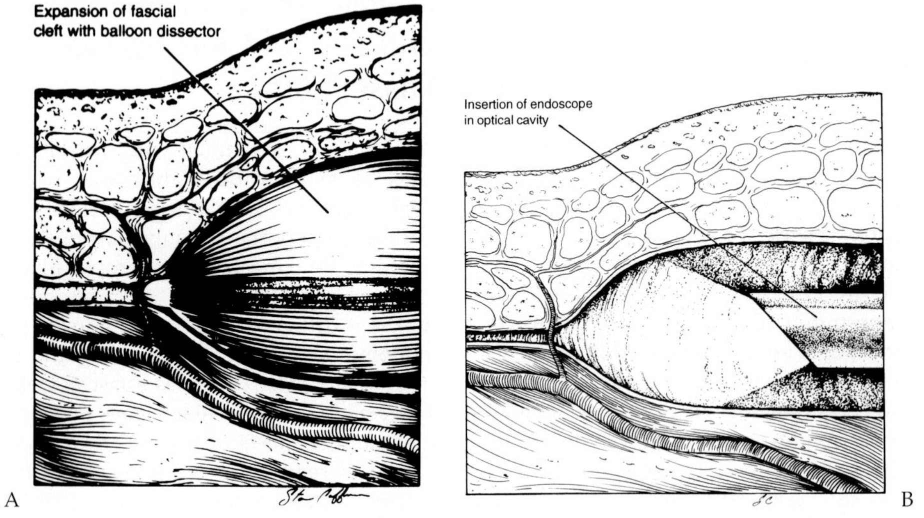

Fig. 58-2. Balloon dissector expanding a superficial fascial cleft (A) into an endoscopic cavity (B).

Endoscopic Facial Rejuvenation

The most common endoscopic procedure performed by plastic surgeons is the endoscopic browlift. The relative ease of developing the endoscopic cavity in this procedure accounts for its being the initial subcutaneous endoscopic procedure. As in many areas of minimally invasive surgery, the primary steps are the same as for the open procedure; the difference lies in the size of the incision. Endoscopic facial rejuvenation is built on the principles of the subperiosteal approach to facelifting. The endoscope removes the need for a long bicoronal incision and replaces it with a few 1.5-cm-long ports. Through these endoscopic ports, the frontal bone, orbital rims, zygomatic arch, and malar eminence

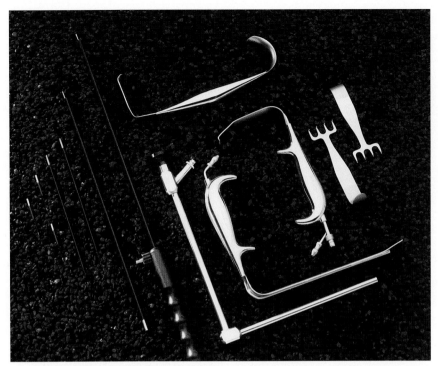

Fig. 58-3. Tebbetts Endoplastic Instrument System (Snowden Pencer, Tucker, Georgia).

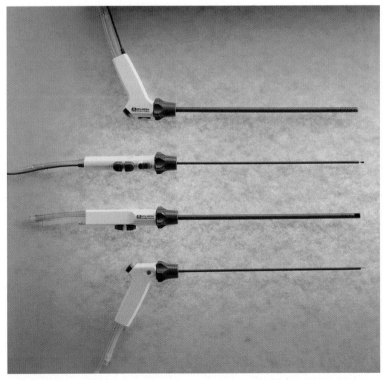

Fig. 58-4. Combined suction, irrigation, and cautery instruments (Probe Plus II, Ethicon Endosurgery, Cincinnati, Ohio).

are exposed in the process of mobilizing the overlying soft tissues of the face prior to their elevation and suspension to the facial skeleton. In properly selected patients, skin excision, with its attendant long scars, is completely avoided (Fig. 58-5).

Anatomic Considerations

The pertinent anatomy for brow- and facelifting is as hotly contested and the techniques are as diversified as those of hernia repair in general surgery. A summary of key points follows.

The soft tissues of the face are held in place through anchorage to the facial skeleton. This is accomplished directly via the muscles of facial expression originating from the periosteum, and indirectly through sheets of connective tissue or fascia that are strategically fixed to the skull. The face is arranged in concentric layers of skin, subcutaneous fat, muscle, and periosteum. The middle lamina, composed of muscle and fat, is sandwiched by a two-ply layer of superficial fascia called the SMAS. This system is connected to the skin by vertical cutaneous retaining ligaments, or retinacula cutis. Below the SMAS layer is the deep fascia and deep structures such as the parotid gland, the muscles of mastication, and the facial nerves. As aging occurs, the middle lamina is pulled downward by gravity, resulting in soft tissue ptosis and the recognizable stigmata of aging (Fig. 58-6). The goal of endoscopic facial rejuvenation is mobilization of the middle lamina of soft tissue from the underlying bone and deep fascia so that it can be resuspended to its youthful relationship to the skull.

Endoscopic Brow-, Face-, and Necklift

Endoscopic cavities are so easily developed in the subgaleal or subperiosteal plane that balloon dissectors are not necessary. The key tools for this procedure are curved periosteal elevators. They are inserted through 1.5-cm incisions (behind the hairline) in sagittal planes just medial to the pupil and above the tail of the brow in the temporal scalp (Fig. 58-7). Blunt periosteal elevators are inserted into the subgaleal cleft, which is easily identified by pulling up on the scalp incision with skin hooks. This separates the galea from the periosteum, which is densely adherent to the skull. Wispy strands of connective tissue between the periosteum and galea are

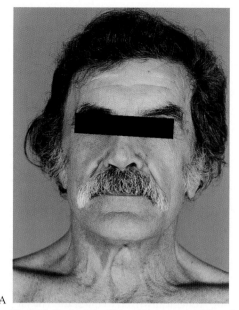
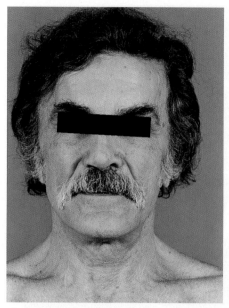

A

B

Fig. 58-5. Preoperative **(A)** and postoperative **(B)** *patient photographs after endoscopic brow-, face-, and necklift in which skin excision was completely avoided.*

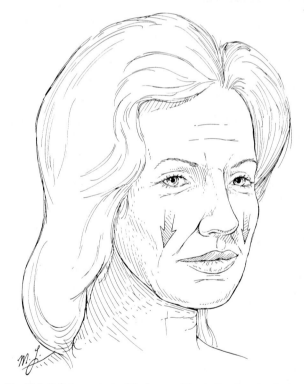

Fig. 58-6. *Soft tissue ptosis of the face resulting in the stigmata of aging.*

rovascular bundle comes into view, running in the sagittal plane directly in front of the medial ports. This blunt dissection is carried to the supraorbital rim but not beyond, thus preventing injury to the supraorbital nerve or disruption of the ocular septum (a periorbital fusion between the SMAS and the periosteum of the orbital rim). The origins of the procerus and corrugator muscles can be avulsed with graspers to weaken them and thus smooth glabellar rhytids.

With the frontal pocket dissection performed, attention is turned to the temporal dissection. Once again, an initial blind dissection is performed with a curved periosteal elevator to establish an endoscopic cavity. As the endoscope is inserted through the temporal port, an elevator is inserted through the same port for blunt dissection of the fascial cleft below the temporoparietal fascia. Medially, it becomes apparent that a barrier exists between the temporal and frontal pockets—the line of fusion between the SMAS and the supratemporal ridge. It is divided bluntly with an elevator or sharply with curved endoscopic scissors held flush against the skull.

Once the temporal and frontal pockets have been connected, the temporal dissection is extended downward toward the zygomatic arch under direct endoscopic vision. Injury to the frontal branch of the facial nerve is avoided in two ways. First, as one advances along the supratemporal line, the plane of dissection goes below the periosteum. This deeper plane of dissection begins at the point where the supratemporal ridge becomes the zygomatic process of the frontal bone. This is easily accomplished by a scraping maneuver on the ridge with a sharp, curved elevator. Further dissection along the lateral orbital rim and the frontal process of the zygomatic bone continues in the subperiosteal plane. Second, if the zygomatic arch is to be exposed, as in endoscopic facelift, the subperiosteal dissection is carried laterally below the innominate fascia down to the zygomatic arch. This deeper plane of dissection in the temporal pocket begins at a level two fingerbreadths above the arch. If only an endoscopic browlift is planned, the subperiosteal dissection is taken to the midportion of the lateral orbital rim, and the dissection below the innominate fascia is unnecessary.

separated blindly with a blunt periosteal elevator along a 3- to 4-cm strip anterior to the incisions. A 4-mm, 30-degree endoscope with an attached retractor is then inserted through one of the medial ports, while a periosteal elevator, inserted through the other, is used to advance the plane of dissection toward the supraorbital rim under direct endoscopic visualization. This frontal cavity is developed by advancing the elevator a short distance at a time with a lifting motion that separates the galea from the periosteum. As one nears the orbital rim, the supraorbital neu-

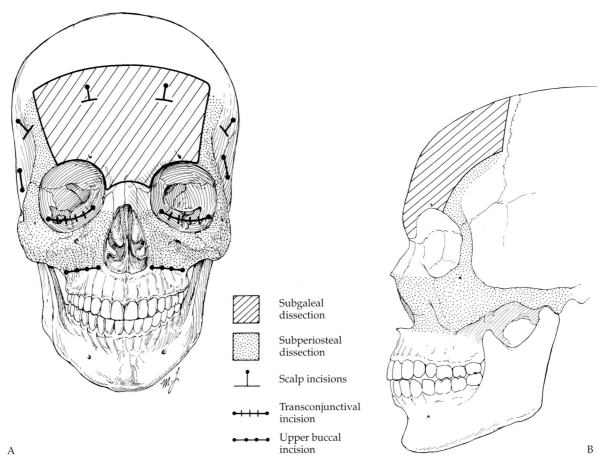

Fig. 58-7. Ports **(A)** and dissection **(B)** for endoscopic facelift.

Subgaleal
dissection

Subperiosteal
dissection

Scalp incisions

Transconjunctival
incision

Upper buccal
incision

A

B

If an endoscopic browlift alone is planned, then the next step is suspension and fixation of the mobilized brow. There are many techniques available to accomplish this, such as screw fixation, suture suspension through cortical tunnels, and external bolster or taping. We prefer another approach—T-to-V closure of the endoscopic ports (see Fig. 58-7)—for two reasons. First, the T incision gives a larger port that is easier to work through. Second, the tension created with closure not only suspends the brow but places a shearing force on the outer lamella of skin and subcutaneous fat. This acts directly on the components of the ptotic brow, allowing the inner lamella of frontalis muscle to relax and therefore smooth horizontal brow rhytids.

The subgaleal approach with T-to-V closure is preferred over the subperiosteal plane of dissection with screw fixation, since it more closely approaches the standard bicoronal browlift. Subperiosteal brow dissection requires releasing incisions of the periosteum at the supraorbital rim to allow elevation of the periosteal flap. This can result in destruction of the ocular septum and elevation of the brow above its natural upper limit of excursion. As a result, the upper eyelid or palpebral skin is stretched rather than the brow skin, resulting in a thin covering of the supraorbital rim. This overelevation of the brow, with attendant startled appearance, has been a problem with early attempts at endoscopic browlift. This was not a problem with the traditional bicoronal approach that maintains the connections of upper lid skin to supraorbital periosteum and relies on tension generated by scalp closure to elevate the brow.

Endoscopic facelifting employs the addition of exposure of the zygoma and zygomatic arch to an endoscopic browlift. Thus, an additional incision is added above the ear in the coronal plane. As previously mentioned, the temporal dissection then proceeds with blunt dissection below the innominate fascia and through the superficial temporal fat pad toward the zygomatic arch. This is performed with curved periosteal elevators after incising the innominate fascia with a scalpel inserted through the supraauricular incision. Once the arch is reached, a sharp periosteal elevator is used to expose the zygoma and arch subperiosteally. This dissection is then joined with the lateral orbital rim dissection already performed as part of the browlift. A large, blunt periosteal dissector is then used to release the periosteum from the inferior aspect of the zygomatic arch. This is a key step in mobilizing the overlying SMAS lamina and thus allowing suspension of the cheeks. Mobilization of a midface subperiosteal flap is then accomplished with an open technique through intraoral and transconjunctival incisions and is joined with the temporal and zygomatic arch dissection above. Once again, release of the periosteum along the inferior border of the maxilla and zygoma is key to upward mobility of the flap. Suspension sutures are then placed through the periosteum and anchored to drill holes in the orbital rim and to deep temporal fascia.

The SMAS forms one continuous layer of mimetic muscle and subcutaneous fat throughout the cheeks and cervical region. Therefore, the above suspension performs an adequate neck lift in patients with minimal platysmal banding and cervical soft tissue excess. However, in patients with additional soft tissue redundancy, an endoscopic necklift can be performed. This is accomplished through a 4- to 5-cm incision behind the ear at the inferior hair line. An open dissection is performed toward the sternocleidomastoid muscle in the subcutaneous plane. Just after the posterior border of the sternocleidomastoid is passed, the endoscope is inserted and the dissection proceeds under endoscopic visualization. At about this time, the greater auricular nerve and external jugular vein are encountered, running in parallel fashion toward the angle of the mandible. They are accompanied by the posterior border of the platysma, which lays just superficial to them. The dissection proceeds below these three structures in the fascial cleft below the platysma. Blunt dissection in this plane continues medially to the midline. Through a submental incision, a standard corset plastysmaplasty is performed. Finally, the platysma–myocutaneous flap is pulled up against the deep cervical structures with suspension sutures from the posterior border of the platysma to the mastoid fascia. If there is a small amount of redundant skin, an ellipse is excised from the postauricular port, which is then closed.

Endoscopic Breast Augmentation

Minimally invasive breast augmentation employs endoscopic technology along with saline breast implants to perform surgery through 2- to 3-cm-long incisions. The minimally invasive approach, however, employs not only small incisions but also incisions placed in ideal locations. The transaxillary approach meets these criteria and, with the aid of endoscopic technology, has the same high level of precision and low level of complications as open techniques.

Anatomic Considerations

The breast is a specialized glandular organ of the skin located over the chest between split layers of superficial fascia. It derives its shape from the overlying skin brassiere and its attachments to the chest wall by the circummammary ligament. This "ligament" is a zone of fusion between the two layers of superficial fascia and the underlying deep fascia of the chest wall (Fig. 58-8). The location of this attachment can be demonstrated by the limits of excursion of the breast on the chest. This is most obvious inferiorly, where gravity pulls the breast downward over the inframammary fold. Roughly, the breast lies over the pectoralis major superiorly and medially. Inferiorly, it covers the rectus abdominis medially and the external oblique and serratus anterior laterally. The circummammary ligament attaches to the deep fascia just lateral to the midline of the sternum, in the sixth intercostal interspace inferiorly, at the anterior axillary line laterally, and just bellow the clavicle superiorly. Within the boundaries of this ligament, a fascial cleft exists between the superficial and deep fascia, known as the retromammary space. The named neurovascular supply, such as the lateral intercostal, internal mammary, thoracoacromial, and lateral thoracic, enters the breast peripherally, making the retromammary space relatively avascular and an ideal location for placement of a breast implant. In thin patients with little breast tissue, saline implants are too noticeable in the retromammary space and are therefore placed behind the pectoralis major muscle.

Operative Technique

The patient is placed in the supine position with arms secured to arm boards at 90 degrees, allowing the patient to be sat up during the procedure. A 3-cm incision is marked in a wrinkle line in the high axilla and should not extend beyond the hairbearing skin. A subcutaneous dissection is

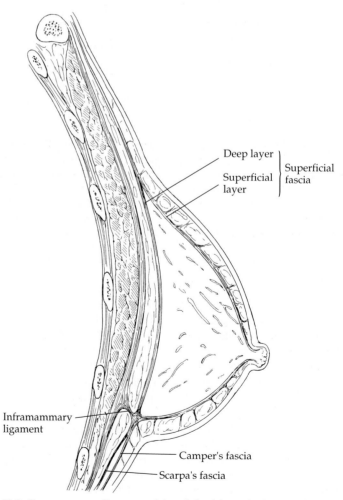

Fig. 58-8. Circummammary ligament and the subglandular and subpectoral fascial clefts.

performed toward the lateral boarder of the pectoralis major, which is identified through open dissection. At this point, a balloon dissector is placed in the fascial cleft above or below the pectoralis major, depending on the desired location for the implant (see Fig. 58-8). In subglandular augmentation, the superficial fascial cleft is identified by a spreading motion with scissors on top of the muscle. This separates the superficial fascia from the deep fascia covering the muscle in a blunt fashion. The balloon dissector is then inserted into this space and pushed across the chest toward the inferomedial aspect of the breast. The balloon is then inflated with saline until the boundaries of the circummammary ligament are demonstrated. On removal of the balloon, the endoscope is inserted into the newly developed endoscopic cavity. A 10-mm, 0- or 30-degree scope is used because more illumination is required for such a large endoscopic cav-

ity. The scope is usually mounted to a hand-held retractor to maintain the space. Given the spatial constraints of working through the axilla, a system whose telescope turns 90 degrees upward and places the camera coupler above the plane of dissection is ideal (see Fig. 58-3).

Since the circummammary ligament is a zone of decussating fascial fibers between the superficial and deep fascia, and not a narrow discrete band, cautery is used to refine the dimensions of the implant pocket created by the balloon dissector. The degree to which this is required depends in large part on the preoperative configuration of the breast and the dimensions to which it will be augmented. Care is taken medially to slowly divide tissue with the cautery on a blend setting as the internal mammary perforators are encountered. Laterally, one must be mindful to avoid injury to the fourth intercostal

nerve, which is the main sensory supply to the nipple. Once the dimensions of the pocket have been established, the scope is removed and the balloon reinserted. It is then inflated with saline to a volume 2 to 2.5 times the volume of the desired implant for a period of 15 minutes. This acts as a form of immediate tissue expansion and relaxes the overlying skin envelope.

Finally, the balloon is sequentially deflated with the patient in the upright position to estimate the optimal size of the final implants. In addition, the pocket dissection is evaluated at this point, and any further modifications of the dissection are made prior to insertion of the implants. The balloons are then removed, and the deflated saline implants are rolled tightly and inserted into the pocket and inflated to their desired volume. It is important to push the rolled implant to the bottom of the pocket prior to inflation, as adjustment

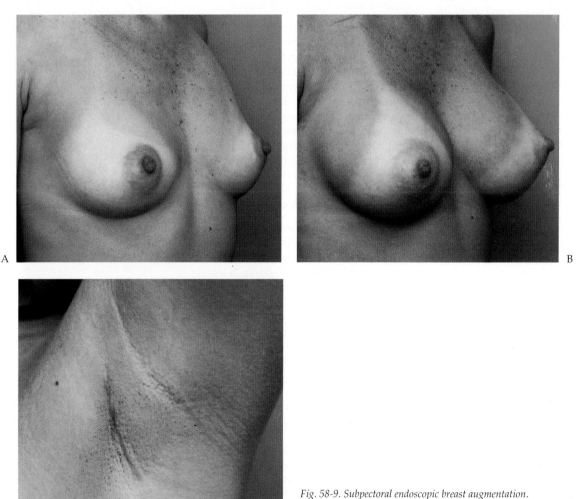

A

B

C

Fig. 58-9. Subpectoral endoscopic breast augmentation.
A: *Preoperative appearance.* **B:** *Postoperative appearance.*
C: *Axillary incision.*

of the implant position is more difficult than in an open approach. The axillary incision is then closed in layers; a drain is infrequently required.

Subpectoral implantation uses the same basic steps below the pectoralis major as those used in the deep fascial cleft. This space is identified once the lateral boarder of the pectoralis is seen through the initial open dissection. The pectoralis major muscle is retracted upward, and scissors are spread just below to bluntly pop through the deep fascia and into the retropectoral space. The surgeon's finger is then inserted, and the smooth surface of the pectoralis major is felt above. Below, the pectoralis minor can be felt superiorly and laterally. Inferiorly and medially, the ribs and intercostal muscles can be felt. Once this proper plane has been identified through palpation, the balloon dissector is inserted and pushed bluntly across the chest wall. This is done with a gentle back-and-forth sweeping motion and slight upward traction. The balloon is inflated to 400 to 500 mL and will dissect to the limits of the pectoralis origins from the clavicle, sternum, and ribs. Once the endoscopic cavity has been dissected, the balloon is removed and the endoscope inserted. Next, the origins of the pectoralis major are released with electrocautery from the lower one-third of the sternum and from the fifth and sixth ribs. This release is performed through the muscle, as well as the overlying deep fascia. It is done approximately 4 mm from the sternum to prevent retraction of mammary perforators as they are divided. It is important to divide the deep fascia lateral to the pectoralis major, where it lies over the serratus anterior and pectoralis minor muscles. This is done by retracting the pectoralis major upward and scoring the deep fascia lateral to it with cautery. Care should be taken not to dissect under the serratus or pectoralis minor. Once the release of the pectoralis major is complete, the endoscope is removed and the balloon dissector inserted once again. It is then inflated to a volume approximately twice that of the final implant volume. This breaks the subpectoral pocket into the retromammary fascial cleft inferior and lateral to the pectoralis major. It completes the blunt dissection to the boundaries of the circummammary ligament. It also performs an immediate tissue expansion of the overlying soft tissue envelope. The remaining steps are completed as in subglandular augmentation (Fig. 58-9).

Endoscopic Latissimus Dorsi Muscle Harvest

The latissimus dorsi muscle is a workhorse flap for reconstruction, including pedicle and microvascular free tissue transfer. Back, proximal upper extremity, breast, thorax, head, and neck anatomic regions are all amenable to latissimus pedicle reconstruction. More distant anatomic sites can be reconstructed using latissimus muscle as a microvascular free tissue transfer (e.g., distal upper extremity and lower extremity). The latissimus muscle flap may be harvested with a skin island (myocutaneous flap); however this obviates a minimally invasive approach due to large skin incisions. Endoscopic technique is therefore reserved for a muscle-only harvest. This muscle has traditionally been harvested through a relatively large back and posterior axillary incision, typically ranging from 20 to 30 cm in length.

Using an endoscopic technique, the latissimus muscle can be harvested through a 6- to 7-cm total incision length. This minimally invasive approach offers several potential advantages over traditional harvesting techniques. Better magnified visualization of the donor site can result in less postoperative hematoma or seroma formation. Shorter incision lengths can result in improved wound healing, less infection, and less unsightly scarring.

Anatomic Considerations

The latissimus dorsi muscle is a large fan-shaped muscle originating from the lower thoracic (T6-12) and lumbar vertebrae, iliac crest, and lumbosacral fascia. It inserts on the proximal humerus and forms the posterior axillary fold. This muscle serves in adduction of the arm. It is a type V muscle with a constant major pedicle (the thoracodorsal artery, vein, and nerve) and several minor segmental vessels. The artery is a branch of the subscapular artery, which originates from the axillary artery, and usually enters the posterior aspect of the latissimus approximately 10 cm distal to the muscle's insertion on the humerus. The latissimus dorsi muscle is also supplied by a relatively constant group of segmental intercostal perforators (usually the ninth to eleventh) entering the muscle approximately 5 cm from the midline in the lower paraspinous region (Fig. 58-10).

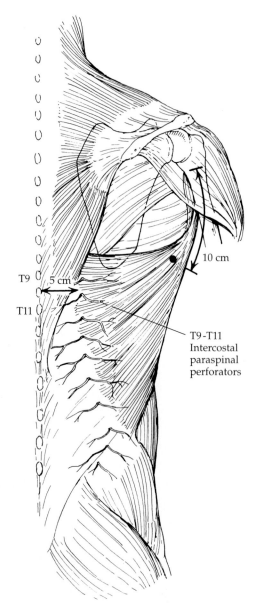

Fig. 58-10. Latissimus dorsi muscle anatomy.

The latissimus has a potential fascial cleft above and below (epimuscular and submuscular). These planes are amenable to balloon dissection for development of endoscopic cavities (Fig. 58-11). The epimuscular fascial cleft is more tenacious than the submuscular cleft but dissects with balloon technique, except for an occasional fibrous band. These bands are easily divided under endoscopic visualization, and their release allows complete balloon dissection. Several port sites may be used for balloon dissector placement. Usually, however, the posterior axillary or auscultatory triangle sites are used.

Operative Technique

The patient is positioned in the lateral decubitus position, with all pressure points adequately cushioned and protected. The patient's arm (donor side) should be prepared into the field with approximately 90-degree extension at the shoulder. The anatomic landmarks are palpated, identified, and marked with a sterile marking pen. These include the anatomic borders of the latissimus muscle, inferior tip of the scapula, posterior border of the axilla, midline of the back, posterior iliac crest, and auscultatory triangle. Utilizing trian-gulation technique, three incisions or port sites are used: (1) a 4- to 5-cm posterior in-fraaxillary incision, (2) a 1.5-cm transverse auscultatory triangle incision, and (3) a 1-cm, low-anterior lateral incision (Fig. 58-12). The posterior infraaxillary incision is made first, and through this incision the lateral border of the latissimus muscle and the thoracodorsal pedicle are identified and dissected. The thoracodorsal pedicle enters the latissimus muscle approximately 10 cm distal to its insertion onto the humerus. It is critical to ascertain this pedicle-entry position prior to placing balloon dissectors in the submuscular fascial cleft.

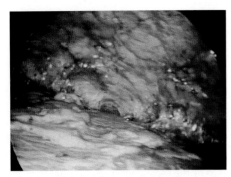

Fig. 58-11. Epimuscular endoscopic cavity (superficial fascial cleft) with subcutaneous fat above and latissimus dorsi muscle below, created by balloon dissector.

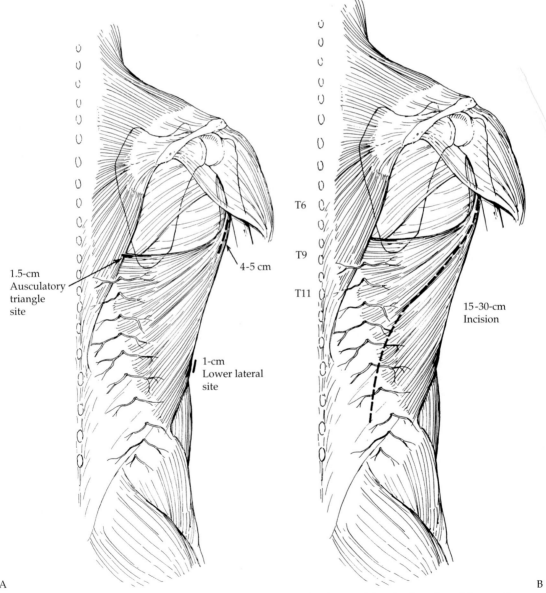

Fig. 58-12. Surgical setup for endoscopic harvest of the latissimus dorsi muscle. **A:** Incision sites for endoscopic harvest. **B:** Incision for traditional open harvest.

If the incision is too proximal, the pedicle is at risk for injury with balloon dissection. If the incision is too distal, the thoracodorsal pedicle dissection toward the axilla becomes increasingly difficult. A minimum 4- to 5-cm incision is required to physically harvest the large latissimus muscle. Because this incision is needed, we recommend open pedicle dissection.

After identification of the lateral border of the latissimus muscle, the epimuscular fascial cleft is identified. This is just on top of the fascia overlying the latissimus muscle. A 750-, 1000-, or 1500-mL balloon dissector is inserted in an inferomedial direction overlying the major central portion of the latissimus muscle. The protective sheath is removed and the balloon inflated with sterile saline. This quickly and atraumatically develops the epimuscular optical cavity. Occasionally, there is a fascial band that can be quickly identified under direct endoscopic visualization and released, thereby allowing complete balloon dissection. The submuscular plane under the latissimus muscle is then identified, and dissection of the thoracodorsal neurovascular pedicle is performed. The proximal dissection depends on the length required for either pedicle mobilization or free tissue anastomosis. Once the pedicle is identified, the submuscular balloon dissector can be placed distal to it, thereby avoiding injury. This balloon dissector is also placed in the inferomedial direction underneath the major central portion of the latissimus muscle. We use the 750-mL balloon dissector in the submuscular fascial cleft and avoid larger balloons that can overdissect the required area. This minimizes unnecessary perforator disruption. When properly placed and positioned, the balloon dissectors greatly speed dissection without disruption of perforating blood vessels.

A 10- to 11-mm endoscopic port is placed within the posterior infraaxillary incision and sealed with a suture. A 10-mm, 0-degree endoscopic camera is inserted, and carbon dioxide (CO_2) is insufflated. The epimuscular optical cavity is now easily visualized. Retractors may be used instead of CO_2 insufflation, but they tend to be less effective and more cumbersome and often require additional port placement. A 10- to 11-mm endoscopic cannula trocar port is inserted under direct visualization via the auscultatory port incision. A 5-mm endoscopic cannula trocar port is also inserted in the lower lateral position. A suction/irrigation catheter device is inserted through the lower border of the suture-closed infraaxillary incision (thus avoiding an additional port incision). The second 10- to 11-mm port in the auscultatory position allows changing of the camera to facilitate muscle dissection and harvest.

A grasper is placed through the lateral 5-mm port and, a pencil-hook Bovie electrocautery is placed through the auscultatory port. With the endoscopic camera in the infraaxillary port, muscle dissection can proceed. The medial edge of the latissimus is divided first. Once this is accomplished, the grasper and the Bovie change port positions. The inferior and lower lateral latissimus borders are then dissected. Finally, the endoscopic camera is repositioned in the auscultatory port, and the grasper is placed in the infraaxillary port. With the Bovie in the lower lateral port, the proximal areas of the latissimus are dissected as the muscle approaches its insertion. Division of the muscle with cautery is performed in the epimuscular optical cavity, with downward dissection until the submuscular cavity is entered. Once this circumferential dissection of the latissimus muscle is completed, the infraaxillary incision is again opened, CO_2 insufflation is stopped, and ports are removed. The muscle is then harvested via the infraaxillary incision. The pedicle can be divided if needed as a free tissue transfer, or mobilized if needed as a pedicle flap. The donor site is then irrigated with sterile saline and inspected for bleeding, and the incisions are closed after a Silastic drain is placed. This technique can be used for complete or partial latissimus muscle harvests.

In addition to the the posterior infraaxillary approach, we have utilized the auscultatory triangle as the port position for balloon dissector placement. Both work effectively if properly positioned. The auscultatory site avoids the potential for pedicle disruption in submuscular-plane balloon dissection and easily avoids the paraspinous and lower lumbar perforators. The disadvantage of this position is that more manual dissection of the optical cavities is required proximally toward the insertion of the latissimus in both epimuscular and submuscular planes. This generally adds time to the procedure and can be avoided by balloon placement via the posterior infraaxillary incision.

Endoscopy-assisted Tissue Expansion

Tissue expansion has seen continued enthusiasm and increasing application since its modern inception by Radovan in the 1970s. Despite significant contributions to reconstructive surgery, tissue expansion is not without some shortcomings. Expander extrusion and insertion-site dehiscence are two of the most common complications in tissue expansion. The need for incision access proximity to the expanded area contributes to these complications. Additionally, expansion must be delayed until the incision has healed sufficiently to accommodate the increased skin tension associated with expansion.

Endoscopic tissue expansion has allowed small, distant access incisions with improved visualization of pocket cavities. Important advantages include immediate expansion at the time of insertion without risk of extrusion and incisional dehiscence.

Anatomic Considerations

Tissue expansion may be performed over many but not all areas of the body. However, one must avoid violating basic anatomic principles (e.g., neurovascular compression, joint impingement/contracture). Fascial clefts are ideally suited for balloon dissection and tissue expansion. Commonly expanded areas utilizing fascial clefts include forehead, scalp, breast, torso, and extremities.

Operative Technique

Careful preoperative planning is essential to an effective tissue-expansion procedure. Proper pocket design, remote access-site placement, and tissue expander and balloon dissector size and shape are all important considerations.

After such planning, the areas are prepared and draped, and appropriate anesthesia is administered. A 1.5-cm incision is made, and dissection to the appropriate fascial cleft/plane is performed. Incision size is limited by port diameter, with pediatric infusion ports being able to be introduced through a 1.5-cm incision. Adult ports require a larger incision, usually 2.5 to 3 cm. The distance of the incision from the expanded area is highly variable, usually between 3 and 20 cm. After identification of the proper plane (usually the fascial cleft between superficial and deep fascia), a balloon dissector is bluntly placed and inflated with sterile saline. After deflation, the cavity is exposed with a retractor, and a 5- or 10-mm, 0- or 30-degree-angle endoscopic camera is inserted, and the dissected optical cavity is inspected (we usually use a 5-mm, 0-degree endoscope). This usually does not require any hemostatic control, but if it is needed, it can easily be performed, as well as any additional pocket dissection. If balloon dissection is not desired, manual dissection of a pocket cavity can be performed with endoscopic instruments (endoscopic scissors, electrocautery, etc.). This often takes additional time, depending on the size and location of the pocket; therefore we usually utilize a balloon dissection technique.

Attention is next directed to the infusion-port pocket. The proximity of the access incision to the port pocket allows an open dissection technique. Care must be taken to provide adequate dissection to accommodate the connection tubing without kinking. Irrigation with sterile saline is performed, and a deflated, cigar-like-rolled tissue expander is bluntly inserted. Manual manipulation is performed for proper placement. The retractor is reinserted, followed by the endoscope to ascertain proper tissue-expander and infusion-port position. Tubing can be modified with a stent and silk ties as needed. Once the tubing is properly positioned, the incision is closed in layered fashion, with care not to injure the underlying infusion port or connecting tubing. The infusion port is then accessed via a sterile needle, and immediate tissue expansion is instituted (usually between 25% and 50% of the total final volume of the tissue expander).

Tissue expansion is an important adjunct in soft tissue reconstruction. Endoscopy-assisted tissue-expander placement can be performed easily with or without balloon fascial cleft dissection technique. This technique has the potential to decrease morbidity from extrusion or wound dehiscence, as well as shortening the total time required to reach full expansion because of the ability to begin expansion at the time of operation.

Endoscopic Abdominoplasty

Many societies view a scaphoid abdomen as aesthetically pleasing. Decreased energy expenditure, a lower metabolic rate, and a sedentary lifestyle generally occur with advancing age. Western diets rich in calories and fat content contribute to obesity and fatty deposition. The anterior and lateral abdomen are prone to fat deposition in both men and women. Changes in postpartum women can include development of abdominal skin striae and elastosis and rectus abdominis muscle diastasis. The traditional approach to abdominal rejuvenation incorporates large, transverse, lower abdominal incisions for skin and pannus redraping and excision. Partly because of significant scarring, the trend has been toward less invasive techniques such as the miniabdominoplasty and liposuction. Unfortunately, large skin excess and marked fatty deposition preclude these less invasive procedures. This applies to endoscopic abdominoplasty as well. However, in selected patients with minimal skin excess, rectus abdominis muscle diastasis, and mild to moderate fat deposition, endoscopic abdominoplasty coupled with liposuction provides a minimally invasive means of achieving a very good aesthetic result.

Anatomic Considerations

The abdomen consists of skin, subcutaneous tissue, underlying musculature with investing fascia (rectus abdominis, external oblique, internal oblique, transversus abdominis), preperitoneal fat, and peritoneum. The anterior abdomen adheres to basic fascial cleft anatomic principles. All dissection in abdominal rejuvenative surgery is superficial to the anterior investing muscular fascia; it is essential to avoid violating the internal abdomen and intraperitoneal cavity. The fascial cleft just superficial to the anterior rectus sheath and external oblique fascia is amenable to balloon dissection.

Operative Technique

After appropriate preoperative evaluation and marking of the abdomen in the upright position, the patient is placed on a flexion-capable operating table in the supine position. Appropriate anesthesia is administered, including, provided that there are no contraindications, dilute lidocaine hydrochloride with epinephrine locally (0.5% lidocaine with 1:200,000 epinephrine).

A 2-cm, transverse, midline incision is made within the pubic hairline. An additional semilunar periumbilical incision and two 5-mm liposuction port sites on the lateral abdomen may be used as well. Liposuction is then performed from the various incision sites selected. Afterward, a 750-, 1000- or 1500-mL balloon dissector is placed via the suprapubic incision and inflated, creating an optical cavity within the fascial cleft overlying the anterior rectus investing fascia (Fig. 58-13). This plane with direct visualization of the rectus musculature is essential for proper diastasis correction. Additional superior dissection can be completed by manual endoscopic dissection or additional balloon dissector placement. The umbilical stalk may be transected (free floating) or left intact to its base. The optical cavity may be maintained by manual retractors or a hydraulic laparoscopic lifting device if available.

Direct endoscopic visualization, usually with a 10-mm, 0-degree endoscope, allows precise tailoring of any irregularities due to the liposuction and control of bleeding with coagulation. Parallel longitudinal plication lines are then marked symmetrically with methylene blue. The amount plicated depends on the degree of diastasis, but generally 1 to 2 cm on either side of the midline are imbricated. A heavy permanent monofilament suture such as no. 0 or no. 1 Prolene is then used to imbricate the anterior rectus in a running fashion beginning near the xiphoid and ending near the pubic symphysis, with the last suture secured as a slip knot and tied outside the abdomen. Additionally, two lateral plications may be performed, and some surgeons use a second midline plication over the first for additional strength. Some surgeons advocate the use of staples using a pull-and-staple technique for their plication. Regardless of the plication technique, a cardinal principle is to take superficial bites, not violating the peritoneum.

After irrigation with sterile saline, attention is directed to reattaching the umbilical stalk to the anterior fascia, if transected initially, usually with a 3-0 Vicryl or 4-0 PDS suture. After external symmetry is ensured, which sometimes requires additional lateral dissection for proper redraping, two Silastic drains are placed and secured, and the incisions are closed in layered fashion. The patient is maintained in the modified Fowler's position postoperatively, allowed ambulation without abdominal straightening the following day, and maintained in an abdominal binder

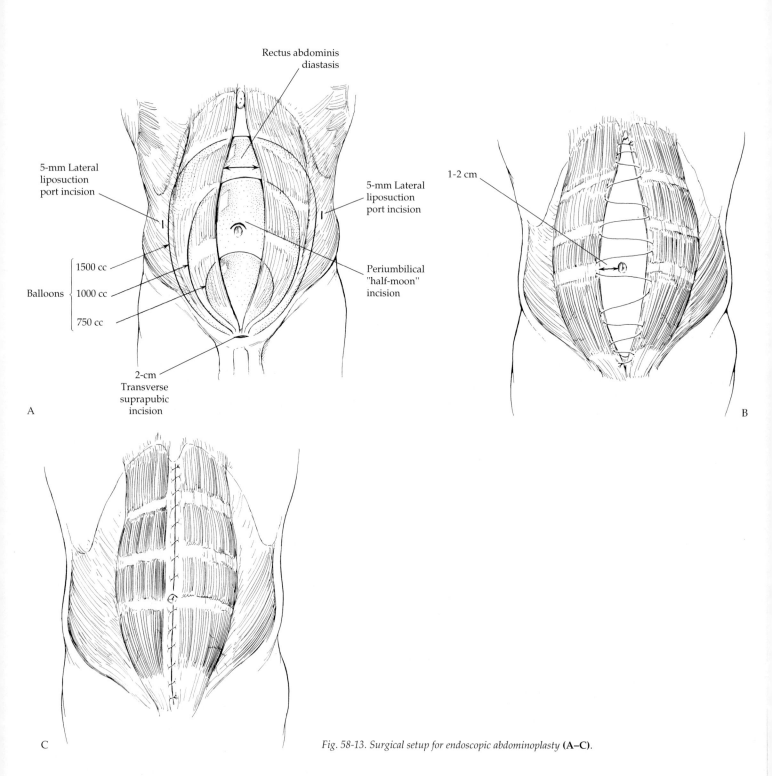

A

Rectus abdominis diastasis

5-mm Lateral liposuction port incision

5-mm Lateral liposuction port incision

1500 cc

Balloons 1000 cc

750 cc

Periumbilical "half-moon" incision

2-cm Transverse suprapubic incision

B

1-2 cm

C

Fig. 58-13. Surgical setup for endoscopic abdominoplasty **(A–C).**

similar to traditional postoperative abdominoplasty management.

In selected patients, particularly those with minimal skin excess, mild to moderate fat deposition, and rectus abdominis muscle diastasis, the minimally invasive approach to abdominal rejuvenation offers the potential for minimal scarring and an excellent aesthetic result.

Conclusion

Our experience, as well as that of many plastic surgeons across the country, has shown the feasibility of performing endoscopic procedures in the subcutaneous and deep spaces throughout the body. These procedures have resulted in outcomes and complication rates comparable to those of open procedures, with incisions and scars that are truly minimal. This evolving field continues to expand, and time will tell its true impact on the field of plastic surgery. It is hoped that this chapter serves as an illustration of the number and variety of techniques that can be performed in a minimally invasive manner outside the visceral cavities.

Suggested Reading

Bostwick J III, Eaves FF III, Nahai F. *Endoscopic plastic surgery*. St. Louis, MO: Quality Medical Publishers, 1995.

Core GB. Endoscopic abdominoplasty. *Oper Tech Plast Reconstr Surg* 1996;3:47–57.

Core GB, Vasconez LO. Minimally invasive techniques in aesthetic and reconstructive surgery. *Clin Plast Surg* 1995;11:59–70.

Eaves FF III, Nahai F, Bostwick J III. The endoscopic neck lift. *Oper Tech Plast Reconstr Surg* 1995;2:145–151.

Levin LS, Rehnke R, Eubanks S. Endoscopic surgery of the upper extremity. *Hand Clin* 1995;22:585–796.

Mackay GJ, Nahai F. The endoscopic forehead lift. *Oper Tech Plast Reconstr Surg* 1995;2:137–144.

Ramirez OM. Endoscopic forehead and face lift: step by step. *Oper Tech Plast Reconstr Surg* 1995; 2:129–136.

EDITOR'S COMMENT

Drs. Rehnke and Van Buskirk provide an insightful overview of the emerging field of minimally invasive plastic surgery. The benefits of less scarring and improved cosmesis make these techniques extremely appealing to plastic surgeons. The development of balloon dissectors for specific plastic and reconstructive needs has led to the ability to perform minimally invasive plastic surgery with minimal blood loss and a reduction in operating-room time.

Current endosurgical instrumentation and techniques for plastic surgery are in the early phases of their evolution. Further advances and refinements are anticipated within the next few years, and significant patient benefits are expected. Plastic surgeons, as well as other surgical subspecialists, would do well to learn from the mistakes made by general surgeons during the early history of laparoscopic cholecystectomy. The timing is appropriate, and opportunities exist for the plastic surgery community to develop credentialing and training standards for these new techniques that could avert unnecessary complications and their associated medical and legal difficulties.

W.S.E

59

Minimally Invasive Spine Surgery

David W. Cloyd and Theodore G. Obenchain

Minimally invasive access to the spine can be achieved by a number of routes. The posterior percutaneous approach as developed by Kambin and Schaffer (1989) has demonstrated that the disc can be safely accessed and discectomy accomplished by a totally percutaneous method. This approach will suffice for simple disc herniation, but more complex procedures, including total discectomy, fusion, instrumentation, or even vertebral body corpectomy, are sometimes required. To achieve these more challenging goals, more complete access to the spine must be obtained. With this in mind, newly developed approaches offered by the laparoscope are reviewed in this chapter. It is estimated that 90% of clinically important disc pathology occurs at the three lowest lumbar levels. Therefore, the emphasis in this chapter will be on lumbar spine access. The principles established, however, apply equally well to the thoracic spine, where access can be achieved through the pleural space.

Anatomic Considerations

The lumbar spine can be accessed laparoscopically by two routes: transperitoneal and retroperitoneal. The anatomy of the two methods is distinct, and each is therefore reviewed separately.

Transperitoneal Approach

Of obvious consideration in the transperitoneal approach is safe bowel retraction. The small intestine in particular must be retracted to permit access to any of the lumbar levels. Steep Trendelenburg or other table positions will assist in this ma-

neuver. Adhesions from prior operations may be present, and a meticulous adhesiolysis may need to be performed to facilitate mobilization of the small bowel out of the pelvis.

The large intestine does not usually need to be specifically mobilized to permit access to the lower lumbar spine. Its broad mesenteric attachment, crossing the left iliac vessels, lies lateral to the usual point of dissection.

At the L5-S1 level, the sacral promontory is readily identified between the vessels. There is a broad area that may be safely approached between the vessels, but it should be recognized that the parasympathetics crossing over the iliac vessels may be injured by overzealous attempts at wide exposure. In the midline, one may encounter the middle sacral artery. Except for this vessel, the zone between the iliac vessels is essentially avascular (Fig. 59-1), consisting of only loose areolar tissue that is easily stripped away to expose the anterior longitudinal ligament and the annulus of the L5-S1 disc. Typically, it is slightly resilient and raised, allowing it to be distinguished by palpation from the hard anterior surfaces of the L-5 and S-1 vertebral bodies immediately above and below. In addition, the annulus can be identified by its typical location at the apex of the angle formed by the sacral promontory.

The L4-5 level is the most frequently involved in disc disease. Unfortunately, the transverse portion of the left iliac vein usually obscures the L4-5 disc, which therefore cannot readily be accessed by the same presacral route (Fig. 59-2). Occasionally, in a patient with an unusually high aortoiliac bifurcation, an exception is pos-

sible. Ordinarily, however, it is safer to approach the L4-5 disc by dissecting lateral to the aorta (Fig. 59-3). This is the same method by which the L3-4 level may be exposed. The left lateral edge of the aorta is the most important landmark, which may be identified by both visual and tactile clues. The proper level must be confirmed fluoroscopically. Both the ureter and the gonadal vessels are located lateral to the aorta on top of the psoas muscle. These are easily avoided if dissection remains immediately adjacent to the aorta and is oriented strictly parallel to the aorta. Periaortic lymph nodes may interfere with the dissection but, unless pathologically enlarged, can typically be handled with little difficulty.

The lower extent of the dissection sometimes may need to extend onto the proximal left common iliac artery. This by itself is of no concern, but it must be recognized that immediately posterior to the artery lies the left common iliac vein, which may be easily injured. It is best to complete the paraaortic dissection cephalad to the iliac artery, with exposure and clear identification of the anterior longitudinal spinous ligament at this point. If fluoroscopy indicates a need for more caudal exposure, the left common iliac vein may be more easily elevated and retracted once the important step of exposing the anterior longitudinal spinous ligament has been accomplished. Wide dissection of the left iliac vessels frequently requires isolation and control of the iliac lumbar vein and artery.

The lateral extent of exposure of the anterior surfaces of the vertebral bodies is defined by the medial border of the iliopsoas muscle. It is not usually necessary to dis-

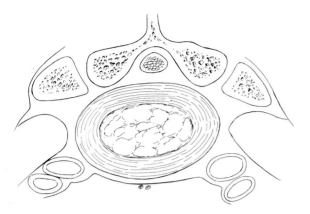

Fig. 59-1. Surgical anatomy at the L5-S1 level. Note the wide area available anteriorly to approach the disc between the iliac veins.

sect these muscle fibers off the vertebral bodies to achieve adequate anterior exposure. Just lateral to the medial edge of the iliopsoas is the lumbar sympathetic chain, which can be damaged by overzealous attempts at dissection of the iliopsoas.

The aorta (and left iliac artery if necessary) must be retracted medially toward the right to adequately expose the anterior surface of the annulus. Lumbar arteries and veins may limit the mobility of the aorta and may have to be clipped and divided, particularly for multilevel disc disease. As with the L5-S1 annulus, the L3-4 and L4-5 discs can be identified by a combination of their slight anterior bulge and their resilience, which is distinct from the rigid vertebral bodies. The fluoroscope is always used to confirm the proper anatomic level.

Retroperitoneal Approach

The retroperitoneal space is most useful for accessing the L3-4, the L4-5, and many other levels. The L5-S1 level is difficult to approach by this route because of both the overlying left iliac vein and the superior edge of the iliac crest, which restricts caudal placement of the working trocars. The L1-2 level is also difficult to approach by this route. The diaphragmatic fibers of the aortic hiatus obscure the spine at this level, and although these may be stripped away, the angle of approach is severely compromised if one attempts to work below the costal margin in a retroperitoneal position. For these reasons, a transthoracic transdiaphragmatic approach, oriented more nearly perpendicular to the target L1-2 disc, is preferable to the retroperitoneal approach, depending on the experience and training of the endoscopist.

At the L2-3 and L3-4 levels, a perpendicular approach can be achieved with little difficulty. The retroperitoneal space is developed with the use of a balloon (see be-

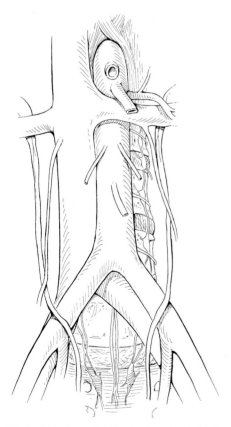

Fig. 59-2. An 8-mm trephine has been inserted into the L5-S1 disc. (Modified from Cloyd and Obenchain, 1995, with permission.)

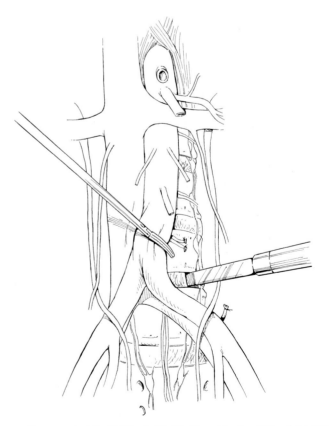

Fig. 59-3. The paraaortic approach at the L4-5 level. (Modified from Cloyd and Obenchain, 1995, with permission.)

low). When correctly positioned, the superficial retroperitoneal structures, including the ureter and descending gonadal vessels, will be lifted anteriorly with the peritoneum, leaving only the sympathetic chain, lateral femoral cutaneous, ilioinguinal, and genitofemoral nerves posteriorly with the iliopsoas muscle.

Diagnostic Considerations/Indications for Procedure

Laparoscopic access to the spine represents a unique collaborative effort, requiring the skills of two surgical specialists for the purpose of conducting an operative procedure that might not otherwise be possible. In this setting, it is not strictly necessary for the laparoscopic surgeon to master the *orthopedic* indications for the contemplated spinal reconstruction. It is felt, however, that the ability of the laparoscopist to participate in the collaborative management of the patient will be enhanced if he or she understands the basic orthopedic principles of patient selection.

Approximately 300,000 patients undergo laminectomy annually for the relief of back pain and/or sciatica. It is useful to classify these patients into those whose predominant symptom is radicular leg pain (sciatica) versus those whose predominant symptom is back pain. Patients with leg pain greater than back pain are more likely to have isolated nerve compression as the source of their pain. This may arise from a bulging or herniated disc. Such disc herniations may arise in the central, lateral, foraminal, or far lateral positions (Fig. 59-4). Herniations may be either *contained*, in which case the posterior longitudinal ligament remains intact, or *extruded* through a defect in the posterior longitudinal ligament. They may also be *sequestered*, which indicates that the fragment has separated from the rest of the disc and is essentially free-floating in the spinal canal.

When symptoms are principally radicular *leg pain* and computed tomography (CT) or magnetic resonance (MR) imaging confirms that the principal pathology is a herniated disc, then the patient may benefit from an isolated discectomy, directed at removing the pathologic herniation (as opposed to a more extensive discectomy and fusion, which is described below)). In this case, the location (central, lateral, far lateral) and the type (contained, extruded, or sequestered) will determine the type of access required by the surgical team. Table 59-1 outlines some of the anterior approaches that might be considered for a variety of combinations of disc disease. Typically, the spine surgeon will choose which angle of approach provides the best access. The laparoscopist in turn must understand the location of the pathologic disc, the alignment or approach that the spine surgeon desires to use, and the best method of attaining that approach. These considerations will lead to selecting a retroperitoneal versus a transperitoneal approach, as well as locating the trocar sites and positioning the endoscopes and instruments. Sequestered disc fragments present a particular challenge to the surgical team and should be approached only after the surgical team has gained experience with simpler disc pathology.

Patients whose symptomatology is *back pain* equal to or greater than leg pain may

Table 59-1. Indications and Approaches for Laparoscopic Anterior Spine Surgery

Indication	Approach
Central disk herniation	Nucleotome discectomy
Radiculopathy/ "internal disc derangement"	Nucleotome discectomy
	Discectomy with fusion
	Discectomy
Spondylolisthesis	Discectomy with fusion
Scoliosis	Multilevel discectomy
Vertebral body disease (tumor, fracture, infection)	Corpectomy and reconstruction or plating

show pathology more extensive than a simple disc herniation. Findings on MR imaging or CT could include loss of disc height and/or spondylolisthesis. These patients may benefit from spinal fusion, which can be accomplished with autologous bone grafts, cadaver bone grafts, or various implant devices. More advanced changes of osteophyte formation, spinal stenosis, or foraminal stenosis may also be present, and probably exceed the capability of currently available endoscopic spinal techniques. Given the rapid advancement of the field, however, it is expected that instruments and techniques will soon be developed to address even these more complex problems.

Laparoscopic considerations also play a role in determining the suitability of the patient for a laparoscopic spinal procedure. Foremost among these are severe cardiopulmonary conditions, which may be aggravated by positive-pressure carbon dioxide (CO_2) insufflation. Some patients may even be better served by open surgery. Prior abdominal procedures can be expected to cause intraperitoneal adhesions, which represent a relative contraindication. It is our opinion that an experienced laparoscopist can almost always still gain safe access to the abdomen and then determine whether or not an adhesiolysis can reasonably be carried out. Known cases of fibroperitoneum would be an obvious exception. Prior retroperitoneal operations have similar adverse implications for retroperitoneal dissections. Also to be considered would be previous episodes of retroperitoneal inflammation. On the right side, appendicitis may alter the ease of retroperitoneal dissection. On the left side, diverticulitis may cause similar problems.

Perioperative Management

In general, laparoscopic spinal access patients should be prepared for surgery in a similar manner to patients undergoing any other laparoscopic procedure. Preoperative antibiotics usually consist of a first-generation cephalosporin administered intravenously. Precautions for deep vein thrombosis are usually warranted. In addition to all the ordinary factors known to place surgical patients at risk of thromboembolic complications, it is felt that increased intraabdominal pressure caused by the pneumoperitoneum may inhibit ve-

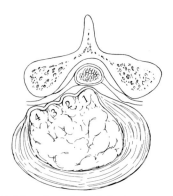

Fig. 59-4. Locations of typical disc herniations (1, central; 2, lateral; 3, foraminal; 4, far lateral).

nous return from the lower extremities and further promote thrombi. Therefore, pulsatile antiembolism stockings are routinely placed. Subcutaneous heparin has not routinely been used but, based on experience with other procedures, could probably be used as a safe alternative.

As with other advanced laparoscopic procedures, these are occasionally lengthy cases. Multiple instrument exchanges, including the use of semiopen techniques for introduction of orthopedic devices, lead to use of large volumes of insufflated gas. CO_2 volume exchanges in excess of 100 L are not uncommon and can cause hypothermia secondary to evaporative losses from the abdominal cavity. Efforts to minimize unnecessary CO_2 losses are indicated. Inspired anesthetic gases should be heated, and additional patient warming can be maintained with the use of air mattress warming blankets.

Nasogastric tubes are rarely necessary either during or after surgery, unless the stomach is inadvertently inflated during mask-assisted ventilation by the anesthesiologist upon induction. If inserted, nasogastric tubes can be removed in the recovery room, as can the Foley catheter. Most patients can resume a limited diet immediately after surgery.

Operative Technique
L5-S1 Transperitoneal Approach

The patient is positioned supine under general anesthesia. Foley catheters are used to decompress the bladder. The operating table must be capable of a steep Trendelenburg position and must permit circumferential access to the fluoroscope at the appropriate level. Monitors are arranged so that the operating surgeon will be able to achieve axial optical alignment of the surgeon, the instruments, the surgical field, and the monitor (Fig. 59-5). After establishment of the pneumoperitoneum through an umbilical trocar, two additional 5-mm trocars are placed in the lower quadrants bilaterally (Fig. 59-6). A steep Trendelenburg is then employed to help deliver the bowel out of the pelvis. If adhesions are present, they must be lysed with care, as an inadvertent enterotomy would likely result in an unacceptably high risk of discitis and force consideration of abandoning the operation.

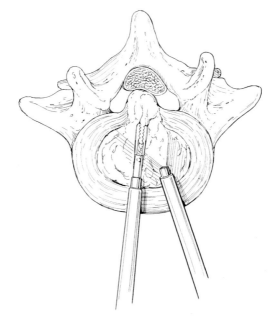

Fig. 59-5. Biportal anterior disc entry accomplished with a 5-mm discoscope and an automated shaver. Observe that the shaver may easily be directed toward the posterior longitudinal ligament, where pathologic disc herniations may be specifically resected under direct vision.

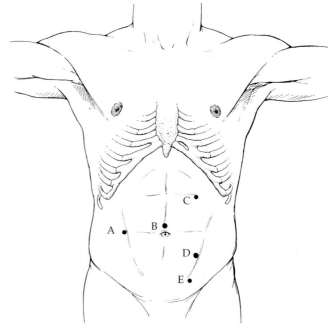

Fig. 59-6. Two 5-mm trocars are placed in the lower quadrants bilaterally. (A, 5-mm port; B, 10-mm port; C, 5-mm port; D, 10-mm port; E, 5-mm port.)

The sacral promontory should be easily visualized and provides an excellent landmark for the L5-S1 disc. Its position is confirmed with the fluoroscope. A 1.5-cm incision is made in the peritoneum immediately over the disc, and blunt dissection is used to strip away the loose adipose and connective tissue of the retroperitoneum. Cautery should be used sparingly, as it will increase the risk of injury to the hy-

pogastric plexus, which can lead to retrograde ejaculation.

Once the annulus is visualized, the position is confirmed again with the fluoroscope. At this time, the location of the working trocar is selected. It should be placed so that a perpendicular entry can be achieved into the disc. It is useful to place an instrument extracorporeally at the patient's side within the beam of the fluoroscope so that it is silhouetted against the anatomy of the spine. This will improve the accuracy of trocar placement at the skin level. The incision for the L5-S1 level will usually be in the midline immediately above the pubis. Care must be taken to avoid the bladder.

The disc can now be entered by several means. If a limited discectomy is to be performed, we have used a specially fabricated trephine to cut a hole in the annulus and provide a closed route of access to the disc itself (Fig. 59-7). The advantage of this method is that once access is established, it is no longer necessary to maintain traction on the bowel. Rongeurs, curettes, shavers, and contact lasers have all been used to tunnel through the disc to the posterior longitudinal ligament. The fluoroscope is used to direct the dissection to the target disc fragment or herniation, as defined by preoperative CT or MR imaging. Simultaneous use of an operating discoscope, similar in design to a rigid cystoscope, allows excellent control of the dissection. It is passed through the trephine and provides a 5-mm working channel. A limited discectomy, directed specifically at the suspected pathologic disc fragment, is then accomplished. If necessary, even sequestered fragments can be extracted through defects in the posterior longitudinal ligament.

At some centers, a more limited entry into the disc is performed, similar in concept and design to the percutaneous posterior approach of Kambin. While Kambin introduced these instruments posteriorly, the same instruments, typically including cannulas of 5- to 6.5-mm diameter, can be introduced through anterior or lateral aspects of the disc following dissection under laparoscopic control. An automated

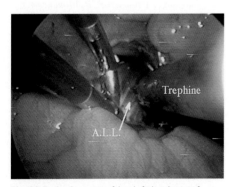

Fig. 59-7. An 8-mm trephine is being inserted through the anterior longitudinal ligament.

shaver is then inserted through the cannula and directed entirely by use of the fluoroscope. This method is most suitable when limited excision of a pathologic disc fragment is desired, with the goal of leaving the remainder of the disc and its supporting ligaments intact.

An alternative method, better suited to cases requiring more extended discectomies or fusions, is to perform an open discotomy. In this technique, the disc entry site is left exposed to the peritoneal cavity. Visualization in this method is maintained by the laparoscope directly. The method most closely approximates that of the traditional open anterior approach and therefore is readily extended to complete discectomy, including resection of the end plates, in preparation for fusion. Autologous or cadaver bone plugs may be inserted, including those premeasured and cut for insertion with the Cloward instrumentation. As an integrated device system, these appear particularly well suited to bridge the gap between traditional open fusion and laparoscopically performed fusion.

When necessary, access to the disc can be further enhanced by prudent use of conversion to either semiopen or gasless techniques at this point in the procedure. This concept is similar to that of laparoscopic-assisted colectomy, in which the dissection is performed with standard pneumoperitoneum and full use of the laparoscope but certain critical steps are performed either extracorporeally or in a semiopen setting. In this instance, once the disc is exposed, the abdominal wall may be stabilized by various lifting devices (e.g., Laparolift, Origin Medsystems, Inc., Menlo Park, CA), which permit release of pneumoperitoneum without loss of exposure. Thereafter, the working trocar site may be enlarged to accommodate larger orthopedic instruments. In addition, release of the abdominal pressure will permit the abdominal wall to fall back to a more normal position. This will shorten the distance from the skin to the disc and reduce the need for reliance on the custom fabrication of longer spinal fusion instruments. It should be remembered that standard-length spine instruments, even though they may fit through a laparoscopic trocar, are usually too short to reach the disc of an adult in the presence of a standard pneumoperitoneum.

L3-4/L4-5 Transperitoneal Approach

Supine positioning and general anesthesia are also used in this approach. Initial trocar entry is usually performed in the infraumbilical position. Accessory trocars, however, must be placed so as to accommodate a working trocar in the left midabdomen and to permit dissection through the retroperitoneum in the lateral paraaortic position. The proposed skin placement of the orthopedic working trocar should be established with the aid of the fluoroscope as previously described, after which the two 5-mm accessory trocars can be positioned. This will usually result in one accessory trocar situated in the left subcostal position and the other in the left hypogastrium, with the space in between left vacant for the working trocar. Due to the need to provide more bowel retraction with this technique, a third 5-mm accessory trocar is often advisable. If a special bowel retractor is to be used, then sometimes a 10- to 12-mm trocar is placed. This is best situated in the right midabdomen so as not to obstruct the working trocar.

The bowel is delivered cephalad, again with the use of a steep Trendelenburg position. If necessary, additional bowel stabilization can be achieved by judicious use of Endoloops (Ethicon, Inc., Somerville, NJ) applied to noncritical parts of the bowel (e.g. epiploic appendage). These sutures can then be drawn through the abdominal wall with the use of a J-hook needle and secured to the skin. This may avoid the troublesome problem of the bowel's falling back into the orthopedic field after the discectomy has been initiated.

The lateral edge of the aorta is palpated and the proper level chosen with the fluoroscope. A 3-cm incision in the peritoneum opens the retroperitoneal space, which is further developed by blunt dissection. It is advisable to stay next to the aorta as the dissection is carried down to the anterior longitudinal ligament. This will reduce the possibility of damaging either the ureter or the descending gonadal vessels. These should be kept to the lateral side of the dissection.

The anterior longitudinal ligament can be exposed broadly by simple blunt dissection. Clips and cautery can be used, if necessary, but this dissection is relatively avascular if proper orientation to dissection planes is maintained. The aorta itself can be moved several centimeters to the right to provide excellent exposure to the underlying annulus, usually without the need to divide lumbar vessels. Known aneurysmal disease or even severe atherosclerotic hardening of the aorta could obviously impede the mobility of the aorta and should be considered with caution whenever this approach is used.

At the L4-5 level, the iliac artery may lie sufficiently far toward the lateral edge of the spine that one may be tempted to dissect on its medial side rather than its lateral edge. This can indeed improve exposure toward the midline of the target disc. However, it must be remembered that the iliac vein will usually lie immediately beneath the artery at this location and can only be moved a short distance because it usually has several small posterior branches. The vein is also tethered by the internal iliac branch. Extreme care must be exercised during mobilization of the iliac vein.

The disc is again entered under a combination of fluoroscopic and laparoscopic control. Fig. 59-8 demonstrates a trephine seated in the L4-5 disc, with the iliac artery being retracted to the right. Some surgeons have advocated use of Steinmann's pins driven percutaneously into the adjacent vertebral body to stabilize retraction of the vessel and free the hands of the laparoscopist. Using the pictured trephine eliminates the need for Steinmann's pins, as once the disc is entered, the bowel and the retroperitoneal structures can safely be allowed to fall back against the trephine. However, if one of the other methods of discectomy is to be employed, and especially if placement of a bone dowel or fusion cage is desired, then Steinmann's pins can be quite useful for providing a stable exposure. Once the disc is entered, a discoscope may be employed to carry out discectomy under direct vision (Fig. 59-9).

L3-4/L4-5 Retroperitoneal Approach

The patient is positioned in a lateral decubitus position on a table that permits circumferential fluoroscopic access (Fig. 59-10). Both right and left sides may be approached with equal ease. Local anesthesia with intravenous sedation may be used if it is felt necessary to monitor nerve root

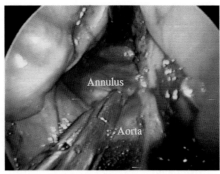

Fig. 59-8. The aorta is retracted to the patient's right during a transperitoneal paraaortic dissection. The annulus of the L4-5 disc is visible.

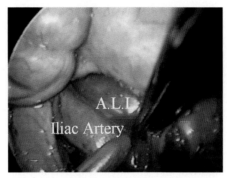

Fig. 59-9. Circumferential dissection of the right iliac artery may provide improved exposure of the anterior longitudinal ligament at the L4-5 level.

stimulation or injury during a transforaminal approach. Otherwise, general anesthesia is utilized.

Initial laparoscopic entry is obtained by a 12-mm incision in the posterior axillary line, midway between the costal margin and the iliac crest (Fig. 59-11). The three layers of the abdominal wall musculature are incised, and the adipose layer immediately beneath the fascia of the transversus abdominis muscle is identified. This space is then developed bluntly. It is important not to inadvertently enter the peritoneum. If this occurs, it will severely limit the effectiveness of the exposure later in the case, as gas will leak into the peritoneum and cause progressive encroachment on the retroperitoneal working space.

A peritoneal balloon distention device (Origin PDB 1000 Peritoneal Balloon Distension System, Origin Medsystems, Inc., Menlo Park, CA) is inserted and inflated. The uniform nature of the pressure applied by the balloon results in a progressive separation of the peritoneum from the retroperitoneum. Up to 1,000 mL may be required to optimally develop the space. Efforts at manually extending the dissection after removal of the balloon should be carried out with caution. The peritoneal membrane is quite fragile and will easily tear. Low-pressure insufflation may im-

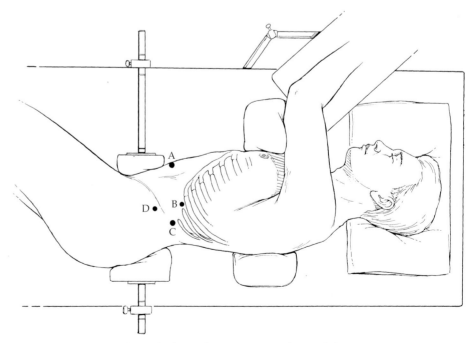

Fig. 59-10. Patient positioning for the L3-4/L4-5 retroperitoneal approach (A, B, C, D, trocar positions).

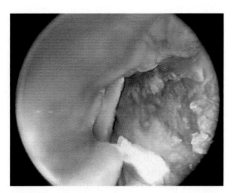

Fig. 59-11. View of the interior of the disc space provided by a discoscope with 3-mm objective lens midway through resection of the disc.

prove the available working space, but much of the exposure results from the fact that the patient is in the lateral decubitus position. The peritoneal contents should simply fall away from the surgically developed retroperitoneal working space, which is in essence self-retracting.

Two additional 5-mm trocars are now inserted, usually in the anterior axillary line. Care must be taken not to transgress the true peritoneal cavity, which usually remains attached along the lateral edge of the rectus sheath, forming a potentially dangerous pseudoreflection. This limits the medial placement of trocars, which in turn will restrict the ability to approach the spine from a true anterior direction. This may have important implications if one desires to fuse the spine with any of the new implantable fusion cages. These devices have usually been implanted in an anteroposterior orientation, sometimes as two parallel devices placed side by side. It remains to be determined whether or not they can be used with the same degree of success when placed from a lateral or oblique approach.

After placement of the accessory trocars, the anterolateral aspect of the spine can be visually inspected. With the aid of the fluoroscope, the proper disc level is identified. As with the L5-S1 disc, the annulus can be palpated with a laparoscopic instrument. Blunt dissection anteriorly will lead promptly to the posterolateral aspect of either the inferior vena cava on the right or the aorta on the left. Additional dissection along these major vessels will broaden the area of exposure of the annulus and the vertebral bodies. Posterolaterally, a layer of fibroconnective tissue can be stripped away to expose more of the annulus. The medial edge of the iliopsoas

will be encountered, and it too can be stripped away to increase the posterior extent of the exposure. Once the disc is exposed, entry and discectomy are identical to those described for the transperitoneal approaches.

Fusion Cages

Perhaps the most exciting aspect of laparoscopic spinal access surgery is the possibility of successful fusion with any of several recently developed fusion cages. These would take maximal advantage of the laparoscopic exposures described above, offering the possibility of reliable laparoscopic-assisted fusion. One of these, the titanium BAK system (Spine-Tech, Inc., Minneapolis, MN), is currently being used in an U.S. Food and Drug Administration–approved I.D.E. trial for implantation laparoscopically at the L5-S1 level. The device was originally developed as a fusion basket to treat equine spinal injuries. It has an established veterinary track record of successful fusion. A version modified for use in the human spine has been tested in baboons and found to have superior bone ingrowth and stability, compared to similar fusions performed with dowels of bone allograft. The cylindrical titanium cage is fenestrated to enhance bone ingrowth and threaded on the outside to allow it to be screwed into place. The implantation system provides a matched set of drills used to tap a threaded hole into the target disc. The titanium cage is then screwed into this threaded discotomy cavity, and the hollow interior of the cage is packed with bone chips to promote fusion.

Surgical Complications

Although we have not yet had a bowel injury in our series of patients, this must certainly be considered as one of the risks of laparoscopic spine access, especially in patients with prior abdominal surgery. The disc space is essentially avascular and cannot be expected to resist infection well if exposed to gastrointestinal flora. If an enterotomy were to occur prior to entry into the disc, one would have to consider whether or not to abandon the discectomy in favor of a second attempt at a later time.

Significant surgical bleeding has been reported in the literature and has caused at least one conversion to open surgery. Iliac vein injury is the most feared event. Even

meticulous blunt dissection may not always avoid this possibility. On one occasion, we noted that the iliac vein had been compressed under a retractor so that the anterior and posterior walls were in direct apposition. Without blood distending the vessel, the vein walls, viewed through the limits of a two-dimensional laparoscope, were initially mistaken for a simple layer of connective tissue overlying the annulus. Fortunately, the mistake was recognized before a serious injury occurred.

Retrograde ejaculation is a known complication of open anterior approaches to the L5-S1 space. We have observed two instances in our series, both of which resolved spontaneously. The hypogastric plexus crosses the iliac vessels just below and lateral to the aortoiliac bifurcation. Dissection in this area, especially during exposure of the L5-S1 disc, places the hypogastric plexus at risk.

Sympathetic injury has also been observed, characterized by a warm leg in the recovery room ipsilateral to the side of dissection. This injury is more likely to occur at the L3-4 or L4-5 levels and is a possibility whether the disc is approached by the transperitoneal paraaortic route or by the retroperitoneal route. The sympathetics can be avoided by restraint from unnecessary dissection of the iliopsoas muscle just lateral to the vertebral body. If exposure in this area is required, it is best to specifically identify the sympathetic chain first, so that it can be preserved during the dissection.

As mentioned above, the disc space is avascular and therefore more prone to infection than many anatomic sites commonly exposed by the laparoscopist. Discitis of infectious origin is possible (one case of staphylococcal discitis in our series) and may actually be related to the use of multiple laparoscopic instruments and multiple entries into the disc space. This is especially true during the developmental or learning phases of an operation, when both operator inexperience and less than perfect instrumentation can contribute to longer procedures and the need for repetitive access to the disc.

Conclusion

Laparoscopic access to the lumbar spine can reliably be obtained by both transperitoneal and retroperitoneal routes. Exposure thus obtained is sufficient to allow lumbar discectomy and fusion. Innovative devices now under investigation promise to expand the ability to perform a wide variety of complex anterior spinal reconstructive procedures while retaining the desirable aspects of minimally invasive surgery. The long-term success rates of discectomy or fusion, including the optimal types of devices (titanium versus carbon fiber versus bone) remains to be determined, and are under active investigation at this time.

Suggested Reading

Cloyd DW, Obenchain TG, Savin M. Transperitoneal laparoscopic approach to lumbar discectomy. *Surg Laparosc Endosc* 1995;5:85–89.

Kambin P, Schaffer JL. Percutaneous lumbar discectomy: review of 100 patients and current practice. *Clin Orthop* 1989;128:24–34.

Regan JJ, McAfee PC, Mack MJ, eds. *Atlas of endoscopic spine surgery.* St. Louis, MO: Quality Medical Publishing, 1995.

Slotman GJ, Stein SC. Laparoscopic lumbar diskectomy: preliminary report of a minimally invasive anterior approach to the herniated L5-S1 disk. *Surg Laparosc Endosc* 1995;5:363–369.

Zelko JR, Misko J, Swanstrom L, Pennings J, Kenyon T. Laparoscopic lumbar discectomy. *Am J Surg* 1995;169:496–498.

EDITOR'S COMMENT

Many spine surgeries lend themselves particularly well to anterior approaches. The anterior approach minimizes the instability resulting from a laminectomy, lessens the chance of nerve root scarring from transforaminal approaches, and avoids the morbidity of mobilizing the large paraspinous muscle groups in posterior midline approaches. Unfortunately, the morbidity of the anterior approach (wound complications, intercostal neuropraxia, ileus, and postoperative pain) made this an approach of last resort. Minimally invasive methods of spine surgery have therefore generated much enthusiasm. These can be posterior (microlaminectomy) or lateral (percutaneous transforaminal discectomy), or, most recently, laparoscopy and thoracoscopy can be used to expose the anterior disc space and vertebral bodies.

These procedures are not for the occasional laparoscopist. Surgeons who perform these exposures should be highly skilled in advanced endoscopic techniques and intimately familiar with the anatomy of the paraspinous retroperitoneum. The potential for catastrophic complication is tremendous both during the access procedure and from the spine procedure itself. The entire effort must be well coordinated between the spine surgeon and the operating room support staff. These are truly a "cosurgery," and the laparoscopist should be involved in assessing the patient's suitability for surgery and be familiar with the indications, techniques, and needs of the spine surgeon. It is important for both surgeons to be present during the entire case. The spine surgeon needs to confirm levels, dictate the degree of exposure, and position the working trocar for effective use. With proper preparation, even extensive exposures of the anterior spine can be achieved safely and effectively.

L.L.S.

Subject Index

Page numbers in *italic* indicate figures. Page numbers followed by "t" indicate tables.